Drug Screening Methods

Drug Screening Methods

THIRD EDITION

Editor

SK Gupta PhD DSc
Professor Emeritus
Department of Pharmacology
Delhi Institute of Pharmaceutical Sciences and
Research, University of Delhi
Pushp Vihar, Sector-3, New Delhi, India
&
National Advisor
Pharmacovigilance Programme of India (PvPI)

Formerly
Professor and Head
Department of Pharmacology
All India Institute of Medical Sciences
Ansari Nagar, New Delhi (India)
and
Dean and Director General
Institute of Clinical Research, India

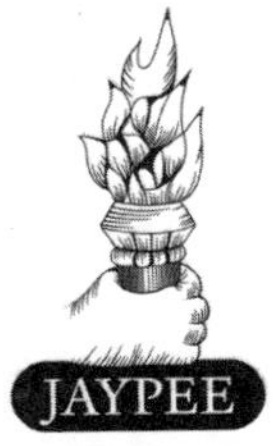

JAYPEE BROTHERS MEDICAL PUBLISHERS
The Health Sciences Publisher
New Delhi | London

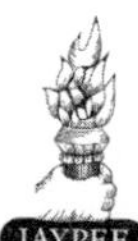

Jaypee Brothers Medical Publishers (P) Ltd

Headquarters

EMCA House, 23/23-B
Ansari Road, Daryaganj
New Delhi 110 002, India
Landline: +91-11-23272143, +91-11-23272703
+91-11-23282021, +91-11-23245672
e-mail: jaypee@jaypeebrothers.com

Corporate Office

4838/24, Ansari Road, Daryaganj
New Delhi 110 002, India
Phone: +91-11-43574357
Fax: +91-11-43574314
e-mail: jaypee@jaypeebrothers.com

Overseas Office

JP Medical Ltd.
83, Victoria Street, London
SW1H 0HW (UK)
Phone: +44-20 3170 8910
e-mail: info@jpmedpub.com

EU GPSR Authorised Representative

Logos Europe, 9 rue Nicolas Poussin
17000, La Rochelle, France
Phone: +33 (0) 6 67 93 73 78
e-mail: contact@logoseurope.eu

Website: www.jaypeebrothers.com
Website: www.jaypeedigital.com

Inquiries for bulk sales may be solicited at: jaypee@jaypeebrothers.com

Drug Screening Methods

First Edition: 2004
Second Edition: 2009
Third Edition: **2016**
Reprint : 2025, **2026**
ISBN: 978-93-5152-982-8

Printed at: Sterling Graphics Pvt. Ltd.

Dedicated to

My Family,
Research Associates and Students...

CONTRIBUTORS

Anna Krasilnikova
Faculty of Medicine
Universiti Teknologi Mara
Sungai Buloh, Malaysia

Binit Kumar PhD
Kresge Eye Institute, School of Medicine
Wayne State University
MI, USA

Deepa Trivedi PhD
HCL Technology
Sector 60, Noida (UP), India

E Anand MD
Clinigene International Ltd
Bengaluru (Karnataka), India

Hanuman Prasad Sharma
Dr Rajendra Prasad Centre for
Ophthalmic Sciences
All India Institute of Medical Sciences
Ansari Nagar, New Delhi, India

Ipseeta Ray Mohanty PhD
Department of Pharmacology
MGM Medical College
Sector-16, Kamothe
Navi Mumbai (Maharashtra), India

Jagdish Jaiswal PhD
Auckland Cancer Society Research Centre
Faculty of Medical and Health Sciences
The University of Auckland
Auckland, New Zealand

Jai Prakash PhD
Indian Pharmacopoeia Commission (IPC)
Ministry of Health and Family Welfare, GOI
Raj Nagar, Ghaziabad (UP), India

Jai Prakash Bansal PhD
Department of Pharmacokinetics and Drug
Delivery, University Centre for Pharmacy
University of Groningen
Groningen, The Netherlands

Klaas Poelstra
Department of Pharmacokinetics and Drug
Delivery, University Centre for Pharmacy
University of Groningen
Groningen, The Netherlands

Leonie Beljaars
Department of Pharmacokinetics and
Drug Delivery
University Centre for Pharmacy
University of Groningen
Groningen, The Netherlands

Monisha Sharma PhD
MSD Pharmaceuticals Private Limited
(Merck & Co. Inc)
Gurgaon, India

Nabanita Halder PhD
Dr Rajendra Prasad Centre for Ophthalmic
Sciences
All India Institute of Medical Sciences
Ansari Nagar, New Delhi, India

Namratta Manhas
Division of Pharmacology
Central Drug Research Institute
Lucknow (UP), India

Niranjan Galpalli PhD
Lupin Bioresearch Center
Pashan, Pune (Maharashtra), India

Pradeep Tyagi PhD
Department of Urology
University of Pittsburgh
Pittsburgh, PA 15217, USA

Priya Mathur PhD
School of Optometry
University of California
Berkeley, USA

Rachna Gupta MD
Department of Pharmacology
University College of Medical Sciences
GTB Hospital, Shahdara, Delhi, India

Rajan Mittal MD
Dr Reddy's Laboratory Ltd
Hyderabad (Andhra Pradesh), India

Rajani Mathur PhD
Department of Pharmacology
Delhi Institute of Pharmaceutical Sciences and Research, University of Delhi
Pushp Vihar, Sector-3, New Delhi, India

Ram Raghubir PhD
Division of Pharmacology
Central Drug Research Institute
Lucknow (UP), India

Ravi Saklani
Department of Pharmacology
Delhi Institute of Pharmaceutical Sciences and Research, University of Delhi
Pushp Vihar, Sector-3, New Delhi, India

Renu Agarwal PhD
Faculty of Medicine
Universiti Teknologi Mara
Selangor, Darul Ehsan, Malaysia

Rishi Sharma PhD
Division of Pharmacology
Central Drug Research Institute
Lucknow (UP), India

RK Bhardwaj PhD
Rutgers University
New Jersey, USA

Rohit Saxena MD
Dr Rajendra Prasad Centre for Ophthalmic Sciences
All India Institute of Medical Sciences
Ansari Nagar, New Delhi, India

Shiladitya Sengupta PhD
Harvard Medical School
Brigham and Women's Hospital
MIT, Rm 317, 65 Landsdowne Street
Cambridge, MA, USA

Shirish Dongare MPharm
Department of Pharmacology
Delhi Institute of Pharmaceutical Sciences and Research, University of Delhi
Pushp Vihar, Sector-3, New Delhi, India

SK Gupta PhD DSc
Professor Emeritus
Department of Pharmacology
Delhi Institute of Pharmaceutical Sciences and Research, University of Delhi
Pushp Vihar, Sector-3, New Delhi, India
and National Advisor
Pharmacovigilance Programme of India (PvPI)

Srinivasan Senthilkumari PhD
Department of Ocular Pharmacology
Aravind Medical Research Foundation (AMRF)
#1, Anna Nagar
Madurai (Tamil Nadu), India

SS Agrawal PhD
Amity University
Sector 125
Noida (UP), India

Subrata Pore PhD
Department of Urology
University of Pittsburgh
Pittsburgh, PA 15217, USA

Sujata Joshi PhD
Department of Pharmacology
All India Institute of Medical Sciences
Ansari Nagar
New Delhi, India

Suresh L Mehta
Division of Pharmacology
Central Drug Research Institute
Lucknow (UP), India

Sushma Srivastava PhD
Department of Pharmacology
Delhi Institute of Pharmaceutical Sciences and Research, University of Delhi
Pushp Vihar, Sector-3, New Delhi, India

T Velpandian PhD
Dr Rajendra Prasad Centre for Ophthalmic Sciences
All India Institute of Medical Sciences
Ansari Nagar, New Delhi, India

V Kalaiselvan PhD
Indian Pharmacopoeia Commission
Ministry of Health and Family Welfare, GOI
Raj Nagar, Ghaziabad (UP), India

PREFACE TO THE THIRD EDITION

I am extremely pleased to introduce the much-awaited third edition of the book *Drug Screening Methods*. Both the previous editions of this book were very well received by the students and professionals from the academia and industry, from across the world. The book was a pioneering endeavor in 2004 and was written keeping in mind the widespread need and limited availability of the consolidated screening methods for biological systems in drug discovery and development. Hence, the techniques of practical importance were discussed in both the 1st and 2nd editions.

I received numerous valuable suggestions and comments for enhancing the quality of the book after publication of first edition and accordingly an improved version was published as the 2nd edition. Subsequently, personal critical evaluation and feedback from readers encouraged me to take up the areas, which were left untouched in both the previous editions, and present this third edition of *Drug Screening Methods*.

Several modifications, additions and deletions have been made in this edition keeping in view the need of the hour. All chapters have been revised to include the latest key studies and updated techniques. One new chapter has been written on antiviral drugs other than HIV. We have again strived to maintain a balance of including the most important information for researchers while keeping the essential backbone. As before, we strongly encourage readers to refer to the primary literature for further details and references not included here. I hope that the clarity of the text makes up for any limitations in its comprehensiveness. I hope that like previous editions, the readers will benefit and appreciate this edition of the book and Drug Screening Methods will continue to be an invaluable resource for postgraduate students, industry professionals and others engaged in the research and drug development at various laboratories.

I would be failing in my duty if I do not express my sincere thanks to Dr Sushma Srivastava, Senior Scientist, for having taken up the responsibility with a smile on her face at all the times and for her editorial assistance from the stage of 1st edition to present 3rd edition of this book. She coordinated effectively and efficiently in bringing out this book.

I am grateful to all the contributing authors, including the new ones, who made an enterprise of this magnitude possible due to their hard work and dedication. As an editor, I express my heartfelt gratitude to the contributors of the chapters. Their names and positions are mentioned.

The publication of the book has been possible due to the hard work put in by the staff of Jaypee Brothers Medical Publishers, New Delhi. The good work done deserves our appreciation to Shri Jitendar Vij, Group Chairman of Jaypee Brothers Medical Publishers, one of the largest Medical Publishers in the world.

SK Gupta

PREFACE TO THE FIRST EDITION

Drug discovery and development is a challenging field of research requiring the synchronized efforts of medicinal chemists, natural chemists, pharmacologists, toxicologists and clinicians, to name a few. The ultimate target of this team is to generate a safe and biologically active drug that is capable of stalling, if not reversing, the pathological events leading to disease condition. In the drug discovery program, the battery of tests and assay systems that evaluate the efficacy and safety of the novel molecule in biological system occupy the center stage. Thus, these assays or 'screening methods' are critical as it is on their basis that the molecule sees the light of the day or is consigned to obscurity.

Advances in the field of drug discovery program has seen the graduation of simple screening methods of yore to automated methods utilizing molecular techniques spanning across *in vitro, in vivo* and clinical systems. There has been an explosion of available information making it essential for the professionals working in this area of research to keep pace with the advancing times. It has become an uphill task for researchers focusing on a particular field to scan realms of literature regarding developments in other fields. This often curtails synchronized research and delays results. At this juncture, it has become of utmost importance to consolidate our present knowledge and review its validity and ascertain the future direction.

In view of this widespread need and limited availability of consolidated screening methods for biological systems, the Herculean task of penning a book on *Drug Screening Methods* was undertaken. It is hoped that the First Edition of this book will enjoy a broad readership ranging from professionals to students of pharmacology.

Keeping in tune with the practically used techniques used in both academia and pharmaceutical industry, this book outlines numerous methods utilizing molecular and fluorescence techniques. A complete section has been devoted to the concept and basic techniques involved in novel drug discovery program. It is hoped that this will at least provide a theoretical exposure to students of pharmacology who may tomorrow be in a position to use them practically. Special attention has been given to novel methods based on genetically modified animals that simulate the human condition as these help in not only understanding the pathogenesis, but also develop targets for therapeutic modalities. Additionally, an overview has been provided for major fields of investigations like drug absorption and metabolism, cancer biology, angiogenesis, apoptosis, AIDS and autoimmune disorders.

As a pharmacology teacher for over 40 years now, I have always felt the need for simple screening procedures that explicitly demonstrate the nuances of sympathetic, parasympathetic nervous system and gut motility to the students, and I hope by way of this book, this lacuna has been addressed. As a researcher, the fields of ocular and cardiovascular pharmacology have been very close to my heart and special care has been taken to develop chapters regarding these areas. Considering the renewed interest in outsourcing novel drugs from natural source, a separate chapter dealing with assay procedures for screening the pharmacological activity of herbal drugs has been written.

Every drug has a therapeutic effect, that is desired, along with an unwanted side effect. This book would be incomplete and lend a myopic view to drug discovery program without the methods for assessing safety of novel molecules. Toxicity studies are critical as it is on their basis that the toxicity and efficacy profile of a novel molecule can be weighed and its future determined.

It is obvious that an enterprise of this magnitude has been possible due to the cooperation and assistance of a large number of individuals across the globe. As the editor, I express my heartfelt gratitude to the authors of the chapters, dedicated team of editorial board and the production staff at M/s Jaypee Brothers Medical Publishers (P) Ltd, New Delhi, who all joined to convert this dream project into reality.

SK Gupta

CONTENTS

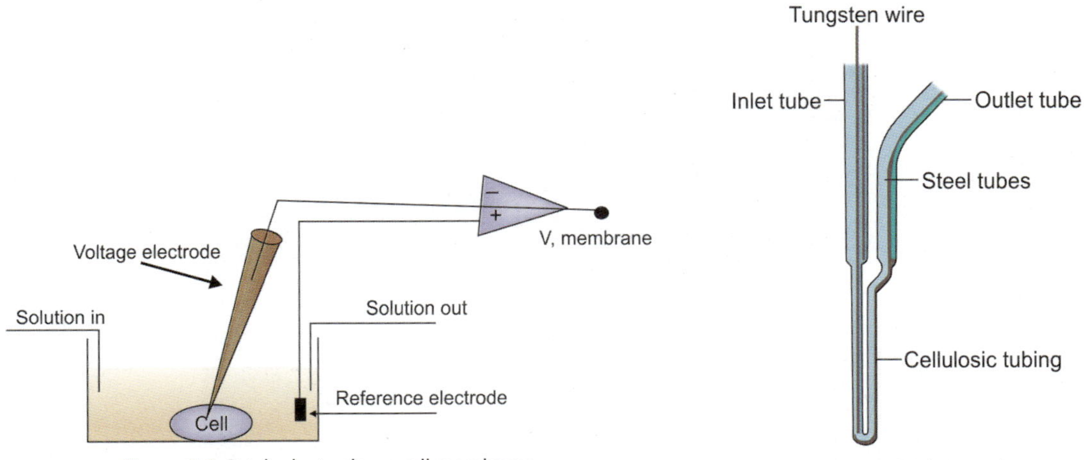

Figure 1.2: Patch electrode on cell membrane

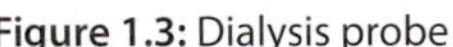

Figure 1.3: Dialysis probe

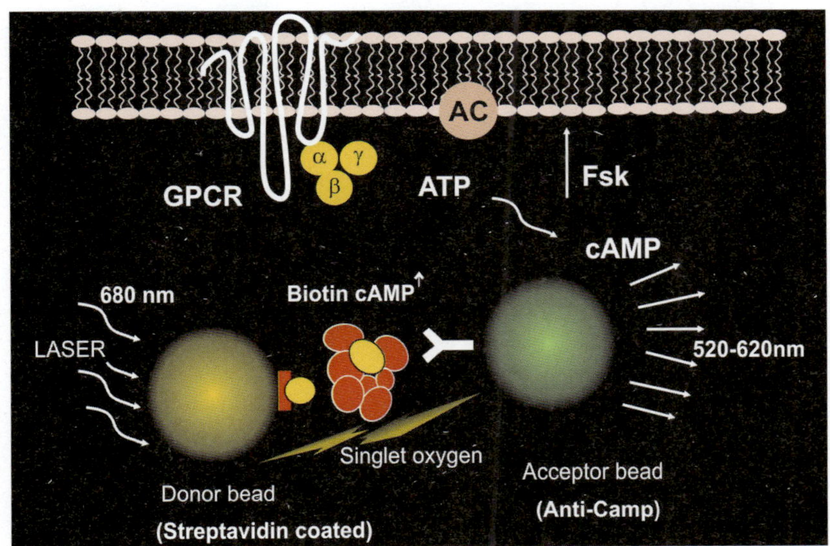

Figure 2.1: cAMP detection using ALPHA screen principle. The ALPHA screen kit includes streptavidin coated donor beads and acceptor beads conjugated with an antibody to cAMP. Biotinylatedc AMP is also included as a positive control and for competition with unlabeled cAMP

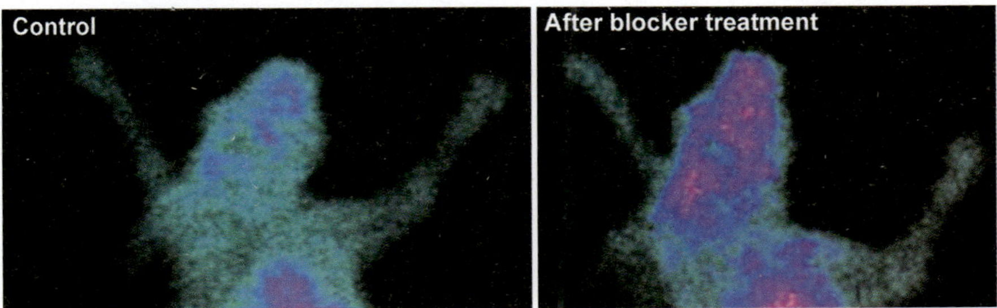

Figure 2.3: Pictures of SPECT-CT showing the intraocular uptake of radiolabeled ciprofloxacin after blocker (verapamil) treatment. Dual head SPECT–CT with collimator-low energy (*Courtesy*: Dept of Ocular Pharmacology & Pharmacy, AIIMS and INMAS, New Delhi)

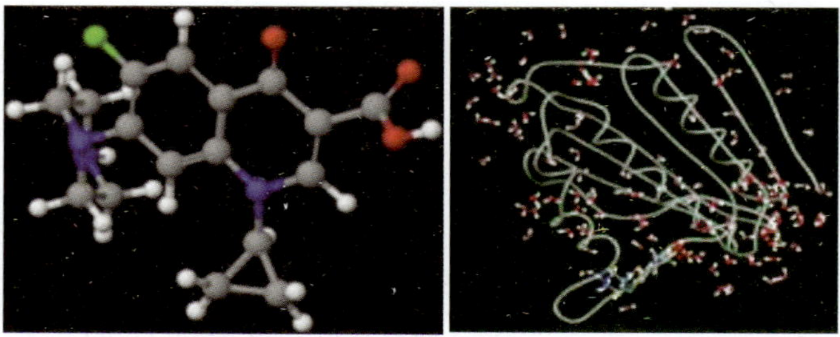

Figure 2.4: Computer-aided molecular design approach

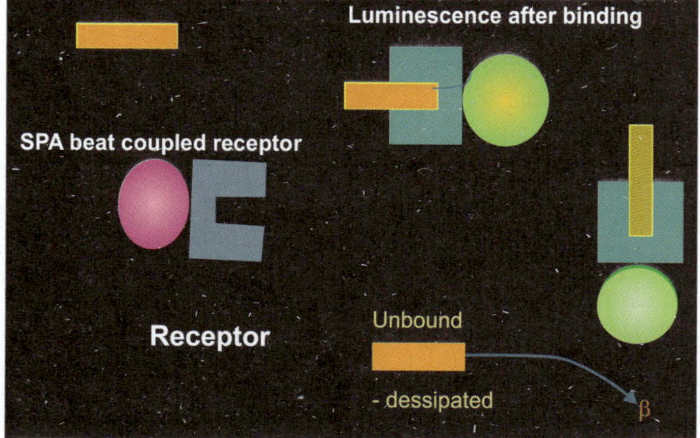

Figure 2.5: Principles of scintillation proximity assay (SPA)

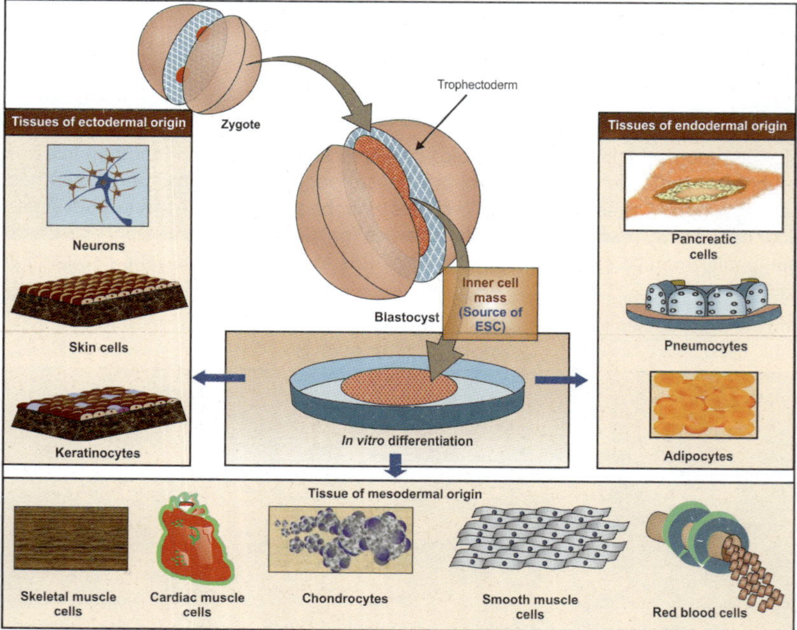

Figure 3.1: Tissues of endodermal, mesodermal and ectodermal origin derived from embryonic stem cells after *in vitro* differentiation

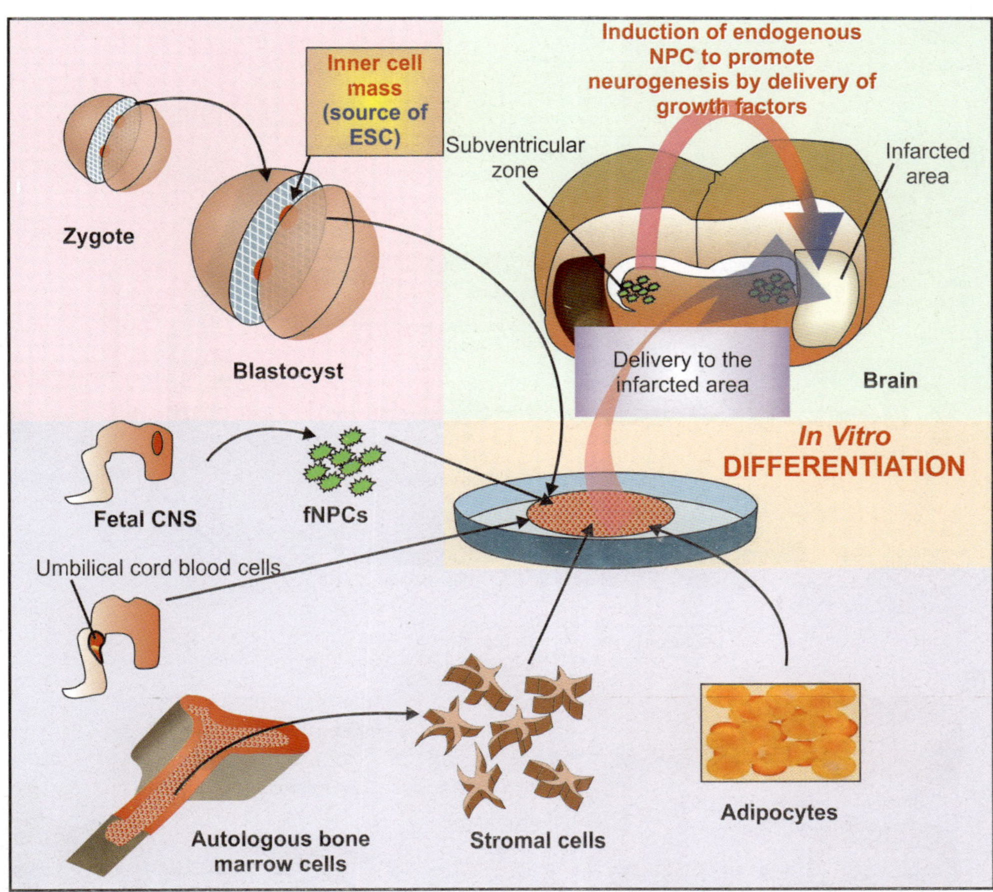

Figure 3.2: Different sources of stem cell employed for cell replacement therapy for the treatment of various neurological disorders

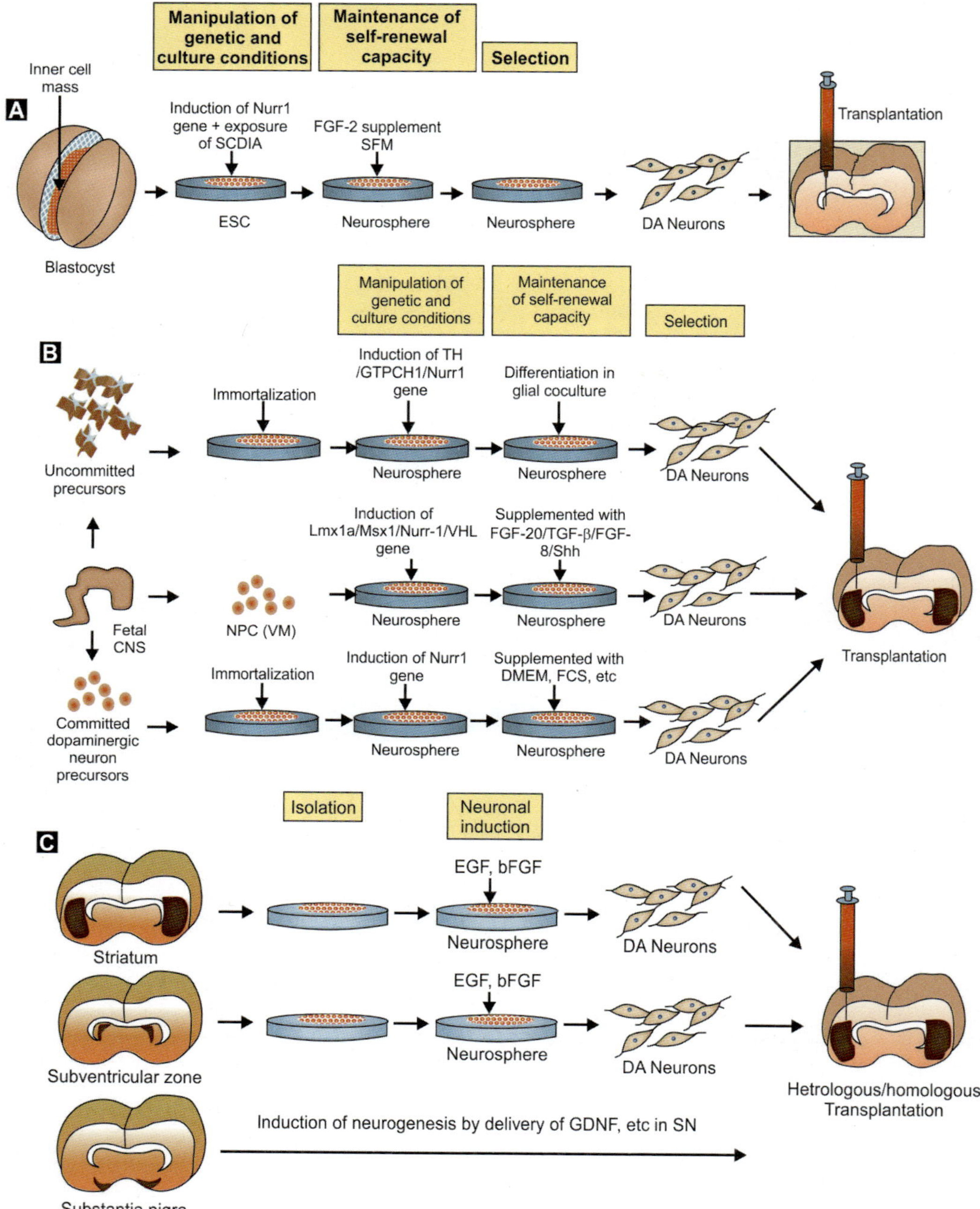

Figures 3.3A to C: Schematic representation of protocols for the generation of dopaminergic neurons for the treatment of parkinson's disease from different sources of stem cells viz Embryonic stem cells (A), Fetal neural progenitor cells (B), Adult neural progenitor cells (C)

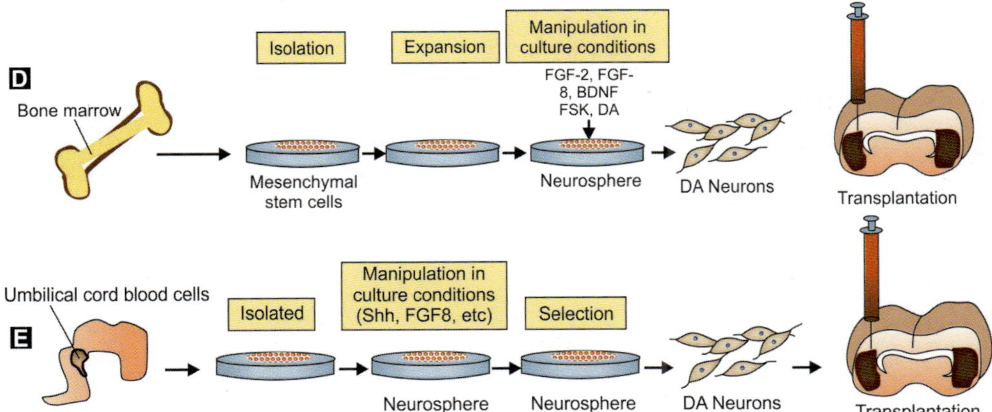

Figures 3.3D and E: Mesenchymal stem cells (D) and umbilical cord blood cells (E)

Abbreviations: SCDIA-stromal cell-derived inducing activity; FGF-2-fibroblast growth factor-2; SFM-serumfree medium; DA-dopaminergic; TH-tyrosine hydroxylase; GTPCH-1-guanidine triphosphate cyclohydrolase- 1; NPC-neural progenitor cells; VM-ventromedial; DMEM-Dulbecco's Modified Eagles' Medium; FCS-fetal calf serum; EGF-epidermal growth factor; bFGF-basic fibroblast growth factor; TGF-tissue growth factor

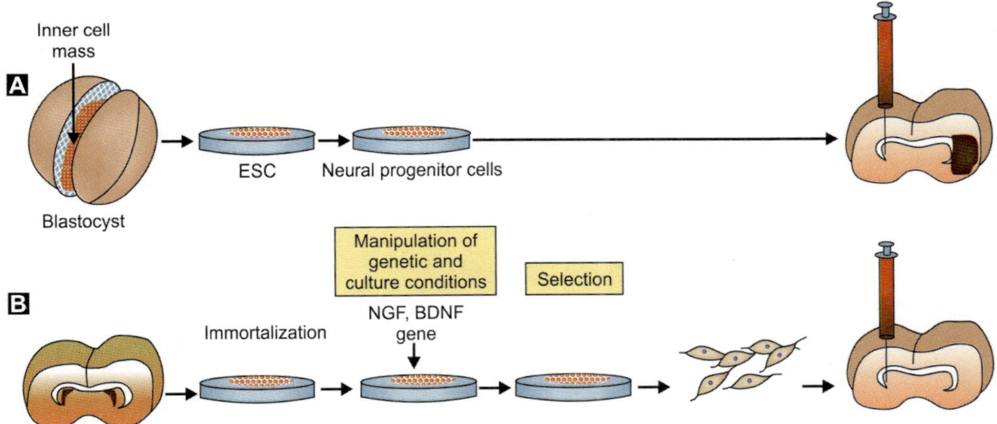

Figures 3.4A and B: Schematic representation showing use of ESC (A) and adult neural stem cells (B) for the generation of neural progenitors cells for the treatment of Huntington's disease

Abbreviations: ESC-embryonic stem cells; NGF-nerve growth factor; BDNF-brain derived neurotrophic factors

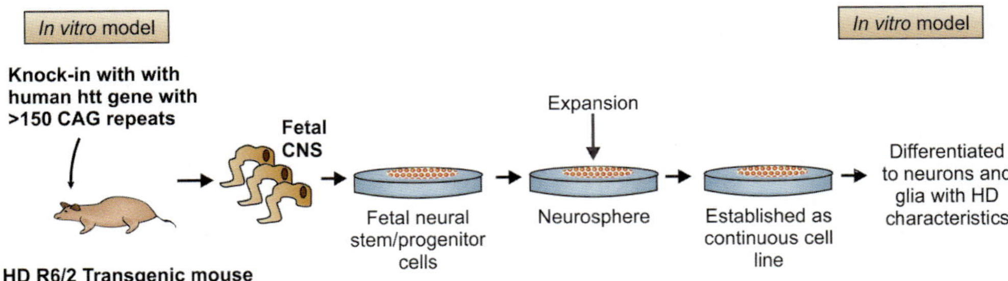

Figure 3.5: Schematic representation showing *in vivo* transgenic mice model carrying a mutated human gene for huntingtin (htt) and a protocol for producing neuronal and glial population with HD phenotype for *in vitro* screening of drugs and stem cell therapy for Huntington's disease

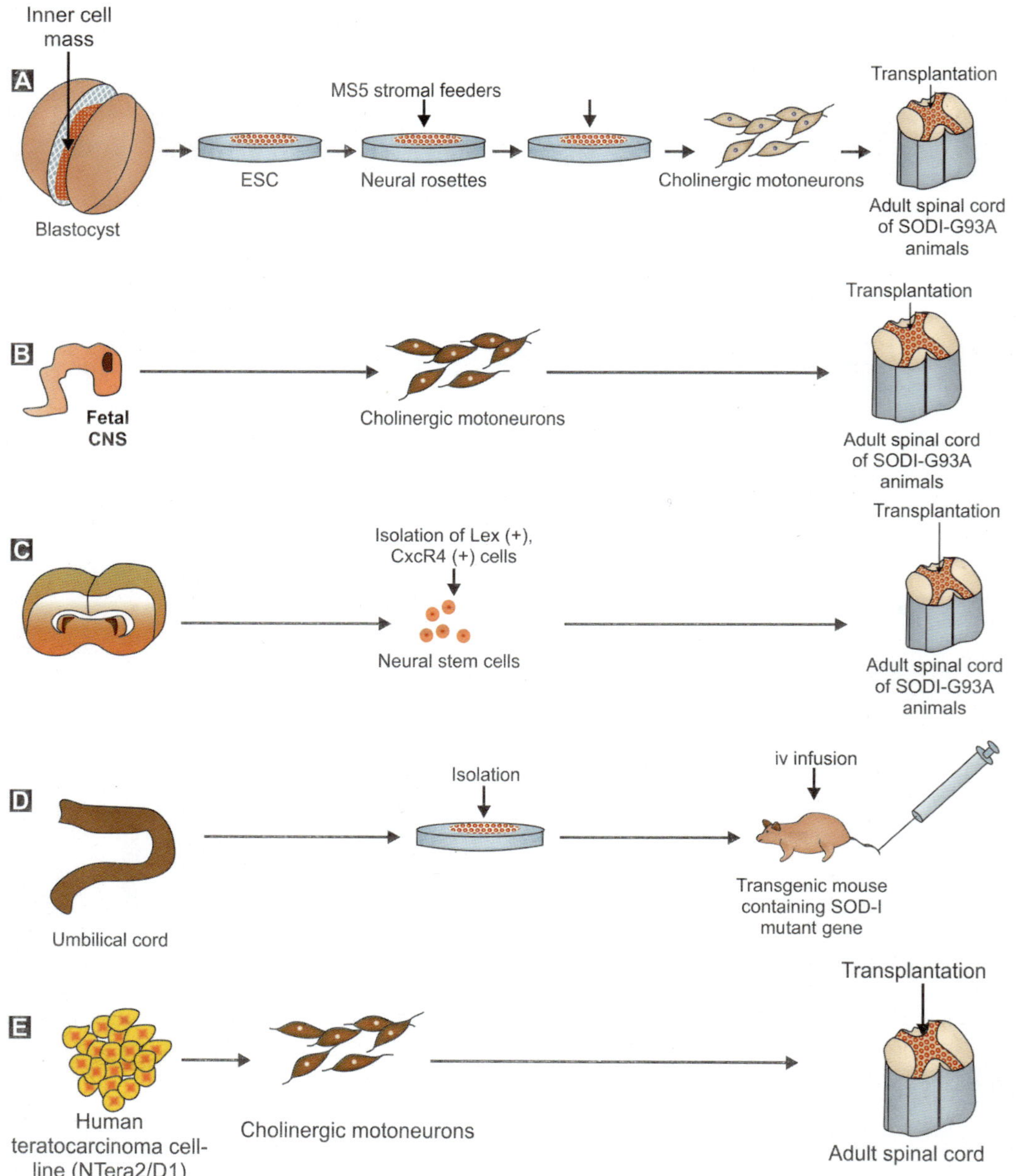

Figure 3.6: Generation of cholinergic motor neurons for ALS
Abbreviation: SOD1-superoxide dismutase-1

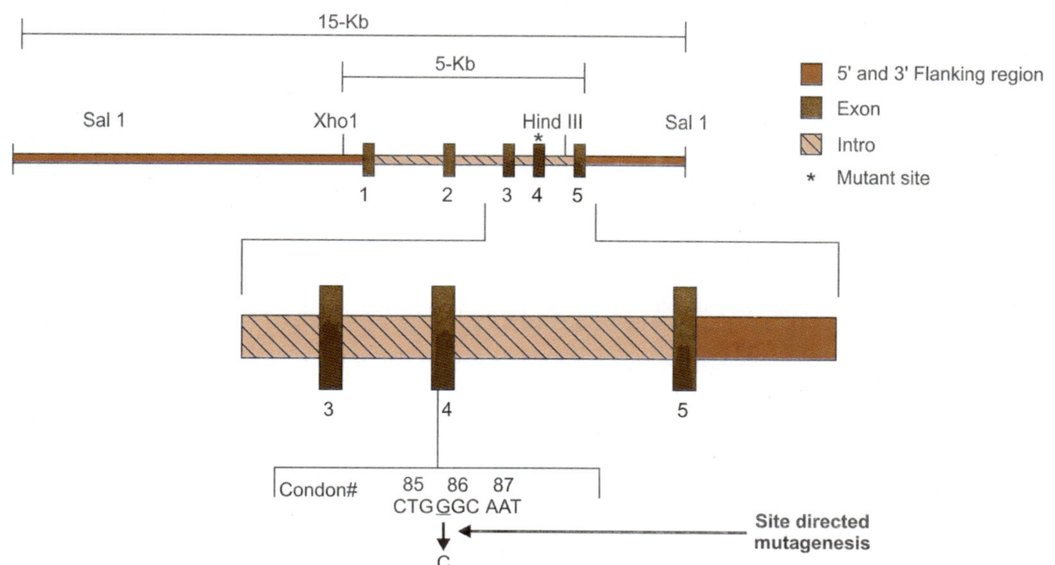

Figure 3.7: Mutagenesis of the mouse SOD-1 gene. The transgene was constructed by introducing a point mutation at the indicated position (*) in exon 4. Nucleotides shown in boldface type form a recognition sequence for Fsp I generated by the mutagenesis procedure

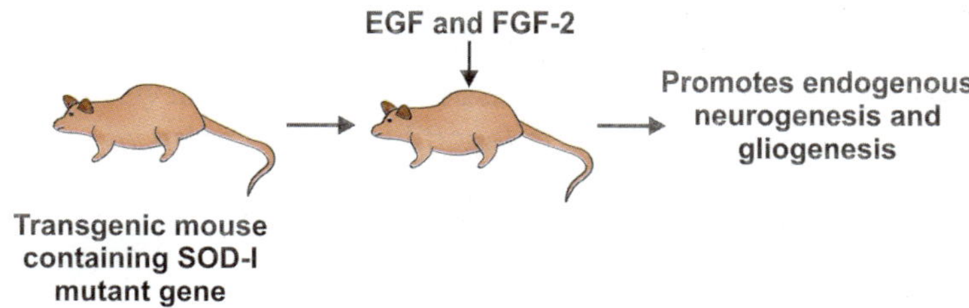

Figure 3.8: Administration of growth factors promotes endogenous regenerative process in ALS mouse model

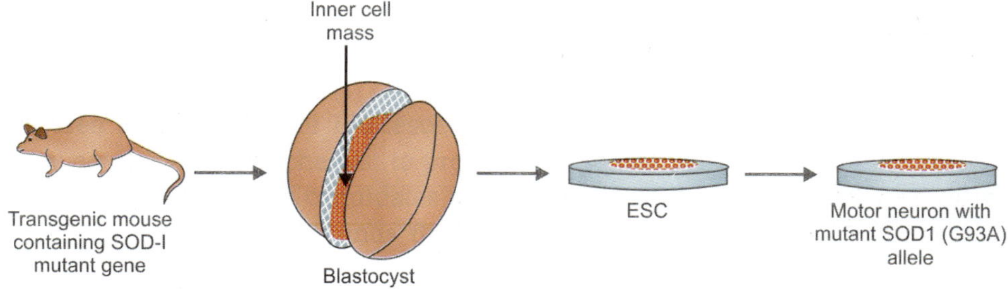

Figure 3.9: *In vitro* model system for studying the mechanisms of neural degeneration and identification of new ALS drugs or alternative stem cell based therapy

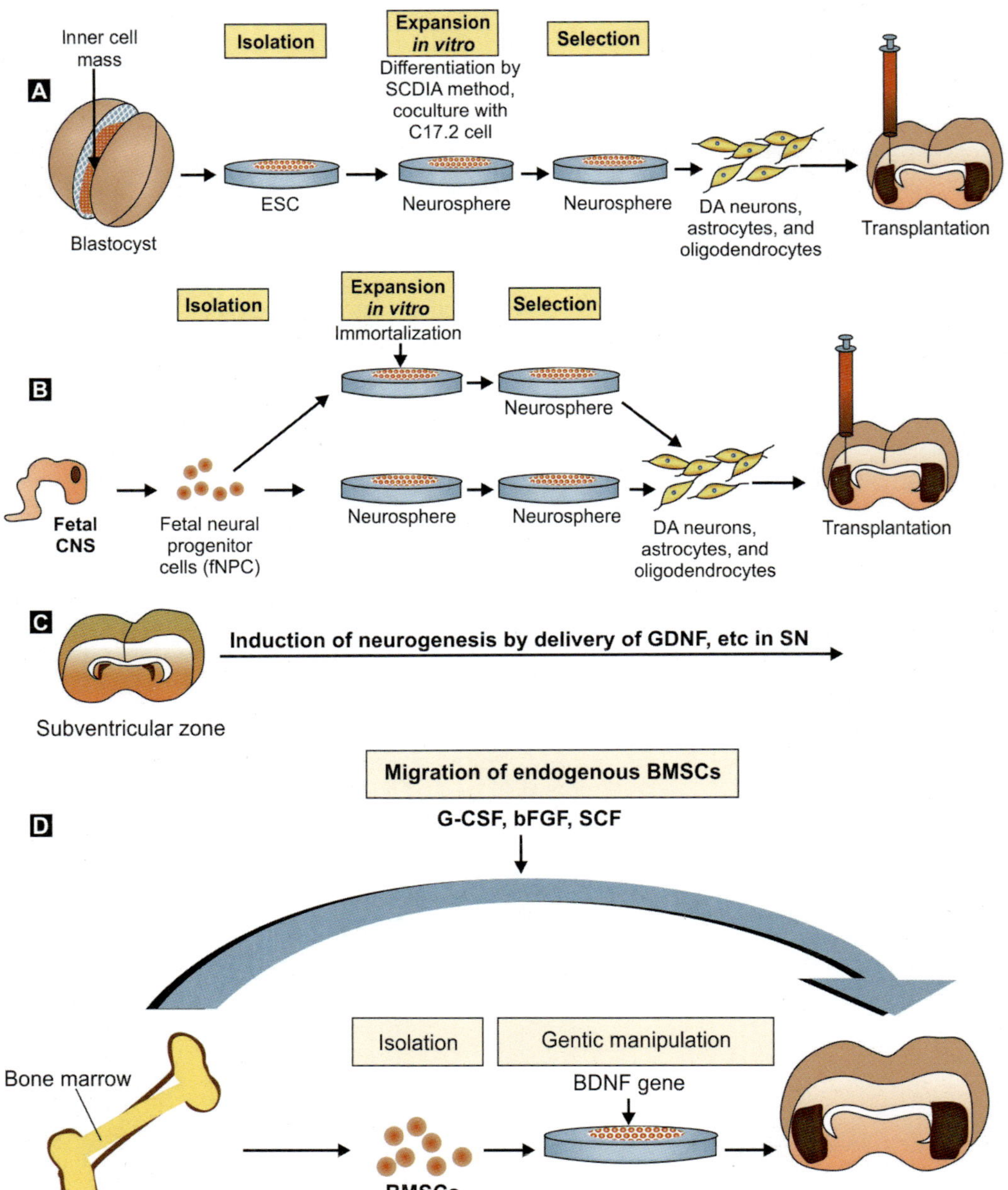

Figure 3.10: Protocols for generation neural and glial population for the treatment of cerebral stroke from different sources of stem cells viz ESCs (A), Fetal neural progenitor cells (B), Adult neural progenitor cells (C), Mesenchymal stem cells (D)

Abbreviations: BMSCs-bone marrow derived stem cells; BDNF-brain derived neurotrophic factors; G-CSF Granulocyte colony stimulating factor; bFGF-basic fibroblast growth factor; SCF-stem cell factor

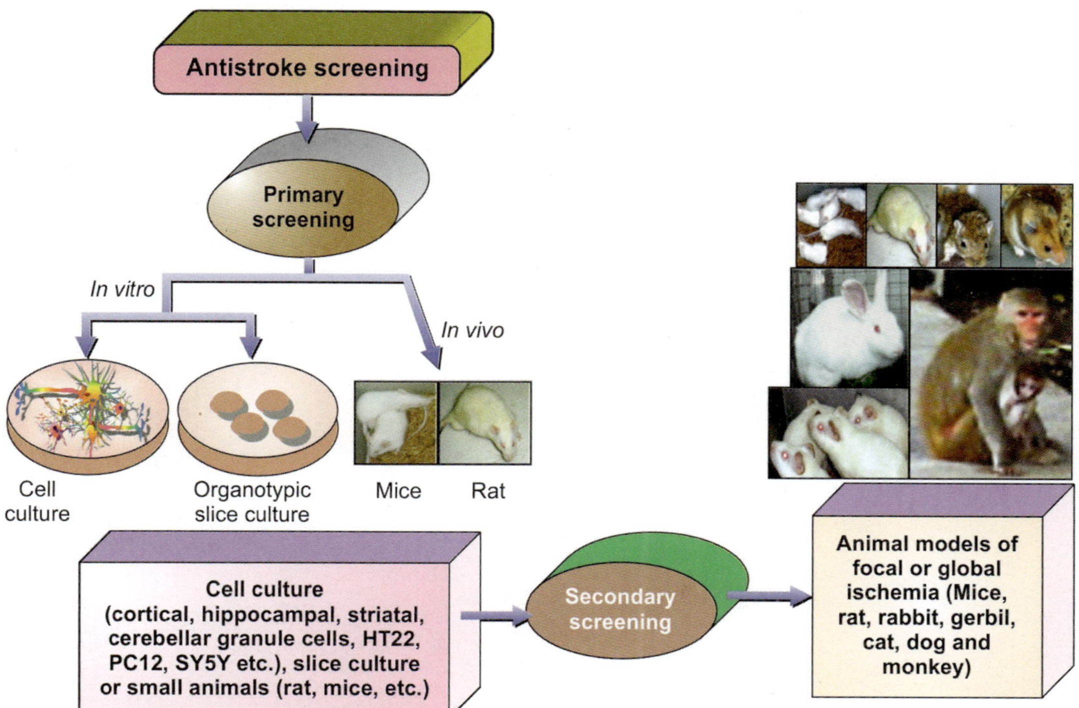

Figure 4.2: Schematic view of primary and secondary screening for antistroke test compounds

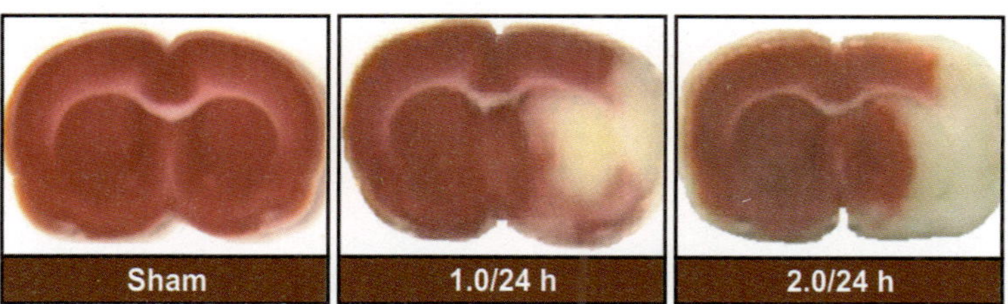

Figure 4.3: TTC stained brain slices after different time point of ischemia/reperfusion

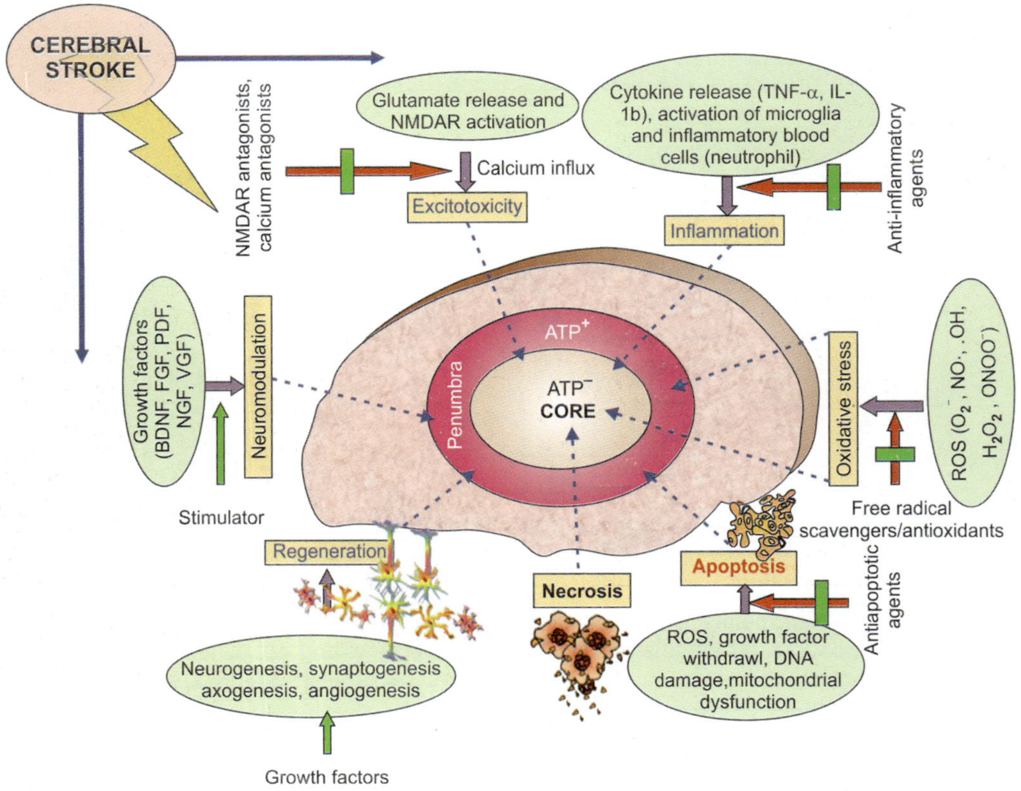

Figure 4.4: Shows various approaches of targeting cerebral stroke

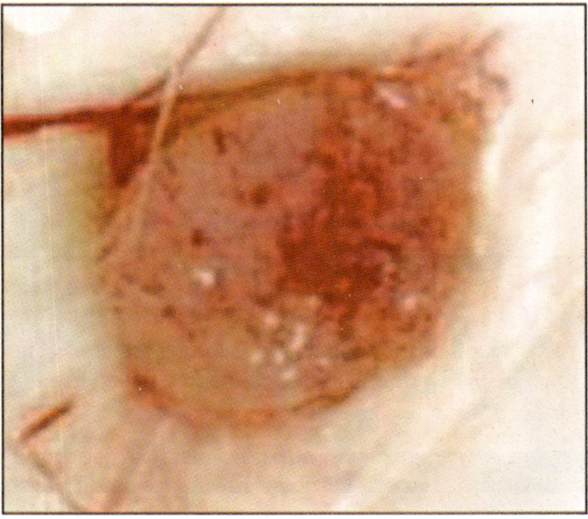

Figure 6.1: Angiogenesis observed in a sponge implanted subcutaneously in the subscapular region in the mouse. Angiogenesis is quantified by measuring the clearance of a dye or radioactive tracer from the sponge or by staining the sections with an antibody against von Willebrand factor that acts as a marker for endothelial cells. Other markers can also be used

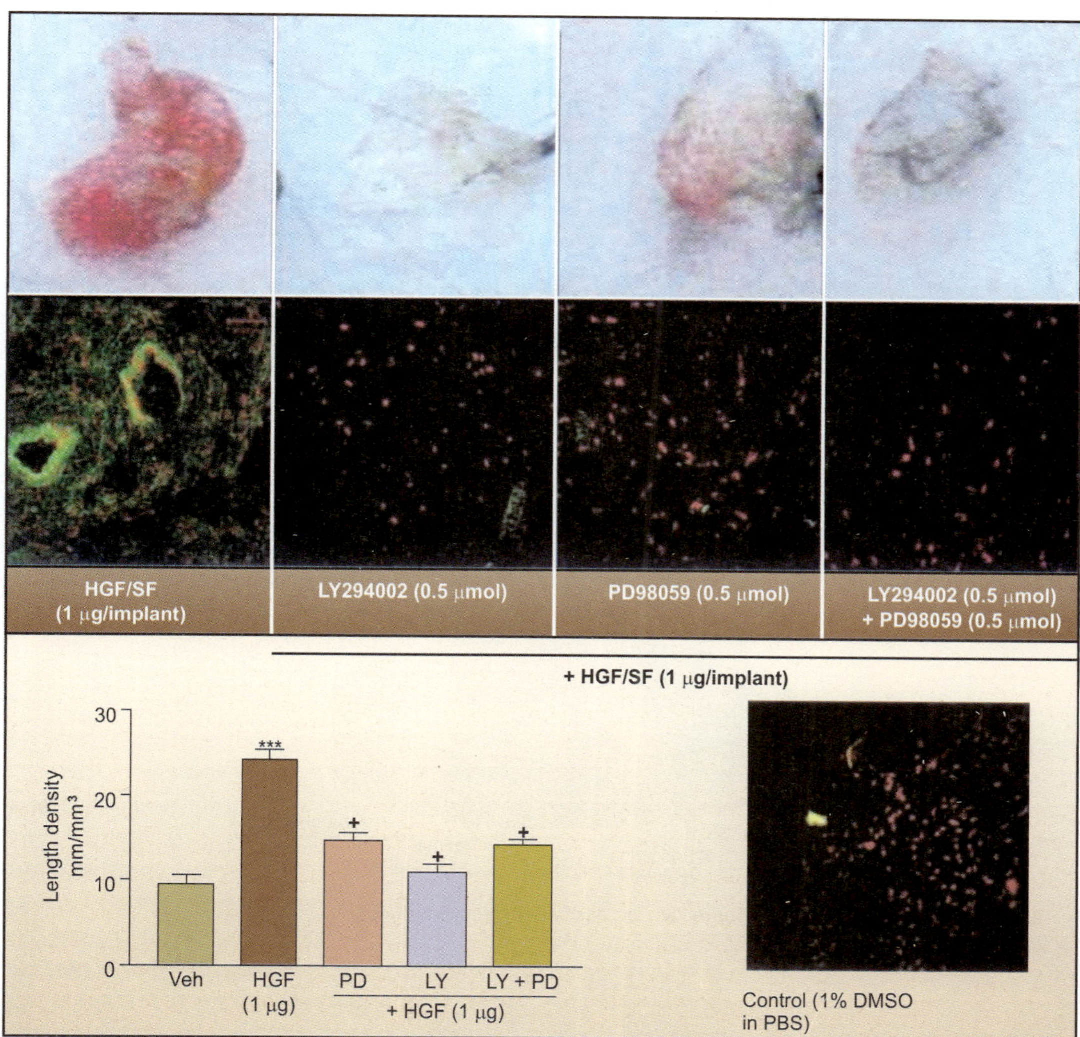

Figure 6.2: Matrigel implant model. Effect of PI3K and MAPK inhibitors on HGF/SF-induced angiogenesis in matrigel implants in vivo. Photomicrographs depict neovascularization induced by HGF/SF and inhibitory effects of PD98059 and LY294002. Upper panel shows gross morphology; lower panel shows cross section with blood vessels delineated with immunolabeling (FITC) for von Willebrand factor. Nuclei were counterstained with propidium iodide and appear blue. Images were captured with resolution of 512 × 512 pixels

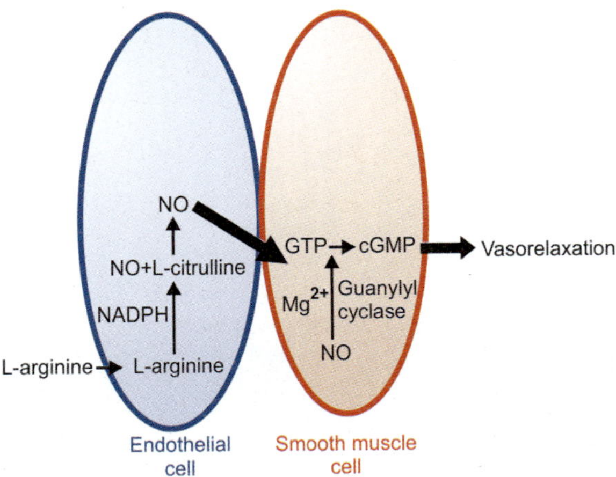

Figure 7.1: Interaction between endothelial cells and smooth muscle of the corpora cavernosa leading to erection

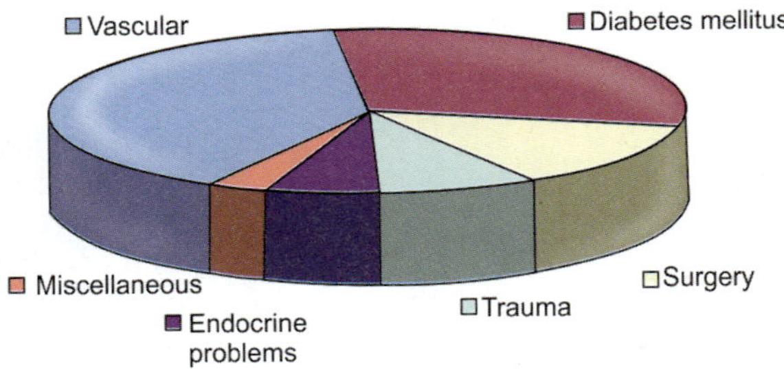

Figure 7.2: Causes of male erectile dysfunction

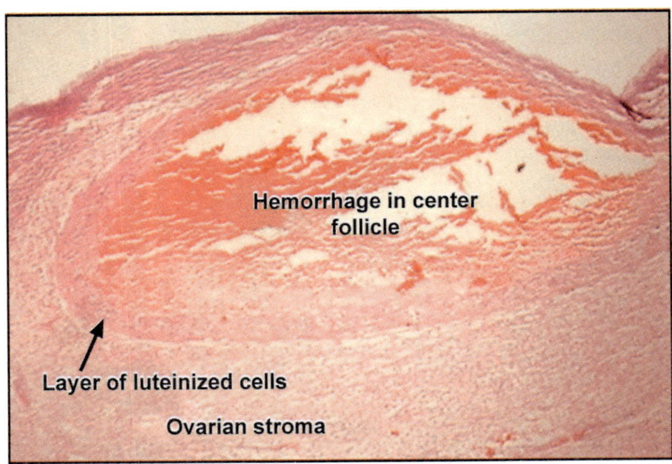

Figure 8.1: Ovulation point in rabbit ovary (HE × 40 ×)

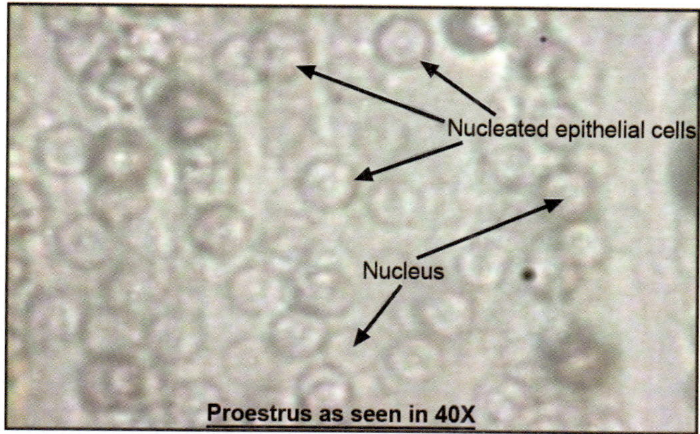

Figure 8.2: Rat vaginal smear at proestrus stage showing nucleated epithelial cells as seen in 40X

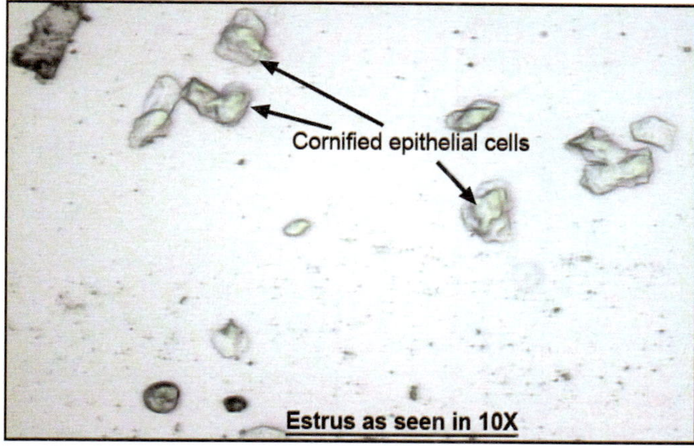

Figure 8.3: Rat vaginal smear at estrus stage showing cornified epithelial cells as seen in 10X

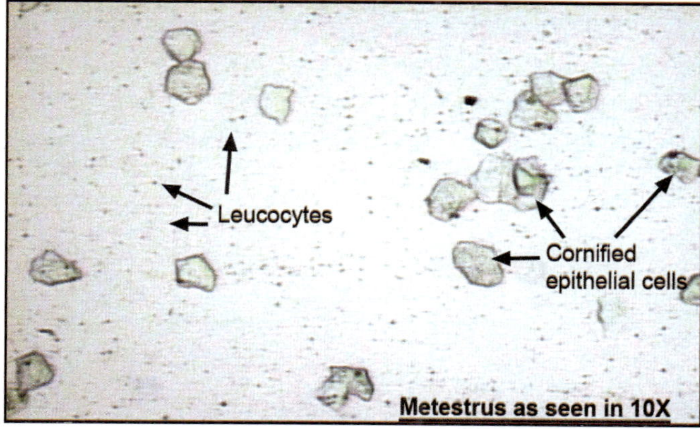

Figure 8.4: Rat vaginal smear at metestrus stage showing both cornified epithelial cells and leukocytes as seen in 10X

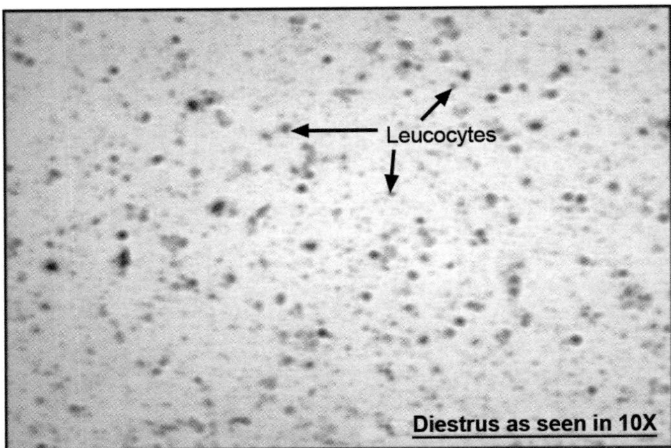

Figure 8.5: Rat vaginal smear at diestrus stage showing only leukocytes as seen in 10X

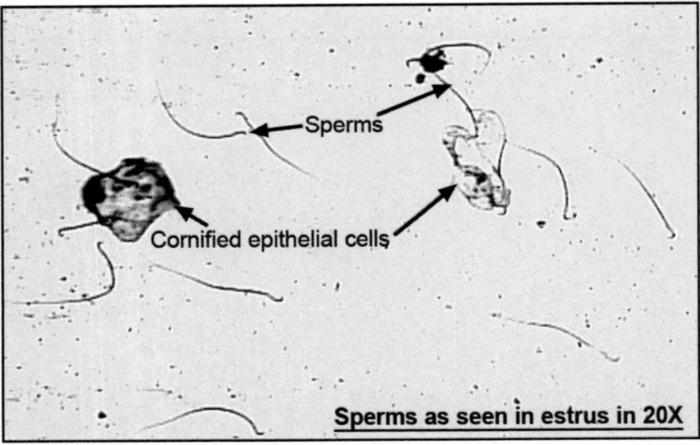

Figure 8.6: Rat vaginal smear of mated animal showing cornified epithelial cells and sperms as seen in 20X

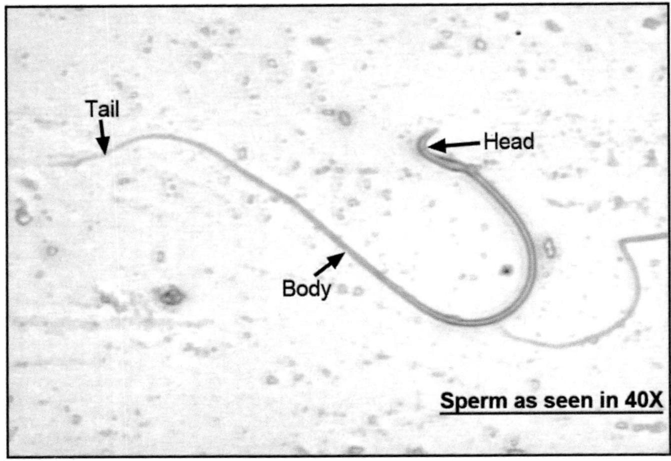

Figure 8.7: Rat vaginal smear of mated animal showing sperms as seen in 40X

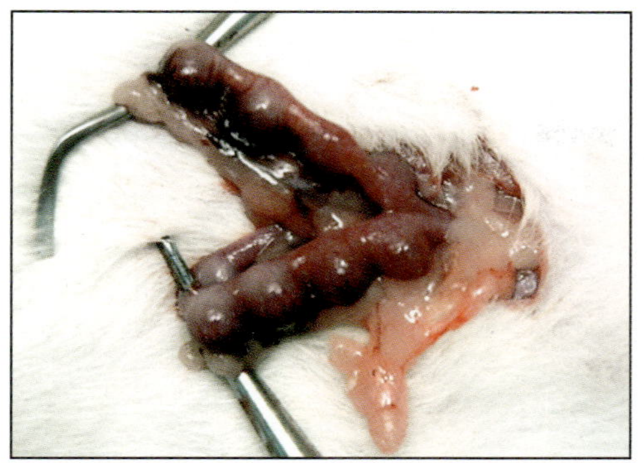

Figure 8.9: Rat uterus showing normal implants on 10th day of pregnancy

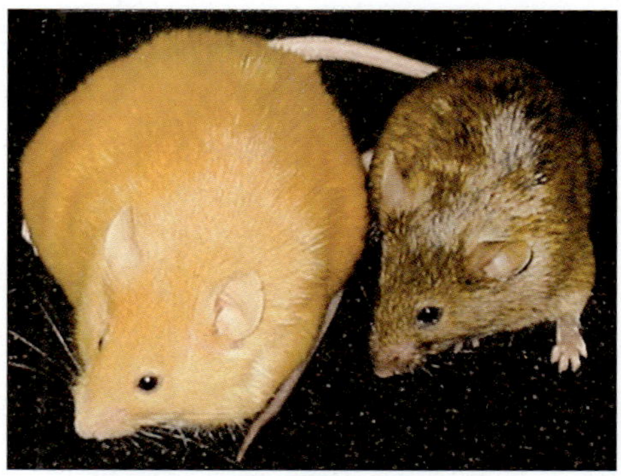

Figure 9.1: Yellow obese ($A^y a$) mice

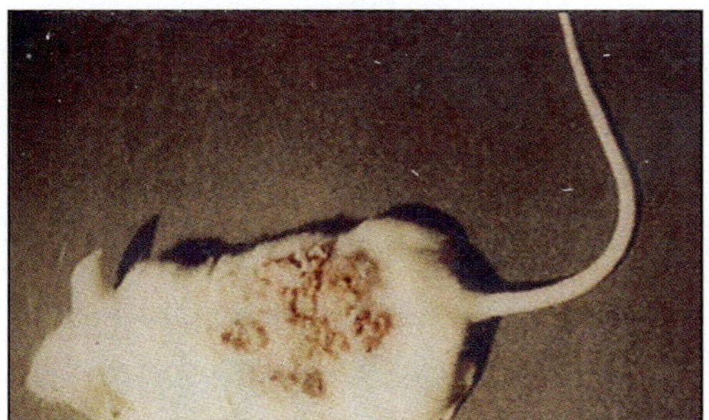

Figure 10.2: DMBA treated Swiss albino mouse (24th week) with papillomas. 100 nmol DMBA/100 µl acetone was applied topically on the depilated back of mouse twice weekly for 8 weeks

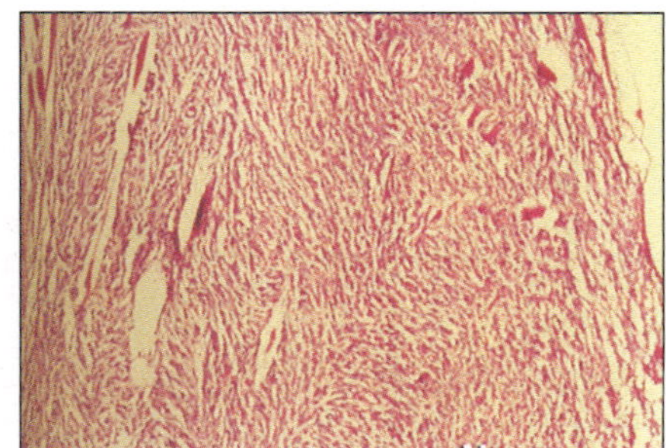

Figure 10.3: 20-Methylcholanthrene induced fibrosarcoma in the subcutaneous tissue of mouse with focal areas of necrosis (N) (H and E × 120). Mouse was injected 200 µg of MCA/100 µl DMSO into the thigh region subcutaneously and sacrificed at the end of 15th week for histopathological analysis

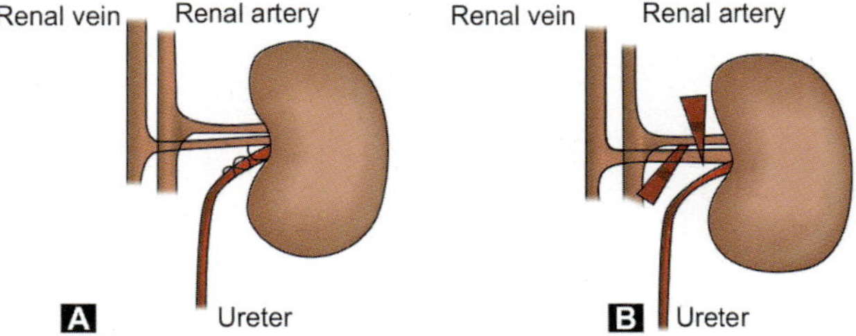

Figure 11.1: Schematic presentation of the ureteral obstruction model showing the placement of two ligations at the ureter (A) and the renal ischemia-reperfusion model showing the blockade of renal artery and vein with clips (B)

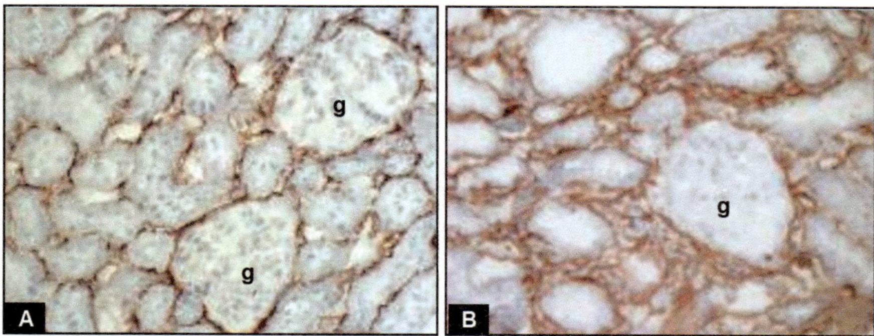

Figure 11.2: Pictures of immunohistochemical staining (red color) for collagen-III in normal kidney (A) and in kidneys with adriamycin-induced nephropathy (B). A single dose of adriamycin (5 mg/kg) was administered in Wistar rats and after 4 weeks staining was performed. Collagen-III deposition in tubulointerstitium was substantially enhanced in adriamycin treatment rats. Sections were counter-stained with hematoxyllin. g = glomerulus. Magnification 20 × 10

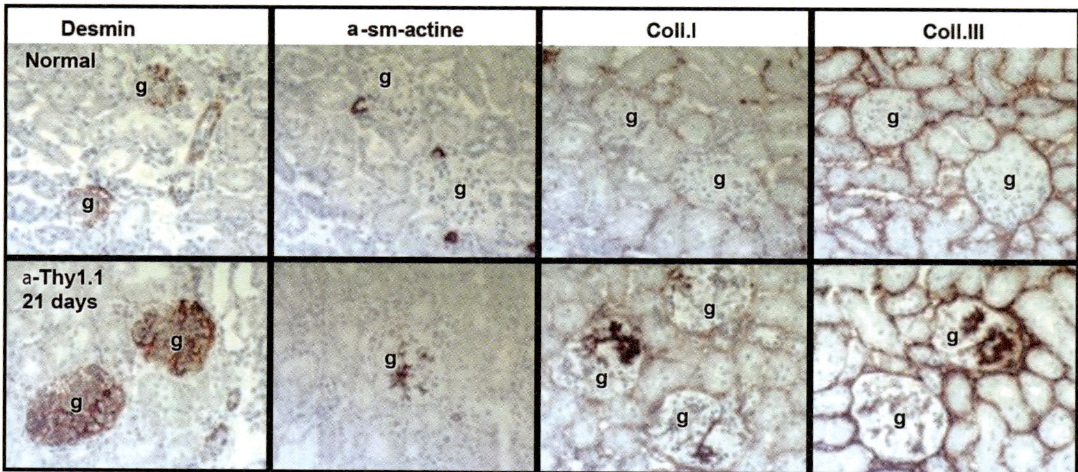

Figure 11.3: Pictures of immunohistochemical stainings (red color) for desmin, alpha-smooth muscle actin collagen type I and collagen type III in normal kidney (upper panel) and in kidneys with anti-Thy1 IgG-induced renal fibrosis (lower panel). A single dose of anti-Thy 1 IgG was administered in Wistar rats and after 21 days staining was performed. The number of fibroblasts (desmin and actin staining) as well as the interstitial matrix deposition (collagens staining) was substantially increased after administration of anti-Thy 1 IgG. Sections were counterstained with hematoxyllin. g = glomerulus. Magnification 20 × 10

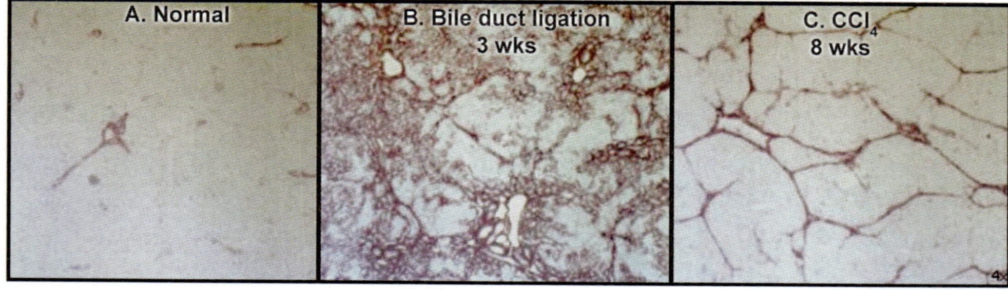

Figure 11.4: Pictures illustrating the enhanced matrix deposition (collagen type III immunostaining) in two important rat models of liver fibrosis as compared to normal livers. (A) normal rat liver (B) rat liver 3 weeks after bile duct ligation, and (C) rat liver 8 weeks after CCl_4 intoxication. Magnification 4 × 10

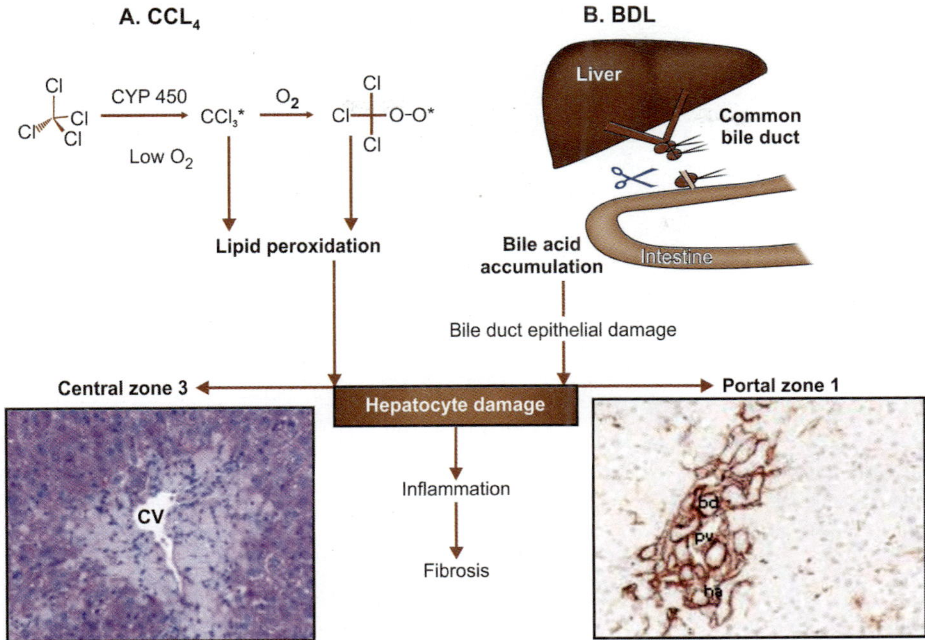

Figure 11.5: Schematic illustration of two different models of liver fibrosis: (A) CCl_4 intoxication and (B) Bile duct ligation (BDL). CCl_4 causes hepatocyte damage predominantly in zone 1 (as illustrated by the PAS stained liver at the left). Ligation of the bile duct causes damage to bile duct epithelial cells and damage is seen in portal area (as illustrated with the collagen I+III stained liver at the right). cv=central vein; bd=bile duct; ha=hepatic artery; pv=portal vein. Magnification 20 × 10

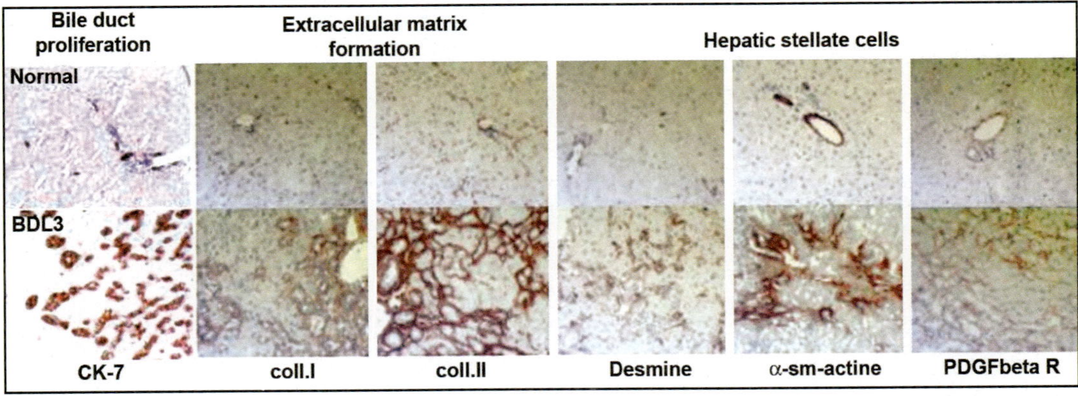

Figure 11.6: Liver fibrosis induced 3 weeks after ligation of the bile duct (BDL3). Pictures of immunohistochemical stainings (red color) for cytokeratin-7 (marker of bile duct epithelial cells), collagen types I and III (matrix formation), desmin (marker for all HSC), and alpha-smooth muscle actin, and PDGFbeta receptor (markers for transformed HSC and myofibroblasts) in normal livers (upper panel) and in BDL3 livers (lower panel). The number of bile duct epithelial cells, myofibroblasts (desmin, actin, and PDGFR staining) as well as the interstitial matrix deposition (collagens staining) was substantially increased after ligation of the bile duct. Sections were counterstained with hematoxyllin. Magnifications 20 × 10

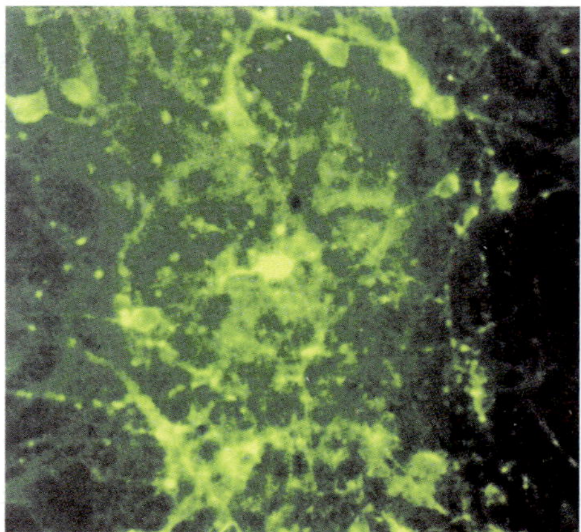

Figure 12.1: Fluorescence microscopy image of 15 weeks gestational age human fetus brain primary cell culture. Cells were stained with Hoechst staining after induction of apoptosis with anti-Fas agonist antibodies. The labeled cells exhibit condensed nuclear fluorescence while viable cells exhibit diffuse nuclear fluorescence. (*Reproduced with permission from J Cell Mol Med 2001;5: 179-87*)

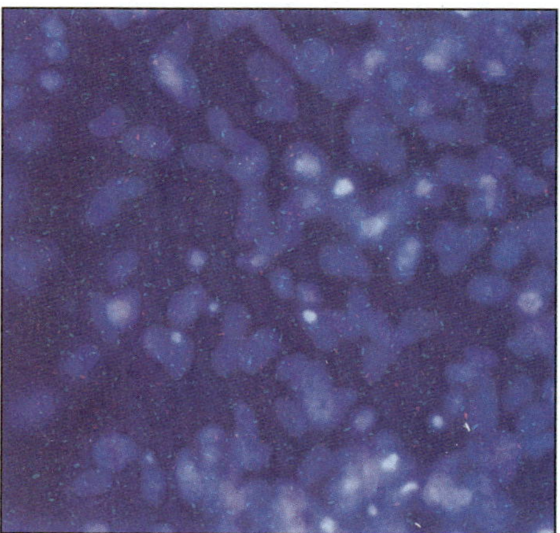

Figure 12.2: Fluorescence microscopy image of 15 weeks gestational age human fetus brain primary cell culture. Cells were stained with annexin V- FITC after induction of apoptosis with anti-Fas agonist antibodies. Labeled cells exhibit condensed nuclear fluorescence while viable cells exhibit diffuse nuclear fluorescence. (*Reproduced with permission from J Cell Mol Med 2001; 5: 179-87*)

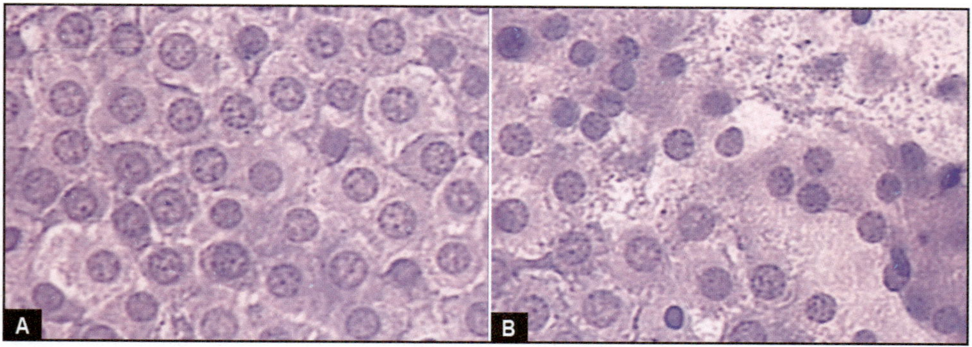

Figure 13.2: Human lens epithelial cells: (A) Normal HLEC cultured in DMEM alone; (B) HLEC cultured in DMEM under oxidative stress

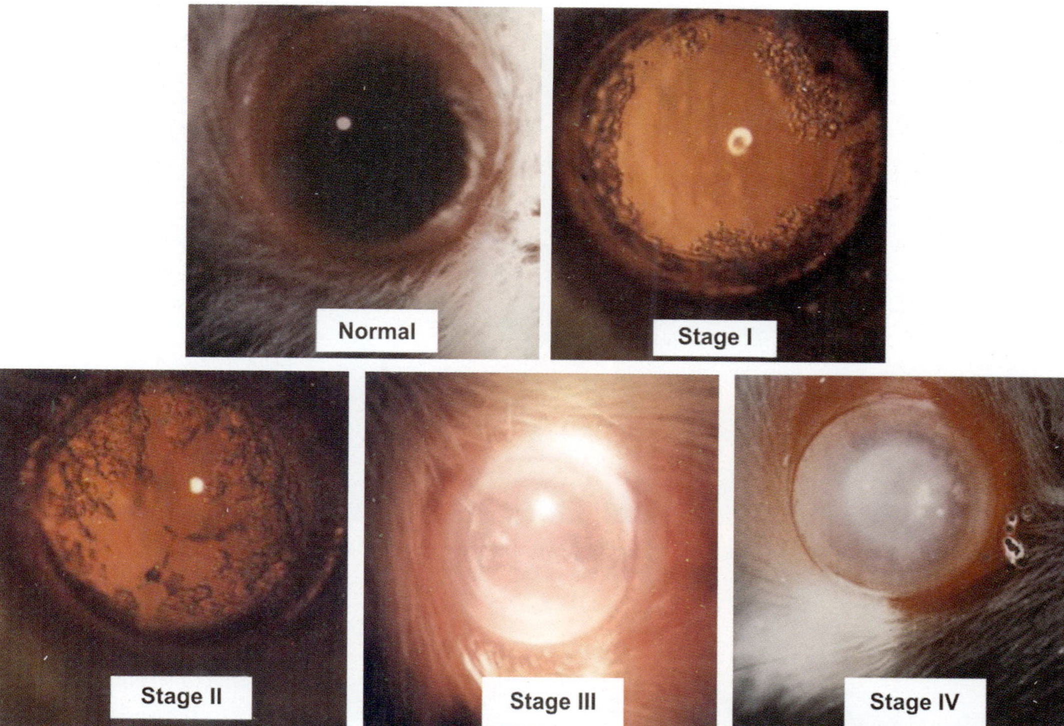

Figure 13.4: Slit lamp photographs of various stages of galactose-induced cataract in rats. Normal: Clear transparent lens; Stage I: Peripheral vacuoles in the lens; Stage II: Vacuoles involving the center of the lens; Stage III: Faint opalescence visible with the naked eye; Stage IV: Mature nuclear cataract. [Reprinted from Nutrition, Vol. 19(9), Suresh Kumar Gupta, Deepa Trivedi, Sushma Srivastava, Sujata Joshi, Nabanita Halder and Shambhu Dayal Verma. 'Lycopene attenuates oxidative stress induced experimental cataract development: An *in vitro* and *in vivo* study', pp 794-9, 2003, with permission from Elsevier]

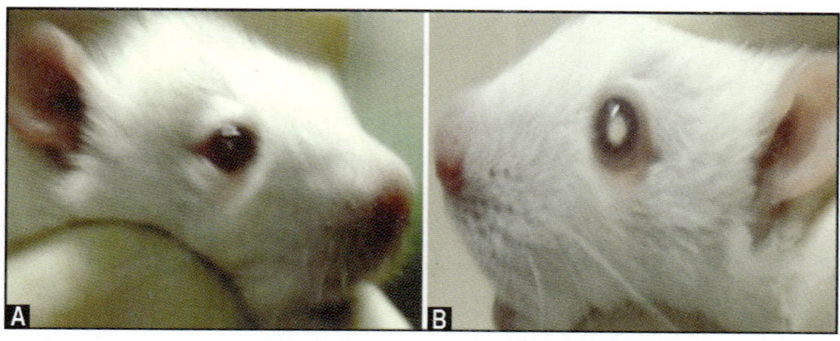

Figure 13.5: Selenite-induced cataract in rat pups: (A) 16-day-old rat pup showing normal eye with clear lens; (B) Rat pup of the same litter injected subcutaneously with sodium selenite showing nuclear cataract

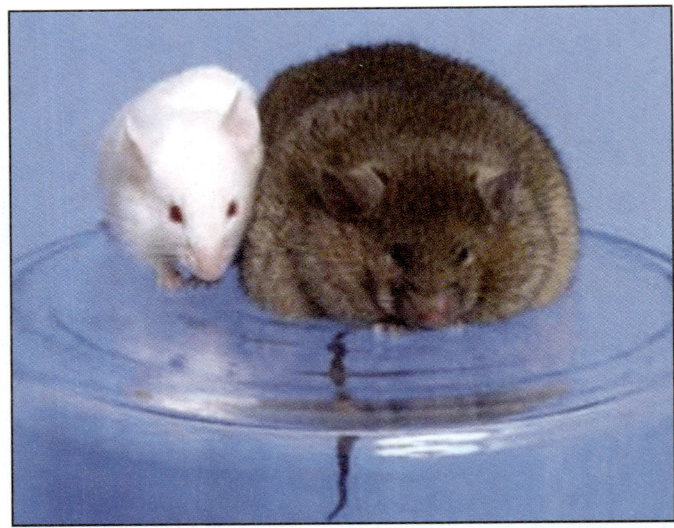

Figure 15.1: Syngeneic mouse-Non-obese diabetic (NOD) mouse as model for screening immune-based disorders

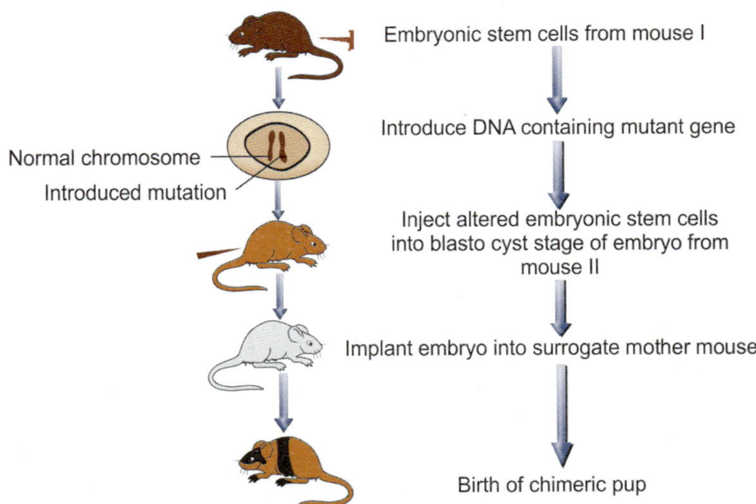

Figure 15.2: Developing knockout mouse

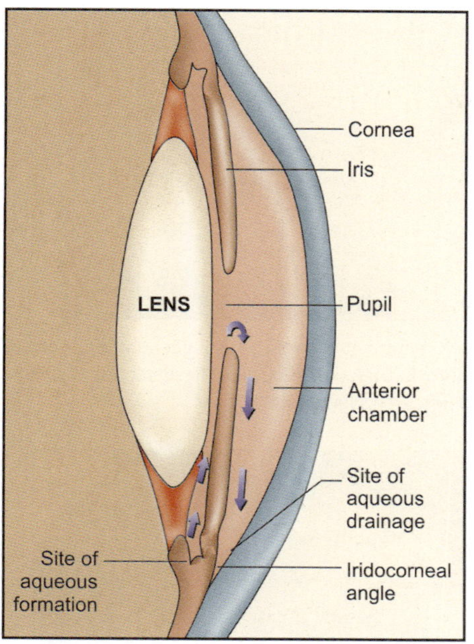

Figure 17.1: Pathway of aqueous flow

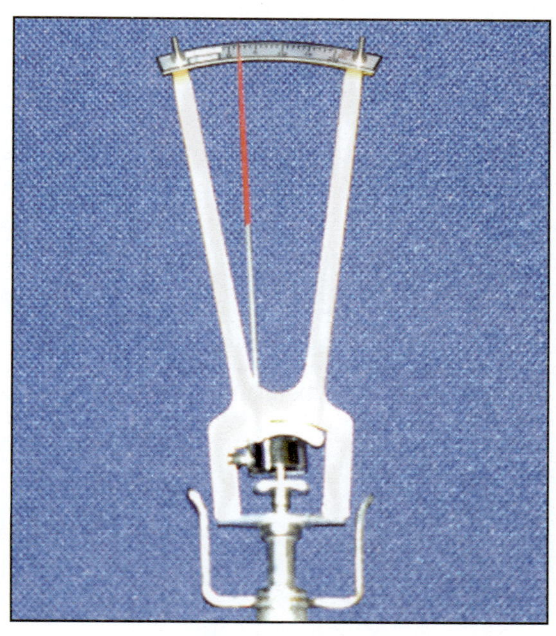

Figure 17.2: Shiotz tonometer

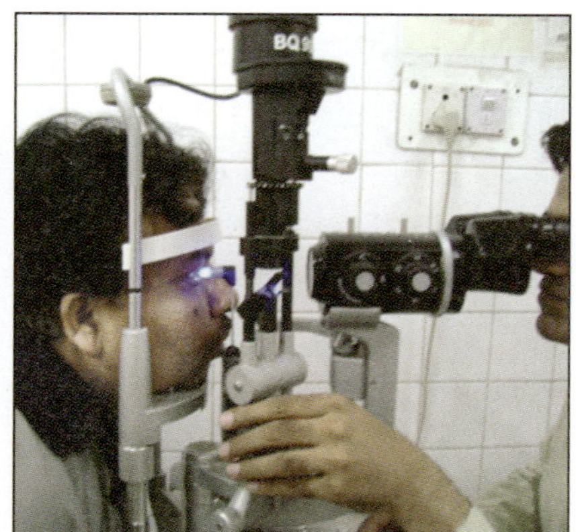

Figure 17.3: Goldman applanation tonometer

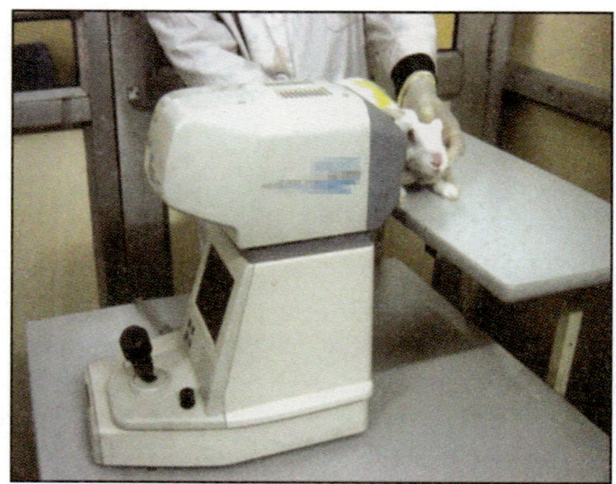

Figure 17.4: Noncontact tonometer

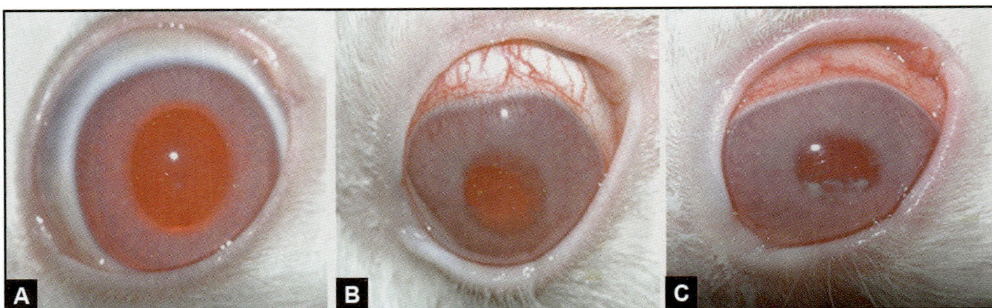

Figure 34.1: Clinical signs of anterior uveitis in control group: (A) Just before intravitreal endotoxin injection; (B) 24 hours post intravitreal endotoxin injection; (C) 72 hours post-intravitreal endotoxin injection (*Courtesy*: Researchers of Ocular Pharmacology Laboratory, Delhi Institute of Pharmaceutical Sciences and Research, New Delhi)

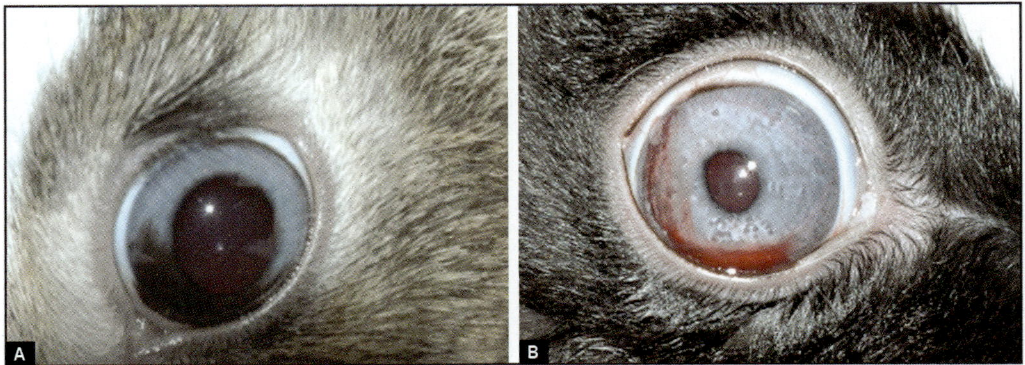

Figure 34.2: Laser treatment in pigmented rabbit eyes: (A) Normal eye (B) Post-laser with hyphema (*Courtesy*: Researchers of Ocular Pharmacology Laboratory, Delhi Institute of Pharmaceutical Sciences and Research, New Delhi)

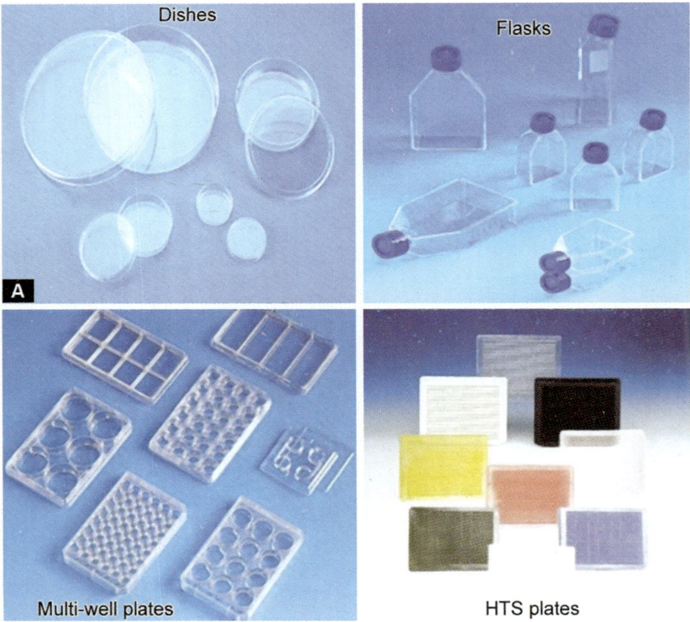

Contd...

Contd...

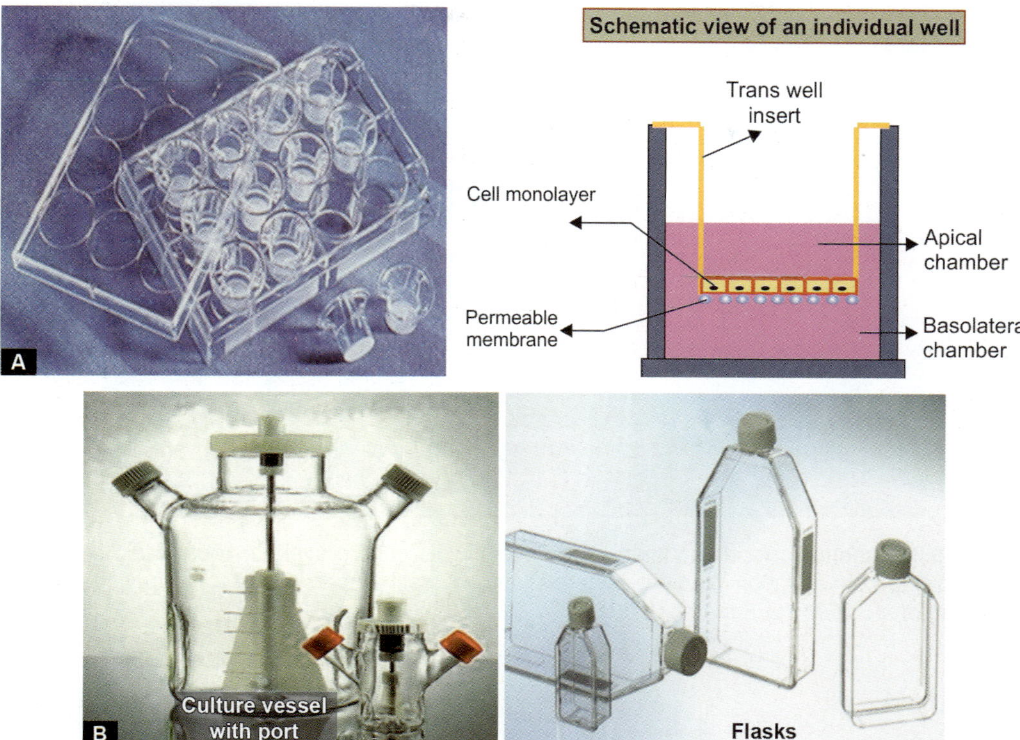

Figure 45.1: Types of vessels for human cell cultures: (A) Adherent Culture System; (B) Suspension Culture System (Ref. www.sigmaaldrich.com)

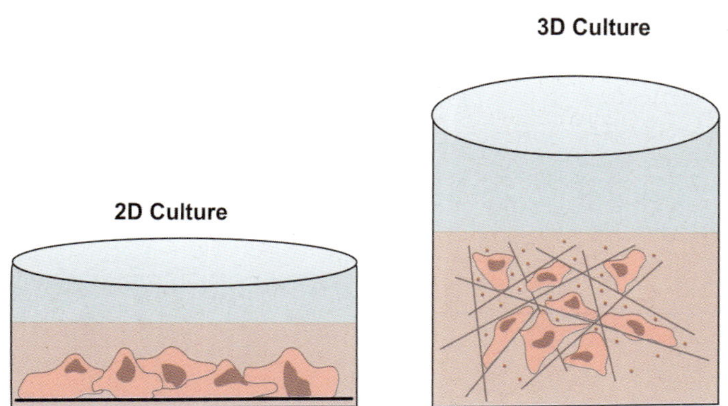

Figure 45.2: Schematic Representation of 2D Vs 3D cultures

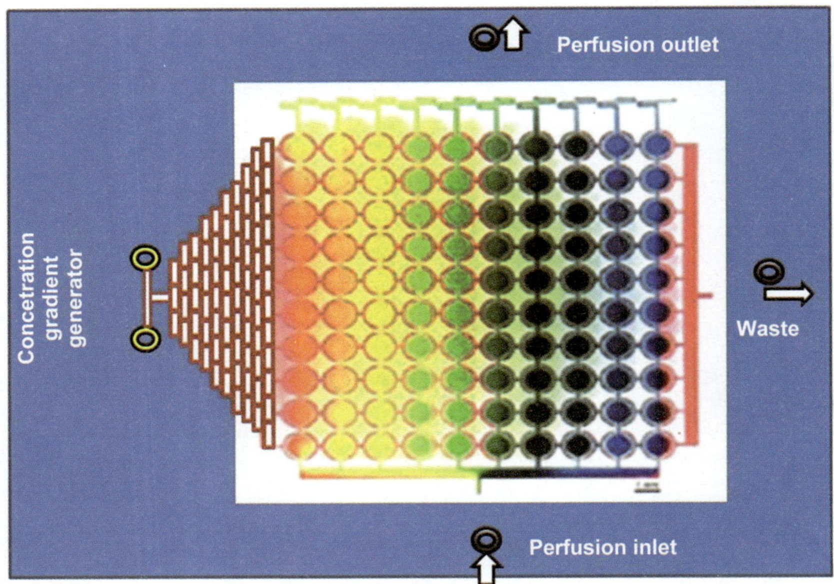

Figure 45.3: Schematic representation of 3D Microfluidic culture system. Microfluidic cell culture array showing concentration gradient generator and microchambers on 2X2 cm device (*Adapted from Hung et al., 2005*[23] *& Zang et al.,2012*[1])

CHAPTER

1

Newer Tools for Drug Screening

INTRODUCTION

The last quarter of the century has seen transformation of the pharmaceutical industry. The advances in the field of information technologies have driven basic research to evolve into fast-track drug discovery and development program that is target oriented while still beating the clock. There is competition within the industry to continuously generate the next billion-dollar selling compound. Market estimates project that the journey of a new molecule from laboratory to market takes well over seven years at an average cost of over $600 m. Consequently there is thrust on developing advances in technologies aiming to reduce the time and the costs involved in bringing a new drug to market. This has lead to the introduction of revolutionary technological advances such as combinatorial chemistry, biochemical assays, genomics, proteomics, miniaturization, automation, robotic systems and computerization, which have cumulatively increased the speed of lead generation manifold.

Just to cite a case, by using way of traditional drug development techniques, it took nearly half-a-century to tap the cholesterol biosynthesis pathway and develop statin drugs, as cholesterol lowering agents. On the other hand, molecular-revelations regarding the role of the HER-2 receptor in breast cancer led to the development of the chemotherapeutic agent, Herceptin® within three years. The advanced techniques of *in silico* molecular modeling, high throughput screening and genomic and proteomic databases, were instrumental in the quick discovery and development of Herceptin.[1]

Some of the screen paradigms that are being rigorously adopted by pharmaceutical companies to speed up the development of next blockbuster drug are discussed in this chapter.

CASSETTE DOSING

As compared to generation of 100 leads that were produced a decade ago, combinatorial chemistry now enables the chemist to produce thousands of leads each year.[2] The problem is no longer of too few drug candidates emerging from the discovery process – in fact the number of quality lead compounds that emerge is much higher. It is being understood that rather than drug discovery, it is drug development that is proving to be the bottleneck (Fig. 1.1). The battery of preclinical tests such as toxicity, bioavailability and pharmacokinetics are extremely critical, time-consuming and costly. Prioritization of leads with regard to

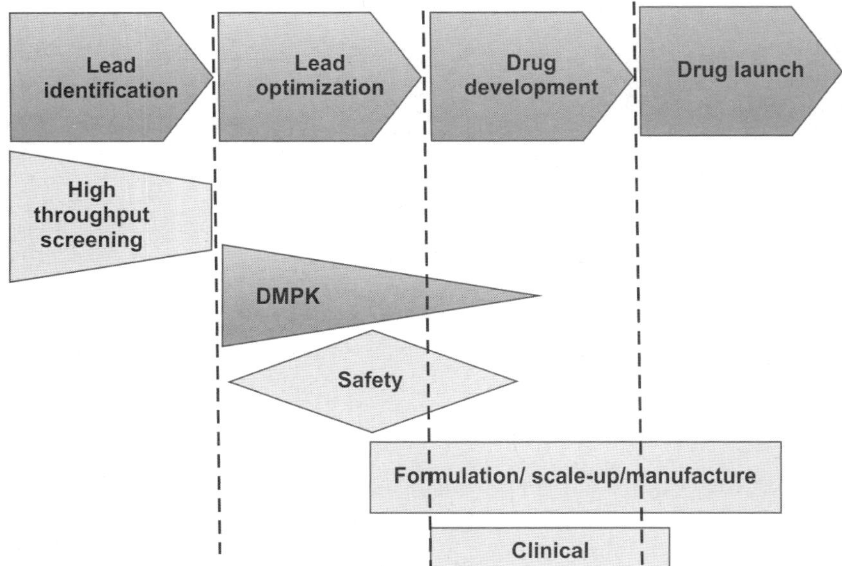

Figure 1.1: Bottleneck at drug development stage reducing the speed of generation of novel drugs

these studies becomes a stumbling block in the selection of viable targets from millions of compounds. Due to several constraints, classical methods are not high throughput and have often impeded the quick development of new drug candidates. This has generated need for high throughput drug development program to be set-up and started in full throttle.[3]

Although pharmacokinetic evaluation is an essential component of drug discovery program, it has proved to be a serious bottleneck during the 'hit-to-lead' and lead optimization phases of drug discovery and development program. The prioritization of leads with regard to drug metabolism and pharmacokinetics (DMPK) assumes importance as it determines the selection of viable targets from millions of compounds. A compound with favorable pharmacokinetics is more likely to be efficacious and safe. Early elimination of pharmacokinetically ineligible candidates helps to sift grain from chaff. For this critical juncture in drug development program, absolute reliance on *in vitro* tests cannot be advocated. As *in vitro* tests can never replicate the complex biological system, they serve as confirmatory tests rather than preliminary tests.[4]

Rodent species (mice, rats) have been classically used for *in vivo* pharmacokinetic studies. As there is a limitation to the amount of blood samples that may be withdrawn per animal, different animals have to be used for each time point, leading to high animal usage. In addition, inter-individual variation of various pharmacokinetic parameters is commonly encountered (up to two-fold) due to the differences in the expression of drug metabolism enzymes and genetic polymorphism. These further complicate data interpretation and slow the progress.[3]

Advances in drug development technology have provided the solution to the problems by providing alternate methods that help the discovery scientists to predict pharmacokinetics within the constraints of real physiological environment, but at the pace of *in vitro* or in silico methods. Cassette dosing is an elegant, inexpensive, nonlabor/time intensive novel technique that has been developed with the aim to rapidly assess pharmacokinetics of a large number of compounds (Table 1.1). Scientists at Glaxo Wellcome have been the pioneers in its development.[3]

In theory, cassette dosing or CD or 'N-in-one dosing' involves the simultaneous administration of several compounds (5-10) to a single animal followed by rapid sample analysis for the compounds and their metabolites by liquid chromatography/tandem mass spectrometry. It is a highly recommended technique as it enhances the efficiency in terms of time, money, manpower while reducing animal usage.[3]

Table 1.1: Estimated reduction in preclinical screening time after adopting cassette dosing

Stage of drug discovery program	*Currently time taken (months)*	*Estimated time taken with cassette dosing (months)*
Preclinical	15	12
Phase I	18	14
Phase II	22	12
Phase III	31.5	17.5
Total estimated time	7.2 years	4.5 years

Cassette dosing is based on the concept of serial bleeding that involves withdrawal of blood samples from the same animal for all the time points, which is estimated to not only dramatically reduce the number of animals used but also increased the quality of the kinetic data for compounds compared in that animal. Furthermore, the volume of blood samples that are withdrawn/animal/time point is miniscule. Literature search brings to fore descriptions of analytical methods that have used only 10-20 µl of whole blood using capillary LC/MS/MS. The onus for the success of this approach has to be granted to the superlative technique of LC/MS/MS, as it would not have been possible with other classical methods of analysis (spectrophotometry and chromatography).

Cassette dosing poses an analytical challenge as it involves simultaneously assaying many compounds in a single sample. In the absence of theoretical guidance, a set of intuitive assumptions has developed regarding the nature of the errors and how to avoid them.[3] These assumptions are:

1. Drug-drug interactions only occur when one of the dosed compounds is a potent inhibitor of drug-metabolizing enzymes.
2. One may guard against competitive inhibition of a shared metabolic enzyme by keeping doses small.
3. The size of the cassette (n) is limited only by the sensitivity of the assay and the solubility of the compounds.
4. Errors can be detected by including a benchmark compound with known pharmacokinetic characteristics.
5. Drug-drug interactions can lead only to false positives, which will be discovered later, and
6. Even if the absolute values are wrong, the correct rank order will be observed.

Although cassette dosing is an advantageous technique in terms of resources and throughput, there are possible complications associated with this approach. The technique of cassette dosing has been under critical review and is subject to high level validation. While using the technique of cassette dosing, inherent limitations of the technique have to be accounted for. Firstly, the potential for compound interactions is increased manifold.[5]

Although cassette dosing has been reported to yield useful results when used as a screen, especially to rank-order drug candidates, it has been shown to be fraught with both theoretical and experimental large errors. Consequently, under no circumstances can the pharmacokinetic parameters derived from cassette dosing be accepted as accurate. Potentially affected parameters include *F*, CL, AUC, *t*½, mean residence time, *Vd*. High-clearance compounds have the greatest potential for screening errors (i.e., false-positive, false-negative). To detect errors, a second dosing episode could be opted, that may in itself defeat the productivity gained from cassette dosing.[5]

A better way to detect errors is to include a benchmark compound with known *in vivo* pharmacokinetics. To minimize the potential for errors, one should use the smallest doses detectable and keep the total number of co-administered compounds small.[4]

Even the looming limitation of drug-drug interactions entailed with cassette dosing is being overcome. With advances in IT and availability of predictive databases, approaches such as structure-metabolism relationship (SMR) are gaining importance. Knowledge about ligand structure, ligand-active site interactions and stereoelectronic factors involved in metabolic transformations, the metabolic pathways that may be involved and corresponding potential metabolites formed can be predicted. Recently, METAPRINT, a metabolic fingerprint has been developed to facilitate in the design of cassette dosing experiments. These approaches will supplement cassette dosing and go a long way in reducing any confounding information especially with regard to drug-drug interactions in cassette dosing.[6]

In another development, a novel method of serial bleeding has been developed to withdraw blood samples from the same animal for all the time points in a pharmacokinetic study. This helps to not only dramatically reduce the number of animals used, but also increased the quality of the kinetic data for compounds compared in that animal. Following protocol has been developed with the approval of Animal Use and Care Committee for conducting *in vivo* experiments.

Male Swiss Webster mice, 7 weeks old (body weight 28-36 g), are used for pharmacokinetic studies. Using a stratified randomization procedure the animals are either administered vehicle, standard or test drug. The route of drug administration may be oral, intraperitoneal or subcutaneous, as per the protocol. After administration, serial tail bled blood samples (5 µl) are collected using heparinized tip at various time points (5 min to 24 h). The samples are transferred to a microcentrifuge tube, weighed with an analytical balance and vortexed with purified water and internal standard.[7]

The samples are extracted with organic solvent (ethyl acetate, methanol or acetonitrile). The organic layer is transferred to a microcentrifuge tube, and dried under nitrogen. The residues can be reconstituted in minimum volume (up to 25 µl) of appropriate solvent (methanol). Aliquots are injected onto LC/MS/MS system for analysis.[7]

The technique has the following distinct advantages:

- Minimizes the number of animals used
- Significantly reduces trauma to the animal that is associated with sample withdrawal
- Marked reduction in inter-individual variation in pharmacokinetic parameters
- Reduces the amount of drug used
- Sample processing time is markedly minimized.

However, care has to be taken, that the small animals are handled with care as serial bleeding may alter the physiological state of the animal. For example, micro sampling increases the amount of inflammatory eicosanoids in blood and may decrease the proportion of cellular components in a sample.[7]

VIRTUAL SCREENING

The rate of synthesis of compounds has increased exponentially owing to the advances in combinatorial chemistry. These compounds have been housed in huge virtual libraries. Numerous such databases have been created, each housing over 10^9 compounds, in each. The obvious question, which arises, is how can this enormous database be filtered to bring forth compounds of utility? To achieve this goal, miniaturized and automated assays have been developed that limit cost, material, time and manpower requirement. As a natural extension high speed computer systems running specialized softwares have been developed that are capable of screening the molecules from the libraries against identified targets.[8]

As the first step the appropriate technique of X-ray crystallography, Nuclear Magnetic Resonance (NMR) are used to determine the 3-D structure of the macromolecular target. This is followed by application of 2D QSAR (2-Dimensional Quantitative Structure Activity Relationship), wherein, the chemical structure is quantitatively correlated against a biological activity so as to predict its biological activity. The compounds are superpositioned on the target site as a function of energy and potential. On the basis of this screen, compounds exhibiting favorable kinetics are selected for "fine tuning" and the rest are eliminated.

While searching a virtual library, maximum output can be generated, if information under following heads is available:

- Information about other known ligands (substrates, agonists, antagonista, etc.) that are bioactive at the target.
- Detailed structural and functional information about the target site on the site, binding thermodynamics, etc.
- Lastly, a thorough knowledge in rules of conformational analysis and a medicinal chemistry 'instinct' proves to be beneficial.[8]

MICROASSAYS

Modern chemical and biological techniques have revolutionized the synthesis of new chemical entities, and have set a pace that was unimaginable with traditional methods of synthesis.

With the advancements in modern science and DNA recombinant biotechnology,[9-12] various novel and sensitive procedures have been developed to determine the side effects, pharmacological action, toxicity, and efficacy of biologically active and clinically important compounds, derived from herbal origin or prepared synthetically. This has provided a much needed impetus to drug development program. Conventional bioassays have been replaced by sensitive ELISA, reverse transcriptional polymerase chain reaction (RT-PCR), ribonuclease protection assays, cDNA microarrays, etc. some of which are briefly described below.

Radioimmunoprecipitation

This elegant procedure is employed to quantitatively estimate the gene expression at the translation level using radiolabeled 35S-methionine.[13-15] The labeled sample is generated as radioimmunoprecipitate which is counted above background using liquid scintillation counter.[8]

Immunoblotting

SDS-polyacrylamide gel electrophoresis is performed to study protein, enzyme, neuro-transmitter or hormone expression of the immunoprecipitated lysates. Slab gel electrophoresis is performed and the autoradiograms are densitometrically analyzed.[13]

RNA Extraction

Cellular monolayer is trypsinized to detach from the bottom of the flask and the cell pellet is obtained by centrifugation. The pellet is suspended in guanidine isothiocyanate (GITC) solution (composition: 0.1 M dithiothretol, 4 M guanidine isothiocyanate, 0.5% (v/v) N-lauryl sarcosine, 20 mM sodium acetate, pH 4.0) and treated according to standard protocol. RNA is pelleted by centrifugation. One µl of the purified RNA sample is diluted to 1 ml. Readings are taken at 260 nm and 280 nm to determine the A260/A280 ratios (pure RNA provides a ratio between 1.6 and 1.8). RNA is resolved in 1% agarose gel containing ethidium bromide at a current strength of 30 mA for 2-3 h (80 volts for 1 h). The gels are visualized on UV eluminator.

Reverse Transcription (First Strand cDNA Preparations)

Reverse transcription of 1 µg of RNA is conducted using either 50-100 ng of poly(A) mRNA or 5-10 µg of total RNA. The volume is adjusted to 38 µl with DEPC-treated water. Three µl of oligo-dT primers (100 ng/µl) or 3 µl of random primers (100 ng/µl) are added and the contents are mixed gently. Both control and experimental tubes are incubated at 65°C. The tubes are cooled slowly at room temperature (10 min) to allow primers to anneal to RNA. First strand cDNA is synthesized by adding the following reagents in the control and experimental tubes in sequence. Five µl (10X) first strand buffer, 1 ml of RNase block (Ribonuclease inhibitor, 40 U/µl), 2 µl of 100 mM dNTPs. One µl of MMLV-RT (50 U/µl). The tubes are mixed gently and incubated at 37°C for 1 h followed by incubation at 90°C for 5 min. The first strand cDNA is kept on ice for use in PCR amplification protocol.

Amplification of First Strand cDNA

One to five µl of first strand cDNA is transferred in autoclaved 500 µl PCR tubes. In control PCR amplification reaction tubes, 10 µl of Taq-DNA polymerase buffer is added along with 0.8 µl of 100 mM dNTPs, 3 µl of control primer set (100 ng/µl) and double distilled water to adjust the final volume to 99.5 µl. In the experimental PCR reaction mixture following reagents are administered in a sequence, 10 µl of 10X Taq DNA polymerase buffer, 0.8 µl of 100 mM dNTPs, 2 µl of 10 µM oligonucleotide (primer 1: Forward: and 2 µl of 10 µl of oligonucleotide) (primer 2. Reverse) primers are added. The final volume of the reaction mixture is adjusted to 99.5 µl. Both control and experimental amplification reaction mixture tubes are placed in a DNA Thermal cycler. Each PCR amplification reaction is heated to 91°C for 5 min and then immediately cooled at 54°C for 5 min. This step is essential to maximize thermal cycling performance. The control and experimental PCR amplification reaction tubes are removed from the Thermal cycler, briefly microcentrifuged and 0.5 μl of Taq-2000 (DNA polymerase) (5 U/μl) to each reaction tube is added. The reaction tubes are briefly centrifuged again. The PCR amplification reaction mixture is overlaid with a drop of mineral oil to prevent evaporation of reaction components during thermal cycling. The PCR amplification reaction tubes are placed in the thermal cycler and processed for amplification. For PCR amplification, programmed thermal cycler is used and experimental parameters are established that are optimal for the oligonucleotide primer set employed. Amplification is usually done depending on the primer length, GC content, and its sequence (usually 25-40 cycles of denaturation for 1 min at 94°C, annealing for 1 min at 54°C, and extension of 2 min at 72°C). The final reaction is done using 72°C for 10 min to complete the amplification. The reaction products are kept at 6°C before the analysis. Ten μl of each PCR amplification reaction is taken from below the mineral oil layer into separate lanes of 1.2% agarose. One Kb DNA ladder is used as molecular weight marker. The amplified products are analyzed densitometer.

Cell Transfection

Cell transfection studies are conducted on healthy cells at subconfluent stage. Usually we have used the cells between 4-5th passage. One μg of antisense oligonucleotide to μ-synuclein: 5'-CCT-TTT-CAT-GAA-CAC-ATC-CAT-GGC-3', Reverse Sense: 5'-GCC-ATG-GAT-GTG-TTC-ATG-AAA-GG-3'; Scrambled: 5'-TAG-CTC-GCT-ACG-TAA-TCA-CCA-CT-3'. Metallothionein-1 antisense: CAC-AGC-ACG-TGC-ACT-TGT-CCG-CCG-CCG-CTT-TGC-AGA-CAC-AGC-C, MT-1 Forward: GTT-CGT-CTC-ACT-GGT-GTG-AGC, MT-1 Reverse: AAA-AGA-AAT-CGA-GGA-AAT-GGC (GIBCO/BRL Life Technologies, USA), mixed with 8 μl of enhancer, and 25 μl of Effectine transfection reagent as per manufacturer's recommendations. The transfected cells are authenticated using Radioimmunoprecipitation, immunoblotting, and RT-PCR using specific primer sets of genes. Spontaneous and drug-induced apoptosis is studied using heat shock, staurosporine (1 μM), serum deprivation, ceramide or other apoptogens including toxic drugs.

Multiple Fluorochrome Comet Assay

This sensitive assay is performed to determine mitochondrial and nuclear DNA damage simultaneously in a single cell in response to various environmental neurotoxins or physiological stress. It can provide basic information regarding condensed, partially condensed, partially fragmented and fully fragmented DNA based on the charge associated with each molecular species of DNA. Thus, this procedure provides information regarding single cell apoptosis. Multiple fluorochrome Comet assay provides more quantitative information regarding the extent of genotoxicity of a compound and that can be determined by quantitatively estimating the Comet tail length, tail intensity, and tail diameter. This procedure is particularly useful to determine the levels of DNA damage in an alkaline medium and is employed particularly in the field of genotoxicology. It is a convenient and more sensitive method for multiple processing and drug screening. It is an assay at the inter-phase between molecular biology and cellular biology and is little more sensitive and specific as compared to conventional DNA fragmentation assay performed on agarose gels. This method is very useful in comparative pharmacological analysis of excitoneurotoxins as well as drugs.[14]

Triple Fluorochrome Analysis

Triple fluorochrome analysis is conducted to assess various stages of apoptosis at the plasma membrane and cytoplasmic level, using 100 nM acridine orange, which stains specifically RNA and proteins, and is very useful to detect apoptotic bodies; to estimate mitochondrial membrane potential and mitochondrial apoptosis, JC-1 and decifer are employed, whereas nuclear apoptosis is detected by fluorochrome.

The neurons are grown in eight-chambered microscopic slides, exposed to either toxins or drugs overnight for seven days, and incubated at 37°C for 45 min in a mixture of fluorochromes. The monolayer is washed with Dulbecco's phosphate buffered saline and the cellular monolayer is mounted, air-dried in the dark chamber, and observed under Fluorescence microscope, equipped with immunofluorescence imaging system. The fluorescence images are digitized using Digital camera and analyzed. For obtaining a detailed analysis of apoptosis and its intermediary events, images captured with different filters are combined and plotted.[15,16]

Multiprobe Ribonuclease Protection Assay (MRPA)

MRPA is a highly sensitive procedure to simultaneously quantify several mRNA species in a single sample of total RNA and can be used for comparative analysis of different mRNA species, which can be compared between samples. MRPA can be performed on total RNA preparations by standard methods from either frozen tissue or cultured cells without further purification of polyA+ RNA. It is highly sensitive procedure for the detection and quantification of gene transcripts, induced in response to neurotoxic insult. It was discovered based on the knowledge about DNA-dependent RNA polymerase from bacteriophage SP6, T7 and T3 and information of their promoter sequences. To synthesize high specific activity RNA probes from DNA templates as they have high degree of fidelity for the promoters, polymerize RNA at high rates, efficiently transcribe long segments, and do not require high concentrations of rNTPs. So a cDNA fragment of interest can be subcloned into a plasmid that contains bacteriophage promoters and the construct can be used as a template for the synthesis of radiolabeled and antisense RNA probes. We use T7 polymerase-directed synthesis of high specific activity 32P labeled anti-sense RNA probe set. The probe set is hybridized in excess to target RNA in solution after which free probe and other single stranded RNA are digested with RNase. The remaining RNase protected probes are purified, and resolved on denaturing PAGE and quantified by autoradiography or phosphor imaging. Quantity of each mRNA species in the original RNA sample can be determined based on the intensity of the properly sized-protected probe segment. The procedure takes usually three days.

Day 1: For probe synthesis and overnight hybridization, Day 2: RNase treatment, purification of protected probe, and Gel Electrophoresis, and Day 3: Autoradiography or phosphor imaging.

cDNA Microarrays for Differential Gene Expression

This is a relatively new research procedure employed to study differential multiple gene expression under the influence of drugs, neurotransmitters, enzymes, or hormones, etc. under investigation. As many as 30,000 genes can be analyzed with this procedure. cDNA Microarray scanning requires cDNA microarray scanner with computer software to investigate the role of various genes involved in drug-induced apoptosis and antioxidants-induced antiapoptosis.

The procedure works hand in hand with DNA sequencing for high throughput screening for exploring point mutations of nuclear and/or mitochondrial origin. Plastic microarrays are relatively economical, and they can be utilized to investigate as low as 1200 genes of interest from the biological samples. cDNA microarray scanning is relatively sensitive procedure and can pinpoint minor yet subtle changes in the gene expression in response to environmental neurotoxins as well as pharmacological drugs of clinical importance (such as anticarcinogenic or antiapoptotic agents). The main objective of these technical procedures is to develop cDNA chips for clinical diagnosis, better prognosis, and effective treatment of various diseases with low undesirable effects.

APPLICATION OF MODERN ANALYTICAL TECHNIQUES IN BIOLOGICAL SYSTEMS

Atomic Absorption Spectroscopy

This method is employed to estimate the concentration of various metal ions of physiological significance, such as Na, K, Ca, Cl, Fe, Cu, and Zn from the biological fluids, tissue extracts, and from the microdialysates. Various atomic absorption spectrometers equipped with graphite furnace and computer software are now available which can analyze more than four metal ions from as small as 20 µl biological sample. Tissue or cell extracts are prepared in 0.3 N perchloric acid by sonication at low wattage and microcentrifuged at 14,000 rpm at 4°C. The supernatants are filtered through the syringe tip filters and the filtered extracts are directly utilized in the atomic absorption spectrometer or high performance liquid chromatography with electrochemical, UV, or fluorescence detector capabilities. Perkin-Elmer Atomic Absorption Spectrometer is equipped with Graphite furnace (which is operated in an argon environment), an autosampler, and computer software for the online data analysis and preparing concentration reports. Usually, pyrolysis at 1,300-1,700°C, and atomization of samples at 2,400-2,800°C, is employed, depending on the metal ion under investigation.[13-15]

Coulter Counting

This procedure is very simple and requires a photocell, which estimates the number of particles present in the photocell. Beckman-Coulter Company (USA) has developed this procedure to determine total number of cells following treatment with a drug. Although it is a single step method and requires only 1:20 dilution of a sample, it does not decipher between live and dead cells. Therefore, Coulter counting is supplemented with hemocytometer reading made using a microscope and Trypan blue exclusion method (the live cells exclude trypan blue, while dead cells are stained with trypan blue).

Fluorescence Activated Cell Sorting (FACS)

This biophysical equipment is utilized to determine differential expression of as many as 6 genes with a capability of estimating 6 more physical parameters of physiological interest, such as number of cells undergoing apoptosis and necrosis, and the number of live cells simultaneously based on the side scatter, forward scatter, and granularity. The FACS machine (flow cytometer) employs lasers (such as He-Ne, Argon lasers, Ruby lasers and Cadmium lasers) microbeams for the determination of fluorescence properties of cells. For measuring intracellular free ionized calcium, UV detectors are employed. The equipment can also sort out genetically engineered cells by a turbo sorter facility. Fluorescence activated cell sorting (FACS) machines are now being utilized to prepare stable transfectants using vectors encoding for green, red, or yellow fluorescence proteins. This approach eliminates the need to perform *in vitro* reporter gene analysis using either X-Gal or luciferase reporter gene assays. pEGFP-N-1 vectors are thus very convenient to study the behavior of various pharmacological agents on genetically engineered cell lines. This approach is being utilized particularly in gene therapy labs. FACS machine is also utilized to detect the efficacy of anticancer drugs based on the extent of DNA damage (apoptosis and/or necrosis) they produce *in vitro*. This machine is also utilized to determine at which phase of the DNA cycle (G1-S, G2-M), the drug might have induced its maximum effect. The cells can be synchronized using chemicals influencing the DNA cell cycle at a particular phase. In addition, this machine is being utilized to study mitochondrial membrane potential, and to determine the production of free radicals in response to a particular drug/agent. Although very useful, this equipment is very costly. Moreover, its maintenance cost is also quite expensive. In addition, the cost of fluorochromes adds to its limited use in many labs all over the world. This equipment requires qualified and trained persons to handle and interpret the experimental data.

Positron Emission Scanning

With the advancements in linear accelerators, cyclotrons, and targets, the preparation of short-lived positron emitters has been facilitated. This procedure is noninvasive and provides information regarding brain regional physiology and biochemistry such as synthesis of DNA, RNA, and proteins *in vivo*. Furthermore, cyclotron-generated positron emitters (15O, t½ 120 sec, 13N t½ 10 min, 11C t½ 20 min, and 18F t½ 110 min) are now being utilized in basic research and clinical practice to study brain regional metabolism and molecular neuroimaging of genes of interest. 18F-DOPA is being employed to examine nigrostriatal dopamine transporter activity, and to discover pleasure centers involved in drug addiction for substances of abuse. 18F-deoxyglucose is being employed for detecting the stages of malignancies. High-resolution microPET scanners (Concorde Microsystems Inc, Knoxville, TN, USA) are now being used to discover new and clinically effective neuroprotective drugs and for an early diagnosis of diseases. CTI Corporation (USA), Physics for Medicine (USA), Seimens-Gamma-Med (German), and Digi-Rad have recently developed high-resolution CT-SPECT fusion scanners for research purpose as well as for clinical applications.

Magnetic Resonance Imaging and Spectroscopy

High-resolution magnetic resonance imaging is utilized in basic and applied research. In particular high-resolution magic angle spinning nano-NMR probes require as small as 40 μl of biological samples in 750 MHz magnets. This equipment can analyze and quantitate biological samples with microgram to nanogram concentrations. Running cost of this equipment could be as high as $800 per hr. This equipment is used to determine the concentration, purity, and structural formula of as many as 80 metabolites from the aliphatic and aromatic regions. Biological compounds including DNA, RNA and proteins contain carbon, hydrogen, and nitrogen atoms. Their nuclei spin at a particular frequency, which can be picked up and detected to evaluate their clinical significance. Usually, brain regional metabolism of amino acid neurotransmitters and metabolites can be explored by these advanced and sophisticated techniques. Various resonances are picked up and computer-analyzed using Fast Fourier transformation (FFT) analysis. From the position of the resonance peak, we identify the compound/metabolite, and from the peak height, we determine the concentration of the compound/metabolite. These advanced research tools are also utilized to determine the structure and purity of various unknown compounds and molecular designing of drugs. Various pharmaceutical industries are interested to determine the structural formula of their product before evaluating its therapeutic potential. High-resolution magnetic resonance imaging is performed on small animals (rats, mice) to determine any space-occupying lesion (such as cyst, infarct, tumor, edema). This equipment measures regional proton density per unit area, which is altered during edema or during water accumulation in the brain in response to neuronal injury or following neurotoxic insult. Thus, MRI is used to correlate and confirm information derived from PET and computerized axial tomography conducted employing soft X-rays.

CELL FREE ASSAYS

Cell-free assays include simple to very complex systems. These biochemical assays include enzyme assays, protein-protein interactions and membrane receptor ligand and soluble receptor-ligand binding assays. The advantages of this kind of assay system includes ready accessibility of the compounds to the target, easy identification of the target of the compound without any ambiguity, a well-defined mechanism of action, the possibility of developing inexpensive screens, the easy adaptability to newer technologies, amenability to miniaturization, and ready automation.[17] These assays can be classified as heterogeneous and homogeneous assays. Heterogeneous assays are multistep assays that include steps of incubations, washings, filtrations, reading of signals etc. as in ELISA. On the other hand, one pot assays that do not involve any transfer or wash steps are known as homogeneous assays, such as, chromogenic, absorbance or fluorescence based assays.[18]

MICROBE-BASED SCREENING ASSAYS

Microbe-based screening has been used to screen antibacterial agents and cytotoxic anticancer agents. Advance biotechnology techniques are used to clone and express target proteins. The mammalian proteins are expressed in microbial cells and stored therein inclusion bodies. These proteins are not useful for the microbial cells. The insoluble aggregates are isolated, dissolved and refolded and if needed, subjected to post-translational modifications. The advantages of this type of assay systems include low cost, simple technique and high yield. Commonly used microbial systems include *E. coli, Saccharomyces* and Yeast. Microbial systems have been adapted to identify agonists and antagonists of GPCRs, detail the mechanism of action of immunosuppressants such as cyclosporin and FK506, screen for K^+ channel openers and blockers and many more.[19-21]

RECEPTOR SCREENS

Langley and Ehrlich described the concept of receptor-ligand interaction.[22] The concept of receptor has been overhauled since then, to include cell membrane, nuclear, ion, voltage gated, tyrosine kinase, tyrosine phosphatase, hematopoietic cytokine, peptide, extracellular calcium sensing, cAMP receptors. The receptors as ligand target represent more than 60% of all drug discovery targets.[23]

Receptor-ligand binding assays using high affinity radiolabeled ligand provide a direct screening approach for detecting specific/non-specific agonists/antagonists. This technique also finds application for quantitation of the potency of competing agents, investigating functional signal transduction pathways, monitoring molecular changes within a single cell, determine functions of orphan receptors.[24]

NANO SCREENS

The face of drug discovery process has been imparted a dramatic lift by combinatorial chemistry, robotics, miniaturization. At the screening rates enabled by ultra-high throughput screening (uHTS) applications, reagent consumption poses as the limiting factor. This calls for means to reduce the cost by reducing the volume of reagent required. This form of miniaturization has given birth to nano screens, wherein assay protocols have been validated using nano volumes (including pipetting, dispensing, and compound retrieval).

To achieve this modular platforms have been specially designed to handle high precision liquid handling and sensitive detection. In these operation systems, piezo technology is used to focus the liquid droplets into accurate volume and well. Moreover, the inherent advantage of amplification by the fluorescence detection systems is utilized at the read-out. NanoStore, EVOscreen, EVOTEC are some of the examples of systems adept at microseparation, detection and analysis.[25]

Patch Clamp Technique: Single Channel Recording

In vitro techniques are crucial to understand the normal physiological processes of synthesis and release, which are ongoing in individual cells. The pivotal patch clamp technique being widely applied today was developed from a series of experiments in frog muscle. Current was passed through individual ion channels activated by ACh and measured with high resolution. This was shown to be a discrete pulse-like event with duration of a few milliseconds. Fluctuation and relaxation measurements of end-plate currents led to the conclusion that the rate of channel opening increases with agonist concentrations, and that the channel, once open, closes spontaneously.[26]

The patch clamp technique has revolutionized cellular physiology since its introduction in the early 1980s. It allows investigators to assess: (i) ionic currents of a whole cell, including the molecular level of single ion channels, (ii) cell membrane potential and (iii) including fusion of a single secretory vesicle.[27] When combined with microfluorimetry and digital imaging techniques, the method can be used to measure the spatio-temporal aspects of intracellular levels and distribution of ions such as calcium, sodium, chloride, changes in pH, production of signaling molecules and movement of these molecules. These techniques help to investigate signaling pathways at the cellular or molecular level in (cell lines, primary and transformed tissue cultures, brain slice preparations transient and/or stable transfections of cells and in primary cells derived from transgenic animals.

Conventional fine tip microelectrodes impale the cell in order to measure potential across the cell membrane, while patch clamp electrodes are too large to be inserted into a cell. The patch pipette is stuck onto the surface of a cell membrane instead of piercing it (Fig. 1.2). If a patch pipette is placed onto the cell surface and gentle suction is applied, a bubble shape of membrane is drawn into the patch pipette. The edges of this patch of membrane adhere tightly to the glass of the patch pipette. The electrical resistance of this seal between pipette glass and membrane is so high (a giga-ohm seal, or gigaseal) that the small patch of membrane underneath the patch pipette is by comparison a low resistance pathway and thus the favored route for current flow. This small patch of membrane may be voltage clamped to a series of potentials and the conductance of the patch calculated from the amount of current required to move from one potential to another. The patch of membrane under the pipette is very small. If the radius of a patch clamp pipette is 1◎m, then the area of the patch under the pipette will be about 3 square picometres. Therefore, opening or closing of a single ion channel will cause a significant alteration in the overall conductance of the patch. Mostly, ion channels are either open or closed and they switch very rapidly from one state to the other. Therefore, the opening of a single ion channel causes an abrupt increase in the conductance of the patch of membrane beneath the pipette. The patch clamp technique involves a step-like increase in current. At a given voltage and ionic environment, the size of the current deflection is directly proportional to the conductance of this channel; the larger the deflection, the greater the conductance. If two channels open simultaneously, then the current is exactly twice as large. Ion channels may be distinguished from one another on the basis of this characteristic unit conductance, the duration of each opening (open time) and on the probability of the channel being open (open probability) under specific experimental conditions.

A patch of membrane from the cell can be removed without breaking the gigaseal and thus measure ion channel openings in an isolated patch of membrane. Besides, the single channel recording modes, the patch clamp technique may be applied to measure the currents that result from ion movements across the membrane of the whole cell. This mode of operation is known as the whole cell configuration. The first step in achieving this configuration is to obtain a high resistance contact between the pipette and the cell membrane (gigaseal). However, the patch of membrane under the pipette, which was the focus of attention in the single channel

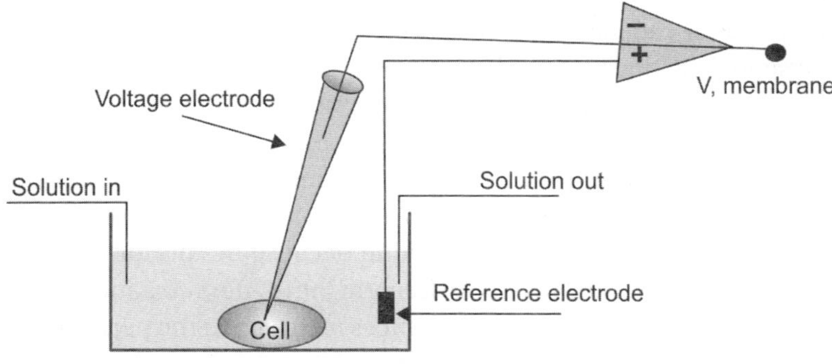

Figure 1.2: Patch electrode on cell membrane (*For color version see Plate 1*)

experiments is, in whole cell experiments, ruptured by application of a short pulse of negative pressure. The tight seal between pipette glass and cell membrane persists and the low resistance route for current flow is now into the cell and across entire cell surface membrane. A second feature of the whole cell configuration is that, following disruption of the patch of membrane under the pipette, the interior of the patch pipette is continuous with the cell interior. Thus, the solution filling the patch pipette will enter into and equilibrate with the cell interior. Small ions equilibrate within seconds of breaking through into the whole cell configuration.[28]

The application of the patch clamp technique has provided so many insights into cellular physiology that its originators, Bert Sakmann and Erwin Neher were awarded the Nobel Prize for Physiology and Medicine in 1991.

Advances in Patch Clamp Technique

More than ten years have passed since the slice-patch-clamp technique was established as a powerful method for the analysis of central synaptic transmission. Although this technique was earlier restricted only to young animal preparations, we can now even apply it to slices obtained from adult animals.

In addition, the advances have made paired whole-cell recording from two or more synaptically connected neurons, recording from dendrites or some presynaptic terminals, possible. Whole-cell patch-clamp technique can help to achieve complete biophysical characterization of an individual neuron, intrinsic, synaptic and spiking properties of cells in either superficial or deep structures, determining the synaptic receptive fields of single cells in anesthetized or awake head-fixed and even freely moving preparations so that synaptic activity may be linked directly to sensory processing and behavior.[29]

Future trends include developments facilitating microscopic analysis such as investigating glutamatergic sensitivities of single dendritic spines in combination with two-photon photolysis of a caged-glutamate compound and physiological function-oriented manner such as investigation of pain perception mechanisms using *in vivo* patch clamp technique.[30]

Microdialysis Technique

The neurobiologists wish to follow moment-by-moment, the sequence of biochemical events in various parts of the brain during a behavior. In this regard, various *in vitro* methods such as incubation of tissue slices and subcellular components have been very successful. Nevertheless, there is a definite need for a chemical technique comparable to the techniques of physiology where functional events can be followed closely over time. So far, the most successful *in vivo* "chemophysiological" techniques have been ventricular perfusions, cup perfusions on the surfaces of the brain, and push-pull perfusions carried out under stereotactic control in various parts of the nervous system.

The technique of microdialysis is a very important tool for *in vivo* studies in neuropsychopharmacology, toxicology, drug delivery, pharmacokinetics and endocrinology. Microdialysis is an extension of the push-pull technique because the perfusion fluid is circulating inside a semipermeable membrane instead of freely in the tissue. Substances in the extracellular fluid will diffuse into the perfusate, while substances included in the perfusate will diffuse into the tissue. This idea was first applied by Delgado and then by Ungerstedt who introduced the use of hollow fibers continuously perfused by a physiological liquid. Physiological processes may be closely followed in anesthetized as well as awake animals.[31]

Principle

Principle of dialysis has been applied for sampling the extracellular fluid of brain, thereby circumventing the problems associated with perfusion solution coming into direct contact with brain tissue. This technique is based on the principle of an artificial blood vessel surgically inserted into the tissue. The diffusion of chemical substances will occur in the direction of the lowest concentration. In this way, substances may be recovered from the organ or added to the organ depending upon their relative concentration in the perfusion fluid. There will be bidirectional molecular and ionic traffic between the interior of the microdialysis probe and the surrounding tissue. This provides the unique possibility of carrying out an entire pharmacological experiment within less than a cubic millimeter of tissue.[31]

Factors Affecting the Microdialysis

A unique feature of microdialysis is the possibility to compare *in vitro* experiments with *in vivo* experiments. The *in vitro* experiments may be performed on a solute contained in a simple beaker. The recovery of individual substances may be studied by determining the relative concentration in the perfusate in comparison with the concentration in the outside medium. The concentration will depend upon the properties of the membrane (most notably its molecular cut-off and its thickness), the speed of the perfusion, and the initial concentration of the compound in the perfusate. By using an appropriate size membrane and a sufficiently low perfusion speed, it is possible to reach 100% recovery.[6]

The dialysis membrane also acts as a filter to prevent the diffusion of large molecules from extracellular fluid into the perfusion medium. This provides certain advantages for the analysis of transmitter content in the dialysate. First, the membrane can prevent large molecules such as enzymes from entering the perfusion solution and thereby halt the continuous enzymatic degradation of neurotransmitters once they have entered the perfusion solution. Also, by virtue of its ability to exclude molecules from the perfusion solution, the membrane partially purifies samples prior to their analysis.[32]

Dialysis Probe

The development of the loop probe provided a means of reducing the extent of surgically induced injury. This probe consists of a loop of dialysis membrane, which is implanted vertically into the brain via a single hole in the skull (Fig. 1.3). Still less damage is produced by a vertical concentric style dialysis probe. This probe consists of a single piece of dialysis tubing blocked off at one end with glue; the inlet and/or outlet portions of the probe pass down into the dialysis tubing.

Adaptations in microdialysis probe designs have made it possible to obtain samples from the extracellular fluid of a variety of tissues with high temporal resolution. The resulting small volume samples, often with low concentration of the analyte(s) of interest, present a particular challenge to the analytical system. Rapid separations can be coupled online with microdialysis to provide near real-time data.[33]

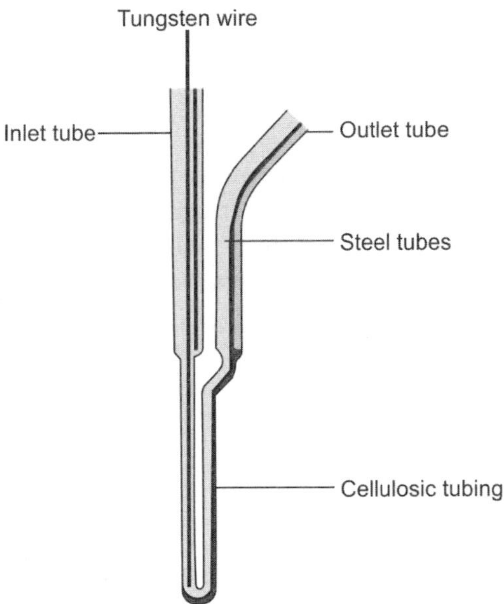

Figure 1.3: Dialysis probe (*For color version see Plate 1*)

Analysis of Sample

In vivo microdialysis in itself is only a sampling technique. The ability to measure compounds within dialysate is entirely dependent upon the sensitivity of an appropriate analytical method. In addition to the postoperative time at which samples are collected, other variables include the ionic composition of the dialysate, and the rate of perfusion affect sample content in the dialysate. Pharmacological tools have been used to compensate for inadequate sensitivity by increasing the level of substance to be analyzed. For example, acetylcholinesterase inhibitors have been used to enable detection of ACh in dialysate.[34] Another approach has been to prelabel neurons by infusing isotopes of the transmitter or precursors and assaying the radiolabeled compounds.[35]

Duration of Experiment

Implantation of the dialysis probe results in several reactions within the CNS tissue. Knowledge of the time course of these events is critical in determining the interval during which microdialysis experiments can be performed with minimal interference from tissue reactions. In general it is thought that dialysis experiments should not be performed either very soon (< 10 h) or very long (several days to weeks) after probe implantation. The optimal interval for performing microdialysis experiments is approximately 16-48 h after implantation of the dialysis probe. Efforts have been made to develop methods whereby sampling can be carried out over many days in a single subject using either chronic implantation of a dialysis probe or implantation of a guide cannula followed by multiple insertions of a probe over days. However, these have generally been unsuccessful.

Microdialysis versus Other Techniques

This technique has advantages over the blood sampling since it provides protein free samples ready to analyze without any loss of blood, permits more frequent sampling and offers an option of simultaneous drug delivery at the same site. Microdialysis can be considered to be superior to biosensors as more than one chemical system can be analyzed while circumventing the electrode contamination.

Present Status of Microdialysis Technique

Microdialysis is now used extensively for the study of several neurotransmitters in the CNS. The two main areas of application of microdialysis are the recovery of endogenous substances (neurotransmitters, catecholamines, neurotrophic factors, cAMP) and the infusion of drugs through the microdialysis cannula (retrodialysis). Clinical applications of microdialysis includes monitoring of ischemic injury, subarachnoid hemorrhage, trauma and epilepsy.[36]

Permutation and combination of novel membrane sampling techniques, ultrafiltration procedures and functional imaging (PET, MRI) have allowed numerous applications of the basic technique in pharmacokinetics, metabolism and/or pharmacodynamics.[37,38] Semi-invasive techniques like microdialysis can be used to measure concentrations of the free, active drug or endogenous compounds in tissues and organs, determine transdermal drug distribution, tissue pharmacokinetics. Thus it gains importance as a widely used sampling technique in clinical drug monitoring, drug development, therapy and disease follow-up. It can play pivotal role in rationalizing drug dosing regimens and influencing the clinical decision-making process.[39]

REFERENCES

1. Augen J. The evolving role of information technology in the drug discovery process. Drug Disc Today 2002;7:315-23.
2. Lazo JS, Wipf P. Combinatorial chemistry and contemporary pharmacology. J Pharmacol Exp Ther 2000;293:705-9.
3. White RE, Manitpisitkul P. Pharmacokinetic theory of cassette dosing in drug discovery screening. Drug Metab Dis 2001;29:957-66.
4. Ramesh KVRNS. Cassette Dosing: rapid in vivo assessment of pharmacokinetics in drug discovery. Pharma Bio World 2007;104-11.
5. Christ DD. Cassette dosing pharmacokinetics: valuable tool or flawed science? Drug Metab Dis 2001;29:935-6.
6. Keseru GM, Molnar L. METAPRINT: a metabolic fingerprint. Application to cassette design for high-throughput ADME screening. J Chem Inf Comput Sci 2002;42:437-44.
7. Watanabe T, Schulz D, Morisseau C, Hammock BD. High-throughput pharmacokinetic method: cassette dosing in mice associated with minuscule serial bleedings and LC/MS/MS analysis. Anal Chim Acta 2006;559:37-44.
8. Walters WP, Stahl MT, Murcko MA. Virtual Screening-an overview. Drug Disc Today 1998;3:160-78.
9. Sambrook J, Fritsch E, Maniatis T. In Molecular Cloning: A Laboratory Manual (2nd ed). Cold Spring Harbor, New York: Cold Spring Harbor Laboratory Press, 1989.

10. Current protocols in molecular biology. Frederick M Ausubel (Ed). Harvard Medical School, Mass. General Hospital. Wiley Interscience, 1989.
11. Leder P, Clayton D, Rubenstein E. In Molecular Medicine. New York: Scientific American Books, 1994.
12. Rabinow P. In Making PCR: A Story of Biotechnology. Chicago: University of Chicago Press, 1996.
13. Sharma S, Kheradpezhou M, Shavali S, et al. Neuroprotective actions of coenzyme q10 in Parkinson's disease. Methods Enzymol 2004;382:488-509.
14. Ebadi M, Sharma S. Peroxynitrite and mitochondrial dysfunction in the pathogenesis of Parkinson's disease. Antioxid Redox Signal 2003;5:319-35.
15. Sharma SK, Ebadi M. Metallothionein attenuates 3-morpholinosydnonimine (sin-1)-induced oxidative stress in dopaminergic neurons. Antioxid Redox Signal 2003;5:251-64.
16. Sharma SK, Carlson E, Ebadi M. Neuroprotective actions selegiline in inhibiting 1-methyl, 4-phenyl, pyridinium ion (mpp+)-induced apoptosis in dopaminergic neurons. J Neurocytol 2003;32(4):329-43.
17. Manly SP. In vitro biochemical screening. J Biomol Screen 1997;2:197-9.
18. Seethala R. Screening platforms. In: Handbook of Drug Screening. (Eds): Seethala R, Fernandes PB. Marcel Dekker AG, Switzerland. 2001;31-67.
19. Cardenas ME, Lorenz M, Hemenway C, Heitman J. Yeast as model T cells. Perspective Drug Discovery Design 1994;2:103-26.
20. King K, Dohlman HG, Thorner J, Caron MG, Lefkowitz RJ. Control of yeast mating signal transduction by a mammalian ◎2-adrenergic receptor and Gs ◎ subunit. Science 1995;250:121-3.
21. Bertin B, Freissmuth M, Jockers R, Strosberg AD, Marullo S. Cellular signaling by an agonist-activated receptor/Gsá fusion protein. Proc Natl Acad Sci USA 1994;14:8827-31.
22. Triggle DJ. Pharmacological receptors: a century of progress. Highlights Recep Res 1984; 1-5.
23. Drews J. Drug discovery: a historical perspective. Science 2000;287:1960-4.
24. Seethala R. Receptor screens for small molecule agonist and antagonist discovery. In Handbook of Drug Screening. (Eds): Seethala R, Fernandes PB. Marcel Dekker AG, Switzerland. 2001;189-64.
25. Turner R, Ullmann D, Sterrer S. Screening in the nanoworld-Single molecule spectroscopy and miniaturized high-throughput screening. In: Handbook of Drug Screening. (Eds): Seethala R, and Fernandes PB. Marcel Dekker AG, Switzerland. 2001;563-82.
26. Sakmann B, Patlak J, Neher E. Single acetylcholine activated channels show burst-kinetics in presence of desensitizing concentrations of agonist. Nature 1980;286:71-3.
27. Sigworth J. The patch clamp is more useful than anyone had expected. Fed Proc 1986;45:2673-7.
28. Sakmann B, Neher E. Patch clamp techniques for studying ionic channels in excitable membranes. Annu Rev Physiol 1984;46:455-72.
29. Momiyama T. Analysis of central synaptic transmission with the slice-patch-clamp technique. Nippon Yakurigaku Zasshi 2003;121:174-80.
30. Rancz EA, Franks KM, Schwarz MK, Pichler B, Schaefer AT, et al. Transfection via whole-cell recording in vivo: bridging single-cell physiology, genetics and connectomics. Nat Neurosci 2011;14(4): 527-32.
31. Ungerstedt U, Hallstrom A. In vivo microdialysis—a new approach to the analysis of neurotransmitters in the brain. Life Sci 1987;41:861-4.
32. Wang PC, De Voe DL, Lee CS. Integration of polymeric membranes with microfluidic networks for bioanalytical applications. Electrophoresis 2001;22:3857-67.

33. Davies MI, Cooper JD, Desmond SS, et al. Analytical considerations for microdialysis sampling. Adv Drug Deliv Rev 2000;45:169-88.
34. Zackheim JA, Abercrombie ED. HPLC/EC detection and quantification of acetylcholine in dialysates. Methods Mol Med 2003;79:433-41.
35. Teng L, Crooks PA, Buxton ST, et al. Nicotinic receptor mediation of S (-) Nornicotine evoked [3H] overflow from rat striatal slices preloaded with [3H] dopamine. J Pharmacol Exp Ther 1997;283:778-87.
36. Bourne JA. Intracerebral microdialysis: 30 years as a tool for the neuroscientist. Clin Exp Pharmacol Physiol 2003;30:16-24.
37. Harrison KE, Pasa SA, Cooper JD, et al. A review of membrane sampling from biological tissues with applications in pharmacokinetics, metabolism and pharmacodynamis. Eur J Pharm Sci 2002;17:1-12.
38. Hutchinson PJ, O'Connell MT, Kirkpatrick PJ, et al. How can we measure substrate, metabolite and neurotransmitter concentrations in the human brain? Physiol Meas 2002;23:R75-109.
39. Azeredo FJ, Dalla Costa T, Derendorf H. Role of microdialysis in pharmacokinetics and pharmacodynamics: current status and future directions. Clin Pharmacokinet 2014;53(3):205-12.

CHAPTER

2

High Throughput Screening for Drug Discovery

INTRODUCTION

The increasing burden of new diseases like cardiovascular disorders, diabetes, immune system related disorders, diverse microbial infections are demanding new drugs to control them in an improved manner. The rise in the occurrence of treatment failure has also increased the strain of the drug discovery scientists for the discovery of novel compounds with better treatment outcomes. As in the case of antibiotics, an innovation gap of almost 50 years came from the rapid discovery era of beta lactam class of antibiotics, still patients are being treated with the congeners of the antibiotics discovered almost 80 years ago. Rapid discoveries of novel drug targets have increased the use of high throughput screening in a potential manner to meet the pace with biochemical or pathological findings.

In the domain of drug research target identification, purification and assay development constitute the initial step. In the next step, the potential compounds are screened against the identified target. Conventionally this has been a slow and tedious manual process requiring huge investment of manpower, time and money. Traditional techniques like test tube analysis and chemical analysis of the intermediate biomolecules may lead to the loss of the precious samples and may not be sensitive enough to capture the minute information that may help in the due course. Consequently, the conventional drug discovery program has been called as a slow process.

WHAT IS HIGH THROUGHPUT SCREENING (HTS)?

The last two decades have seen astonishing innovations in technology that have helped the manual low speed screening to evolve into an automated, microprocessor controlled robotic process called 'High Throughput Screening (HTS)'. This recent process is a synergy of chemistry, biology, engineering and informatics. HTS has helped to speed up conventional languid process and now over 50,000-1,00,000 compounds can be screened per week, against the validated biological target. Further advancements are making it possible to screen 10,000-100,000 compounds within 24 h time and the process is called as ultra-high throughput screening (uHTS). High throughput synthesis of large number of test compounds in a lesser time is also a reality now. Simultaneous development in other areas such as drug synthesis, toxicity screening, drug metabolism and pharmacokinetics studies (DMPK) are helping the process to achieve its ultimate speed in new drug development (NDD). After the fundamental biological research, the effective target is identified and validated for its function. Then the method development takes a few months to initiate screening process. In HTS, the trend is to replace radio labeling by simple luminescence and fluorescent techniques. Since the yield of target protein or purified biological target is generally low (often obtained only in a few milligrams), technologies that permit screening with reduced volumes (3-20 μl) and reduced protein/ligand have played a pivotal role in facilitating HTS. Development of detection techniques having ultra high precisions are used in these assays to give more valuable information about the ligand-protein interaction. The conventional 96-well plates have been replaced with 384-well plates and subsequently by 1536-well plates with low internal volume to make the screening possible at a high speed. Nowadays, rapid development of negative screening method is also in place for earlier detection of the ligand affinity with known targets leading to adverse reactions, drug interaction, altered intestinal permeation, etc. Revolution in every individual process towards drug development is bridging the gap between older concepts with newly optimized robust and technology enabled methods for its quick and economic implementation in drug discovery platform.

HTS—POSITIVE AND NEGATIVE SCREENING

In the drug development screening **Hit** and **Lead** are two frequently used terminologies. **Hit** is explained as: "a molecule with confirmed activity from primary HTS assay with a good profile in secondary assays and with confirmed structure," and **Lead** is explained as**:** "a hit series exhibiting the Structure Activity Relationship (SAR) and demonstrating activities both *in vitro* and *in vivo*."

IN VITRO INTERACTION STUDIES (ARRAY BASED)

In vitro assays have now been miniaturized from the test tubes to well plates having capacity of assaying samples starting from traditional 96 well format to 1536 wells. Microfluidics has impacted the interaction study area in a surprising way and has drastically decreased the need of both reagents and samples. Chemical analysis on the microarray plate for the quick and economic identification of the biological target is evolving as a good tool.[1] The accuracy and speed of the system has made these techniques a great success. Still the system is not completely free from errors

1. Different chemicals have different functional groups
2. Difference in the diffusivity of the samples

Chemical microarray technology has come up with great successes in the evaluation of chemical-protein interactions, enzyme activity inhibition, target identification, signal pathway elucidation and cell-based functional analysis. Their success can easily be seen from the Genomic and proteomic studies where almost 10,000 targets for the drug activities have been found out; however, less than 500 of these targets have turned up in approved drug candidates.

Chip based microarray: Chip based microarrays have started becoming popular these days. They are made in the same way as semiconductors. The microfluidics helps in the mixing of samples with the targets bound on the chip, finally signals are read by the analyzers that can be fluorescent or simple UV or visible signals.

Other microarrays: So many other microarrays are also available in the market. These arrays are specific for some of the important biomolecules in the physiological or pathological pathways, e.g. Cytokine based kits, angiogenesis responsive bimolecular kits, transcription factor analysis kits, etc. They work on the principle of the binding of the biological samples with the antibodies bound to the array membrane, incubation, binding to the secondary antibodies and finally tagging of the secondary antibody with the signal emitting molecules such as dyes.

FLUORESCENCE TECHNIQUES IN HTS

Fluorescence (FU) based detection of the compounds, analytes or genetic materials has now become a well-established technique (Table 2.1). In HTS the interaction of ligand with the biological compartment is elucidated by luminescence-based binding assays. Various fluorescence techniques like Fluorescence Anisotropy (FA), Fluorescence Correlation Spectroscopy (FCS), Fluorescence Intensity (FI), Fluorescence Lifetime Imaging Microscopy (FLIM), Fluorescence Resonance Energy Transfer (FRET), Total Internal Reflection Fluorescence (TIRF) and Time Resolved Resonance Anisotropy (TRRA) are used. Along with these techniques, certain specific nano bead-based techniques like Scintillation Proximity Assay (SPA), Amplified Luminescence Proximity Homogeneous Assay (ALPHA) are also used (Fig. 2.1).

Detection system for the fluorescent based assays has also developed hand in hand with the techniques. Currently the instruments are available which are capable of screening a single reaction well for different modes starting from UV, Visible to FU and chemiluminescence. These instruments are known as multimode readers (Fig. 2.2). These instruments are cartridge based and having the advantage of replacing the cartridge as per the need. FU microscopes

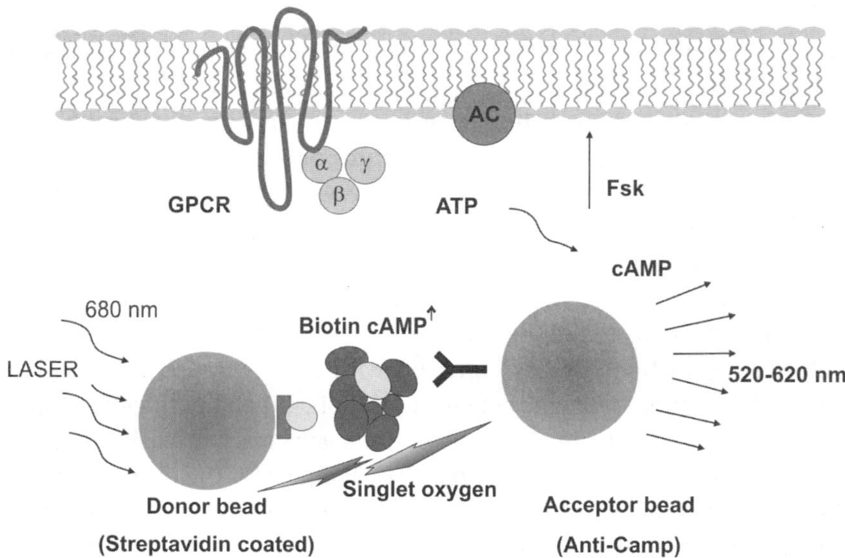

Figure 2.1: cAMP detection using ALPHA screen principle. The ALPHA screen kit includes streptavidin coated donor beads and acceptor beads conjugated with an antibody to cAMP. Biotinylated cAMP is also included as a positive control and for competition with unlabeled cAMP (*For color version see Plate 1*)

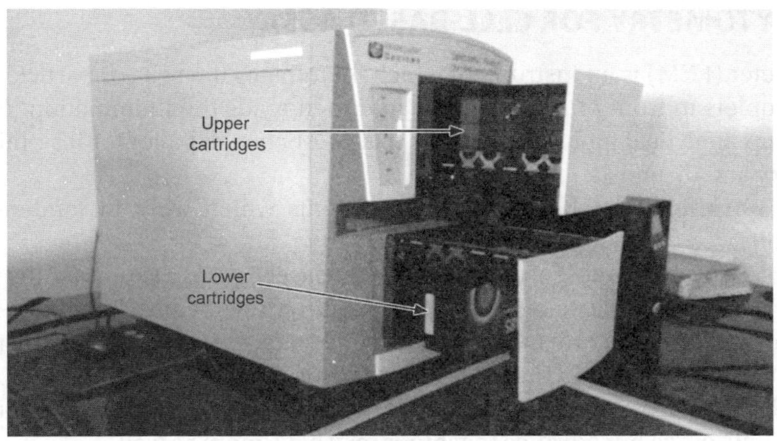

Figure 2.2: Photograph showing multimode reader (*Courtesy* – Ocular Pharmacology & Pharmacy; Dr RP Centre, AIIMS)

are also playing a big role in the drug development. FU microscopes help in the identification of the entry of the fluorescent tagged compound at the desired site in the cell. FU microscope also helps in the identification of the drug effect on to a particular cellular component or biomolecule. Immunofluorescent technique depends on the FU microscope for the detection of the fluorescent bound antibody on the tissue sectioned glass slide.

Table 2.1: Fluorescent techniques used in drug discovery process

Technique	*Principle of working*	*Area of application*
Fluorescence anisotropy (FA) or fluorescence polarization (FP)	Fluoroprobe is exited using plane polarized light and emission is recorded parallel to plane polarized light. Binding of the fluoroprobe with receptor would restrict the rotational mobility of it and would exhibit a higher polarization.	Receptor ligand binding assay[2,3]
Time resolved fluorescence anisotropy (TRFA)	Records the change in the rotational diffusion of phosphorescent-labeled membrane receptor when they bind to a ligand. Also delivers information on protein structural fluctuations	Screening of chemical compounds[4]
Fluorescence correlation spectroscopy (FCS)	Used for mass-Dependent and independent fluorescent assays. Can be used to study the protein-ligand interactions on the membrane bound receptors in live cells	Screening of chemical compounds
Fluorescence resonance energy transfer (FRET)	Works on the interaction of two different chromophores via dipole-dipole mechanism, excited donor chromophore transfers its excitation energy to a closely located acceptor chromophore	Interaction of the chemicals or drugs with biomolecules[5]
Time resolved Fluorescence resonance energy transfer (TR - FRET)	Combines the advantage of fluorescence resonance energy transfer along with the time	Interaction of the chemicals or drugs with biomolecules[6,7]
Fluorescence microscopy	Based on the excitation of the fluorescent molecule bound to the cellular surface and visualizing under a magnifying object lens	Cellular or tissue structural analysis
Real time PCR	Works on the ability of the dyes to emit fluorescence signals via binding to a double stranded DNA	Gene expression analysis
Fluorescence Lifetime Imaging Microscopy (FLIM)	Sample is illuminated with a pulsed laser and the lifetime of the fluorescent probe is determined from the phase shift between the modulation of the excitation light and the emission of fluorescence	Analysis of the cellular components[8]

FLOW CYTOMETRY FOR CELL-BASED ASSAY

A flow cytometer (FCM) is an instrument which illuminates the cells or particles as they flow in form of droplets in front of a light source and then reads the illumination. FCM was first described as an analytical tool in 1960. After that FCM changed a lot for it's utilization in the drug discovery and diagnosis.

Principle of working: FCM has several components which work in tandem to produce desirable results.

1. ***Light source:*** Nowadays most of the FCMs contain laser light as a source for the illumination. Lasers are preferred because of their intense and narrow beams. They may be gas lasers (e.g. argon ion laser or helium neon laser) or solid state lasers (e.g. red or green diode laser, new blue and violet lasers). These lasers would be generating defined and fixed type of wavelengths (e.g. 488 nm for argon ion laser). Usually a flow cytometer would be having one laser light source but advance machines may have more as well.
2. ***Fluidics:*** In FCMs particles need to be suspended in the fluid so that a single particle can be analyzed at a time. Concentrated cell suspension may form aggregates of the cells, even so called single cell suspension cells may form clumps. Hence fluidics is designed in a way to decrease the chances of aggregation and to facilitate similar illumination of each cell. The strategy used by Crosland-Taylor for the confinement of the cells in a focused, narrow flow stream (known as hydrodynamic focusing) is applied to achieve this. The sample stream is injected into the rapidly flowing stream (sheath stream) in a "flow cell" which has a narrow exit orifice. This difference in the diameter increases the velocity of the entire stream and confined the path of the cells tightly to the center of the laser beam.
3. ***Detectors:*** Photodiode is fitted in the line of the illuminating laser beam with an obscuration bar in front of it. The laser light which has been bent by the cell can only reach the detector after avoiding the obscuration bar, it is known as forward scatter. The forward scatter light is not well defined in the terms of biology or chemistry of the cells because of the confusion in the refractive indices of the live or dead cells and the medium. One lens is fitted to the right angle to the direction of the laser beam and light collected by it is known as side scatter light or 90° light scatter.

- **Applications**: Since the development of the first FCM in 1960s, a tremendous work has been carried out in the hematological discoveries. One or two color FCMs helped in the identification of cellular (T-cells) and humoral (B-cells) cells lineages, followed by CD3, CD4 and CD8 identification by multicolor flow cytometer.[9,10] These days flow cytometry has also been utilized in the vaccine development by intracellular cytokine staining assays and further cell sorting for their genomic as well as transcriptional analysis.[11] In previous 10 years possibilities of the *in vivo* flow cytometry has also been tried by several research groups from around the world. By using very high speed, high resolution, continuous CCD or CMOS cameras, images have been taken from the rat mesenteric blood and lymphatic vessels.[10] Several compounds have been tested in the *in vivo* flow cytometric analysis of the blood and lymphatic vessels. Natural property of the lymph vessel and valve function has also been studied by the *in vivo* flow cytometry.[12]

THERMAL SHIFT ANALYSIS FOR HTS

Thermal shift analysis of the proteins has now become a good tool for the identification of the ligand interaction with the proteins in a rapid and high throughput manner. This method needs a fluorescent dye which associates and dissociates from the protein with the change in the temperature of the reaction. It is based on the principle of binding of the ligand to a protein and stabilizing or destabilizing its structure which ultimately changes the melting temperature (Tm) of the protein. Sypro orange is such a dye which binds to the protein in a temperature dependent manner. Fluorescence of sypro orange is quenched in the aqueous environment but when protein unfolds and expresses its hydrophobic core then dye binds to it and starts emitting fluorescence. Finally fluorescence is monitored and plotted versus temperature. Thermal shift analysis can be used to assess the following:

1. Role of inhibitor in the binding affinity of the ligand with protein.
2. Stability of the protein at different pH and salt conditions.
3. Ligand screening for the binding with the protein for the lead identification.

Thermal shift assay has helped in the identification of the inhibitors of the carbonic anhydrase enzyme.[13,14] Carbonic anhydrase is a zinc metal containing enzyme which is involved in the dehydration of the bicarbonate. This enzyme is also involved in the several pathologies like glaucoma, epilepsy, Alzheimer's and Parkinson's disease hence serves as a potential drug target. Thermal shift assay has also helped in the identification of the estrogen receptor antagonists (Toremifene and tamoxifen) as anti-cryptococcal agents. The assay showed that these drugs directly bound to the calmodulin (cam1) which was purified from *Cryptococcus neoformans* and prevented it from binding to its substrate calcineurin (Cna1) and blocked its activation.[15] Further thermal shift assay helped in the evaluation of the mitogen activated protein kinase inhibitor 4 (MAP2K4) which activates pro-invasion signaling pathways in the prostate cancer.[16]

ROLE OF MASS SPECTROMETRY IN THE HIGH THROUGHPUT SCREENING

Mass spectrometry is an important tool in the clinical and medical development area. Almost hundred years have passed when Nobel laureate Sir J. J. Thomson first described about mass spectrometer in Cambridge Philosophical Society. From the time of its initial development, mass spectrometer changed a lot but became suitable for the biological field only after the development of the electrospray ionization (ESI) technique by John Fenn which fetched him a Nobel Prize in 2002. After this development mass spectrometer evolved as an important tool in the field of biology. Coupling the separation capabilities of the liquid chromatography with the structural analysis abilities of mass spectrometer gave a third dimension for the quick and accurate identification and quantification of the compounds. Information dependent acquisition (IDA) available with some of the mass spectrometers gives the freedom of the identification of the unknown from the pool of several molecules by available mass spectras of the known one. Thus the mass spectrometer has now become an essential tool for the drug development in a rapid and accurate manner.

Phytochemical extract analysis: Analysis of the natural product extracts has always been a tedious task. This process needs the identification of the gross chemical group, purification, enrichment and structure elucidation of the final compound. Once the process is done, the compound is again screened pharmacologically. This process is having one drawback that compound recovered at the end may fail to show any pharmacological activity. The reason behind this is that the separated and enriched compound might not be responsible for the pharmacological activity found with crude extract at the beginning. Mass spectrometry has given a solution for the above problem—information dependent scans of the extract and identification of the hit. It works on the basis of the available structural and functional (pharmacological) information for the similar natural product group compounds. Once the pharmacological activity on the crude extract is done, the library is constructed for the compounds similar in the pharmacological activity and from the similar natural product group. The extract is screened for the diverse mass ranges (from few Daltons to almost one thousand Dalton) and the fragmentation pattern of the similar molecular mass compounds (hit) is matched with the available mass spectra of the known compounds. The same technique was used by Kyadari et al for the identification of lyngbyatoxin-A and malyngamide-J in the marine algae extracts.[17]

Purity analysis of the drugs or synthesized compounds: Mass spectrometry can very well be used for the purity analysis of the compounds. Purity analysis of the drug formulation or the synthesized molecules gives important information regarding the improvement in the formulation or synthesis process. In case of drug formulation impurities may lead to therapeutic failure or even adverse events due to toxic metabolites or contaminants. The stability and impurity profile of latanoprost drug formulation was evaluated by Velpandian et al using LC-MS/MS.[18]

IN VIVO IMAGING OF DRUG ACTION (NEAR INFRARED IMAGING)

It is a newly added method to evaluate the drug action and quantification without killing the animal. Rapid development in this technology is expected to revolutionize the *in vivo* studies that warrant the killing of the experimental animals. Fundamental of this technique is using molecules capable of emitting light in higher wavelength near IR region thereby, it gains the capability of crossing biological membrane and to be detected by sensitive camera turned for near IR region. For this application an exogenous contrast agent like indocyanine green (ICG) is used. *In vivo* near IR fluorescence imaging has been successfully utilized in vascular mapping, and tissue perfusion studies, to image vasculature of brain, for conducting angiograms of eye, imaging tumors, biodistribution studies, gastrointestinal tract (using endoscopic optics), inflammation, atherosclerosis, cell death, and osteoblastic activity, etc.[19] For all the studies excitation was achieved by using pulsed diode laser having different fluence rate above 700 nm and emission was recorded using powerful cooled CCD capable of monitoring near IR emission radiation.

Recently, GFP (Green fluorescent protein) or Ds Red2 genes are making a rapid entry in the biological research. For tumor imaging Ds Red2 expressing CR8 Lewis-lung carcinoma cells were injected into nu/ne mice. Seven to ten days after inoculation of cells Cy-annexin V conjugate was injected intravenously to the mice bearing tumors and submitted for imaging near infrared signal. Using cyclophosphamide, Petrovsky et al[20] evaluated the usefulness of active Cy-annexin that can be used as a near infrared probe to image apoptosis from outside an intact living animal and facilitate the antiproliferative drug screening.

Other Whole Body Imaging Techniques

Single photon emission computed tomography (SPECT) is a highly sensitive nuclear medicine tomographic imaging technique using gamma rays. It is very similar to conventional nuclear medicine planar imaging using a gamma camera. However, it is able to provide true

3D information. This information is typically presented as cross-sectional slices through the organism, but can be freely reformatted or manipulated as required.

SPECT uses gamma-emitting nuclides, which undergo a radioactive decay with the emission of gamma radiation. In order to attain a nuclear stability, the nucleus of an unstable atom undergoes a process of transition in which neutrons are converted to protons and vice versa. This process leads to the formation of daughter nucleus in an excited state. This state is unstable; therefore, it reverts back to the ground state and loses some form of energy in terms of electromagnetic radiation or gamma radiation, e.g. Technetium-99m (^{99m}Tc), Iodine-123 (^{123}I), cobalt-60 (^{60}Co).

SPECT imaging involves the administration of radiotracers into the biological system and the radiations emitted from the radiotracer in the body are captured by the gamma cameras with sodium iodide crystal detector and photomultiplier tube (PMT) in which the radiations are converted into scintillating photons and amplified and the images at different angles are reconstructed by the computer in such a way that the imaging of the organ of interest is achieved.

Recently, SPECT has been utilized in the study of involvement of drug efflux transporters like multidrug resistance associated protein (MRP), P-glycoprotein (P-gp) and lung resistance protein (LRP) as a contribtuting factor for multidrug resistance in cancer therapy in patients.[21] In research, due to the ease of small animal imaging with SPECT, it is been utilized to evaluate and to visualize the modulation of P-gp or MRP using (99m) Tc - sestamib as a model substrate.

For the first time from our laboratory, SPECT imaging has been utilized to explore the intraocular uptake of fluoroquinolones following systemic administration by such drug efflux transporter (Fig. 2.3) in the eye using ciprofloxacin labelled^{99m}Tc as a radiotracer in rabbits.[22] This study was carried out in presence of GF 120918, which is a P-gp modulator and verapamil, a known P-gp as well as OCT inhibitor.

VIRTUAL SCREENING (*IN SILICO* DRUG DEVELOPMENT OR DRY LAB)

It is totally an indirect approach using advanced computer technology to screen newer compounds based on virtual coordinates of receptor and ligands. Computer-aided molecular design (CAMD) approach involves computational analysis of large data set in order to highlight those compounds most likely to be active in the actual assay, so that a focused

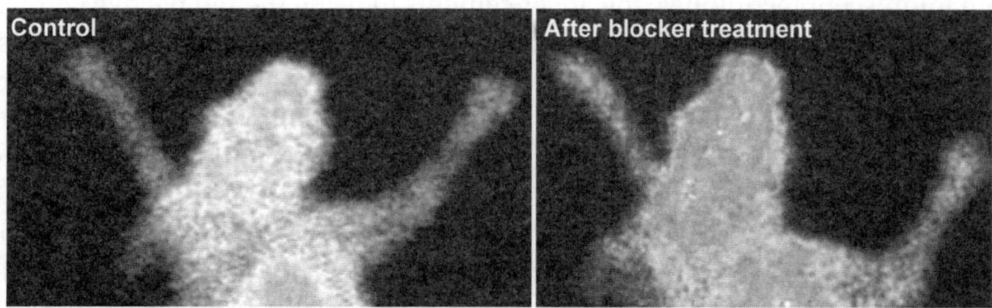

Figure 2.3: Pictures of SPECT-CT showing the intraocular uptake of radiolabeled ciprofloxacin after blocker (verapamil) treatment. Dual head SPECT–CT with collimator-low energy (*Courtesy*: Dept. of Ocular Pharmacology & Pharmacy, AIIMS and INMAS, New Delhi) (*For color version see Plate 1*)

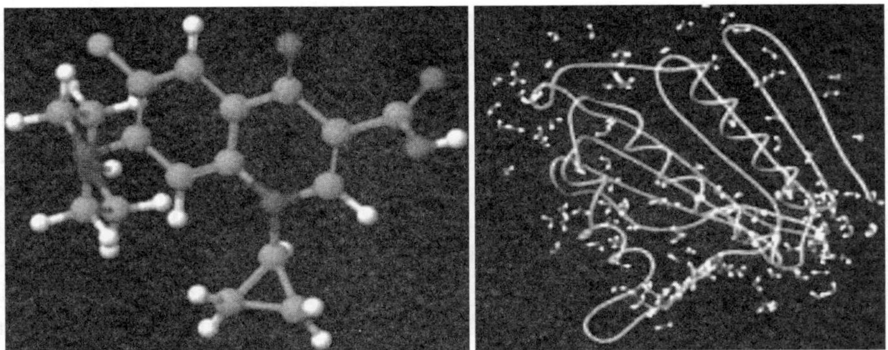

Figure 2.4: Computer-aided molecular design approach (*For color version see Plate 2*)

subset of compounds can be selected. CAMD covers a wide range of technologies leading to very fast property predictions through more computationally elaborate modeling of drug-receptor binding. Using receptor-based properties, such as binding affinity and receptor selectivity, CAMD calculates to propose a broad range of properties that are likely to be useful in drug design—from physical properties like molecular size and solubility to indicators of developmental issues like metabolic fate and toxicity, etc. Therefore, virtual screening can filter out undesirable compounds on the basis of a wide variety of criteria, depending on the problem in hand. Virtual screening needs the 3D molecular structure of the receptor along with the 3D structure of ligands to perform docking. However, this approach is highly applicable for the lead optimization process since for many newly isolated receptor's conformational data may not be available. Moreover, the techniques like X-ray crystallography and NMR studies are necessary for the information about spatial arrangement and virtual coordinates of targets and ligands.[23] Figure 2.4 showing the docking of ciprofloxacin on DNA gyrase using CaChe (Ver.6.1, Fujitsu, Japan).

The applicability of computer models has also used completely empirical and statistical model like the Rule of Five or Lipinski's rule. According to this rule, a drug like compound looks like a molecule with a molecular weight less than 500, OH and NH groups less than 5, the sum of N and O atoms less than 10 and log P value less than 5 for a better absorption in the intestine.

HTS-SCINTILLATION METHODS IN DRUG SCREENING

Apart from fluorescent techniques, the advancements in using the radioactive compounds to understand molecular mechanisms are also very interesting. One of such attempts is named as scintillation proximity assay (SPA). This system uses the principle that an antibody or a receptor molecule, which is bound to a bead, emits light when beta emission from an isotope occurs in close proximity, i.e. when a radiolabeled ligand binds to the bead with receptor or antibody (Fig. 2.5). Amersham has introduced several advancements in these techniques leading to make it as a successful high throughput screen. The basic technology of the SPA is based on the fluorescent signal produced by a scintillant-dyed polystyrene or polyvinyl toluene microsphere that could be excited by the proximity of a radiolabeled molecule. The scintillant-dyed microspheres are in the size range of < 2 μm in diameter. The recent improvements in this technique are yttrium silicate and yttrium oxide beads which enable the use of higher number

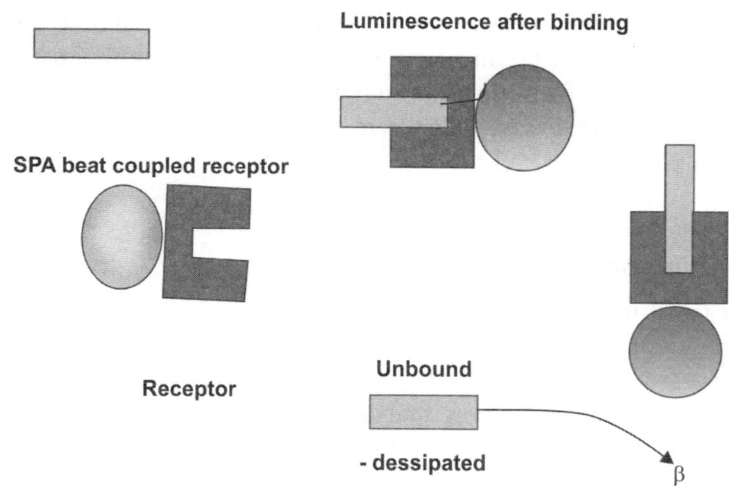

Figure 2.5: Principles of scintillation proximity assay (SPA) (*For color version see Plate 2*)

of wells in which the signal can be picked up by highly sensitive readers containing CCD camera instead of classical photomultiplier tubes. So far, this technology is applied in several attempts in drug discovery processes like evaluation of kinetics of protein kinase inhibitors, to evaluate neurotransmitter transporter inhibitors, to evaluate novel farnesyltransferase inhibitors, to identify poly (ADP-ribose) polymerase-1 inhibitors (enzyme involved in DNA repair), evaluation of HIV-I reverse transcriptase inhibitors, etc. SPA is a homogeneous, rapid, versatile and amenable to automation, which can also simplify the screening protocol in the drug discovery process.

UNCONVENTIONAL RAPID PHARMACOLOGICAL AND TOXICITY TESTING MODELS

Zebrafish (Danio rerio) and Gold Fish (Carassius auratus auratus)

Drugs working on the central nervous system (CNS) are having a choice of being tested on the marine organisms like fishes. Antipsychotic class of drugs have been discovered without having any target approach. Still mechanism is unknown for many of them. For these classes rational approach may not work but behavioral approaches may work for the screening of newer compounds. Gold fishes have mainly been used for the CNS depressant and stimulant drug analysis. It was an attempt of the Vijayakumar et al[24] to develop a model for the screening of the drugs for their effect on CNS. Gold fishes were exposed to the low concentration of known CNS depressant and stimulant drugs and their swimming pattern (optomotor response) was assessed along the gyro-dots of different colors. Similarly, toxicity of the ethambutol on the eye was also evaluated using the gold fishes.

Zebrafishes are used mainly for the angiogenic and anti-angiogenic effects of the compounds on the vasculature of this marine organism. The reason of the extensive use of the zebrafish is the development of optically clear embryo provides the opportunity of the visual inspections and very high egg laying capacity of the female zebrafish.[25] Zebrafish has been utilized for the better understanding of the Alzheimer's disease.[26] Zebrafish has been used in the hematology research because of the conserved genetic factors regulating blood development and visualization of the circulating erythrocytes with only a dissecting microscope. Their organ regeneration capacity made them popular model in the regeneration experiments like heart regeneration.[27] As zebrafish express cytokines, macrophages, neutrophils, dendritic cells, mast cells, eosinophil, T-cells, and B-cells; it has also been used in the host pathogen interaction studies as well.[28]

Chick (Gallus gallus domesticus)

Use of chick for the drug screening is now a well applied model in the drug development. Extraembryonic membrane serving gas exchange known as Chorioallantoic membrane has a network of blood vessels (Fig. 2.6A). Chorioallantoic membrane can be used for the evaluation of the angiogenic or antiangiogenic potential of the compounds. One important factor for the use of chick for these studies is the non-requirement of the ethical approval. Fertilized egg can be obtained from the hatchery and can further be developed as per need in the incubator at the laboratory. Several marine isolates have been studied for their anti-angiogenic effect on the chorioallantoic membrane of the chick.[29]

The size of the lens and the time taken for the development of the model has made hydrocortisone-induced cataract in the chick a good model (Fig. 2.6B). This model has been used for the screening of the larger groups of the compounds for their anti-cataract activity on the lens. Several polyherbals have also successfully been studied using the same technique.[30,31]

Caenorhabditis elegans

Currently in toxicity and pharmacological studies *C. elegans* are being utilized extensively. Availability of whole Genome sequence, transparency of the tissues at all the developmental stages, availability of large mutant species and shorter life span has made *C. elegans* a very good model for biological as well as disease and drug effect research. *C. elegans* was used for the evaluation of the Genistein for its life span enhancement ability by Lee et al (2015). Genistein is a dietary phytoestrogen present in the seeds of Vigna angularis cultivated in East Asia. The phytoestrogen was tested on the nematode *C. elegans* in both normal and stress conditions

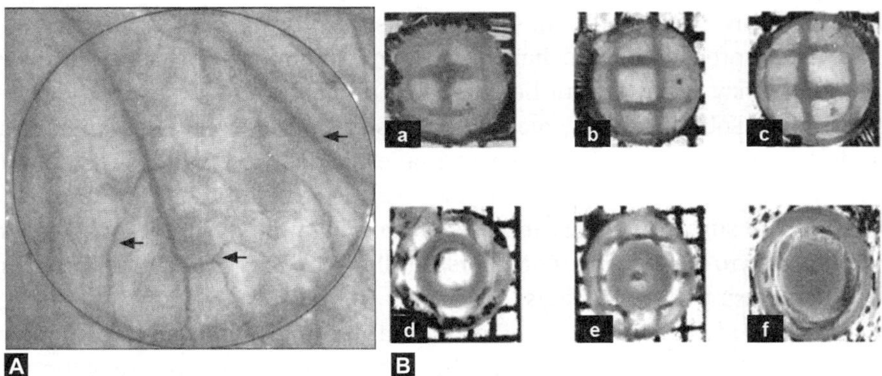

Figure 2.6: Photographs showing use of chick for pharmacological screening of compounds: (A) Black arrows showing developing blood vessels in the chorio allantoic membrane of the chick under a coverslip (black circle). (*Courtesy*: Gupta et al (2014); (B) Figures a,b and c are showing normal lenses; d—stage 2 cataract; e—stage 3 cataract; f—stage 5 cataract; *Courtesy* Velpandian et al (2003)

produced by heat and oxidation. Genistein could able to enhance the life span of the nematode in both the conditions.[32] In another study the growth retardation effect of caffeine on the fetus was assessed on the larvae of the *C. elegans* by Min et al. They found that the caffeine was able to hinder development at most of the stages in a dose dependent manner.[33]

HTS PHARMACOKINETIC STUDIES

HTS-absorption Studies

Oral route is a preferred way of drug administration. In the drug development process it is very important to screen the drugs for gastrointestinal absorption. Conventionally, it is a very lengthy and time-consuming process. Moreover, this process also requires a large number of animals. Intestinal absorption is mainly due to the concentration dependent diffusion. If the drug passes through paracellular route, then there is not much of a hurdle. Some compounds, like cyclosporine and digoxin, are substrates of well recognized P-gp transporters, which belong to the ATP Binding Cassette (ABC) transporters having Walker's motives. P-gp substrates were found to have variable bioavailability. Therefore, it is necessary to screen the drug candidates during the developmental stage to ensure that they are not substrates for P-gp. Colon cancer cell lines (CaCo) grow confluently and form a monolayer upon polycarbonate support or collagen coated polycarbonate support.[34] They are quite suitable for performing intestinal permeation studies and to elucidate the drug candidates susceptible for P-gp efflux mechanism in the intestine. Moreover, they also express CYP3A4 enzyme allowing prediction of intestinal metabolism. This process can be automated to examine the intestinal absorption characteristics of drugs in a shortest possible period to decrease the incidence of failure in the Phase I clinical trial in human volunteers.

PARALLEL ARTIFICIAL MEMBRANE PERMEABILITY ASSAY (PAMPA)

In order to assess the intestinal permeation, apart from cell-based assays like CaCo monolayer cells, PAMPA is an alternative. It is a passive-permeability screen with focus on the simulation of transcellular processes. It is reported to be an excellent compliment to cellular models in absorption, distribution, metabolism, excretion (ADME) screening of research compounds. It is a fast, versatile and low-cost method that is compelling and biologically relevant model of transport. Its principle is based on the application of physicochemical properties of molecules to predict intestinal permeability.[35] In PAMPA, a 96 well microtiter plate completely filled with aqueous buffer solutions is covered with a hydrophobic filter coated with lipids in an organic solvent solution in a sandwich construction. Typically, Hwang et al[36] prepared the membrane by wetting with 5 μl of the artificial membrane solution (0.8% egg lecithin in n-dodecane). The donor and recipient solutions consisted of phosphate-buffered saline (pH 5.5 or 7.4) with 2% DMSO (donor contained 200 μM test compound in each well). These plates were incubated for 2 hours at room temperature with gentle shaking, following which drug concentrations in the receiving solutions were assayed by HPLC. Percentage transport across the lipid bilayer (%T) was calculated by %T= 100 x Ar/Ad (Ar and Ad correspond to the HPLC peak areas of the receiving solution and initial donor solution). Using this method they have predicted their model drug supposed to be absorbed via passive diffusion across the human gastrointestinal tract following oral administration. Different membranes used for the prediction of absorption from intestinal,[36] blood brain barrier[37] and skin[38] are listed in the Table 2.2.

Table 2.2: Membranes used for prediction of absorption in PAMPA

Membranes used	*Predicted absorption in PAMPA*
Egg-lecithin + N-dodecane	Intestinal permeability
Egg-lecithin + 1,9, decadiene	Intestinal permeability
Composition of lipids + 1,7-octadiene	Intestinal permeability
Porcine polar brain lipid + dodecane	Blood-brain barrier permeability
70% silicone + 30% isopropyl myristate	Skin permeability

HTS Metabolism Studies

In order to increase the speed of metabolism studies or to decrease the animal utilization in the metabolism studies, *in vitro* techniques were developed. Isolated human or animal liver microsomes are incubated along with the drug of interest and at periodical interval the aliquots are subjected for LC-MS or LC-NMR to elucidate the metabolites. Sometimes the major metabolites are isolated and subjected to primary *in vitro* screening to elucidate whether they are active metabolites or not. Liver microsomes are prepared by the homogenization of a liver, followed by centrifugation of the homogenate at 10000 g to obtain a supernatant fraction known as S10 fraction. The S10 fraction at 100,000 g pellets out smooth endoplasmic reticulum where the enzymes responsible for Phase I oxidation, including the CYP450 monooxygenases reside. However, most of the Phase II enzymes are cytosolic and are absent from the liver microsomes. Apart from microsomes, isolated hepatocytes (or hepatocytes-derived microsomes), cDNA-expressed enzymes and liver slices are also used to study the metabolic stability of drugs. The screening of metabolic stability with liver microsomes or human hepatocytes can be performed in 96-well plates to enhance throughput.

HTS-cytochrome (CYP) Inhibition and Induction Studies

During the drug development process, pharmacokinetic drug-drug interaction can also be an undesirable factor. For example, ketoconazole, a potent inhibitor of CYP3A4, causes drug-drug interaction with drugs that are substrates for the same enzyme. Cryopreserved hepatocytes retain both Phase I and II drug metabolizing enzyme activities and, therefore, are used extensively for drug interaction studies. To get more information about the newly developed compound's metabolic interaction in specific cytochrome, liver microsome incubation studies are carried out using specific inhibitors. For this study phenacetin (for CYP1A2), coumarin (for CYP2A6), tolbutamide (for CYP2C9), s-mephenytoin (for CYP2C19), dextromethorphan (for CYP2D6), chlorzoxazone (for CYP2E1) and testosterone (for CYP3A4) are used. For HTS enzyme induction studies, the mechanism of CYP3A4 induction has been defined. Compounds, which are capable of inducing CYP3A4, also induce pregnane-X-receptor (PXR), that bind to the response element in the CYP3A4 gene called the pregnane-X-receptor response element (PXRE). An HTS method has been developed using a genetically engineered cell line that expresses a PXRE-luciferase reporter gene. In this method, the induction of CYP3A4 by the xenobiotic-mediated binding of PXR to PXRE leads to the activation of luciferase synthesis, which can be quantified using a chemiluminescent substrate (luciferin).

HTS Hepatotoxicity Studies

The isolated hepatocytes are also used to study the possible xenobiotic induced hepatotoxicity *in vitro*. After the incubation of hepatocytes along with the drug candidate, the hepatocytes are subjected for measurement of ATP content in microtiter plates using chemiluminescence with the help of a luciferin-luciferase assay. MTT [3-(4,5-dimethylthiazol-2-yl)-2,5-diphenyl tetrazolium bromide] assay is performed to quantify mitochondrial toxicity. LDH measurement, neutral red uptake test, thymidine uptake test and estimation of glutathione give more information on the possible hepatotoxicity of the xenobiotics.

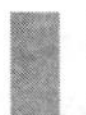

HIGH SPEED DRUG SYNTHESIS PROCESS 'COMBINATORIAL CHEMISTRY' (COMBICHEM)

High-speed primary screening for 'hits' require the support from chemistry to feed the prolific requirement. This is achieved by combinatorial chemistry using parallel synthesis technology. Traditional synthesis of organic compounds is a very slow process as compared to the present day technologies adopted for high speed combichem synthesis to meet the requirement of compound libraries for HTS and lead optimization. The first combinatorial chemistry methods were presented by Geysen and coworkers[39] for peptide synthesis. Later, this has been utilized for classical heterocyclic and other small molecule organic compounds.[40] The intervention of microwave flash-heating chemistry in dramatically reducing reaction times (reduced from days and hours to minutes and seconds) has been well recognized.[41] Conventional round bottom flask is replaced with polymer (like Tentagel™) attached reactants in columns to make easy elution after the reaction. This process can also reduce the time involved in purification of the final product from the unreacted reactants. Automated organic synthesizers are on rapid development to further support this effort.

High Speed Natural Product Isolation Techniques

Natural products (NP) are the most successful sources of leads to the evolutionary development of biologically active metabolic byproducts. Out of 520 new drugs developed and approved between 1983-1994, 39% of them were either NP or their derivatives.[42] However, the long-pending problems with the NP are the isolation and identification of the active ingredients as well as ensuring their pharmacological properties. Seasonal, regional, geographical, taxonomical variations and processing methods make traditional activity guided NP development very long. Many pharmaceutical giants stopped using whole natural product extract for biological activities. Due to the development of successful two-dimensional high performance isolation units like SEPBOX (SEPIAtec, GmbH, Germany) for multiparallel HPLC, it is now possible to load up to 5 gm of NP extract and to isolate all compounds in 70-80% purity within 24 hr and in amounts sufficient and in microtiter formats amenable for direct HTS.

This SEPBOX system works by using gradient elution and polarity based trapping in solid phase extraction (SPE) trap columns. After the successful entrapment of compounds, they are eluted to obtain pure compounds. Coupling the SEPBOX to photodiode array (PDA) detector (enhanced UV detector), and evaporative light-scattering detector (ESD) in series enables the identification and quantification of the significant compounds. NMR or mass spectroscopy is further used for the complete identification and structure elucidation. NP database containing about 10000 different structurally characterized compounds is being commercialized [Chapman and Hall Dictionary of Natural Products (DNP), Ver. 7:2, 8:2 on CD-ROM and Antibase, Ver 3.0] using a combination of mass spectroscopy and 1 and 2 D NMR.

A study was conducted jointly by Aventis Pharma AG (Vitrysur Seine, France) and AnalytiCon Discovery (Berlin, Germany) to test the feasibility of high-throughput profiling, isolation and structure-elucidation technology for NP. A project named Megabolite was initiated to get minimum 5 mg samples of 4000 pure compounds from microbes and plants. They have used the above (SEPBOX) technology for the isolation of the active compounds. The plants were selected from the families of Leguminosae, Euphorbiaceae, Umbelliferae, Solanaceae, Borganiaceae, Compositeae, Labiatae, Apocynaceae, Rubiaceae, Meliaceae and Araliaceae. A total of 2242 compounds from microorganisms and 1758 compounds from plants were isolated in the course of the project. About 2400 pure compounds isolated from NP were tested against biological targets using HTS assays (scintillation proximity assay and homogeneous time-resolved fluorescence). The compounds isolated from NP gave a higher confirmation rate as compared to the Rhone-Poulenc Rorer synthetic compound collection (>50000 single compounds) and combinatorial library (> 50000 single compounds). Therefore, the development of advanced HPLC techniques can go beyond the synthetic process in making drugs with higher success rate in screens.[43]

NATURAL PRODUCTS COMBICHEM—A NEWER DIMENSION

Crude natural product isolation and testing their activity using different pharmacological assays is a way to identify thehit from the mixture of the biodiverse compounds. An outstanding example of the richness of the resources available is the Natural Products Repository of the National Cancer Institute, comprising >180,000 extracts from > 50,000 organisms. Other organizations maintain similar, often focused libraries of natural product extracts, including the Spanish Fundación Medina, with a large collection of microbial samples, the Korean Research Institute of Bioscience and Biotechnology, with a Korean plant extract bank (http://www.kribb.re.kr/eng/sub02/sub02_07_02.jsp), and the Eskitis Institute in Australia, with Australian plants and marine invertebrates.[44,45]

It is a combined strength of natural products optimization with combinatorial chemistry for getting the successful bioactive ligands to quicken the success rate. The most powerful bioactive compounds obtained from natural sources could be due to the revolutionary transformation of prey-predator concept to acquire unique feature to escape from being destroyed. For example, Datura is not eaten by cattles only due to the presence of the bioactive alkaloids. Similarly, thousands of examples can be explained from plants for having bioactive compounds. One of the key factors for this secret is the enrichment of stereochemistry within the scaffolds of such molecules. This classically differs from man made compounds having heterocyclic rings as basic blocks. Simple alkaloid morphine is obtained from opium poppy takes 40 organic synthetic steps to synthesis. The major structural differences between natural and combinatorial compounds originate mainly from properties introduced to make combinatorial synthesis more efficient. These include the number of chiral centers, the prevalence of aromatic rings, the introduction of complex ring systems, and the degree of the saturation of the molecule as well as the number and ratios of different heteroatoms. As drug molecules derive from both natural and synthetic sources, they cover a joint area in property space of natural and combinatorial compounds. A principal component analysis compares random selection of combinatorial compounds from commercial suppliers against a natural product and drug database.[46,47]

OTHER ROLES OF HTS

Role of high throughput techniques in the analysis of the toxins: Currently the increasing utilization of the natural sources especially for sea foods has posed a potential risk of the exposure of the consumers to marine toxins. Pollution of drinking water from the marine toxins is also a big problem. Palytoxins, Ciguatoxins, Cyclic imines and Tetrodotoxins are few of the marine toxins which are having their impact on the sea food as well as on the water also. Scientists have started using the techniques of the high throughput screening for the rapid identification of the contaminants. European Commission and the European Food Safety Authority (EFSA) have emphasized the potential of these toxins. Earlier Mouse bioassays (MBAs) have been used for years as important tools to manage seafood safety. Currently the debate over utilization of the animals for the toxicological analysis has also impacted marine toxin testing. For the lipophilic marine toxin identification the LC-MS/MS technique is the reference used by the European Union in an approach to completely remove the use of MBA. Immunoassay techniques have also been employed for the identification of the marine toxins. Cell based approaches using the Ouabain and Veratridine as agonist or antagonists have been utilized for the identification owing the action of toxins on the physiology, morphology or viability of the cells. Biosensors have also shown promising approaches for the detection of the marine toxins.[48]

CONCLUSION

High throughput screening is one of the most prominent domains in terms of drug discovery which has a pivotal contribution for a new molecule to turn into a therapeutic entity. Emergence of new diseases and failing treatments for existing diseases has increased the importance of high throughput screening in a greater extent. Availability of multiplex systems and cellular imaging systems has made the live screening of the compound a reality. The approach has again turned towards natural sources for the discoveries of the new molecules in a high throughput manner. Rapid development in the instrumentation has also helped to fasten up the process of drug discovery. The combinatorial approach of the drug development scientists and engineering experts has made the never approaching dream a reality. Learning experiences and out of box thoughts are still waiting so many changes in this area. This amalgamation of technology in every field is expected to increase to multiple folds in the next decade and would be creating a method through which more and more safe drugs would be discovered for almost all the diseases.

REFERENCES

1. Ma H1, Horiuchi KY. Chemical microarray: A new tool for drug screening and discovery. Drug Discov Today 2006;11(13-14):661-8.
2. Chicchi GG, Cascieri MA, Graziano MP, et al. Fluorescein-Trp25-exendin-4, a biologically active fluorescent probe for the human GLP-1 receptor. Peptides 1997;18:319-21.
3. Lee J, Pilch PF, Shoelson SE, et al. Conformational changes of the insulin receptor upon insulin binding and activation as monitored by fluorescence spectroscopy. Biochemistry 1997;36:2701-8.
4. Ho C, Slater SJ, Stagliano BA, et al. Conformation of the C1 phorbol-ester-binding domain participates in the activating conformational change of protein kinase C. Biochem J 1999;344:451-60.
5. Stenroos K, Hurskainen P, Eriksson S, et al. Homogeneous time-resolved IL-2-IL-2R alpha assay using fluorescence resonance energy transfer. Cytokine 1998;10:495-9.
6. Achard S, Jean A, Lorphelin D, Amoravain M, Claret EJ. Homogeneous assays allow direct "in well" Cytokine level quantification. Assay Drug Dev Technol 2003;1:181-5.
7. Yang X, Li P, Feldberg L, Kim SC, Bowman M, Hollander I, Mallon R, Wolf SF. A directly labeled TR-FRET assay for monitoring phosphoinositide-3-kinase activity. Comb Chem High Throughput Screen 2006;9:565-70.
8. Farah OI, Cuiling L, Jiaojiao W, et al. Use of fluorescent dyes for readily recognizing sperm damage. J Reprod Infertil 2013;14(3):120-5.
9. Jaye DL, Bray RA, Gebel HM, et al. Translational applications of flow cytometry in clinical practice. J Immunol 2012:188(10).
10. De Rosa SC, Herzenberg LA, Herzenberg LA, et al. 11-color, 13-parameter flow cytometry: identification of human naive T cells by phenotype, function, and T-cell receptor diversity. Nat Med 2001;7(2):245-8.
11. De Rosa SC. Vaccine applications of flow cytometry. Methods 2012;57(3):383-91.
12. Tuchin VV1, Tárnok A, Zharov VP. In vivo flow cytometry: a horizon of opportunities. Cytometry A 2011;79(10):737-45.
13. Kišonaitė M, Zubrienė A, Capkauskaitė E, et al. Intrinsic thermodynamics and structure correlation of benzenesulfonamides with a pyrimidine moiety binding to carbonic anhydrases I, II, VII, XII, and XIII. PLoS One 2014;9(12).
14. Rutkauskas K, Zubrienė A, Tumosienė I, et al. 4-amino-substituted benzene sulfonamides as inhibitors of human carbonic anhydrases. Molecules 2014;19(11).
15. Butts A, Koselny K, Chabrier-Roselló Y, et al. Estrogen receptor antagonists are anti-cryptococcal agents that directly bind EF hand proteins and synergizę with fluconazole in vivo. mBio 2014;5(1).
16. Krishna SN, Luan CH, Mishra RK, et al. A fluorescence-based thermal shift assay identifies inhibitors of mitogen activated protein kinase kinase 4. PLoS One 2013;8(12).
17. Kyadari M, Fatma T, Velpandian T, et al. Antiangiogenic and antiproliferative assessment of cyanobacteria.Indian J Exp Biol 2014 Aug;52(8):835-42.
18. Velpandian T, Kotnala A, Halder N, et al. Stability of latanoprost in generic formulations using controlled degradation and patient usage simulation studies. Curr Eye Res 2014 Dec 11:1-11.
19. Frangioni JV. In vivo near IR fluorescence imaging. Curr Opion Chem Biol 2003;7:626-34.
20. Petrovsky A Schellenberger E, Josephson L, Weissleder R, Bogdanov A. Near -Infrared fluorescent imaging of tumor apoptosis. Can Res 2003;63:1936-42.

21. Zhou J, Higashi K, Ueda Y, Kodama Y, Guo D, Jisaki F, et al. Expression of multidrug resistance protein and messenger RNA correlate with (99m)Tc-MIBI imaging in patients with lung cancer. J Nucl Med 2001;42:1476-83.
22. Hendrikse NH. Monitoring interactions at ATP-dependent drug efflux pumps. Curr Pharm Des 2000;6:1653-68.
23. Walters WP, Stahl MT, Murcko MA. Virtual screening—an overview. Drug Discov Today 1998;3: 160-78.
24. Vijayakumar AR, Velpandian T, Biswas NR, et al. Development and evaluation of gyro-dot optomotor response in goldfish to predict drugs affecting vision perception. In IERG-ARVO-IC 20th Annual meeting at Hyderabad (July 2012).
25. Carroll KJ, North TE. Oceans of opportunity: exploring vertebrate hematopoiesis in zebrafish. Exp Hematol 2014;42(8):684-96.
26. Newman M, Ebrahimie E, Lardelli M. Using the zebrafish model for Alzheimer's disease research. Front Genet 2014;5:189.
27. Kikuchi K. Advances in understanding the mechanism of zebrafish heart regeneration. Stem Cell Res. 2014;13(3PB):542-55.
28. Harwood CG, Rao RP. Host pathogen relations: exploring animal models for fungal pathogens. Pathogens 2014;3(3):549-62.
29. Gupta P, Arumugam M, Azad RV, et al. Screening of antiangiogenic potential of twenty two marine invertebrate extracts of phylum Mollusca from South East Coast of India. Asian Pac J Trop Biomed 2014;4(Suppl 1):S129-38.
30. Velpandian T, Gupta P, Ravi AK, et al. Evaluation of pharmacological activities and assessment of intraocular penetration of an ayurvedic polyherbal eye drop (Itone™) in experimental models. BMC Complement Altern Med 2013 Jan 2;13:1.
31. Velpandian T1, Nirmal J, Gupta P, et al. Evaluation of calcium dobesilate for its anti-cataract potential in experimental animal models. Methods Find Exp Clin Pharmacol 2010 Apr;32(3):171-9.
32. Lee EB, Ahn D, Kim BJ, et al. Genistein from Vigna angularis extends lifespan in Caenorhabditis elegans. Biomol Ther (Seoul). 2015 Jan;23(1):77-83.
33. Min H, Kawasaki I, Gong J, et al. Caffeine induces high expression of cyp-35A family genes and inhibits the early larval development in Caenorhabditis elegans. Mol Cells 2015 Jan 16.
34. Li AP. Screening for human ADME/Tox drug properties in drug discovery. Drug Discov Today 2001;6:357-66.
35. Kansy M, Avdeef A, Fischer H. Advances in screening for membrane permeability: high-resolution PAMPA for medicinal chemists. Drug Discov Today: Technologies 2004;1:349-55.
36. Hwang K, Martin NE, Jiang L. Permeation prediction of M100240 using the parallel artificial membrane permeability assay. J Pharm Pharmaceut Sci 2003;6:315-20.
37. Di L, Kerns EH, Fan K, McConnell OJ, Carter GT. High throughput artificial membrane permeability assay for blood-brain barrier. Eur J Med Chem 2003;38:223-32.
38. Ottaviani G, Martel S, Carrupt PA. In silico and in vitro filters for the fast estimation of skin permeation and distribution of new chemical entities. J Med Chem 2007;50:742-8.
39. Geysen HM, Meloen RH, Barteling SJ. Use of peptide synthesis to probe viral antigens for epitopes to a resolution of a single amino acid. Proc Natl Acad Sci USA 1984;81:3998-4002.
40. Crowley JI, Rapoport H. Solid phase organic synthesis: novelty or fundamental concept? Acc Chem Res 1976;9:135-44.

41. Larhed M, Hallberg A. Microwave-assisted high-speed chemistry: a new technique in drug discovery. DDT 2001;6:406-15.
42. Cragg GM, Newman DJ, Snader KM. Natural products in drug discovery and development. J Nat Prod 1997;60:52-60.
43. Bindseil KU, Jakupovic J, Wolf D, et al. Pure compound libraries: A new perspective for natural product based drug discovery. Drug Discov Today 2001;6:840-47.
44. Genilloud O, González I, Salazar O, et al. Current approaches to exploit actinomycetes as a source of novel natural products. J Ind Microbiol Biotechnol 2011;38(3):375-89.
45. Camp D, Davis RA, Evans-Illidge EA, et al. Guiding principles for natural product drug discovery. Future Med Chem 2012;4(9):1067-84.
46. Feher M, Schmidt JM. Property distributions: differences between drugs, natural products, and Molecules from combinatorial chemistry. J Chem Inf Comput Sci 2003;43:218-27.
47. Ortholand JY, Ganesan A. Natural products and combinatorial chemistry: back to the future. Curr Opin Chem Biol 2004;8:271-80.
48. Reverté L, Soliño L, Carnicer O, et al. Alternative methods for the detection of emerging marine toxins: biosensors, biochemical assays and cell-based assays. Mar Drugs 2014;12(12):5719-63.

CHAPTER

3

Models for Studying Stem Cell Therapy

STEM CELLS: AN INTRODUCTION

The science of stem cell therapy, evolved through an imperative phase of research and development, could possibly bring about unprecedented cures and palliative treatments. Successful culturing of human stem cells may further illustrate the feasibility and possibility offered by stem cell derived therapies. Although, the new drug development and advancements in the biomedical sciences has provided enormous benefits to the individuals as well as society, yet devastating illnesses such as heart diseases, diabetes, cancer, and neurological disorders such as Alzheimer's disease renders enduring challenges to the health and well-being of people world over. Such disorders have imposed a high economic and psychological burden virtually on every citizen directly or indirectly. The total costs of treating diabetes, for example is approaching $100 billion in the United States alone. The existing evidence from animal studies suggests that stem cells can be made to differentiate into cells of choice, and that these cells will act properly in their transplanted environment. The transplants of hematopoietic stem cells for the treatments of cancer, in human beings have been used for years now. *Ex-vivo* expansion and transplantation of limbal epithelial stem cells to the corneas to treat blinding ocular surface disease was one of the first stem cell therapies to be exploited clinically. It is only through controlled scientific research that the role of stem cell biology in benefiting various degenerative, metabolic, cardiovascular and cerebrovascular disorders can be evaluated in animal models as a proof-of-concept and that the true promise of stem cell therapy will become a boon for incurable diseases.

TYPES OF STEM CELLS

There are several types of stem cells viz:

- Embryonic stem cells
- Fetal neural stem/progenitor cells
- Adult neural stem/progenitor cells
- Mesenchymal stem cells
- Umbilical cord blood cells
- Adipose tissue.

Embryonic Stem Cells

Human embryonic stem cells (ESCs) are pluripotent or endlessly dividing cells that represent an inexhaustible source of precursor cells as they can differentiate into any cell type. The capacity of multipotency and self-renewal makes these cells a valuable experimental tool. The development of ESCs from the human blastocysts and their subsequent differentiation involves a complex interplay of several technical manipulations.[1-7] The human ES cell lines were derived from embryos produced by IVF for infertility treatment. Cryopreserved embryos were thawed, cultured to the blastocyst stage (5-6 days) and the pluripotent stem cells from the ICM were isolated. The stem cells were most commonly cultured on mouse embryonic fibroblast feeder cell layer to prevent differentiation and to promote the proliferation of the stem cells.[8] Several lineages have been developed using this technique, for example, endothelial and hematopoietic progenitor cells,[9] and neural stem cells.[10] Different strategies have also been adopted to eliminate the use of mouse feeders and maintain the human ESCs in an undifferentiated state.[11-18]

Since, the key factor responsible for the differentiation of ESCs is still unknown, several trial and error approach have been adopted to direct them to differentiate into a desired lineage as shown in Figure 3.1. There are evidences that most of the undifferentiated cells in the EBs express receptors for the growth factors.[19] Hence, supplementation of the human ES cell culture

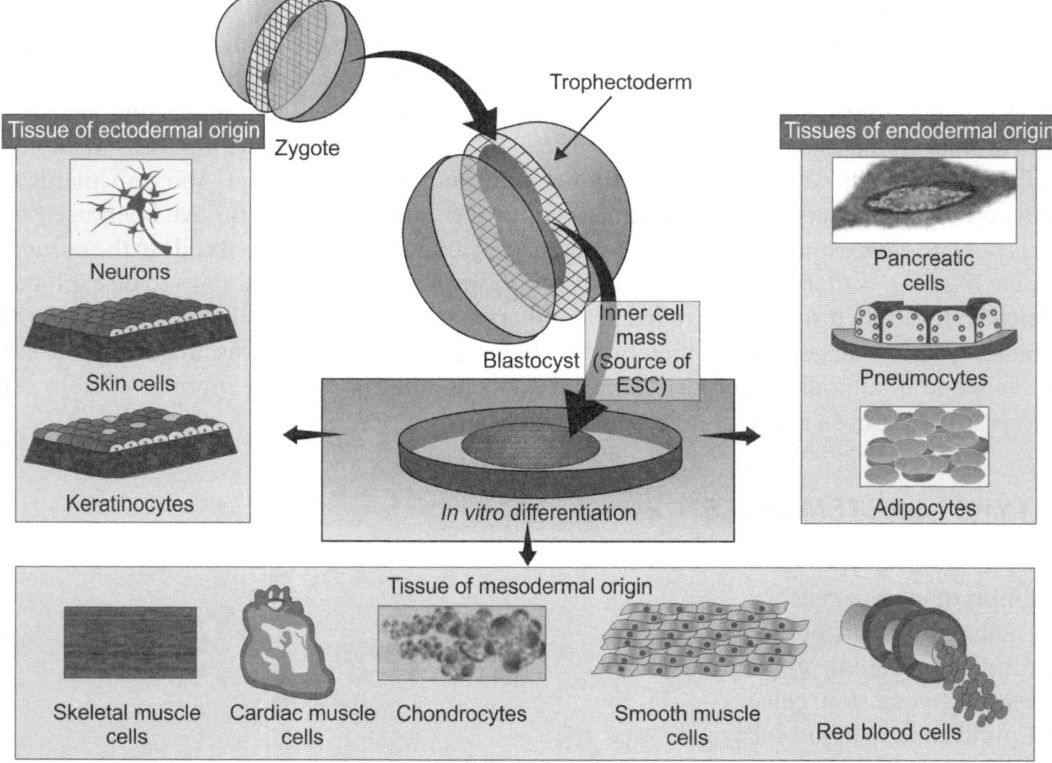

Figure 3.1: Tissues of endodermal, mesodermal and ectodermal origin derived from embryonic stem cells after *in vitro* differentiation (*For color version see Plate 2*)

with different growth factors altered the expression profile of an array of tissue-restricted gene. With this technique a variety of cell and tissue types have been derived from ESCs (Table 3.1).

Although, many studies using embryonic or fetal stem cells have shown cell maturation and successful engraftment, yet there are several difficulties in using human ESCs. The first one is the ethical issue surrounding the use of human ES cells.[50] Secondly, ES cells are allogenic, and immunosuppressive therapy might be needed. This problem could be alleviated by establishing ES cell banks containing the full range of major histocompatibility antigens.[51] However, this may be a futuristic approach since the establishment of human cell lines[52] has been more difficult than murine ones.[53] Thirdly, increased cell death due to ischemia has been observed, when ES cell-derived cardiomyocytes were grafted into a normal myocardium. Finally, human ESCs have also been shown to have the potential to form teratomas, when injected into an immunocompromised mouse.[52] These drawbacks have lead researchers to seek alternative undifferentiated cells for cell replacement therapy.

Fetal Neural Stem/Progenitor Cells

Neuronal progenitor cells (NPC) derived from ventral mesencephalon (VM) are particularly suited as the target population for genetic and cellular therapy of neurological disorders. Recently, continuously dividing immortalized cell lines of neural stem cells (NSCs) have been generated by introduction of oncogenes and these immortalized NSC lines have advantageous characteristics for basic studies on neural development and cell replacement therapy or gene

Table 3.1: Differentiated cell types from mouse and human ESCs *in vitro*

S. No.	*Mouse*	*Human*
1.	Adipocytes[20]	Hematopoietic colony-forming cells[43]
2.	Astrocytes[21]	Dopaminergic neurons[44]
3.	Cardiomyocytes[22]	Myocytes[45]
4.	Chondrocyte[23]	Pancreatic cells[46]
5.	Primitive and Definitive hematopoietic cells[24]	Different cells of spinal cord[47]
6.	Dendritic cells[25]	Cardiomyocytes[48]
7.	Endothelial cells[26]	Endothelial cells[49]
8.	Keratinocytes[27]	
9.	Lymphoid precursor cells[28]	
10.	Mast cells[29]	
11.	Neurons[30, 31]	
12.	Oligodendrocytes[32, 33]	
13.	Osteoblasts[34]	
14.	Insulin secreting cells[35, 36]	
15.	Smooth muscle cells[37]	
16.	Skeletal muscle cells[38]	
17.	Melanocytes[39]	
18.	Hepatocytes[40, 41]	
19.	Pneumocytes[42]	

therapy studies because: (a) NSC cell line can be expanded to large numbers in culture in short time (24–36 h doubling time); (b) NSC cells are homogeneous, since they were generated from a single clone; (c) stable expression of therapeutic genes can be achieved readily.[54-57] Immortalized NSCs were shown to have genetically manipulated *in vitro*, survive, integrate into host tissues and differentiate into both neurons and glial cells after transplantation to the intact or damaged brain.[58,59] More recently, new lines of immortalized human NSCs, were developed with the ability to self-renew, differentiate into cells of neuronal and glial lineages both *in vivo*[60] and *in vitro*.[61] Following transplantation into the brain of animal models of focal ischemia,[62, 63] intracerebral hemorrhage,[64] Huntington disease[65,66] and Parkinson's disease.[67] HB1.F3 human NSCs successfully integrated into host brain parenchyma and provided functional recovery in these experimental animals.

Adult Neural Stem/Progenitor Cells

Recent, studies have confirmed that the adult mammalian brain, including that of primates and humans, harbors stem cell populations. Adult NPC in the nigrostriatal dopaminergic system have the ability to respond to the lesion or when exposed to appropriate environmental signals to repopulate missing cells in neurodegenerative disorders such as Parkinson's disease.[68-71] Manipulations of NPCs in culture can be made for therapeutic transplantation or for mobilizing endogenous precursors to repair diseased or injured brain.[72,73]

Mesenchymal Stem Cells

Mesenchymal stem cells (MSCs), also referred to as marrow stromal cells, can be isolated from several tissues but easily accessible bone marrow (BM) seems to be the most common source. These cells isolated from BM can be induced *in vitro* and *in vivo* to differentiate into neuronal cell population.[74] The multilineage potential of MSCs,[75,76] their ability to elude detection by the host's immune system as expression of costimulatory molecules like B7-1 (CD80), B7-2 (CD86) and CD40 are lacking in them, which are necessary for instigation of T-cell proliferation.[77-79] Recently, it was shown that human MSCs isolated by their adherence to plastic were transplanted[80,81] or infused[82-86] into the corpus striatum and successful engraftment was achieved.

Umbilical Cord Blood Stem Cells (UCBSC)

The multipotent-stem-cell-rich blood found in the umbilical cord has proven useful, as they are less prone to rejection than either BM or peripheral blood stem cells. This is probably because the cells have not yet developed the features that can be recognized and attacked by the recipient's immune system. Also, because umbilical cord blood lacks well-developed immune cells, there is less chance that the transplanted cells will show immune reaction with the recipient's body. Both the versatility and availability of umbilical cord blood stem cells makes them a promising source for transplant therapies.

Adipose Tissue

Primary cultures of adipose tissue are a heterogeneous collection of hematopoietic cells, pericytes, endothelial cells, and smooth muscle cells. Several passages in cultures yields stromal cells that exhibit cell-surface markers consistent with mesenchymal stem cells.[87,88]

STEM CELL THERAPY FOR NEUROLOGICAL DISORDERS

Chronic degenerative diseases and traumatic injuries are responsible for a decline in neuronal function and transplantation of stem cells or their derivatives, and mobilization of endogenous stem cells within the adult brain has been proposed as future therapies for such neural disorders (Table 3.2), and many kinds of cells including ESCs and NSC have been considered as candidates for transplantation therapy (Fig. 3.2).

Parkinson's Disease

Parkinson's disease (PD) is caused by the degeneration of dopaminergic bundle originating from SN pars compacta (SNpc) leading to diminished tone exerted by dopamine which elicits the characteristic parkinsonian movement disorder. Currently, the stem cells from various sources are induced to acquire a mesodiencephalic dopaminergic (mdDA) phenotype.

The protocols summarized in Figure 3.3 briefly describe the methods for *in vitro* expansion, manipulation of genetic as well as culture conditions of stem cells. Out of the various PD models, 6-OHDA and MPTP induced PD has been widely used to assess the therapeutic potential of stem cells.

In Vivo Models

a. **6-OHDA Model:** The 6-OHDA is the first chemical agent discovered that has specific neurotoxic effects on catecholaminergic pathways.[139] To specifically target the nigrostriatal DA pathway, 6-OHDA must be injected steriotactically into the SN, the nigrostriatal tract or the striatum.[140] Following injections, DA neurons start degenerating within 24 h after, and striatal dopamine is depleted 2 to 3 days later. [141]

   There is ample evidence for the involvement of oxidative stress in 6-OHDA-induced neurotoxic effects.[142-147] The 6-OHDA lesion model has been used to ascertain the efficacy of antiparkinsonian compounds.[148] Additionally, this experimental model has been useful for evaluating the efficacy of cell transplantation, and for testing neurotrophic factors, compounds that promote survival of the degenerated dopaminergic nigral neurons in PD.[149]

b. **The MPTP Model:** Inadvertent injection of MPTP resulted in clinical symptoms remarkably similar to sporadic PD in humans[150] by selectively affecting DA neurons.[151] The mechanism of action of MPTP suggests a role of mitochondrial dysfunction in typical PD.[152,153] MPTP administration is one of the most common animal models used to study PD and various doses and regimens of MPTP administration are used by different laboratories.[154-156]

Gene-knockout and Transgenic Animals

Recent transgenic strategies have generated several mouse lines with mutations in the DA system.[157,160] D2-receptor-deficient mice,[161] in contrast to D1[162] and D3[163] receptors exhibit PD-like symptoms without neuronal death and Lewy bodies' formation. Mutations in the gene encoding a-synuclein, found in Lewy bodies, are related to PD in some species.[164,165] However, transgenic mice overexpressing either wild-type or mutant asynuclein have generated inconsistent results.[166,167]

Table 3.2: Use of different stem cells in various animal models of neurological disorders

Types of stem cells	*Cerebral stroke*		*Alzheimer's disease*		*Parkinson's*		*Huntington's*		*Amyotrophic lateral*	
	Models	*Species*	*Models*	*Species*	*Models*	*Species*	*Models*	*Species*	*Models*	*Species*
Embryonic stem cells	MCAO	R[89,90]	Nucleus basalis of Meynert (NBM) lesion	M[103]	6-OHDA Model	R[106]	Quinolinic acid induced lesion in striatum	R[116]	Transgenic animals	M[129]
Embryonic carcinoma cells					6-OHDA Model	R[107]			Transgenic animals	R[130]
Adult neural stem/ Progenitor cells	MCAO	SprhR[91], R[92, 93]	Transgenic animals	M[104]	6-OHDA Model	R[108-110]	Quinolinic acid induced -lesion in striatum, Transgenic animals	M[117-119] R[120-123]	Transgenic animals	R[131]
Fetal neural stem/ Progenitor cells	MCAO	M[94, 95,] CM[96], R[97], MG[98]	Nucleus basalis of Meynert (NBM) lesion	M[105]	6-OHDA Model	R[111-113]	Quinolinic acid induced -lesion in striatum	R[124-126, 66]	Transgenic animals	R[132-134]
Mesenchymal stem cells or Marrow stromal cells	MCAO	R[99]			6-OHDA Model, MPTP-Model	R80, 86, 114, M81, 115	Quinolinic acid induced -lesion in striatum	R[127], M[128]	Familial ALS model, Transgenic animals	M[135,] R[136]
Hematopoietic stem cells									Motoneuron degeneration model	M[137]
Umbilical cord	MCAO	R[100, 101]			6-OHDA Model				Transgenic animals	R[138]
Adipose tissue derived stem cells	MCAO	M[102]		6-OHDA Model						

MCAO-middle cerebral artery occlusion; R-rat; M-mouse; 6-OHDA-6-hydroxy dopamine; Sprh R-Spontaneously hypertensive rats; CM-cynomolgus monkeys; MG-Mongolian gerbils; MPTP-1-methyl-4-1, 2, 3, 6- tetrahydropyridine; ALS-amyotrophic lateral sclerosis

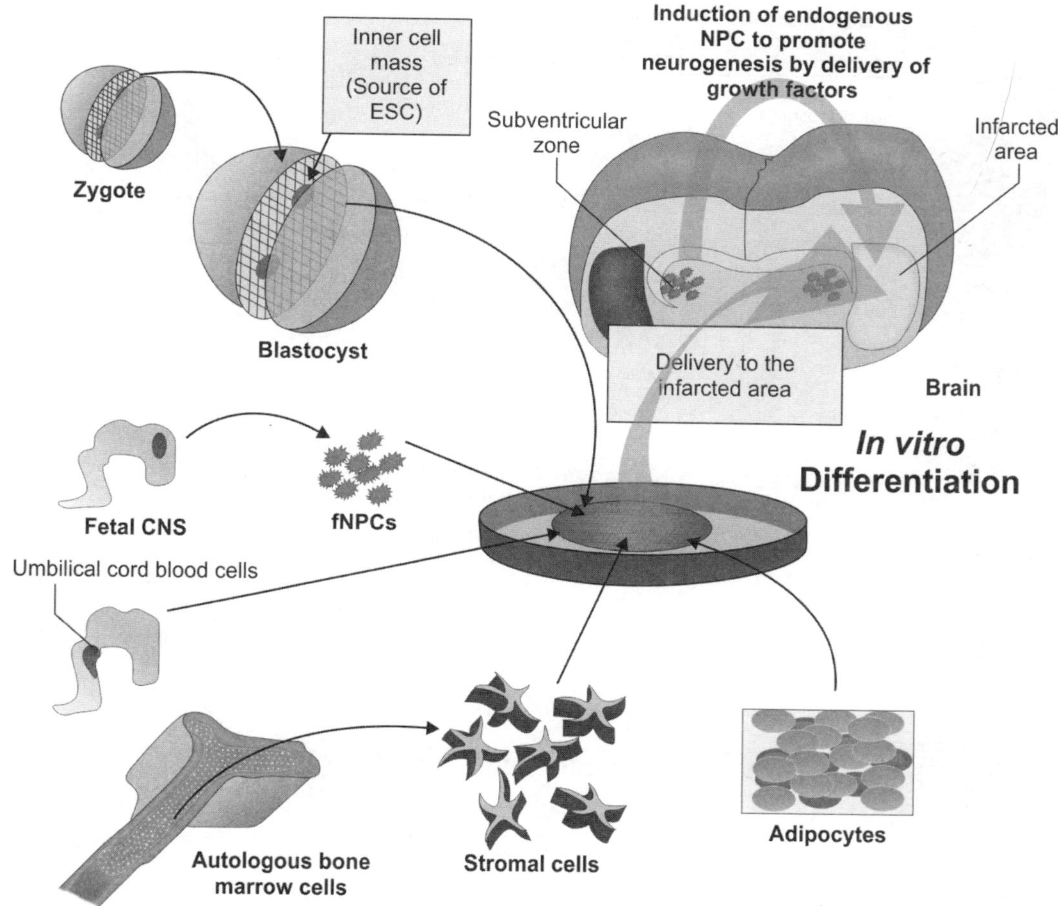

Figure 3.2: Different sources of stem cell employed for cell replacement therapy for the treatment of various neurological disorders (*For color version see Plate 3*)

In Vitro Models

Cultures of dissociated mesencephalic neurons from fetal rats[168] and human neuroblastoma SH-SY5Y cells[169] are suitable models of PD.

The restorative potential of successful transplantation of stem cells may be assessed by subjecting the animals to the battery of neurobehavioral tests such as amphetamine/apomorphine-induced rotation,[170] rotarod test,[171] cylinder test[172] and elevated body swing test.[173]

Alzheimer's Disease

Alzheimer's disease is a neurological disorder characterized by the presence of neurofibrillary tangles, neuritic plaques and dystrophic neurites in susceptible areas of the brain. The adult mammalian brain contains populations of stem cells that can proliferate and then differentiate. The highest concentration of such neural progenitor cells (NPC) is located in the SVZ and provide a cellular reservoir in the aged and AD brain, both the pool of NPC and

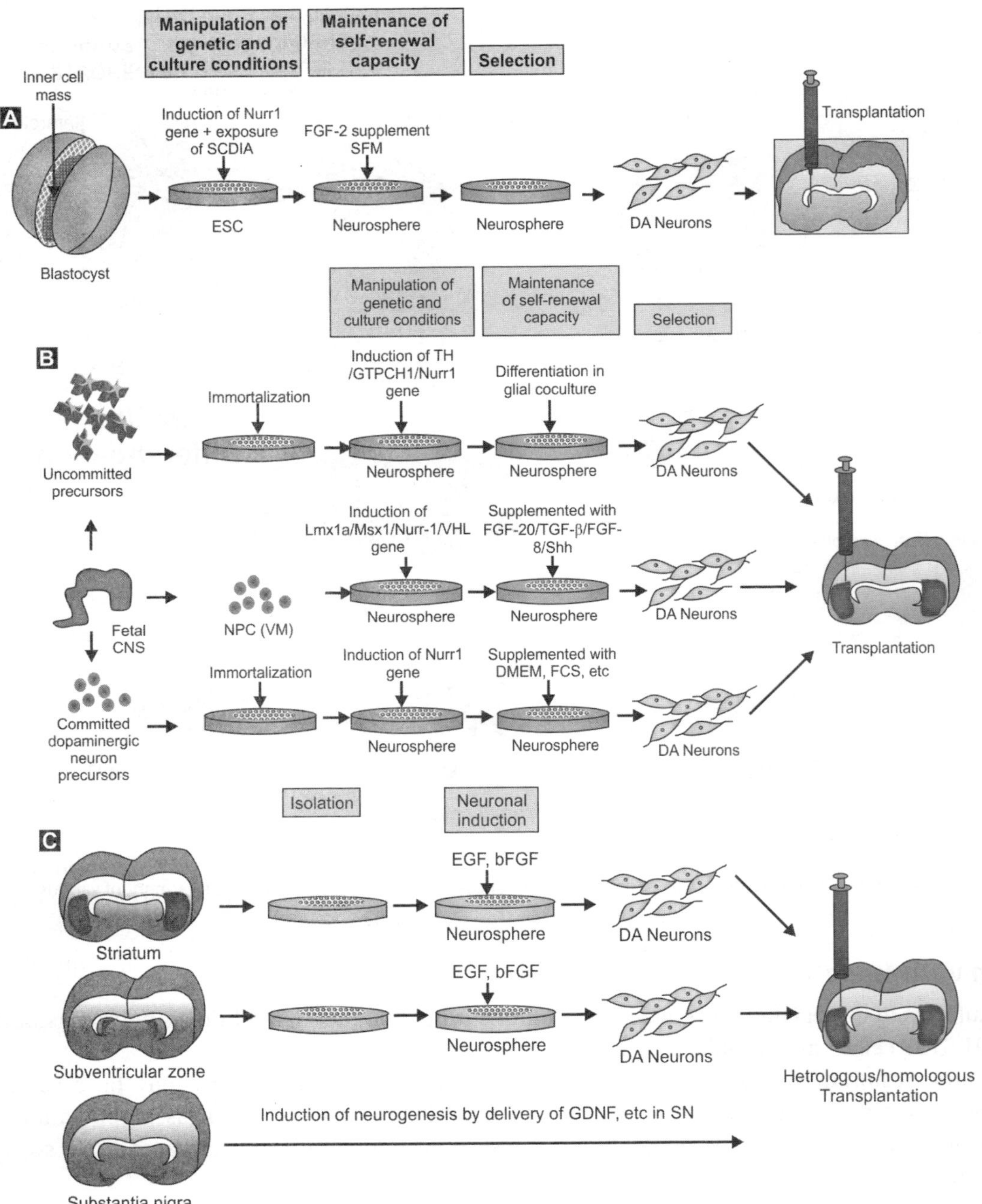

Figures 3.3A to C: Schematic representation of protocols for the generation of dopaminergic neurons for the treatment of parkinson's disease from different sources of stem cells viz Embryonic stem cells (A), Fetal neural progenitor cells (B), Adult neural progenitor cells (C) (*For color version see Plate 4*)

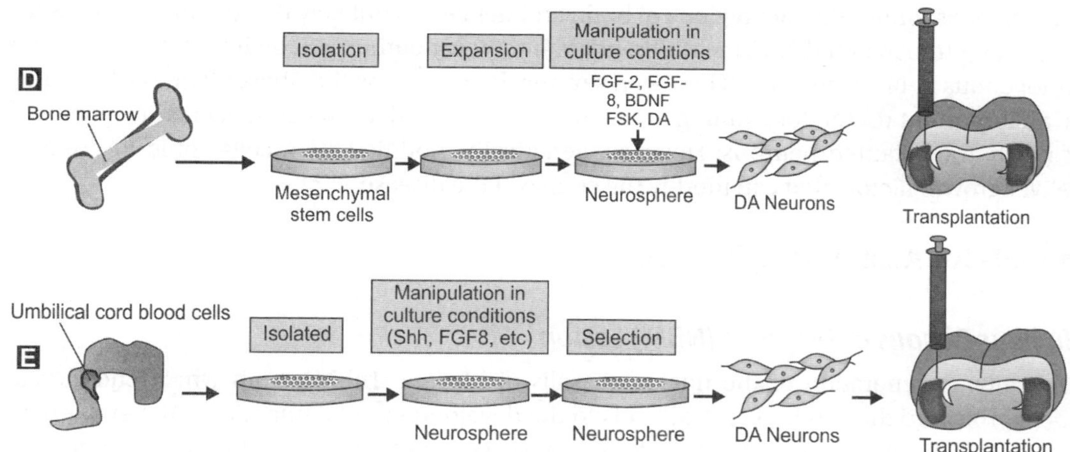

Figures 3.3D and E: Mesenchymal stem cells (D) and umbilical cord blood cells (E). (*For color version see Plate 5*)

Abbreviations: SCDIA-stromal cell-derived inducing activity; FGF-2-fibroblast growth factor-2; SFM-serumfree medium; DA-dopaminergic; TH-tyrosine hydroxylase; GTPCH-1-guanidine triphosphate cyclohydrolase- 1; NPC-neural progenitor cells; VM-ventromedial; DMEM-Dulbecco's Modified Eagles' Medium; FCS-fetal calf serum; EGF-epidermal growth factor; bFGF-basic fibroblast growth factor; TGF-tissue growth factor

their proliferative potential is markedly diminished. It was reported that Abeta itself can impair neurogenesis in the SVZ/cerebral cortex of adult mice and in human cortical NPC in culture. The proliferation and migration of NPC in the SVZ of APP mutant mice, and in mice receiving an intraventricular infusion of Abeta, were greatly decreased compared to control mice. Studies of NPC neurosphere cultures derived from human embryonic cerebral cortex showed that Abeta can suppress NPC proliferation and differentiation, and can induce apoptosis. The adverse effects of Abeta on neurogenesis were associated with a disruption of calcium regulation[174] and high oxidative stress.[175] It has been recently discovered that Seladin-1 (**sel**ective **A**lzheimer's **d**isease **i**ndicator-1) abundantly expressed by stem cells is an antiapoptotic gene, which is down-regulated in brain regions affected by Alzheimer's disease (AD).[176,177] However, recently it has been shown that alpha-secretase-cleaved fragment of the amyloid precursor protein (sAPPalpha), a potent neurotrophic factor, potentiates the NGF/retinoic acid (RA) induced transdifferentiation of bone marrow-derived adult progenitor cells (MAPCs) into neural progenitor cells and, more specifically, enhances their terminal differentiation into a cholinergic-like neuronal phenotype.[178] Further, a neurosteroid alloprognanolone (APalpha) was discovered, which showed potential to promote neurogenesis in the aged brain and restore neuronal populations in brains recovering from neurodegenerative disease or injury.[179,180]

Mammalian presenilins (PS) consist of two highly homologous proteins, PS1 and PS2. Because of their indispensable activity in the gamma-secretase cleavage of APP to generate Abeta peptides, inhibition of PS gamma-secretase activity is considered a potential therapy for Abeta blockage and AD intervention. In addition to its well-established role in gamma-secretase cleavage, presenilin (PS) also plays a role in regulating the stability of cytosolic beta-catenin, a protein involved in Wnt signaling in familial Alzheimer's disease, mutation in the presenilin-1 (PS1) or APP gene and abnormally elevated levels of FGF-2[181] is responsible for the development of early-onset of vascular pathology[182] and altered neurogenesis in the adult hippocampus.[183,184]

As mentioned above, the pathological changes seen in AD display an extremely problematic situation for cell replacement. The widespread damage found in the AD brain usually incorporates distinct regions of brain and hence it is unlikely that the mechanisms for instructing transplanted NSCs to differentiate into new neurons will be intact. Moreover, the endogenous neurogenesis itself has been severely hampered by the Abeta plaques which may be an important reason for running out of the nitch required for the growth and development of newly transplanted neurons. However, genetically modified stem cells could be used to deliver growth factors that can modify the course of the disease.

Models for Alzheimer's Disease

Nucleus Basalis of Meynert (NBM) Lesion

Clinically, degeneration of the nucleus basalis of Meynert (nbM), from which cholinergic fibers project to the cerebral cortex, leads to the development of dementia of Alzheimer type (DAT).[185-191] To obtain more selective lesion in the substantia innominata (SI), ibotenic acid injection rather than kainic acid injection or electrocoagulation techniques[192,193] are employed.

Transgenic Animals

Overexpression of the gene encoding the beta-amyloid precursor protein (APP) may have a key role in the pathogenesis of both Alzheimer's disease (AD). Because it has been difficult to overexpress APP by using conventional transgenic technologies, Lamb et al[194] have recently used yeast artificial chromosome(s)/ESC (YAC-ES) technologies to create a dosage imbalance and overexpression of APP in mice.

A 650 kb YAC that contained the entire unrearranged 400 kb APP gene was transferred into ES cells by lipid mediated transfection; ES cells that expressed human APP were introduced into mouse blastocytes to generate a number of chimeric mice. Subsequent breeding efforts resulted in mice that harbor human sequences in the germ line.

Huntington's Disease

Huntington's disease (HD) is an autosomal dominant genetic disease, which results in progressive neuronal degeneration in the neostriatum and neocortex, and the mechanism by which this leads to neuronal cell death is still a mystry. Huntingtin (Htt) gene plays a fundamental role in embryogenesis,[195] growth and development and, is essential for the normal nuclear (nucleoli, transcription factor-speckles) and perinuclear membrane (mitochondria, endoplasmic reticulum, Golgi and recycling endosomes) organelles and for proper regulation of the iron pathway.[196] One proposed mechanism by which mutant htt causes dysfunction of striatal enkephalinergic neurons is the downregulation of BDNF.[197] NSC may become the tissue/cell source necessary for developing the therapeutic potential of neural transplantation (Fig. 3.4).

Models for Huntington's Disease

1. **Quinolinic Acid Induced Lesion in Striatum**
   The leading animal models of HD have involved injection of neurotoxins into the striatum of rats, which causes local destruction of this area of the brain. Neurotoxins such as kainic

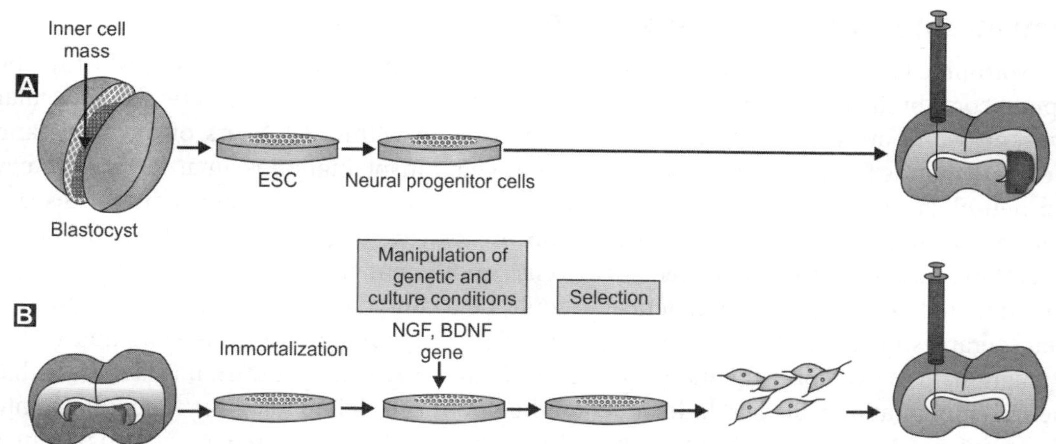

Figures 3.4A and B: Schematic representation showing use of ESC (A) and adult neural stem cells (B) for the generation of neural progenitors cells for the treatment of Huntington's disease (*For color version see Plate 5*)
Abbreviations: ESC-embryonic stem cells; NGF-nerve growth factor; BDNF-brain derived neurotrophic factors

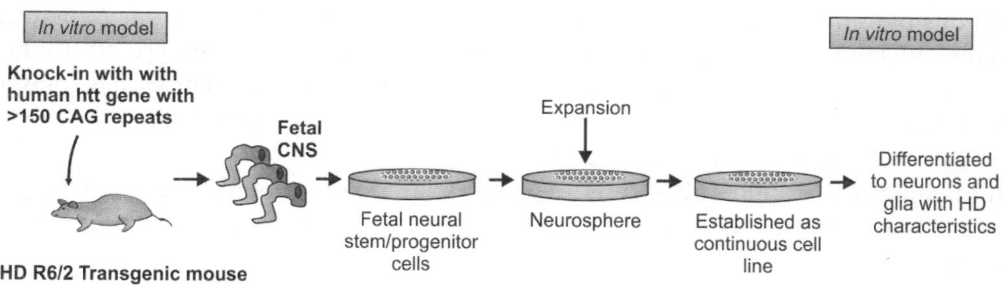

Figure 3.5: Schematic representation showing *in vivo* transgenic mice model carrying a mutated human gene for huntingtin (htt) and a protocol for producing neuronal and glial population with HD phenotype for *in vitro* screening of drugs and stem cell therapy for Huntington's disease (*For color version see Plate 5*)

acid[198] and ibotenic acid,[199] lead to excitotoxic death. In 1983, Schwarcz group found that injection of quinolinic acid (QA) into the striatum of rats produced a similar excitotoxic effect.[200-206]

2. **Transgenic Models**

The transgenic mouse model R6/2 expresses exon 1 of the human huntingtin gene with >150 CAG repeats, which produces mutant HD protein with an expanded poly-glutamine tract. For *in vitro* models, neuronal stem cell system deriving from transgenic HD R6/2 neonatal brains can be used as a renewable source for neurons and glia to facilitate studies of HD neuropathology and therapies. These R6/2 stem cell cultures can be cryopreserved and revived. Thawed neural progenitors can be expanded, established as continuous cell lines, and induced to differentiate into glia and neurons[207, 208] (Fig. 3.5). The restorative potential of successful transplantation of stem cells may be assessed by subjecting the animals to the battery of neurobehavioral tests such as amphetamine/apomorphine-induced rotation,[170] water-maze test,[209] beam-walk test,[210] staircase (skilled-limb use) test.[211]

Amyotrophic Lateral Sclerosis (Lou Gehrig's Disease)

Amyotrophic lateral sclerosis (ALS) is a fatal degenerative motor neuron disease affecting the spinal cord, brainstem, and cortex. This disease clinically manifests as progressive muscular weakness and atrophy, leading to paralysis and death within 3–5 years of diagnosis and hence demands for an effective treatment. Stem-cell transplantation is an attractive strategy for neurological diseases and early successes in animal models of neurodegenerative disease generated optimism about restoring function or delaying degeneration in human beings. Therefore, autologous or allogeneic stem cells, undifferentiated or transdifferentiated and manipulated epigenetically or genetically, could be a candidate source for local or systemic cell therapies in ALS (Fig. 3.6). The attraction of cell implantation or transplantation is that it might help to overcome the inability of the CNS to replace lost neurons. It is also clear that neural implantation will yield little benefit if the donor cells fail to integrate functionally into the recipient CNS circuitry. The recent breakthroughs in stem cell research provide possibilities for neural implantation and cell replacement therapy for patients with ALS.

Models for Amyotrophic Lateral Sclerosis

1. Transgenic Model

Mutations of human Cu, Zn superoxide dismutase (SOD) are found in about 20 percent of patients with familial ALS. Expression of high levels of human SOD containing a substitution of glycine to alanine at position 93 in chromosome 4, causes motor neuron disease in transgenic mice. The mice became paralyzed in one or more limbs as a result of motor neuron loss from the spinal cord and died at 5 to 6 months of age.

The familial mouse model of ALS was prepared as described in Figure 3.7, and the completed construct was then excised with Sal I and electroeluted from agarose for microinjection[212-214] into zygotes.

There are evidences of widespread regenerative response in the spinal cord of amyotrophic lateral sclerosis transgenic (Tg) mice.[215-217] However, this regenerative response appears to be largely unproductive and it has been shown that proliferation and migration of neural precursor cells to the ventral horns is greatly activated in symptomatic Tg mice and is further enhanced by EGF and FGF2 treatment.[31] (Fig. 3.8)

2. *In Vitro* Model

In vitro model has been developed for studying the molecular and cellular mechanisms that underlie the neurodegenerative disease ALS[213] (Fig. 3.9). ESCs derived from mice carrying normal or mutant transgenic alleles of the human SOD1 gene were used to generate motor neurons by *in vitro* differentiation. These motor neurons could be maintained in long-term coculture either with additional cells that arose during differentiation or with primary glial cells. Motor neurons carrying either the nonpathological human SOD1 transgene or the mutant SOD1(G93A) allele showed neurodegenerative properties when cocultured with SOD1(G93A) glial cells. The glial cells carrying a human SOD1(G93A) mutation have a direct, non-cell autonomous effect on motor neuron survival. More generally, ESC-based models of disease provide a powerful tool for studying the mechanisms of neural degeneration. These phenotypes displayed in culture could provide cell-based assays for the identification of new ALS drugs or alternative stem cell based therapy.

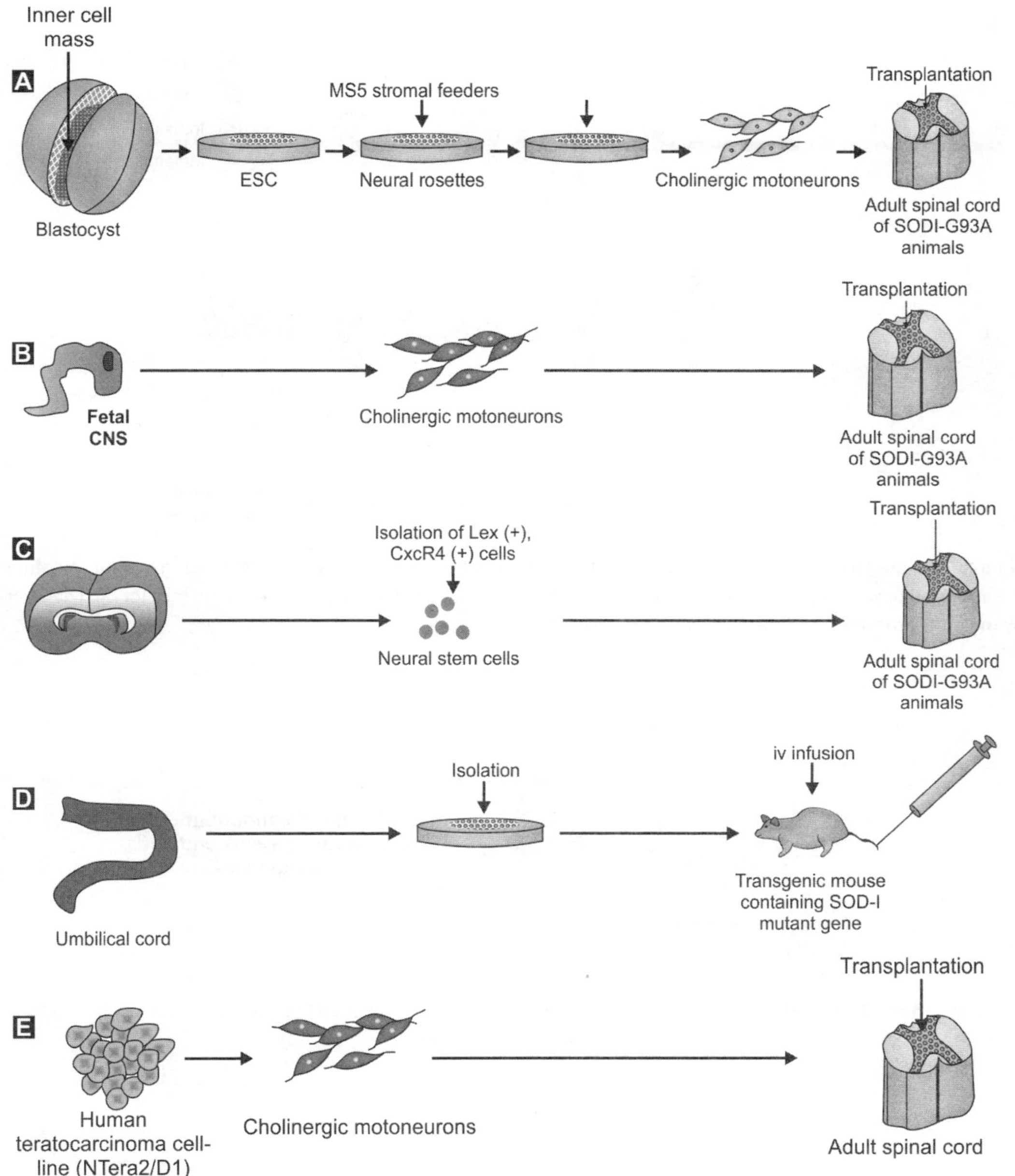

Figure 3.6: Generation of cholinergic motor neurons for ALS (*For color version see Plate 6*)

Abbreviation: SOD1-superoxide dismutase-1

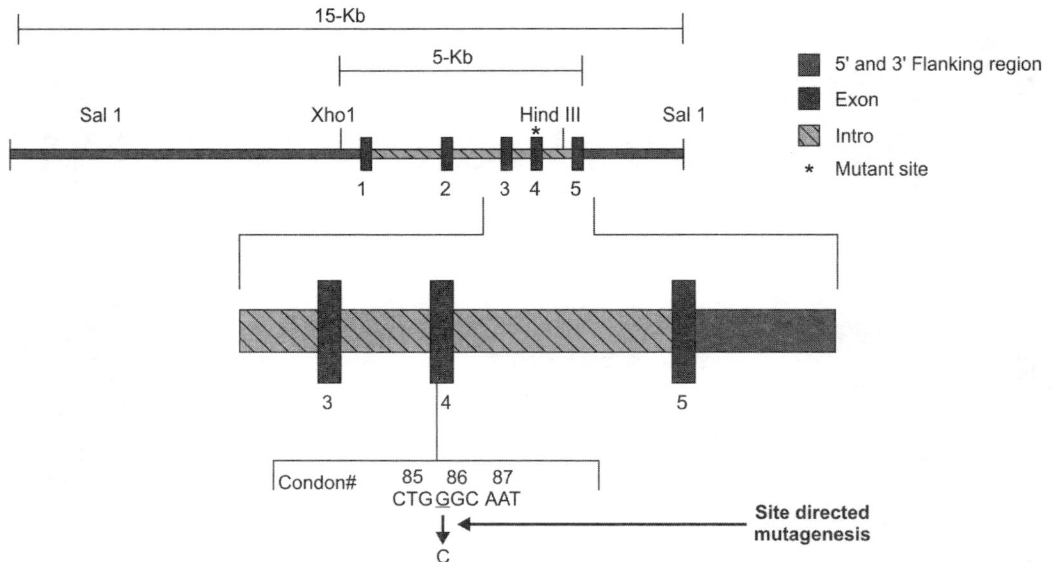

Figure 3.7: Mutagenesis of the mouse SOD-1 gene. The transgene was constructed by introducing a point mutation at the indicated position (*) in exon 4. Nucleotides shown in boldface type form a recognition sequence for Fsp I generated by the mutagenesis procedure (*For color version see Plate 7*)

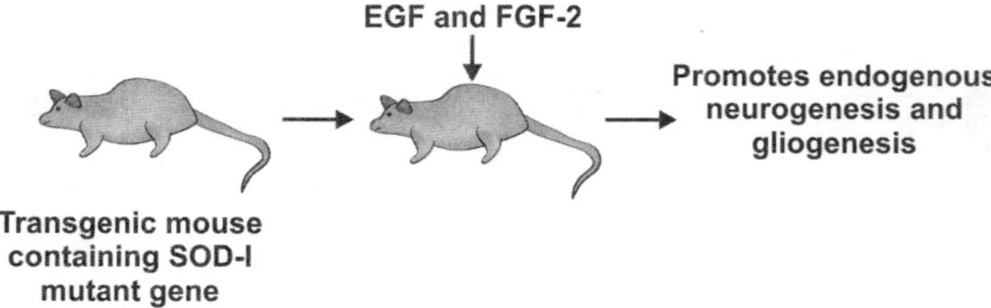

Figure 3.8: Administration of growth factors promotes endogenous regenerative process in ALS mouse model (*For color version see Plate 7*)

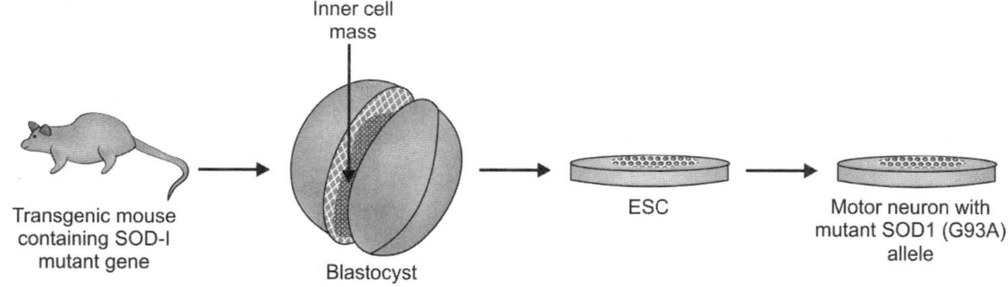

Figure 3.9: *In vitro* model system for studying the mechanisms of neural degeneration and identification of new ALS drugs or alternative stem cell based therapy (*For color version see Plate 7*)

STEM CELL THERAPY FOR CARDIO- AND CEREBROVASCULAR DISORDERS

Congestive heart failure (CHF) due to myocardial infarction (MI, or heart attack) often has scar tissue in the heart, which limits the heart's ability to pump blood which may be characterized by dyspnea, edema and disability. In MI, the infarcted tissue does not contribute to the generation of mechanical activity and the compensatory forced contractile movements uncouples the excitation contractile function of surrounding viable myocardium through a series of events known as left ventricular remodeling. Treating physicians may now have the opportunity to successfully replace scarred heart tissue with healthy muscle via intracardiac injections of stem cells taken from the patient's own body. By using a catheter and transplanting the stem cells into scarred tissue, myocardium can be regenerated with limited risk to the patient. Since, the transplanted stem cells are harvested from the patient's own body, the cells are compatible with the body, avoiding possible immune system and tissue compatibility complications.

Myocardial Infarction

There is growing evidence, which suggests that the heart has the ability to regenerate through the activation of resident cardiac stem cells or through the recruitment of stem cell population from other tissues such as bone marrow. Hence, stem cell therapy appears as a promising new approach for myocardial repair.

Experimental models were extensively used to study the stem cell potential in regenerating cardiomyocytes.[218] Therapeutic intervention like supply of endothelial stem cell[219] or angiogenic factors like the cytokine vascular endothelial growth factor (VEGF) and the bFGF have also been successfully tested.[220] Lyseggen et al[221] used an open chest dog heart model to document echocardiographic indices of potential use during evaluation of reperfused myocardium. This model provides means to evaluate post-ischemic viability and therefore whether reperfusion was successful on the basis of echocardiography, sonomicrometry, intraventricular pressure measurements, tissue staining for necrosis and coronary perfusion measurements using radionucleotid microspheres for microvascular perfusion.

In Vivo Model

Coronary Artery Ligation in Mice

Ischemia is achieved by occluding LAD by using 8-0 silk suture, with a 1 mm section of polyethylene (PE)-10 tubing placed on top of the LAD, 1 to 3 mm from the tip of the normally positioned left atrium. After occlusion for a specified duration, reperfusion is allowed to occur by releasing the ligature and removing the PE-10 tubing. Blood flow is confirmed by visualization of the return of a bright red color in the previously pale region. Hearts are harvested after desired period of reperfusion.[222, 223]

In Vitro Models

a. *Isolated perfused heart*: Hearts are excised from heparinized mice and prepared according to the standard Lagendorrf preparation for retrograde perfusion.[224] The hearts are subjected to global ischemia by clamping the perfusion line. After ischemia of desired duration, the perfusion line is released, and hearts are reperfused. Cardiac contractile performance and coronary flow are recorded during stabilization, ischemia, and reperfusion.

b. *Cardiomyocytes*: Cardiomyocytes can be isolated acutely from hearts of all species and manipulated to simulate ischemia. By applying confocal laser scanning microscopy-based cell imaging technique to study isolated adult rat cardiomyocytes, mitochondrial function and integrity intact cells.[225]
c. *Cell culture techniques*: Neonatal mice heart cell cultures can be harvested from genetically engineered mice hearts; transfection techniques as well as silencing RNA technique can be used in cell cultures. HL-1 cells are immortalized cells derived from an atrial tumor (myoma) in female mice.[226, 227] Compared to the use of primary isolation of ventricular myocytes, the advantages of having a good immortalized cell culture model for use in ischemia studies involve the following: (i) no animal use and care, (ii) no costly and lengthy preparation time before any experiments can take place, (iii) no variable and limited yield for high-throughput approaches and (iv) no problems with heterogeneous cell population. The HL-1 cells and the following generations of these cells have been used successfully for ischemia related experiments; overall results correlate well with results obtained, for example, isolated hearts.[228-231]

In Silico Models

There is limited tradition for *in silico* models in ischemic heart research. One exception is the electrophysiological modeling of the consequences of changes in ion balance with ischemia. Important input in these models includes potassium loss to the extracellular space, intracellular proton accumulation and opening of ATP dependent potassium channels, cellular electrical uncoupling and delayed conduction, diastolic calcium overload and increase in cellular sodium.[232,233]

Cerebral Stroke

The major causes of stroke include ischemia and intracerebral hemorrhage (ICH) and it affects multiple different neuronal phenotypes like oligodendrocytes, astrocytes, and endothelial cells. Medical therapy against stroke remains limited, hence prompting an alternative approach.[234] No approach has been successful in replacing the lost neurons, improving the deteriorated functions, or reducing the long-term sequelae.[235] There have been previously several reports of cell transplantation in the brain of ischemic animal models. Stem cells from various sources such as ESCs, MSCs,[236] immortalized NPCs[237,238] and adult stem cells were grafted into the ischemic brain as shown in Figure 3.10, and reduced the neurological deficits induced by experimental brain ischemia. Specific types of cells with restricted fates may limit their use as potential sources for implantation in stroke. For maximal functional recovery, however, regenerative therapy may need multifaceted approaches, which may include cell replacement, trophic support, protection from oxidative stress, and the neutralization of the growth-inhibitory components for endogenous neuronal stem cells.

Models for Cerebral stroke

To instigate better understanding of the underlying pathology, and neurological and behavioral consequences of cerebral ischemia, it is mandatory that physiologically controlled and highly reproducible *in vivo* models be developed.[239-257]

Several methods have been adopted to achieve clinical manifestations as close as possible, as shown in Table 3.3.

Table 3.3: Some common models of cerebral ischemia

Types of model	*Representative models*	*Notes*
Focal ischemia	Middle cerebral artery occlusion	Several species used:
	• Transient	• Uses clips, intraluminal thread and snare
	• Permanent	• Uses intraluminal thread, clips and coagulation
	• Thrombotic	• Injection of either microspheres or clots into cerebral vessels including MCA
Global ischemia	Bilateral carotid occlusion	• Primarily in gerbils
	Two vessel plus hypotension	• Normally in rats
	Four vessel occlusion	• Normally in rats
Hemorrhagic	Infusion of collagenase into brain	

CONCLUSION AND FUTURE PERSPECTIVES

The hope of stem cell-based therapy against irreversible cellular damage in organs with limited regenerative capacity has opened up new vistas for the treatment of several debilitating disorders. However, American Association of Advancement of Science (AAAS) and the Institute of Civil Society (ICS) have recognized that varied ethical, religious, legal and social view points are to be considered before carrying out research on tissues derived from embryonic and fetal stem cells. Although, the concept of transdifferentiation and reprogramming had resolved several long-standing issues such as teratoma formation, immune rejection, etc. yet successful functional and anatomical integration of transplanted cells with the host environment needs several technical manipulation. These include isolation of desired stem cells from a mixed population and alteration in growth medium during *in vitro* differentiation in order to obtain a repertoire of specific types of cells for replacement. Moreover, transfer of new genetic material to stem cells and expression of the gene product in daughter cells is an exiting approach to make cells compatible for the host environment. Recently, researchers have explored self-repair mechanism in organs earlier thought of as post-mitotic one, by identifying resident stem cells which could also be induced to migrate to the damaged site for repair. However, there is still a long way to go before exploiting them clinically since many basic issues remain to be resolved, and we need to move forward with caution while undertaking clinical trials. Hence, overall stem cell-based therapy is a promising, yet to improve, strategy for the treatment of several degenerative disorders.

To aid in further progress toward the clinics, animal models that closely mimic the human disease have been used. Such models will allow us to assess and balance potential risks and benefits of stem cell therapies before their application in humans. Moreover, transgenic animals expressing wild-type or mutated genes which may be responsible for any disease phenotype are currently being used which provide an important opportunity to study the involvement of specific gene/s in particular disorder and derive a relation between genetic mutations and environmental exposures. Moreover, current *in vivo* test methods are laborious, costly and

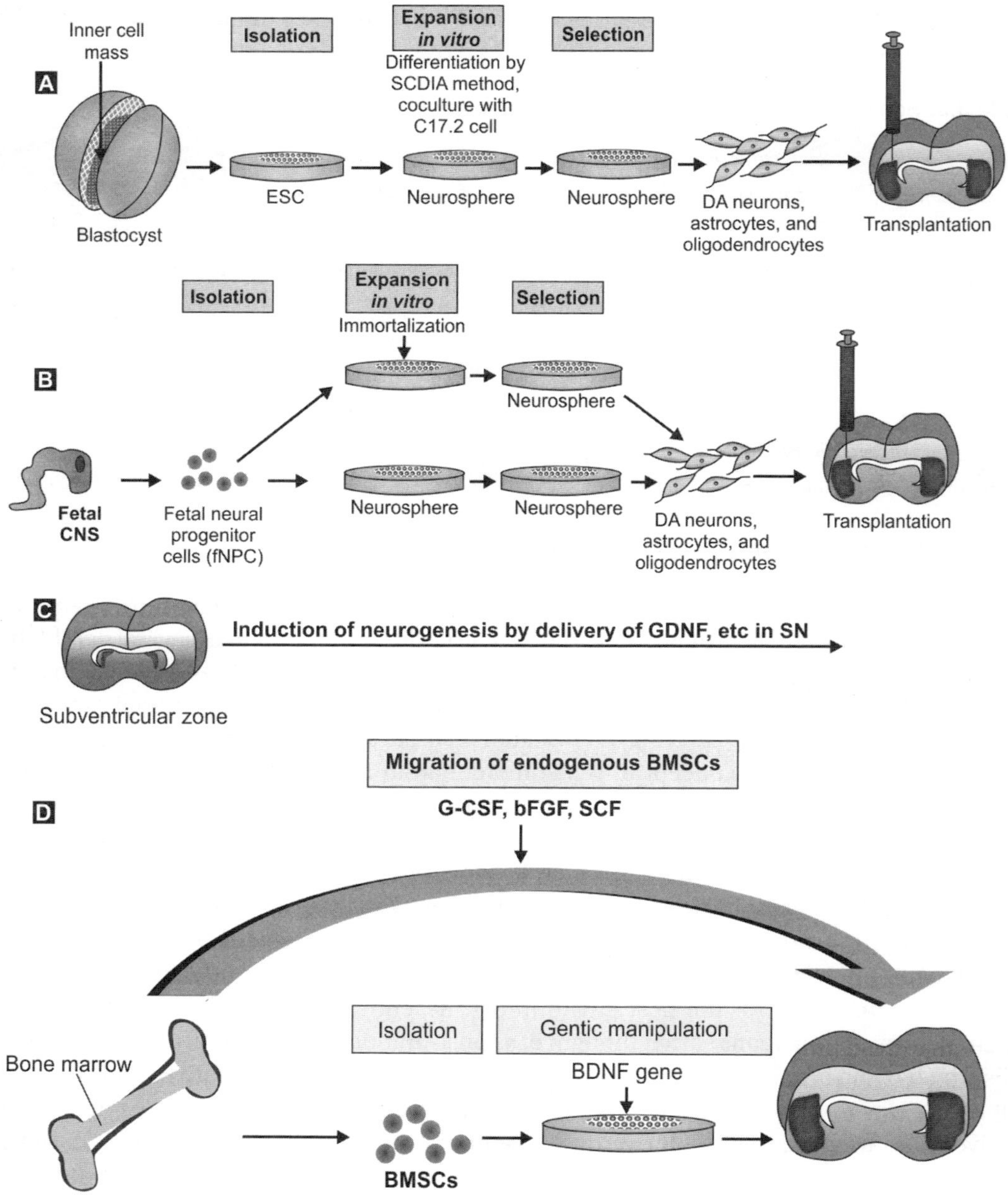

Figure 3.10: Protocols for generation neural and glial population for the treatment of cerebral stroke from different sources of stem cells viz ESCs (A), Fetal neural progenitor cells (B), Adult neural progenitor cells (C), Mesenchymal stem cells (D) (*For color version see Plate 8*)

Abbreviations: BMSCs-bone marrow derived stem cells; BDNF-brain derived neurotrophic factors; G-CSF Granulocyte colony stimulating factor; bFGF-basic fibroblast growth factor; SCF-stem cell factor

require use of large numbers of laboratory animals which necessitates the use of *in vitro* model system. Likewise, we need to improve noninvasive *in vivo* imaging technologies so that we can track down the migration of stem cells to the damaged site and monitor regenerative processes subsequent to stem cell-based approaches in animals and humans.

REFERENCES

1. Reubinoff BE, Pera MF, Vajta G, et al. Effective cryopreservation of human embryonic stem cells by the open pulled straw vitrification method. Hum Reprod 2001;16:2187-94.
2. Gropp M, Itsykson P, Singer O, et al. Stable genetic modification of human embryonic stem cells by lentiviral vectors. Mol Ther 2003;7:281-7.
3. Doetschman TC, Eistetter H, Katz M, et al. The in vitro development of blastocyst-derived embryonic stem cell lines: formation of visceral yolk sac, blood islands and myocardium. J Embryol Exp Morphol 1985;87:27-45.
4. Wobus AM, Wallukat G, Hescheler J. Pluripotent mouse embryonic stem cells are able to differentiate into cardiomyocytes expressing chronotropic responses to adrenergic and cholinergic agents and Ca2+ channel blockers. Differentiation 1991;48:173-82.
5. Bishop AE, Buttery LD, Polak JM. Embryonic stem cells. J Pathol 2002;197:424-9.
6. Kawasaki H, Suemori H, Mizuseki K, et al. Generation of dopaminergic neurons and pigmented epithelia from primate ES cells by stromal cell-derived inducing activity. Proc Natl Acad Sci USA 2002;99:1580-5.
7. Itsykson P, Ilouz N, Turetsky T, et al. Derivation of neural precursors from human embryonic stem cells in the presence of noggin. Mol Cell Neurosci 2005;30:24-36.
8. Thomson JA, Marshall VS. Primate embryonic stem cells. Curr Top Dev Biol 1998;38:133-65.
9. Nishikawa SI, Nishikawa S, Hirashima M, et al. Progressive lineage analysis by cell sorting and culture identifies FLK1+VE-cadherin+ cells at a diverging point of endothelial and hemopoietic lineages. Development 1998;125:1747-57.
10. Tropepe V, Hitoshi S, Sirard C, et al. Direct neural fate specification from embryonic stem cells: a primitive mammalian neural stem cell stage acquired through a default mechanism. Neuron 2001;30:65-78.
11. Xu C, Inokuma MS, Denham J, et al. Feeder-free growth of undifferentiated human embryonic stem cells. Nat Biotechnol 2001;19:971-4.
12. Richards M, Fong CY, Chan WK, et al. Human feeders support prolonged undifferentiated growth of human inner cell masses and embryonic stem cells. Nat Biotechnol 2002;20:933-6.
13. Amit M, Margulets V, Segev H, et al. Human feeder layers for human embryonic stem cells. Biol Reprod 2003;68:2150-6.
14. Amit M, Shariki C, Margulets V, et al. Feeder layer- and serum-free culture of human embryonic stem cells. Biol Reprod 2004;70:837-45.
15. Sato N, Meijer L, Skaltsounis L, et al. Maintenance of pluripotency in human and mouse embryonic stem cells through activation of Wnt signaling by a pharmacological GSK-3-specific inhibitor. Nat Med 2004;10:55-63.
16. Genbacev O, Krtolica A, Zdravkovic T, et al. Serum-free derivation of human embryonic stem cell lines on human placental fibroblast feeders. Fertil Steril 2005;83:1517-29.

17. Xu C, Rosler E, Jiang J, et al. Basic fibroblast growth factor supports undifferentiated human embryonic stem cell growth without conditioned medium. Stem Cells 2005;23:315-23.
18. Ludwig TE, Bergendahl V, Levenstein ME, et al. Feeder-independent culture of human embryonic stem cells. Nat Methods 2006;3:637-46.
19. Schuldiner M, Yanuka O, Itskovitz-Eldor J, et al. Effects of eight growth factors on the differentiation of cells derived from human embryonic stem cells. Proc Natl Acad Sci USA 2000;97:11307-12.
20. Dani C, Smith AG, Dessolin S, et al. Differentiation of embryonic stem cells into adipocytes in vitro. J Cell Sci 1997;110:1279-85.
21. Fraichard A, Chassande O, Bilbaut G, et al. In vitro differentiation of embryonic stem cells into glial cells and functional neurons. J Cell Sci 1995;108:3181-8.
22. Maltsev VA, Rohwedel J, Hescheler J, et al. Embryonic stem cells differentiate in vitro into cardiomyocytes representing sinusnodal, atrial and ventricular cell types. Mech Dev 1993;44:41-50.
23. Kramer J, Klinger M, Kruse C, et al. Ultrastructural analysis of mouse embryonic stem cell-derived chondrocytes. Anat Embryol (Berl) 2005;210:175-85.
24. Wiles MV, Keller G. Multiple hematopoietic lineages develop from embryonic stem (ES) cells in culture. Development 1991;111:259-67.
25. Fairchild PJ, Brook FA, Gardner RL, et al. Directed differentiation of dendritic cells from mouse embryonic stem cells. Curr Biol 2000;10:1515-8.
26. Risau W, Sariola H, Zerwes HG, et al. Vasculogenesis and angiogenesis in embryonic-stem-cell-derived embryoid bodies. Development 1988;102:471-8.
27. Bagutti C, Wobus AM, Fassler R, et al. Differentiation of embryonal stem cells into keratinocytes: comparison of wild-type and beta 1 integrin-deficient cells. Dev Biol 1996;179:184-96.
28. Potocnik AJ, Nielsen PJ, Eichmann K. In vitro generation of lymphoid precursors from embryonic stem cells. EMBO J 1994;13:5274-83.
29. Tsai M, Wedemeyer J, Ganiatsas S, et al. In vivo immunological function of mast cells derived from embryonic stem cells: an approach for the rapid analysis of even embryonic lethal mutations in adult mice in vivo. Proc Natl Acad Sci USA 2000;97:9186-90.
30. Bain G, Kitchens D, Yao M, et al. Embryonic stem cells express neuronal properties in vitro. Dev Biol 1995;168:342-57.
31. Strubing C, Ahnert-Hilger G, Shan J, et al. Differentiation of pluripotent embryonic stem cells into the neuronal lineage in vitro gives rise to mature inhibitory and excitatory neurons. Mech Dev 1995;53:275-87.
32. Brustle O, Jones KN, Learish RD, et al. Embryonic stem cell-derived glial precursors: a source of myelinating transplants. Science 1999;285:754-6.
33. Liu S, Qu Y, Stewart TJ, et al. Embryonic stem cells differentiate into oligodendrocytes and myelinate in culture and after spinal cord transplantation. Proc Natl Acad Sci USA 2000;97:6126-31.
34. Buttery LD, Bourne S, Xynos JD, et al. Differentiation of osteoblasts and in vitro bone formation from murine embryonic stem cells. Tissue Eng 2001;7:89-99.
35. Lumelsky N, Blondel O, Laeng P, et al. Differentiation of embryonic stem cells to insulin-secreting structures similar to pancreatic islets. Science 2001;292:1389-94.
36. Soria B, Roche E, Berna G, et al. Insulin-secreting cells derived from embryonic stem cells normalize glycemia in streptozotocin-induced diabetic mice. Diabetes 2000;49:157-62.
37. Yamashita J, Itoh H, Hirashima M, et al. Flk1-positive cells derived from embryonic stem cells serves as vascular progenitors. Nature 2000;408:92-6.

38. Rohwedel J, Maltsev V, Bober E ,et al. Muscle cell differentiation of embryonic stem cells reflects myogenesis in vivo: developmentally regulated expression of myogenic determination genes and functional expression of ionic currents. Dev Biol 1994;164:87-101.
39. Yamane T, Hayashi S, Mizoguchi M, et al. Derivation of melanocytes from embryonic stem cells in culture. Dev Dyn 1999;216:450-8.
40. Hamazaki T, Iiboshi Y, Oka M, et al. Hepatic maturation in differentiating embryonic stem cells in vitro. FEBS Lett 2001;497:15-9.
41. Jones EA, Tosh D, Wilson DI, et al. Hepatic differentiation of murine embryonic stem cells. Exp Cell Res 2002;272:15-22.
42. Ali NN, Edgar AJ, Samadikuchaksaraei A, et al. Derivation of type II alveolar epithelial cells from murine embryonic stem cells. Tissue Eng 2002;8:541-50.
43. Kaufman DS, Hanson ET, Lewis RL, et al. Hematopoietic colony-forming cells derived from human embryonic stem cells. Proc Natl Acad Sci USA 2001;98:10716-21.
44. Savatier P, Lapillonne H, Van Grunsven, et al. Withdrawal of differentiation inhibitory activity/ leukemia inhibitory factor up-regulates D-type cyclins and cyclin-dependent kinase inhibitors in mouse embryonic stem cells. Oncogene 1996;12:309-22.
45. Menasché P. Stem cells: where we stand. Dialogues Cardiovasc Med 2003;8:123-33.
46. Assady S, Maor G, Amit M, et al. Insulin production by human embryonic stem cells. Diabetes 2001;50:1691-7.
47. McDonald JW, Liu XZ, Qu Y, et al. Transplanted embryonic stem cells survive, differentiate and promote recovery in injured rat spinal cord. Nat Med 1999;5:1410-12.
48. Odorico JS, Kaufman DS, Thomson JA. Multilineage differentiation from human embryonic stem cell lines. Stem Cells 2001;19:193-204.
49. Levenberg S, Golub JS, Amit M, et al. Endothelial cells derived from human embryonic stem cells. Proc Natl Acad Sci USA 2002;99:4391-6.
50. Weissman IL. Stem cells—scientific, medical, and political issues. N Engl J Med 2002;346:1576-9.
51. Gearhart J. New potential for human embryonic stem cells. Science 1998;282:1061-2.
52. Thomson JA, Itskovitz-Eldor J, Shapiro SS, et al. Embryonic stem cell lines derived from human blastocysts. Science 1998;282:1145-7.
53. Evans MJ, Kaufman MH. Establishment in culture of pluripotential cells from mouse embryos. Nature 1981;292:154-6.
54. Martinez-Serrano A, Bjorklund A. Immortalized neural progenitor cells for CNS gene transfer and repair. Trends Neurosci 1997;20:530-8.
55. Uchida N, Buck DW, He D, et al. Direct isolation of human central nervous system stem cells. Proc Natl Acad Sci USA 2000;97:14720-25.
56. Snyder EY, Deitcher DL, Walsh C, et al. Multipotent neural cell lines can engraft and participate in development of mouse cerebellum. Cell 1992;68:33-51.
57. Hoshimaru M, Ray J, Sah DW, et al. Differentiation of the immortalized adult neuronal progenitor cell line HC2S2 into neurons by regulatable suppression of the v-myc oncogene. Proc Natl Acad Sci USA 1996;93:1518-23.
58. Flax JD, Aurora S, Yang C, et al. Engraftable human neural stem cells respond to developmental cues, replace neurons, and express foreign genes. Nat Biotechnol 1998;16:1033-9.
59. Renfranz PJ, Cunningham MG, McKay RD. Region-specific differentiation of the hippocampal stem cell line HiB5 upon implantation into the developing mammalian brain. Cell 1991;66:713-29.

60. Cho T, Bae JH, Choi HB, et al. Human neural stem cells: electrophysiological properties of voltage-gated ion channels. Neuroreport 2002;13:1447-52.
61. Ryu JK, Choi HB, Hatori K, et al. Adenosine triphosphate induces proliferation of human neural stem cells: Role of calcium and p70 ribosomal protein S6 kinase. J Neurosci Res 2003;72:352-62.
62. Chu K, Kim M, Jeong SW et al. Human neural stem cells can migrate, differentiate, and integrate after intravenous transplantation in adult rats with transient forebrain ischemia. Neurosci Lett 2003;343:129-33.
63. Chu K, Kim M, Park KI, et al. Human neural stem cells improve sensorimotor deficits in the adult rat brain with experimental focal ischemia. Brain Res 2004;1016:145-53.
64. Jeong SW, Chu K, Jung KH, et al. Human neural stem cell transplantation promotes functional recovery in rats with experimental intracerebral hemorrhage. Stroke 2003;34:2258-63.
65. Ryu JK, Kim J, Cho SJ et al. Proactive transplantation of human neural stem cells prevents degeneration of striatal neurons in a rat model of Huntington disease. Neurobiol Dis 2004;16:68-77.
66. Lee ST, Chu K, Park JE, et al. Intravenous administration of human neural stem cells induces functional recovery in Huntington's disease rat model. Neurosci Res 2005;52:243-9.
67. Kim SU, Park IH, Kim TH, et al. Brain transplantation of human neural stem cells transduced with tyrosine hydroxylase and GTP cyclohydrolase 1 provides functional improvement in animal models of Parkinson disease. Neuropathology 2006;26:129-40.
68. Mao L, Wang JQ. Adult neural stem/progenitor cells in neurodegenerative repair. Sheng Li Xue Bao 2003;55:233-44.
69. Lie DC, Dziewczapolski G, Willhoite AR, et al. The adult substantia nigra contains progenitor cells with neurogenic potential. J Neurosci 2002;22:6639-49.
70. Ostenfeld T, Svendsen CN. Recent advances in stem cell neurobiology. Adv Tech Stand Neurosurg 2003;28:3-89.
71. Zhao M, Momma S, Delfani K, et al. Evidence for neurogenesis in the adult mammalian substantia nigra. Proc Natl Acad Sci USA 2003;100:7925-30.
72. Lim DA, Huang YC, Alvarez-Buylla A. The adult neural stem cell niche: lessons for future neural cell replacement strategies. Neurosurg Clin N Am 2007;18:81-92.
73. Hermann A, Maisel M, Wegner F, et al. Multipotent neural stem cells from the adult tegmentum with dopaminergic potential develop essential properties of functional neurons. Stem Cells 2006;24:949-64.
74. Pisati F, Bossolasco P, Meregalli M, et al. Induction of neurotrophin expression via human adult mesenchymal stem cells: implication for cell therapy in neurodegenerative diseases. Cell Transplant 2007;16:41-55.
75. Song L, Tuan RS. Transdifferentiation potential of human mesenchymal stem cells derived from bone marrow. FASEB J 2004;18:980-2.
76. Tropel P, Noel D, Platet N, et al. Isolation and characterisation of mesenchymal stem cells from adult mouse bone marrow. Exp Cell Res 2004;295:395-406.
77. Beyth S, Borovsky Z, Mevorach D, et al. Human mesenchymal stem cells alter antigen-presenting cell maturation and induce T-cell unresponsiveness. Blood 2005;105:2214-9.
78. Bartholomew A, Sturgeon C, Siatskas M, et al. Mesenchymal stem cells suppress lymphocyte proliferation in vitro and prolong skin graft survival in vivo. Exp Hematol 2002;30:42-8.
79. Tse WT, Pendleton JD, Beyer WM, et al. Suppression of allogeneic T-cell proliferation by human marrow stromal cells: implications in transplantation. Transplantation 2003;75:389-97.

80. Hellmann MA, Panet H, Barhum Y, et al. Increased survival and migration of engrafted mesenchymal bone marrow stem cells in 6-hydroxydopamine-lesioned rodents. Neurosci Lett 2006;395:124-8.
81. Li Y, Chen J, Wang L, et al. Intracerebral transplantation of bone marrow stromal cells in a 1-methyl-4- phenyl-1,2,3,6-tetrahydropyridine mouse model of Parkinson's disease. Neurosci Lett 2001;316:67-70.
82. Azizi SA, Stokes D, Augelli BJ, et al. Engraftment and migration of human bone marrow stromal cells implanted in the brains of albino rats—similarities to astrocyte grafts. Proc Natl Acad Sci USA 1998;95:3908-13.
83. Kan I, Ben Zur T, Barhum Y, et al. Dopaminergic differentiation of human mesenchymal stem cells-Utilization of bioassay for tyrosine hydroxylase expression. Neurosci Lett 2007;419:28-33.
84. Chai LH, Wu SX, Yan WH, et al. [Human bone marrow mesenchymal stem cells differentiated into dopaminergenic neurons in vitro]. Sheng Wu Gong Cheng Xue Bao 2007;23:252-6.
85. Dezawa M. [Future views and challenges to the peripheral nerve regeneration by cell based therapy]. Rinsho Shinkeigaku 2005;45:877-9.
86. Lu L, Zhao C, Liu Y, et al. Therapeutic benefit of TH-engineered mesenchymal stem cells for Parkinson's disease. Brain Res Brain Res Protoc 2005;15:46-51.
87. Gronthos S, Franklin DM, Leddy HA, et al. Surface protein characterization of human adipose tissue derived stromal cells. J Cell Physiol 2001;189:54-63.
88. Kang SK, Lee DH, Bae YC, et al. Improvement of neurological deficits by intracerebral transplantation of human adipose tissue-derived stromal cells after cerebral ischemia in rats. Exp Neurol 2003;183:355-66.
89. Buhnemann C, Scholz A, Bernreuther C, et al. Neuronal differentiation of transplanted embryonic stem cell-derived precursors in stroke lesions of adult rats. Brain 2006;129:3238-48.
90. Yanagisawa D, Qi M, Kim DH, et al. Improvement of focal ischemia-induced rat dopaminergic dysfunction by striatal transplantation of mouse embryonic stem cells. Neurosci Lett 2006;407:74-9.
91. He YD, Zeng JS, Yu J, et al. [EphB2-Fc promotes activation of endogenous neural stem cells after cerebral cortex infarction: experimental with hypertensive rats]. Zhonghua Yi Xue Za Zhi 2005;85:2395-9.
92. Zhang B, Wang RZ, Yao Y, et al. Proliferation and differentiation of neural stem cells in adult rats after cerebral infarction. Chin Med Sci J 2004;19:73-7.
93. Zhang B, Wang RZ, Li GL, et al. [Experimental study on the proliferation and plasticity of neural stem cells in situ in adult rats after cerebral infarction]. Zhongguo Yi Xue Ke Xue Yuan Xue Bao 2004;26:8-11.
94. Lee HJ, Kim KS, Park IH, et al. Human neural stem cells over-expressing VEGF provide neuroprotection, angiogenesis and functional recovery in mouse stroke model. PLoS ONE 2007;2:e156.
95. Lee HJ, Kim KS, Kim EJ, et al. Brain transplantation of immortalized human neural stem cells promotes functional recovery in mouse intracerebral hemorrhage stroke model. Stem Cells 2007;25:1204-12.
96. Roitberg BZ, Mangubat E, Chen EY, et al. Survival and early differentiation of human neural stem cells transplanted in a nonhuman primate model of stroke. J Neurosurg 2006;105:96-102.
97. Chu K, Kim M, Chae SH, et al. Distribution and in situ proliferation patterns of intravenously injected immortalized human neural stem-like cells in rats with focal cerebral ischemia. Neurosci Res 2004;50:459-65.

98. Ishibashi S, Sakaguchi M, Kuroiwa T, et al. Human neural stem/progenitor cells, expanded in long-term neurosphere culture, promote functional recovery after focal ischemia in Mongolian gerbils. J Neurosci Res 2004;78:215-23.
99. Wei JJ, Zeng LF, Fan XT, et al. Treatment of stroke in rats with bone marrow mesenchymal stem cells. Zhonghua Yi Xue Za Zhi 2007;87:184-9.
100. Xiao J, Nan Z, Motooka Y, et al. Transplantation of a novel cell line population of umbilical cord blood stem cells ameliorates neurological deficits associated with ischemic brain injury. Stem Cells Dev 2005;14:722-33.
101. Willing AE, Lixian J, Milliken M, et al. Intravenous versus intrastriatal cord blood administration in a rodent model of stroke. J Neurosci Res 2003;73:296-307.
102. Rice HE, Hsu EW, Sheng H, et al. Superparamagnetic iron oxide labeling and transplantation of adipose derived stem cells in middle cerebral artery occlusion-injured mice. AJR Am J Roentgenol 2007;188:1101-8.
103. Wang Q, Matsumoto Y, Shindo T, et al. Neural stem cells transplantation in cortex in a mouse model of Alzheimer's disease. J Med Invest 2006;53:61-9.
104. Wang QH, Xu RX, Nagao S. Transplantation of cholinergic neural stem cells in a mouse model of Alzheimer's disease. Chin Med J (Engl) 2005;118:508-11.
105. Brinton RD, Wang JM. Preclinical analyses of the therapeutic potential of allopregnanolone to promote neurogenesis in vitro and in vivo in transgenic mouse model of Alzheimer's disease. Curr Alzheimer Res 2006;3:11-7.
106. Iacovitti L, Donaldson AE, Marshall CE, et al. A protocol for the differentiation of human embryonic stem cells into dopaminergic neurons using only chemically defined human additives: studies in vitro and in vivo. Brain Res 2007;1127:19-25.
107. Nakao N, Yokote H, Nakai K, et al. Promotion of survival and regeneration of nigral dopamine neurons in a rat model of Parkinson's disease after implantation of embryonal carcinoma-derived neurons genetically engineered to produce glial cell line-derived neurotrophic factor. J Neurosurg 2000;92:659-70.
108. Richardson RM, Broaddus WC, Holloway KL et al. Grafts of adult subependymal zone neuronal progenitor cells rescue hemiparkinsonian behavioral decline. Brain Res 2005;1032:11-22.
109. Cooper O, Isacson O. Intrastriatal transforming growth factor alpha delivery to a model of Parkinson's disease induces proliferation and migration of endogenous adult neural progenitor cells without differentiation into dopaminergic neurons. J Neurosci 2004;24:8924-31.
110. Grothe C, Timmer M, Scholz T, et al. Fibroblast growth factor-20 promotes the differentiation of Nurr1- overexpressing neural stem cells into tyrosine hydroxylase-positive neurons. Neurobiol Dis 2004;17:163-70.
111. Zhou C, Wen ZX, Wang ZP, et al. Green fluorescent protein-labeled mapping of neural stem cells migrating towards damaged areas in the adult central nervous system. Cell Biol Int 2003;27:943-5.
112. Wang X, Lu Y, Zhang H, et al. Distinct efficacy of pre-differentiated versus intact fetal mesencephalon-derived human neural progenitor cells in alleviating rat model of Parkinson's disease. Int J Dev Neurosci 2004;22:175-83.
113. Sun ZH, Lai YL, Zeng WW, et al. Neural stem/progenitor cells survive and differentiate better in PD rats than in normal rats. Acta Neurochir Suppl 2003;87:169-74.
114. Suon S, Yang M, Iacovitti L. Adult human bone marrow stromal spheres express neuronal traits in vitro and in a rat model of Parkinson's disease. Brain Res 2006;1106:46-51.

115. Park KW, Eglitis MA, Mouradian MM. Protection of nigral neurons by GDNF-engineered marrow cell transplantation. Neurosci Res 2001;40:315-23.
116. Jordan JD, Ming GL, Song H. Adult neurogenesis as a potential therapy for neurodegenerative diseases. Discov Med 2006;6:144-7.
117. Batista CM, Kippin TE, Willaime-Morawek S, et al. A progressive and cell non-autonomous increase in striatal neural stem cells in the Huntington's disease R6/2 mouse. J Neurosci 2006;26:10452-60.
118. Johann V, Schiefer J, Sass C, et al. Time of transplantation and cell preparation determine neural stem cell survival in a mouse model of Huntington's disease. Exp Brain Res 2007;177:458-70.
119. Pineda JR, Rubio N, Akerud P, et al. Neuroprotection by GDNF-secreting stem cells in a Huntington's disease model: optical neuroimage tracking of brain-grafted cells. Gene Ther 2007;14:118-28.
120. Tattersfield AS, Croon RJ, Liu YW, et al. Neurogenesis in the striatum of the quinolinic acid lesion model of Huntington's disease. Neuroscience 2004;127:319-32.
121. Bottcher T, Mix E, Koczan D, et al. Gene expression profiling of ciliary neurotrophic factor-overexpressing rat striatal progenitor cells (ST14A) indicates improved stress response during the early stage of differentiation. J Neurosci Res 2003;73:42-53.
122. Weinelt S, Peters S, Bauer P, et al. Ciliary neurotrophic factor overexpression in neural progenitor cells (ST14A) increases proliferation, metabolic activity, and resistance to stress during differentiation. J Neurosci Res 2003;71:228-36.
123. Martinez-Serrano A, Bjorklund A. Protection of the neostriatum against excitotoxic damage by neurotrophin-producing, genetically modified neural stem cells. J Neurosci 1996;16:4604-16.
124. Roberts TJ, Price J, Williams SC, et al. Preservation of striatal tissue and behavioral function after neural stem cell transplantation in a rat model of Huntington's disease. Neuroscience 2006;139:1187-99.
125. Lee ST, Park JE, Lee K, et al. Noninvasive method of immortalized neural stem-like cell transplantation in an experimental model of Huntington's disease. J Neurosci Methods 2006;152:250-4.
126. McBride JL, Behrstock SP, Chen EY, et al. Human neural stem cell transplants improve motor function in a rat model of Huntington's disease. J Comp Neurol 2004;475:211-9.
127. Lescaudron L, Unni D, Dunbar GL. Autologous adult bone marrow stem cell transplantation in an animal model of huntington's disease: behavioral and morphological outcomes. Int J Neurosci 2003;113:945-56.
128. Dunbar GL, Sandstrom MI, Rossignol J, et al. Neurotrophic enhancers as therapy for behavioral deficits in rodent models of Huntington's disease: use of gangliosides, substituted pyrimidines, and mesenchymal stem cells. Behav Cogn Neurosci Rev 2006;5:63-79.
129. Ohta Y, Nagai M, Nagata T, et al. Intrathecal injection of epidermal growth factor and fibroblast growth factor 2 promotes proliferation of neural precursor cells in the spinal cords of mice with mutant human SOD1 gene. J Neurosci Res 2006;84:980-92.
130. Garbuzova-Davis S, Willing AE, Milliken M, et al. Positive effect of transplantation of hNT neurons (NTera 2/D1 cell-line) in a model of familial amyotrophic lateral sclerosis. Exp Neurol 2002;174:169-80.
131. de H, I, Boucherie C, Pochet R, et al. Unilateral induction of progenitors in the spinal cord of hSOD1(G93A) transgenic rats correlates with an asymmetrical hind limb paralysis. Neurosci Lett 2006;401:25-9.
132. Corti S, Locatelli F, Papadimitriou D, et al. Neural stem cells LewisX+ CXCR4+ modify disease progression in an amyotrophic lateral sclerosis model. Brain 2007;130:1289-305.

133. Yan J, Xu L, Welsh AM, et al. Combined immunosuppressive agents or CD4 antibodies prolong survival of human neural stem cell grafts and improve disease outcomes in amyotrophic lateral sclerosis transgenic mice. Stem Cells 2006;24:1976-85.
134. Klein SM, Behrstock S, McHugh J, et al. GDNF delivery using human neural progenitor cells in a rat model of ALS. Hum Gene Ther 2005;16:509-21.
135. Huang H, Zhang C, Zhao CP, et al. [Effect of transplantation of wild-type bone marrow stem cells in mouse model of familial amyotrophic lateral sclerosis]. Zhongguo Yi Xue Ke Xue Yuan Xue Bao 2006;28:562-66.
136. Corti S, Locatelli F, Donadoni C, et al. Wild-type bone marrow cells ameliorate the phenotype of SOD1- G93A ALS mice and contribute to CNS, heart and skeletal muscle tissues. Brain 2004;127:2518-32.
137. Cabanes C, Bonilla S, Tabares L, et al. Neuroprotective effect of adult hematopoietic stem cells in a mouse model of motoneuron degeneration. Neurobiol Dis 2007;26:408-18.
138. Garbuzova-Davis S, Willing AE, Zigova T, et al. Intravenous administration of human umbilical cord blood cells in a mouse model of amyotrophic lateral sclerosis: distribution, migration, and differentiation. J Hematother Stem Cell Res 2003;12:255-70.
139. Ungerstedt U. 6-Hydroxy-dopamine induced degeneration of central monoamine neurons. Eur J Pharmacol 1968;5:107-10.
140. Perese DA, Ulman J, Viola J, et al. A 6-hydroxydopamine-induced selective parkinsonian rat model. Brain Res 1989;494:285-93.
141. Przedborski S, Jackson-Lewis V, Popilskis S, et al. Unilateral MPTP-induced parkinsonism in monkeys. A quantitative autoradiographic study of dopamine D1 and D2 receptors and re-uptake sites. Neurochirurgie 1991;37:377-82.
142. Sachs C, Jonsson G. Mechanisms of action of 6-hydroxydopamine. Biochem Pharmacol 1975;24:1-8.
143. Ben Shachar D, Eshel G, Finberg JP, et al. The iron chelator desferrioxamine (Desferal) retards 6- hydroxydopamine-induced degeneration of nigrostriatal dopamine neurons. J Neurochem 1991;56:1441-4.
144. Perumal AS, Gopal VB, Tordzro WK, et al. Vitamin E attenuates the toxic effects of 6-hydroxydopamine on free radical scavenging systems in rat brain. Brain Res Bull 1992;29:699-701.
145. Kumar R, Agarwal AK, Seth PK. Free radical-generated neurotoxicity of 6-hydroxydopamine. J Neurochem 1995;64:1703-7.
146. Cleeter MW, Cooper JM, Schapira AH. Irreversible inhibition of mitochondrial complex I by 1-methyl-4- phenylpyridinium: evidence for free radical involvement. J Neurochem 1992;58:786-9.
147. Ben Shachar D, Youdim MB. Intranigral iron injection induces behavioral and biochemical "parkinsonism" in rats. J Neurochem 1991;57:2133-5.
148. Schwarting RK, Huston JP. Unilateral 6-hydroxydopamine lesions of meso-striatal dopamine neurons and their physiological sequelae. Prog Neurobiol 1996;49:215-66.
149. Dunnett SB, Bjorklund A, Stenevi U, et al. Behavioural recovery following transplantation of substantia nigra in rats subjected to 6-OHDA lesions of the nigrostriatal pathway. II. Bilateral lesions. Brain Res 1981;229:457-70.
150. Langston JW, Forno LS, Tetrud J, et al. Evidence of active nerve cell degeneration in the substantia nigra of humans years after 1-methyl-4-phenyl-1,2,3,6-tetrahydropyridine exposure. Ann Neurol 1999;46:598-605.

151. Javitch JA, D'Amato RJ, Strittmatter SM, et al. Parkinsonism-inducing neurotoxin, N-methyl-4-phenyl- 1,2,3,6 -tetrahydropyridine: uptake of the metabolite N-methyl-4-phenylpyridine by dopamine neurons explains selective toxicity. Proc Natl Acad Sci USA 1985;82:2173-7.
152. Tipton KF, Singer TP. Advances in our understanding of the mechanisms of the neurotoxicity of MPTP and related compounds. J Neurochem 1993;61:1191-206.
153. Shoffner JM, Watts RL, Juncos JL, et al. Mitochondrial oxidative phosphorylation defects in Parkinson's disease. Ann Neurol 1991;30:332-9.
154. Zigmond MJ, Stricker EM. Animal models of parkinsonism using selective neurotoxins: clinical and basic implications. Int Rev Neurobiol 1989;31:1-79.
155. Petzinger GM, Langston JW. The MPTP-lesioned non-human primate: a model of Parkinson's disease. In Marwah J, Teiltelbaum H, (Eds): Advances in Neurodegenerative Disorders. Parkinson's Disease. Scottsdale: Prominent Press.1998;113-48.
156. Przedborski S, Jackson-Lewis V, Naini AB, et al. The parkinsonian toxin 1-methyl-4-phenyl-1,2,3,6-tetrahydropyridine (MPTP): a technical review of its utility and safety. J Neurochem 2001;76:1265-74.
157. Jankowsky JL, Savonenko A, Schilling G, et al. Transgenic mouse models of neurodegenerative disease: opportunities for therapeutic development. Curr Neurol Neurosci Rep 2002;2:457-64.
158. Zetterstrom RH, Solomin L, Jansson L, et al. Dopamine neuron agenesis in Nurr1-deficient mice. Science 1997;276:248-50.
159. Zhou QY, Quaife CJ, Palmiter RD. Targeted disruption of the tyrosine hydroxylase gene reveals that catecholamines are required for mouse fetal development. Nature 1995;374:640-3.
160. Zhou QY, Palmiter RD. Dopamine-deficient mice are severely hypoactive, adipsic, and aphagic. Cell 1995;83:1197-209.
161. Baik JH, Picetti R, Saiardi A, et al. Parkinsonian-like locomotor impairment in mice lacking dopamine D2 receptors. Nature 1995;377:424-8.
162. Xu M, Moratalla R, Gold LH, et al. Dopamine D1 receptor mutant mice are deficient in striatal expression of dynorphin and in dopamine-mediated behavioral responses. Cell 1994;79:729-42.
163. Accili D, Fishburn CS, Drago J, et al. A targeted mutation of the D3 dopamine receptor gene is associated with hyperactivity in mice. Proc Natl Acad Sci USA 1996;93:1945-9.
164. Vila M, Wu DC, Przedborski S. Engineered modeling and the secrets of Parkinson's disease. Trends Neurosci 2001;24:S49-5.
165. Abeliovich A, Schmitz Y, Farinas I, et al. Mice lacking alpha-synuclein display functional deficits in the nigrostriatal dopamine system. Neuron 2000;25:239-52.
166. Beal MF. Experimental models of Parkinson's disease. Nat Rev Neurosci 2001;2:325-34.
167. Masliah E, Rockenstein E, Veinbergs I, et al. Dopaminergic loss and inclusion body formation in alpha synuclein mice: implications for neurodegenerative disorders. Science 2000;287:1265-9.
168. Sawada H, Shimohama S, Kawamura T, et al. Mechanism of resistance to NO-induced neurotoxicity in cultured rat dopaminergic neurons. J Neurosci Res 1996;46:509-18.
169. Kitamura Y, Kosaka T, Kakimura JI, et al. Protective effects of the antiparkinsonian drugs talipexole and pramipexole against 1-methyl-4-phenylpyridinium-induced apoptotic death in human neuroblastoma SH-SY5Y cells. Mol Pharmacol 1998;54:1046-54.
170. Mandel RJ, Spratt SK, Snyder RO, et al. Midbrain injection of recombinant adeno-associated virus encoding rat glial cell line-derived neurotrophic factor protects nigral neurons in a progressive 6-hydroxydopamine-induced degeneration model of Parkinson's disease in rats. Proc Natl Acad Sci USA 1997;94:14083-8.

171. Rozas G, Guerra MJ, Labandeira-Garcia JL. An automated rotarod method for quantitative drug-free evaluation of overall motor deficits in rat models of parkinsonism. Brain Res Brain Res Protoc 1997;2:75-84.
172. Schallert T, Fleming SM, Leasure JL, et al. CNS plasticity and assessment of forelimb sensorimotor outcome in unilateral rat models of stroke, cortical ablation, parkinsonism and spinal cord injury. Neuropharmacology 2000;39:777-87.
173. Borlongan CV, Sanberg PR. Elevated body swing test: a new behavioral parameter for rats with 6-hydroxydopamine-induced hemiparkinsonism. J Neurosci 1995;15:5372-8.
174. Haughey NJ, Liu D, Nath A, et al. Disruption of neurogenesis in the subventricular zone of adult mice, and in human cortical neuronal precursor cells in culture, by amyloid beta-peptide: implications for the pathogenesis of Alzheimer's disease. Neuromolecular Med 2002;1:125-35.
175. Mazur-Kolecka B, Golabek A, Nowicki K, et al. Amyloid-beta impairs development of neuronal progenitor cells by oxidative mechanisms. Neurobiol Aging 2006;27:1181-92.
176. Benvenuti S, Saccardi R, Luciani P, et al. Neuronal differentiation of human mesenchymal stem cells: changes in the expression of the Alzheimer's disease-related gene seladin-1. Exp Cell Res 2006;312:2592-604.
177. Kwak YD, Brannen CL, Qu T, et al. Amyloid precursor protein regulates differentiation of human neural stem cells. Stem Cells Dev 2006;15:381-9.
178. Chen CW, Boiteau RM, Lai WF, et al. sAPPalpha enhances the transdifferentiation of adult bone marrow progenitor cells to neuronal phenotypes. Curr Alzheimer Res 2006;3:63-70.
179. Brinton RD, Wang JM. Therapeutic potential of neurogenesis for prevention and recovery from Alzheimer's disease: allopregnanolone as a proof of concept neurogenic agent. Curr Alzheimer Res 2006;3:185-90.
180. Brinton RD, Wang JM. Preclinical analyses of the therapeutic potential of allopregnanolone to promote neurogenesis in vitro and in vivo in transgenic mouse model of Alzheimer's disease. Curr Alzheimer Res 2006;3:11-7.
181. Wick G, Berger P, Jansen-Durr P, et al. A Darwinian-evolutionary concept of age-related diseases. Exp Gerontol 2003;38:13-25.
182. Nakajima M, Ogawa M, Shimoda Y, et al. Presenilin-1 controls the growth and differentiation of endothelial progenitor cells through its beta-catenin-binding region. Cell Biol Int 2006;30:239-43.
183. Wen PH, Hof PR, Chen X, et al. The presenilin-1 familial Alzheimer disease mutant P117L impairs neurogenesis in the hippocampus of adult mice. Exp Neurol 2004;188:224-37.
184. Chevallier NL, Soriano S, Kang DE, et al. Perturbed neurogenesis in the adult hippocampus associated with presenilin-1 A246E mutation. Am J Pathol 2005;167:151-9.
185. Whitehouse PJ, Price DL, Struble RG, et al. Alzheimer's disease and senile dementia: loss of neurons in the basal forebrain. Science 1982;215:1237-9.
186. Ichimiya Y, Arai H, Kosaka K, et al. Morphological and biochemical changes in the cholinergic and monoaminergic systems in Alzheimer-type dementia. Acta Neuropathol (Berl) 1986;70:112-6.
187. Gottfries CG, Adolfsson R, Aquilonius SM, et al. Biochemical changes in dementia disorders of Alzheimer type (AD/SDAT). Neurobiol Aging 1983;4:261-71.
188. Reinikainen KJ, Soininen H, Riekkinen PJ. Neurotransmitter changes in Alzheimer's disease: implications to diagnostics and therapy. J Neurosci Res 1990;27:576-86.
189. Wenk H, Bigl V, Meyer U. Cholinergic projections from magnocellular nuclei of the basal forebrain to cortical areas in rats. Brain Res 1980;2:295.

190. Haroutunian V, Mantin R, Kanof PD. Frontal cortex as the site of action of physostigmine in nbM-lesioned rats. Physiol Behav 1990;47:203-6.
191. Haroutunian V, Kanof PD, Tsuboyama G, et al. Restoration of cholinomimetic activity by clonidine in cholinergic plus noradrenergic lesioned rats. Brain Res 1990;507:261-6.
192. Jaskiw GE, Karoum F, Freed WJ, et al. Effect of ibotenic acid lesions of the medial prefrontal cortex on amphetamine-induced locomotion and regional brain catecholamine concentrations in the rat. Brain Res 1990;534:263-72.
193. Contestabile A, Migani P, Poli A, et al. Recent advances in the use of selective neuron-destroying agents for neurobiological research. Experientia 1984;40:524-34.
194. Lamb BT, Sisodia SS, Lawler AM, et al. Introduction and expression of the 400 kilobase amyloid precursor protein gene in transgenic mice [corrected]. Nat Genet 1993;5:22-30.
195. Reiner A, Dragatsis I, Zeitlin S, et al. Wild-type huntingtin plays a role in brain development and neuronal survival. Mol Neurobiol 2003;28:259-76.
196. Hilditch-Maguire P, Trettel F, Passani LA, et al. Huntingtin: an iron-regulated protein essential for normal nuclear and perinuclear organelles. Hum Mol Genet 2000;9:2789-97.
197. Canals JM, Pineda JR, Torres-Peraza JF, et al. Brain-derived neurotrophic factor regulates the onset and severity of motor dysfunction associated with enkephalinergic neuronal degeneration in Huntington's disease. J Neurosci 2004;24:7727-39.
198. Coyle JT, Schwarcz R. Lesion of striatal neurones with kainic acid provides a model for Huntington's chorea. Nature 1976;263:244-6.
199. Schwarcz R, Hokfelt T, Fuxe K, et al. Ibotenic acid-induced neuronal degeneration: a morphological and neurochemical study. Exp Brain Res 1979;37:199-216.
200. Schwarcz R, Whetsell WO, Jr., Mangano RM. Quinolinic acid: an endogenous metabolite that produces axon-sparing lesions in rat brain. Science 1983;219:316-8.
201. Wolfensberger M, Amsler U, Cuenod M, et al. Identification of quinolinic acid in rat and human brain tissue. Neurosci Lett 1983;41:247-52.
202. Beal MF, Kowall NW, Ellison DW, et al. Replication of the neurochemical characteristics of Huntington's disease by quinolinic acid. Nature 1986;321:168-71.
203. Beal MF, Kowall NW, Swartz KJ, et al. Systemic approaches to modifying quinolinic acid striatal lesions in rats. J Neurosci 1988;8:3901-8.
204. Davies SW, Roberts PJ. No evidence for preservation of somatostatin-containing neurons after intrastriatal injections of quinolinic acid. Nature 1987;327:326-9.
205. Davies SW, Roberts PJ. Sparing of cholinergic neurons following quinolinic acid lesions of the rat striatum. Neuroscience 1988;26:387-93.
206. Boegman RJ, Smith Y, Parent A. Quinolinic acid does not spare striatal neuropeptide Y-immunoreactive neurons. Brain Res 1987;415:178-82.
207. Chu-LaGraff Q, Kang X, Messer A. Expression of the Huntington's disease transgene in neural stem cell cultures from R6/2 transgenic mice. Brain Res Bull 2001;56:307-12.
208. Levine MS, Klapstein GJ, Koppel A , et al. Enhanced sensitivity to N-methyl-D-aspartate receptor activation in transgenic and knockin mouse models of Huntington's disease. J Neurosci Res 1999;58:515-32.
209. Morris R. Developments of a water-maze procedure for studying spatial learning in the rat. J Neurosci Methods 1984;11:47-60.

210. Schallert T, Woodlee MT, Fleming SM. Disentangling multiple types of recovery from brain injury. In: Kreiglstein J, Klumpp S (Eds). Pharmacol of Cerebral Ischaemia. Stuttgart: Medpharm Scientific Publishers 2002:201–16.
211. Montoya CP, Campbell-Hope LJ, Pemberton KD, et al. The "staircase test": a measure of independent forelimb reaching and grasping abilities in rats. J Neurosci Methods 1991;36:219-28.
212. Erie EA, Shim H, Smith AL, et al. Mice deficient in the ALS2 gene exhibit lymphopenia and abnormal hematopietic function. J Neuroimmunol 2007;182:226-31.
213. Di Giorgio FP, Carrasco MA, Siao MC, et al. Non-cell autonomous effect of glia on motor neurons in an embryonic stem cell-based ALS model. Nat Neurosci 2007;10:608-14.
214. Braat DD, Mummery CL, Schattenberg AV, et al. [Freezing umbilical-cord blood and bone marrow for one's own use: present-day quackery?]. Ned Tijdschr Geneeskd 2006;150:2410-14.
215. Guan YJ, Wang X, Wang HY, et al. Increased stem cell proliferation in the spinal cord of adult amyotrophic lateral sclerosis transgenic mice. J Neurochem 2007;102:1125-38.
216. de H, I, Boucherie C, Pochet R et al. Unilateral induction of progenitors in the spinal cord of hSOD1(G93A) transgenic rats correlates with an asymmetrical hind limb paralysis. Neurosci Lett 2006;401:25-9.
217. Chi L, Ke Y, Luo C, et al. Motor neuron degeneration promotes neural progenitor cell proliferation, migration, and neurogenesis in the spinal cords of amyotrophic lateral sclerosis mice. Stem Cells 2006;24:34-43.
218. Xing D, Martins JB. Myocardial ischemia-reperfusion damage impacts occurrence of ventricular fibrillation in dogs. Am J Physiol Heart Circ Physiol 2001;280:H684-92.
219. Silva GV, Litovsky S, Assad JA , et al. Mesenchymal stem cells differentiate into an endothelial phenotype, enhance vascular density, and improve heart function in a canine chronic ischemia model. Circulation 2005;111:150-56.
220. Liu Y, Sun L, Huan Y, et al. Effects of basic fibroblast growth factor microspheres on angiogenesis in ischemic myocardium and cardiac function: analysis with dobutamine cardiovascular magnetic resonance tagging. Eur J Cardiothorac Surg 2006;30:103-7.
221. Lyseggen E, Skulstad H, Helle-Valle T, et al. Myocardial strain analysis in acute coronary occlusion: a tool to assess myocardial viability and reperfusion. Circulation 2005;112:3901-10.
222. Michael LH, Ballantyne CM, Zachariah JP, et al. Myocardial infarction and remodeling in mice: effect of reperfusion. Am J Physiol 1999;277:H660-8.
223. Michael LH, Entman ML, Hartley CJ, et al. Myocardial ischemia and reperfusion: a murine model. Am J Physiol 1995;269:H2147-54.
224. Tian R, Miao W, Spindler M, et al. Long-term expression of protein kinase C in adult mouse hearts improves postischemic recovery. Proc Natl Acad Sci USA 1999;96:13536-41.
225. Juhaszova M, Zorov DB, Kim SH, et al. Glycogen synthase kinase-3beta mediates convergence of protection signaling to inhibit the mitochondrial permeability transition pore. J Clin Invest 2004;113:1535-49.
226. Okada T, Otani H, Wu Y, et al. Integrated pharmacological preconditioning and memory of cardioprotection: role of protein kinase C and phosphatidylinositol 3-kinase. Am J Physiol Heart Circ Physiol 2005;289:H761-7.
227. Claycomb WC, Lanson NA, Jr., Stallworth BS, et al. HL-1 cells: a cardiac muscle cell line that contracts and retains phenotypic characteristics of the adult cardiomyocyte. Proc Natl Acad Sci USA 1998;95:2979-84.

228. Gross ER, Hsu AK, Gross GJ. The JAK/STAT pathway is essential for opioid-induced cardioprotection: JAK2 as a mediator of STAT3, Akt, and GSK-3 beta. Am J Physiol Heart Circ Physiol 2006; 291: H827-34.
229. Seymour EM, Wu SY, Kovach MA et al. HL-1 myocytes exhibit PKC and K(ATP) channel-dependent delta opioid preconditioning. J Surg Res 2003;114:187-94.
230. Tantini B, Fiumana E, Cetrullo S, et al. Involvement of polyamines in apoptosis of cardiac myoblasts in a model of simulated ischemia. J Mol Cell Cardiol 2006;40:775-82.
231. Tanno M, Bassi R, Gorog DA, et al. Diverse mechanisms of myocardial p38 mitogen-activated protein kinase activation: evidence for MKK-independent activation by a TAB1-associated mechanism contributing to injury during myocardial ischemia. Circ Res 2003;93:254-61.
232. Nygren A, Baczko I, Giles WR. Measurements of electrophysiological effects of components of acute ischemia in Langendorff-perfused rat hearts using voltage-sensitive dye mapping. J Cardiovasc Electrophysiol 2006;17 (Suppl 1):S113-23.
233. Keener JP. Model for the onset of fibrillation following coronary artery occlusion. J Cardiovasc Electrophysiol 2003;14:1225-32.
234. Gebel JM, Broderick JP. Intracerebral hemorrhage. Neurol Clin 2000;18:419-38.
235. Savitz SI, Rosenbaum DM, Dinsmore JH, et al. Cell transplantation for stroke. Ann Neurol 2002;52:266-75.
236. Zhao LR, Duan WM, Reyes M, et al. Human bone marrow stem cells exhibit neural phenotypes and ameliorate neurological deficits after grafting into the ischemic brain of rats. Exp Neurol 2002;174: 11-20.
237. Veizovic T, Beech JS, Stroemer RP, et al. Resolution of stroke deficits following contralateral grafts of conditionally immortal neuroepithelial stem cells. Stroke 2001;32:1012-9.
238. Modo M, Rezaie P, Heuschling P, et al. Transplantation of neural stem cells in a rat model of stroke: assessment of short-term graft survival and acute host immunological response. Brain Res 2002;958:70- 82.
239. Garcia JH. Experimental ischemic stroke: a review. Stroke 1984;15:5-14.
240. Robinson RG, Shoemaker WJ, Schlumpf M, et al. Effect of experimental cerebral infarction in rat brain on catecholamines and behaviour. Nature 1975;255:332-4.
241. Tamura A, Graham DI, McCulloch J, et al. Focal cerebral ischaemia in the rat: 2. Regional cerebral blood flow determined by [14C] iodoantipyrine autoradiography following middle cerebral artery occlusion. J Cereb Blood Flow Metab 1981;1:61-9.
242. Ringelstein EB, Biniek R, Weiller C, et al. Type and extent of hemispheric brain infarctions and clinical outcome in early and delayed middle cerebral artery recanalization. Neurology 1992;42:289-98.
243. Buchan AM, Xue D, Slivka A. A new model of temporary focal neocortical ischemia in the rat. Stroke 1992;23:273-9.
244. Markgraf CG, Green EJ, Watson B, et al. Recovery of sensorimotor function after distal middle cerebral artery photothrombotic occlusion in rats. Stroke 1994;25:153-9.
245. Longa EZ, Weinstein PR, Carlson S, et al. Reversible middle cerebral artery occlusion without craniectomy in rats. Stroke 1989;20:84-91.
246. Kudo M, Aoyama A, Ichimori S, et al. An animal model of cerebral infarction. Homologous blood clot emboli in rats. Stroke 1982;13:505-8.
247. Zhang Z, Zhang RL, Jiang Q, et al. A new rat model of thrombotic focal cerebral ischemia. J Cereb Blood Flow Metab 1997;17:123-35.

248. Gerriets T, Li F, Silva MD, et al. The macrosphere model: evaluation of a new stroke model for permanent middle cerebral artery occlusion in rats. J Neurosci Methods 2003;122:201-11.
249. Mayzel-Oreg O, Omae T, Kazemi M, et al. Microsphere-induced embolic stroke: an MRI study. Magn Reson Med 2004;51:1232-8.
250. Schmid-Elsaesser R, Zausinger S, Hungerhuber E, et al. A critical reevaluation of the intraluminal thread model of focal cerebral ischemia: evidence of inadvertent premature reperfusion and subarachnoid hemorrhage in rats by laser-Doppler flowmetry. Stroke 1998;29:2162-70.
251. Gerriets T, Stolz E, Walberer M, et al. Complications and pitfalls in rat stroke models for middle cerebral artery occlusion: a comparison between the suture and the macrosphere model using magnetic resonance angiography. Stroke 2004;35:2372-7.
252. Dittmar MS, Vatankhah B, Fehm NP, et al. Fischer-344 rats are unsuitable for the MCAO filament model due to their cerebrovascular anatomy. J Neurosci Methods 2006;156:50-4.
253. Tamura A, Graham DI, McCulloch J, et al. Focal cerebral ischaemia in the rat: description of technique and early neuropathological consequences following middle cerebral artery occlusion. J Cereb Blood Flow Metab 1981;1:53-60.
254. Watson BD, Dietrich WD, Busto R, et al. Induction of reproducible brain infarction by photochemically initiated thrombosis. Ann Neurol 1985;17:497-504.
255. Bederson JB, Pitts LH, Tsuji M, et al. Rat middle cerebral artery occlusion: evaluation of the model and development of a neurologic examination. Stroke 1986;17:472-6.
256. Olsson M, Nikkhah G, Bentlage C, et al. Forelimb akinesia in the rat Parkinson model: differential effects of dopamine agonists and nigral transplants as assessed by a new stepping test. J Neurosci 1995;15:3863-75.
257. Schallert T, Lindner MD. Rescuing neurons from trans-synaptic degeneration after brain damage: helpful, harmful, or neutral in recovery of function?. Can J Psychol 1990;44:276-92.

CHAPTER 4

Antistroke Agents

INTRODUCTION

Stroke, or "brain attack," is a clinical syndrome caused by impairment of cerebral blood flow (CBF) leading to acute cerebral deficit. It is the second commonest cause of death with an estimated 5·7 million deaths in 2005 and 87% of these deaths were in poor and developing countries.[1-4]

Brain receives effective perfusion about 55 ml/100 g/min through finely distributed blood vessels and their collaterals in order to cope with the high metabolic demands of the brain. The inability of brain unlike other organs to store oxygen and energy substrates makes it highly sensitive to CBF changes and any disruption of blood supply to the brain tissue if persists for more than three to four minutes, neuronal cells are at the thresholds of damage.[5]

Neuronal injury in stroke is thought to results following reduction in the blood supply predominating at the center of ischemic zone (core) and at the penumbra of ischemic damage, and is dependent on the severity and duration of ischemic insult. The oxidative damage does not occur in isolation but in a complex interplay between excitotoxicity, apoptosis, inflammation and extent of reperfusion.[6] The cellular and molecular basis of these events is highlighted by us in a recent review with a focus on numerous molecular targets.[7]

The energy failure following CBF reduction results in neuronal depolarization and subsequent activation of glutamate receptors. This in turn alters ionic gradient across membranes and activate complex survival/damage signaling mechanisms. However, a particular threshold exists for various cellular/molecular events leading to failure of synaptic function, when CBF falls below 16-18 ml/100 g/min and at a lower threshold (10-12 ml/100 g/min), the membrane failure ensues due to breakdown of cellular ionic homeostasis.[5,8] Further, the most brain lesions that develop after cerebral ischemia evolve from an initial stage of reversible to an infarct at the core, where most neurons become necrotic, while cellular damage in penumbral zone is mediated via apoptotic pathway although secondary necrosis may occur if the CBF is not restored early. Necrosis occurs in an indiscriminate fashion due to loss of osmotic homeostasis and rupture of plasma membrane. On the other hand apoptosis becomes activated following cerebral ischemia by variety of death signals such as production of free radicals and tumor necrosis factor, deficiency of growth factor, DNA damage, and mitochondrial dysfunction.[9,10] It is characterized by a series of well-defined distinct morphological and biochemical changes.[11-13]

Apoptosis is fundamentally mediated by caspases, a family of cysteine proteases that are synthesized as proenzymes and cleaved into active form. Caspase activation ultimately leads to break down of cellular framework, DNA cleavage and chromatin condensation, which is the hallmark of apoptosis. The caspase cascade is initiated either by death receptor belonging to tumor necrosis factor receptor (TNFR) superfamily proteins (extrinsic), mitochondrial dysfunction or endoplasmic stress (intrinsic).[12,14,15] The crosstalk between extrinsic and intrinsic apoptosis occurs at various stages.

Neuroprotection remains a key goal for stroke therapy and rt-PA is the only current pharmacological option clinically available.[16] However, the use of rt-PA has been limited only to less than 5% of ischemic stroke patients owing to its narrow therapeutic window and chances of hemorrhagic transformation. Further, the announcement by AstraZeneca of withdrawal of nitrone radical trapping agent disodium 2,4-disulfophenyl-N-tert-butylnitrone (NXY-059) from clinical trials due to the poor results at most of the endpoints is the latest setback to the development of effective neuroprotective therapy and has joined the list of unsuccessful 114 compounds that have gone under clinical trials. To avoid this ever increasing widespread failure of neuroprotective drugs, a meeting of experts from academia and industry was held to formulate the guidelines for the preclinical evaluation of candidate neuroprotective drugs.[17,18] Despite these efforts in translational research, the failure of NXY-059 and other have further raised the doubts on future trial.[18-20] Recommendations of the Stroke Therapy Academic Industry Roundtable (STAIR) for development of preclinical neuroprotectant for clinical advancements.[17,18]

- The candidate drug should be evaluated in permanent and transient focal occlusion models and subsequently in primate models.
- Time window studies confirming efficacy at both pre- and post-treatment dose regimen, dose response effect over a reasonable time window.
- Appropriate physiological monitoring of animals undertaken.
- Histological and functional short and long-term outcome should be assessed with prolonged survival and protection of subcortical as well as cortical structures.
- Results should be replicated in different animal models and in various laboratories.
- Data should be published both positive and negative in peer-reviewed journal.

Moreover, a single neuroprotective agent working on only one aspect of the ischemic cascade is not likely to exert a substantial beneficial effect on the size of infarct or functional outcome. Thus, it is speculated that combination therapies[21,22] or single agent that acts on multiple pathways of the ischemic cascade[23] might have a greater chance of success in providing neuroprotection.

TYPES OF STROKE

Stroke may be classified as ischemic accounting for ~85% of all stroke cases and hemorrhagic only by 15% (Fig. 4.1). Ischemic stroke is induced by total hypofusion as during cardiac arrest, near drowning, carbon dioxide poisoning, massive bleeding or focal loss of regional CBF due to atherosclerotic or embolic blockade of an artery. Whereas, hemorrhagic stroke occurs, when there is focal loss of blood flow may be due to vasospasm, which is caused by rupture of blood vessels within the brain (primary subarachnoid) or on the surface (primary intracerebral).

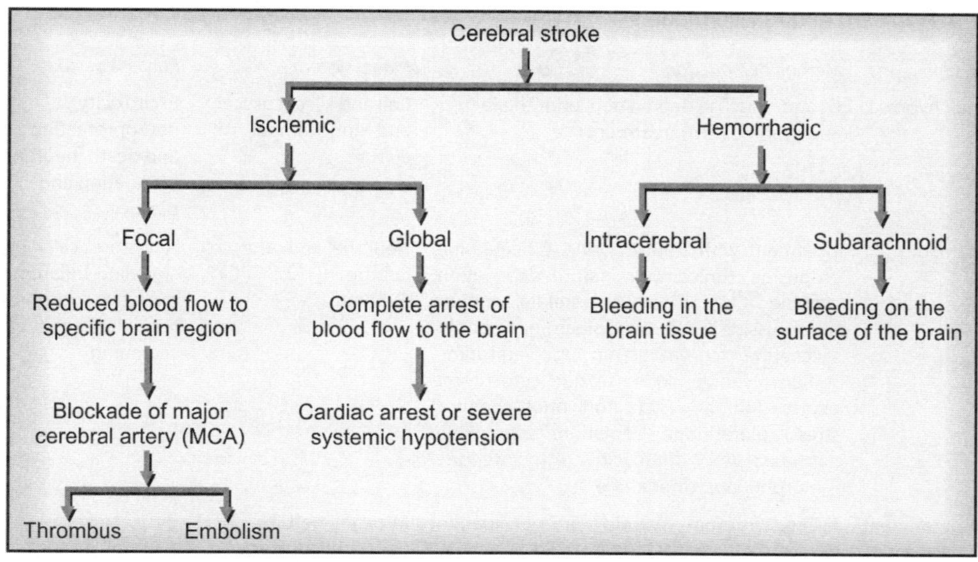

Figure 4.1: Schematic presentation of different types of stroke

SELECTION OF MODEL

The contribution of the various signaling mechanisms to the extent of the final infarct in human is still not very clear, therefore, *in vitro* and *in vivo* models have been developed to mimic human stroke pathophysiology to develop the effective neuroprotective strategies. Their inclusion in the stroke and related study depends upon the anatomic homogeneity, complexity, reproducibility or simulation of physiological and pathophysiological events. These models can be classified as focal or global, complete or incomplete and transient or permanent (Table 4.1).

However, appropriate selection of model system is imperative prerequisite for drug development for any pathology including stroke. Therefore, designing any neuroprotective strategy, STAIR recommendations should be taken into consideration in order to achieve a drug with fruitful outcome (Fig. 4.2).

In Vitro Models

The effect of cerebral ischemia *in vitro* can be visualized using primary culture of cerebral capillary endothelial cells, astrocytes, microglia, neurons (cortical, hippocampal, striatal, cerebellar granule cells, etc.), cell lines (HT22, PC12, SY5Y, etc.). The cells, for example, postmitotic neurons, from different brain regions such as cortex, striatum, hippocampus, etc. of 16 to 18 day old mouse or rat embryos can be isolated and grown for several days as 10 to 14 days. These cells are then deprived from oxygen and glucose referred as oxygen-glucose deprivation (OGD) model and induced chemical hypoxia through 3NPA, CN- and deoxyglucose. Moreover, stroke related changes can be also studied *in vitro* using organotypic cortical or hippocampal brain slices (acute and culture),[24-29] since, it is believed that complexity in a system decreases the screening capacity and high throughput screening is easiest to perform in cell free systems. Therefore, cultured brain slices have advantages over cell culture as it retain many

Table 4.1: *In vitro* and *in vivo* models

Model type	*Method of induction*	*Model system*	*Purpose of study*
Anoxia, hypoxia, OGD	O_2 and/ glucose deprivation, endothelin-1 and cyanide (CN^-) treatment	Cell and slice (cortical and hippocampal) culture	Excitoxicity, neuroprotection and death, neuronal maturation and plasticity
Cell damage	Treatment with staurosporine, C2-ceramide, etoposide, tunicamycin, serum deprivation, cyanide (CN^-), bleomycin sulfate, sodium nitroprusside (SNP), thapsigargin, lipopoly-saccharide, chromogranin A, veratridine, sodium cyanide, sodium azide cytochrome oxidase inhibitor H_2O_2, iron, photochemical stress, glutathione depletion, superoxide, naphthazarin, antimycin A, rotenone, 3-morpholinosydnonimine	Neuronal and other cell culture (HT22, PC12, SY5Y, etc.)	Apoptosis, calcium signaling, inflammation, oxidative stress and candidate agent screening
Focal permanent ischemia	MCAo, internal carotid artery ligation, intracarotid perfusion with wax, polyvinyl acetate, single/multiple clip, electrocautery, thrombic or embolic.	Mice, rat, gerbil, cat, rabbit, dog and monkey	Basic stroke pathophysiology study and neuroprotective compound screening
Focal transient ischemia	MCAo, internal carotid artery ligation, single/ multiple clip, electrocautery, thrombic or embolic (microsphere, macrosphere, autologous clot, fibrin clot, polyvinyl acetate) Chemical by endothelin-1, Rose Bengal photochemical dye, arachidonic acid, adenosine 5-phosphate and epinephrine, $FeCl_3$, subarachnoid hemorrhage		
Global ischemia complete	Respiratory block by cyanide (CN-), asphyxia, carbon dioxide, nitrogen, electrocauterization by clip, tourniquet, balloon compression, decapitation, ligation, intracranial pressure elevation, cardiac arrest, aortic occlusion, drowning, neck puff.	Mice, rat, gerbil, cat, rabbit, dog and monkey	Stroke pathophysiology study and neuroprotective compound screening
Global ischemia incomplete	2, 3 or 4-VO, intracranial hypertension, hemorrhage, cervical compression.		

essential organizational features of the host tissue, such as neuronal connectivity, relatively well preserved cellular stoichiometry and complex glial-neuronal interactions.[26] These slices are made ischemic by incubating with 95% N_2/5% CO_2 without glucose and can be replaced with 95% O_2/5% CO_2 to simulate a reperfusion period. Therefore, cellular damage that occurs depends on the duration and severity of the insult and can be detected by morphological, biochemical or molecular markers.

These models can be used to screen putative neuroprotective agents at high throughput scale for various parameters such as ionomycin cell lesion, glutamate mediated excitotoxicity, rotenone induced oxidative stress, lipopolysaccharide induced inflammation, serum withdrawal and apoptosis with apoptosis inducing agents (staurosporine, ceramide, etoposide, tunicamycin, etc.). Further, advances in automation, genomics and proteomics technology have also considerably amplified the number of potentially interesting targets that can be used for drug development.

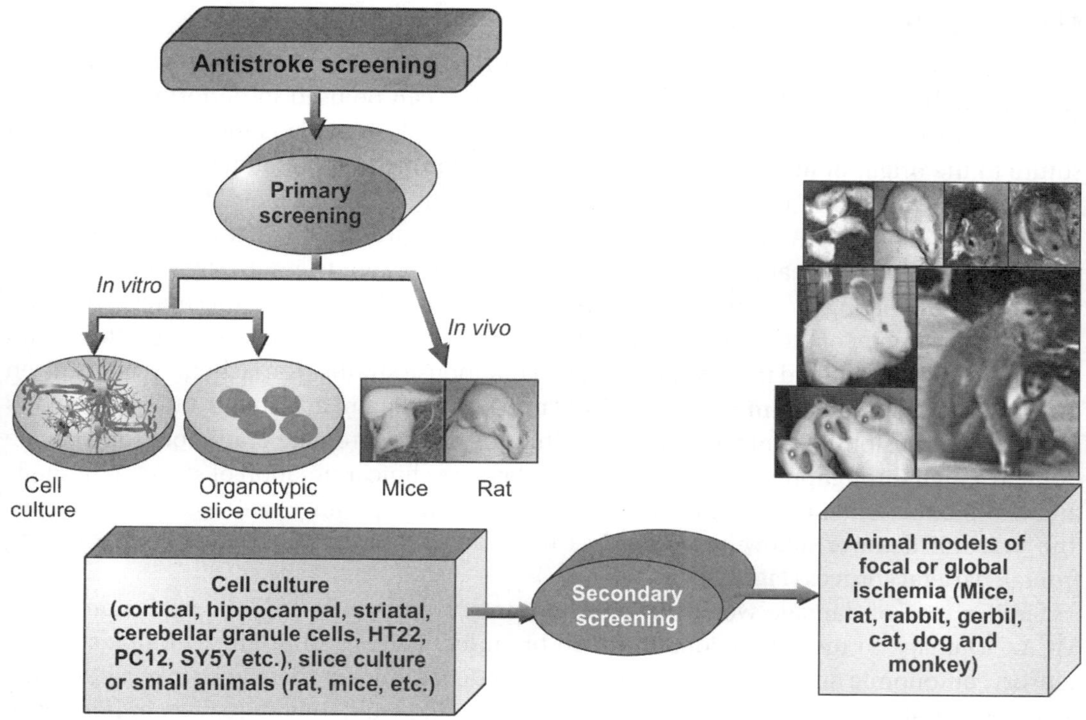

Figure 4.2: Schematic view of primary and secondary screening for antistroke test compounds

(*For color version see Plate 9*)

In Vivo Models

Besides *in vitro* model of stroke, several *in vivo* focal and global animal models have been developed in various animal species (mice, rats, gerbils, rabbits, cats, dogs, monkeys and baboons). However, the rat and mice strain are usually preferred for stroke study. The use of rat in stroke and related studies owes its resemblance to human cerebrovascular anatomy and physiology, easiness in handling due to moderate size, homogeneity in various strains and importantly reproducibility of stroke damage. Mice bear the special advantage of being its easiness for genetic manipulation.[30] Therefore, its application in studying various molecular mechanisms has been largely attributed. Despite rodents models, it is recommended that neuroprotective studies must be replicated in higher animals particularly nonhuman primates[17] due to their closer resemblance to brain of human in term of behavior and sensorimotor function. These model systems, therefore, can be used to screen molecules with thrombolytic, neuroprotective and neurorestorative potential.

Focal Ischemic Model

Experimentally focal cerebral ischemia can be induced by occluding middle cerebral artery (MCA) with intraluminal suture or with a vascular clip either transiently or permanently, mimicking stroke in humans.[31] Depending upon the type of occlusive method used, the damage occurs in cortex or striatum. Further, occlusive model can also simulate the reperfusion injury situation in humans, which may be due to lysis of a thrombo-embolic clot.

Middle Cerebral Artery Occlusion (MCAo)

The middle cerebral artery occlusion (MCAo) in rat is considered to be the most reliable and acceptable model of stroke. It is less invasive and can be used to perform transient or permanent ischemia in controlled manner. Focal cerebral ischemia is induced by inserting suture to the origin of middle cerebral artery (MCA) through the proximal external cerebral artery and advanced via internal carotid artery (ICA) until it blocks blood flow to MCA. The intraluminal suture MCAo model is most widely used in rats and mice. It was introduced by Kozuimi et al.,[32] and thereafter modified to avoid the subarachnoid hemorrhage and premature reperfusion by coating the suture either with silicone or poly-L-lysine.[33-35] These factors besides length and diameter of the suture affect the lesion size. This model has also been extended and used in genetically altered transgenic and knockout mouse strains. The ischemia can be given for a variable duration of time 60, 90, and 120 min or permanent and then suture removed to produce reperfusion. Advantageously, this technique does not require craniotomy and can be done in a high throughput manner.[36] It can simulate the clinical situation of stroke in humans and is therefore, often used in the preclinical evaluation of putative neuroprotective agents. The cerebral damage following MCAo has been demonstrated in striatum and overlying frontal, parietal cortices (Fig. 4.3).

Similar type of damage would be seen in human thrombotic-embolic occlusion of the MCA.[37] Damage to these functionally varied brain loci is likely to produce complex motor, sensory, autonomic and perhaps cognitive deficits depending upon a number of factors that includes mainly the intensity and duration of ischemic insult. Therefore, it is important to study neurobehavioral alterations and histologic endpoints over a limited time frame. Hence, determining the true potential of an intervention requires a set of behavioral analysis that can depict the true functional outcome in terms of sensorimotor and cognitive deficits.

Embolic Model

Embolic models of focal cerebral ischemia can be produced by injecting homologous small clot or fibrin-rich autologous clots, collagen, viscous silicone, polyvinylsiloxane, retractable silver ball and heterologous atheroemboli into extracranial arteries such as the external carotid artery to reach the more distal intracranial arteries most commonly in rats but also in larger animals although many studies often used non-clot embolus models produced by microsphereinduced embolization.[38-44] Similarly, ischemia may also be produced by photoactive dye most often Rose Bengal that when exposed to radiations generate singlet

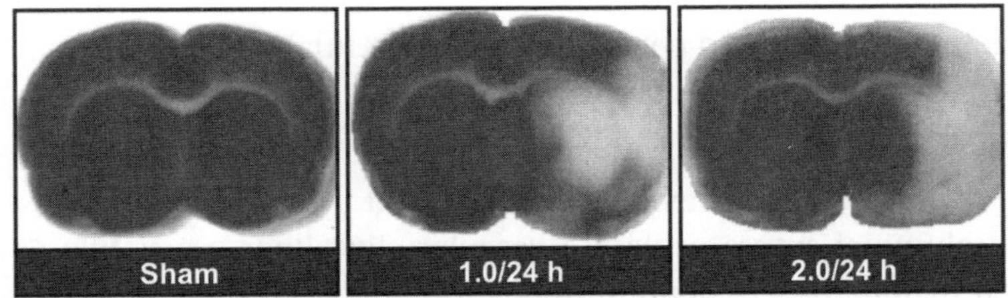

Figure 4.3: TTC stained brain slices after different time point of ischemia/reperfusion

(For color version see Plate 9)

oxygen and leads to focal endothelial damage and platelet activation. Thus, thromboembolic ischemia developed may produce damage around the territory affected by occlusion. The advantages of these types of models are their potential to test thrombolytic, neuroprotective and indeed combination therapies.

In addition to above focal models, endothelin-1, a potent vasoconstrictor can be used to induce stroke by applying endothelin-1 directly onto the exposed MCA or adjacent to the MCA by stereotaxic intracerebral injection. The lesion developed, thus, mimic ischemic damage produced by MCAo.

Global Ischemic Model

The global model on the other hand is more relevant to human cardiac arrest and involves brief bilateral occlusion of carotid and vertebral arteries. It is believed that global ischemia follows selective neuronal necrosis, whereas focal cerebral ischemia is more likely to develop infarction with pannecrosis. The various global ischemic model viz., two-vessel occlusion (2-VO) by transient bilateral common carotid artery (CCA) occlusions plus hypotension, fourvessel occlusion (4-VO) by transient bilateral CCA occlusions plus permanent vertebral artery occlusions, decapitation without recirculation, neck tourniquet, neck cuff inflation, ventricular fibrillation, cardiopulmonary resuscitation (CPR), has been developed to study the various aspects of brain damage. The global cerebral ischemia is generally induced for a brief period (5-15 min) to allow near complete cessation of CBF, followed by reperfusion. The 2-VO in rat and gerbil is the simplest and most often used global model for screening novel neuroprotactants although 4-VO is can also be valuable to drug discovery and development.[31,45] Gerbil lacks the posterior communicating arteries necessary to complete the circle of Willis, which allows collateral blood flow in humans and rats, therefore, gerbil is the preferred animal to study the effect of ischemia on hippocampal area.

The foremost property of a potentially therapeutic compound should be to restore or maintain the normal brain function. Thus, a systematic study of the effect of a putative neuroprotective agent at various dose regimens, administered before ischemia (pretreatment) or after ischemia and or reperfusion (post-treatment) such as, it can be applied at 0.0, 3.0, 6.0, 12.0, etc. hours post-ischemia, is required. It is also important to determine the therapeutic window of the agent administered, since any drug with broader therapeutic window will obviously have greater chances to combat the fatal disorder and will be available to larger population affected by stroke unlike rt-PA. Various putative agents with antiexcitotoxicity, anti-inflammatory, free radical scavenger/antioxidant, antiapoptotic, restorative/regenerative, calcium antagonists, adrenergic modulators, antihypertensive, nootropic/stimulator, thrombolytic properties can be screened using these models (Fig. 4.4).

TARGET SELECTION FOR DRUG SCREENING

The difficulty in distinguishing and evaluating early the reversible cellular changes from irreversible brain damage needs the identification of appropriate potential reliable soluble markers of brain damage in blood and cerebrospinal fluid (CSF) that can be used as a fast screening tool during early ischemic period[46,47] such as neuronal specific enolase (NSE), myelin basic protein (MBP), S100 protein and a brain endothelial membrane protein viz.

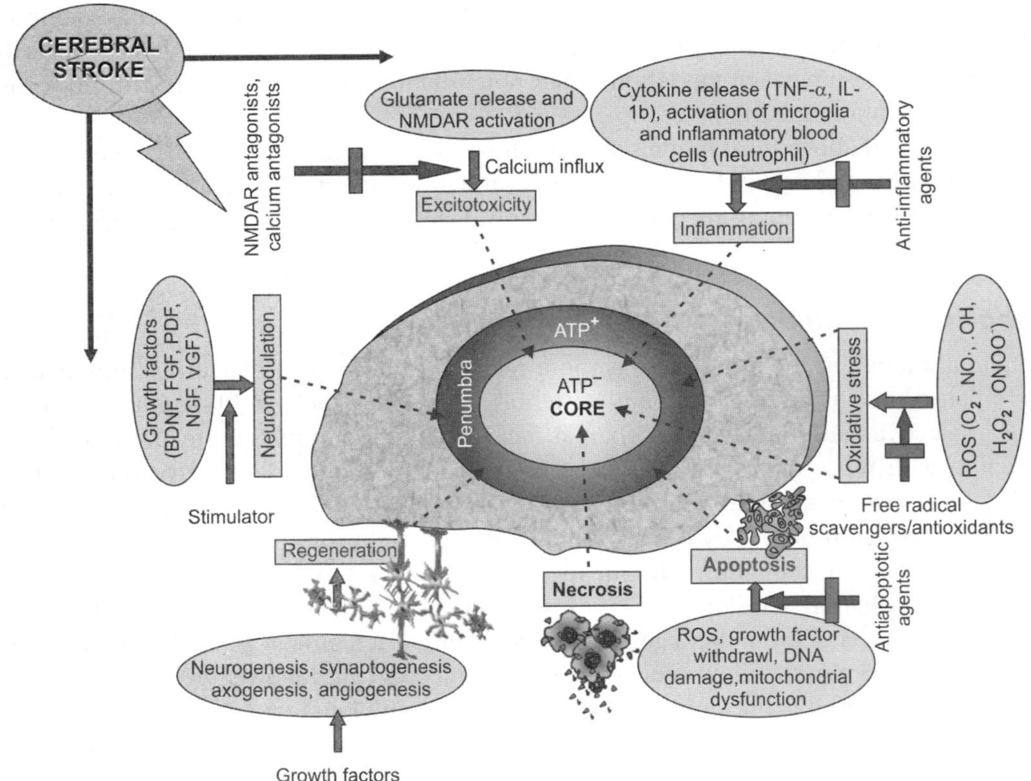

Figure 4.4: Shows various approaches of targeting cerebral stroke (*For color version see Plate 10*)

thrombomodulin or a similar molecule, based upon ischemic injury to different brain cell types. NSE is a dimeric isoenzyme of the glycolytic enzyme enolase, localized mainly within neurons and cells of neuroendocrine origin. MBP, on the other hand, is an abundant myelin membrane proteolipid produced by oligodendroglia cells. S100 is an abundant cytosolic calcium-binding protein isoforms, primarily found in glial and Schwann cells. The characteristic features: low molecular size, high organ specificity and a high degree of solubility of isoforms S100ß of S100 bear the desirable advantage to be considered as a potential biochemical marker. Further, thrombomodulin is an endothelial cell membrane-bound glycoprotein that binds thrombin, producing an anticoagulant effect. The deregulation of these marker help to presume the stroke induced injury to brain cells and their presence in blood plasma/serum and CSF make them available for early damage prediction and drug evaluation.

These markers can be easily detected with immunoassays involving western blotting, immunocytochemistry and enzyme-linked immunosorbent assay (ELISA). ELISA bears the special attention since it is rapid, highly sensitive and specific, and can estimate nano to picogram concentration in serum. The basic principle of an ELISA is to use an enzyme bound to antibody (Ab) to detect the antigen (Ag) present in the sample. The reaction can be read with the ELISA plate reader upon conversion of colorless substrate (chromogen) to a colored product by enzyme, indicating the presence of Ag:Ab complex.

METHODS OF ASSESSMENT

In Vitro Methods

Receptor Binding Assay

Glutamate mediated excitotoxicity through glutamate receptors, such as NMDA receptor, is one of the early event in cerebral ischemic cascade. Characterizations and anatomical distribution of these receptor can be analyzed with radioligand receptor binding assays. The receptor-based screening system normally uses a cell-free system or cells from a mammal. Radioligand binding assay require preparation of receptor of interest that is incubated with a suitable radioligand for an appropriate period of time and then radioactivity bound to the receptor is determined. The three major types of experiment that can be performed with this assay are saturation, kinetic and inhibition. A saturation curve is generated by keeping the amount of receptor constant and varying the concentration of radioligand. This experiment is widely used to measure receptor density (B_{max}) and affinity of the receptor for the radioligand [dissociation constant (K_d)] through quantitative autoradiography or phosphor-imaging and β/ω emission detector. The kinetic experiment on the other hand involves variable time, constant receptor and radioligand, therefore, used to determine the reverse rate constant. The inclusion of variable nonradioactive competitor in the experiment can be used to determine the affinity (Ki) of that drug for the receptor by radioligand.[48] So, what is required for the assay is crude or isolated receptors and appropriate radiolabeled or unlabeled agonist/ antagonist. Most receptor preparations can be stored at–20°C or at -80°C for extended periods of time. The important factors that should be considered to perform assay are time, buffer, concentration of radioligand, receptor and nonradioactive drug. This is also important to determine the specific binding to the receptor from nonspecific binding in the presence of an appropriate excess of unlabeled drug. However, the selectivity of a receptor may vary depending on the post-translational modifications, its state of presence, i.e. homodimers or heterodimers and association with other proteins. However, when experiments are properly conducted and appropriately interpreted, these assays can be an extremely powerful tool for the study of receptors although *in vivo* imaging are beginning to allow receptor binding to be studied at the level of intact organs or whole animals including humans and can be thus used to screen potential unlabeled neuroprotective compounds.

Methods of Oxidative Stress Measurement

Flow Cytometric Determination of ROS

The reactive oxygen species (ROS) is one of the hallmark mechanisms of brain damage following cerebral ischemia. Its estimation is therefore critical for both evaluating the cerebral damage and effectiveness of antioxidants. ROS generation can be detected by flow cytometry in cells using 2'-7'-dichlorofluorescein (DCF) and ethidium (ETH), which are the oxidation products of 2', 7'-dichlorodihydrofluorescein (DCDHF) and dihydroethidium (DHE) with a sensitivity for H_2O_2/NO-based radicals and O_2^- respectively.[49] DHE reacts with ROS and forms red fluorescent ETH. ETH binds to DNA, causing amplification of the red fluorescence signal. For the assay, single cell suspension or primary culture form various brain loci viz., cortex, striatum and hippocampus can be obtained by a combination of mechanical and enzymatic (collagenase or trypsin) dissociation methods. The enzymatic dissociation is terminated by washing the cells with phosphate buffered saline (PBS). Isolated 1×10^6 cells may be incubated with DCF or DHE in the dark and subjected to flow cytometeric estimation for signal recording at 530 nm (FL-1 channel) or 610 nm (FL-2 channel).

TBARS Reactive Substances
Brain tissue contains large amounts of polyunsaturated fatty acids (PUFA), which are particularly vulnerable to free radical attacks. An important indicator of the lipid peroxidation is conjugated diene (CD), formed from the molecular rearrangement of the carbon-centered radicals,[50] malondialdehyde (MDA) or its enol form, 4-hydoxynonenal. These products are toxic to neurons and white matter as it can induce apoptosis.[51,52] Therefore, specific quantitation of these markers is useful to reveal the extent of lipid damage as a result of oxidative stress in stroke.

Lipid peroxidation can be measured by the thiobarbituric acid test for malondialdehyde.[53-55] The pink colored MDA-TBA complex formed at low pH and high temperature may be measured at 532 nm by spectrophotometer.

Brain Glutathione Level
Glutathione is a central component in the antioxidant defences of cells present in both cytoplasmic and mitochondrial compartments. It is a tripeptide (g-L-glutamyl-L-cysteinylglycine) that is the reductant for glutathione peroxidase. Oxidation of the cysteine sulfhydryl groups joins two glutathione (GSH) molecules with a disulfide bridge to form glutathione disulfide (GSSG). Glutathione, directly detoxify reactive oxygen species and also act as a substrate for several peroxidases.[56,57] Normally, the brain maintains a high ratio of GSH/GSSG for antioxidant defence. Depletion of total glutathione and a decreased GSH/GSSG ratio are markers for oxidative stress in ischemic brain. Brain glutathione levels can be measured by the 5, 5'dithiobis-(2-nitrobenzoic acid) (DTNB)-glutathione reductase coupled assay essentially.[58] The yellow colored chromogen formed by reaction of GSH with DTNB may be read at 412 nm with spectrophotometer.

Superoxide Dismutase (SOD)
SOD activity can be measured according to the method described by Fridovich[59,60] based on the principle that xanthine and xanthine oxidase generate superoxide radicals that react with p-iodonitrotetrazolium violet (INT) to form a red formazan dye that can be measured at 505 nm or the inhibition of autoxidation of epinephrine.[61] SOD activity is expressed as U/mg protein in tissue samples.

Catalase
Similarly, catalase is one of the antioxidant enzymes responsible for scavenging free radical and can be used to as a marker of oxidative stress. Catalase activities can be determined by measuring the decrease in hydrogen peroxide concentration at 230 nm[62-64] and is expressed as U/mg protein in tissue samples.

Cerebral Infarcts Analysis Using 2,3,5-Triphenyltetrazolium Chloride (TTC)

Cerebral infarct depicts the region of brain tissue under irreversible cellular damage and can be analyzed using TTC staining (see Fig. 4.2). For the staining, animals are sacrificed after completion of ischemia or ischemia/reperfusion. The brain should be removed immediately and cut into 2 mm thick coronal slices. The brain slices should be immersed in 0.5-2% solution of 2,3,5-triphenyltetrazolium chloride in normal saline/PBS at 37 °C for 15-30 min and then fixed in 10% phosphate-buffered formalin at 4°C.[65,66] Images of brain can be captured with digital camera-based imaging and infarct volume can be analyzed by image-analysis software system, by multiplying the area of the lesion with the slice thickness. Enlargement of the infracted tissue by edema results in overestimation of infarct volume, therefore, calculation of corrected infarct volume may be used to compensate for the effect of brain edema.[67,68]

Assessment of Cellular Damage by Hematoxylin and Eosin (H and E) Staining

The cellular changes following cerebral ischemia/reperfusion injury can be analyzed with hematoxylin and eosin (H and E) staining. This is a differential stain used for detailed histological morphology analysis of intact, injured, necrotic and apoptotic cells in thin brain tissue sections with light microscopy. Hematoxylin is a base that preferentially stains acidic (nucleus containing DNA and RNA) components of the cell blue, whereas, eosin stain the basic components of cell (cytoplasm) pink. The paraffin embedded or fresh frozen cryostat brain sections are stained with H and E. The sections are dehydrated, mounted with DPX (Deoxyplasticizer Xylene) and examined under light microscope. Histological features that can be used to identify the ischemic lesion includes: diffuse pallor of the eosinophilic background, alterations in the shape, size and stainability of cellular perikarya, and vacuolation (sponginess) of the neuropil.[69]

Annexin V/PI Apoptosis/Necrosis Detection Assay

Apoptosis and necrosis are the two routes of cell loss resulting due to metabolic derangement, genomic fragmentation and ultimately a collapse of cellular infrastructure. Therefore, various changes, viz. morphological, biochemical and genomic are important factors to discriminate between apoptosis and necrosis during progression of ischemic lesion, since, it is believed that penumbral region, which is the site of apoptotic damage may be rescued with the application of appropriate therapy. One of the methods, Annexin V/PI apoptosis/necrosis detection assay, is used to detect the early changes due to apoptotic cell damage. It is based on the observation that during early stage of apoptosis induction, phosphatidylserine (PS) is translocated from the inner leaflet to the outer leaflet of the plasma membrane. PS exposure acts as a signal for elimination of apoptotic cells by phagocytic cells such as microglial in case of brain. Annexin V is a 35 kDa $Ca^{2\pm}$-binding protein with high affinity to PS.[70] Its conjugation to fluorochromes allows for the use of this assay with fluorescent microscopy, flow cytometry and real-time imaging although dyes for light and electron microscopy are also available for the use of annexin V. However, annexin V can also label necrotic cells rather makes this method less specific. But this assay, when used with vital dye propidium iodide (PI), is quite sensitive in detection of apoptosis at early stage.

TUNEL Staining

The most commonly used technique to quantify apoptosis in cells, fresh or fixed tissues is the terminal transferase-mediated dUTP nick end-labeling (TUNEL) method.[71,72] It takes advantage of the multiple free DNA ends generated by activated endonucleases to insert labeled dUTP that can be later detected by light or fluorescence microscopy. The enzyme, terminal deoxynuclotidyl transferase (TdT) specifically binds to 3'-OH ends and incorporate X-dUTP (X = biotin, DIG, or fluorescein) at sites of DNA breaks following proteolytic treatment of histological sections. Termini modified nucleotides, Avidin-peroxidase amplifies the signal and allows for examination of labeled cells under light or fluorescent microscopy, flow cytometry, or immunohistochemistry. However, a serious drawback of TUNEL remains in its ability to stain, in certain conditions, necrotic cells that can also have free DNA ends, especially after oxidant and toxic injury. But use of vital dye propidium iodide (PI) particularly in single cells study makes TUNEL assay a sensitive technique to detect apoptosis, although it should be confirmed with other reliable test methods.

Electron Microscopy

The differences in the specific morphological changes such as apoptosis or necrosis and changes in early and late apoptosis can be detected using electron microscopy (EM). It is a highly specific and sensitive test for the detection of apoptosis and can be enhanced by staining DNA fragmentation by using EM-TUNEL. Cells or brain tissue need to be fixed, stained, dehydrated, embedded, and cut into thin sections with an ultramicrotome. Sections are picked up on copper grids, post-stained, then viewed under electron microscope. This technique although is cumbersome, expensive time consuming and requires specialized training but is the gold standard in apoptosis detection.

In Vivo Methods

Neurobehavioral Assessment

The neurobehavioral break-down correlation to extent of histologically-determined stroke damage in animal models is the key event in drug development program. However, it is not always easy to interpret the behavioral recovery due to neuroprotective agent administration and from self-improvement with time. Nevertheless, inclusion of behavioral end-points in experimental stroke studies represents an important step for preclinical intervention. Therefore, to investigate interventions that at least show clinical promise, an extensive battery of behavioral tests are required. At a minimum, the tests should be able to distinguish among the levels of injury and also should also be capable of detecting beneficial effects during recovery phase. Additionally, whenever possible, procedures should be used that are not influenced by recurrent testing.

Gross neurological dysfunction of animals following cerebral ischemia (MCAo) can be evaluated based on the assessment of spontaneous motor functions on a 5-point scale (0: no deficit; 1: failure to extend left forepaw fully; 2: circling to the left; 3: falling to the left (hemiparesis); 4: non-spontaneous walking) as demonstrated by Longa et al.[33] or score that includes testing of lateral instability as 5: no deficit; 4: consistent flexion of the left forelimb; 3: reduced resistance to lateral push toward the paretic side; 2: circling to the left when held by the tail; 1: spontaneous circling to the left; 0: no spontaneous motion.[73]

In addition other behavioral tests that assess MCAo-induced deficits such as versions of the water maze (radial arm maze (RAM) or morris water maze (MWM)), hemi-neglect and sensorimotor integration, forelimb use for vertical-lateral exploration, vibrissae-evoked forelimb placing and passive and active avoidance can be performed to assure the proper evaluation of putative neuroprotective agents.[74-76] However, it is especially important to distinguish between a test compound's ability to speed up normal recovery from its ability to produce recovery of functions otherwise lost.

Imaging of Cerebral Ischemic Damage

Magnetic resonance imaging (MRI)

The infarct volume produced as a result of final outcome following ischemic stroke can be easily demarcated by various histological techniques, however, *in vivo* magnetic resonance imaging (MRI) not only measure the final infarct size, but it is also applicable to investigate the temporal evolution of ischemic lesion, differentiation of ischemic over hemorrhagic transformation and prediction of stroke severity. Neuroimaging, particularly with diffusion and perfusion MRI has been advanced to the extent that even the minute disturbances in brain following stroke in humans as well as experimental animals can be detected. Diffusion weighted imaging (DWI) is the most sensitive and accurate method for stroke detection and when linked with perfusion-weighted imaging (PWI), it can be used to review the functional status of the ischemic brain. Further, MRI when used together with the X-ray computed tomography (CT) may be helpful to demarcate the core and penumbra. Although, the frequent use of imaging techniques is not possible for routine drug screening but may be used as a standard for drug effect conformation. Therefore, it is presently considered as a gold standard in therapeutic decision making and is used as one of the paradigm in clinical trial studies for evaluation of neuroprotective agents.[77,78]

Molecular Techniques

Other methods that can be used to detect apoptosis are: DNA laddering, caspase assay, immmuno-detection of apoptotic proteins such as caspases, apoptosis inducing factor (AIF), poly (ADP-ribose) polymerase (PARP), Bcl-2 family proteins etc.[79] Besides these methods, other fast screen methods may also be used and developed *in vitro* and *in vivo* so that stroke research, particularly development of antistroke drugs becomes a reality. Studying in such lines, recently, Wang and colleagues[80] have developed an ultra-high-content chemical genetic screening assay of rat brain slices transfected with the gene for yellow fluorescent protein and subjected to OGD. The yellow fluorescent protein labeled a subset of cortical neurons that acted as sentinels in providing a measure of neuronal survival. They screened a collection of 1,200 small-molecules with known pharmacologies for potential neuroprotective properties.

CONCLUSION

Cerebral stroke is a heterogeneous neurological disorder with a complex pathophysiology and serious long-term disability. Therefore, proper understanding of the molecular mechanisms of stroke damage is imperative for bioevaluation of antistroke agents that interferes with specific or multiple mechanisms of injury, which may serve as critical determinant in drug discovery and development. However, the failures of various neuroprotective agents in clinical settings warrant the rigorous assessment of test substance having thrombolytic, neuroprotective and neurorestorative properties. The various novel putative antistroke agents can be tested preclinically using suitable *in vitro* and *in vivo* models mimicking closely the clinical situation. The testing of short- and long-term functional outcome should also be assessed in primate models as well besides rodents for optimizing efficacy and clinical safety of candidate drugs as per STAIR recommendations.

REFERENCES

1. Bonita R, Mendis S, Truelsen T, et al. The global stroke initiative. Lancet Neurol 2004;3:391-3.
2. Lopez AD, Mathers CD, Ezzati M, et al. Global and regional burden of diseases and risk factors, 2001: systematic analysis of population health data. Lancet 2006;367:1747-57.
3. Brainin M, Teuschl Y, Kalra L. Acute treatment and long-term management of stroke in developing countries. Lancet Neurol 2007;6:553-61.
4. Strong K, Mathers C, Bonita R. Preventing stroke: saving lives around the world. Lancet Neurol 2007;6:182-7.
5. Markus H S. Cerebral perfusion and stroke. J Neurol Neurosurg Psychiatry 2004:75:353-61.
6. McCulloch J, Dewar D. A radical approach to stroke therapy. Proc Natl Acad Sci USA 2001;98:10989-91.
7. Mehta SL, Manhas N, Raghubir R. Molecular targets in cerebral ischemia for developing novel therapeutics. Brain Res Rev 2007;54:34-66.
8. Hossmann KA. Thresholds of ischemic injury. In Ginsberg MD, Bogousslavsky J (Ed): Cerebrovascular Disease: Pathophysiology, Diagnosis, and Treatment. Blackwell Science, Malden, MA, USA 1998;193-204.
9. MacManus JP, Linnik MD. Gene expression induced by cerebral ischemia: an apoptotic perspective. J Cereb Blood Flow Metab 1997;17:815-32.
10. Chan PH. Reactive oxygen radicals in signaling and damage in the ischemic brain. J Cereb Blood Flow Metab 2001;21:2-14.
11. Choi DW. Ischemia-induced neuronal apoptosis. Curr Opin Neurobiol 1996;6:667-72.
12. Love S. Apoptosis and brain ischaemia. Prog Neuropsychopharmacol Biol Psychiatry 2003;27:267-82.
13. Zhang F, Yin W, Chen J. Apoptosis in cerebral ischemia: executional and regulatory signaling mechanisms. Neurol Res 2004;26:835-45.
14. Filchenkov AA, Zalessky VN. Apoptosis of cortical neurons in ischemic insult. Neurophysiol 2002; 34:468-84.
15. Danial NN, Korsmeyer SJ. Cell death: critical control points. Cell 2004;116:205-19.
16. Adams HP, del Zoppo G, Alberts MJ, et al. Guidelines for the early management of adults with ischemic stroke: a guideline from the American Heart Association/American Stroke Association Stroke Council, Clinical Cardiology Council, Cardiovascular Radiology and Intervention Council, and the Atherosclerotic Peripheral Vascular Disease and Quality of Care Outcomes in Research Interdisciplinary Working Groups: The American Academy of Neurology affirms the value of this guideline as an educational tool for neurologists. Stroke 2007;38:1655-711.
17. Stroke Therapy Academic Industry Roundtable (STAIR). Recommendations for standards regarding preclinical neuroprotective and restorative development. Stroke 1999;30:2752-8.
18. Savitz SI, Fisher M. Future of neuroprotection for acute stroke: in the aftermath of the SAINT trials. Ann Neurol 2007;61:396-402.

19. O'Collins VE, Macleod MR, Donnan GA, et al. 1026 experimental treatments in acute stroke. Ann Neurol 2006;59:467-77.
20. Savitz SI. A critical appraisal of the NXY-059 neuroprotection studies for acute stroke: a need for more rigorous testing of neuroprotective agents in animal models of stroke. Exp Neurol 2007;205:20-5.
21. Liu D, Cheng T, Guo H, et al. Tissue plasminogen activator neurovascular toxicity is controlled by activated protein C. Nat Med 2004;10:1379-83.
22. Lo EH. Combination stroke therapy: easy as APC? Nat Med 2004;10:1295-6.
23. Jiang ZG, Lu XC, Nelson V, et al. A multifunctional cytoprotective agent that reduces neurodegeneration after ischemia. Proc Natl Acad Sci USA 2006;103:1581-6.
24. Gahwiler BH. Organotypic monolayer cultures of nervous tissue. J Neurosci Methods 1981;4:329-42.
25. Stoppini L, Buchs PA, Muller D. A simple method for organotypic cultures of nervous tissue. J Neurosci Methods 1991;37:173-82.
26. Gahwiler BH, Capogna M, Debanne D, et al. Organotypic slice cultures: a technique has come of age. Trends Neurosci 1997;20:471-7.
27. Sarnowska A. Application of organotypic hippocampal culture for study of selective neuronal death. Folia Neuropathol 2002;40:101-6.
28. Sundstrom L, Morrison IIIB, Bradley M, et al. Organotypic cultures as tools for functional screening in the CNS. DDT 2005;10:993-1000.
29. Holopainen IE. Organotypic hippocampal slice cultures: a model system to study basic cellular and molecular mechanisms of neuronal cell death, neuroprotection, and synaptic plasticity. Neurochem Res 2005;30:1521-8.
30. Durukan A, Tatlisumak T. Acute ischemic stroke: overview of major experimental rodent models, pathophysiology, and therapy of focal cerebral ischemia. Pharmacol Biochem Behavior 2007;87:179-97.
31. Traystman RJ. Animal models of focal and global cerebral ischemia. ILAR J 2003;44:85-95.
32. Koizumi J, Yoshida Y, Nakazawa T, et al. Experimental studies of ischemic brain edema: 1. A new experimental model of cerebral embolism in rats in which recirculation can be introduced in the ischemic area. Jpn J Stroke 1986;8:1-8.
33. Longa EZ, Weinstein PR, Carlson S, et al. Reversible middle cerebral artery occlusion without craniectomy in rats. Stroke 1989;20:84-91.
34. Belayev L, Alonso OF, Busto R, et al. Middle cerebral artery occlusion in the rat by intraluminal suture. Neurological and pathological evaluation of an improved model. Stroke 1996; 27:1616-22.
35. Schmid-Elsaesser R, Zausinger S, Hungerhuber E, et al. A critical reevaluation of the intraluminal thread model of focal cerebral ischemia: evidence of inadvertent premature reperfusion and subarachnoid hemorrhage in rats by laser-Doppler flowmetry. Stroke 1998;29:2162-70.
36. Carmichael ST. Rodent models of focal stroke: size, mechanism, and purpose. NeuroRx 2005;2:396-409.
37. Hudzik TJ, Borrelli A, Bialobok P, et al. Long-term functional end points following middle cerebral artery occlusion in the rat. Pharmacol Biochem Behav 2000;65:553-62.
38. Lauer KK, Shen H, Stein EA, et al. Focal cerebral ischemia in rats produced by intracarotid embolization with viscous silicone. Neurol Res 2002;24:181-90.
39. Purdy PD, Devous Sr MD, Batjer HH, et al. Microfibrillar collagen model of canine cerebral infarction. Stroke 1989;20:1361-7.
40. Yang Y, Yang T, Li Q, et al. A new reproducible focal cerebral ischemia model by introduction of polyvinylsiloxane into the middle cerebral artery: a comparison study. J Neurosci Methods 2002;118: 199-206.

41. Molnar L, Hegedus K, Fekete I. A new model for inducing transient cerebral ischemia and subsequent reperfusion in rabbits without craniectomy. Stroke 1988;19:1262-6.
42. Rapp JH, Pan XM, Yu B, et al. Cerebral ischemia and infarction from atheroemboli b100 micron in size. Stroke 2003;34:1976-80.
43. Ringer AJ, Guterman LR, Hopkins LN. Site-specific thromboembolism: a novel animal model for stroke. AJNR Am J Neuroradiol 2004;25:329-32.
44. Henninger N, Eberius KH, Sicard KM, et al. A new model of thromboembolic stroke in the posterior circulation of the rat. J Neurosci Methods 2006;156:1-9.
45. Small DL, Buchan AM. Animal models. Br Med Bull 2000;56:307-17.
46. Reynolds MA, Kirchick HJ, Dahlen JR, et al. Early biomarkers of stroke. Clin Chem 2003;49:1733-9.
47. Lynch JR, Blessing R, White WD, et al. Novel diagnostic test for acute stroke. Stroke 2004;35:57-63.
48. Bylund DB, Toews ML. Radioligand binding methods: practical guide and tips. Am J Physiol 1993; 265:L421-9.
49. Korystov YN, Shaposhnikova VV, Korystova AF, et al. Detection of reactive oxygen species induced by radiation in cells using the dichlorofluorescein assay. Radiat Res 2007;168:226-32.
50. Gutteridge JM. Lipid peroxidation and antioxidants as biomarkers of tissue damage. Clin Chem 1995;41:1819-28.
51. Bruce-Keller AJ, Li YJ, Lovell MA, et al. 4-Hydroxynonenal, a product of lipid peroxidation, damages cholinergic neurons and impairs visuospatial memory in rats. J Neuropathol Exp Neurol 1998;57:257-67.
52. Montine TJ, Amarnath V, Martin ME, et al. E-4-hydroxy-2-nonenal is cytotoxic and cross-links cytoskeletal proteins in P19 neuroglial cultures. Am J Pathol 1996;148:89-93.
53. Ohkawa H, Ohishi N, Yagi K. Assay for lipid peroxides in animal tissues by thiobarbituric acid reaction. Anal Biochem 1979;95:351-8.
54. Das NP, Ratty AK. Studies on the effects of the narcotic alkaloids, cocaine, morphine, and codeine on nonenzymatic lipid peroxidation in rat brain mitochondria. Biochem Med Metab Biol 1987;37:258-64.
55. Colado MI, O'Shea E, Granados R, et al. A study of the neurotoxic effect of MDMA ('ecstasy') on 5-HT neurones in the brains of mothers and neonates following administration of the drug during pregnancy. Br J Pharmacol 1997;121:827-33.
56. Dringen R. Metabolism and functions of glutathione in brain. Prog Neurobiol 2000a;62:649-71.
57. Dringen R. Glutathione metabolism and oxidative stress in neurodegeneration. Eur J Biochem 2000b;267:4903-3.
58. Anderson ME. Determination of glutathione and glutathione disulfide in biological samples. Methods Enzymol 1985;113:548-55.
59. Fridovich I. The biology of oxygen radicals. Science 1978;201:875-80.
60. Fridovich I. Superoxide dismutases: defence against endogenous superoxide radical. Ciba Found Symp 1978;77-93.
61. Misra HP, Fridovich I. The role of superoxide anion in the autoxidation of epinephrine and a simple assay for superoxide dismutase. J Biol Chem 1972;247:3170-5.
62. Beutler E, Catalase. In Beutler E, Editor. Red Cell Metabolism: a manual of biochemical methods. Grune & Stratton, New York 1975;p. 105.
63. Aebi H. Catalase in vitro. Methods Enzymol 1984;105:121-6.
64. Luck H. Catalase methods of enzymatic analysis. Measurement of enzyme activtiy. 1963;885-8.

65. Bederson JB, Pitts LH, Germano SM, et al. Evaluation of 2,3,5-Triphenyltetrazolium chloride as a stain for detection and quantification of experimental cerebral infarction in rats. Stroke 1986;17:1304-8.
66. Benedek A, Moricz K, Zsolt Juranyia Z, et al. Use of TTC staining for the evaluation of tissue injury in the early phases of reperfusion after focal cerebral ischemia in rats. Brain Res 2006;116:159-65.
67. Takano K, Tatlisumak T, Formato JE, et al. Glycine site antagonist attenuates infarct size in experimental focal ischemia. Postmortem and diffusion mapping studies. Stroke 1997;28:1255-62.
68. Tatlisumak T, Takano K, Carano RA, et al. Delayed treatment with an adenosine kinase inhibitor, GP683, attenuates infarct size in rats with temporary middle cerebral artery occlusion. Stroke 1998;29:1952-8.
69. Li Y, Powersa C, Jianga N et al. Intact, injured, necrotic and apoptotic cells after focal cerebral ischemia in the rat. J Neurol Sci 1998;156:119-32.
70. Martin SJ, Reutelingsperger CP, McGahon AJ, et al. Early redistribution of plasma membrane phosphatidylserine is a general feature of apoptosis regardless of the initiating stimulus: Inhibition by overexpression of Bcl-2 and Abl. J Exp Med 1995;182:1545-56.
71. Labat-Moleur F, Guillermet C, Lorimier P, et al. TUNEL apoptotic cell detection in tissue sections: critical evaluation and improvement. J Histochem Cytochem 1998;46:327-34.
72. Kelly KJ, Sandoval RM, Dunn KW, et al. A novel method to determine specificity and sensitivity of the TUNEL reaction in the quantitation of apoptosis. Am J Physiol Cell Physiol 2003;284:C1309-18.
73. Zausinger S, Hungerhuber E, Baethmann A , et al. Neurological impairment in rats after transient middle cerebral artery occlusion: a comparative study under various treatment paradigms. Brain Res 2000;863:94-105.
74. DeVries AC, Nelson RJ, Traystman RJ, et al. Cognitive and behavioral assessment in experimental stroke research: will it prove useful? Neurosci Biobehav Rev 2001;25:325-42.
75. Schallert T. Behavioral tests for preclinical intervention assessment. NeuroRx 2006;3:497-504.
76. Bouet V, Freret T, Toutain J, et al. Sensorimotor and cognitive deficits after transient middle cerebral artery occlusion in the mouse. Exp Neurol 2007;203:555-67.
77. Sa de Camargo EC, Koroshetz WJ. Neuroimaging of ischemia and infarction. NeuroRx 2005;2:265-76.
78. Muir KW, Buchan A, von Kummer R, et al. Imaging of acute stroke. Lancet Neurol 2006;5:755-68.
79. Huerta S, Goulet EJ, Huerta-Yepez S, et al. Screening and detection of apoptosis. J Surg Res 2007;139:143-56.
80. Wang JK, Portbury S, Thomas MB, et al. Cardiac glycosides provide neuroprotection against ischemic stroke: discovery by a brain slice-based compound screening platform. Proc Natl Acad Sci USA 2006;103:10461-6.

CHAPTER

5

Anti-HIV Agents

INTRODUCTION

Acquired immunodeficiency syndrome (AIDS) is a viral disease caused by human immunodeficiency virus type-1 (HIV-1) and type-2 (HIV-2). Both of these are retroviruses. Since the detection of first case of AIDS in USA in 1981,[1] AIDS has spread world over acquiring pandemic proportions. It is estimated that 6 new infections occur every minute[2] and globally there are over 33 million cases of HIV infection, with AIDS now being the fourth leading cause of death worldwide.[3]

HIV infection is characterized by an acute HIV syndrome, which occurs 3-6 weeks after the primary infection, followed by a period of clinical latency and finally clinical disease after a long latency of 8-10 years. The characteristic feature of AIDS is decline in CD4+ T-cell count, which leads to severe immunodeficiency and death due to a variety of opportunistic infections.

Although a large number of highly effective antiretroviral drugs are available but their high cost, need for lifelong therapy, toxicity and emergence of resistant strains of virus have limited the use of these drugs. Also, in spite of development of various vaccine strategies, none have proved to be efficacious either in the preclinical or in the clinical phases of vaccine development.[4,5]

Therefore, there is an urgent need for safer anti-HIV drugs and a cheap and effective vaccine. The answer to all these issues can be acquired by extensive research in suitable *in vivo* and *in vitro* screening procedures. Some of the important animal models and *in vitro* methods employed in the screening of antiretroviral drugs and vaccine are described here.

IN VIVO MODELS

NONHUMAN PRIMATE MODELS FOR AIDS

Nonhuman primates have provided us with invaluable information about AIDS pathogenesis. Depending on the virus and species of the nonhuman primate, a disease resembling AIDS can be produced in these animals. Decline in CD4+ cell count and viral load are used as surrogate markers for AIDS in these models.[6] These animals can be utilized for understanding the hitherto unknown aspects about AIDS or for preclinical evaluation of potential anti-retroviral compounds and vaccine strategies.

HIV-1 virus, as such, causes infection only in chimpanzees and pigtailed macaques, besides human beings. However, with the discovery and isolation of simian immunodeficiency virus (SIV), a lentivirus, from a rhesus macaque by MD Daniel, et al[7] and subsequent demonstration that certain SIV strains could cause a disease very similar to AIDS, most of the studies regarding AIDS have been conducted in macaques using SIV as surrogate virus for HIV-1. SIV has been obtained from a number of primate species like African green monkeys, chimpanzees and sooty mangabeys.[8-10] Molecular cloning of SIV and demonstration of pathogenecity of a molecular clone, SIVmac239, has been a big advancement in the study of AIDS pathogenesis.[11]

In spite of all the similarities between SIV and HIV-1, the two differ in their envelope glycoproteins, which can lead to differing immune responses.[12] Therefore, in order to study the behavior of HIV-1 genes in SIV animal models, SIV and HIV-1 hybrid virus, i.e. SHIV (simian human immunodeficiency virus) was designed. It consists of HIV-1 genes like env, tat or rev inserted into SIV genetic background.[13,14] SHIV has been shown to be pathogenic for pigtailed macaques and rhesus monkeys.[15,16] Biggest advantage with SHIV infection is that since the envelope glycoproteins are of HIV-1 origin, SHIV infection of macaques can be used to evaluate HIV-1 envelope based vaccines.[13-17]

HIV-2 virus has also been used to study AIDS pathogenesis by infection of a variety of primates like baboons (Papio cynocephalus), pigtailed macaques (Macaca nemestrina), rhesus macaques (Macaca mulatta), cynomolgus monkeys (Macaca fascicularis) and the mangabey monkeys.[2,18-20]

At present we have a large number of nonhuman primate models of AIDS utilizing different animal species or strains of the virus. Some important models include the following:

Chimpanzees (Pan Troglodytes)

Chimpanzees have been proposed to be the most likely origin of AIDS in humans.[21] They offer the best animal model for studying AIDS as they have been shown to be infectable with HIV-1.[22] Although infectable with HIV-1, the primary infection in chimpanzees is associated with only mild symptoms and no clinical disease or immune impairment is apparent.[23] However, Novembre et al have reported the development of AIDS in a chimpanzee over 10 years post-infection. The disease was characterized by plasma viremia, CD4+ T-cell decline, opportunistic infections and the infection could be transmitted to other chimpanzees by blood transfusion.[24]

Shibata et al have reported the cultivation of a HIV-1 strain, HIV-$1_{DH12,}$ from a patient of AIDS that can establish infection in chimpanzees. They isolated viruses from 23 patients by cell free infection of fresh activated human peripheral blood mononuclear cells (PBMCs). Out of these, three strains viz. HIV-$1_{DH12,}$ HIV-1_{DH20} and HIV-1_{DH29} could infect the chimpanzee PBMCs. Further screening with PBMCs from other chimpanzees showed that HIV-1_{DH12} produced rapid and highly cytopathic infection and exhibited a dual tropism for T-cells and macrophages. Injection of HIV-1_{DH12} isolate into a chimpanzee led to establishment of infection within 1 week, with virus being recoverable by cocultivation of chimpanzee PBMCs with human PBMCs. The animal also developed lymphadenopathy and disseminated rash during the acute phase and levels of viremia during the acute phase and 6 months post-infection were similar to that observed in humans.[25]

Chimpanzees have greater than 98% genetic identity to the humans[26] and are infectable with HIV-1 virus. Therefore, they have played a crucial role in the development of our current concepts about HIV-1, like modes of transmission, the immune response to infection and various other aspects about AIDS pathogenesis. Chimpanzees are also suited for preclinical evaluation of antiretroviral drugs and vaccines.

However, being endangered species, the number of chimpanzees available for study is limited and their maintenance is expensive. Thus ethical and practical problems can limit their use.

Pigtailed Macaques (*Macaca Nemestrina*)

Pigtailed macaques are the only nonhuman primates, other than chimpanzees, which can be infected with HIV-1. Agy et al showed that HIV-1 infection could lead to acute and persistent infection in pigtailed macaques. The animals developed lymphadenopathy and rash over the abdominal and inguinal regions, HIV DNA could be detected in PBMC and seroconversion was observed in these animals.[27] However, Frumkin et al observed that although pigtailed macaques could be infected with HIV-1, the virus could not be recovered from the infected animals after 2 months and there were no disturbances in immune system.[28] It has, therefore, been proposed that use of HIV-1/2 chimeric viruses or SHIV chimeras for infecting these animals may be able to overcome the block in replication normally seen in these animals.[18-29] Pigtailed macaques are also infectable with HIV-2.[18]

Pigtailed macaques have been used to study different routes of transmission of HIV-1 like vertical, oral, anal and intravenous.[30,31] These animals have also been employed in preclinical studies of antiretroviral drugs like AZT.[28] These animals can give important insights into the acquired immune response to HIV-1 and have been used for anti-HIV vaccine testing.[32]

The advantages offered by pigtailed macaques are that they are not endangered species, available in large number and are not expensive to maintain.

Baboons (Papio Cynocephalus)

Baboons have been shown to develop a disease, very similar to human AIDS, by HIV-2. Virus isolate and baboon subspecies dictate the development of AIDS like disease in baboons with disease being produced by HIV-2_{UC2} isolate in hamadryas subspecies of baboons.[17] The disease progression in baboons is similar to that observed in the chronic HIV-1 infection in humans and is characterized by an acute phase, lasting up to 20 weeks, followed by a clinically healthy phase lasting 4-7 years and subsequently development of AIDS like disease. Lymphadenopathy, petechial rash over abdomen and back of the animal, high plasma viremia, a decline in CD4+ cell count and subsequent development of cytotoxic T-lymphocyte (CTL) response and neutralizing antibodies characterize the acute phase. In the clinically healthy phase, the plasma viremia is low but the onset of AIDS like disease is associated with increase in plasma viremia, fall in level of CD4+ T-cell counts and it manifests as gingivitis, hair loss, interstitial pneumonia, cachexia and Kaposi's sarcoma like lesions on limbs.[2]

Due to similarity of disease progression in the humans and baboons, it is possible to study pathogenesis of AIDS in baboons including the immunobiology of viral latency, mechanisms of disease progression, the lymphatic tissue pathogenesis, the dynamics of viral-host interactions, the acquired immune response and also the modes of transmission of HIV. Baboons are especially suitable for preclinical assessment of efficacy of antiviral drugs and vaccines.[2]

A variety of advantages are offered by baboons as animal model for AIDS:

- Baboons are not endangered species and available in sufficient numbers to carry out studies.
- They are physiologically and genetically related to humans[33] and have similar immune response, so are more suitable for preclinical vaccine efficacy studies.
- Since the HIV infection in baboon subspecies are virus isolate specific, mechanisms of innate and acquired resistance to HIV infection can be studied in these animals. This will be helpful in developing new targets for vaccine and therapeutics.

However, lack of infectivity of baboons with HIV-1 is a significant disadvantage of these animals.

Rhesus Macaques (Macaca Mulatta)

Asian rhesus macaques are readily infectable with SIV and have been widely used for AIDS studies. Rhesus monkeys are also infectable with HIV-220 and SHIV.[34] With marked similarity in the disease caused by SIV and HIV-1, rhesus macaques infected with SIV have been used to assess almost all aspects about the pathogenesis of AIDS like modes of transmission, genetics of lentiviruses, the host immune response, potential antiretroviral drugs and vaccination strategies.[17]

However, as referred to above, SIV differs from HIV-1 in its envelope glycoproteins, so efficacy of envelope-based vaccines in these animals may not be reflective of their efficacy in humans. Also since protease inhibitors are not effective against SIV proteases, therefore, it is not possible to study combination therapy in these SIV infected animals.[6]

SEVERE COMBINED IMMUNODEFICIENCY (SCID) MICE MODELS

SCID mice were first described in 1983 by Bosma et al.[35] These mice have an autosomal recessive mutation that impairs the rearrangement of B and T-cell receptor genes and thus immunocompetancy of these animals.[35] As a result, the SCID mice are not able to produce antibodies or reject foreign tissue grafts. It is, therefore, possible to transplant human tissues into these mice without the elicitation of graft-versus-host disease. Taking this lead a variety of human immune tissues capable of being infected with HIV-1 have been xenotransplanted into the SCID mice to study important aspects of the HIV-1 infection like its pathogenesis, modes of transmission, safety and efficacy of antiretroviral drugs and vaccines, etc.

SCID-hu Mice (Thy/Liv Model)

SCID-hu mice are constructed by co-transplantation of human fetal thymus and liver fragments under the renal capsule of 2-3 months old SCID mice. These liver and thymic fragments fuse to form a conjoined organ in which the fetal liver acts as a source of multipotent hemopoietic stem cells while thymus provides the appropriate environment for maturation of T and B-cells.[36] Human thymopoiesis can take place for over a year in these mice and phenotypically normal and functional T and B-cells of human origin can be detected in the peripheral circulation of these mice.[36-38] These T-cells, in the process of maturation, become tolerant to the major histocompatibility complex (MHC) background of the mice and thus do not mount any host vs graft attack.[39]

The SCID-hu mice are infected by direct injection of HIV-1 isolate into the graft tissue, 3-4 months after transplantation. The pathological changes induced by HIV-1 infection can then be studied by analyzing the grafts and the circulating peripheral T-cells at varying times after infection using various methods like *in situ* hybridization, immunohistochemistry, PCR, ELISA, etc. The animals can be treated with anti-HIV drugs at any time before or after the infection and their effects are studied using suitable analytical parameters.[37]

The advantages offered by SCID-hu mice for studies on AIDS include:

- SCID-hu mice provide excellent *in vivo* environment for studying the efficacy and toxicity of antiretroviral drugs. A number of anti-HIV drugs like zidovudine, nevirapine and bicyclam have been shown to be efficacious in this model.[40-42]
- SCID-hu mice can be used to identify new targets for therapeutic intervention.
- Active human thymopoiesis can occur for extended periods of time in these mice.

However, some potential disadvantages of these mice are:

- Due to the immunocompromized nature of these animals, the upkeep of these animals requires very stringent, pathogen-free conditions thus posing difficulties in maintenance.
- Good surgical skills are required for construction of these mice.
- The study may be confounded by physiological variables of the mice. Cytokines and other growth factors required for growth and optimal function of the engrafted cells are lacking in these mice.
- HIV infection can only be produced by intragraft injection and the infection is mainly limited to the graft tissue. Thus peripheral immune system cannot be studied.
- The data obtained from these mice may not be generalizable to adults as only human fetal tissue is transplanted.
- Some SCID/SCID mice have been shown to produce antibodies and mature lymphocytes due to somatic reversion events. This may interfere with engraftment.[43,44]

Modifications

In order to enhance the efficacy of Thy/Liv graft in populating the peripheral lymphoid organs with T-cells, Kollmann et al transplanted the fetal human thymus and liver fragments under both the renal capsules of the mice. This led to increased number of circulating T-cells and offered the advantage of infection of the animal by intraperitoneal route, in addition to the intragraft route. Disseminated infection was also observed in these mice.[45]

Hu-PBL-SCID Mice

Hu-PBL-SCID mice are constructed by injecting human peripheral blood leucocytes (PBL) into the SCID mice. The PBL are taken from a HIV-1 negative, Ebstein Barr Virus (EBV)-negative donor and injected intraperitoneally into the mice, 2 weeks prior to exposure with the virus isolates. The cells, being of adult human origin, get activated in the mice and thus are easily infectable with HIV-1 virus.[46] Intraperitoneal injection of HIV-1 isolate leads to high titers of plasma viremia and depending on the tropism of the virus injected, a decline in the CD4+ T-cells. Thus this model provides good *in vivo* environment for studying the pathogenesis of HIV.

Further, Mosier et al have shown that donors who have been vaccinated with anti-gp160 vaccines can pass on the resistance to the hu-PBL-SCID mice.[47] These mice can therefore serve as a model for preclinical evaluation of anti-HIV vaccines. Hu-PBL-SCID mice can also be used to study the efficacy of antiviral drugs and immunomodulators.[48]

Human-CBL-nSCID Mice

Human-Cord Blood Leukocyte-neonatal SCID mice were developed to mimic pediatric HIV infection. These mice are constructed by intraperitoneally injecting human cord blood leukocytes (hu-CBL) into 1-4 days old neonatal C.B-17 SCID/SCID mice. These cells contain immature T and B-cells, more CD4+ than CD8+ T-cells and few memory cells. Following injection, these cells engraft in the spleen, lymph nodes and are also present in high number in the peripheral circulation and can be detected for upto 8 weeks postimplantation. Two weeks after the CBL injection, the mice are injected with HIV-1 isolates, intraperitoneally. At various time points after infection, blood samples can be collected to study the viral antigenemia and effect of HIV-1 on the blood cell counts or the animals can be sacrificed and their organs subjected to various analytical procedures like coculturing and PCR analyses to establish pathological changes induced by HIV-1 infection. These mice can be used to study the peculiarities of pediatric AIDS and test strategies for prevention of HIV-1 infection of the neonates.[49]

NOD/SCID BLT Mice

Non-obese diabetic (NOD)/SCID bone marrow-liver-thymus (BLT) mice are constructed by transplanting of human bone marrow, liver and the thymus under the kidney capsule. NOD/SCID mice are characterized by reduced NK cell levels and transplantation of the liver, and thymus enhances the reconstitution of the human immune system. This model is used for the studies of HIV latency and could be very helpful in antiretroviral drug screening.[50]

U-937-SCID Mice

U-937-SCID mice are constructed by injecting human U-937 tumor cells, subcutaneously, into 4-5 week old C.B-17 SCID/SCID female mice. In order to increase the take of grafted tissue the mice are treated with either polyclonal sheep antimurine IFNα/β or antimouse granulocyte mAb given 1 day before and on days 3 and 7 after tumor cell injection. Various protocols are followed for HIV-1 infection of these mice. The infection can be accomplished by injecting either *in vitro* HIV-1 infected human PBMCs or cell free HIV-1 isolates simultaneously with the tumor cells or the tumor cells can be injected with cell free HIV-1, 20 days postimplantation. A long lasting HIV-1 infection (for up to 3 months), with high levels of infectious particles at the tumor site and p24 antigenemia, is seen. It was shown that treatment of these animals with AZT could dramatically reduce the p24 antigenemia and serum level of HIV-1 RNA copies as well as suppress the HIV-1 infection at the tumor level.[51]

This model offers the advantage of high reproducibility, ease of establishment of the tumor cells, high levels of viremia, well defined viral kinetics and long-lasting HIV-1 infection which can be very valuable for the screening of potential antiretroviral compounds. This model also allows the serial implantation of the tumor cells from HIV-1 infected and drug treated mice to other naïve mice and thus long-term selection of resistant infections can be studied.[51]

MO-MSV INDUCED TUMORS IN NMRI MICE

Antiretroviral compounds can be screened by studying the inhibitory effect of these compounds on Moloney-MSV (Mo-MSV) induced tumor formation in NMRI mice. Briefly, inject 2-3 day old NMRI mice with 100 focus-forming units of Mo-MSV subcutaneously in the left leg and treat the animals with test compound for 5 days. Treatment is started 2-4 hr prior to the inoculation with MSV. Antiretroviral potential is estimated by noting the effect on time to appearance of visible tumor formation and time to death of animal. In normal course, the virus causes tumor formation within 4-5 days and leads to death within 10-12 days postinfection.[52-54]

TRANSGENIC ANIMAL MODELS

Transgenic Mice

Transgenic mice expressing individual HIV-1 viral genes like *gag, pol, nef, env* or even full length HIV-1 DNA have provided substantial evidence about the role played by these genes in the pathogenesis of AIDS. Some of the important insights gained using transgenic mice are described below.

Hanna et al constructed transgenic mice expressing full-length proviral DNA of HIV-1. These animals developed severe immune disease resembling AIDS in humans. The disease was characterized with thymic atrophy, depletion of CD4+ cells, architectural changes in lymphoid organs, wasting and failure to thrive, diarrhea, interstitial lymphocytic pneumonitis, tubular interstitial nephritis and early death.[55] It has further been shown that *nef* gene is a major determinant of pathogenecity of HIV virus and severity of disease is positively correlated with the level of expression of *nef* gene.[56]

The role of *tat* gene in the development of Kaposi's sarcoma has been confirmed by studies on *tat* transgenic mice.[57] It has also been shown that *tat* causes upregulation of TNFα in activated T-cells, which may play a role in AIDS pathogenesis.[58] *env* gene has been shown to be important in the development of neurological lesions associated with AIDS.[59,60]

The potential role of transgenic mice in the development of anti-HIV drugs that target specific genes like *nef* or *tat* is rapidly emerging and these animals will play a significant role in the future in the better understanding of HIV pathogenesis as well as in drug development.

Humanized Transgenic Mice

There are several transgenic murine lines humanized to enhance their ability to maintain HIV replication. Such models can be infected up to a year and are used as chronic models of HIV infection.

The Rag2-/-γc-/- mice are double knockout mice that lack T, B and NK cells. This allows easy transplantation of human stem cells which are often rejected by NK cells. Humanization with hematopoietic stem cells, leads to development of human T, B, and dendritic cells in the blood, lymphoid and mucosal tissues and allows mice to be infected intrarectally or intravaginally that mimics natural way of HIV transmission.[61]

Transgenic Rats

Human CD4 and CCR5 (hCD4/hCCR5)-transgenic rats are genetically constructed on an outbred *Sprague-Dawley* rats by the introduction of hCD4 and hCCR5 vectors. hCD4/hCCR5 rats express the HIV-1 receptor complex on CD4 T cells, macrophages, and microglia and are susceptible to HIV-1 infection expressing viral gene products and even displaying a low-level viremia.[62] This model has shown to be well suited for the screening of new antiviral compounds targeting viral entry or reverse transcriptase.[63]

Transgenic Rabbits

Transgenic rabbits expressing human CD4 receptors have been developed. These can be used to study the pathogenesis of disease as well as for testing of potential antiretroviral drug.[44]

IN VITRO MODELS

Mono Mac 1-Cell Line

Mononuclear cells (monocyte/macrophage) are major targets for HIV. Mono Mac 1-cell line exhibits all the properties of mature monocytes including phagocytosis, surface marker expression, etc.[64] Therefore, Mono Mac 1 is being considered as an appropriate model system to study the HIV-1 infection of the mononuclear cells.[65]

Procedure: Mono Mac 1-cell line is cultured in RPM1 1640 medium containing 10% heat inactivated fetal bovine serum, penicillin-streptomycin, L-glutamine, nonessential amino acids and sodium pyruvic acid. Bacterial Lipopolysaccharides (LPS) or phorbol 12-myristate 13-acetate (PMA) are added in the culture for differentiation of Mono Mac 1-cells into a more mature phenotype i.e. macrophage. After this flow cytometric analysis is performed and untreated and LPS treated cells are incubated for 30 min on ice with saturation of monoclonal antibodies against CD4 (SIM.d), CCR5 (clone 2D7), CXCR4 (clone 12G5), CCR3 (clone 7B11) and CD14 (clone CRIS-6). Cells are again incubated for 30 min on ice with concentration of a secondary antibody of R-phycoerythrin-conjugated goat antimouse immunoglobulin G. Cells are resuspended in phosphate buffered saline (PBS). Controls consist of commercial isotype-matched murine monoclonal antibodies.[66]

After this virus stocks are prepared using NL4-3 luciferase backbone (pNL4-3-luc-ER) and pc DNA/Amp based vectors coding for HIV-1 ADA (R5), JR-FL(R-5) or amphotropic murine leukemia virus (AMLV) envelope proteins.[66] Infectivity experiments are done using recombinant luciferase-encoding and infectious viruses to confirm increased virus production in differentiated Mono Mac 1 cells.

To perform viral infection assay, treated and LPS-treated cells are seeded in 96-well dishes in culture medium and infected with luciferase-encoding virions (10 ng of p24). After 72 hr supernatant is removed and incubation is performed with cell culture lysis buffer [triphosphate, dithiothereitol (DTT), triton, glycerol] for 30 min at room temperature. An aliquot (20 ml) from lysate is mixed with luciferase assay buffer. Luciferase activity is measured by microplate luminometer. After that undifferentiated Mono Mac 1-cells are infected with HIV-1 (X4) or HIV-1 (R5) (100 ng of p24) in culture medium for at least two hours at 37°C. Cells are washed with ice-cold PBS and resuspended in cold RPMI 10 consisting of pronase for 5 min at 40°C. Later pronase is eliminated from cells by washing these cells with ice-cold RPMI 10 (with 10%) Fetal Bovine Serum and with ice-cold PBS. Semiquantitative PCR analysis is done to detect viral (HIV-1) DNA levels.[67]

Visna Virus Model

Visna virus is a nononcogenic retrovirus that causes chronic diseases of sheep including pneumonia, neurological diseases, etc. and affects mononuclear cells.[68,69] As this virus is closely related to HIV and nonpathogenic to humans, it is used to study HIV replication *in vitro* and to inhibit reverse transcriptase as well as to identify novel potential agents for the treatment of HIV. [70, 71]

Method: A line of sheep choroids plexus (SCP) cells is established from a newborn lamb as described by Sundquist and Larner[72] and monolayer cultures are maintained in EMEM containing 10% fetal bovine serum. Visna virus (strain 1514) is used to infect the cells. SCP cell monolayers are washed with PBS and viruses adsorbed at 37°C for 1 hr in serum free EMEM. After this EMEM is added with 1% heat inactivated lamb serum and gentamicin is added. Medium is changed after 2 days and incubated till marked virus induced pathology is observed. After that cells and supernatant are stored at –70° C. Titration of virus is done in six-well SCP cell cultures by plaque assay. Using phosphate-buffered saline cells are rinsed and infected with virus (200 µl vol). After one hour these cells are cultured in EMEM, which contains 1% heat-inactivated lamb serum, 25 µg of gentamicin/ml and 0.5% agarose. After 6 days, cell monolayers are stained with 1% crystal violet in 20% ethanol.

Plaque reduction assays are performed in six-well SCP plates.[73] Viruses that can produce 100 to 200 plaques are exposed to test compound for 10 days and then plaques are counted. Cytopathic effect (CPE) inhibition assays are performed in 96-well SCP microtiter plates.[74] Cells are infected prior to addition of test compound. After 5 days of incubation, CPE in untreated cultures and treated cultures are compared. Reverse transcriptase assay is performed for reverse transcriptase activity.[75]

Human Lymphocytes

CEM Cells

Lymphoblastoid leukemia cell line (CEM) was obtained from a Caucasian patient with acute T-lymphoblastic leukemia and is widely used.

HIV induces giant cell formation in these cell cultures. Antiretroviral activity can be assessed by observing the inhibition of giant cell formation. Briefly, 2-3 × 10^5 cultured cells per ml are seeded in wells of a 96 well microtiter plate. The test compounds are added after dissolving in cell culture medium. Four days after infecting the cells with 100 CCID50 (50% cell culture infective dose) of HIV-1 or HIV-2, giant cell formation is observed microscopically.[53]

MT-4 Cells

MT-4 cells are human T cells isolated from a patient with adult T-cell leukemia. Protection against HIV induced cytopathogenicity in MT-4 cells is an important *in vitro* screening test for antiretroviral drugs. Briefly, MT-4 cells are infected with 100 CCID50 of HIV viruses in a microtiter plate and incubated at 37°C for 90 min. Now, 5×10^4 infected MT-4 cells are transferred to wells of a 96-well microplate that contain 100 microliter of various concentrations of test compounds. These are then incubated for 5 days at 37°C. Whole of the procedure is carried out in parallel with mock-infected MT-4 cells. After the 5 days incubation, cells from both the groups are stained with trypan blue and number of viable cells determined in a blood cell counting chamber. Concentration of compound that protects 50% of HIV infected cells (ED50) and concentration of compound that reduces viability of mock-infected cells by 50% (CD50) are determined.[52,76]

C8166 Cells

C8166 cells are primary umbilical cord blood T lymphocytes immortalized by human T cell leukemia virus (HTLV-1) from adult T cell leukemia. These cells are commonly used as an *in vitro* model for antiretroviral drug screening, because of their ability to form syncytia in the presence of HIV. Briefly, C8166 cells (4×10^4 cells per well), infected with HIV are seeded on 96-well plate in the absence or presence of various concentrations of tested compounds in triplicate. Cells are incubated at 37°C for different time periods and the cytopathic effect (CPE) is measured by counting the number of syncytia under an inverted microscope. Then EC50 is calculated.[77,78]

Murine C3H-3T3 Embryo Fibroblast Cells

Antiretroviral compounds can be screened for activity against MSV by studying their inhibitory effect on Moloney-MSV (Mo-MSV) induced transformation of murine C3H-3T3 embryo fibroblast cells. Procedure, as described by Balzarini et al (1989) is briefly described. 5×10^5 C3H-3T3 embryo fibroblast cells per ml are seeded into wells of a microplate and grown to confluency. Twenty four hours later, these are infected with 80 focus forming units of Mo-MSV for 60-90 min at 37°C. Subsequently, the medium in the microplate is replaced with fresh culture medium containing various concentrations of the test compound. Six days later, transformation of cell culture is examined under microscope and ED_{50} (concentration of compound that inhibits Mo-MSV induced cell transformation by 50%) is calculated.[52,53,76]

Human PBMC Cultures

Peripheral blood mononuclear cells are collected from healthy donors and cultured for 3 days at 37°C after stimulating with phytohemagglutinin. Subsequently 0.5×10^6 cells are seeded into wells of a 48 well microplate. Test compounds are added in various concentrations after dissolving in cell culture medium and the wells are infected with HIV-1 virus. On day 12, the cell supernatant is collected and analyzed for HIV-1 core antigen using a p24 antigen ELISA kit. EC_{50} (concentration of compound required to inhibit viral replication, i.e. p24 production in PBMC culture by 50%) and EC_{90} (concentration of compound required to inhibit viral replication, i.e. p24 production in PBMC culture by 90%) are calculated.[53]

Human Embryonic Stem Cells

H9 (WA09) is one of the most widely used human embryonic stem (HES) cell lines. HES cells are derived from the inner cell mass of blastocyst-stage human embryos and are widely used for antiviral drug screening.[79]

IN VITRO MODEL SYSTEMS FOR HIV IN THE CNS

Blood-Brain Barrier (BBB) Models

The failure of blood-brain barrier (BBB) structural integrity and its functions play a pivotal role in the development of HIV induced CNS destruction. Various *in vitro* models of the BBB have been developed to reproduce the key physical and biochemical properties of the mammalian BBB. These models are used to investigate various aspects of HIV infection including the infectivity of the endothelial cell of the BBB by HIV and mechanisms of transendothelial migration of monocytes.[80]

Macaque BBB Model

Microvascular brain endothelial cells (MBEC) are isolated from rhesus macaque at necropsy [80] and cultured in medium containing M 199, 10% FCS, 5% human serum, 15 mg/ml endothelial cell growth supplement, insulin-transferring-selenium premix and antibiotics. After one week, distinct colonies are transferred to 2% gelatin coated tissue culture flasks.

Autologous astrocytes are cultured.[81] Small pieces of brain are incubated for 30 min in the presence of trypsin and DNAse. Fetal calf serum is added to inhibit trypsin. Cells are then passed through a 120 μm nylon mesh, pelleted (1000 rpm) and plated at 10^5/ml in M199, 5% FCS. Medium is replaced on the next day. EDTA washing and quick trypsinization is performed for removal of astrocytes. Astrocytes are subcultured at a ratio of 1:4.

MBEC are grown onto 3 μm PET filter inserts precoated with fibronectin in 2% gelatin solution. After 5 days, monolayers are stained with hematoxylin and eosin to observe confluence and astrocytes are then transferred onto the lower layer of the filter. Astrocytes are allowed to adhere for 2 hr in a humidified atmosphere and MBEC are added to the upper well and astrocytes to the lower well. After 5 days in culture, immunocytochemical analysis is done to confirm the presence of the markers, i.e. GLUT-1, CD 147.[82]

Cultured Brain Microvascular Endothelial Cells

In this model human endothelial cells are taken from umbilical cord and astrocytes from human cerebrum. These cells are cocultured *on opposite* sides of a porous (3 mm diameter pores) tissue culture support. Astrocytes penetrate the tissue culture barrier through these pores and come in contact with endothelial cells. In this model system BBB protein, brain type glucose transporter and glutamyl transpeptidase are expressed.[83]

Modification

In this model human umbilical cord endothelial cells and rat fetal astrocytes are used and cocultured.[84]

DIV-BBB MODEL

Brain or peripheral microvascular endothelial cells (BMEC) are cultured in hollow fiber capillaries inside a sealed chamber and endothelial cells are grown intraluminally in the presence of astrocytes, which are cultured albuminally. The hollow fiber cartridge system is made up of artificial capillaries that are in contact with luminal pulsatile flow. A high transendothelial electrical resistance of 1500-2000 ohms/cm^2 is used that mimics *in vivo*. In this model HIV infection is maintained for a longer period in BMEC.[85,86]

This model is used to study the mechanisms of viral persistence, viral entry into the CNS through the BBB and viral interference with tight junction formation.

REFERENCES

1. Gottlieb MS, Schroff R, Schanker HM, et al. Pneumocystis carinii pneumonia and mucosal candidiasis in previously healthy homosexual men: Evidence of a new acquired cellular immunodeficiency. N Engl J Med 1981;305:1425-31.
2. Locher CP, Witt SA, Herndier BG, et al. Baboons as an animal model for human immunodeficiency virus pathogenesis and vaccine development. Immunol Rev 2001;183:127-40.
3. Fauci AS, Lane HC. Human immunodeficiency virus (HIV) disease: AIDS and related disorders. In: Braunwald E, Fauci AS, Kasper DL, Hauser SL, Longo DL, Jameson JL (Eds). Harrison's Principles of Internal Medicine. New York: McGraw Hill 2001;1852-1912.
4. Graham BS, McElrath JM, Connor RI, et al. Analysis of intercurrent human immunodeficiency type-1 infections in phase I and II trials of candidate AIDS vaccines. J Infect Dis 1998;177:310-9.
5. Walker MC, Fast PE. Clinical trials of candidate AIDS vaccines. AIDS 1994;8:S213-36.
6. Haigwood NL. Progress and challenges in therapies for AIDS in nonhuman primate models. J Med Primatol 1999;28:154-63.
7. Daniel MD, Letvin NL, King NW, et al. Isolation of T-cell tropic HTLV-III-like retrovirus from macaques. Science 1985;228:1201-4.
8. Ohta Y, Masuda T, Tsujimoto H, et al. Isolation of simian immunodeficiency virus from African green monkeys and seroepidemiologic survey of the virus in various nonhuman primates. Int J Cancer 1988;41:115-22.
9. Peeters M, Honore C, Huet T, et al. Isolation and partial characterization of an HIV-related virus occurring naturally in chimpanzees in Gabon. AIDS 1989;3:625-30.
10. Fultz PN, McClure HM, Anderson DC, et al. Isolation of a T-lymphotropic retrovirus from naturally infected sooty mangabey monkeys (Cercocebus atys). Proc Natl Acad Sci USA 1986;83:5286-90.
11. Kestler HW, Kodama T, Ringer D, et al. Induction of AIDS in rhesus monkeys by molecularly cloned simian immunodeficiency virus. Science 1990;248:1109-12.
12. Weiss RA, Clapham PR, Weber JN, et al. Variable and conserved neutralization antigens of human immunodeficiency virus. Nature 1986;324:572-5.
13. Lu Y, Salvato MS, Pauza CD, et al. Utility of SHIV for testing HIV-1 vaccine candidates in macaques. J Acquir Immune Defic Syndr Hum Retrovirol 1996;12:99-106.
14. Li J, Lord CI, Haseltine WA, et al. Infection of cynomolgus monkeys with a chimeric HIV-1/SIVmac virus that expresses the HIV-1 envelope glycoproteins. J Acquir Immune Defic Syndr 1992;5:639-46.
15. Joag SV, Li Z, Foresman L, et al. Chimeric simian/human immunodeficiency virus that causes progressive loss of CD4+ T cells and AIDS in pig-tailed macaques. J Virol 1996;70:3189-97.

16. Reimann KA, Li JT, Voss G, et al. An env gene derived from a primary human immunodeficiency virus type-1 isolate confers high in vivo replicative capacity to a chimeric simian/human immunodeficiency virus in rhesus monkeys. J Virol 1996;70:3198-206.
17. Locher CP, Barnett SW, Herndier BG, et al. Human immunodeficiency virus-2 infection in baboons is an animal model for human immunodeficiency virus pathogenesis in humans. Arch Pathol Lab Med 1998;122:523-33.
18. Otten RA, Brown BG, Simon M, et al. Differential replication and pathogenic effects of HIV-1 and HIV-2 in Macaca nemestrina. AIDS 1994;8:297-306.
19. Putkonen P, Bottiger B, Warstedt K, et al. Experimental infection of cynomolgus monkeys (Macaca fascicularis) with HIV-2. J Acquir Immune Defic Syndr 1989;2:366-73.
20. Nicol I, Flamminio-Zola G, Dubouch P, et al. Persistent HIV-2 infection of rhesus macaque, baboon, mangabeys. Intervirology 1989;30:258-67.
21. Gao F, Bailes E, Robertson DL, et al. Origin of HIV-1 in the chimpanzee Pan troglodytes troglodytes. Nature 1999;397:436-41.
22. Fultz PN, McClure HM, Swenson CR, et al. Persistent infection of chimpanzees with human T-lymphotropic virus type III/lymphadenopathy-associated virus: A potential model for acquired immunodeficiency syndrome. J Virol 1986;58:116-24.
23. Fultz PN. Nonhuman primate models for AIDS. Clin Infect Dis 1993;17:S230-35.
24. Novembre FJ, Saucier M, Anderson DC, et al. Development of AIDS in a chimpanzee infected with human immunodeficiency virus type-1. J Virol 1997;71:4086-91.
25. Shibata R, Hoggan MD, Broscius C, et al. Isolation and characterization of a syncytium-inducing, macrophage/T-cell line-tropic human immunodeficiency virus type-1 isolate that readily infects chimpanzee cells in vitro and in vivo. J Virol 1995;69:4453-62.
26. King MC, Wilson AC. Evolution at two levels in humans and chimpanzees. Science 1975;188:107-16.
27. Agy MB, Frumkin LR, Corey L, et al. Infection of Macaca nemestrina by human immunodeficiency virus type-1. Science 1992;257:103-6.
28. Frumkin LR, Agy MB, Coombs RW, et al. Acute infection of Macaca nemestrina by human immunodeficiency virus type-1. Virology 1993;195:422-31.
29. Kimball LE, Bosch ML. In vitro HIV-1 infection in Macaca nemestrina PBMCs is blocked at a step beyond reverse transcription. J Med Primatol 1998;27:99-103.
30. Ochs HD, Morton WR, Kuller LD, et al. Intra-amniotic inoculation of pigtailed macaque (Macaca nemestrina) fetuses with SIV and HIV-1. J Med Primatol 1993;22:162-8.
31. Bosch ML, Schmidt A, Agy MB, et al. Infection of Macaca nemestrina neonates with HIV-1 via different routes of inoculation. AIDS 1997;11:1555-63.
32. Kent SJ, Zhao A, Best SJ, et al. Enhanced T-cell immunogenicity and protective efficacy of a human immunodeficiency virus type-1 vaccine regimen consisting of consecutive priming with DNA and boosting with recombinant fowlpox virus. J Virol 1998;72:10180-8.
33. Rogers J, Hixson JE. Baboons as an animal model for genetic studies of common human disease. Am J Hum Genet 1997;61:489-93.
34. Bogers WM, Dubbes R, ten Haaft P, et al. Comparison of in vitro and in vivo infectivity of different clade B HIV- 1 envelope chimeric simian/human immunodeficiency viruses in Macaca mulatta. Virology 1997; 236:110-7.
35. Bosma GC, Custer RP, Bosma MJ. A severe combined immunodeficiency mutation in the mouse. Nature 1983;301:527-30.

36. Namikawa R, Weilbaecher KN, Kaneshima H, et al. Long term human hematopoiesis in the SCID-hu mouse. J Exp Med 1990;172:1055-63.
37. Bonyhadi ML, Kaneshima H. The SCID-hu mouse: An in vivo model for HIV-1 infection in humans. Mol Med Today 1997;3:246-53.
38. Krowka JF, Sarin S, Namikawa R, et al. Human T-cells in the SCID-hu mouse are phenotypically normal and functionally competent. J Immunol 1991;146:3751-6.
39. Vandekerckhove BA, Namikawa R, Bacchetta R, et al. Human hematopoietic cells and thymic epithelial cells induce tolerance via different mechanisms in the SCID-hu mouse thymus. J Exp Med 1992;175:1033-43.
40. McCune JM, Namikawa R, Shih CC, et al. Suppression of HIV infection in AZT-treated SCID-hu mice. Science 1990;247:564-6.
41. Rabin L, Hincenbergs M, Moreno MB, et al. Use of standardized SCID-hu Thy/Liv mouse model for preclinical efficacy testing of anti-human immunodeficiency virus type-1 compounds. Antimicrob Agents Chemother 1996;40:755-62.
42. Datema R, Rabin L, Hincenbergs M, et al. Antiviral efficacy in vivo of the anti-human immunodeficiency virus bicyclam SDZ SID 791 (JM 3100), an inhibitor of infectious cell entry. Antimicrob Agents Chemother 1996;40:750-4.
43. Bosma GC, Fried M, Custer RP, et al. Evidence of functional lymphocytes in some (leaky) scid mice. J Exp Med 1988;167:1016-33.
44. McCune JM. Animal models of HIV-1 disease. Science 1997;278:2141-2.
45. Kollmann TR, Pettoello-Mantovani M, Zhuang X, et al. Disseminated human immunodeficiency virus-1 (HIV-1) infection in SCID-hu Mice after peripheral inoculation with HIV-1. J Exp Med 1994;179:513-22.
46. Picchio GR, Gulizia RJ, Wehrly K, et al. The cell tropism of human immunodeficiency virus type-1 determines the kinetics of plasma viremia in SCID mice reconstituted with human peripheral blood leukocytes. J Virol 1998;72:2002-9.
47. Mosier DE, Gulizia RJ, MacIsaac PD, et al. Resistance to human immunodeficiency virus-1 infection of SCID mice reconstituted with peripheral blood leukocytes from donors vaccinated with vaccinia gp160 and recombinant gp160. Proc Natl Acad Sci USA 1993;90:2443-7.
48. Del Real G, Llorente M, Bosca L, et al. Suppression of HIV-1 infection in linomide-treated SCID-hu-PBL mice. AIDS 1998;12:865-72.
49. Reinhardt B, Torbett BE, Gulizia RJ, et al. Human immunodeficiency virus type-1 infection of neonatal severe combined immunodeficient mice xenografted with human cord blood cells. AIDS Res Hum Retroviruses 1994;10:131-41.
50. Pace MJ, Agosto L, Graf EH, O'Doherty U. HIV reservoirs and latency models. Virology 2011; 411:344–54.
51. Lapenta C, Fais S, Rizza P, et al. U937-SCID mouse xenografts: A new model for acute in vivo HIV-1 infection suitable to test antiviral strategies. Antiviral Res 1997;36:81-90.
52. Balzarini J, Naesens L, Herdewijn P, et al. Marked in vivo antiretrovirus activity of 9(2-phosphonyl methoxyethyl) adenine, a selective anti-human immunodeficiency virus agent. Proc Natl Acad Sci USA 1989;86:332-6.
53. Balzarini J, Schols D, Laethem KV, et al. Pronounced in vitro and in vivo antiretroviral activity of 5-substituted 2,4-diamino-6-[2-(phosphonomethoxy)ethoxy] pyrimidines. J Antimicrob Chemother 2007;59:80-6.

54. Balzarini J, Holy A, Jindrich J, et al. 9-[(2RS)-3-Fluoro-2-phosphonylmethoxypropyl] derivatives of purines: a class of highly selective antiretroviral agents in vitro and in vivo. Proc Natl Acad Sci USA 1991;88:4961-5.
55. Hanna Z, Kay DG, Cool M, et al. Transgenic mice expressing human immunodeficiency virus type-1 in immune cells develop a severe AIDS-like disease. J Virol 1998;72:121-32.
56. Hanna Z, Kay DG, Rebai N, et al. Nef harbors a major determinant of pathogenicity for an AIDS-like disease induced by HIV-1 in transgenic mice. Cell 1998;95:163-75.
57. Vogel J, Hinrichs SH, Reynolds RK, et al. The HIV tat gene induces dermal lesions resembling Kaposi's sarcoma in transgenic mice. Nature 1988;335:606-11.
58. Brady HJ, Abraham DJ, Pennington DJ, et al. Altered cytokine expression in T lymphocytes from human immunodeficiency virus Tat transgenic mice. J Virol 1995;69:7622-9.
59. Berrada F, Ma D, Michaud J, et al. Neuronal expression of human immunodeficiency virus type-1 env proteins in transgenic mice: Distribution in the central nervous system and pathological alterations. J Virol 1995;69:6770-8.
60. Thomas FP, Chalk C, Lalonde R, et al. Expression of human immunodeficiency virus type-1 in the nervous system of transgenic mice leads to neurological disease. J Virol 1994;68:7099-107.
61. Denton PW, Garcia JV. Humanized mouse models of HIV infection. AIDS Rev 2011;13(3):135–48.
62. Keppler OT, Welte FJ, Ngo TA, Chin PS, Patton KS, Tsou CL, et al. Progress toward a human CD4/CCR5 transgenic rat model for de novo iInfection by human immunodeficiency virus type 1. J Exp Med 2002;195(6):719–36.
63. Goffinet C, Allespach I, Keppler OT. HIV-susceptible transgenic rats allow rapid preclinical testing of antiviral compounds targeting virus entry or reverse transcription. Proc Natl Acad Sci USA 2007;104(3):1015-20.
64. Steube KG, Teepe D, Meyer C, et al. A model system in hematology and immunology: The human monocytic line MONO-MAC 1. Leuk Res 1997;21:327-35.
65. Genois N, Robichaud GA, Tremblay MJ. Mono Mac 1: A new in vitro model system to study HIV-1 infection in human cells of the mononuclear phagocyte series. J Leukoc Biol 2000;68:854-64.
66. Deng H, Liu R, Ellmeie W, et al. Identification of a major coreceptor for primary isolates of HIV-1. Nature 1996;381:661-6.
67. Zack JA, Arrigo SJ, Weitsman SR, et al. HIV-1 entry into quiescent primary lymphocytes: Molecular analysis reveals a labile, latent viral structure. Cell 1990;61:213-22.
68. Geballe AP, Ventura P, Stowring L, et al. Quantitative analysis of Visna virus replication in vivo. Virology 1985;141:148-54.
69. Haase AT. Pathogenesis of lentivirus infections. Nature 1986;322:130-6.
70. Chiu IM, Yaniv A, Dahlberg A, et al. Nucleotide sequence evidence for relationship of AIDS retrovirus to lentiviruses. Nature 1985;317:366-8.
71. Sonigo P, Alizon M, Staskus K, et al. Nucleotide sequence of Visna lentivirus: Relationship to the AIDS virus. Cell 1985;42:369-82.
72. Sundquist B, Larner E. Phosphophonophormate inhibition of visna virus replication. J Virol 1977;30:847-51.
73. Smee DF, Martin JC, Verheyden JPH, et al. Anti Herpes virus activity of acyclic nucleoside 9-guanine. Antimicrob Agents Chemother 1983;23:676-82.
74. Smee DF, Sidwell RW, Barnett BB, et al. A bioassay system for determining ribavarin levels in human serum and urine. Chemotherapy1981;27:1-11.

75. Vrang L, Oberg B. PPi analogs as inhibitors of human T-lymphotropic virus type III reverse transcriptase. Antimicrob Agents Chemother 1986;29:867-72.
76. Pauwels R, Balzarini J, Schols D, et al. Phosphonylmethoxyethyl purine derivatives, a new class of anti-human immunodeficiency virus agents. Antimicrob Agents Chemother 1988;32:1025-30.
77. Zhang X, Yang LM, Liu GM, Liu YJ, Zheng CB, Lv YJ, et al. Potent anti-HIV activities and mechanisms of action of a pine cone extract from Pinus yunnanensis. Molecules 2012;17:6916-29.
78. Wang RR, Yang LM, Wang YH, Pang W, Tam SC, Tien P, Zheng YT. Sifuvirtide, a potent HIV fusion inhibitor peptide. Biochem Biophys Res Commun 2009;382:540–4.
79. Cen S, Peng ZG, Li XY, Li ZR, Ma J, Wang YM, et al. Small molecular compounds inhibit HIV-1 replication through specifically stabilizing APOBEC3G. J Biol Chem 2010;285:16546-52.
80. Maclean AG, Orandle MS, Alvarez X, et al. Rhesus macaque brain microvessel endothelial cells behave in a manner phenotypically distinct from umbilical endothelial cells. J Neuroimmunol 2001;118:223-32.
81. Guillemin G, Boussin FD, Croitoru J, et al. Obtention and characterization of primary astrocyte and microglial cultures from adult monkey brains. J Neurosci Res 1997;49:576-91.
82. Maclean AG, Orandle MS, Mackey J, et al. Characterization of an in vitro rhesus macaque blood brain barrier. J Neuroimmunol 2002;131:98-103.
83. Hurwitz AJ, Berman J, Rashbaum W, et al. Human fetal astrocytes induce the expression of blood brain barrier specific proteins by autologous endothelial cells. Brain Res 1993;625:238-43.
84. Hayashi Y, Nomura M, Yamagishi SI, et al. Induction of various blood brain barrier properties in nonneuronal endothelial cells by close apposition to cocultured astrocytes. Glia 1997;19:13-26.
85. Janigro D, Strewlow L, Grant G, et al. In vitro blood-brain barrier model for HIV- induced CNS disease. NeuroAIDS 1 1998. http://www.aidscience.org/neuroaids/articles/Neuro1(H).asp.
86. Chackerian B, Haigwood NL, Overbaugh J. Characterization of CD4 expressing macaque cell line that can detect virus after a single replication cycle and can be infected by diverse simian immunodeficiency virus isolates. Virology 1995;213:386-94.

CHAPTER

6

Angiogenesis

INTRODUCTION

Blood vessels perfuse the entire body and are structurally and functionally highly heterogeneous in order to meet the metabolic demands of tissues that are exposed to different microenvironments. The basic components of blood vessels include an endothelial cell monolayer known as the endothelium, which is surrounded by organ-specific mural cells and an extracellular matrix.[1,2] These vessels serve many crucial physiological roles, including the separation of blood and tissues, regulation of leukocyte adhesion, regulation of organ blood flow, coagulation, vasodilation and angiogenesis.[2]

In all vertebrates, both vasculogenesis and angiogenesis are required for normal development of the vascular system in the developing embryo. While vasculogenesis entails *de novo* formation of blood vessels from the mesoderm during early embryogenesis, all other vessels arise from this vasculature by angiogenesis, a process that persists throughout adult life. In the adult, angiogenesis is essential to maintain homeostasis, such as during wound healing and menses, whereas uncontrolled angiogenesis underlies a plethora of diseases.[3] As such, excessive angiogenesis can lead to tumor growth and metastasis, psoriasis, retinal vasculopathy and arthritis,[4-7] whereas insufficient angiogenesis is observed in ischemia, strokes and myocardial infarctions.[8-11] At the molecular level, angiogenesis is mediated to a large extent by endothelial cell-specific tyrosine kinase receptors, such as Flk-1/KDR and Tie-2, receptors for vascular endothelial growth factor (VEGF) and the novel angiopoietin family (Ang-1, -2, -3 and -4), respectively.[12]

TUMOR ANGIOGENESIS

In 1991, Judah Folkman et al. were the first to propose that tumor growth and metastasis correlate with the extent of angiogenesis.[13] This finding revolutionized anticancer therapeutics, as it suggested that blood vessels, rather than the cancer cells themselves, should preferentially be targeted in tumor settings. Effectively, it has since been established that without angiogenesis, tumors can not grow more than 2 mm in diameter.[14-16] Tumor angiogenesis entails the same sequence of events as physiological angiogenesis, namely endothelial cell invasion into the surrounding matrix, proliferation, migration and tube formation; however, these events proceed in an uncontrolled and excessive manner.[15] Due to the complexity of this disease, as well as its associated morbidity and mortality, most *in vitro* and *in vivo* angiogenesis models have focused on investigating tumor angiogenesis.

Although *in vitro* models of angiogenesis are crucial to quantitate discrete steps of angiogenesis, e.g. migration, proliferation, etc., they can not mimic the effects of the microenvironment and spatiotemporal cues on vessel phenotype that occur *in vivo*. For instance, it is well-established that microenvironment cues help define the type and number of vessels being formed, explaining why for instance, liver vessels are functionally and structurally distinct from cardiovascular vessels.[17] In addition, due to the complex 3-dimensional vessels structures observed *in vivo*, effective modeling of vessels is only possible in whole animals versus cell cultures. A main limitation of animal models of angiogenesis, as compared to cell culture models, involves lack of sensitivity, accuracy and reproducibility in quantifying angiogenesis. These limitations are mainly due to the fact that the heterogeneous microenvironment can not be controlled and kept static in animal models as it can under tissue culture conditions. In addition, *in vivo* approaches are generally much more time consuming and expensive than cell culture assays. Hence, there is an urgent need to improve existing *in vivo* models, or even create new ones, so that animal assays will one day be as cost and time-effective, quantitative and reproducible as *in vitro* assays. Being able to modulate angiogenesis in laboratory animals is crucial for understanding the underlying mechanisms of angiogenesis in order to find suitable targets which will translate to humans.

This review will describe the most established models, as well as emerging ones, focusing on their respective advantages and limitations. For clarification purposes, these models are classified into four categories: (i) tissue excision models, (ii) implant models, (iii) translucent models, and (iv) non-mammalian models.

Tissue Excision Models

The models presented here require that a piece of tissue be removed from the animal either after (xenografts, cancer tissue arrays) or prior (ischemic hind limb model) induction of angiogenesis.

Xenografts

One of the most popular methods for studying tumor angiogenesis and anticancerous drugs are xenografts, whereby cells or tissues from one animal (donor) are transplanted into an immunodeficient animal from another species (recipient).[18] When transplantation involves the same tissue type between donor and recipient, then this is termed an "orthologous xenograft". Xenograft models allow morphometric and immunohistological measurements to be performed which reflect the role of the heterogeneous microenvironment on the vasculature.[19] For instance, injecting breast tumor cells in the mammary gland of mice results in less angiogenesis than when these cells are injected in the cranial window.[20] These results are clinically relevant, as they imply that various types and stages of human cancers can be mimicked by alternating the grafts sites, which in turn will help identify markers of disease progression.

Xenografts can also be performed between mammalian and non-mammalian systems, such as between mammals and fish, by grafting human or mice tumor cells close to the subintestinal vessels of 2 days-old zebrafish embryos.[17] This model is useful for studying the mechanisms of tumor angiogenesis and antitumor drugs at a large scale, as zebrafish are easily manipulated and can be studied hundreds at a time (see below). Although extensively used, this method is time-consuming, but does not require extensive surgical skills.

Syngeneic Grafts

Syngeneic grafts, also called allografts,[21] are performed between a donor and recipient belonging to identical species, thus negating the need for an immunodeficient recipient.[22] For example, Lewis Lung Carcinoma cells or B16/F10 melanoma cells can be implanted into C57/Bl6 mouse, and leads to robust tumor growth with vigorous angiogenesis. This property makes the syngeneic graft the ideal *in vivo* model for studying the complex interactions that occur between tumor cells and host cells.[22] More recently, this model has found widespread application for investigating murine stem cell transplantation for therapeutic strategies during cardiovascular diseases and diabetes.[21,23]

The main advantages of tumor allografts, as compared with xenografts, are that they are less costly[24] and metastasis can be induced more readily.[22,25] The latter is explained by the lack of natural killer cells in nude mice, which often impairs the metastatic potential of the injected tumor cells. This limitation, however, has been partly addressed by injecting immunodeficient mice with human peripheral blood or bone marrow cells from the donors (e.g. humanized mice) and then challenging them with the donor tumor cells or tissue.[26] The main disadvantage of allografts when compared with the latter is that human tumors can not be studied, hence limiting its clinical usefulness, especially in terms of drug responsiveness.[22,26] In order to study as many parameters of cancer as possible, it would, hence, be advantageous to combine both xenografts and allografts, allowing the investigator to obtain more data than using either model alone.

Cancer Tissue Arrays

A new twist on immunohistochemistry, inspired by DNA microarrays in that they allow for high throughput analyses, was recently introduced as "cancer tissue arrays". These arrays have gained considerable popularity in the past 7 years and have proved a valuable tool in the discovery of potential tumor markers. Each array can accommodate up to 600 "spots" of cancer tissues or corresponding non-neoplastic controls (of around 0.6 diameter per spot) which are embedded in paraffin on a glass slide.[27,28] This model has the advantages of analyzing clinically relevant human samples, and to simultaneously allow for the analysis of many different types of tumors, or different grades of the same tumor type, thus bypassing the needs for animal models in some cases and saving considerable time and money.[27,28]

However, as histochemistry is semiquantitative, tissue arrays still need to be validated using more sensitive techniques, such as ELISA.[27] Although not well-documented, it should be noted that these arrays can introduce gender and ethnic biases, as it does not reflect population heterogeneity and it is a well-known fact that tumor markers differ among sexes and ethnic groups.[29] Although tissue arrays are currently used for cancer research, it will be interesting to construct protein arrays to study other diseases in the future, such as diabetes and cardiovascular diseases.

Ischemic Hind Limb Model

The models described thus far are mainly useful to study diseases of excessive angiogenesis, hence their usefulness in cancer studies. However, models to study insufficient angiogenesis remain scarce. The best known and used of such models is the ischemic hind limb muscle model, which has successfully been used since 1994 to study ischemia-induced vessel regression.[30] In this model, a segment of the proximal femoral artery and vein are excised from one leg of the animal, generally a rabbit or rodent, and the remaining collateral vessels (emanating mainly from the internal and external iliac artery) are ligated in order to induce unilateral hind limb ischemia.[30-32] This procedure yields ischemia-induced vessel regression in about 10-14 days, thus mimicking cardiovascular disease-induced ischemia in patients. To investigate the roles of pro-angiogenic factors in treating ischemic symptoms, various angiogenic agents or drugs can be administered at low doses to the animal using various routes (e.g. local injection in the collateral vessels or oral administration) and vascular recovery monitored in real-time. Although this is a technically-demanding and time-consuming assay, it has the advantages of being highly quantitative and reproducible. In addition, since vessel growth is easily quantified in the live animal using angiography and Doppler flowmetry, for instance, this minimizes the number of animals, and hence, the costs associated with this assay.

Implant Models

Various models have been developed in order to deliver continual and slow release of angiogenic factors or tumors cells implanted at localized sites. These models rely on the encapsulation of these factors or cells in avascular matrices prior to implantation in the animal, allowing vessel infiltration in the matrices to be easily recovered from the implant sites and quantified by microscopy. These assays require an inert matrix devoid of endogenous angiogenic/angiostatic activities and are useful to quantitate not only the effects of the angiogenic modulators or tumors, but also to assess the pharmacokinetic profiles of drugs.[33,34] As described in the next section, these types of models offer much diversity simply by playing with the nature and design of the sponge.

Sponge Implant Model

In this model, a sterile polyester sponge containing the angiogenic modulator under study is attached to a cannula and subcutaneously implanted in the animal (usually a mouse or rat), with only the cannula protruding from the skin (Fig. 6.1).[18,35,36] The protruding cannula can then be easily injected with a tracer (the radioisotope133Xe) and vessel infiltration into the sponge, indicative of blood flow and hence angiogenesis, is quantified by measuring radioisotope (133Xe) clearance from the sponge or from the tail blood.[18,36] In addition, the sponge can be excised and vessel density correlated to blood flow histologically. This

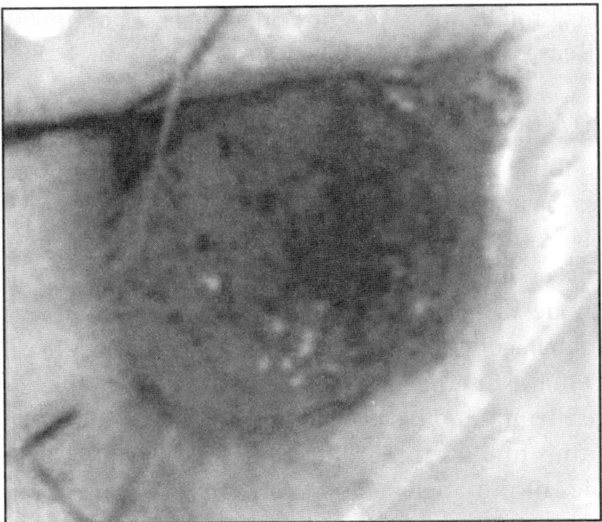

Figure 6.1: Angiogenesis observed in a sponge implanted subcutaneously in the subscapular region in the mouse. Angiogenesis is quantified by measuring the clearance of a dye or radioactive tracer from the sponge or by staining the sections with an antibody against von Willebrand factor that acts as a marker for endothelial cells. Other markers can also be used (*For color version see Plate 10*)

assay offers several advantages. For instance, the small size of the sponges allows them to be implanted in various sites in the animal, thus allowing vascularization to be assessed in heterogeneous microenvironments. This model is technically simple, inexpensive and the exposed canula allows for repeated real-time measurements to be performed. A major limitation of this model, however, is that since sponges are encapsulated by granulation tissue at the site of implant, inflammation-induced angiogenesis is a main source of false-positive results. Also, sponge-to-sponge compositional variability, by influencing the degree of inflammation, can also create false positive results.[18] Radioactivity is another limitation, due to the increased risk of toxicity as well as the increased monetary cost associated with it. This latter issue has been remedied by substituting 133 Xe with the fluorometric dye sodium fluorescein.[34]

Matrigel Plug

Matrigel is an extracellular-rich tumor basement membrane extract which becomes rapidly vascularized *in vivo* without the requirement for surgery, thus allowing vessel infiltration into the Matrigel plug to be quickly visualized (Fig. 6.2).[35,37] Matrigel is a solution at 4°C, but polymerizes at body temperature into a gel-like structure. Its major disadvantages are that the composition of Matrigel is poorly defined, histological analysis of the plug is time-consuming due to its inhomogeneous structure and low reproducibility, since different Matrigel plugs tend to have variable 3-dimensional structures.[38] These disadvantages can be partly minimized by

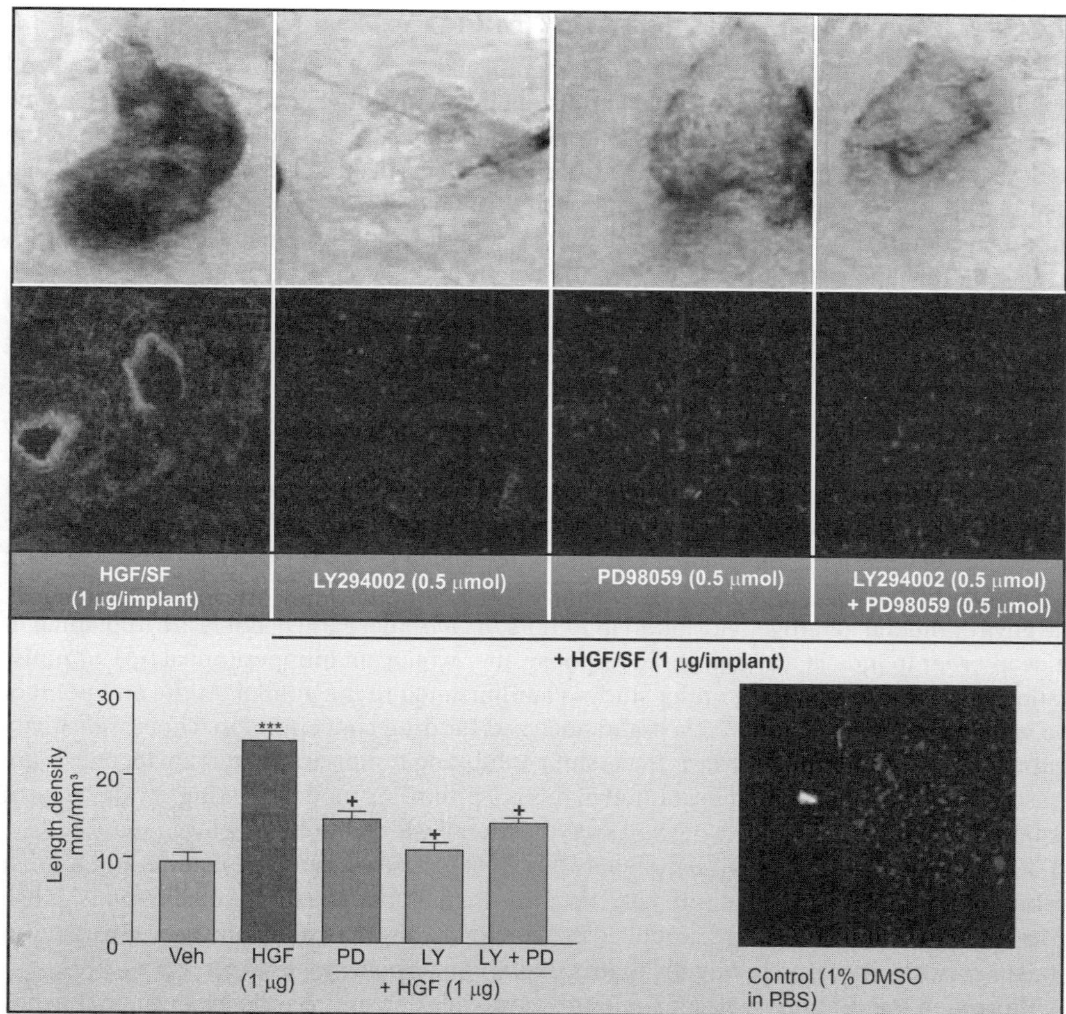

Figure 6.2: Matrigel implant model. Effect of PI3K and MAPK inhibitors on HGF/SF-induced angiogenesis in matrigel implants in vivo. Photomicrographs depict neovascularization induced by HGF/SF and inhibitory effects of PD98059 and LY294002. Upper panel shows gross morphology; lower panel shows cross section with blood vessels delineated with immunolabeling (FITC) for von Willebrand factor. Nuclei were counterstained with propidium iodide and appear blue. Images were captured with resolution of 512 × 512 pixels (*For color version see Plate 11*)

using growth factor reduced Matrigel and quantifying blood flow in the plugs by ultrasound measurements, rather than by histology.[39]

Disc Assay (DAS)

DAS consists of polyvinyl alcohol sponges sandwiched between two "Millipore" filters.[33,40] It is a generally useful model for investigating tumor-mediated angiogenesis, but is very lengthy (7-12 days to detect significant angiogenesis).

The Directed in Vivo Angiogenesis Assay (DIVAA)

DIVAA involves semi-closed silicone cylinders plugged at one end with a stainless steel rod or silicone (angioreactor). The angioreactor is filled with the angiogenic agents under study, which are themselves encapsulated in Matrigel. Following subcutaneous implantation of the angioreactor in the animal, a fluorogenic dye such as FITC-dextran is systemically injected in the tail vein. Vessel density is then quantified in the angioreactor by measuring fluorescence. For all its complexity, this is a poorly accurate model due to the subjectivity associated with vessel quantification, the use of Matrigel, the length of the assay (it typically takes 9 days to detect significant angiogenesis), the low amount of angiogenic factor that can be added to the bioreactor (18 µl) and the fact that this model only quantifies the effect of pro-angiogenic agents, but not inhibitors of angiogenesis nor xenografts.[41,42]

Hollow Fiber Solid Tumor Model

The hollow fiber solid tumor model was initially created at the National Cancer Institute to screen for anticancer drugs prior to performing xenograft experiments, in order to minimize the cost associated with the latters.[43-45] In this model, well-characterized tumor cell lines are first propagated in biocompatible polyvinylidene fluoride (PVDF) fibers, in order to reproduce the environmental heterogeneity found in tumors *in vivo*. These PVDF fibers are implanted in mice in order to induce an angiogenic response after which, an intraperitoneal (ip) administration of the anticancer drug under study is administered to the animal. At the end point of the experiment, the fiber is removed and analyzed for drug concentration, chemosensitivity and vessel infiltration. Only drugs successfully inhibiting tumor-associated angiogenesis are subsequently tested in xenografts. Although this is a promising model covering a wide range of variables for cancer drug screening, it is costly, extremely lengthy (14 days for *in vitro* studies, 28-32 days for *in vivo* studies), requires extensive expertise in both cell culture and animal techniques and often culminates in false negatives results.[43,45] Due to these limitations, it has scarcely been used since being introduced in 1994 and has instead been substituted with more straight-forward assays including the matrix implants (see below).[43]

Altogether, the usefulness of sponge implant models depends on the experimental needs of the investigator. For instance, the Matrigel plug allows for the most rapid quantification of tumor angiogenesis, but provides less reproducibility than the other models. Hence, combining implant models could offer more advantages than using each method alone. Effectively, it was recently demonstrated that combining the sponge implant model with the Matrigel plug increases sensitivity of vessel quantification.[46] The main disadvantage that these implant models all share is that they do not allow for real-time observations to be made. This disadvantage is partly remedied in the subsequent section.

Translucent Models

These models rely on physiological or artificially-induced translucent structures in order to facilitate vessel visualization and quantification, usually in real-time. In general, quantification of vessel growth in these models has been greatly aided by imaging using intravital microscopy. Intravital, meaning "in the living animal", is highly useful for real-time measurements in chamber and windows models, but is also used to quantify vessels in tissues taken from sacrificed animals.[47] Intravital microscopy, often combined with video and computer technology techniques (e.g. videomicroscopy), relies on oblique trans-illumination and fluorescence epi-illumination in order to quantify vessel architecture according to vascular volume per unit area.[47-49]

Hamster Cheek Pouch Model

The first established model of naturally-occurring transparent structure is the hamster cheek pouch assay, which has been used since 1950.[50-52] This is a localized model of angiogenesis which is mainly used to investigate angiogenic mechanisms related to buccal cancers. This is an ideal model to study tobacco-related carcinogenesis, where the carcinogen under study is directly placed on or inside the cheek pouch. Although vessel growth can be quantified in real-time, the animal generally has to be sacrificed for measurements to be taken, as the pouch is not readily accessible.

Corneal Micropocket Model

The corneal micropocket model, introduced in 1974 in rabbits, provides a more readily accessible organ to study real-time angiogenesis than the cheek pouch. This assay relies on the fact that the cornea is an avascular tissue under homeostatic conditions, and hence, inducing angiogenesis can be easily quantified in real-time using light microscopy.[53,54] This is accomplished by making several incisions (pockets) in the corneal stroma and implanting pellets containing the angiogenic modulators or drugs under study in these pockets. Since the cornea is initially isolated from potential angiogenic factors present in blood, this model has the immense advantage of only allowing the factors present in the pellets to be studied. However, this model is costly, although this can be partly remedied using smaller animals such as mice or rats, is highly time-consuming and requires intricate surgical expertise, especially in smaller corneas (e.g. rats versus rabbits).[53] For these reasons, only a small number of animals can be studied for a given experiment. In addition, great care must be taken by the surgeon to minimize an inflammatory response, as this would lead to artifactual angiogenesis.

Mesentery Model

The mesentery is a thin connective membrane, which extends from the dorsal body wall to the small gut. Under physiological conditions, it is sparsely vascular and transparent, similarly to the cornea, thus allowing vessel density to be easily quantified by light microscopy.[55] In the mesenteric window model of angiogenesis, the animal is usually injected ip with a mast cell-activating agent in order to induce inflammation-mediated angiogenesis. Other methods used to stimulate angiogenesis include ip injections of inflammatory mediators (e.g. interleukins) or potent growth factors (e.g. VEGF), as well as perforating the mesenteric window.[56-58] The mesentery, along with the small intestine, is then collected and spread out on objective slides at the desired time points. The small intestine is excised and the membranous part of the mesentery examined under the microscope in order to quantitate microvessel density. The main advantage of this model is that the large numbers of mesenteric windows per animal, for example up to 45 windows in the rat, allow multiple observations to be made in only one animal. The main disadvantages of this method are that it relies on inflammation-induced angiogenesis, thus restricting the types of angiogenic inducers that can be studied, and that the animal must be injected with the angiogenic inducer for several days in order to detect angiogenesis, thus increasing the time and monetary cost of this assay.

Chamber and Rat Dorsal Air Sac Models

In the chamber assay, a piece of tissue is excised from the animal in order to expose translucent structures where angiogenesis can be easily visualized. This assay is generally performed on rabbit ears or on the dorsal skinfold or cranium of rodents.[18,38,59] Following the removal of skin or skull from the animal, a matrix containing the tumor cells or angiogenic factors under study is layered on the exposed surface and covered by a glass coverslip, hence the name of this assay.[18,38] This assay has a major advantage over most other *in vivo* models, in that it quantifies angiogenesis in 3-dimensions, thus more accurately representing the intricate complexity of blood vessels than 2-dimensional measurements.[49] The main disadvantages of this model are that it is invasive, technically demanding, costly and can result in false positives due to significant inflammation-induced angiogenesis following implantation of the glass window.[18,38,60]

The rat dorsal air sac assay (also called pouch or blister assay) creates an artificial transparent chamber by subcutaneously injecting air in the back of the animal, resulting in a sizeable air sac within 8 to 10 days.[61] Neovascularization in the air sac is then induced by implantation of angiogenic factors or tumor cells, either in solvent or matrices, under or into the sac.[61,62] Although this model is invasive and time-consuming, it is technically simple to perform.

Angiomouse/Metamouse

Thus far, the major limitations with the above models are that animals are subjected to intense discomfort or even sacrificed in order for angiogenesis to be quantified, and that false positive results often occur (e.g. artificial chambers). These limitations are due to the scarcity of physiological translucent structures, to inflammation induced by artificially created chambers and to the requirement of surgically altering the animal in order to expose the tissues of interest (e.g. mesentery). In order to remedy these limitations, a novel experimental model, the Angiomouse (or Metamouse) was recently introduced.

In this model, mice are either injected systemically or grafted with human or rodent tumor cells stably expressing green fluorescent protein (GFP) and the metastasized tumor cells visualized in real-time, without the need to sacrifice or further alter the animal.[63,64] This is a very promising model where many variations are possible. For instance, conditional GFP promoters can be used in order to investigate the roles of specific growth factors during cancer progression, as was recently done using the VEGF promoter.[49] Growth and infiltration of tumor cells into the mouse vasculature can be measured in real-time using a trans-illuminated epi-fluorescence microscope, a multiphoton laser-scanning microscope or a fluorescence light box.[49,63] The tumor cells can be visualized in depths and appear intensely green, whereas the mouse's endogenous vasculature appears as well-defined dark networks. This model offers the immense advantage of allowing for rapid, technically simple, non-invasive and real-time whole-body measurements of tumor metastasis for prolonged time periods and, unlike most models presented thus far, does not induce an inflammatory response.[63] The main limitation of this method is that the short wavelength of GFP (520 nm) is highly scattered by surrounding tissues, thus reducing sensitivity of the assay.[63] Although the experimental set-up is initially more expensive than most other methods, in the end, the reduced numbers of animals (since no sacrifice is necessary) and analysis (no need to excise tissues and count vessels) make this an ideal and cost-effective method for studying tumor angiogenesis and for testing anti-tumor drugs.[64]

Non-mammalian Models

The models reviewed thus far were performed on various mammals (e.g. mice, rats or rabbits) in order to closely mimic human vascular phenotypes and genotypes. However, non-mammalian models can also provide valuable angiogenesis tools, especially with regards to studying developmental angiogenesis. These animal models include the extensively used chick chorioallantoic membrane (CAM) and *Danio rerio* (zebrafish) models, as well as the *Xenopus Laevis* tadpole, and more surprisingly, the common medicinal leech, *Hirudo medicinalis*.

As opposed to the larger mammalian models previously described, these small animal models of angiogenesis are technically simple to maintain and manipulate, as these animals are easily bread and produce large quantities of offsprings in a rapid amount of time. These models hence allow high throughput experiments to be performed, explaining their use for high scale genomics. Their main disadvantages are that they are embryonic by nature, and hence, care must be taken when extrapolating results to adult vasculatures. In addition, the zebrafish model in particular is costly as it requires expensive housing. The use of these animals as angiogenesis models is hereby presented in terms of chronological order.

Chick Chorioallantoic Membrane (CAM)

CAM is one of the most widely used *in vivo* angiogenesis model, owing mainly to its requirements for minimal technical handling, as well as time (eggs hatch in 18 days) and money.[65] It involves removing a small part of the fertilized egg's shell (windowed method) in order to expose the extraembryonic CAM membrane. The membrane is then overlaid with the angiogenic modulators, cancer cells or tissues grafts under study and vessel density is assessed by light microscopy.[65,66] Limitations with this model are that some angiogenic factors produce opposite phenotypes on CAM vessels as compared with mammalian vessels, resulting in non-negligible artefacts.[18,38] These limitations are due to the fact the CAM model is an embryonic avian model, whose vasculature hence has different physiological requirements than adult mammalian vessels. Furthermore, overestimation of vascular growth often occurs in CAM models, resulting from non-specific angiogenesis induced by inflammation or changes in oxygen tension. Another limitation with this method is the highly subjective quantification of vessel growth, due to the presence of an existing vasculature prior to the addition of carriers or grafts, which make it harder to distinguish newly formed vessels from pre-existing ones.65 Numerous methods have been developed to overcome the latter limitation, including morphometric analyses of vessels, metabolic labeling of endothelial cells with thymidine, or more recently, mathematical modeling based on fractal 2-dimensional analyses or imaging using 3-dimensional probing techniques.[65-69]

Xenopus laevis

Although the *Xenopus laevis* tadpole is not as widely used as the zebrafish model, one model by no means replaces the other, and using both models could actually complement angiogenic studies. Early embryos are partly transparent (e.g. tail fin), thus allowing angiogenesis to be monitored in real-time.[70,71] Compared to zebrafish, tadpoles have several disadvantages, explaining why they have been largely replaced by the zebrafish model. As such, as opposed to zebrafish, albino or pigment-deficient (e.g. not completely albinic) tadpoles are required for better overall visualization of the vasculature, handling of the tadpoles is more time-consuming and tadpoles transgenics are not as easily generated, requiring alternative approaches such as retrovirus infection, which can lead to deleterious side effects.[70] However, tadpoles have the major advantage over zebrafish, as well as many other species, of being exceptionally disease-resistant, thus minimizing long-term costs. Xenopus are also better suited to study lymphogenesis than zebrafish. Hence, combining zebrafish and Xenopus models would give an overall better estimate of vascular and lymphatic mechanisms than using either model alone.

Danio rerio

Among all animal models of angiogenesis, the small (3-4 cm long in adults) tropical zebrafish has become the most widely used model since 1999.[70] This is primarily due to the unique characteristics of zebrafish embryos of being completely translucent, thus allowing highly accurate quantification of the vasculature to be made in real-time. This quantification is further improved by fluorescent techniques, such as injecting fluorescent markers in the cardinal vein of zebrafish or generating GFP stable transfectants (Fig. 6.3).[70,72] Although more genetically divergent from humans than tadpoles, increasing evidence suggests that most zebrafish genes have human orthologues.[70] In addition, zebrafish is one of the easiest system to modify for both forward and reverse genetics, translating in a plethora of knock-down and transgenics models of vascular pathologies by simple injection (e.g. morpholino antisense oligonucleotides) into single to four-cell stage embryos.[72] It is also a model of choice for drug screening, as the drug can simply be added to the fish embryo culture media and the vascular phenotype monitored by intravital microscopy.[73] The main disadvantage of this system is that zebrafish are highly susceptibility to parasites, which can alter embryo development and easily spread between laboratories.[74]

Angiogenesis in the Regenerating Zebrafish Fin

Adult zebrafish have a remarkable regenerative capability. Many tissues which may not be regenerated in mammals are quickly regenerated in zebrafish. Among these are the heart,

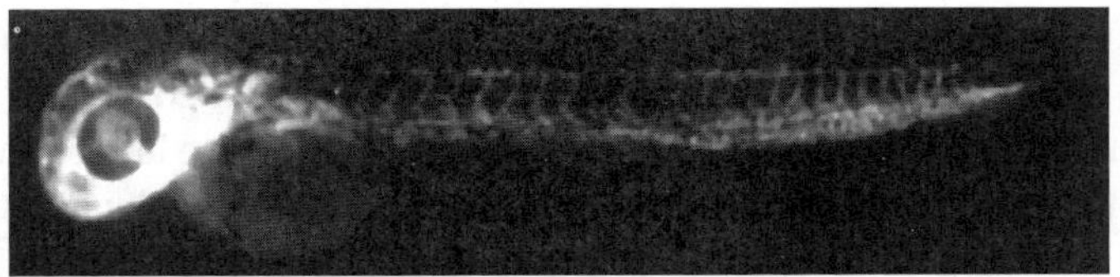

Figure 6.3: Fluorescence image of 48-hour post-fertilization zebrafish larvae expressing GFP under a Fli-1 promoter. Fli is preferentially expressed on the endothelial cells

retina, maxillary barbell and fins.[75] Importantly, as they regenerate, new blood and lymph vessels grow into the regenerating tissue - which enables studies on regenerative angiogenesis. One commonly used assay in the adult zebrafish, based on this principle is the regenerating tail fin. After amputation, the tail fin will re-grow and after approximately 1 month, the fin is back to its original size.[76] This process of fin regeneration encompasses many of the same mechanisms as in human wound healing and regeneration, and is therefore a good model of regenerative angiogenesis. As the fin is largely transparent, and as morpholinos can be introduced by microinjection and electroporation, this assay is almost as versatile as the zebrafish developmental angiogenesis assays, the major difference being that it is performed in an adult animal. Also in the fins, the vasculature is remarkably simple, and as the fin grows back various levels of vascular remodeling can be observed and therefore studied in detail.[75] This regeneration model is probably the most commonly used, adult zebrafish angiogenesis model, and is considered to be complementary to the developmental angiogenesis models.

Hirudo Medicinalis

The leech *Hirudo medicinalis*, well-known for its blood-sucking feeding habits, was recently proposed to be a promising model of angiogenesis for the following reasons: its vasculature responds to treatment of human pro- (e.g. VEGF) and anti-angiogenic factors, as well as to the anti-cancer drug mitomycin, following injection in the body wall.[77] These results indicate a surprisingly high degree of vascular homology between leeches and mammalian systems. Although this model has not gained popularity in the scientific community, we propose it could serve as a complementary method to quantify angiogenesis, as it is a simple system which is initially largely avascular, like the cornea, and which can be studied in both embryos and adults.[77,78] Blood vessel growth in the leech is also faster than in other animal models, as its whole body wall (2 mm thick) can be vascularized in only 24 hours. In addition, leeches are very easily manipulated. For instance, to monitor endothelial cell proliferation in real-time, leeches are simply dipped in BrdU-containing solution and then examined by electron microscopy.[77] Since leeches feed on blood, it is also tempting to speculate that adding angiogenic modulators or drugs in blood, rather than injecting them, would provide easier and quicker methods of assaying their angiogenic potentials.

Genetic Models

Ob/ob Mice

In 1950, obese mice carrying the mutation obese (ob) were described for the first time.[79] The ob mutation was later shown to be located in the gene coding for a hormone known as leptin. Leptin is important in the regulation of appetite and food intake. Leptin signaling is mediated via binding to the leptin receptor (Ob-R) and subsequent signaling to the hypothalamus. Via this pathway, food uptake, energy expenditure as well as fat and glucose metabolism are regulated. Heterozygotes on the other hand do not display any phenotype as the mutation is recessive. The leptin deficient mouse can be used as an excellent model to study the role of angiogenesis in adipose tissue expansion.[80] Obesity in these mice can be prevented by treatment with anti-angiogenic drugs. Since these mice are comparable to morbidly obese humans regarding the obesity phenotype, using this model might be helpful to identify potential novel targets to treat obesity and obesity-related metabolic disorders in the future.

Db/db mice

The autosomal recessive mutation diabetes (db) was first described in 1966 in the mouse strain C57BL/KsJ.[81] These mice are deficient for the leptin receptor. Animals which are homozygous for this mutation, exhibit a phenotype that resembles human diabetes mellitus. This mutant strain is also characterized by an obese phenotype. Furthermore, homozygous mutants are infertile and hyperglycemic while heterozygotes are phenotypically indistinguishable from wild type littermates. These mice are excellent models for studying mechanisms of obesity-related diabetes and insulin insensitivity, and the role of angiogenesis in this regard.

CONCLUSION

In conclusion, with so many different *in vivo* angiogenesis models available, it can become overwhelming to know which one to use. The choice of model would depend on laboratory resources, technical expertise, type of disease being investigated and budget. The ultimate goal would be to combine the high throughput potential and ease of use of zebrafish to mammalian models, in order to more sensitively and reproducibly quantify angiogenesis, ultimately saving time and money. Furthermore, studying angiogenesis *in vivo* should not rely on a single, global experimental approach, but rather, should combine assays depending on the parameters (e.g. antitumor drugs and metastatic potential of tumor xenografts) and/or disease (e.g. tumor versus infarctions) under study. Just as each disease in humans has distinct, yet overlapping phenotypes, so should animal models of angiogenesis.

REFERENCES

1. Cleaver O, Melton DA. Endothelial signaling during development. Nat Med 2003;9:661-8.
2. Jain RK. Molecular regulation of vessel maturation. Nat Med 2003;9:685-93.
3. Folkman J. Angiogenesis in cancer, vascular, rheumatoid and other disease. Nat Med 1995;1:27-31.
4. Sengupta S, et al. Temporal targeting of tumour cells and neovasculature with a nanoscale delivery system. Nature 2005;436:568-72.
5. Kerbel R, Folkman J. Clinical translation of angiogenesis inhibitors. Nat Rev Cancer 2002;2:727-39.
6. Ward NL, Dumont DJ. The angiopoietins and Tie-2/Tek: adding to the complexity of cardiovascular development. Semin Cell Dev Biol 2002;13:19-27.
7. Carmeliet P, Jain RK. Angiogenesis in cancer and other diseases. Nature 2000;407:249-57.
8. Couffinhal T, et al. Impaired collateral vessel development associated with reduced expression of vascular endothelial growth factor in ApoE-/- mice. Circulation 1999;99:3188-98.
9. Rivard A, et al. Age-dependent impairment of angiogenesis. Circulation 1999;99:111-20.
10. Rivard A, et al. Rescue of diabetes-related impairment of angiogenesis by intramuscular gene therapy with adeno-VEGF. Am J Pathol 1999;154:355-63.
11. Van BE, et al. Hypercholesterolemia attenuates angiogenesis but does not preclude augmentation by angiogenic cytokines. Circulation 1997;96:2667-74.

12. Sato TN, Qin Y, Kozak CA, Audus KL. Tie-1 and tie-2 define another class of putative receptor tyrosine kinase genes expressed in early embryonic vascular system. Proc Natl Acad Sci USA 1993;90:9355-8.
13. Weidner N, Semple JP, Welch WR, Folkman J. Tumor angiogenesis and metastasis: correlation in invasive breast carcinoma. N Engl J Med 1991;324:1-8.
14. Folkman J. Tumor angiogenesis: therapeutic implications. N Engl J Med 1971;285:1182-6.
15. Chaplain MA. Mathematical modeling of angiogenesis. J Neurooncol 2000;50:37-51.
16. Singletary SE, Greene FL. Revision of breast cancer staging: the 6th edition of the TNM Classification. Semin Surg Oncol 2003;21:53-9.
17. Hansen-Smith FM. Capillary network patterning during angiogenesis. Clin Exp Pharmacol Physiol 2000;27:830-5.
18. Staton CA, et al. Current methods for assaying angiogenesis in vitro and in vivo. Int J Exp Pathol 2004;85:233-48.
19. Kallinowski F, et al. Blood flow, metabolism, cellular microenvironment, and growth rate of human tumor xenografts. Cancer Res 1989;49:3759-64.
20. Cohen MM., Jr. Vascular update: morphogenesis, tumors, malformations and molecular dimensions. Am J Med Genet 2006;A 140:2013-38.
21. Drukker M, Benvenisty N. The immunogenicity of human embryonic stem-derived cells. Trends Biotechnol 2004;22:136-41.
22. Smith LP, Thomas GR. Animal models for the study of squamous cell carcinoma of the upper aerodigestive tract: a historical perspective with review of their utility and limitations. Part A. Chemically-induced de novo cancer, syngeneic animal models of HNSCC, animal models of transplanted xenogeneic human tumors. Int J Cancer 2006;118:2111-22.
23. Stojkovic M, Lako M, Strachan T, Murdoch A. Derivation, growth and applications of human embryonic stem cells. Reproduction 2004;128:259-67.
24. Teicher BA. Tumor models for efficacy determination. Mol Cancer Ther 2006;5:2435-43.
25. Kirchner C, et al. Cytotoxicity of colloidal CdSe and CdSe/ZnS nanoparticles. Nano Lett 2005;5:331-8.
26. Talmadge JE, Singh RK, Fidler IJ, Raz A. Murine models to evaluate novel and conventional therapeutic strategies for cancer. Am J Pathol 2007;170:793-804.
27. Ryden L, et al, Tumor specific VEGF-A and VEGFR2/KDR protein are co-expressed in breast cancer. Breast Cancer Res Treat 2003;82:147-54.
28. Charpin C, et al, Tumor neoangiogenesis by CD31 and CD105 expression evaluation in breast carcinoma tissue microarrays. Clin Cancer Res 2004;10:5815-9.
29. Rebbeck TR. Inherited genetic markers and cancer outcomes: personalized medicine in the postgenome era. J Clin Oncol 2006;24:1972-4.
30. Takeshita S, et al, Therapeutic angiogenesis. A single intraarterial bolus of vascular endothelial growth factor augments revascularization in a rabbit ischemic hind limb model. J Clin Invest 1994;93:662-70.
31. Duan J, et al. Hyperhomocysteinemia impairs angiogenesis in response to hindlimb ischemia. Arterioscler Thromb Vasc Biol 2000;20:2579-85.
32. Asano T, et al. Hyperbaric oxygen induces basic fibroblast growth factor and hepatocyte growth factor expression, and enhances blood perfusion and muscle regeneration in mouse ischemic hind limbs. Circ J 2007;71:405-11.
33. Nelson MJ, Conley FK, Fajardo LF. Application of the disc angiogenesis system to tumor-induced neovascularization. Exp Mol Pathol 1993;58:105-13.

34. Andrade SP, et al. Sponge-induced angiogenesis in mice and the pharmacological reactivity of the neovasculature quantitated by a fluorimetric method. Microvasc Res 1997;54:253-61.
35. Sengupta S, et al. Modulating angiogenesis: the yin and the yang in ginseng. Circulation 2004;110:1219-25.
36. Andrade SP, Fan TP, Lewis GP. Quantitative in-vivo studies on angiogenesis in a rat sponge model. Br J Exp Pathol 1987;68:755-66.
37. Passaniti A, et al. A simple, quantitative method for assessing angiogenesis and antiangiogenic agents using reconstituted basement membrane, heparin, and fibroblast growth factor. Lab Invest 1992;67:519-28.
38. Auerbach R, Akhtar N, Lewis RL, Shinners BL. Angiogenesis assays: problems and pitfalls. Cancer Metastasis Rev 2000;19:167-72.
39. Stieger SM, et al. Ultrasound assessment of angiogenesis in a matrigel model in rats. Ultrasound Med Biol 2006;32:673-81.
40. Fajardo LF, Kowalski J, Kwan HH, Prionas SD, Allison AC. The disc angiogenesis system. Lab Invest 1988;58:718-24.
41. Guedez L, et al. Quantitative assessment of angiogenic responses by the directed in vivo angiogenesis assay. Am J Pathol 2003;162:1431-9.
42. Wang T, et al. CD97, An adhesion receptor on inflammatory cells, stimulates angiogenesis through binding integrin counter receptors on endothelial cells. Blood 2005;105:2836-44.
43. Gelmon KA, Eisenhauer EA, Harris AL, Ratain MJ, Workman P. Anticancer agents targeting signaling molecules and cancer cell environment: challenges for drug development? J Natl Cancer Inst 1999;91:1281-7.
44. Casciari JJ, et al. Growth and chemotherapeutic response of cells in a hollow-fiber in vitro solid tumor model. J Natl Cancer Inst 1994;86:1846-52.
45. Phillips RM, et al. Angiogenesis in the hollow fiber tumor model influences drug delivery to tumor cells: implications for anticancer drug screening programs. Cancer Res 1998;58:5263-6.
46. Akhtar N, Dickerson EB, Auerbach R. The sponge/Matrigel angiogenesis assay. Angiogenesis 2002;5:75-80.
47. MacDonald IC, Groom AC, Chambers AF. Cancer spread and micrometastasis development: quantitative approaches for in vivo models. Bioessays 2002;24:885-93.
48. Vajkoczy P, Ullrich A, Menger MD. Intravital fluorescence videomicroscopy to study tumor angiogenesis and microcirculation. Neoplasia 2000;2:53-61.
49. Brown EB, et al. In vivo measurement of gene expression, angiogenesis and physiological function in tumors using multiphoton laser scanning microscopy. Nat Med 2001;7:864-8.
50. Lutz BR, Fulton GP, Patt DI, Handler AH, Stevens DF. The cheek pouch of the hamster as a site for the transplantation of a methyl-cholanthrene-induced sarcoma. Cancer Res 1951;11:64-6.
51. Shubik P, Feldman R, Garcia H, Warren BA. Vascularization induced in the cheek pouch of the Syrian hamster by tumor and nontumor substances. J Natl Cancer Inst 1976;57:769-74.
52. Chandra Mohan KV, Devaraj H, Prathiba D, Hara Y, Nagini S. Antiproliferative and apoptosis inducing effect of lactoferrin and black tea polyphenol combination on hamster buccal pouch carcinogenesis. Biochim Biophys Acta 2006;1760:1536-44.
53. Fournier GA, Lutty GA, Watt S, Fenselau A, Patz A. A corneal micropocket assay for angiogenesis in the rat eye. Invest Ophthalmol Vis Sci 1981;21:351-4.

54. Gimbrone MA Jr, Cotran RS, Leapman SB, Folkman J. Tumor growth and neovascularization: an experimental model using the rabbit cornea. J Natl Cancer Inst 1974;52:413-27.
55. Norrby K, Jakobsson A, Sorbo J. Mast-cell-mediated angiogenesis: a novel experimental model using the rat mesentery. Virchows Arch B Cell Pathol Incl Mol Pathol 1986;52:195-206.
56. Norrby K. Microvascular density in terms of number and length of microvessel segments per unit tissue volume in mammalian angiogenesis. Microvasc Res 1998;55:43-53.
57. Norrby K, Jakobsson A, Sorbo J. Quantitative angiogenesis in spreads of intact rat mesenteric windows. Microvasc Res 1990;39:341-8.
58. Malcherek P, Franzen L. A new model for the study of angiogenesis in connective tissue repair. Microvasc Res 1991;42:217-23.
59. Stehbens WE. Observations on the microcirculation in the rabbit ear chamber. Q J Exp Physiol Cogn Med Sci 1967;52:150-6.
60. Szentirmai O, et al. Noninvasive bioluminescence imaging of luciferase expressing intracranial U87 xenografts: correlation with magnetic resonance imaging determined tumor volume and longitudinal use in assessing tumor growth and antiangiogenic treatment effect. Neurosurgery 2006;58:365-72.
61. Lichtenberg J, et al. The rat subcutaneous air sac model: a new and simple method for in vivo screening of antiangiogenesis. Pharmacol Toxicol 1997;81:280-4.
62. Cavallo T, Sade R, Folkman J, Cotran RS. Tumor angiogenesis. Rapid induction of endothelial mitoses demonstrated by autoradiography. J Cell Biol 1972;54:408-20.
63. Yang M, et al. Whole-body optical imaging of green fluorescent protein-expressing tumors and metastases. Proc Natl Acad Sci USA 2000;97:1206-11.
64. Yang M, et al. Whole-body and intravital optical imaging of angiogenesis in orthotopically implanted tumors. Proc Natl Acad Sci USA 2001;98:2616-21.
65. Ribatti D, et al. Chorioallantoic membrane capillary bed: a useful target for studying angiogenesis and antiangiogenesis in vivo. Anat Rec 2001;264:317-24.
66. Ausprunk DH, Knighton DR, Folkman J. Differentiation of vascular endothelium in the chick chorioallantois: a structural and autoradiographic study. Dev Biol 1974;38:237-48.
67. Shing Y, et al. Angiogenesis is stimulated by a tumor-derived endothelial cell growth factor. J Cell Biochem 1985;29:275-87.
68. Vico PG, Kyriacos S, Heymans O, Louryan S, Cartilier L. Dynamic study of the extraembryonic vascular network of the chick embryo by fractal analysis. J Theor Biol 1998;195:525-32.
69. Ejaz S, Chekarova I, Ashraf M, Lim CW. A novel 3-d model of chick chorioallantoic membrane for ameliorated studies in angiogenesis. Cancer Invest 2006;24:567-75.
70. Ny A, Autiero M, Carmeliet P. Zebrafish and Xenopus tadpoles: small animal models to study angiogenesis and lymphangiogenesis. Exp Cell Res 2006;312:684-93.
71. Tiedeken JJ III, Rovainen CM. Fluorescent imaging in vivo of developing blood vessels on the optic tectum of Xenopus laevis. Microvasc Res 1991;41:376-89.
72. Nasevicius A, Larson J, Ekker SC. Distinct requirements for zebrafish angiogenesis revealed by a VEGF-A morphant. Yeast 2000;17:294-301.
73. Serbedzija GN, Flynn E, Willett CE. Zebrafish angiogenesis: a new model for drug screening. Angiogenesis 1999;3:353-9.
74. Whipps CM, Kent ML. Polymerase chain reaction detection of Pseudoloma neurophilia, a common microsporidian of zebrafish (Danio rerio) reared in research laboratories. J Am Assoc Lab Anim Sci 2006;45:36-9.

75. Poss KD, Wilson LG, Keating MT. Heart regeneration in zebrafish. Science 2002;298:5601,2188-90.
76. Vihtelic TS, Hyde DR. Light-induced rod and cone cell death and regeneration in the adult albino zebrafish (Danio rerio) retina. J Neurobiol 2000;44(3):289-307.
77. De EM, et al. Hirudo medicinalis: a new model for testing activators and inhibitors of angiogenesis. Angiogenesis 2001;4:299-312.
78. De EM, et al. Leeches: immune response, angiogenesis and biomedical applications. Curr Pharm Des 2003;9:133-47.
79. Ingalls JM, Dickie MM, Snell GD. Obese, a new mutation in the house mouse. J Hered 1950;41:317-8.
80. Friedman JM, Halaas JL. Leptin and the regulation of body weight in mammals. Nature 1998;395, 6704:763-70.
81. Hummel KP, Dickie MM, Coleman DL. Diabetes, a new mutation in the mouse. Science 1966;153, 740:1127-8.

CHAPTER

7

Sexual Dysfunction

INTRODUCTION

Although sexual dysfunction has been well recognized both in male and female, male erectile dysfunction has been studied in greater detail as compared to female. After the introduction of phosphodiesterase V inhibitors, drug therapy for sexual dysfunction created a lot of commercial interest in developing newer and safe drugs. Penile erection is a complex neurohumoral-hemodynamic phenomenon.[1,2] Stimulation of sacral parasympathetic or cavernous nerves causes erection. Various neurotransmitters (acetylcholine, norepinephrine) and neuropeptides (vasoactive intestinal peptide, substance P) are known to be key mediators of erection.[3,4] Nonadrenergic, noncholinergic (NANC) neurotransmission is also a critical player in penile erection. During sexual arousal nitric oxide is produced in corpus cavernosum leading to relaxation of smooth muscle and engorgement of sinusoids with blood and penile erection (Fig. 7.1).[5-7] Male erectile dysfunction (MED) is multifactorial in origin wherein; stress, hypertension, hypercholesterolemia, diabetes mellitus, cigarette smoking and aging have been implicated (Fig. 7.2).[8-10] Different treatment options available are: psychosexual counseling, use of external vacuum devices, vascular surgery, penile prosthesis, intracavernous

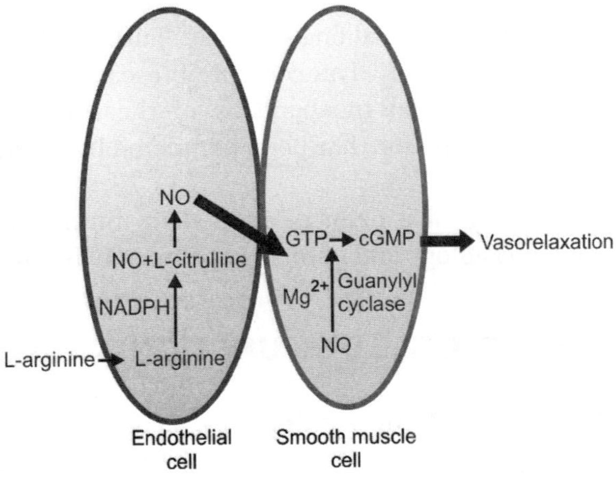

Figure 7.1: Interaction between endothelial cells and smooth muscle of the corpora cavernosa leading to erection (*For color version see Plate 12*)

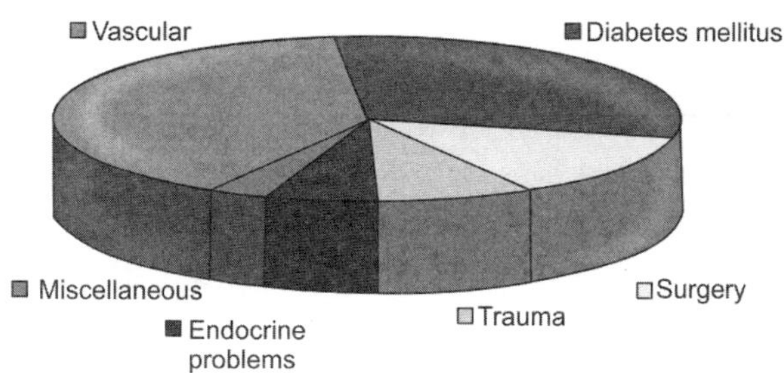

Figure 7.2: Causes of male erectile dysfunction (*For color version see Plate 12*)

injection therapy and medication. Majority of the drugs currently used are the result of serendipitous discovery rather than systematic research. Vascular smooth muscle relaxants like papaverine, prostaglandin E1 or an adrenoceptor antagonists like phentolamine, when injected intracavernously, cause increase in arterial inflow of blood, distention of sinusoids and consequently penile erection. However, these drugs do not act through any of normal physiological pathways or address the underlying pathology of erectile dysfunction and are ridden with numerous morbid side-effects like pain during injection, priapism, prolonged erection and cavernous fibrosis.

Metabolic syndrome (MetS) is a cluster of risk factors (hyperglycemia/diabetes, abdominal obesity, hypertriglyceridemia, low HDL cholesterol and hypertension), which identifies subjects at high risk for type 2 diabetes mellitus (T2DM) and CVD. Recently, MetS has been associated with ED and unresponsiveness to PDE5 inhibitors. The prevalence of ED in subjects with MetS ranges from 27% to 80% and is strictly associated with the number of MetS components and endothelial function impairment.[11]

The models for mimicking female sexual dysfunction (FSD) are more complex than male sexual dysfunction. FSD is currently categorized according to disorders of desire, arousal, orgasm and sexual pain.[12] The female sexual response cycle is initiated by nonadrenergic/ noncholinergic neurotransmitters (vasoactive intestinal polypeptide, nitric oxide) that maintain vascular and non-vascular smooth muscle relaxation resulting in increased pelvic blood flow, vaginal lubrication, and labial engorgement. Furthermore, hormonal status may influence female sexual function.[13] The advancement of research defining the physiological, pathophysiological and psychological mechanisms of these disorders, and to develop treatments for female sexual dysfunction, has been hampered by the paucity of experimental paradigms and animal models.

Bioassay and animal models have been developed in mice, rats, rabbits and dogs to understand the underlying physiology and pathology of erectile dysfunction, respectively.

MODELS FOR MALE ERECTILE DYSFUNCTION

Isolated Tension Studies in Organ Bath

Sexually mature male (22 to 26 weeks old) New Zealand rabbits weighing between 3.75–4.5 kg are used for the bioassay studies. Under intramuscular anesthesia of ketamine/xylazine and nembutal (25 mg/kg), the penis is isolated at the level of attachment of the corporal bodies to the ischium. The corpus cavernosum (total length—20 mm) is sharply dissected free from the tunica albuginea. Two longitudinal strips with a resting length of about 10 mm are made from its proximal portion, within Tyrode's solution gassed continuously with 95% oxygen and 5% CO_2 and maintained at 37°C. The tissue is mounted into the organ bath of 10 ml capacity and allowed to equilibrate for 30 minute under 2 g mechanical tension. The other end of the tissue is connected to a force displacement transducer and the change in muscle tension is recorded using polygraph.

Each strip is prestimulated with 100 µl of 200 µM phenylephrine to produce maximal contraction. Field stimulation method using a field stimulator is used to deliver biphasic square wave pulses of 80 V, 1 msec duration and 1-64 Hz frequencies. The relaxant effect of test agents is studied on the phenylephrine-stimulated contraction.[14]

Similarly, human corpus cavernosum strips obtained from patients undergoing penile prosthesis implant or penectomy can also be used to test *in vitro* effect of drugs on human tissue.[15] As a modification, corpus cavernosum of diabetic rabbit can also be used to understand the pathology of diabetic impotence and explore pharmacological interventions for it.[16]

An obvious limitation of *in vitro* models is the complete physiological mechanisms of cellular transport, tissue distribution and metabolism. Hormonal effects do not come into play and the results need to be interpreted with caution. In isolated tissue preparations, the turnover rate of cyclic nucleotide is low and a high concentration of phosphodiesterase (PDE) inhibitors is required to achieve significant response. PDE inhibitors show better efficacy in *in vivo* systems than in this model.[17]

In Vivo Model for Vasculogenic Impotence

Penile erection is a consequence of three simultaneous hemodynamic events, *viz*: increased arterial flow, sinusoidal relaxation and venous outflow restriction. Vasculogenic impotence is an important clinical issue, which demands thorough investigation. In such patients, vascular smooth muscle relaxants, like papaverine, prostaglandin E1 or a-adrenoceptor antagonists like phentolamine, have proved to be efficacious. Studies have been designed to evaluate the effect of impairment of each hemodynamic event alone, or in combination, on erectile function.

Adult male Sprague-Dawley rats weighing 200–300 g are used for the experiment. On the day of experiment, the animals are anesthetized with intraperitoneal pentobarbital sodium (50 mg/kg). Trachea, femoral artery and vein are cannulated for maintaining airway, measuring arterial pressure and drug administration, respectively.

With a midline perineal incision, followed by blunt dissection of the overlying striated muscles, entrance to the tunica albuginea of the crus corpus cavernosum is achieved. Needle prefilled with heparinized saline, attached to polyethylene catheter and connected to a pressure transducer, is inserted into corpus cavernosum to monitor intracavernous pressure. The needle has to be accurately inserted to avoid it from protruding from the corpus cavernosum. Standard drug like papaverine or prostaglandin E1 can be used to evaluate the robustness of the set-up. Test drugs and vehicle are injected intracavernously either subsequent to or in combination with papaverine for pharmacological evaluation. The dose response at various concentrations can be plotted to achieve dose response curve and ED.[50] Peak effect, peak time, initiation of response, duration of response and the ratio of peak intracavernous pressure to systemic blood pressure are the other paradigms which are evaluated.[18]

For electrical stimulation, cavernous nerve should be selected. The appropriate submaximal electrical stimulation correlates the increase or decrease in intracavernous pressure for the evaluation. On electrical stimulation, the difference between basal and peak intracavernous pressure, ratio of peak intracavernous to systemic blood pressure and the slopes of tumescence and detumescence are evaluated.

Rats provide suitable model for the evaluation of penile erection in small laboratory animals. Although penile elongation and intracavernous pressure can be recorded, erectile angle is not feasible due to congenital angulation of penis in the rat. Also, the engorgement during erection is not prominent.[18]

Monitoring intracavernous pressure is an objective, accurate and quantitative assessment for penile erection. Moreover, in this model neuraxis is intact and neurophysiological and pharmacological studies can be conveniently conducted.[18]

Model for Arteriogenic Impotence

Penile vascular smooth muscle relaxation increases the inflow of arterial blood and distension of sinusoids leading to erection. Low cavernosal artery perfusion pressure can lead to erectile dysfunction. Arteriogenic impotence is clinically manifested as slowly developing, inadequately rigid erections for satisfactory sexual intercourse.[19] To elucidate the effect of obstruction of internal iliacs on erectile function, models with acute and chronic occlusion have been designed in dogs. In the acute model, the penile artery can be clamped with non-crushing clamps unilaterally or bilaterally.[20]

Arteriogenic impotence is induced in adult male dogs weighing between 15–20 kg. The penile arteries are ligated just proximal to the crus of the penis. The cavernous vein and penile artery are anastomosed proximal to the site of ligation and the pudendal vein is ligated proximally to prevent the diversion of arterial blood away from the penis. The intracavernosal pressure is recorded through a 21-gauge butterfly needle inserted into the cavernosum and connected to a pressure transducer. Electrodes are planted around cavernous nerves and erection is induced by electrostimulation. Alternatively, erection may also be induced by intracavernous injection of papaverine. The effect of the drugs is studied by comparing the erectile response before and after cavernous vein arterializations. The following parameters are studied: blood flow rate through penile artery and intracavernosal pressure. After completion of the drug treatment, selective pudendal artery angiography can also be conducted. The animals are sacrificed under excess ether and the tissue is assessed histopathologically.[21]

Acute mechanical ligation of both right and left internal iliacs, or pudendal arteries in dogs, reduces the cavernosal blood supply by 50% and 60% fall in intracavernosal pressure.[20,22] However, chronic obstruction of penile blood vessels has minimal effect on erectile function due to the development of collaterals around the penis.[20]

Model for Atherosclerotic Impotence

Studies have associated obstruction of the arterial supply to the corporal bodies due to atherosclerotic vascular disease to impotence in humans.[23] Rabbit model, simulating erectile dysfunction due to atherosclerotic lesions, has been validated by Azadzoi and Goldstein.[24]

Six to seven months old male White New Zealand rabbits, weighing between 3 and 3.5 kg are used for the experiment. The animals are divided into two groups. The control group is fed with normal diet. The test group is administered pentobarbital anesthesia and a catheter is passed through femoral arteriotomies into the abdominal aorta. A balloon is inflated with 0.2 ml normal saline to fit the abdominal aorta, and subsequently withdrawn to femoral artery. The exercise is repeated thrice and endothelial injury inflicted on the iliacs. After balloon de-endothelialization, the animals receive 1.6% cholesterol mixed with 4% peanut oil for 8 weeks. After 8 weeks, the arterial blood is analyzed for cholesterol, triglycerides, high density lipoprotein, low density lipoprotein along with angiographic analysis. The percentage of arterial narrowing of iliacs is evaluated and intracavernosal effects are also studied. Under anesthesia, the carotid artery is cannulated and connected to pressure transducer to monitor systemic blood pressure. A 21-gauge needle connected to catheter is inserted into the corporal body for recording intracavernosal pressure. A second 21-gauge needle is placed into contralateral corporal body for intracavernosal drug administration. Penile erections are induced by 5 mg intracavernosal papaverine. The test and vehicle are injected either concomitantly or subsequent to papaverine administration. The parameters studied are: ratio of intracavernosal to systemic blood pressure, systemic systolic and diastolic arterial blood pressure. After the conclusion of the experiment, the animals are sacrificed and the tissue is studied histopathologically.[24]

Attempts to induce atherosclerotic arteriogenic impotence in dogs using ligatures or occluding rings, have failed to achieve any hemodynamic impairment or local vascular and erectile abnormalities.[24] The rabbit model is more appropriate to study the effect of hypercholesterolemia and atherosclerosis on erectile function. Moreover, the effects manifest within 6 weeks in rabbits, while dogs and monkeys may take one to five years to exhibit the same.[25] However, there are some pathologic differences evident in the atherosclerotic lesions between rabbits and humans.[24]

Model for Post-traumatic Arteriogenic Erectile Dysfunction

Pelvic or perineal trauma from bicycle accidents are known to cause focal lesion of the common penile or cavernous artery, leading to post-traumatic arteriogenic erectile dysfunction. Rat model has been developed to simulate traumatic arteriogenic erectile dysfunction by ligating each internal iliac artery of the animal.[26]

The experiment protocol requires 3-month-old male Sprague-Dawley rats weighing between 350–400 g. Under intraperitoneal pentobarbitone (35 mg/kg) anesthesia, a midline laparotomy is done and iliac vessels identified. In the test group the internal iliac artery is ligated at its origin, whereas, in the sham group only exploration is conducted. Intracavernous pressure is recorded using a needle inserted into crus and connected to a pressure monitor. The wound is closed and animal observed for 6 weeks.

The cavernous nerve is stimulated using bipolar platinum wire electrodes. The exposed end of the electrodes is hooked around the nerve and stimulated with positive electrode positioned proximally and the negative electrode 2-3 mm distally. The stimulus parameters used are 1.5 V, frequency 20 pulses/second pulse width 0.2 msec and duration 50 second.

After the study, the animals are sacrificed and the tissue can be used for immunohisto-chemical staining and electron microscopy.

Arteriogenic erectile dysfunction develops immediately in these animals with no gross ischemic changes in pelvic organs or genitalia. This model has many advantages. The nerves of the rat can be easily identified and stimulated. The rats are resilient and less prone to infection and anesthesia related complications. However, as the internal iliac artery of the rat is small, the surgical procedure has to be conducted under operating microscope with constant monitoring of intracavernous pressure.[26]

Cavernous Nerve Injury Model of Erectile Dysfunction

The rat model of cavernous nerve (CN) injury has been developed in an effort to define the functional and structural consequences of neural trauma in the corpus cavernosum. However, many methods were reported in the literature to induce cavernous nerve injury in rats viz. neurotomy,[27] nerve crush,[28] and hemostat nerve crush bilateral nerve freezing,[27] etc. Mullered et al.[29] induced cavernous nerve injury using various techniques in an effort to compare the hemodynamic sequelae of these injuries. They compared the effect of different procedures on the intracavernosal pressure in adult male Sprague-Dawley rats to standardize this model.

1. Control: laparotomy only.
2. Exposure: laparotomy and exposure of cavernous nerves bilaterally without nerve manipulation.
3. Neurotomy: bilateral neurotomy.
4. Bulldog crush: bilateral nerve crush with bulldog vascular clamp.
5. Hemostat nerve crush: bilateral nerve crush with a hemostat.

Ten days later, a second surgery was performed during which systemic mean arterial pressure (MAP) and intracavernosal pressure (ICP) was measured in response to cavernosal nerve stimulation proximal to the site of injury. This study reported that ICP/MAP ratios were significantly reduced in all cavernosal nerve injury groups as compared with control group. No significant difference existed in ICP/MAP ratios between the injury groups. Moreover, the rates of tumescence and detumescence were significantly reduced in all groups as compared with the control group, without any significant difference in the magnitude and consistency of hemodynamic alterations. Using the cavernous nerve injury model, Allaf and co-workers studied the effect of erythropoietin in promoting the recovery of the cavernous nerve injury.[30]

Model for Venous Incompetence Induced Impotence

Venous incompetence leads to organic impotence and was first reported by Lowsley and Bray in 1936.[31]

Adult healthy male mongrel dogs weighing between 20 and 30 kg are used in this study. The animals are anesthetized using intravenous pentobarbitone (30 mg/kg). An intravenous line for fluid infusion (2 ml/kg/hr) is also given. Surgery involves a midline incision and prostate exposure. The cavernous nerve is identified by electrostimulation and bipolar cuff electrodes are placed around it for inducing erection. Saline prefilled needle is carefully inserted into the corpus cavernosum and connected to a pressure transducer to monitor intracavernous pressure. Ipsilateral pudendal artery is cannulated to monitor blood flow. Systemic blood pressure is monitored via catheter placed in femoral artery.

After all cannulations are made, a stabilization time of 30 minute is allocated and baseline reading of following paradigms recorded: peak and maintenance of penile blood flow, latency period to achieve maximal intracavernous pressure, rise in intracavernous pressure and duration of detumescence. The cavernous nerve is stimulated to elicit erection and above-mentioned paradigms are recorded again.

To simulate the pathological condition of erectile dysfunction due to venous leakage, different sized heparinized needles are inserted in corpus cavernosum and venous blood is allowed to leak. Cavernous nerves are re-stimulated and the aforementioned paradigms are re-estimated. In addition, the volume of blood lost is also recorded. The effect of test, vehicle and standard is recorded and the data analyzed statistically.

This model helps to gain insight into the physiology and interplay of various mechanisms of penile erection. In a healthy animal with robust arterial flow, minor venous leakage does not have prominent impact on erectile response. This model sheds light on the assessment criteria set for the diagnosis of vasculogenic impotence in humans.

Psychical Model of Erectile Dysfunction

It is now well established hypothesis that stress deters sexual function and this hypothesis has been demonstrated in animal model of psychical erectile dysfunction wherein, emotional stress has been correlated to the sexual performance of the animals.[32] Male rats with normal sexual function were divided into normal group and model group randomly according to their weights. Stress was applied to the rats in the model group by suspending them upside down in midair over the water and irritated repeatedly. Two weeks later, the sexual abilities of all rats, i.e. the times of mounting and intromitting the estrus female rats, the latent period of mounting, intromission and ejaculation, were recorded, and the number of rats that had sexual activities were also counted. They have also measured hemorheology indices of the rats. This study has also compared the sexual behavior of demasculinized rats subjected to the same stress. The authors observed that as compared to normal rats, the latency of mounting and intromission of the model rats were longer ($p < 0.01$), with the shortening of latency of ejaculation ($p < 0.05$). They have also reported that intromission times of model rats were lower than that of the normal rats ($p < 0.01$). Compared with the normal rats, the sexual activity incidence of the model rats (mounting: 58.3%, intromission: 33.3%, ejaculation: 16.7%) was significantly lower than that of the normal rats (100%) ($p < 0.01$). But, there was no significant difference in the sexual ability between the model and the demasculinized rats ($p > 0.05$). This could be one of the available models to study the drug, which can reduce stress on the sexual behavior.

Model for Diabetes Mellitus Induced Impotence

Due to unhealthy lifestyle, the prevalence of diabetes and its complications is increasing. Diabetes mellitus is a significant risk factor in the development of erectile function and animal models have been developed to study this complications.

Neonate C57BL6 (bl6) mice are randomly divided into different groups of treated and control. The treatment-group rats are fed a high-fat (45% of total calories) diet for either 4, 8, 12, 16, or 22 weeks. The animals in control group are fed normal diet. At the end of the study, under excess ether anesthesia, the corporal tissues from the animals is harvested and studied for various parameters including vasoreactivity, endothelial and smooth muscle cell content. Corporal tissue from mice with diet-induced diabetes mellitus demonstrate many of the major functional, structural, and biochemical changes found in humans with erectile dysfunction. This model serves as a valuable tool for studying the role of diabetes mellitus in the pathogenesis of ED.[33]

High-fat Diet (HFD)-induced Metabolic Syndrome and Complication of Erectile Dysfunction

Male New Zealand white rabbits are provided with either high-fat-diet (0.5% cholesterol and 4% peanut oil) or regular diet for 12 weeks. The animals develop alterations in hormonal and endothelial function that chronically manifests as erectile dysfunction. The penile tissue from rabbits from the different groups can be compared on the basis of morphology and function of endothelial and smooth muscle cells of the vascular bed and cavernous spaces.[11,34]

Genetically Modified Mice

The development of sterility in the inbred male mice homozygous for the stubby gene mutation has been reported. Chubb and Henry reported the utilization of stubby gene mutated mice as an animal model for the study of impotence.[35] The autosomal gene mutation is reported to be a responsible factor for the primary effect on male sexual behavior in this model. The utility of this model was not found in subsequent literature for the screening of MED.

ANIMAL MODELS FOR FEMALE SEXUAL DYSFUNCTION

Female sexual dysfunction (FSD) is a significant and highly prevalent problem that affects a substantial number of women that causes personal distress and has negative effects on quality of life and interpersonal relationships. The experimental models of female sexual dysfunction (FSD) have involved a range of *in vitro* to *in vivo* methodologies. Specifically, the *in vitro* and *in situ* models include vaginal or clitoral smooth muscle preparations, histological evaluation and vaginal blood flow assessments.

Vaginal or Clitoral Smooth Muscle Preparations (Bio-Assay)

Female rabbits were anesthetized with sodium thiopental (30 mg/kg intravenously) and exsanguinated. The entire clitoris including vagina was excised rapidly. The vaginal wall was dissected free from the clitoral body. The clitoral cavernosum tissue was then carefully dissected free from the surrounding tunica albuginea under dissecting microscope and two strips along the longitudinal axis (about 0.5 × 0.5 mm) were obtained. During the preparation, care was taken not to damage the functional endothelium or overstretch the tissue. A strip of the rabbit clitoris was vertically placed in 2 ml organ chamber, with one end connected with a cotton thread to the prong of force transducer and the other end secured with a cotton thread to a holder for isometric tension measurements. The bath chambers contained the appropriate HEPES buffer solution (37°C) and constantly aerated with 100% O_2. Isometric force was measured and recorded using a polygraph. After mounting, strips were equilibrated for 60 minute with several adjustments of length until a baseline force stabilized at 1 g and oxygenated medium was replaced every 20 minute. This preparation was contracted with phenylephrine and relaxed with acetylcholine. Using the above procedure and preparation, Park and coworkers[36] studied the effect of angiotensin peptides in the regulation of clitoral cavernosum smooth muscle tone.

Pelvic Nerve Electrical Stimulation in Female Dogs

Angulo et al[37] evaluated the effects of vardenafil on the increase of blood flow into the vagina and clitoris induced by Pelvic Nerve Electrical Stimulation (PNES) in female dogs. Application of PNES produced consistent and frequency-related increased blood flow into the vagina and clitoris of anesthetized female dogs. The magnitude and duration of the blood flow responses to PNES were variable among the different animals but remained stable over time within the same animal. In this model, they have evaluated the effect of vardenafil, a phosphodiesterase -V inhibitor, by monitoring blood flow produced by PNES into the vagina and clitoris after drug administration. Similarly, effect of sildenafil facilitated female genital sexual arousal was studied in female rabbits[38] after pelvic nerve stimulation. After pelvic nerve stimulation at 4, 16, and 32 Hz, hemoglobin concentration and oxygen saturation in female genital (vaginal, labial, clitoral) tissues is evaluated by laser oximetry. Clitoral blood flow is recorded by laser Doppler flowmetry, vaginal luminal pressure by a balloon catheter pressure transducer and vaginal lubrication by tampon.

CONCLUSION

Continued upsurge in the insight towards human sexual functions, behavior and innovative approaches in understanding molecular mechanisms in this field, triggered researchers to develop and validate suitable *in vitro* and *in vivo* models. The models enable effective screening of molecules for the management of male and female sexual dysfunction.

REFERENCES

1. Lue TF, Takamura R, Schmid RA, et al. Hemodynamics of erection in the monkey. J Urol 1983;130:1237-41.
2. Adaikan PG, Ratnam SS. Pharmacology of penile erection in humans. Cardiovasc Intervent Radiol 1988;11:191-4.
3. De Groat WC, Steers WD. Neuroanatomy and neurophysiology of penile erection. In Tanagho EA, Lue TF (Eds): Contemporary Management of Impotence and Infertility. Baltimore : Williams and Wilkins, 1988:3-27.
4. Polak JM, Gu J, Mina S, et al. Vipergic nerves in the penis. Lancet 1981;2:217-9.
5. Kim N, Azadzoi KM, Goldstein I, et al. A nitric oxide-like factor mediates nonadrenergic, noncholinergic neurogenic relaxation of penile corpus cavernosum smooth muscle. J Clin Invest 1991;88:112-8.
6. Rajfer J, Aronson WJ, Bush PA, et al. Nitric oxide as a mediator of relaxation of the corpus cavernosum in response to nonadrenergic, noncholinergic neurotransmission. N Engl J Med 1992;326:90-4.
7. Burnett AL, Lowenstein CJ, Bredt DS, et al. Nitric oxide: a physiologic mediator of penile erection. Science 1992;257:401-3.
8. Goldstein I, Feldman MI, Deckers PJ, et al. Radiation-associated impotence: a clinical study of its mechanism. JAMA 1984;251:903-10.
9. Rosen MP, Greenfield AJ, Walker TG, et al. Arteriogenic impotence: findings in 195 impotent men examined with selective internal pudendal angiography. Radiology 1990;174:1043-8.

10. Levine FJ, Greenfield AJ, Goldstein I. Arteriographically determined occlusive disease within the hypogastric cavernous bed in impotent patients following blunt perineal and pelvic trauma. J Urol 1990;144:1147-53.
11. Maneschi E, Vignozzi L, Morelli A, Mello T, Filippi S, Cellai I et al. FXR activation normalizes insulin sensitivity in visceral preadipocytes of a rabbit model of MetS. J Endocrinol 2013;218(2):215-31.
12. Hale TM, Heaton JP, Adams MA. A framework for the present and future development of experimental models of female sexual dysfunction. Int J Impot Res 2003;15 Suppl 5:S75.
13. Verit FF, Yeni E, Kafali H. Progress in female sexual dysfunction. Urol Int 2006;76(1):1-10.
14. Liu SP, Hass MA, Horan P, et al. Physiological effects of macrocycle 1 on the rabbit corpus cavernosum. Pharmacology 1998;56:144-9.
15. Stief CG, Uckert S, Becker AJ, et al. The effect of the specific phosphodiesterase (PDE) inhibitors on human and rabbit cavernous tissue in vitro and in vivo. J Urol 1998;159:1390-3.
16. Utkan T, Yildirim MK, Yildirim S, et al. Effects of the specific phosphodiesterase inhibitors on alloxan-induced diabetic rabbit cavernous tissue in vitro. Int J Impot Res 2001;13:24-30.
17. Nicholson CD, Challiss RA, Shahid M. Differential modulation of tissue function and therapeutic potential of selective inhibitors of cyclic nucleotide phosphodiesterase isoenzymes. Trends Pharmacol Sci 1991;12:19-27.
18. Chen KK, Chan JY, Chang LS, et al. Intracavernous pressure as an experimental index in a rat model for the evaluation of penile erection. J Urol 1992;147:1124-8.
19. Vardi Y, Siroky MB. Hemodynamics of pelvic nerve induced erection in a canine model.I. Pressure and flow. J Urol 1990;44:794-7.
20. Aboseif SR, Breza J, Orvis BR, et al. Erectile response to acute and chronic occlusion of the internal pudendal and penile arteries. J Urol 1989;141:398-402.
21. Breza J, Aboseif SR, Lue TF, et al. Cavernous vein arterialization of vasculogenic impotence: an animal model. Urology 1990;35:513-8.
22. Takagane H, Matsuzaka J, Aoki H, et al. Hemodynamic studies of penile erection in dogs blood flow changes in the corpus cavernosum caused by arterial ligation. Proceedings of the sixth Biennial International Symposium on Corpus Cavernosum Revascularization and Third Biennial World Meeting on Impotence, Boston, Massachusetts, 13, October, 1988.
23. Virag R. Impotence: a new field in angiology. Int Angio 1984;3:217-9.
24. Azadzoi KM, Goldstein I. Erectile dysfunction due to atherosclerotic vascular disease: The development of an animal model. J Urol 1992;147:1675-81.
25. Wissler RW, Vesselinovitch D. Evaluation of animal models for the study of the pathogenesis of atherosclerosis. In International Symposium on the State of Prevention and Therapy in Human Arteriosclerosis in Animal Models, in Mèunster/Westfalen, June 22nd to June 25th 1977.
26. Lee MC, El-Sakka AL, Graziottin TM, et al. The effect of vascular endothelial growth factor on the rat model of traumatic arteriogenic erectile dysfunction. J Urol 2002;167:761-7.
27. Kato R, Wolfe D, Coyle CH, Wechuck JB, Tyagi P, Tsukamoto T et al. Herpes simplex virus vector-mediated delivery of neurturin rescues erectile dysfunction of cavernous nerve injury. Gene Ther 2009 Jan;16(1):26-33.
28. Hayashi N, Minor TX, Carrion R, Price R, Nunes L, Lue TF. The effect of FK1706 on erectile function following bilateral cavernous nerve crush injury in a rat model. J Urol 2006 Aug;176(2):824-9.
29. Mullerad M, Donohue JF, Li PS, Scardino PT, Mulhall JP. Functional sequelae of cavernous nerve injury in the rat: is there model dependency. J Sex Med 2006 Jan;3(1):77-83.

30. Allaf ME, Hoke A, Burnett AL. Erythropoietin promotes the recovery of erectile function following cavernous nerve injury. J Urol 2005 Nov;174(5):2060-4.
31. Lowsley OS, Bray JC. The surgical relief of impotence: Further experiences with a new operative procedure. JAMA 1936;107:2029-35.
32. Wang QL, Wang SR, Duan J.Establishment of rat model of psychical erectile dysfunction. Zhonghua Nan Ke Xue 2006;12:43-5;49.
33. Xie D, Odronic SI, Wu F, Pippen A, Donatucci CF, Annex BH. Mouse model of erectile dysfunction due to diet-induced diabetes mellitus. Urology 2007;70:196-201.
34. Morelli A, Vignozzi L, Maggi M, Adorini L. Farnesoid X receptor activation improves erectile dysfunction in models of metabolic syndrome and diabetes. Biochim Biophys Acta 2011 Aug;1812(8):859-66.
35. Chubb C, Henry L. Impotence induced by a single gene mutation. Biol Reprod 1987;36:557-61.
36. Park JK, Kim SZ, Kim JU, Kim YG, Kim SM, Cho KW. Comparison of effects of angiotensin peptides in the regulation of clitoral cavernosum smooth muscle tone. Int J Impot Res 2002;14:72-80.
37. Angulo J, Cuevas P, Cuevas B, Bischoff E, Sáenz de Tejada I. Vardenafil enhances clitoral and vaginal blood flow responses to pelvic nerve stimulation in female dogs. Int J Impot Res 2003;15:137-41.
38. Min K, Kim NN, McAuley I, Stankowicz M, Goldstein I, Traish AM. Sildenafil augments pelvic nerve-mediated female genital sexual arousal in the anesthetized rabbit. Int J Impot Res 2000;12:S32-9.

CHAPTER

8

Antifertility Agents

INTRODUCTION

Antifertility agents are the agents, which prevent the fertility by interfering with various normal reproductive mechanisms, in both males and females. Development of newer methods/agents for fertility control and research in this direction are imperative, particularly, in the developing nations. If an ideal contraceptive were available, that contraceptive would be 100% effective, safe, and easy to use; its effect would be reversible. It would be aesthetically and personally acceptable in a variety of social, political and religious settings. It would be suitable culturally in terms of local attitudes concerning sexuality, reproduction, menstruation and the roles and responsibilities of men and women, and it would be applicable in terms of the health status of widely differing populations. It would be affordable, readily available and legal. Finally, it would be appropriate for use at all stages of reproduction. As yet, no single method of contraception meet all of these criteria, but each of the presently available methods meet at least a few, and some methods meet many of them.[1]

METHODS FOR FEMALES

Female antifertility agents might be acting through following mechanisms:

1. Inhibition of ovulation.
2. Prevention of fertilization.
3. Interference with transport of ova from oviduct to endometrium of the uterus.
4. Interference with the implantation of fertilized ovum.
5. Distraction of early implanted embryo.

Antiovulatory Activity

HCG-induced Ovulation in Rats

Immature female albino rats do not ovulate spontaneously and do not show cyclic changes of the vaginal epithelium. Priming with human chorionic gonadotropin (HCG) induces follicular maturation, followed by spontaneous ovulation 2 days later. Injection of antiovulatory drugs, prior to the induction procedure will prevent ovulation. This principle is used for the screening of anti-ovulatory agents.[2]

Procedure: Immature female albino rats 24-26 days of age are used for the experiment. The animals are treated with various test drugs in a different dose levels. After the administration of the test drug, HCG is given exogenously for ovulation. After 2 days, animals are sacrificed, ovaries are dissected out, preserved in 10% buffered formalin and subjected to histopathological evaluation. The results are compared with the control group.

Cupric Acetate-induced Ovulation in Rabbits

The rabbits are reflex ovulators. They ovulate within a few hours after mating or after mechanical stimulation of vagina or sometimes even mere presence of males, or administration of certain chemicals like cupric acetate. In this method, cupric acetate is used for the induction of ovulation. The rabbit ovulates within a few hours after injection of cupric acetate (0.3 mg/kg i.v. of 1% cupric acetate in 0.9% saline). Injection of antiovulatory drugs, 24 hours before the induction procedure prevents ovulation.[3]

Procedure: Sexually mature female albino rabbits, weighing 3-4 kg, are used for the study. Animals are kept in isolation for at least 21 days to ensure, they are not pregnant and to prevent the induction of ovulation by mating. They are treated with test drug and 24 hours later cupric acetate is given. The rabbits are sacrificed and ovaries are examined 18-24 hours later. The total number of ovulation points on both ovaries are recorded for each animal. Then the ovaries and uterus are excised out and preserved in 10% buffered formalin and subjected to histopathological evaluation (Fig. 8.1).[4]

Estrogenic Activity

A primary therapeutic use of estrogen is in contraception. The rationale for these preparations is that excess exogenous estrogen inhibits FSH and LH, thus prevents ovulation.

In Vivo Methods

Vaginal Opening

This assay is based on the principle that vaginal opening occurs in immature female albino mice and rats by treating with estrogenic compounds. The sign of complete vaginal opening is observed as a sign of estrogenic activity.

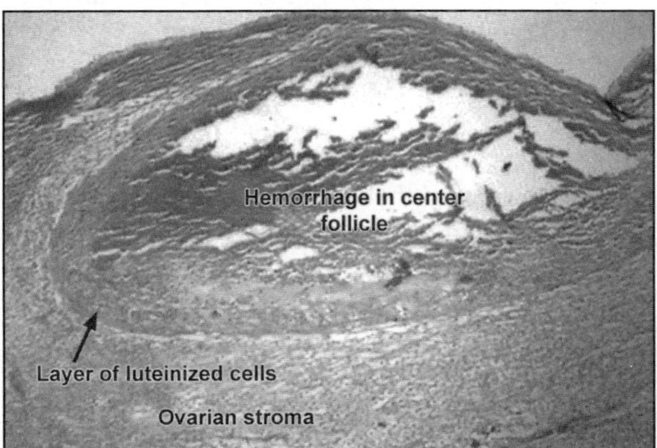

Figure 8.1: Ovulation point in rabbit ovary (HE × 40 ×) *(For color version see Plate 12)*

Procedure: Immature female animals (18-day-old mice, 21-day-old rats) are used for the study. The test and standard drugs are administered to the animals intramuscularly in cotton seed oil. The time of complete vaginal opening can be observed as a sign of estrogenic activity.[3]

Assay for Water Uptake

The principle of the assay is based on the observation that the uterus responds to estrogens by increased uptake and retention of water. A peak for water uptake is observed at 6 hours after administration.[3]

Procedure: Ovariectomized animals may be used, because this assay employs the uterine weight increase as the response, the uterus must remain intact during ovariectomy. It is simpler to use immature 18-day-old mice or 22-day-old rats obtained 2 days prior to the beginning of the experiment. The animals are randomly grouped. The control group is given 0.1 ml of cotton seed oil subcutaneously. The estrogen control group is given a range doses (0.01–0.1 μg) to establish a dose response curve. The test compound is given to groups in the initial test at a high and low dose. In subsequent tests it is given over a range of doses to provide the dose response curve. All doses are given in 0.1 ml of cotton seed oil. Five hours after treatment, the animals are killed by cervical dislocation and the uteri are quickly excised. The operation is begun by a longitudinal slit through the skin of abdomen and through the body wall. The uterus is picked up with the forceps and severed from vagina. The uterine horns are separated from the connective tissues and are then cut at constriction near the ovary. The uteri are kept damp by placing them on (not wet) filter paper and by covering them with moist filter paper. They are then rapidly weighed in a sensitive balance. The uteri are dried in an oven at 100°C, for 24 hour and are reweighed. The percentage increase in water over control can be calculated, and can be compared with the values of other groups.

Ovariectomy: The animals are slightly anesthetized with ether. A single transverse incision is made in the skin of the back. That incision can be shifted readily from one side to the other, so as to lie over each ovary in turn. A small puncture is then made over the site of the ovary, which can be seen through the abdominal wall, embedded in a pad of fat. The top of a pair of fine forceps is introduced and the fat around the ovary was grasped, care being taken not to rupture the capsule around the ovary itself. The tip of the uterine horn is then crushed with a pair of artery forceps, and the ovary together with the fallopian tube is removed with a single cut by a pair of fine scissors. Usually, no bleeding is observed.

The muscular wound is closed by absorbable sutures and outer skin wound is closed by nylon suture.

Four-day Uterine Weight Assay

This assay is based on the observation that estrogens cause an increase in protein synthesis, and thus, bring about an increase in uterine weight. A peak in uterine weight is observed in about 40 hours.[3]

Procedure: Immature or adult ovariectomized albino mice or rats can be given test drug intramuscularly in cotton seed oil for three consecutive days. On the fourth day, animals are killed by cervical fracture, the uteri are rapidly excised, and the uterine contents are gently squeezed out (results are unreliable if the uterine contents are not removed). The uteri are weighed immediately in the wet state. The uteri may be dehydrated in an oven at 100° C for 24 hour and reweighed to obtain the dry weight increase. The log dose, plotted against the wet weight, produces a sigmoid curve, and the ED50 can be determined for comparison of the test compound with estradiol.

Vaginal Cornification

On the basis of the observation of cyclic vaginal cornification in guinea pigs by Stockard and Papanicolaou (1917),[5] the Allen-Doisy (1923)[6] found the vaginal cornification in rodents.

This assay is based on the fact that rats and mice exhibit a cyclical ovulation with associated changes in the secretion of hormones, this lead to the changes in the vaginal epithelial cells. The estrus cycle is classified into proestrus, estrus, metestrus and diestrus. Drugs with estrogenic activity change the animals into estrus stage.

Procedure: Adult female albino rats having regular estrus cycle are used for the study. Animals are treated with various test and standard drugs. Changes in the vagina can be observed by taking vaginal smears, and examining these for cornified cells, leukocytes and epithelial cells in the normal animals, and treated animals twice daily over a period of 4 days. The drug, which changes the animals into estrus stage skipping other stages, is considered to have estrogenic activity.[3,7]

Stages of the estrus cycle in rats: The estrus cycle is a cascade of hormonal and behavioral events, which are highly synchronized and repetitive.

The short and precise estrus cycle of the laboratory rats has been a useful model for reproductive studies. The laboratory rat is a spontaneous ovulating, nonseasonal, polyestrus animal. It ovulates every 4–5 days throughout the year unless interrupted by pregnancy or pseudopregnancy. A century ago, the English scientist Walter Heape described the progressive stages of the estrus cycle. The cycle itself is divided into four stages, centered around the period proceeding estrus "proestrus", which signifies the period of follicular growth in the ovary, and he termed the period succeeding estrus "metestrus" and recovery period following ovulation and "diestrus", a period when the ovarian secretions from the corpus luteum prepare the uterus for implantation. The estrus cycle of a rat is usually completed in 4–5 days.

Proestrus: It is the beginning of new cycle. The follicles of the ovary start to mature under the influence of gonadotropic hormones and estrogen secretion start increasing; the smear is characterized by nucleated epithelial cells, the stage last for about 12 hours.

Estrus: In this stage, the uterus is enlarged and extended due to fluid accumulation, estrogen secretion is at its peak. In estrus stage, the smear shows presence of squamous cornified cells (hexagonal or pentagonal cells). Estrus means period of heat and is characterized as a period of sexual receptivity, when the female allows copulation. During this stage, there is increased running activity. This stage lasts for 12 hours.

Metestrus: The ovary contains corpora lutea, secreting progesterone. This stage is indicated by the presence of a mixture of cornified epithelial cells and leukocytes indicating the postovulatory stage and desquamation of the epithelial cells. Metestrus stage lasts for about 21 hours.

Diestrus: The corpus lutea regress and the declining secretion of estrogen and progesterone causes regression of the uterus. The smear shows only leukocytes. This stage is the longest phase of the estrus cycle and has duration of about 57 hours (Figs 8.2 to 8.7).

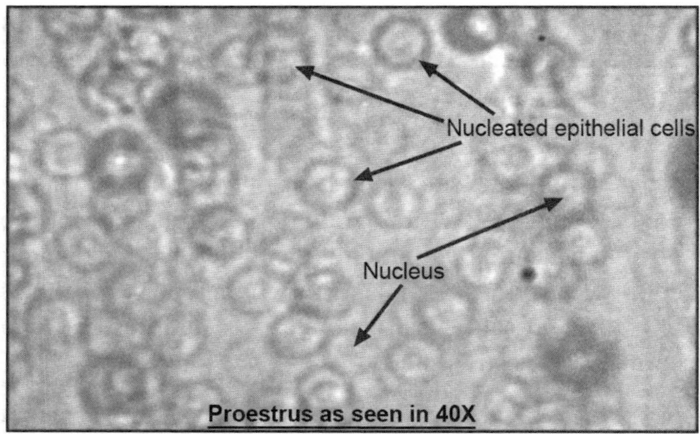

Figure 8.2: Rat vaginal smear at proestrus stage showing nucleated epithelial cells as seen in 40X (*For color version see Plate 13*)

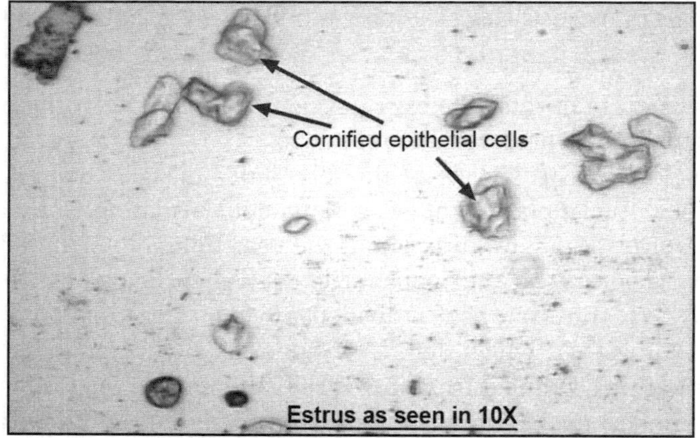

Figure 8.3: Rat vaginal smear at estrus stage showing cornified epithelial cells as seen in 10X (*For color version see Plate 13*)

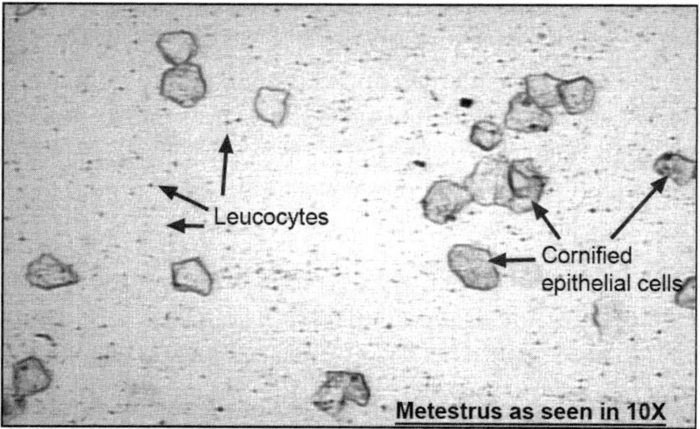

Figure 8.4: Rat vaginal smear at metestrus stage showing both cornified epithelial cells and leukocytes as seen in 10X (*For color version see Plate 13*)

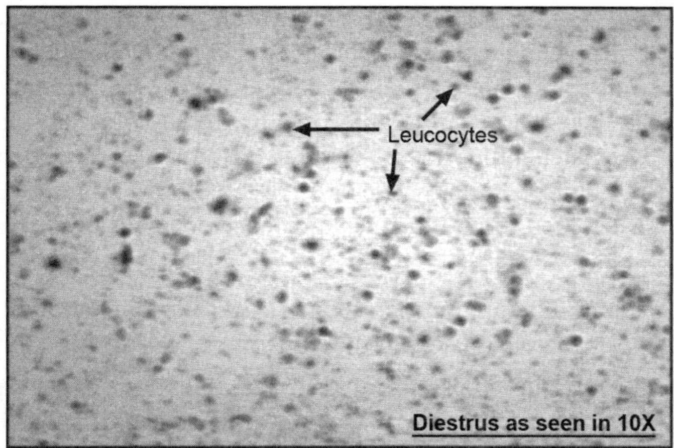

Figure 8.5: Rat vaginal smear at diestrus stage showing only leukocytes as seen in 10X (*For color version see Plate 14*)

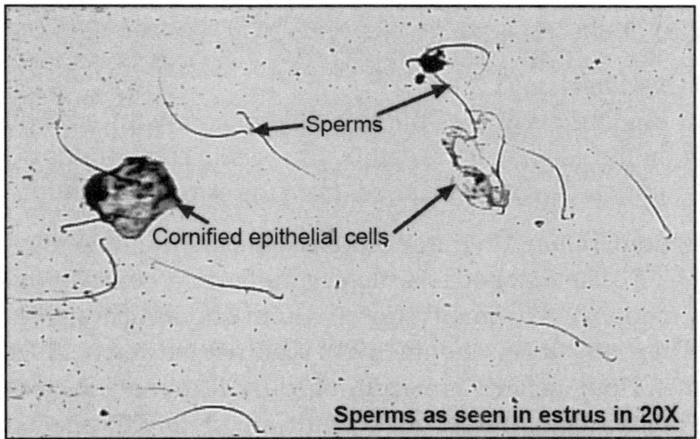

Figure 8.6: Rat vaginal smear of mated animal showing cornified epithelial cells and sperms as seen in 20X (*For color version see Plate 14*)

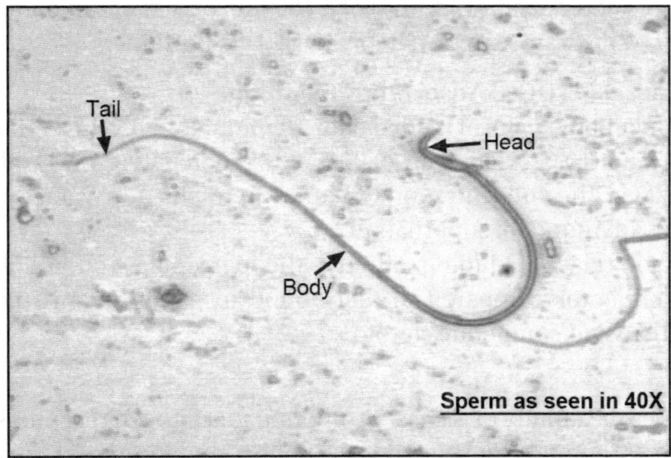

Figure 8.7: Rat vaginal smear of mated animal showing sperms as seen in 40X (*For color version see Plate 14*)

Preparation of vaginal smears: Hold the animal with the ventral side up, a drop of normal saline is inserted into the vagina with a Pasteur pipette. Care must be taken to avoid damage or injury to vagina so as to prevent pseudopregnancy. The drop of normal saline should be aspirated and replaced several times and transferred to a microscopic slide and allowed to dry. The smears are fixed by placing the slide in absolute alcohol for 5 second, allowing it to dry, and staining it with a 5% aqueous methylene blue solution for 10 minutes. The excess stain is washed off with tap water and the slide is dried and observed using low power of microscope.[8]

Chick Oviduct Method

The weight of the oviduct of young chicken is increased dose-dependently by natural and synthetic estrogen. This principle is used for the screening of estrogenic compound.[7]

Procedure: Seven days old pullet chicks are injected subcutaneously, twice daily with solutions of the test compound in various doses for 6 days. Doses between 0.02 and 0.5 μg 17 β-estradiol per animal serve as standard. Six to ten chicks are used for each dosage group. On the day after the last injection, the animals are sacrificed and weight of the body and oviduct is determined.

In Vitro Methods

Estrogenic Receptor-binding Assay

Estrogenic receptor binding assay uses the principle of competitive binding of labeled and unlabeled estrogen on the estrogenic receptors. Estrogenic compounds displace the labeled estrogen in a concentration dependent manner from the estrogen receptor.[7]

Procedure: Cytosol preparation: Uteri from 18-day-old female albino mice are removed and homogenized at 0°C in 1:50 (w/v) of Tris-sucrose buffer in a conical homogenizer. Human endometrium from menopausal women is frozen within 2 hours of hysterectomy and stored in liquid nitrogen until use. The frozen endometrium is pulverized and homogenized in 1:5 (w/v) of Tris-Sucrose buffer. Homogenates are centrifuged for 1 hour at 1,05,000 g. Determination of specific binding in mouse uterus cytosol as a function of steroid concentration, incubation time and temperature. Triplicate aliquots of 125 ml of cytosol are incubated with 5 or 25 nM labeled steroid either for 2 or 24 hour at 0°C or for 2 or 5 hours at 25°C in the absence (total binding) or presence (non-specific binding) of a 100 fold excess of radio inert steroid. Bound steroid is measured by dextran coated charcoal (DCC) adsorption.

Dextran-coated Charcoal (DCC) Adsorption Technique

A 100 μl aliquot of incubated cytosol is stirred for 10 minutes at 0°C in a micro titer plate with 100 μl of DCC suspension (0.625% dextran 80,000, 1.25% charcoal Norit A) and then centrifuged for 10 minutes at 800 g. The concentration of bound steroid is determined by measuring the radioactivity in a 100 μl Aliquot of supernatant.

For calculation of relative binding affinity, the percentage of radioligand bound in the presence of competitor compared to that bound in its absence is plotted against the concentration of unlabeled competing steroid.

Potency Assay

This assay determines the affinity of the test compound for estrogen receptor sites in the uterus (rats, rabbits, mice). The uptake of titrated estradiol by immature uteri must be established, and then the inhibition of this uptake by pretreatment with a test compound will indicate the estrogenic potency of the compound. The procedure for this assay is based on the work of Terenius (1965, 1966)[9,10] and Johnsson and Terenius (1965).[11]

Procedure: Four immature female mice (20-day old) are killed. The uteri are quickly excised and are placed in Krebs'-Ringer phosphate buffer. Pieces of diaphragm are taken from each animal to serve as control tissue for nonspecific uptake of estradiol. The uteri are divided at the cervix into two horns; in this way one horn is used as the control and the other for testing the compound. The tissues are placed in vials containing 5.0 ml of Krebs'-Ringer phosphate buffer, incubated, and shaken at 37°C with 95% oxygen, and 5% carbon dioxide is bubbled through. The radiochemical purity of the 3H-estradial can be checked chromatographically. Buffer solution of radioactive estradiol is made up so that each 5 ml of buffer contains 0.0016 µg of radioactive estradiol (0.25 µCi). A stock solution can be made and kept refrigerated for up to 6 weeks. The excised tissues are treated as follows:

- **Control**: Four pieces of diaphragm are incubated and shaken with 5 ml of buffer solution for 15 minutes at 37°C and are then shaken for 1 hour with 5 ml of buffer containing the radioactive estradiol and 2% w/v bovine albumin.
- **Experimental**: Four uterine horns are incubated and are shaken in 5 ml of buffer at 37°C for 15 minutes. Then they are incubated and shaken with 5 ml of buffer containing 2% of albumin and radioactive estradiol at 37°C for 1 hour. Both control and experimental tissue are removed and washed with buffer at 37°C for 5 minutes, kept in damped filter paper, and weighed. The tissues are then prepared for counting. Samples of 100 µl of the incubation solution are also taken for counting.

Treatment of tissues for counting: The tissues are dried for constant weight and the dry weight is recorded. Each piece of tissue is placed in a glass counting vial and incubated at 60°C in a shaking water bath with 0.5 ml of hyamine hydrochloride 10x until the tissue has completely dissolved. If the solution is discolored 50 µl of 20% hydrogen peroxide may be added. 50 µl of concentrated HCl and 15 ml of phosphor solution are added to each vial. The vials are allowed to equilibrate in the packed liquid scintillation counter and counts are taken. Counting efficiency is determined by the addition of an internal standard. The results are expressed as disintegrations per minute per unit of wet weight (dpm/mg). Test compounds can be incubated with the labeled estrogen in assaying their effectiveness in competing for the receptors in the uterus.[3]

Anti-estrogenic Activity

In Vivo Methods

Antagonism of Physiological Effects of Estrogen

Anti-estrogenic compounds will inhibit some or all of the physiological effect of estrogen such as water uptake of uterus, uterotrophy and vaginal cornification. This principle is used for the screening of anti-estrogenic activity.[7]

Procedure: The assay techniques used for anti-estrogens are modifications of the estrogenic assays. The dose of estrogen used is that which is required to produce 50% of the maximum possible response. The test compound can be injected simultaneously or at varying times before or after the estrogen. The procedure for assays of water uptake, uterotrophy and vaginal cornification are followed as described earlier, except that the test compounds are given along with the estrogen.

In Vitro Methods

Aromatase Inhibition

This assay is based on the principle that compounds which inhibit aromatase (estrogen synthase) possess anti-estrogenic activity. Anti-estrogenic activity of compounds can be evaluated indirectly by evaluating aromatase-inhibiting ability.[7]

Procedure: Ovarian tissue from adult golden hamsters is used. Estrus cycle is monitored for at least three consecutive 4 days estrus cycle prior to the experiment. The experiments for evaluating inhibitor effects are performed with ovaries obtained from animals sacrificed on day 4 (pro-estrus). The ovaries are excised freed from adhering fat tissue and quartered. The quarters are transferred into plastic incubation flasks with 2 ml of Kreb's Ringer bicarbonate salt (KBR) solution pH 7.6, containing 8.4 mM glucose. The flasks are gassed with O_2/CO_2 (95%/5%) tightly closed and placed in a shaker/water bath (37°C) for incubation of the fragments. The incubation media are replaced with fresh KBR after pre incubation for 1 hour. The ovaries are further incubated for 4 hour in the presence or absence of inhibitors. 4-OH androstendione is used as standard in concentrations between 0.33 and 330 μM/L. At the end of the experiment the incubation media are removed and centrifuged. In the supernatant estrogen, progesterone and testosterone are determined by radioimmunoassays. The data of control and test groups are compared with suitable statistical analysis.

Progestational Activity

In Vivo Methods

Pregnancy Maintenance Test

Progesterone is responsible for the maintenance of pregnancy. This principle is used for the screening of progestational compound.[7]

Procedure: Ovariectomy is done on day 5/10/15 of pregnancy in different groups of pregnant rats. The animals are treated with different test and standard drugs. Pregnant rats are killed 5/10/15 days later. An average of living fetuses at the end of the experiment is compared with the standard and the control group (without ovariectomy). The ED50 of progesterone is 5 mg/day in rat and less than 0.5 mg/day in mouse.

Proliferation of Uterine Endometrium in Estrogen-primed Rabbits (Clauberg Mcphail Test)

Female rabbits weighing between 800–1,000 g are primed with estradiol and followed by the administration of progestational compound, leading to the proliferation of endometrium and converted into secretary phase. This principle is used for the screening of progestational compounds.[3,7,13]

Procedure: Female rabbits weighing 800–1,000 g are primed with injection of estradiol 0.5 mcg/ml in aqueous solution daily. On day 7 drug treatment is begun. The total dose is given in five equally divided fraction daily over 5 days. Twenty-four hours after the last injection, animals are killed and uteri are dissected out and frozen sections of segment of middle portion of one horn is prepared and examined for histological interpretation. For interpretation of progestational proliferation of endometrium, beginning of glandular development may be graded 1 and endometrium consisting only of glandular tissue may be graded 4.

Carbonic Anhydrase Activity in Rabbit's Endometrium

There is a linear dose response relationship between dose of progestogens and carbonic anhydrase activity in rabbit endometrium. This principle is used for the screening of progestational compounds.[3,7]

Procedure: Immature female albino rabbits are used in this study. The animals are primed with estradiol and followed by the administration of test and standard drugs. After the drug treatment, animals are sacrificed and uteri are removed. The endometrial extract of the uterus is evaluated for the carbonic anhydrase activity calorimetrically.

Deciduoma Reaction in Rats

This study is based on the principle of maternal/placental tumor formation by progestational drugs in traumatized uterus of ovariectomized rats. This phenomenon is used for the screening of progestational compounds.[3]

Procedure: The ovariectomized adult female albino rats weighing between 150–200 g are used for the study. The rats are primed with four injection of 1 µg of estrone/estradiol. This is followed by 9 days of drug therapy. On day 5, one uterine horn is exposed and 1 mg of histamine dihydrochloride is injected into the lumen. Twenty-four hours after the last dose of drug, animals are killed, uterine horns are cut off and weighed and histologically examined.

Prevention of Abortion in Oxytocin Treated Pregnant Rabbits

Intravenous administration of oxytocin to the pregnant rabbits on 30th day of pregnancy causes abortion. Prior administration of progestational compound prevent the abortion. This principle is used for the detection and screening of progestational compounds.

Procedure: Ten units of oxytocin are administered intravenously to pregnant rabbits on day 30 of pregnancy. Twenty-four hours before oxytocin, test and standard drugs in oil are injected. Control animal not receiving drug abort within 2–30 minutes after oxytocin. The drugs, which are having progestational activity, prevent abortion.[12]

In Vitro Methods

Progesterone Receptor-binding Assay

Progesterone receptor binding assay uses the principle of competitive binding of labeled and unlabeled progesterone on the progesteronic receptors. Progesteronic compounds displace the labeled progesterone in a concentration dependent manner from the progesterone receptor.[7,14,15]

Procedure: Human uteri obtained after hysterectomy is frozen in liquid nitrogen and stored at –80°C until use. For cytosol preparation uterine tissues are minced and homogenized with a homogenizer at 0–4°C in ice-cold buffer composed of 10 mM KH_2PO_4, 10 mM K_2HPO_4, 1.5 mM EDTA, 3 mM NaN_3, 10% glycerol, pH 7.5 (PENG buffer). The homogenates are then centrifuged at 10,500 g at 4°C for 30 minutes. The supernatant is taken as cytosol.

The cytosol preparations are incubated with 3H-R5020 as radioligand at a concentration of 8 nmol/L and increased concentrations (1 × 10-10 to 1 × 10-5 mol/L) of the competitor steroid overnight at 4°C. Then unbound steroids are adsorbed by incubating with 0.5 ml of DCC (0.5% Norit A, 0.05% dextran T400 in PENG buffer) for 10 minute at 4°C. After centrifugation (10 minute at 1,500 g at 4°C) 0.5 ml of the supernatant is withdrawn and counted for radioactivity. To calculate the relative binding affinity, the percentage of radioligand bound in the presence of competitor compared to that bound in its absence is plotted against the concentration of unlabeled competing steroid.

Anti-progestational Activity

The anti-progestational compound inhibits some or all the physiological effect of progesterones. This principle is used to screen the anti-progestational activity.[7] The procedure for assay of Clauberg/McPhail and deciduoma formation is followed, except that the test compounds are given along with the progesterone.

Anti-progestational Activity in Immature Rabbits (Mc Ginty Test)

Mc Ginty method is used to determine the local progestational activity of the test drugs. It determines the degree of endometrial proliferation and transformation in immature rabbits, initially primed with estradiol and subsequently treated with the test substances. Antagonistic properties may be evaluated by the co-administration with progesterone.

Procedure: Local progestational test involves a direct injection of progesterone into a uterine segment. The test is performed in immature rabbits (700–950 g) primed for 6 days with estrogen. Estradiol at a dose of 1 μg/kg/rabbit is injected by subcutaneous route to the rabbits of positive control and test groups.[16] The rabbits of negative control group received only the vehicle (0.5% CMC) by subcutaneous route for 6 days. On the 7th day, the rabbit is anesthetized by intramuscular injection of ketamine hydrochloride (dose 35 mg/kg). The abdomen is opened and the uterus is exposed by laparotomy. The upper middle segment of each horn is ligated without disturbance of blood circulation. In the positive control group, 0.1 ml of progesterone was injected alone in the right uterine horn (concentration 0.1 mg/ml).[17] In the opposite horn, only 0.1 ml of the vehicle is injected (0.5% C.M.C). In the test groups, a solution of the progesterone and the test drugs in 0.5% C.M.C is injected into the left lumen of segment through the lower ligature, which is drawn right after the injection. Progesterone is injected alone in the right uterine horn. In the negative control group, progesterone alone is injected in the right uterine horn. In the opposite horn, only vehicle is injected. After the injection, the lower ligature can be tightened. Three days later, the animals were sacrificed. The uteri were excised, weighed, fixed in buffered formalin. The sections of the horn are evaluated histologically according to Mc Phail scores.[17,18]

Evaluation: Compared to the vehicle treated animals, the rabbits treated with estradiol benzoate have an increased uterine weight. In estimating the degree of proliferation the six sections of each uterus are examined and the average proliferation judged as accurately as possible, taken as the result. Variation in different parts of the same uterus often exceeded one

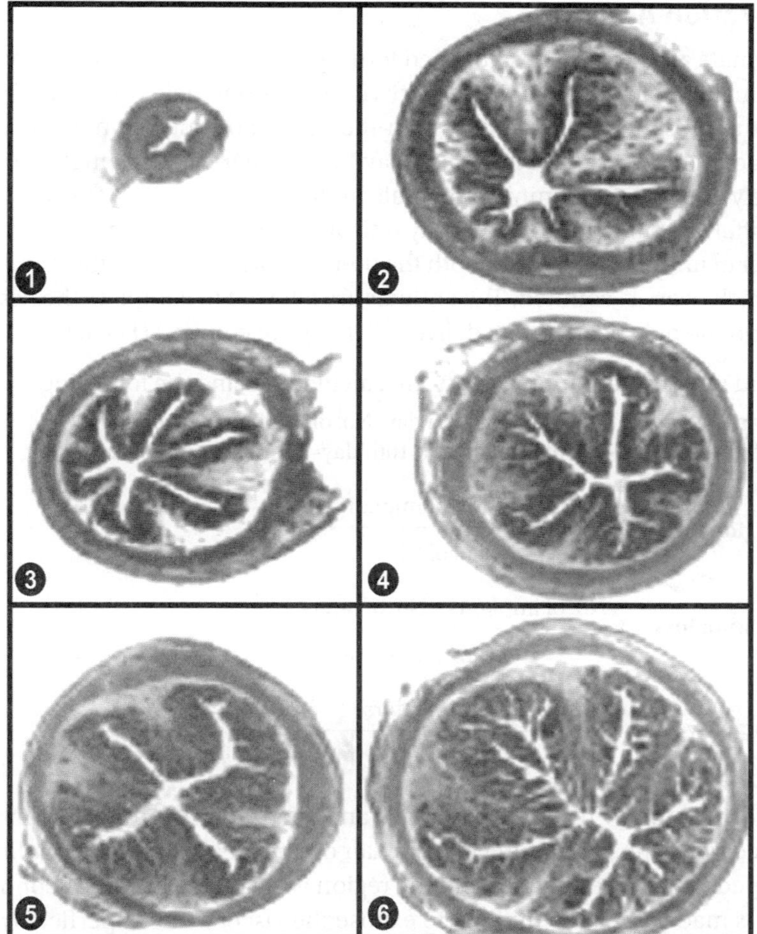

Figure 8.8: Uteri of immature rabbits showing the standard scale of progestational proliferation (x17) **(1)** no treatment; **(2)** estrin only, reaction 0; **(3-6)** estrin followed by progestin, reaction 1,2,3 and 4, respectively. (Adopted from original article "The assay of progestin" by Mc Phail, 1934)[13]

stage. The average of all reactions in a group of animals is reached as the proliferation index. Inhibition by test compounds for the proliferation ability is the index of antiprogestational activity. The following Mc Phail scores are used for evaluating the degree of proliferation (Fig. 8.8).

Scores:

Score 0—Ramification of the uterine mucosa but no proliferation (estrogen treatment only).

Score 1—Slight proliferation of the uterine mucosa.

Score 2 —Medium proliferation of the uterus mucosa, slight additional ramification.

Score 3—Pronounced proliferation of the uterine mucosa.

Score 4—Very pronounced, proliferation of the uterus mucosa, pronounced proliferation of the uterus mucosa, pronounced ramification.

The scores from each dosage group are averaged.

Anti-implantation Activity

Procedure: Female albino rats of established fertility in proestrous or estrous stage are mated with matured male rats of established fertility (in the ratio female 3:1 male). Each female is examined for the presence of spermatozoa in the early morning vaginal smear. The day on which this sign of mating is seen is taken as a day 1 of pregnancy. The female is then separated and caged singly and drug is administered orally to the animals once daily on specific days of pregnancy at different concentrations. On day 10th of pregnancy, the animals are laparotomized and the number of implants present in both the uterine horns as well as the number of corpora lutea (CL) on each ovary is counted. The animals are allowed to complete the gestation period (21–23 days) and the number of litters delivered, if any are counted (Fig. 8.9).[19,20]

Pre-post- and anti-implantation activity are calculated using the following formula.[21]

Pre-implantation loss = No. of CL on 10th day–No. of implants on 10th day.
Post-implantation loss = No. of implants on 10th day–No. of litters delivered.

$$\textbf{\% Pre-implantation loss} = \frac{\text{No. of CL - No. of implants}}{\text{No. of CL}} \times 100$$

$$\textbf{\% Post-implantation loss} = \frac{\text{No. of implants - No. of litters}}{\text{No. of implants}} \times 100$$

$$\textbf{\% Antifertility activity} = \frac{\text{No. of CL - No. of litters}}{\text{No. of CL}} \times 100$$

Procedure for laparotomy: The animal is lightly anesthetized with ether and limbs are tied to a rat board (waxed) with the ventral side up. The hair on the area around the midline abdominal region are clipped with curved scissor and the region is cleaned with 70% alcohol. An incision of 2 cm length is made along the midline to expose the viscera. The superficially lying coils of ileum are lifted to expose the two uterine horns. The horns are examined for implantation sites. Implants are visible as clear swellings on the uterine horns giving the uterine tube a beaded appearance. Embryos with bright-red dish aspect and a clear margin are considered to be

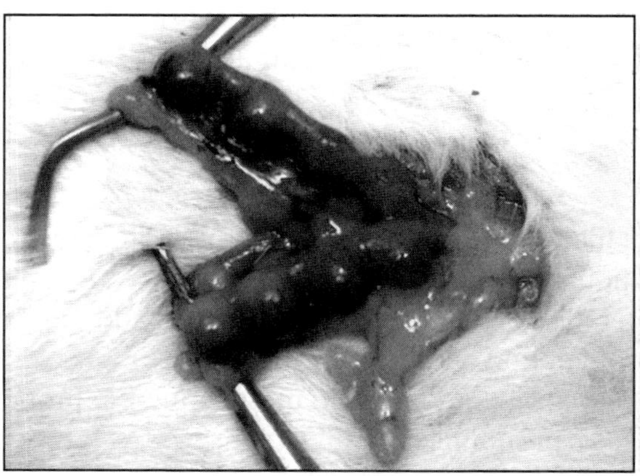

Figure 8.9: Rat uterus showing normal implants on 10th day of pregnancy (*For color version see Plate 15*)

healthy. Those with dull blue color, with no clear margin and orientation with some exudates are considered resorbing. The number of implants and resorption sites per horn are counted. The ovaries, which lie on the upper end of the uterine horns, show corpora lutea as yellow spots over the surface. The number of corpora lutea present on each ovary is also noted.

After counting, the organs are replaced back. A small quantity of neosporin powder is sprinkled over the organs to prevent any infection. The incision through muscular layer is closed with continuous suture using absorbable catguts and skin layer with continuous sutures using silk thread. An antiseptic, povidone iodine solution is applied on the sutured area after wiping with 70% alcohol. After laparotomy, the rats are transferred to a warm place till they recover from the anesthesia.

Abortifacient Activity

Procedure: Adult female albino rabbits are used for the study. The pregnancy date is counted from the date of observed mating. The existence of pregnancy may be confirmed by palpation after 12th day of pregnancy. Intra-amniotic and intraplacental injections are performed on rabbits under ether anesthesia on day 20 of pregnancy. The uterus is exposed through the midline incision, a particular site is chosen for injection and its various parts are identified by transillumination from a strong source of light. Then material is injected in 0.1 ml of solvent into the amniotic fluid or in 0.05 ml of solvent into the placenta. Alternatively, the drugs can be given through any route and duration from day 20 of pregnancy. The effect of drug is determined by looking for vaginal bleeding, changes in weight, abdominal palpation and by postmortem examination.[12,22]

METHODS FOR MALES

Developing male antifertility agent involves interference with spermatogenesis without loss of libido and secondary sexual characteristics.

Emergent Spermatozoa Made Nonfunctional/Oligospermia/Aspermia

In Vivo Methods

Cohabitation Test

This test determines the time interval for litter production after placing treated males with 2 females. The date of mating is calculated from the date of parturition. This method is suitable for drugs known to cause several weeks sterility.

Procedure: Adult female and male albino rats of proven fertility are used for the study. They are kept for mating in the ratio of 2:1 till both females deliver the litters. The date of mating is calculated from the date of parturition. The time interval for litter production after placing treated males with two females is calculated.

Fertility Test

Fertility test is based on the evaluation of average litter size. Antifertility agents negatively affect the average litter size.

Procedure: Groups of 5–10 male rats of proven fertility are treated with drug and are paired with fertile females in the ratio of 1:3. Daily vaginal smears are examined for the presence of sperms. All females passed through 1 estrus cycle must have mated. The mated animals are kept separately till the completion of the gestational period. The litters are counted, and using the following formula average litter size is calculated:

$$\text{Average litter size} = \frac{\text{Total no. of litters}}{\text{No. of females mated}}$$

If vaginal smear shows leukocytes for 10–14 days, pseudopregnancy is confirmed. If insemination is not detected, then inhibition of libido or aspermic copulation might be the cause. Fertility patterns can be obtained from changes in average litter size.[12]

Subsidiary Test

This test determines the changes in spermatozoa count with time. The antifertility drugs affect the spermatozoa count negatively.

Procedure: Adult male albino rats weighing between 150–250 g are used for the study. They are kept in a cage containing artificial or animal vagina. Artificial vagina is the cylindrical plastic jacket with the rubber liner, filled with water at 5°C. 0.5 ml of ejaculate is diluted with saline containing traces of formalin. Resulting suspension counted on hemocytometer.[12]

In Vitro Methods

Spermicidal Activity

Procedure: Spermicidal drugs are diluted with normal saline and serial dilutions are made in 0.2 ml of human seminal fluid with 1 ml of spermicidal solution. Then the mixture is incubated at 37°C for 30 minutes. A drop of the mixture is placed immediately on a slide and at least five fields were microscopically observed under high power (400X) for assessment of sperm morphological changes and motility. Effective agents can immobilize and kill the sperms.[23]

Immobilization Assay

Procedure: The cauda portion of epididymes of ram is isolated and minced in 0.9% saline solution (pH 7.5) and filtered through a piece of cheese cloth to get sperm suspension. For human sample, ejaculates (n=10) from normal subjects, after 72–96 h of sexual abstinence, are subjected to routine semen analysis following liquefaction at 37°C. Sperm count above 100 million/ml and viability above 60% with normal morphology, rapid and progressive motility is employed for the test. Ram epididymal sperm suspension (100 million/ml to 200 million/ ml) or human ejaculate (100 million/ml to 150 million/ml) is mixed thoroughly in 1:1 ratio with different concentration of drugs. A drop of the mixture is placed immediately on a slide and at least five fields were microscopically observed under high power (400×) for assessment of sperm motility. The mixture is then incubated at 37°C for 30 minutes and the above process is repeated.[23]

Nonspecific Aggregation Estimation

Procedure: Different concentrations of drugs are treated with ram sperm suspension in 1:1 ratio and kept at 37°C for 1 hour. Then from the bottom of the micro centrifuge tube, one drop of the sedimented sperm is placed on a slide and the percent aggregation was examined microscopically under 400X magnification. Considering that the non-aggregated spermatozoa will remain in the supernatant, the latter is collected and the turbidity determined spectrophotometrically at 545 nm. The aggregation is indirectly proportional to the sperm viability.[23]

Sperm Revival Test

This assay determines the extent of spermicidal and immobilization capability of drugs by evaluating the revival of sperm motility.

Procedure: To study the revival of sperm motility, after completion of the immobilization assay, the spermatozoa are washed twice in physiological saline and incubated once again in the same medium, free of drug at 37°C for 30 minute to observe the reversal of sperm motility.[23]

Assessment of Plasma Membrane Integrity

Procedure: To assess the sperm plasma membrane integrity, ram sperm suspension (100 million/ml to 200 million/ml) or human ejaculated sperm (100 million/ml to 150 million/ml) are mixed with drug at the minimum effective concentration, respectively, at a ratio of 1:1 and incubated for 30 minutes at 37°C. Similarly, sperm samples in saline served as the controls. For viability assessment, one drop each of 1% aqueous solution of eosin Y and of 10% aqueous solution of nigrosin was placed in a micro centrifuge tube. A drop of well-mixed sperm sample is added to it and mixed thoroughly. The mixture is dropped onto a glass slide and observed under 400X magnification.

For hypo-osmotic swelling test (HOS) 0.1 ml of aliquot is taken from each of the treated and control sample, mixed thoroughly with 1 ml of HOS medium (1.47% fructose and 2.7% sodium citrate at 1:1 ratio), incubated for 30 minutes at 37°C and the curling tails were examined under phase contrast microscope using 100X magnification.

5-nucleotidase is released possibly due to destabilization of plasma membrane. This can be estimated to find the effect of drug on plasma membrane integrity of sperm. The activity of 5'-nucleotidase can be determined by measuring the rate of release of inorganic phosphate from adenosine 5'-monophosphate. After incubating the sperm suspension with drug, the sperm pellet is collected by centrifugation at 3,000 g at 37°C. Then it is washed twice in 0.9% saline and then suspended in 0.1 mol/L Tris-HCl buffer (pH 8.5) with each reaction system containing 100–200 million spermatozoa. An aliquot of 0.1 ml suspension of sperm is added to 0.9 ml of buffered substrate containing 3-mmol/L adenosine 5'-monophosphate and 50 mmol/L $MgCl_2$ dissolved in 0.1 mol/L Tris-HCl buffer. The tubes are incubated at 37°C for 30 minutes and 0.5 ml 20% TCA (0°C–4°C) is added to the mixture to stop the reaction. The mixture was then centrifuged at 10,000 g at 4°C. The pellet is discarded and the supernatant was kept for phosphate estimation. The activity of 5'-nucleotidase was expressed in terms of μg of phosphate released. The activity of 5'-nucleotidase is indirectly proportional to the plasma membrane integrity.[23]

Evaluation of Acrosomal Status

Acrosome is the cap like structure on the head of spermatozoa. It breaks down just before fertilization, releasing a number of enzymes that assist penetration between the follicle cells that still surround the ovum. This method evaluated the acrosomal status of sperm. The most widely studied acrosomal enzyme is the acrosin that has been shown to be associated with acrosomes of all mammalian spermatozoa, and the highest substrate specificity was obtained with BAEE (N-benzoyl-L-arginine ethyl ester).

Procedure: Different concentrations of drugs are mixed with ram sperm suspension in 1:1 ratio and kept at 37°C for 1 hour. The suspension is centrifuged and the pellets are collected. The pellets are extracted with 3 mmol/L HCl at pH 3 and the enzyme activity is measured, following the hydrolysis of 0.5 mmol/L BAEE dissolved in 0.05 mol/L Tris HCl buffer containing 0.05 mol/L $CaCl_2$ at pH 8. The activity of acrosin is expressed in terms of m IU. One m IU activity means the amount of enzyme, which causes the hydrolysis of one nanomole of BAEE in one minute at 25°C. The activity of acrosin is directly proportional to the fertilizing capability of sperms.[23]

Androgenic Activity

In Vivo Methods

Chicken Comb Method

This assay is based on the principle of growth of cap on comb by androgenic compounds. This method has been useful for the isolation and structural elucidation of natural androgens.[24]

Procedure: In the beginning of the assay, the sum of the length plus height of each individual comb is determined by measurement with a millimeter rule placed directly on the comb. The capons are injected daily intramuscularly for 5 consecutive days with a solution or suspension of the test compound or the standard in 1 ml olive oil. Twenty four hours after the last injection, the comb is re-measured and the growth of the comb is expressed as the sum of the length and height in millimeter. Groups of eight animals are used for at least two doses of the test compound and the compound. The weight of control and test group is compared with suitable statistical analysis.[7]

Weight of Ventral Prostate, Seminal Vesicles and Musculus Levator Ani

This assay is based on the principle that the androgens affect the secondary sex organs in male individual. In the rats, the growth of the ventral prostate, the seminal vesicle and the musculus levator ani depend on the presence of male sexual hormones.

Procedure: Immature male rats weighing about 55 g are orchidectomized. The animals are treated with the test compounds in various doses orally in 0.5 ml 0.5% carboxymethyl cellulose or 0.2 ml sesame oil suspension daily over a period of 10 days. Testosterone given subcutaneously in doses of 0.02, 0.1 and 0.5 mg per animal, or methyl testosterone in doses of 0.25, 1.5, and 5 mg per animal, serve as standard. Controls receive the vehicle only. On the eleventh day, the animals are sacrificed and the seminal vesicles, the ventral prostate, and the musculus levator ani carefully dissected and weighed. The weight of control and test group is compared with suitable statistical analysis.[7]

Nitrogen Retention
The assay is based on the principle that the anabolic agents induce positive nitrogen balance in the rats. Anabolic agents decrease the nitrogen excretion in the castrated rats fed a liquid diet and in nitrogen balance.[25]

Procedure: Twenty-five-day-old rats are castrated and kept untreated for 67 days, reaching about 300 mg body weight on normal laboratory diet. After 67 days they are changed to liquid diet force-feeding regime. Besides carbohydrates and fat, the diet contains casein and brewer's yeast as nitrogen source. At the start, the rats receive 10 ml per day, and this is increased to 26 ml per day. This feeding is continued for 30 days with simultaneous administration of the test drug once a day. Twenty-four hour urine specimens are collected 3 times weekly and analyzed for total nitrogen.[7]

Anti-androgenic Activity

In Vivo Methods

Chicken Comb Method
This assay is based on the principle of inhibition of growth of capon comb by anti-androgenic compounds.

Procedure: One to 3 days old male or female white leghorn chicks are housed at constant temperature in a heated incubator. Testosterone is incorporated into the finely ground chick starting mash at a concentration of 80 mg per kilogram food. The chicks are placed on this diet for day one. The test compound is dissolved in sesame oil. Each day for 4 days 0.1 ml of the oil solution is injected subcutaneously. Control chicks receive only the vehicle. Twenty-four hour after the last injection, the animals are sacrificed, the combs removed and after blotting of the cut edge, weighed rapidly to the nearest 0.5 mg. The weight of control and test groups are compared using suitable statistical method.[7]

Antagonisim of Effect of Testosterone on Weight of Ventral Prostate, Seminal Vesicles and Musculus Levator Ani
In the rats, the growth of the ventral prostate, the seminal vesicle and the musculus levator ani is stimulated by testosterone, anti-androgenic compound inhibits this effect.

Procedure: Male rats weighing 50–70 g are castrated and one day after surgery, the rats are injected once daily for 7 days with 0.15 mg testosterone propionate in 0.1 ml sesame oil. The test compound also dissolved or suspended in sesame oil at various doses and injected subcutaneously daily at a separate site for 7 days. Controls receive testosterone injections only. On 8th day, the animals are sacrificed and weights of ventral prostate, seminal vesicles and musculus levator ani weighed. The weight of control and test group is compared with suitable statistical analysis.[7]

Anti-androgenic Activity in Female Rats
This assay is based on the principle of antagonism of the anti-androgens against the tropical effect of testosterone on uterine and preputial growth.

Procedure: Female rats weighing 40–45 g are ovariectomized, one week later the treatment is started over a period of 12 days with daily subcutaneous injection of 0.3 mg testosterone propionate and various doses of the antagonist. Controls receive testosterone propionate only. On the 13th day, the animals are sacrificed and the uteri and preputial glands weighed. Weight increase of female accessory sexual organs due to testosterone treatment is dose despondent reduced by an anti-androgens.[7]

REFERENCES

1. Sciarra JJ. The continuing need for contraceptive research. Fertil Steril 1981;36:697–8.
2. Kostyk SK, Dropcho EJ, Moltz H, Swartwout JR. Ovulation in immature rats in relation to the time and dose of injected human chorionic gonadotropin or pregnant mare serum gonadotrophin. Biol Reprod 1978;19:1102-7.
3. Turner RA. Screening methods in pharmacology. New York: Academic Press 1971:85-118.
4. Kapoor M, Garg SK, Mathur VS. Antiovulatory activity of five indigenous plants in rabbits. Ind J Med Res 1974;62:1225-7.
5. Stockard CR, Papanicolaou GN. The existence of a typical estrus cycle in the guinea pig with the study of its histological and physiological changes. Am J Anat 1917;22:225-83.
6. Allen E, Doisy EA. An ovarian hormone. Preliminary report on its localization, extraction and partial purification and action in test animals. J Am Med Ass 1923;81:819-21.
7. Vogel HG, Vogel WH, Editors. Drugs Discovery and Evaluation. Berlin: Springer 1997.
8. Agrawal SS, Paridhavi M. Herbal Drug Technology. Hyderabad: Universities Press 2007.
9. Terenius L. Uptake of radioactive estradiol in some organs of immature mice. Acta Endocrinol (Copenh) 1965;50:584-96.
10. Terenius L. The uptake of radioactive isomers of synthetic estrogens in various organs in immature mice. Acta Endocrinol (Copenh) 1966;53:84-92.
11. Jonsson CE, Terenius L. Uptake of radioactive estrogen in the chicken oviduct and some other organs. Acta Endocrinol (Copenh) 1965;50:289-300.
12. Ghosh R. Modern concept on pharmacology and therapeutics. (24th ed). Calcutta, Hilton and Co, 1991.
13. Mc Phail MK. The assay of progestin. J Physiol 1934;83:1545-56.
14. Verma U, Laumas KR. Screening of antiprogestins using in vitro human uterine progesterone receptor assay system. Steroid Biochem 1981;14:733-40.
15. Bayard F, Damilano S, Robel P, Baulieu EE. Cytoplasmic and nuclear estradiol and progesterone receptors in human endometrium. J Clin Endocrinol Metab 1978;46:635-48.
16. Brooks JR, Babiarz EA, Berman C, Primka RL, Rasmusson GH. Some endocrinological and anti-fertility properties of an androstane cyanohydrin derivative in the rat. Biol Reprod 1978;18:186-92.
17. Mc Ginty DA, Anderson LP, Mc Collough NB. Effect of local application of progesterone on the rabbit uterus. Endocrinology 1939;24:829-32.
18. Tayama T, Mtoyama T, Ohono Y, Ide N, Turusaki T, Okada H. Local progestational and antiprogestational effects of steroids and their metabolites on the rabbit uterus. Jpn J Feril Steril 1979;24:48-51.
19. Agrawal SS, Aravinda S. Anti-implantation activity of H2 receptor blockers. Indian J Pharmacol 1995;27:40-42.
20. Shafiq N, Malhotra S, Pandhi P. Comparison of nonselective cyclo-oxygenase (COX) inhibitor and selective COX-2 inhibitors on preimplantation loss and duration of gestation: an experimental study. Contraception 2004;69:71-75.

21. Agrawal SS, Gatak N, Arora RB. Antifertility activity of roots of Abrus precatorius Linn. Pharmacol Res Commun 1970;2:159-62.
22. Turner RA. Screening methods in pharmacology. New York: Academic Press, 1965:270-73.
23. Chakrabati K, Pal S, Battacharyyya AK. Sperm immobilization activity of Allium sativum L. and other plant extracts. Asian J Androl 2003;5:131-5.
24. Dorfman RI. Studies on the bioassay of hormones. The assay of testosterone propionate and androsterone by a chick inunction method. Endocrinology 1948;48:1-6.
25. Stafford RO, Bowman BJ, Olson KJ. Influence of 19-nortestosterone cyclopentyl-propionate on urinary nitrogen of castrate male rats. Proc Soc Exp Biol Med 1954;86:322-6.

CHAPTER

9

Antiobesity Agents

INTRODUCTION

When energy intake exceeds energy expenditure, obesity develops. Obesity is characterized by an excessive development of fat mass, which is a consequence of increased size of adipocytes and/or increased number of adipocytes. It increases the risk of developing diabetes, hypertension, dyslipidemia, certain forms of cancer and osteoarthritis, etc.

Obesity is a multifactorial disease. It arises as a result of interaction among numerous behavioral, environmental and genetic factors and associated with the dysregulation of energy homeostasis, normally maintained by the hypothalamic neuroendocrine/neurotransmitter network. Signaling factors, like leptin and various neuropeptides, are important components of this complex network. Leptin is synthesized and secreted primarily from adipocytes and acts centrally in the hypothalamus by binding to the leptin receptor. Circulating levels of leptin are highly correlated with the level of body fat. Insulin and glucocorticoids can stimulate production of leptin by adipocytes. Low plasma concentrations of leptin and insulin, e.g. during fasting and weight loss, increase food intake and decrease energy expenditure by stimulating neuropeptide Y (NPY) synthesis, and perhaps by inhibiting sympathetic activity and other catabolic pathways. High leptin and insulin concentrations, e.g. during feeding and weight gain, decrease food intake and increase energy expenditure through release of melanocortin and corticotropin-releasing hormone (CRH). Stimulation of the leptin receptor can lead to changes in the expression of a variety of neuropeptides.

Neuropeptides that are involved in energy homeostasis can be orexigenic (appetite stimulating) and anorectic as shown in Table 9.1.[1] The involvement of most of these neuropeptides in maintaining energy homeostasis was deduced from transgenic animal studies and spontaneous mutations.

β_3-adrenoceptor also has an important role in the regulation of lipid metabolism and obesity. However, the physiological function of β_3-adrenoceptor in humans has not yet been established.

ANIMAL MODELS FOR THE STUDY OF ANTIOBESITY DRUGS

The animal models of obesity have been either of spontaneous origin or the result of experimental manipulation of the environment or hypothalamic centers that regulate food

Table 9.1: Orexigenic and anorectic neuropeptides involved in energy homeostasis

Orexigenic peptides	*Anorectic peptides*
NeuropeptideY (NPY)	Corticotropin-Releasing Hormone
Agouti-related peptide (AgRP)	Melanocyte Stimulating Hormone
Orexins A and B	Cholecystokinin
Galanin	Glucagon-like peptide1
β endorphin	Calcitonin gene-related peptide
Norepinephrine	Bombesin
Growth Hormone-Releasing Hormone	
Melanin concentrating hormone	

intake and energy balance. The identification of gene mutations that cause obesity and the use of transgenic techniques have provided new insights into the physiologic and molecular mechanisms underlying obesity. However, much remains to be studied in this complex field of research.

In animal models of obesity some parameters are studied:
- Food intake
- Body weight
- Adipose tissue cell size and number
- Body composition
- Locomotor/physical activity
- Plasma lipids, insulin and glucose levels.

Food intake and weight gain: Food intake and weight gains are recorded in control and experimental group daily at a fixed time, preferably in the morning. For measurement of food intake, spilled food is collected by suspending a paper under the cage and the amounts of spillage are also determined after drying. Food intake measurements are also important to study the anorectic activity of various compounds.[2]

Adipose tissue cell size and number: Number and size of adipose tissue cell is determined by osmium fixation method.[3]

Body composition: Body composition is estimated by determining the water content of the carcasses by oven drying at 95°C for 6–9 days until constant weight is reached. Lipid content is measured in gonadal and retroperitoneal fat pads. For this, adipose tissue is homogenized with a 2:1 chloroform-methanol mixture and extract is washed by addition of water. The resulting mixture separates into two phases. Lower phase consists of pure lipid extract, which is measured.[4,5]

Locomotor/physical activity: Generally, locomotor/physical activity is reduced in obese animal.

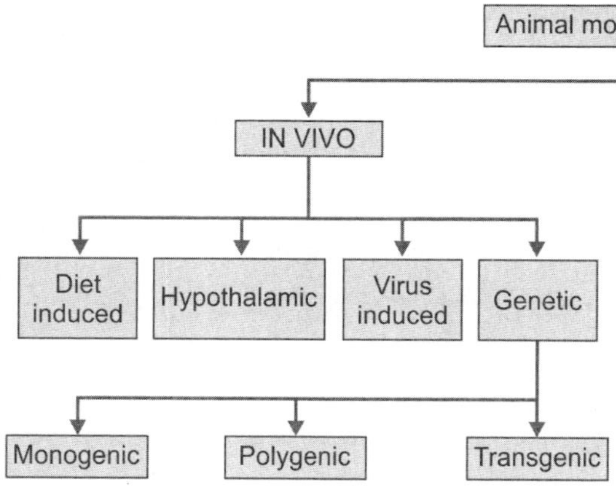

Animal models of obesity
IN VIVO
IN VITRO
Diet induced
Hypothalamic
Virus induced
Genetic
Monogenic
Polygenic
Transgenic

Diet-induced Obesity

Procedure

Adult female rats, weighing approximately 230 g, are housed individually in wire mesh cages under controlled temperature and artificial light/dark cycle. Animals are divided into two groups. First group receives ordinary purina chow and the other group is given in addition to chow, a high fat diet, sweetened condensed milk and a number of supermarket foods like cookies, cheese, milk chocolate, peanut, butter, etc. (cafeteria diet). Body weight, food intake, locomoter activity and serum insulin levels are measured and compared in both the groups. After three months, rats are sacrificed by decapitation and adipose tissue cell size and number, body composition and lipid content in fat pads are determined, and comparison is made between the groups.[6,7]

Hypothalamic Obesity

Hypothalamus regulates food intake by interaction of a lateral feeding center and a medial satiety center. Ventromedial hypothalamic lesions are found to increase food intake followed by increased body weight and obesity after 3–4 months. Injury to hypothalamus can be produced by surgical methods and by chemical agents (such as gold thioglucose, mono sodium glutamate, etc.) in the animals especially rodents, which can result into obesity.

Surgically-induced Hypothalamic Obesity

Procedure

Female Sprague Dawley rats, weighing approximately 190 g are fed a high fat diet for 5–9 days. After this, rats are anesthetized with 35 mg/kg pentobarbital sodium along with 1 mg atropine methyl nitrate administered intraperitoneally.

To produce hypothalamic lesions, bilateral knife cuts are stereotaxically made in the hypothalamus of rats. Incision bar is positioned at -3.0 mm and parasagittal cuts are made in between the lateral and medial hypothalamus using a retractable wire knife.[8] The cuts are made 1.0 mm lateral to the midline and extended from 8.5 to 5.5 mm anterior to the ear bars and from 3.0 mm dorsally from the base of the brain.

Sham-operated rats serve as control.[9,10] Food intake, body weight and other parameters are recorded for comparison in between the groups.

Chemically-induced Hypothalamic Obesity

Monosodium Glutamate-induced Hypothalamic Obesity in Mice

Mice are injected daily with mono sodium-L-glutamate subcutaneously in the doses of 2 g/kg for 5 consecutive days in early stages of life. In control group, physiological saline is administered.

All mice are housed under maintained temperature and artificial light/dark cycle and provided with chow and water ad libitum. Food consumption, weight gain and other parameters (as mentioned above) are recorded and comparison is made between the groups.[11]

Modification:Young albino rats between the age of 2–40 days are used and treated with either single or repeated doses of 0.1–6.0 mg/g body weight of monosodium-L-glutamate.[12]

Gold Thioglucose Induced Hypothalamic Obesity in Mice

Six weeks old Swiss albino mice of either sex are given a single intraperitoneal injection of gold-thioglucose in the doses of 30–40 mg/kg. After that body weight is recorded for 3 months and compared with untreated controls.[13]

Modification: Gold thioglucose implants in the hypothalamus of rats, are used to induce obesity.[14]

Other Chemical Compounds

Besides these, several other chemical compounds have been reported to produce obesity in mice, such as single intraperitoneal injection of bipiperidyl mustard in doses between 5–50 mg/kg and single intracerebral injection with 4-nitroquinoline-1-oxide.[15,16]

Virus-induced Obesity

Mice infected with canine distemper virus, a morbillivirus antigenically related to measles virus, develop obesity. Obesity is seen after 8–10 weeks of viral infection. Canine distemper virus targets certain brain structures, including the hypothalamus followed by virus-induced disruption of critical brain catecholamine pathways as a result of which obesity is developed.[17]

Other viruses that can cause obesity in animals[18-22] are shown in Table 9.2.

Table 9.2: Viruses causing obesity in animals

Viruses	*Animals*
Canine distemper virus	Mice
Borna disease virus	Rats
Rous-associated virus-7	Chickens
Avian adenovirus SMAM-I	Chickens
Ad-36 (human adenovirus)	Chickens, mice, nonhuman primates

The exact mechanism of obesity caused by these viruses is unclear.[23]

Genetic Models of Obesity

Obesity is a phenotype that is readily observable, and mice with naturally arising mutations causing this phenotype have been extensively characterized. Genetic models can be monogenic, polygenic and transgenic.[24]

Monogenic Models (Table 9.3)

Mice with naturally arising mutations causing obesity have been extensively characterized.The oldest of these mutations is the agouti gene, whereas the most well-known are mutations in the genes of the hormone leptin and its receptor, ob and db, respectively. Naturally occurring single gene mutations producing obesity (Table 9.4) form the basis for a candidate gene approach to identify the genes responsible for human obesity. Several human counterparts of these rodent obesity syndromes have been identified.

Table 9.3: Monogenic and polygenic models of obesity

Monogenic	*Polygenic*
Yellow obese (Aya) mouse	Japanese K K mouse
Obese (ob/ob) mouse	NZO mouse
Diabetes (db/db) mouse	Otsuka-Long_Evans-Tokushima-Fatty rats
Fat mouse	BSB model
Tubby mouse	AKR/J × SWR/J model
Fatty (fa/fa) rat	M16 mouse
Obese SHR rat	
JCR: LA- Corpulent rat	
WDF/TA-FA Rat	

Table 9.4: Obesity mutations in rodents and mutant proteins

	Mutation	*Gene*	*Inheritance (Autosomal)*	*Mutant protein*
Mouse	Agouti	*Ay*	Dominant	ASP
	Diabetes	*db*	Recessive	Lepr
	Fat	*fat*	Recessive	Carboxypeptidase
	Obese	*ob*	Recessive	Phosphodiesterase
Rat	Fatty	*fa*	Recessive	Lepr

Yellow Obese (Aya) Mouse

The yellow obese mouse was discovered as early as 1883 by Lataste and in 1905 by Cuenot.[25,26] An agouti mutation results into obese yellow mice. Yellow obese mouse is the only example of obesity inherited through a dominant gene, located on chromosome 2 at linkage group 5, the agouti locus. Since genes controlling obesity and the agouti coat colors are closely linked, the obesity is associated with a change of pigmentation of hair from black to yellow. This association allows the early identification of pre-obese mice as soon as the coat hair begins to

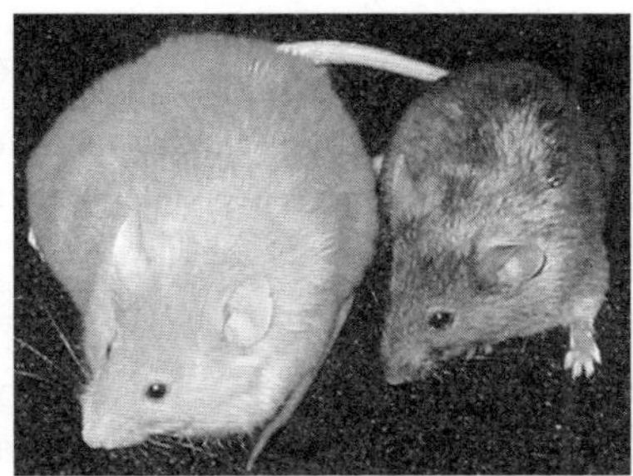

Figure 9.1: Yellow obese ($A^y a$) mice (*For color version see Plate 15*)

grow. The homozygous (A^y/A^y) alleles are lethal in utero and several different alleles (A^{vy}/A^{vy}, A^{iy}/A^{iy}) have appeared at the agouti locus, in which the degree of obesity is linked directly to the level of yellow pigmentation in the coat.

Yellow ($A^y a$) mice exhibit moderate form of obesity and diabetes. Body weight starts increasing at the time of puberty (8–12 week) and reaches maximum up to 40 g.[27,28]

In 1992, agouti gene was cloned and it was the first obesity gene characterized at the molecular level.[29] The molecular categorization of agouti was responsible for elucidation of the melanocortin system's involvement in weight regulation, due to its resemblance to agouti-related protein activity in the hypothalamus. The melanocortin receptor family comprises five G-protein-coupled proteins, melanocortin 1 receptor (Mc1r) to Mc5r, which demonstrate tissue-specific patterns of expression. Mc4r is expressed in the hypothalamus and plays a key role in the regulation of feeding and metabolism and is normally antagonized by agouti-related protein.[30]

Obese (ob/ob) Mouse

The obese mouse, first described by Ingalls et al. in 1950, inherits its obesity as autosomal recessive mutation on chromosome 6. This obese (OB) mutation has been maintained as inbred stock on the C57BL/6J strain. Obese mouse is characterized by obesity, hyperglycemia and insulin resistance. Animal is visually detectable as obese by 25–28 days.[31,32]

The mutant gene responsible for the phenotype in Lepob mice encodes a protein termed leptin, which is deficient in these animals. The gene encoding human leptin has been studied extensively.

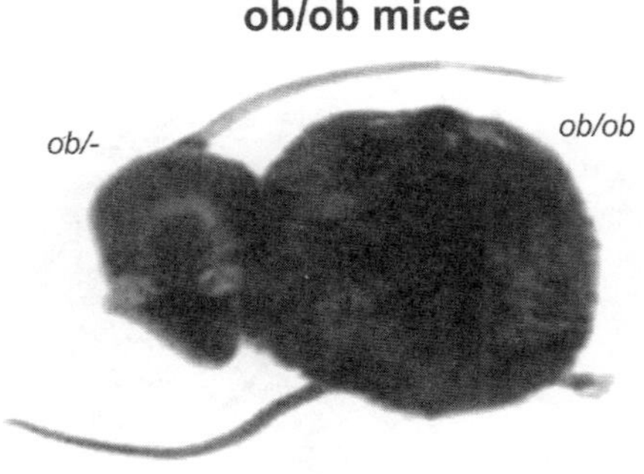

Figure 9.2: Ob/ob mice

Diabetes (db/db) Mouse

The diabetes (db) mutation arose in the C57BL/KsJ strain on chromosome 4. It is an autosomal recessive gene with full penetrance. Diabetes mouse exhibits marked obesity and hyperglycemia associated with insulin resistance. Overt obesity is observed shortly after weaning, after that body weight increases rapidly.[33] db/db mice have a mutation in leptin receptor as mentioned above.

Fat Mouse

The fat mouse (fat/fat or Cpe^{fat}/ Cpe^{fat}) is a model of a late-onset form of obesity. Obesity is inherited as autosomal recessive mutation known as fat mutation, located on chromosome 8 as coding for carboxypeptidase E (CPE). CPE is involved in the final stages of processing of insulin, POMC and other hormones. Mouse is characterized by pronounced early onset hyperinsulinemia, obesity and infertility. Fat mouse develops obesity between 6–8 weeks of age and attains body weight of 60–70 g by 24 weeks.[34-35]

Tubby Mouse

The tub mutation was discovered for the first time in a C57BL/6J male mouse and tubby colony was bred from this mouse. Mutation is autosomal recessive. Tubby mouse exhibits slow onset obesity; means phenotype cannot be recognized until 9–12 weeks of age and average weight is 46 g at 24 weeks. This animal also develops sensorineural hearing loss and retinal degeneration.[36]

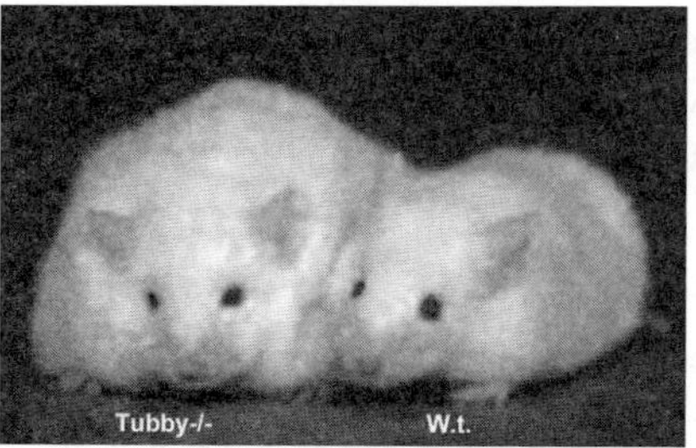

Figure 9.3: Tubby mouse

Fatty (fa/fa) Rat

The Zucker fatty (fa/fa) rat is the best known and most widely used rat model of genetic obesity. The fa mutation was discovered by Zucker and Zucker (1961) in crosses between Sherman and Merck stock M rats. The affected rats are characterized by obesity, hyperinsulinemia and insulin resistance. The obesity is inherited as an autosomal recessive mutation. Rats homozygous for the fa allele become noticeably obese by 3–5 weeks of age.[37, 38]

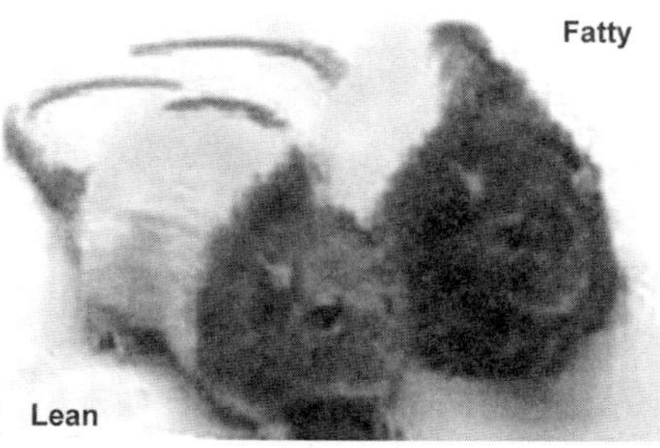

Figure 9.4: Fatty (fa/fa) rat

Obese SHR Rat

Obese SHR rat was developed by mating a spontaneous hypertensive female rat (Kyoto-Wistar strain) with a normotensive Sprague-Dawley male rat. After several generations of selective inbreeding, rats exhibited obesity, hypertension and hyperlipidemia.[39]

JCR: LA- Corpulent Rat

JCR: LA-corpulent rat was developed as a substrain from obese SHR rats. This rat is characterized by obesity, hyperinsulinemia with impaired glucose tolerance and hyperlipidemia.[40]

WDF/TA-FA Rat

WDF/TA-FA rat is also known as Wistar Fatty rat. This strain was established by transfer of the fatty (fa) gene from the Zuker rat to the Wistar Kyoto rat. WDF/TA-FA rat is characterized by hyperinsulinemia, glucose intolerance, hyperphagia and obesity.[41]

Polygenic Models (Table 9.3)

The polygenic models of obesity have allowed identification of multiple genetic loci within individual strains that modify obesity, plasma cholesterol levels, specific deposition of body fat depots, and propensity toward development of obesity on a high-fat diet. These polygenic models more closely resemble the human obesity phenotypes than single gene models. These models are described below:

Japanese KK mouse

Japanese KK is one of the most suitable polygenic mouse models of obesity. Konello et al. first described it in Japan in a strain of mice bred for large body size mice. The dominant gene for yellow obesity (Ay) has also been transferred into the Japanese KK strain and the resultant animals are named as yellow KK mice (KK-Ay). In KK mouse onset of obesity is late, body weight begins to rise after 2–3 months of age and slowly attains a maximum up to 40–50 g by 6–9 months of age. The mouse also develops hyperinsulinemia, hyperphagia and moderate hyperglycemia.[42]

NZO Mouse

The New Zealand obese (NZO) mouse was first described in 1953 by Bielschowsky and Bielschowsky.[36, 43] NZO mouse develops obesity, mild hyperglycemia and insulin resistance. The adult NZO attains a body weight of 50–70 g by 6–8 months. After this age, weight gain occurs slowly. By 6 months of age this mouse develops renal disease and other autoimmune disorders.[44]

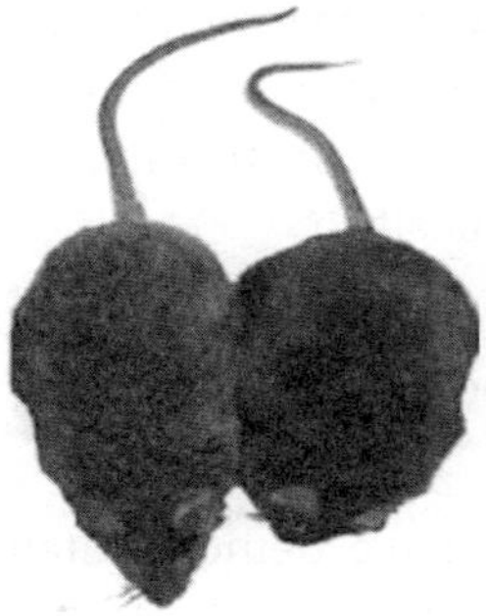

Figure 9.5: NZO mouse

Otsuka-Long-Evans-Tokushima-Fatty (OLETF) Rats

OLETF rat strain is developed from outbred colony of Long-Evans rats by selective breeding. It has since been maintained at the Tokushima Research Institute, Japan. OLETF rat is characterized by mild obesity, hyperglycemia, polyuria and polydipsia. Weight begins to rise two weeks after weaning.[45]

The M16 Mouse

The M16 mouse is an outbred animal model of polygenic obesity. Selection for increased 3–6 weeks postweaning gain in the M16 line of mice was first reported by Hanrahan et al.[46] M16 is the result of long-term selection for 3–6 weeks weight gain from an ICR base population. M16 mice are heavier, fatter, hyperphagic, hyperinsulinemic, and hyperleptinemic relative to ICR.

M16 mice represent an excellent polygenic model to study the genetics of growth, obesity, and type 2 diabetes. Relaxed selection over to facilitate gene discovery and pathway regulation controlling early onset polygenic obesity and type 2 diabetic phenotypes. These phenotypes, observed at young age (early onset), closely mimic current trends in humans.[47]

Transgenic or Knockout Animal Models

In these animal models, genes regulating energy homeostasis are manipulated. Gene manipulations are targeted either to a specific tissue or to more ubiquitous expression such as: **Knockout of β_3 adrenergic receptor gene** in white and brown adipose tissue.[48]

Knockout of uncoupling protein in brown adipose tissue: Transgenic toxigene approach is used to create transgenic mice. In this approach, targeted expression of a gene for diphtheria toxin A chain is used to knockout selectively functional activity of brown adipose tissue. By linking the gene to uncoupling protein gene expression, brown adipose tissue thermogenic function is abolished and mice become obese and develop hyperphagia.[49]

Knockout mice lacking steroidogenic factor I (SF-I): Knockout (KO) mice lacking steroidogenic factor I (SF-I) exhibit a phenotype that is characterized by abnormalities of ventromedial hypothalamic nucleus, gonadal agenesis and impaired gonadotropin expression. SF-1 KO mouse become obese by 8 weeks of age and represents late-onset obesity.[50]

Barden and colleagues incorporated a type II glucocorticoid receptor antisense RNA construct into mice and focused its expression primarily to neural tissues by linking the construct to a human neurofilament gene promoter sequence 4. All transgenic offspring developed obesity (two fold increase in body weight) by 6 months of age.[51,52]

Knockout of the Mc4r gene in mice is observed to result in early-onset obesity, non-insulin-dependent diabetes, and other obesity-associated syndromes. These symptoms are in parallel to the yellow agouti mouse syndrome, indicating that agouti expression in the hypothalamus inhibits Mc4r function, leading to obesity.[53]

Targeted deletion of the Mc3r gene also results in a late-onset obesity phenotype, but regulation of appetite and metabolism remains intact. Mc3r transgenic mouse are also susceptible to diet-induced obesity.[53]

NPY Y5 receptor knockout mice have demonstrated that mutants lacking this receptor develop mild late-onset obesity characterized by increased food intake, weight gain, and increased body fat mass.[54]

Serotonin receptor type-2C null mutant mouse is developed to understand serotonin receptor functions, since this single-gene-mutation produced a mouse which is predisposed to obesity. The serotonin type-2C null mutant exhibits excessive feeding behavior (hyperphagia) without concurrent hyperinsulinemia. The hyperphagia observed in the null mutants preceded development of obesity and reduced sensitivity to insulin and leptin.[55]

Melanin-concentrating hormone overexpression in transgenic mice: Melanin-concentrating hormone (MCH) is known to play an important role in feeding behavior. In the brain, MCH is expressed in the lateral hypothalamus and responds to nutritional signals, including fasting and leptin deficiency. Thus, expression is increased with fasting.

Transgenic mice that overexpress MCH (MCH-OE) in the lateral hypothalamus, around two-fold higher levels than normal mice, are produced on the FVB genetic background. Homozygous transgenic animals are found to be heavier at 13 weeks of age when fed a high-fat diet than wild-type animals along with higher systemic leptin levels. MCH-OE animals were hyperphagic, hyperleptinemic, and had higher blood glucose levels. MCH-OE animals also develop hyperinsulinemia and insulin-resistance.[56] When transgene was bred onto obesity-prone genetic background, the C57BL/6J, heterozygote C57BL/6J mice expressing the transgene showed increased body weight on a standard diet, confirming that MCH overexpression can lead to obesity.[57]

Other transgenic mice models of over expression of genes include—over expression of corticotropin releasing factor gene, GLUT-4 gene, human agouti-related protein complementry DNA.[58-60]

Transgenic mice overexpressing 11beta HSD-1: Model of visceral obesity: Glucocorticoids can be produced locally from inactive 11-keto forms by an enzyme 11beta hydroxysteroid dehydrogenase type 1 (11beta HSD-1). Increased glucocorticoid levels are known to produce visceral obesity. Transgenic mice overexpressing 11beta HSD-1 selectively in adipose tissue (similar to that found in adipose tissue of obese humans) are created. These mice had elevated levels of corticosterone in adipose tissue and developed visceral obesity. The mice also exhibited insulin-resistant diabetes, hyperlipidemia, hyperphagia and hyperleptinemia.[61]

IN VITRO ASSAYS ON ISOLATED ADIPOSE TISSUE CELLS

To Study Metabolic Activity in Brown Adipose Tissue

Brown adipose tissue (BAT) is an important site for energy expenditure or thermogenesis. BAT activity is associated with uncoupling proteins (UCP), which are mitochondrial carrier proteins and dissipate the hydrogen ion gradient in the oxidative respiration chain, releasing energy as heat. UCP1 is expressed in brown adipose tissue, UCP2 is widely expressed and UCP3 is found in skeletal muscle and brown adipose tissue. Brown adipose tissue activity is increased by leptin activity through the sympathetic nervous system. Uncoupling proteins and GLUT 4 are indicators of thermogenic activity of brown adipose tissue.

Assay for Uncoupling Protein and GLUT 4 in Brown Adipose Tissue

Procedure

Male fatty (OLETF fatty) rats, 10 weeks of age are given subcutaneous injection of test compound or solvent once daily. Rats are sacrificed after 14 weeks of treatment and brown and white adipose tissue are removed. Uncoupling proteins and glucose transporter 4 (GLUT-4) are determined by protein analysis or Western blot analysis.[62]

To carry out this analysis, adipose tissue is homogenized in 5–10 volumes of a solution, which contains 10 mmol/1 Tris-HCl and 1 mmol/1 EDTA (pH 7.4) for 30 sec with a Polytron. After that centrifugation is performed at 1,500 g for 5 min and the infranatant (fat-free extract) is used to measure the proteins. The fat free extracts (10 μg protein of brown adipose tissue, 20 μg of white adipose tissue) are solubilized. The solubilized tissue is subjected to sodium dodecyl sulfate-polyacrylamide gel electrophoresis and transferred to a nitrocellulose filter. After blocking with 5% non-fat dry milk, the filter is incubated with rabbit antiserum against rat uncoupling protein or GLUT. The rabbit antisera against rat uncoupling protein and GLUT4 are prepared by immunizing purified rat uncoupling protein[63] and a 12-amino acid peptide corresponding to GLUT4 (residues 498–509, TELEYLGPDEND), respectively, that is coupled with keyhole limpet hemocyanin.[64] Then the filter is incubated with [^{125}I] protein A. Autoradiography is done by exposing dry blot to an X-ray film and to an imaging plate of BASI 000 (Fuji film) for quantitative analysis.

Assay to Study Activity of β_3 Agonists

β_3 adrenoceptors have been cloned and well characterized in animals and humans. They are expressed mainly in brown adipose tissue and in white adipose tissue. In obese rodents, β_3 agonists induce weight loss, without reducing food intake, which may be due to increased thermogenesis in brown adipose tissue, increased lipolysis in white adipose tissue and suppression of leptin gene expression and serum leptin levels.

c-AMP Response Element-luciferase Receptor Gene Assay for β_3 Adrenoceptor

Using the human β_3 adrenoceptor gene, a Chinese hamster ovary (CHO), cell transfection system is developed. Human β_1, β_2 and β_3 adrenoceptors are expressed in CHO cells. These cells are transfected with cAMP response element-luciferase plasmids using electroporation with a single 70 ms, 150 V pulse.[65] The transfected cells are seeded at a density of 40,000/well in 96-well microtiter plates and allowed to grow for 20 h. After 20 h the cells receive varying drug concentrations (10^{-11} to 10^{-4} M) for 4 h, which result in lysis of the cells. Luciferase activity is measured using the LucLite assay kit. Changes in light production are measured using a Topcount luminometer.[66]

Assay for Neuropeptide Y (NPY)

Neuropeptide Y is the most widely distributed neuropeptide in the brain as well as in the peripheral nervous system, playing an important role in the weight regulation. NPY is a potent stimulant of appetite. Six receptors of neuropeptide Y have been identified: Y_1, Y_2, Y_3, Y_4, Y_5, and Y_6. Neuropeptide Y antagonists (Y_5, Y_1) are being evaluated as new therapeutic targets for the treatment of obesity. Bioassays have also been performed for neuropeptide Y receptors characterization.[67]

To Study Role of Leptin in Obesity

Ob gene product has been identified and named as leptin. It is expressed in adipose tissue and enters the brain where it functions to reduce food intake, serum glucose and insulin levels and increases metabolic rate, ultimately leading to a reduction in body weight. Leptin mediate its effects through a specific receptor OB-R (lepr). Five different isoforms of leptin receptors have been identified. In OB/OB mice, obesity is due to mutation in Ob (lep) gene associated with deficiency of leptin, whereas in db/db mice and fa/fa rats, mutations in the leptin receptor (lepr) lead to obesity. Human homologue of mouse obese gene has been cloned and it is 84% homologous to the mouse protein (leptin). Leptin and leptin mRNA levels are correlated with the percentage of body fat. Generally, obese rodents and humans show increased levels of these in blood.

In Vitro Assay for Leptin mRNA Level in Adipose Tissue

Leptin mRNA levels in adipose tissue are determined by Northern blot analysis.[68]

Procedure

Male Wistar rats around 230 g body weight are administered with test drug for 14 days and then sacrificed by decapitation. Liver, epididymal white adipose tissue and brown adipose tissue (intracapsular) are rapidly removed and freezed in liquid nitrogen. Total RNA is extracted from frozen tissues by a guanidiniumthiocyanate-phenol/chloroform method.[69] The RNA (10 µg per lane) is fractionated by horizontal gel electrophoresis and transferred to a positively charged nylon membrane and fixed with UV-light.

Prehybridization is performed at 42°C in prehybridization solution containing 7% sodium dodecyl sulfate, 50% formamide, 5X saline-sodium citrate buffer, 2% blocking reagent, 50 mM sodium phosphate (pH 7.0) and 0.1% N-laurylsarcosine for 45 min. After that hybridization is performed at 42°C in prehybridization solution containing oligonucleotide probe (25 ng/ml) specific to leptin, malic enzyme or 185 RNA. This is followed by post-hybridization washes, i.e. twice for 15 min in 0.1% saline-sodium citrate buffer/0.1% sodium dodecyl sulfate (at room temperature) and twice for 5 min in 2% saline-sodium citrate buffer, 0.1% sodium dodecyl sulfate (at 48°C). The membranes are washed with washing buffer. At room temperature, they are blocked with blocking buffer by incubation for 30 min and again incubated (at the same conditions as above) with blocking buffer containing a polyclonal antibody against digoxigenin conjugated to alkaline phosphate. Then washing is done twice with washing buffer for 15 min. The membranes are rinsed with detection buffer (1 M Tris-Cl. pH 9.5, 0.1 M NaCl) for 5 min and immersed in CDP star solution for 5 min. Membranes are exposed to Kodak XAR film for 15 min to 1 h.[70] The mRNA level is determined by using Peak Fit software.

Radioimmunoassay for Measurement of Plasma Leptin

Procedure

The peptide VPIQKVQDDTKTLIKTIVT represents the first twenty amino acids of the predicted sequence of mature leptin protein (leptin 1-20), which is synthesized with 9-fluorenyl methyl oxycarbonyl-(Fmoc)-protected L-amino acids on an applied biosystems peptide synthesizer and purified by HPLC on a Dynamax column developed with a 0.1% trifluoroacetic acid (TFA)/ H_2O/acetonitrile (8-40%) gradient. By using carbodiimide as coupling reagent the peptide is conjugated to thyroglobulin. Rabbits are immunized by injections given intradermally and boosted at 4 weeks intervals.

A synthetic peptide identical to the one used for antibody generation, except for a tyrosine residue added to the C-terminal end, is labelled with ^{125}I using the oxidizing agent iodogen and purified on HPLC. For radioimmunoassay, the buffer consists of Tris-HCl 1 M, pH 7.4; 0.1% Triton X-100, and 0.01% NaN_3. Unlabelled ob peptide is used as standard. 100 µl of standard or unknown, 200 µl buffer, 100 µl ^{125}I-leptin peptide (approximately 5000 cpm) is added to polystyrene tubes and incubation is performed for 48 h at 4°C. Separation of antibody-bound and unbound peptides is done by addition of goat-rabbit immunoglobulin antibody followed by centrifugation.

The precipitates are counted on a computer-linked gamma-counter and the leptin concentrations of the samples are recorded using the "RIA-Calc" program.[71,72]

Isolated Adipocytes Cell-lines for Leptin and Leptin m-RNA

Rat Preadipocytes

Epididymal fat pad is removed after killing the rats by decapitation. The fat is minced and digested with collegenase [1 mg/ml in Hanks balanced salt solution]. Stromalvascular cells from adipose tissue are isolated by centrifugation at 800 g for 10 min and plated in 100 mm culture in Eagle's medium supplemented with 10% (v/v) fetal calf serum, 100 IU/ml penicillin and 100 µg/ml streptomycin (Basal medium). After 12 h, the adherent cells are washed 3 times with Hanks balanced salt solution, treated with trypsin and counted. Cells are plated for 12 h before replating to permit separation of the preadipocytes from other cell types. 95% cells isolated by this procedure are preadipocytes.[73]

Rat Primary Cultured Mature Adipocytes

Male Sprague-Dawley rats weighing 180–200 g are killed by decapitation. The epididymal fat pads are removed, minced and digested with collagenase1. Cell preparation is performed at 37°C in Krebs-Ringer bicarbonate HEPES buffer (pH 7.4) containing 10 mmol/L $NaHCO_3$, 30 mmol/L HEPES and 1% bovine serum albumin. Incubations are performed at 37°C in DMEM (Dulbecco's Modified Eagle's Medium) supplemented with 5% bovine serum albumin, glutamine, 200 mmol/L adenosine, 50 µg/ml gentamicin and 100 mg/dl glucose. Isolated adipose cells are distributed equally into plastic dishes to a final incubation volume of 10 ml. Using these primary cultured mature adipocytes, leptin protein level and leptin m-RNA level can be measured.[74]

3T3-L1 Adipocytes

3T3-L1 adipocytes are derived from mouse fibroblast 3T3 line. 3T3-L1 cells are cultured in basal medium (Dulbecco's Modified Eagle's Medium) (DMEM), fetal bovine serum (10%), penicillin (100 units/ml and streptomycin 100 μg/ml) for 2 days post-confluence. To induce differentiation cells are exposed to basal medium supplemented with MDI [methylisobutylxanthine (120 μg/ml), dexamethasone (0.39 μg/ml) and insulin (10 μg/ml)]. Cells are washed 2 days later and exposed to insulin (2.5 μg/ml) with basal medium.[75]

Human Mesenchymal Stem Cells (hMSCs): New Model for the Study of Human Adipogenesis

Janderov et al. evaluated human mesenchymal stem cells (hMSCs) as an *in vitro* model for human adipogenesis. hMSCs can be differentiated into adipocytes by exposure to insulin, dexamethasone, indomethacin, and 3-isobutyl-1-methylxanthine three times for three days each. hMSCs differentiated into adipocytes to a different extent depending on the experimental conditions. Differentiation medium based on medium 199 and containing 170 nM insulin, 0.5 mM 3-isobutyl-1-methylxanthine, 0.2 mM indomethacin, 1 mM dexamethasone, and 5% fetal bovine serum was optimal. The gene expression during adipogenic conversion is assessed by reverse-transcription polymerase chain reaction, real-time reverse-transcription polymerase chain reaction, and Western blotting.[76]

CONCLUSION

The development of animal models for obesity is important in the development of treatments for obesity. The mouse is an ideal model because it has similar genetics and development as humans and genetic manipulation techniques are now routine.

Obesity is a particularly challenging medical condition to treat because of its complex etiology involving behavior, energy expenditure, and genetics. No single animal model could be able to represent all these factors. However, research using rodent models of obesity has led to a significant expansion in our knowledge of the physiological mechanisms of this disease. Various animal models have been developed for better understanding of the anatomical, neurochemical and endocrine systems regulating food intake and energy expenditure. Behavioral and environmental factors are represented in animal models of dietary obesity. Hence, dietary obesity model could be more appropriate model for human obesity. As far as genetic models are concerned, they are useful in providing tools to study the genetics of obesity because identification of the genes involved in rodent genetic obesity has implications for understanding the genetics of human obesity. Human geneticists have used the candidate gene approach, using known genes identified from their obesity effects on animal models, in the search for potential human obesity genes. Other genetic mutations in candidate genes have been found in obese humans, including mutations in the genes encoding leptin, leptin receptor, and carboxypeptidase E. However, the frequency in obese humans exhibiting these single genetic mutations is exceedingly low, and therefore, are not suspected to be the key genetic factors responsible for the most common forms of obesity.

The genetic alterations leading to obesity appear to be much more complex than single-gene mutations, since few cases of single-gene mutations in obese human subjects have been identified. Many individuals may have a combination of genetic alterations, which may predispose them to obesity.

Since, human obesity is polygenic having significant genetic heterogeneity, therefore polygenic models are known to be good models to characterize genetic mechanisms of complex human obesity. Genetic models have revealed several genes involved in human obesity that help us providing new therapeutic targets for obesity treatment. For example: leptin, leptin receptor, α-melanocyte stimulating hormone, melanocortin 4-receptor, Agouti-related protein, TUB, neuropeptide Y receptor, $\beta_3$adrenoreceptor, uncoupling proteins that are being extensively studied and being evaluated for their role in the treatment of obesity.

Recombinant leptin is also being developed as both an appetite suppressant and a mobilizer of fat mass. This is a powerful approach, since this therapy has the potential to decrease appetite, increase metabolic rate, and reduce body fat levels. In the future, small molecule therapeutics may be developed as leptin receptor stimulators (agonists). These therapeutics may be more effective in combating obesity, since obese human subjects have decreased receptor responsiveness to leptin, despite having hyperleptinemia.[77] It will be important to identify the molecular determinants causing leptin insensitivity in order to identify future drug targets.

REFERENCES

1. Kalra SP, Dube MG, Pu S, et al. Interacting appetite-regulating pathways in the hypothalamic regulation of body weight. Endocrinol Rev 1999;20:68-100.
2. Rolls BJ, Rowe RA, Turner RC. Persistent obesity in rats following a period of consumption of a mixed, high-energy diet. J Physiol 1980;298:415-27.
3. Han PW, Young T. Obesity in rats without hyperphagia following hypothalamic operations. Chin J Physiol 1964;19:143-54.
4. Folch J, Lees M, Sloane-Stanley GH. A simple method for the isolation and purification of total lipids from animal tissue. J Biol Chem 1957;226:497-509.
5. Hirsch J, Gallian E. Method for determination of adipose cell size in man and animals. J Lipid Res 1968;9:110-9.
6. Scalfani A, Springer D. Dietary obesity in adult rats: similarities to hypothalamic and human obesity syndromes. Physiol Behav 1976;17:461-71.
7. Hill JO, Lin D, Yakubu F, et al. Development of dietary obesity in rats: influence of amount and composition of dietary fat. Int J Obes 1992;16:321-33.
8. Gold RM, Kapatos G, Carey RJ. A retracting wire knife for stereotaxic brain surgery made from a microliter syringe. Physiol Behav 1973;10:813-5.
9. Bray GA, York DA. Hypothalamic and genetic obesity in experimental animals: An autonomic and endocrine hypothesis. Physiol Rev 1979;59:719-809.
10. Funahashi T, Shimomura I, Hiraoka H, et al. Enhanced expression of rat obese gene in adipose tissue of ventromedial hypothalamus (VMH) - lesioned rats. Biochem Biophys Res Commun 1995; 211:469-75.

11. Olney JW. Brain lesions, obesity and other disturbances in mice treated with monosodium glutamate. Science 1969;164:719-21.
12. Seress L. Divergent effects of acute and chronic monosodium L-glutamate treatment on the anterior and posterior parts of arcuate nucleus. Neuroscience 1982;7:2207-16.
13. Perry JH, Liebelt RA. Extra-hypothalamic lesions associated with gold-thioglucose induced obesity. Proc Soc Exp Biol Med 1961;106:55-7.
14. Smith CJV, Britt DL. Obesity in the rat induced by hypothalamic implants of gold thioglucose. Physiol Behav 1971;7:7-10.
15. Rutman RJ, Lewis FS, Bloomer WD. Bipiperidyl mustard, a new obesifying agent in the mouse. Science 1966;153:1000-2.
16. Mizutani T. Characterization of obesity in mice induced with 4-nitroquinoline 1-oxide. Jap J Vet Sci 1977;39:141-7.
17. Lyons MJ, Faust IM, Hemmes RB, et al. A virally induced obesity syndrome in mice. Science 1982;216:82-5.
18. Carter JK, Ow CL, Smith RE. Rous-associated virus type 7 induces a syndrome in chickens characterized by stunting and obesity. Infect Immunol 1983;39:410-22.
19. Carter JK, Garlich JD, Donaldson WT, Smith RE. In Quence of diet on a retrovirus induced obesity and stunting syndrome. Avian Dis 1983;27:317-22.
20. Gosztonyi G, Ludwig H. Borna disease: neuropathology and pathogenesis. Curr Top Microbiol Immunol 1995;190:39-73.
21. Dhurandhar NV, Kulkarni PR, Ajinkya SM, Sherikar AA. Effect of adenovirus infection on adiposity in chickens. Vet Microbiol 1992;31:101-7.
22. Dhurandhar NV, Israel BA, Kolesar JM, Mayhew GF, Cook ME and Atkinson RL. Increased adiposity in animals due to a human virus International Journal of Obesity 2000;24:989-96.
23. Dhurandhar NV. Infectobesity: obesity of infections origin. J Nutr 2001;131:2794-7.
24. West DB. Genetics of obesity in humans and animal models. Endocrin Metab Clin North Am 1996;25:801-13.
25. Lataste F. Trois questions: naturaliste. Bull Sci du Dep du Nord 1883;8:364.
26. Cuenot L. Les races puresetleur combination chez les souris. Arch Zool Exp Gen 1905;122:123-32.
27. Carpenter KJ, Mayer J. Physiological observation on yellow obesity in the mouse. Am J Physiol 1958;193:499-504.
28. Hellman BL, Thalender. Postnatal growth of epididymal adipose tissue in yellow obese mice.Acta Anat 1963;55:286-94.
29. Bultman SJ, Michaud EJ, Woychik RP, Molecular characterization of the mouse agouti locus. Cell 1992;71:1195–204.
30. Cone RD, Lu D, Koppula S. The melanocortin receptors: agonists, antagonists, and the hormonal control of pigmentation. Recent Prog Horm Res 1996;51:287-318.
31. Ingalls AM, Dickie MM, Snell GD. Obesity, new mutation in the mouse. J Hered 1950;41:317-8.
32. Thurlby PL, Trayhurn P. The development of obesity in preweanling (ob/ob) mice. Br J Nutr 1978;39:397-402.
33. Coleman DL. Obesity and diabetes, two mutant gene causing diabetes-obesity syndromes in mice. Diabetologia 1978;14:141-8.
34. Coleman DL, Eicher EM. Fat (fat) and tubby (tub): two autosomal recessive mutations causing obesity syndromes in the mouse. J Hered 1990;88:424-7.

35. Naggert JK, Fricker DL, Varlamov O, et al. Hyperinsulinemia in obese fat/fat mice associated with a carboxy peptidase E mutation that reduces enzyme activity. Nat Genet 1995;10:135-42.
36. Kleyn Pw, Fan W, Kovats SG, et al. Identification and characterization of the mouse gene tubby: a member of a novel gene family. Cell 1996;85:281-90.
37. Zucker LM, Zucker TF. Fatty, a new mutation in the rat. J Hered 1961;52:275-8.
38. Bray GA. The Zucker-fatty rat: a review. Federation Proc. 1977;36:148-53.
39. Ernsberger P, Koletsky RJ, Friedman JE. Molecular pathology in the obese spontaneous hypertensive koletsky rat: a model of syndrome X. Ann New York Acad Sci 1999;892:272-88.
40. Russel JC, Graham S, Hameed M. Abnormal insulin and glucose metabolism in JCR: LA corpulent rat. Metabolism 1999;43:538-43.
41. Ikeda H, Shino A, Matsue T, et al. A new genetically obese-hyperglycemia rat (Wistar fatty). Diabetes 1981;30:1045-50.
42. Konello KK, Nozawa TT, Ezaki K. Inbred strains resulting from Japanese mice. Bull Exp Animal 1957;6:107-12.
43. Bielschowsky M, Bielschowsky F. A new strain of mice with hereditary obesity. Proc Uni Otago Med School 1953;31:29-31.
44. Cofford OB, Davis CK. Growth characteristics, glucose tolerance and insulin sensitivity of New Zealand Obese mice. Metabolism 1965;14:271-80.
45. Kawano K, Hirashima T, Mori S, et al. A new rat strain with non-insulin dependent diabetes mellitus "OLETF". Rat News Lett 1991;25:24-6.
46. Hanrahan JP, Eisen EJ, Legates JE. Effects of population size and selection intensity on short-term selection for post-weaning gain in mice Genetics 1973;73:513-30.
47. Allan MF, Eisen EJ, Pomp D. The M16 mouse: an outbred animal model of early onset polygenic obesity and diabesity. Obes Res 2004;12:1397-407.
48. Susalic VS, Ito M, Ghrujic D, et al. Knockout of β_3-adrenergic receptor gene. Obesity Res Suppl 1995;3:319.
49. Lowell BB, S-Susulic V, Hamann A, et al. Development of obesity in transgenic mice after genetic ablation of brown adipose tissue. Nature 1993;366:740-42.
50. Majdic G, Young M, Gomez-Sanchez E, et al. Knockout mice lacking steroidogenic factor are a novel genetic model of hypothalamic obesity. Endocrinol 2002;143:607-14.
51. Barden N, Pepin MC. Decreased glucocorticoid receptor activity following glucocorticoid receptor antisense RNA gene fragment transfection. Mol Cell Biol 1991;11:1647-53.
52. Richard D, Chapdelaine S, Deshaies Y, et al. Energy balance and lipid metabolism in transgenic mice bearing an antisense GCR gene construct. Am J Physiol 1993;265:R146-50.
53. Butler AA, Cone RD, The melanocortin receptors: lessons from knockout models. Neuropeptides 2002;36:77–84.
54. Marsh DJ, Hollopeter G, Kafer KE, Palmiter RD. Role of the Y5 neuropeptide Y receptor in feeding and obesity. Nature Med 1998;4:671-2.
55. Nonagaki K, StrackAM, Dallman MF, Tecott LH. Leptin-independent hyperphagia and type 2 diabetes in mice with a mutated serotonin 5-HT2C receptor gene. Nature Med 1998;4:1152-6.
56. Ludwig DS, Tritos NA, Mastaitis JW, Kulkarni R, Kokkotou E, Elmquist J, Lowell B, Flier JS, Maratos-Fliet E. Melanin-concentrating hormone overexpression in transgenic mice leads to obesity and insulin resistance. J Clin Invest 2001;107:379-86.

57. Bergen HT, Mizuno T, Taylor J, Mobbs CV. Resistance to diet-induced obesity is associated with increased pro-opiomelanocortin mRNA and decreased neuropeptide Y mRNA in the hypothalamus. Brain Res 1999;851:198-203.
58. Stenzel-Moore MP, Cemeron VA, Vauqham J, et al. Development of Cushing's syndrome in corticotrophin-releasing factor transgenic mice. Endocrinology 1992;130:3378-86.
59. Shepherd PR, Gnudi L, Tozzo E, et al. Adipose cell hyperplasia and enhanced glucose disposal in transgenic mice over expressing GLUT4 selectively in adipose tissue. J Biol Chem 1993;268:22243-6.
60. Ollman MM, Wilson BD, Yang YK, et al. Antagonism of central melanocortin receptors in vitro and in vivo by agonist-related protein. Science 1997;278:135-8.
61. Masuzaki H, Paterson J, Shinyama H, Morton NM, Mullins JJ, Seckl JR, Flier JS. A transgenic model of visceral obesity and the metabolic syndrome. Science 2001;294:2071-2.
62. Umekawa T, Yoshida T, Sakane N, et al. Anti-obesity and anti-diabetic effects of CL316, 243, a highly specific β_3 agonist in Otsuka Long-Evans Tokushima Fatty rats: induction of uncoupling protein and activation of GLUTA4 in white fat. Eur J Endocrinol 1997;136:429-37.
63. Lin CS, Klingenberg M. Isolation of the uncoupling protein from brown adipose tissue mitochondria. FEB S Lett 1980;133:299-303.
64. Shimizu Y, Nikami H, Isukazaki K, et al. Increased expression of glucose transporter GLUT-4 in brown adipose tissue of fasted rats after cold exposure. Am J Physiol 1993;264:E890-5.
65. Vansal SS, Fellner DR. An efficient cyclic AMP assay for the functional elevation of β-adrenergic receptor ligands. J Receptor Signal Transduc Res 1999;19:853-63.
66. He Y, Nikulin VI, Vansal SS, et al. Synthesis and human β_3 adrenoceptor activity of 1-(3,5 diiodo-4-methoxybenzyl)-1,2,3,4-tetrahydroiso-quinolin-6-ol derivatives in vitro. J Med Chem 2000;43:591-598.
67. Pheng LH, Regoli D. Bioassays for NPY receptors: Old and new. Regul Pept 1998;75-76:79-87.
68. Frederich RC, Lollmann B, Hamann A, et al. Expression of obesity mRNA and its encoded protein in rodents: Impact of nutrition and obesity. J Clin Invest 1995;96:1658-63.
69. Chanczynski P, Sacchi N. Single-step methods of RNA isolation by acid guanidinionthiocyanate-phenol-chloroform extraction. Anal Biochem 1987;162:156-9.
70. Karbowska J, Kochan Z, Zelewski L, et al. Tissue-specific effect of clofibrate on rat lipogenic enzyme gene expression. Eur J Pharmacol 1999;370:329-36.
71. McGregor GP, Desaqa JF, Ehleng K, et al. Radioimmunological measurement of leptin in plasma of obese and diabetic human subjects. Endocrinol 1996;137:1501-4.
72. Considine RV, Sinha MK, Heiman ML, et al. Serum immunoreactive leptin concentrations in normal weight and obese humans. N Eng J Med 1996;334:292-6.
73. Brown NF, Hill JK, Esser V, et al. Mouse white adipocytes and 3T3-LI cells display an anomalous pattern of carnitinepalmitoyltransferease (CPT) I isoform expression during differentiation. Biochem J 1997;327:225-31.
74. Shintani M, Nishimura H, Yonemitsu S, et al. Down regulation of Leptin by free fatty acids in Rat Adipocytes: Effects of Trianein C, Palmitate and 2-Bromopalbitate. Metabolism 2000;49:326-30.
75. Wen GVO, Ji-Kyung Choi, James L Kirkland. Esterification of free fatty acids in adipocytes: a comparison between octanoate and oleate. Biochem J 2000;349:463-71.
76. Janderov A, LENKA, Michele M, Angela NM, Randall LM, Steven RS. Human mesenchymal stem cells as an in vitro model for human adipogenesis.Obes Res 2003;11:65-74.
77. Campfield LA, Smith FJ, Burn P. Strategies and potential molecular targets for obesity treatment. Science 1998;280:1383-7.

CHAPTER

10

Anticancer Agents

INTRODUCTION

Cancer is a disease characterized by uncontrolled proliferation of cells that have transformed from the normal cells of the body. On a worldwide basis cancer represents the single largest cause of death both in men and women. Oral cavity cancer is amongst the most prevalent cancers worldwide and incidence rates are higher in men than women.[1] Apart from this, other cancers burden is also very high. As per latest press release of WHO (International Agency for Research on Cancer),[2] with 528,000 new cases every year, cervical cancer is the fourth most common cancer affecting women worldwide, after breast, colorectal, and lung cancers with almost 70% of the global burden falling in areas with lower levels of development, and more than one-fifth of all new cases are diagnosed in India.

There are more than 100 different types of cancer.[3] It is a multifactorial disease, the biology of which is not yet fully understood. However, the induction of proto-oncogenes and inhibition of tumor suppressor genes has been implicated in the pathogenesis of cancer. Apart from this, angiogenesis plays an important role in the pathogenesis of cancer and is a common target for most chemopreventive agents. Angiogenesis is a highly coordinated process regulated by a variety of molecules. Vascular endothelial growth factor (VEGF) is the major regulator of tumor associated angiogenesis in lung adenocarcinoma, responsible for promoting tumor growth and metastasis.[4] VEGF-A is considered to be the most prominent angiogenic factor in human lung cancer. The over expression of pituitary tumor-transforming gene-1 (PTTG1) has also been reported in a variety of tumors.[5] Down regulation of Forkhead transcription factor (FOXO1) has been associated with promotion of cell proliferation in cervical cancer.[6] As a result of continuous research newer molecular targets are being identified and it has facilitated the anticancer drug development process.

The cancer cells can invade the adjacent and distant tissues via the circulation. In advanced stages cancer patient may die as a result of either improper diagnosis and treatment or treatment failure. One of the causes of treatment failure is the development of resistance to anticancer agents. The mechanisms of cellular resistance to anticancer agents have been dealt in detail by Kruh et al. 2003[7] and therefore not explained here. Cancer is one of the thrust area for which effective drugs at affordable prices are not available as yet probably due to lack in understanding the cancer pathophysiology. For such a dreadful disease, anticancer drugs have been developed from a variety of sources ranging from natural products (plants and microbes) to synthetic molecules. Over the past decade, drugs for cancer have become a large therapeutic market, third only after central nervous system and cardiovascular drugs, and it is continuously growing. The number of blockbuster anticancer drugs with sales of $1 billion or more increased from 19 in 2007 to 24 in 2008.[8]

However, the widely used drugs that are cancer chemotherapeutic agents suffer from drawback of high toxicity such as bone marrow suppression, alopecia, nausea and vomiting and are not within the reach of a common man. Therefore, the challenging task at this moment is to identify the quick and novel methods that can identify and develop, which can be of therapeutic value in human cancers. This urgently necessitates screening of a large number of compounds. For this purpose both, the *in vitro* and *in vivo* models are employed for systematic screening of an anticancer drug. In this chapter, screening methods for anticancer drug discovery are described with a focus on their strength and limitations.

IN VITRO METHODS

Though animal models provide more predictable results, *in vitro* testing is still preferred prior to *in vivo* testing of a potential chemotherapeutic agent. There are following advantages of *in vitro* models over *in vivo* models.

1. These are less time consuming.
2. More cost effective.
3. Small quantities of, and large number of compounds can be tested.
4. These are easier to manage.

In addition, *in vitro* cultures can be cultivated under a controlled environment (pH, temperature, humidity, oxygen/carbon dioxide balance, etc.) resulting in homogenous batches of cells and thus minimizing experimental errors.

The *in vitro* methods are not free from disadvantages also and they often furnish false positive results (compounds show no activity *in vivo*) and false negative results (compounds show no activity *in vitro* but show activity *in vivo* as they need to be biotransformed *in vivo* to a pharmacologically active compound).[4] A second pitfall is that the role of pharmacokinetics in determining drug effects cannot be evaluated *in vitro*. In addition, geometry of solid tumors *in vivo* is very different from that of cells growing *in vitro* in suspension or monolayer cultures.

Ideal Characteristics of an *in Vitro* Screening Method

An ideal *in vitro* screening method should be simple, economical, reproducible, rapid and sensitive. The assay should be applicable to large number of tumor types and test compounds. The choice of the cell lines should be representative of clinical situation as close as possible. The range of drug concentrations used *in vitro* should be comparable to that expected for *in vivo* treatment. The assay should be able to process a large number of samples quickly and in an automated fashion. Data acquisition should be simple, easily interpreted and applied. At present no such system is available. Even the most extensively studied assays will more often identify agents that will not work in an individual patient. However, the chemosensitivity assays contribute to an active area of research and are routinely used for the screening of anticancer drugs.[9]

The goal of a screening assay is to test the ability of a compound to kill cells, at the same time, the assay should be able to discriminate between replicating cells and non-replicating cells (quiescent cells that are dead or dying (apoptosis). Different assays take advantage of various properties of cells as mentioned below.

S. No.	*Cell properties*	*Assay*
1.	Enzymatic properties	Tetrazolium salt assay (MTT)
2.	Protein content/synthesis	Sulphorhodamine B assay
3.	DNA content/synthesis	^{3}H-Thymidine uptake Newer fluorescent analogues with flow cytometry
4.	Membrane integrity	Dye exclusion tests
5.	Clonogenic properties	Clonogenic assay
6.	Cell division	Cell counting assay

Tetrazolium Salt Assay (Microculture Tetrazolium Test or MTT)

MTT assay is an internationally accepted *in vitro* method for anticancer drug screening. Though viable cells can be measured using several other staining procedures also but these procedures suffer from drawbacks that they require washing steps thereby increasing processing time and sample variation. The multiwell plate scanning spectrophotometers can quickly measure large number of samples with a high degree of precision and accuracy. Ideally, a colorimetric assay for living cells should utilize a colorless substrate that is modified to a colored product by any living cell, but not by non-viable or dead cells or culture medium. However, the MTT assay utilizes a color reaction as a measure of viable cells.[10] The assay is dependent on the cellular reduction of 3-(4,5-dimethylthiazol-2-yl)-2,5-diphenyltetrazolium bromide, a tetrazolium salt to a blue formazan product by the mitochondrial dehydrogenase of viable cells/metabolically active cells. The intensity of blue colored formazan produced is directly proportional to the cell viability.

The cells from a particular cell line when in log phase of growth are trypsinized, counted in a hemocytometer and adjusted to appropriate density in a suitable medium and then inoculated in different multiwell plates (usually 96-well plates). The cells are treated with various concentrations (in replicates) of drugs for specified duration (usually 1 to 4 days), after which MTT dye is added in each well and plates are incubated at 37°C for 4 h in a CO_2 incubator. The plates are then taken out of incubator and dark blue colored formazan crystals are thoroughly dissolved in isopropanol/DMSO at room temperature. The plates are then read on an ELISA Reader at 570 nm. The percent cell viability with respect to control is calculated using the formula:

$$\% \text{ Cell viability} = \frac{\text{OD of treated cells}}{\text{OD of control cells}} \times 100$$

This assay has been successfully used by us.[11] The DMSO as a solvent rapidly solubilizes the serum as well as formazan and use of spectrophotometric grade DMSO gives stable "background" absorbance levels. Other solvents like isopropanol, propanol, hexane and dimethylformamide though used, do not solubilize serum at concentrations exceeding 0.0625 %.[12]

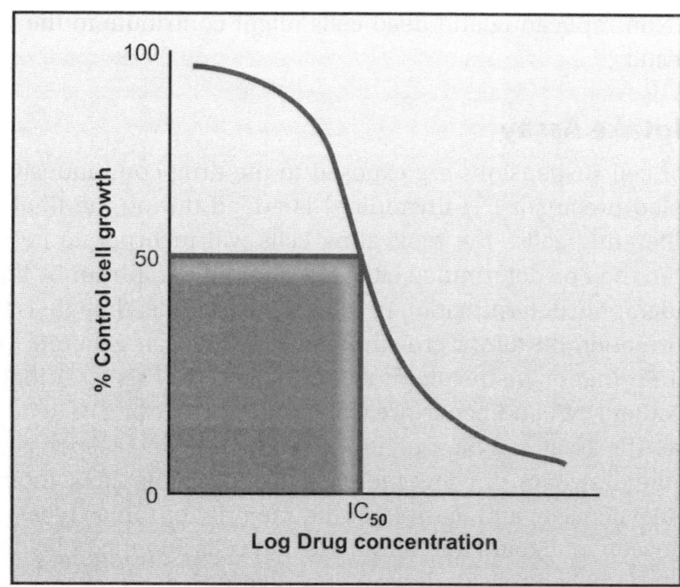

Figure 10.1: Dose response curve

The advantage of this assay is that it can be run on microtiter dishes on hundreds of cell samples at one time so that the various drug concentrations can be used to get an idea of the dose response relationship for each drug tested. As a result, this assay can be adopted for the determination of IC_{50} of drugs (concentration of drug required to inhibit 50% cell growth) (Fig. 10.1).

Further this assay is relatively simple and therefore easy to perform. It can be used for both adherent and suspension cell lines. This method is cheap, requires low number of cells, manageable and a large number of drugs can be quickly screened for antiproliferative activity. However, the assay suffers from the drawback of giving false results due to the inclusion of cells that might be metabolically active but not capable of dividing (nonreplicating). In addition, drugs whose mechanism of action might spare mitochondria may not yield positive results in this assay, especially for short incubation times. Also, use of DMSO warrants safe handling by laboratory personnel.

Sulphorhodamine B Assay

The sulphorhodamine B (SRB) assay measures whole-culture protein content, which should be proportional to the cell number.[13] Cell cultures are stained with a protein staining dye, SRB. SRB is a bright pink anionic dye that binds to basic amino acids of cells. Unbound dye is then removed by washing with acetic acid, and protein-bound dye extracted using unbuffered. Tris base for determination of optical density in a computer-interfaced, 96-well microtiter plate reader. Since, dead cells either lyse or are lost during the procedure, the amount of SRB binding is proportional to the number of live cells left in a culture after drug. This assay can be used to measure the cellular protein content of both adherent and suspension cultures. Screening capacity, reproducibility and quality control all appear to be enhanced in this assay relative to the tetrazolium salt assays. The assay is more cumbersome and time consuming compared to the MTT assay. Non-replicating and dead cells might contribute to the total protein and interfere with the results.[11]

^{3}H-thymidine Uptake Assay

In this assay, tumor cell suspensions are exposed to the drug continuously for 5 days, after which a radio-labeled precursor (^{3}H-thymidine) is added during the final 48 hours of the assay to label proliferating cells. The replicating cells will incorporate [^{3}H]-thymidine into their DNA, which can then be determined either by autoradiography or by liquid scintillation counting. Autoradiographic determination of the [^{3}H]-thymidine, though, is time-consuming but it provides information on tumor growth kinetics.[14] This can generate DNA histograms, which can provide information on the ploidy status of the cells. This assay looks at cells, which have actively replicating DNA and hence are viable. Non-replicating or dead cells will not be counted in this case. The assay can be used for both adherent and suspension cell- lines. The assay suffers from the drawback of using radioactivity and being labor intensive. This assay is rapid, relatively inexpensive, and feasible in the majority of tumor types. However, it will not differentiate between malignant and nonmalignant cells and might lead to false-negative predictions if lethally damaged cells undergo a final division.

Fluorescence

Fluorescent dyes may be used in conjunction with microscopic evaluation methods as an *in vitro* chemosensitivity assay.[15] Cells are exposed to fluorescent-labeled precursors after drug-exposure. The replicating cells will incorporate labeled precursor into their DNA and the resulting fluorescence is then measured by flow cytometry. This assay also looks at actively replicating cells and hence dead or nonreplicating cells are not counted. In addition, the assay does not involve the use of radioactivity and is useful for adherent and suspension cell-lines. Also using flow cytometry it is possible to determine that in what phase of the cell cycle the cells are. The quantitation of apoptotic cells is also possible. However this, assay requires the data to be analyzed by an expensive and sophisticated fluorescence activated cell-sorter (FACS) instrument. Because of technical difficulties in applying flow cytometry to primary tumor specimens, data on the predictive value for clinical response for this assay are too scarce to permit definitive conclusions.

Dye Exclusion Tests

Early attempts to use exclusion of vital dyes like trypan blue, eosin, or nigrosin to predict chemosensitivity were unsuccessful. These assays relied on the structural integrity of the cells. Dead cells would have lost membrane integrity and hence would take up vital dyes like trypan blue. This method was mainly used because of its technical simplicity and ease of handling a number of specimens.[16] More recently, Weisenthal and colleagues have used a novel combination of fast green dye and eosin-hematoxylin [called the differential staining cytotoxicity (DiSC) assay] with more promising results, particularly in patients with hematologic malignancies such as chronic lymphocytic leukemia (CLL).[17-19] No prospective trials of these assays have yet been performed, however, to demonstrate their ability to predict for response or lack of response. The DiSC assay is drug sensitive assay, which relies on structural integrity of the cells. In this assay, cells are incubated with drugs for 4 days. Dead cells are stained in suspension with fast green dye with or without nigrosin. The specimen is centrifuged and disks of cells are collected in the microscopic slides. Live cells are then stained with hematoxylin-eosin. As control duck erythrocytes are used. The end point of the study is the morphologic identification of tumor-cell cytotoxicity compared with the internal control standard of duck erythrocytes. The DiSC assay measures cell kill in both dividing and nondividing tumor cell population.

Clonogenic Assays

A concern in the use of antiproliferative assays is that they measure growth inhibition rather than cell killing. This is particularly important for drugs that act by arresting cells at checkpoints in the cells cycle. Checkpoint arrest is a survival response of cells that allows repair of DNA damage and is therefore not directly related to the induction of cell death. Thus, cells that act by arresting cells at checkpoints may show lower IC_{50} but increased survival. Clonogenic survival assays on the other hand, measure loss of tumor cell reproductive viability (i.e. the ability of a single cell to form colonies). It is the most direct method of measuring cytotoxic activity of a drug. In clonogenic assays single-cell suspension are prepared from tumor biopsies and exposed to anticancer agents to be tested. Cells are then rinsed and plated in a semisolid medium (agar or methyl cellulose), a medium that precludes proliferation of nonmalignant cells in the specimen.[20] After 14 to 28 days, some cells will have undergone several divisions and will have formed tumor colonies, which can be quantified in a visual or semi-automated fashion. Non-replicating and dead cells are not counted in this case. The number of colonies from the treated cells is compared with the number of colonies from the untreated control cells and the fraction of control growth provides an index of drug activity. Traditional clonogenic systems suffer from a number of significant technical problems like long incubation time (at least 14 days) before results can be made available to the clinician. The assay is labor-intensive, costly, and cannot be used for suspension cell-lines.

Cell Counting Assay

Cells are cultured in the presence of drug for 2-5 culture-doubling times, after which the cell number is estimated using a hemocytometer or a cell counter. The assay is easy to perform, rapid and can be used for both adherent and suspension cell lines. However, dead and non-replicating cells can be counted in this assay by the cell counter. The IC_{50} values can be calculated in all the above assays.

3D Tumor Models

3D *in vitro* models have revolutionized cancer research in recent years due to its biomimetic property and the ability to accurately depict the *in vivo* situation for drug screening. 3D models are advantageous over the complexity of animal models and the spatial limitations of the cell culture models.

In 3D cancer models appropriate matrix components found *in vivo* can be obtained. Cancer cells can be cocultured in a spatially relevant manner with endothelial cells and other cells associated with the *in vivo* scenario. It makes it possible to monitor and control the oxygen levels to mimic the levels of angiogenic factors released by cancer cells in response to hypoxia in native tumors. 3D models provide promising *in vitro* platform for aggregation and clustering of cancer cells, migration and proliferation, release of angiogenic factors and formation of hypoxia within tumor masses which assist in preclinical evaluation of the efficacy and molecular mechanism of the anticancer drugs.[21]

An automated assay for 3D models, such as SpheroChip system has been developed by Kwapiszewska et al. (2014).[22] It is a relatively new microfluidic-based platform for long-term 3D cell culture and analysis compatible with commercially available microplate readers. This chip provides a continuous *in situ* monitoring of cultured tumor spheroids cultured on a chip where the dynamic changes in the metabolic activity of the cells can be observed after subsequent drug doses. They compared the penetration of doxorubicin, quantum dots, and synthetic micelles into 3D HeLa spheroid versus HeLa cells grown in a traditional two-dimensional culturing system.

Ma et al. (2012)[23] developed a flexible and highly reproducible method using three-dimensional (3D) multicellular tumor spheroids derived from HeLa cell to quantify chemotherapeutic and nanoparticle penetration properties *in vitro*. They compared the penetration of doxorubicin, quantum dots, and synthetic micelles into 3D HeLa spheroid versus HeLa cells grown in a traditional two-dimensional culturing system. Their data revealed that 3D cultured HeLa cells acquired several clinically relevant morphologic and cellular characteristics (such as resistance to chemotherapeutics) often found in human solid tumors which could not be captured using conventional two-dimensional cell culture techniques. The development of this image-based, reproducible, and quantifiable *in vitro* HeLa spheroid screening tool will greatly aid future exploration of chemotherapeutics and nanoparticle delivery into solid tumors.

4D Tumor Models

In a more recent research, Mishra et al. (2014)[24] developed an *ex vivo* lung cancer model (four dimensional, 4D) that forms perfusable tumor nodules on a lung matrix mimicking human lung cancer histopathology and protease secretion pattern. In their study they compared the gene expression profile (Human One Array v5 chip) of A549 cells, a human lung cancer cell line, grown in a petri dish (two-dimensional, 2D), and of the same cells grown in the matrix of *ex vivo* model (4D). They also compared the 3D expression profile with that of 4D. Gene ontology (GO) analysis showed up-regulation of several genes associated with extracellular matrix, polarity and cell fate and development. The *ex vivo* 4D model may be a good mimic of natural progression of tumor growth in lung cancer patients with larger tumors having worse rate of survival.

National Cancer Institute's *in Vitro* Screening Program

There are nine broad categories of cancer cells covered in NCI-60, a panel of 60 diverse human cancer cell lines. The drugs are screened against this diverse panel of cell lines, including lung, colon, CNS, leukemia, pancreatic, melanoma, prostate, ovarian, cancer of breast and kidney cancer cell lines, at five different doses and allowed to incubate for 48 hours.[25] Drug-resistant tumors are specifically included in the screen. These include the human breast carcinoma selected for multiple drug resistance (MDR) and P-388 murine leukemia resistant to natural products, both of which potentially provide additional identification of new agents with particular activity against potentially resistant tumors.[26,27] As many as 200 compounds per week, or 10,000 per year can be tested in the screening facilities. National Cancer Institute (NCI) has planned to implement full-scale screen with a capacity for testing new substances at a rate > 10,000 per year against a broadly representative panel of 100 or more human tumor cell lines.[28] If the drug is unique in some way-kills preferentially one or more of the tumor cell lines, has unique structure or mechanism of action, or can kill tumors at a very small concentration, testing will proceed to the next stage. About 2% of those screened will be recommended for the next stage of testing in mice. Blower et al. 2007 have studied the MicroRNA expression profiles for NCI-60 cancer cell panel and have incorporated the resulting data into the CellMiner program package for integrative analysis.[29] They showed that cell line groupings based on microRNA expression were generally consistent with tissue type and with cell line clustering based on microRNA expression. However, mRNA expression seemed to be somewhat more informative among tissue types than was microRNA expression.

In addition, there did not seem to be a significant correlation between microRNA expression patterns and those of known target transcripts. Comparison of microRNA expression patterns and compound-potency patterns showed significant correlations suggesting that microRNAs might play a role in chemoresistance. These investigators have suggested that combined with gene expression and other biological data using multivariate analysis, microRNA expression profiles may provide a critical link for understanding mechanisms involved in chemosensitivity and chemoresistance.

IN VIVO METHODS

In vivo models are advantageous over *in vitro* models in the sense that they detect host-mediated activity, are relatively predictable and estimate therapeutic ratio. However, as compared with *in vitro* systems, their sensitivity is low, are costly, time consuming and large number of samples cannot be handled and are difficult to manage. After all, animal models are used both for toxicological studies and for detecting preclinical anticancer efficacy. They are able to detect agents irrespective of their mechanism of action. The drugs with high degree of efficacy and broad spectrum of activity in animal models are usually expected to be effective in clinical cancer, however, there are exceptions also[30] which could be due to metabolic differences and heterogeneity of cancer cells between human and rodents. Despite these differences animal models are widely used to support the results obtained from *in vitro* studies. The most promising candidate compound is tested in more than one animal model. Dose response relationship, combined effect of drugs, modes of their anticancer action and organ specificity are established. Varied drug dosage forms, doses and animal strains and animals of a particular age group may be used. The selected animal models should be representative of high incidence of human cancers.[31] The *in vivo* anticancer drug screening methods are described under the following headings:

A. Chemically induced tumor models
B. Models involving cell line/tumor pieces implantation.

Chemically Induced Tumor Models

Chemical carcinogens are well-known to account for about 80% of all cancers and are used to induce cancer in animal models. Carcinogens require metabolic activation before inducing carcinogenesis. The epidemiological studies indicate that human carcinogenesis occurs through multiple steps in the same way as in mouse skin. The concept of multistep carcinogenesis was first of all developed in rodent skin models in 1940s and applies to cancers to many species and cell types. Experimental carcinogenesis involves following three steps:

i. *Initiation* is due to exposure to carcinogens transforming the normal cell to a cancer cell.
ii. *Promotion* is due to the triggering of uncontrolled growth of the transformed cell.
iii. *Malignant conversion* is caused due to unlodging of cancer cells from the original site, its transportation by circulation and the establishment of secondary tumors in the body.

The exact sequence of cellular, biochemical and molecular genetic events may differ between tissues and species, the overall concept seems to be directly applicable to clinical cancer and thus in future multistage mouse skin carcinogenesis model will be of immense utility for further understanding the mechanisms of epithelial carcinomas in human beings.[32] The with over one-half of the chemotherapeutic drugs currently in use. This institute is systematically experiment is well designed; dose of the carcinogen as well as drug treatment schedule is standardized by conducting pilot studies. This helps in accurate evaluation of the test compound.

National Cancer Institute's *in Vivo* Screening Program

National Cancer Institute (NCI) is playing an active role in the development of anticancer drugs for last over 50 years with over one-half of the chemotherapeutic drugs currently in use. This institute is systematically screening a large number of compounds for anticancer activity using *in vitro* (cancer cells grown in culture dishes in the laboratory) and *in vitro* systems (animal models).

About 80,000 compounds have been screened by NCI since 1990. The chemoprevention branch of NCI has been using the following chemically induced tumor models, which represent high incidence of human cancers.[31]

DMBA-induced Mouse Skin Papillomas

This is a classical two-stage experimental carcinogenesis model. Mouse skin is generally most sensitive to epidermal carcinogenesis. Rats, hamsters and rabbits are less sensitive and guinea pig is very resistant.[32] SENCAR mice are highly sensitive to DMBA-induced skin tumors. Swiss albino mice are relatively less susceptible to tumor induction. DMBA acts as an initiator and 12-O-tetradecanoyl-phorbol-13-acetate (TPA) is used as a promoter to induce skin papillomas and squamous cell carcinomas. Mice are topically applied a single dose of 2.5 μg DMBA in acetone on the shaved back, followed by 5-10 μg of TPA in 0.2 ml acetone twice weekly on the same site starting one week after DMBA application. Papillomas begin to appear after 6 to 7 weeks of application of TPA. Weekly observations are made to monitor tumor development till the experiment terminates after 18 weeks. Percent tumor incidence and multiplicity of treatment group is compared with DMBA control group. Drug under test can be administered either topically or by oral route. The tumor incidence in this model is usually about 100% in

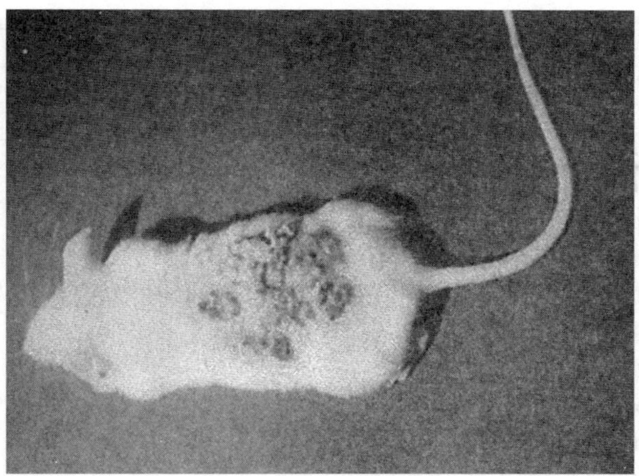

Figure 10.2: DMBA treated Swiss albino mouse (24th week) with papillomas. 100 nmol DMBA/100 μl acetone was applied topically on the depilated back of mouse twice weekly for 8 weeks (*For color version see Plate 15*)

DMBA controls. In various laboratories, however, repeated topical application of DMBA alone has also been shown to induce carcinogenesis.[33,34] The development of papillomas in DMBA treated Swiss albino mouse (24th week) is represented in Figure 10.2.

N-methyl, N-nitrosourea (MNU)-induced Rat Mammary Gland Carcinogenesis

MNU induces hormone dependent tumors. In MNU-induced rat mammary gland cancer model, single intravenous injection of 50 mg/kg body weight of MNU (pH 5.0) is given to Sprague-Dawley rats, usually at 50 days of age. In some tests, carcinogen has been administered to 120 days old animals (a better model). The incidence of tumors produced in this model is 75-95% within 180 days post-carcinogen. MNU-induced tumors are invasive and predominantly adenocarcinomas. Because MNU does not require metabolic activation, this model cannot detect inhibition of carcinogen activation. This model is a better model of human breast cancer. Drug efficacy is measured as percent reduction in adenoma incidence, multiplicity or percent increase in adenocarcinoma latency compared with that of carcinogen control. The usual tumor multiplicity ranges from 2-4 in this model. Tumor latency is about 65 to 80 days.

DMBA-induced Rat Mammary Gland Carcinogenesis

In DMBA-induced model, female Sprague-Dawley rats are given single intragastric injection of 12 mg/kg DMBA at 50 days of age. This dose results in 80-100% incidence of total mammary tumors (adenocarcinoma, adenoma and fibroadenoma) within 120 days post-carcinogen. This model can detect the agents/drugs inhibiting carcinogen activation (for example, those inhibiting cytochrome P-450).

DMBA produces encapsulated tumors with high incidence (adenomas and fibroadenomas). In addition, tumors are associated with activated *ras* gene. Drug efficacy is measured as percent reduction in adenoma incidence, multiplicity or percent increase in adenocarcinoma latency compared with that of carcinogen control. The usual tumor multiplicity ranges from 3-4.4 in DMBA controls. Tumor latency is about 65 to 80 days.

Mechanism of mammary tumorigenesis: The molecular mechanism of mammary tumorigenesis is not yet fully understood. Currier et al. 2005 have examined oncogenic signaling pathways that are activated in mammary tumors in mice treated with the DMBA.[35] In female FVB mice given 6 doses of 1 mg of DMBA by weekly gavage beginning at 5 weeks of age, all of the mice developed tumors by 34 weeks of age (median 20 weeks after beginning DMBA); 75% mice had mammary tumor, DMBA induced mammary tumors exhibited elevated expression of the aryl hydrocarbon receptor (AhR), c-myc, Cyclin D1 and hyperphosphorylated retinoblastoma (Rb) protein. The elements of Wnt signaling pathway, the NF-kB pathway and the prolyl isomerase Pin-1 were found to be frequently upregulated in the tumors when compared to normal mammary gland controls suggesting that environmental carcinogens can produce long lasting alterations in growth and anti-apoptotic pathways, leading to mammary tumorigenesis.

In another study, Wang et al. (2014)[36] were able to induce stable breast premalignant lesions in SD (Sprague-Dawley) rats by administration of DMBA (15 mg/kg, administered three times) followed by administration of female hormones (estrogen and progesterone) 5-day cycle. The premalignant breast lesions were confirmed by ultrasound and palpation.

MNU-induced Tracheal Squamous Cell Carcinoma in Hamster

In this model, 5% solution of MNU in normal saline is administered once a week for 15 weeks using specially designed catheter, which exposes a defined area of the trachea of male Syrian golden hamsters to the carcinogen. Fifteen weeks MNU administration produces tumors in 40-50% animals within 6 months. Test drug efficacy is measured as percentage reduction of tumor incidence compared with carcinogen control.

MNU-induced Prostate Cancer in Gerbils

Goncalves et al (2013)[37] developed a new rodent model of chemically induced prostate carcinogenesis in which prostate cancer progression occurs differentially in the dorsolateral (DL) and ventral lobes (VL). In their study adult gerbils were treated with MNU alone or associated with testosterone for 3 or 6 months of treatment. DL developed tumors exclusively in the periurethral area and showed intense AR, PCNA (proliferating cell nuclear antigen), and MGMT immunostaining. Moreover, VL lesions emerged throughout the entire lobe. MNU-induced lesions presented markers indicative of an aggressive phenotype: lack of basal cells, rupture of the smooth muscle cell layer, loss of E-cadherin, and high MGMT staining. The investigators propose this as a good model for prostate cancer as it allowed the investigation of advanced steps of carcinogenesis with shorter latency periods in both lobes.

N, N-Diethylnitrosamine (DEN)-induced Lung Adenocarcinoma in Hamster

In this model, 17.8 mg DEN/kg body weight twice weekly by subcutaneous injection for 20 weeks starting at age 7 to 8 weeks usually produces tracheal tumors in 90-100% and lung tumors in 40-50% of male Syrian hamsters. The studies have shown that lung tumors originate from pulmonary Clara and endocrine cells while the tracheal tumors are derived from the basal cells of the respiratory epithelium. The percentage reduction in tumor incidence in treatment group is compared with that of control group animals.

1,2-Dimethylhydralazine (DMH)-induced Colorectal Adenocarcinoma in Rat and Mouse

Intraperitoneal injection of DMH, a procarcinogen, produces colorectal adenocarcinoma both in rats and mice. DMH is first activated to azoxymethane (AOM) and then to ultimate carcinogen methylazoxymethanol (MAM). In rat model, a single subcutaneous dose of 30 mg/kg body weight given to 7-week-old F-344 male rats produces colon adenomas and adenocarcinomas within 40 weeks. The total tumor incidence is approximately 70%. In the mouse model, 9-11-week-old female CF1 mice are injected intraperitoneally MAM four times in 11 days (low dose) and 8 times in 22 days (high dose). Colon tumors have been reported to appear within 38 weeks after dosing.

Azoxymethane (AOM)-induced Aberrant Crypt Foci in Rat

Azoxymethane is a commonly used colon carcinogen in rodents inducing aberrant crypt foci. Aberrant crypt foci are single and multiple colonic crypts containing cells exhibiting dysplasia. These are potential precancerous lesions and are being evaluated as intermediate biomarkers for colon cancers in rodents. These crypts foci can be produced by single injection of 30 mg AOM/kg body weight in rats. Drug treatment schedules can vary depending on the selection. At the end of the treatment, animals are sacrificed and frequency of aberrant crypt foci are determined by histopathologic examination (larger size and increased stain uptake, increased distance from luminal to basal surface of crypt cells and enlarged pericryptical zone compared with normal crypts after staining with methylene blue.

N-Butyl-N-(4-hydroxybutyl)-nitrosamine (OH-BBN)-induced Bladder Carcinoma in Mouse

OH-BBN induces urinary bladder invasive transitional cell carcinomas that are morphologically similar to that of human variant of advanced urinary bladder transitional cell carcinomas. In this model male BDF (C57 BL/6 × DBS/2-F1) mice are administered 8 weekly doses of 7.5 mg OH-BBN by intragastric instillation beginning at 50 days of age. Drug effectiveness is measured as percent reduction in incidence of transitional cell carcinoma compared with carcinogen control group. This model induces about 40% tumor incidence during 180 days of experimental period in control animals.

Other Models

Apart from animal models used at NCI, a few other important models of chemical carcinogenesis are as follows.

DMBA-induced Oral Cancer in Hamster

Oral cancer can be induced in male Syrian hamsters by painting right buccal mucosa, 3 times/week for 16 weeks with 0.5% solution of DMBA in liquid paraffin (approximately 10 µl containing 100 µg). Tumor size, number and tumor burden of drug treated animals can be compared with that of control animals at the termination of the experiment.[38]

DMBA Sustained release suture technique

Wami et al. (2001)[39] induced squamous cell carcinoma in cheek pouch of Syrian hamsters using DMBA sustained-release suture technique followed by application of a promoter (arecaidine). In 80.6% of hamsters, squamous cell carcinoma reached a size of 100 mm^2. The mortality was observed in 15.8% and severe inflammation in 3.6% animals. This model is useful to study upper aerodigestive tract tumors.

3-Methylcholanthrene-induced Fibrosarcoma Tumors in Mouse

3-Methylcholanthrene is also known as 20-Methylcholanthrene (MCA). In this model, single dose of 200 µg of MCA/100 µl of DMSO is injected subcutaneously into the thigh region. Tumor incidence occurs approximately 6 to 7 weeks after MCA injection and reaches approximately 90% within 15 weeks. Tumor growth delay and tumor volume of control animals are compared with that of drug treated animals. Weekly fibrosarcoma incidence is also observed in both treated and control animals during the 15-week experimental period.

MCA has been shown to produce 100% fibrosarcoma incidence within 15 weeks.[40] Almost similar incidence has been observed in our studies also.[41] The MCA injected mice were diagnosed as having fibrosarcoma in the subcutaneous tissue with focal areas of necrosis (Fig. 10.3).

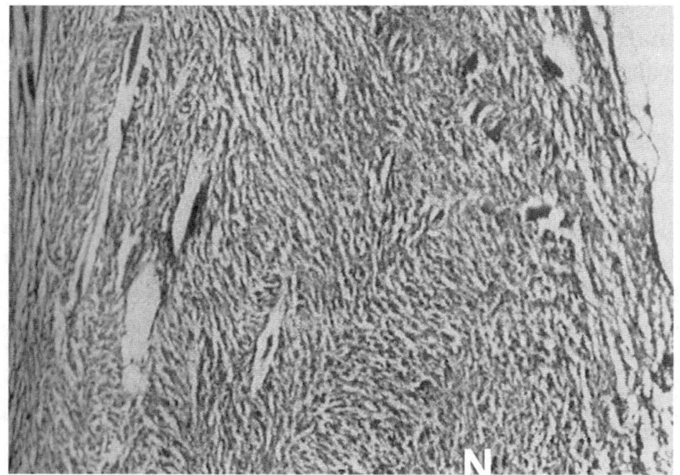

Figure 10.3: 20-Methylcholanthrene induced fibrosarcoma in the subcutaneous tissue of mouse with focal areas of necrosis (N) (H and E × 120). Mouse was injected 200 µg of MCA/100 µl DMSO into the thigh region subcutaneously and sacrificed at the end of 15th week for histopathological analysis (*For color version see Plate 15*)

3-Methylcholanthrene-induced Skin Tumors in Mouse

Skin tumors can be induced with 0.05 ml of 0.3% twice weekly topical application of MCA on the shaved back of ddY mice till appearance of visible tumors. Tumor incidence and multiplicity in drug treated and control group is observed during the 15 weeks period of the experiment. Tumor incidence in this model has been found to be approximately 85%.[42]

Benzopyrene-induced Forestomach Tumors in Mouse

Benzopyrene, a tremendously potent carcinogen, occurs widely as an environmental pollutant. The presence of methyl group constitutes the principal pathway of its metabolism, which is similar to a number of other polycyclic hydrocarbons found in the environment.

Benzopyrene induces tumors when given by gavage to mice (1 mg of benzopyrene in 0.1 ml peanut oil) twice weekly for 4 weeks. Tumor incidence and tumor burden in drug treated animals can be observed and compared with carcinogen control animals at the end of the experiment. It has been shown to induce 100% incidence of fore stomach tumors in benzopyrene control mice.[33]

Hepatocellular Carcinoma

Hepatocellular carcinoma (HCC) can be readily induced using various chemicals.[43] There are several animal models of HCC which are well established, including those which are naturally occurring such as wood chucks infected with the wood chuck hepatitis virus and Long-Evans cinnamon rats with a copper- storage condition analogous to Wilson's disease [44,45] and chemically-induced carcinogenesis.[46] Wood chuck infected with wood chucks hepatitis virus is the only reliable animal model of HCC[44] however; these animals are difficult to maintain.

Di Bisceglie et al. (2005) have used male B6C3F1 mice and induced hepatocellular carcinoma and associated lesions just by single intraperitonial dose of 120 μg/kg of ENU (Ethylnitrourea) and killed the animals 60 weeks after injection of ENU.[47]

The advantages of using these animals are:

1. Maintenance is easy.
2. For the sake of consistency of results.
3. HCC is more common in males than females.
4. Model is suitable for screening chemopreventive agents (substantial incidence of HCC).
5. Long duration of study (60 weeks) comparable to human situation as HCC most often develops after prolonged necroinflammation and fibrosis resulting from viral hepatitis or non-viral liver disease.

Estrogen receptors have been demonstrated by Alagaratnam et al. 1987 in chemically induced HCCs in rodents.[48]

Hepatocarcinogenesis in MDR2 knockout mice: It is a model of inflammation associated hepatocellular carcinoma. MDR-KO mice lack P-glycoprotein responsible for phosphatidylcholine transport across the bile canalicular membrane. Absence of phospholipids from bile results in bile regurgitation and portal inflammation followed by development of hepatocyte dysplasia and hepatocellular carcinoma.[49-51]

Katzenellenbogen et al. (2006) have shown induction of antioxidant protection systems and stimulation of hepatocyte DNA replication in the liver of MDR2-KO mice at the age of 3 months. PCNA and cyclin D1 expression was highly increased. However, the hepatocyte mitotic activity was blocked at this stage. In the later stage of the disease, although inflammation was less prominent, and the total antioxidant capacity of liver tissue returned to normal level, mitotic activity of hepatocyte was increased.[52]

High fat diet induced NAFLD/NASH model in mouse

Nakamura et al. (2013)[53] have shown that long-term (60 weeks) high fat (HF) diet induced obesity and insulin resistance in C57BL/6J male mice leading to non-alcoholic steatohepatitis (NASH) caused hepatocellular carcinoma. The results showed the natural course of non-alcoholic fatty liver disease (NAFLD)/NASH i.e. steatosis development in healthy livers, release of cytokines triggering inflammatory process and oxidative stress which leads to hepatocellular degeneration, fibrosis and tumorigenesis. This model also showed some atypical features as compared to human NASH.

Pancreatic Cancer Models

Dramatic progress has been made over the last few years in the development of animal models of pancreatic cancer, in particular the genetically engineered mutant mouse models (GEMs) of exocrine pancreatic cancer. Thirteen GEMs of exocrine pancreatic dysplasia and neoplasia, including a new model of chronic pancreatitis were presented by 11 investigators during a 3-day conference cosponsored by the National Cancer Institute Mouse Models of Human Cancer Consortium and the Abramson Cancer Centre of the University of Pennsylvania, at Philadelphia, Pennsylvania, in December 2004. The models were characterized histologically and immunohistochemically. However, it is yet unproven whether GEMs will more closely predict therapeutic efficacy in pancreatic cancer patients than the current FDA standard of tumor xenografts. The infrastructural facilities similar to those necessary for the proper conduct of investigational human clinical trials have also been suggested.[54]

Angiogenesis Assays

Various *in vitro* and *in vivo* angiogenesis assays used in anticancer drug research have been reviewed recently by Phung and Dass (2006)[55] involving testing on other transplantable tumors. Some other cell lines which can be inoculated.

METHODS INVOLVING CELL LINE/TUMOR PIECES IMPLANTATION

1. If the specified number of cells of a particular cell line are inoculated into sensitive mouse strain, tumors can be developed rapidly as compared to chemical carcinogen-induced tumors and time can be saved using this model system. Usually, L-1210 and P-388 cell lines are used. These cell lines are derived from mouse lymphocytic leukemia and have 100% growth fraction and tumor implanted animal dies on reaching the tumor burden to 10^9 cells. So, the death time of the animal implanted with specified number of L-1210 or P-388 cells can be predicted. The effective drug would retard the tumor growth and increase the life span of the animal. A drug, which prolongs the lifespan of the animal by 20%, is taken for subsequent studies involving testing on other transplantable tumors. Some other cell lines which can be inoculated to induce tumors are B-16 (melanoma), Lewis lung carcinoma and sarcoma-180, etc. The host mouse strain for above type of cell lines is BDF_1 except Swiss for sarcoma-180. P-388 and L-1210 cell lines are inoculated intraperitoneally, B-16 as intraperitoneally and subcutaneously, Lewis lung carcinomas as intramuscularly and sarcoma-180 as subcutaneously. The experiment takes about 10 days for completion.[56]

Mean survival time (MST) is calculated as:

$$T/C\,\% = \frac{\text{MST of treated animals (T)}}{\text{MST of control animals (C)}} \times 100$$

For sarcoma 180 tumors, reduction of tumor size (tumor weight) is used to find out the tumor inhibiting activity of solid tumors as follows:

$$\text{Tumor inhibiting activity (TIA)} = \frac{\text{Average tumor weight of the treated animals (T)}}{\text{Average tumor weight of the control animals (C)}} \times 100$$

2. **Hollow-fiber technique:** Small hollow fibers (tubes 1 millimeter in diameter and 2 centimeters long made of a plastic, polyvinylidene fluoride), containing cells from human tumors are inserted underneath the skin and in the body cavity of the mouse. Each candidate drug is administered at two dosages and is tested against 12 target tumor cells in different hollow fibers. A total of about 20 compounds per week are screened by this method. Compounds that retard the growth of the cells are recommended for the next level of testing. The average length of this test is four days.

   The assays using hollow fiber techniques have been optimized for human cancers originating from the lung, breast, colon, ovary, brain gastric and hepatocellular cancer mouse cell lines. The gastric and hepatocelluar cell lines have been found to be useful in screening small molecules.[57]
3. **Use of xenografts:** Human tumors are injected directly below the skin of mice. Candidate drugs, which have evidence of activity in the hollow fibers, are administered to the mice at various dosages, and those compounds that kill or slowdown the growth of specific tumors with minimal toxicity to the animal will proceed to the next stage of testing. The average length of this test is about 30 days.

   Spheroid culture of LuCaP 147-induced prostate cancer
   Saar et al. (2014)[58] for the first time developed a prostate cancer model by serially passaging spheroid cultures of several LuCaP 003147 xenografts, demonstrating capabilities for high-throughput drug screening and anticancer agents-induced cell cycle arrest and apoptosis in spheroid cultures. Their study showed that cells formed tumors when re-introduced into mice, providing an authentic *in vitro-in vivo* preclinical model of a subtype of prostate cancer with a hypermutator phenotype and an SPOP mutation.

   Integration free-induced pluripotent stem cells (iPSCs) model
   Liu et al. (2014)[59] derived an integration free-induced pluripotent stem cells (iPSCs) from an FA (Fanconi anaemia) patient without genetic complementation and reported in situ gene correction in FA-iPSCs and generated isogenic FANCA (Fanconi anaemia, complementation group A)-deficient human embryonic stem cell (ESC) lines. This model can be used as a drug-screening platform by identifying several compounds that improve hematopoietic differentiation of FA-iPSCs.
4. **Nude mouse model:** Nude mice have been widely used to test the tumorigenicity of cells or for testing of anticancer drugs. These mice are immunologically incompetent because of absence of thymus. They neither show mitotic response in mixed lymphocyte reaction, nor

generate cytotoxic effector cell. Lack of helper T and suppressor T cells alters the antibody response of the animals to antigen. They do not show contact sensitivity and do not reject the transplanted material. They are required to be maintained under strictly sterile conditions and in a warm environment (26-28°C). Some other points regarding their use are:

a. Certain tumors like melanomas and colon carcinomas grow very well in nude mice, whereas prostate carcinomas and most types of leukemia grow very poorly.
b. Large numbers of cells, usually > 10^6 are required to be inoculated beneath the skin to get a successful tumor take.
c. Metastases are rarely observed.
d. Overall maintenance is very expensive.

5. **Newborn rat model:** Newborn rat pups can be used for transplantation of tumors as an alternate for nude mice because they are cost effective and their maintenance is easy. Transplantable tumor cell line can be maintained with ease using rat pups. Rat pups are especially useful to study neural tumors. As an example, 1×10^6 viable C6 glioma cells in 10 µl of phosphate buffered saline can be injected into the left side of the pup under sterile conditions. The animals are checked for palpable tumors twice weekly. C6 glioma tumors transplanted in Sprague-Dawley rats come to palpable stage within 15-20 days.[60]
6. **Transgenic mouse model:** Cancer is known to be a disease of genome and a large number of human cancers arise from mutations in one or more oncogene or tumor suppressor gene. Therefore, inactivation of a particular gene within specific tissues of adult mouse may confer an excellent model of somatic mutational events characteristic of human cancer. The genetically engineered mouse may serve both as a model of disease as well as a model for possible gene therapy. Such mice can be generated either by pronuclear injection of DNA or by gene targeting.[61]

Metamouse, a genetically engineered animal has got US patent in the recent past. In this mouse, tumor pieces of patients are transplanted into the organ of primary growth, in contrast to conventional models in which single cell suspension from tumor cell line is injected underneath the skin of nude mice. In this particular mouse, metastasis and weight loss occurs in the same way as that in humans. The conventional mouse models rarely show metastasis (because metastasis either occurs very slowly or not at all). This limitation contributes to the failure of so many drugs, which are active in such systems to become the approved anticancer drugs. In words of Tetsuro Kubota, tumors require cell-to-cell contact to grow. In suspension form tumor breaking enzymes are expected to destroy the cell surface receptors mediating such cell-cell contact to grow. Certain human cancers, which can develop well in metamouse, include liver, pancreas, head and neck, bladder, stomach, ovarian, colon cancer and lymphomas. It is the only relevant model of mesothelioma. The metastasis of breast and prostate cancer is very slow in this mouse. The important indication of metamouse is to test new routes, doses and indications of old drugs. It can serve as surrogate marker in cancer patient and prognosis of the patient is also possible. The model is very useful to clinicians to make better therapeutic choice by first testing the drugs on patients tumor grown in metamouse. The disadvantages of such studies are that they require prolonged time.[62]

CONCLUSION AND FUTURE PERSPECTIVES

Basic research in cancer biology has provided new targets for cancer drug development and has brought older targets into sharper focus, leading to new and novel approaches to cancer prevention and treatment. The conventional methods of drug screening are continuously being refined or replaced with newer methods and thereby accelerating the drug development. Newer smart approaches are now being sought to screen potential anticancer drugs in the postgenomic era. The trend is directed towards the application of robotics and miniaturization to achieve high throughputs.[63] The pharmaceutical companies are focusing their efforts towards more rational screening of agents that target a specific predefined locus of action. In cancer field for example, the efforts are being directed to identify molecular abnormalities, which are responsible for cancer causation and progression. Of particular interest are signal transduction pathways involved in cell proliferation, which are deregulated in most human cancers.[64] In addition, relevant genes that are mutated or aberrantly expressed in cancer cells and their corresponding proteins targets are increasingly being realized as interesting candidates. Some success in this area has been achieved with discovery of inhibitors of EGF-receptor tyrosine kinase.[65] 3D and 4D models of personalized therapy as well as the genetically engineered mouse models have revolutionized the cancer research and help understanding the tumorgenesis process in a better way than earlier and thus facilitating the anticancer drug discovery for clinical benefit. It is inevitable that in the years to come we will see high technology, high-speed, high-volume and information-intensive approaches to the identification of novel targets genes, proteins and drugs. However, the importance of basic research in the molecular biology and pharmacotherapy of cancer remains critical.

ACKNOWLEDGMENT

The encouragement and guidance from Dr GN Singh, Indian Pharmacopoeia Commission, Ghaziabad, during the course of preparation of this manuscript is gratefully acknowledged. The efforts of Amandeep Bhatia in preparing the manuscript is acknowledged.

REFERENCES

1. http://www.who.int/oral_health/publications/cancer_maps/en/
2. Press Release N°223. International Agency for Research on Cancer, WHO. 12 December 2013. http://www.iarc.fr/en/media-centre/pr/2013/pdfs/pr223_E.pdf
3. http://www.cancer.gov/cancertopics/cancerlibrary/what-is-cancer
4. Fukumura D, Xavier R, Sugiura T. Tumor induction of VEGF promoter activity in stromal cells. Cell 1998;94:715-25.
5. Vlotides G, Eigler T, Melmed S. Pituitary tumor transforming gene: physiology and implications for tumorigenesis. Endocr Rev 2007;28:165-86.
6. Prasad SB, Yadav SS, Das M, et al. Down regulation of FOXO1 promotes cell proliferation in cervical cancer. Cancer 2014;5(8):655-62.
7. Kruh GD, Belinsky M, Chen ZS, et al. Mechanisms of cellular resistance to anticancer agents. Fox Chase Cancer Center 2003 Scientific Report: 1-6.

8. In: M.A. Rudek et al (eds.), Handbook of Anticancer Pharmacokinetics and Pharmacodynamics, Cancer Drug Discovery and Development, 2nd Ed 2014; Humana Press New York.
9. Thayer PS, cordon HL, Macdonald M. In vitro growth inhibition by 3837 compounds tested for antitumor activity: comparison of tumor cell culture and microbial assays. Cancer Chemother Rep 1971;2:27-55.
10. Mosmann T. Rapid calorimetric assay for cellular growth and survival: application to proliferation and cytotoxicity assays. Immunol Meth 1983;64:55-63.
11. Prakash J, Gupta SK, Singh N, et al. Antiproliferative and chemopreventive activity of *Ocimum* sanctum Linn. Int J Med Biol Environ 1999;27:165-71.
12. Alley MC, Scudiero DA, Monks A, et al. Feasibility of drug screening with panels of human tumor cell lines using a microculture tetrazolium assay. Cancer Res 1988;48:589-601.
13. Skehan P, Storeng R, Scudiero, et al. New colorimetric cytotoxicity assay for anticancer-drug screening. J Natl Cancer Inst 1990;82:1107-12.
14. Houghton PJ, Taylor DM. Fractional incorporation of [^{3}H] Thymidine and DNA specific activity as assays of inhibition of tumour growth. Br J Cancer 1977:35(1);68-77.
15. Rotman B. Fluorescent cytoprinting: a simple nondestructive process for assessing chemosensitivity in microorgan cultures. Proc Am Assoc Cancer Res 1989;30:654.
16. Isomura JI, Yoshimatsu K, Ikeda T, et al. A dye uptake method using cultured human cancer cells and its application to sensitivity test for anticancer drugs. Yakugaku Zasshi 1981;101:227-31.
17. Weisenthal LM, Dill PL, Kurnick NB, et al. Comparison of dye exclusion assays with a clonogenic assay in the determination of drug-induced cytotoxicity. Cancer Res 1983;43:258-64.
18. Weisenthal LM, Marsden JA, Dill PL, et al. A novel dye exclusion method for testing in vitro chemosensitivity of human tumors. Cancer Res 1983;43:749-57.
19. Bosanquet AG. Correlations between therapeutic response of leukemias and in vitro drug-sensitivity assay. Lancet 1991;337:711-4.
20. Von Hoff DD, Kronmal R, Salmon SE, et al. A Southwest Oncology group study on the use of human tumor cloning assay for predicting response in patients with ovarian cancer. Cancer 1991;67:20-7.
21. Nyga A, Cheema U, Loizidou M. 3D tumour models: novel in vitro approaches to cancer studies. J Cell Commun Signal 2011;5(3):239–48.
22. Kwapiszewska K, Michalczuk A, Rybka M, et al. A microfluidic-based platform for tumour spheroid culture, monitoring and drug screening. Lab Chip 2014;14(12):2096-104.
23. Ma HL, Jiang Q, Han S, Wu Y, Cui Tomshine J, et al. Multicellular tumor spheroids as an in vivo-like tumor model for three-dimensional imaging of chemotherapeutic and nano material cellular penetration. Mol Imaging 2012;11(6):487-98.
24. Mishra DK, Creighton CJ, Zhang Y, et al. Gene expression profile of A549 cells from tissue of 4D model predicts poor prognosis in lung cancer patients. Int J Cancer 2014;134(4):789-98.
25. Boyd M, Shomemaker R, McLemore T, et al. New drug development. In Roth J, Ruckdescel J, Weisberger T (Eds). Thoracic Oncology. Philadelphia: Saunders, 1989.
26. Danks MK, Yalowich JC, Beck WT. A typical multiple drug resistance in a human leukemic cell line selected for resistance to teniposide (VM-26). Cancer Res 1987;47:1297-301.
27. Gupta RS. Genetic, biochemical, and cross-resistance studies with mutants of Chinese hamster ovary cells resistant to the anticancer drugs, VM-26 and VP16-213. Cancer Res 1983;43:1568-74.
28. Monks A, Scudiero D, Skehan P, et al. Feasibility of a high-flux anticancer drug screen utilizing a diverse panel of cultured human tumor cell lines. J Natl Cancer Inst 1991;83:757-66.

29. Blower PE, Verducci JS, Lin S, Zhou J, Chung JH, Dai Z, et al. MicroRNA expression profiles for NCI-60 cancer panel. Mol Cancer Ther 2007;6:1483-91.
30. Johnson RK. Screening methods in antineoplastic drug discovery. J Natl Cancer Inst 1990;82:1082-3.
31. Steele VE, Moon RC, Lubet RA, et al. Preclinical efficacy evaluation of potential chemopreventive agents in animal carcinogenesis models and results from the NCI chemoprevention drug development program. J Cell Biochem 1994;20:32-54.
32. Di Giovanni J. Multistage carcinogenesis in mouse skin. Pharmacol Ther 1992;54:63-128.
33. Azuine MA, Bhide SV. Chemopreventive effect of turmeric against stomach and skin tumors-induced by chemical carcinogens in Swiss albino mice. Nutr Cancer 1992;17:77-83.
34. Prakash J, Gupta SK, Dinda AK. Withania somnifera root extract prevents DMBA-induced squamous cell carcinoma of skin in Swiss albino mice. Nutr Cancer 2002;42:91-7.
35. Currier N, Solomon SE, Demicco EG, Chang DLF, Farago M, Ying H, et al. Oncogenic signaling pathways activated in DMBA-induced mouse mammary tumors. Toxicologic Pathol 2005;33:726-37.
36. Wang F, Ma Z, Wang F, Fu Q, Fang Y, Zhang Q, et al. Establishment of novel rat models for premalignant breast disease. Chin Med J (Engl) 2014;127(11):2147-52.
37. Gonçalves BF, de Campos SG, Zanetoni C, Scarano WR, Falleiros LR, jr, et al. A new proposed rodent model of chemically induced prostate carcinogenesis: distinct time-course prostatecancer progression in the dorsolateral and ventral lobes. Prostate 2013;73 (11):1202-13.
38. Balasubramanian S, Elangovan V, Govindasamy S. Fluorescence spectroscopic identification of 7, 12-dimethylbenz (a) anthracene-induced hamster buccal pouch carcinogenesis. Carcinogenesis 1995;16:2461-5.
39. Wami M K, Yarber R H, Ahmed A, et al. Cancer induction in the DMBA hamster cheek pouch: a modified technique using a promoter. Laryngoscope 2001;111(2):204-6.
40. Elangovan V, Sekar N, Govindasamy S. Chemopreventive potential of dietary bioflavonoids against 20-methylcholanthrene-induced tumorigenesis. Cancer Lett 1994;87:107-13.
41. Prakash J, Gupta SK. Chemopreventive activity of Ocimum sanctum seed oil. J Ethnopharmacol 2000;72:29-34.
42. Ohkoshi M, Fujii S. Effect of the synthetic protease inhibitor [N, N-dimethylcarbamoyl-methyl 4-(4-guanidinobenzoyloxy)-phenylacetate]-methanesulfate on carcinogenesis by 3-methylcholanthrene in mouse skin. J Natl Cancer Inst 1983;71:1053-7.
43. Bannasch P, Zerban H. Experimental hepatocarcinogenesis. Molecular mechanisms of hepato-carcinogenesis. In: Okuda K, Tabor E (Eds): Liver Cancer. New York, NY: Churchill Livingstone 1997:213-54.
44. Tennant BC. Animal models of hepadnavirus-associated hepatocellular carcinoma. Clin Liver Dis 2001;5:43-68.
45. Yoon S, Kazusaka A, Fujita S. Accumulation of diacylglycerol in the liver membrane of the Long-Evans Cinnamon (LEC) rat with hepatitis: FT-IR spectroscopic and HPLC detection. Cancer Lett 2000;151:19-24.
46. Vesselinovich SD. Perinatal mouse liver carcinogenesis model and the role of the sex hormonal environment in tumor development. In: Stevenson, Donald E (Eds): Mouse Liver Carcinogenesis: Mechanisms and Species Comparisons. New York, NY: Alan R, Liss 1990:53-68.
47. Di Bisceglie AM, Osmack P, Brunt EM. Chemoprevention of hepatocellular carcinoma: use of tamoxifen in an animal model of hepatocarcinogenesis. J Lab Clin Med 2005;145:134-8.

48. Alagaratnam TT, Wei W, Wong J. Oestradiol binding activity in rat liver tumors and in human hepatocellular carcinoma. Aust N Z J Surg 1987;57:477-9.
49. Smit JJ, Schinkel AH, Oude Elferink RP, et al. Homozygous disruption of the murine MDR P-glycoprotein gene leads to a complete absence of phospholipids from bile and to liver disease. Cell 1993;75:451-62.
50. Fickert P, Fuchsbichler A, Wagner M, et al. Regurgitation of bile acids from leaky bile ducts causes sclerosing cholangitis in Mdr2 (Abcb4) knockout mice. Gastroenterol 2004;127:261-74.
51. Mauad TH, van Nieuwkerk CM, Dingemans KP, et al. Mice with homozygous disruption of the MDR2 P-glycoprotein gene. A novel animal model for studies of nonsuppurative inflammatory cholangitis and hepatocarcinogenesis. Am J Pathol 1994;145:1237-45.
52. Katzenellenbogen M, Pappo P, Barash H, et al. Multiple adaptive mechanisms to chronic liver disease revealed at early stages of liver carcinogenesis in the Mdr2-knockout mice. Cancer Res 2006;66:4001-10.
53. Nakamura A, Terauchi Y. Lessons from Mouse Models of High-Fat Diet-Induced NAFLD. Int J Mol Sc 2013;14(11):21240-57.
54. Hruban RH, Rustgi AK, Brentnall TA, Tempero MA, Wright CV, Tuveson DA. Pancreatic cancer in mice and man: The Penn Workshop 2007. Cancer Res 2006;66:14-7.
55. Phung MW, Dass CR. In vitro and in-vivo assays for angiogenesis modulating drug discovery and development. J Pharm Pharmacol 2006;58:153-60.
56. Indap MA. Chemotherapy: screening of anticancer drug. In Seshadri R, Mulherkar R, Mukhopadhyay R (Eds): Techniques in Cancer Research: A Laboratory Manual, Bombay, Cancer Research Institute, Tata Memorial Centre, Parel 1995;343-5.
57. Park JW, Baek NS, Lee SC, Oh SJ, Jang SH, Kim IH, et al. Preclinical efficacy testing for stomach and liver cancers. Cancer Res Treat 2014 Apr; 46(2):186-93.
58. Saar M, Zhao H, Nolley R, Young SR, Coleman I, Nelson PS, et al. Spheroid culture of LuCaP 147 as an authentic preclinical model of prostate cancer subtype with SPOP mutation and hypermutator phenotype. Cancer Lett 2014;351(2):272-80.
59. Liu GH, Suzuki K, Li M, Qu J, Montserrat N, Tarantino C, et al. Modelling Fanconi anemia pathogenesis and therapeutics using integration-free patient-derived iPSCs. Nat Commun 2014 7;5:4330.
60. Seshadri R. Use of newborn rats for transplantation of tumors. In Seshadri R, Mulherkar R, Mukhopadhyay R (Eds). Techniques in Cancer Research: A Laboratory Manual. Bombay, Cancer Research Institute, Tata Memorial Centre, Parel 1995;352.
61. Lovejoy EA, Clarke AR, Harrison DJ. Animal models and the molecular pathology of cancer. J Path 1997;181:130-5.
62. Holzman D. Of mice and metastasis: a new for-profit model emerges. J Natl Cancer Inst 1996;88:396-7.
63. Bevan P, Ryder H, Shaw I. Identifying small-molecule lead compounds: the screening approach to drug discovery. Trends Biotechnol 1995;13:115-21.
64. Brunton VG, Workman P. Cells-signaling targets for antitumour drug development. Cancer Chemother Pharmacol 1993;32:1-19.
65. Fry DW, Kraker AJ, McMichael A, et al. A specific inhibitor of epidermal growth factor receptor tyrosine kinase. Science 1994;265:1093-5.

CHAPTER

11

Screening Methods for Renal and Liver Fibrosis

INTRODUCTION

Fibrotic diseases are characterized by an increasing amount of connective tissue deposited in the afflicted organ. Fibrosis can occur in a variety of organs including the liver, kidney, lung, intestine, heart and skin. The underlying mechanism of fibrosis in all of these particular organs involves the proliferation of mesenchymal cells that posses a myofibroblast—like phenotype and the subsequent deposition of interstitial collagens and other extracellular matrix proteins by these cells leading to progressive scarring and loss of organ function.[1,2] In general, the fibrotic process is a physiological response to chronic and persistent tissue injury and the pattern shows similarities with the wound healing process, which occurs after acute damage to an organ. In the current chapter, we will focus on fibrosis in the kidney and in the liver and we will discuss the most widely used models for screening of experimental drugs.

THE PATHOGENESIS OF RENAL FIBROSIS

Renal fibrosis is a final common process of many chronic renal diseases. It is characterized by over-deposition of the extracellular matrix, which eventually leads to the end-stage renal disease.[3] Several renal disorders such as diabetic nephropathy, chronic glomerulonephritis, tubulointerstitial fibrosis and hypertensive nephrosclerosis can result into end-stage renal disease.[4] Nephrons, the major unit of kidney, comprise of two major parts, i.e. the glomerulus and the tubulus. Renal fibrosis can be initiated through the injury either at glomerular cells such as mesangial cells, basement membrane, podocytes or at tubular cells. In many pathological conditions, systemically-produced immune complexes bind to glomerular cells and cause inflammation called glomerulonephritis. Persistent occurrence of such events can lead to glomerulosclerosis during which process scar tissues is formed.[5]

Proteinuria, i.e. excessive excretion of proteins in urine, is a hallmark of renal injury. After a renal insult, either by immunologic or non-immunologic events, several molecules such as albumin, immunoglobulins, complement factors, growth factors, angiotensin-II, cytokines and high glucose concentrations filter through the glomerulus and subsequently activate renal tubular cells.[6] In addition, hypoxia, oxidative stress, and many other factors which are induced during pathological conditions, stimulate pro-inflammatory and profibrotic pathways in tubular cells. In response of these activating agents, tubular cells produce growth factors, chemokines and adhesion molecules. Chemokines such as monocyte chemoattractant protein-1 (MCP-1) attract monocytes/macrophages from the systemic circulation. These infiltrated macrophages subsequently produce several growth factors such as transforming growth factor- beta (TGF-β) which stimulate native fibroblast cells. Recent evidence has shown that tubular cells can be activated with TGF-β and undergo epithelial mesenchymal transdifferentiation (EMT) and transform into fibroblasts.[7] Activated fibroblasts called myofibroblasts generate extracellular matrix (ECM) proteins including fibronectin and collagens in the interstitial space which eventually cause tubulointerstitial fibrosis.[8] In this chapter, we will explain the most commonly used animal models for renal fibrosis to test antifibrotic drugs. Although these models are representative for renal fibrosis, many issues such as type and etiology of the disease may differentiate for their applicability.

THE PATHOGENESIS OF LIVER CIRRHOSIS AND THE CRUCIAL ROLE OF HEPATIC STELLATE CELLS (HSC)

Liver cirrhosis is a slowly progressing disease that develops gradually over a period of about 20 years without major symptoms in these patients. In contrast to renal function, which can be monitored by urinary protein excretion, there is a lack of early markers to screen for liver fibrosis. The disease is initiated after repeated and chronic damage to hepatic cells. This damage can be caused by viruses (hepatitis B and C virus), chronic alcohol abuse, toxic injury, biliary problems, but it is also induced by genetic and metabolic liver disorders. Liver cirrhosis, the end-stage of the fibrotic process, is characterized by insufficient liver functioning. In general, three different processes contribute to the gradual loss of liver function; [1] chronic inflammation that causes damage to hepatocytes and activates other resident hepatic cells, [2] capillarization that leads to portal hypertension and shunting of blood which impairs proper blood flow through the liver sinusoids, and [3] *fibrosis* that leads to the excessive deposition of scar tissue within the liver which affects the liver architecture and nutrient exchange.[9-11]

Various hepatic cell types are involved in the processes of initiation and perpetuation of fibrosis. Often, inciting stimuli damage the hepatocytes that subsequently release factors that activate other resident hepatic cells such as Kupffer cells and sinusoidal endothelial cells. Simultaneously, inflammatory cells are recruited from the general circulation. All these cells in turn produce various cytokines and growth factors that activate the HSC and these cells will subsequently proliferate and differentiate into myofibroblasts. It is the chronic activation of this inflammatory process that leads to an irreversible accumulation of extracellular matrix constituents. Several autocriene and paracriene positive feedback loops further stimulate activation of sinusoidal endothelial cells, Kupffer cells, HSC and myofibroblasts. Eventually, this leads to a perpetuation of the disease independently of the presence of the inciting stimulus. Nowadays, the HSC are considered as the crucial cells in the development of liver fibrosis and are therefore viewed upon as the central target cell for drugs aiming at an attenuation of the fibrogenic process.[12,13] HSC and myofibroblasts are the major producers of collagens and other extracellular matrix constituents in the fibrotic liver. These myofibroblasts are of various origin from inside and outside the liver: transformed HSC, portal fibroblasts, stem cells,[14-16] and recent evidence indicate origination from epithelial cells such as hepatocytes and bile duct epithelial cells.[17,18] This latter process is called epithelialmesenchymal transition (EMT).

Since, the current pharmacotherapeutic treatment of fibrosis in the clinic is not effective, the need for novel therapies to treat liver fibrosis is high. Amongst others, research groups nowadays focus on the development of potent and safe antifibrotic agents that interfere with the various activities of HSC. These include inhibition of HSC proliferation and activation, inhibition of cytokine and growth factor production, inhibition of matrix production, promotion of matrix degradation, inhibition of vasoconstriction and promotion of HSC apoptosis. A number of comprehensive overviews of these novel experimental therapies have been published.[10,13,19,20]

To evaluate the effects of potential antifibrotic compounds, animal models are indispensable. The disease involves namely many hepatic cell types and several different processes act in concert with each other, which will occur only *in vivo*. Furthermore, animal models allow easy testing of compounds in various stages of the disease provided that the proper model is chosen. In addition, *in vitro* models can be useful to study cell-specific aspects of the drug-of-interest. However, final efficacy studies should always be performed *in vivo* since all hepatic cell types contribute to the disease progression and their contribution to the disease changes in time. Therefore, in section 2.2 various animal models will be discussed that are used to asses drug efficacy in liver fibrosis, but also two *in vitro* systems with its options and limitations will be outlined.

MODELS OF RENAL FIBROSIS

Since, progression of fibrosis is a long-term process, in most of the animal models renal fibrosis develops during weeks to months. There have been many attempts to design quick models to test antifibrotic drugs in short time. In addition, several animal models have been described on the basis of the etiology of the renal disease. Renal injury can be induced by physical/surgical damage (e.g. subtotal nephrectomy, ureteral obstruction and renal ischemia/reperfusion injury) and biochemical stimuli (e.g. adriamycin and puromycin) as well as it can be instigated by metabolic diseases (e.g. diabetes mellitus and hyperlipidemia) or immune-mediated diseases (anti GBM-nephritis, anti-Thy1 nephritis, and Heymann nephritis). In addition, these models can lead to fibrosis after injuring primarily either the glomerulus (subtotal nephrectomy model), the tubule (ureteral obstruction model) or both (protein overload model). A specific animal model can be selected to screen an antifibrotic compound for its activity in specific type (s) of renal fibrosis, e.g. glomeruloscelerosis, tubulointerstitial fibrosis or both. In addition, antifibrotic drugs can display their pharmacological activity with different modes of action; therefore different animal models can be selected on the basis of etiology to the disease. For instance, the anti-hypertensive drug carvedilol has been found to inhibit fibrosis by reducing blood pressure in spontaneously hypertensive rats with adriamycin nephropathy.[21] Moreover, selection of animal model may depend on the duration of the disease, since some models develop renal fibrosis rapidly e.g. ureteral obstruction model (1-2 weeks) while other takes several weeks e.g. adriamycin, Anti-Thy1 or protein overload induced nephropathy. Furthermore, reproducibility in the level of disease is an important criterion to choose the animal model.

Unilateral Ureteral Obstruction Model

Unilateral ureteral obstruction (UUO) model is characterized by tissue loss, atrophy of tubular epithelial cells, and the development of tubulointerstitial inflammation and fibrosis.[22] This

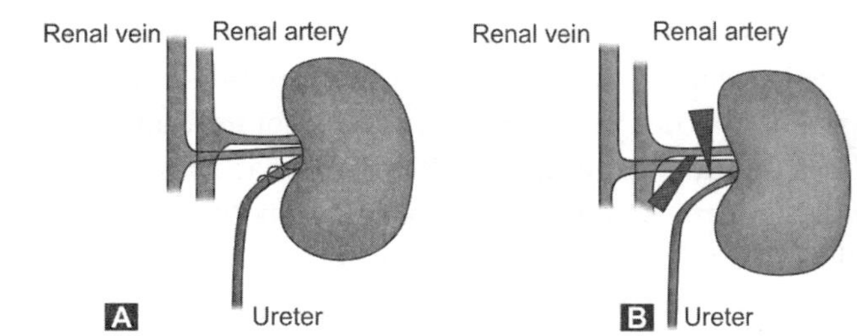

Figure 11.1: Schematic presentation of the ureteral obstruction model showing the placement of two ligations at the ureter (A) and the renal ischemia-reperfusion model showing the blockade of renal artery and vein with clips (B) *(For color version see Plate 15)*

model resembles conditions seen in human obstructive nephropathy. In the UUO model, one ureter is ligated to block the flow of urine from kidneys to urinary bladder. The accumulated urine in kidneys activates renal tubular cells, which eventually leads to fibrosis in the obstructed kidney whereas the contralateral kidney can regulate renal function at some extent. The UUO model is widely performed in mice and rats.

Animals are preferably anesthetized with general anesthesia (2 % isoflurane in 2:1 O_2/N_2O, 1 L.min-1) for their rapid recovery after operation. Alternatively, ketamine chloride (100 mg/kg) and xylazine sulfate (10 mg/kg) intraperitoneally can be used. Left kidneys and ureter are exposed via a flank-incision. Then the ureter is ligated near the hilum at two sites with silk suture (i.e. 4-0) for reliable ligation (Fig. 11.1). Abdominal muscle and skin are stitched separately layer-by-layer. After recovery from anesthesia, animals are put back in cages and animals are treated with postsurgical analgesic buprenorphine (0.05 mg/kg, subcutaneously) after every 12 h for 48 h. In this model, renal fibrosis is visible on day 3 at the earliest and extensive fibrosis occurs after 2-3 weeks.[23] This animal model has been used from 3 days to 21 days but 14 days is an optimum time to test antifibrotic drugs. Samples from the obstructed kidney can be used to determine the extent of fibrosis whereas the contralateral kidney can serve as a control. However, one should be careful in using contralateral kidneys as control as they are not completely normal. Immunohistochemical analyses are performed on kidney sections to determine tubulointerstitial collagen deposition (collagen I and III), activation of fibroblasts (alpha-smooth muscle actin, α-SMA) and tubular cell apoptosis (TUNEL or caspase-3 assay). Yamate et al.[24] have explained some crucial immunostainings in long-term UUO model. Kidney cortex pieces can be used to study gene expression for inflammatory (MCP-1, RANTES, etc.) and fibrotic (TGF-β_1, α-SMA, TIMP-1, procollagen-Iα1) factors.

This model is quite consistent and takes relatively little time to develop fibrosis. However, this model is only suitable to study antifibrotic effects on tubulointerstitial fibrosis and not on glomerulosclerosis.

Subtotal Nephrectomy

The 5/6 subtotal nephrectomy (SNx) or subtotal renal ablation is a model for chronic renal disease which develops proteinuria, hypertension, and ECM deposition with a fall in glomerular filtration rate. SNx is induced by right nephrectomy and partial left nephrectomy (upper and lower poles excision).[25,26]

In general, male Wistar rats are used for this model. To perform 5/6 subtotal nephrectomy, rats are operated by incising at the flank under anesthesia (halothane or isoflurane). The right kidney is exposed and the adrenal gland is separated from the upper pole, and the kidney is decapsulated. The renal pedicle is ligated and the right kidney is removed. Thereafter, the left kidney is also exposed through a flank incision. The adrenal gland is separated from the upper pole and the kidney is decapsulated. Ligatures are placed around the upper and lower poles and the poles are excised. Abdominal muscle and skin are stitched separately layer-by-layer with silk sutures. After recovery from anesthesia, animals are put back in cages. Animals are treated with postsurgical analgesic buprenorphine (0.05 mg/kg, subcutaneously) after every 12 h for 48 h. In SNx model, animals develops mild tubular atrophy at day 7 which gradually increases until day 150 with 75% tubules damage. Glomerular damage and interstitial ECM accumulation are visible after 15 days which increase at the highest level after 150 days.[27] Moreover, 12 weeks time point has been widely used to test antifibrotic drugs. The progression of the disease can be followed by monitoring proteinuria and renal functions.

This model has advantages to analyze both glomerular and tubular damage in the same model and the development of the disease can be followed during the study by analyzing proteinuria and renal function. But it has drawbacks of tedious surgical procedure, high variability and long time for establishment of the disease.

Adriamycin-induced Nephropathy

Adriamycin or doxorubicin-induced nephropathy model is characterized to develop proteinuria, focal segmental glomerulosclerosis and tubulointerstitial fibrosis.[28] This model mimics the proteinuric condition in patients and is considered as an experimental analogue of human focal glomerulosclerosis. Adriamycin is an anti-neoplastic agent and causes nephrotoxicity through many mechanisms such as by inducing oxidative stress and by affecting water and urea transporters in renal medulla.[29] This model is usually performed in mice and rats.

Animals are injected intravenously with a single dose of adriamycin (2 to 7 mg/kg in rats and 10 to 13 mg/kg in mice)[28,30,31] The rate of the renal damage and the development of fibrosis increases with the increase of the adriamycin dose. To examine the extent of disease, urine is collected at different time points and analyzed for urinary protein levels. Animals can be stratified on the basis of the proteinuria levels. The renal damage starts after 1 to 2 weeks and progresses continuously for several weeks. During this period of time, renal functions drop and ECM proteins gradually accumulate in glomeruli and tubulointerstitium (Fig. 11.2). At the end of the studied time point, animals are sacrificed and kidneys are studied for tubular injury, inflammation and fibrosis using the immunohistochemical and gene expression analyses as discussed earlier. This model has been used to evaluate several drugs such as angiotensin converting enzyme inhibitor captopril, angiotensin receptor antagonist losartan and different kinase inhibitors.[32-34] In addition, we have used this model to examine the affectivity of renal-specific delivered captopril-lysozyme conjugate on proteinuria.[35]

Adriamycin-induced nephropathy model has many advantages, e.g. it mimics the clinical situation of proteinuria; it is easy to induce; it develops both glomerular and tubulointerstitial fibrosis; variation can be reduced by stratifying animals on the basis of their proteinuria levels; and development of the disease can be followed during the study by measuring proteinuria

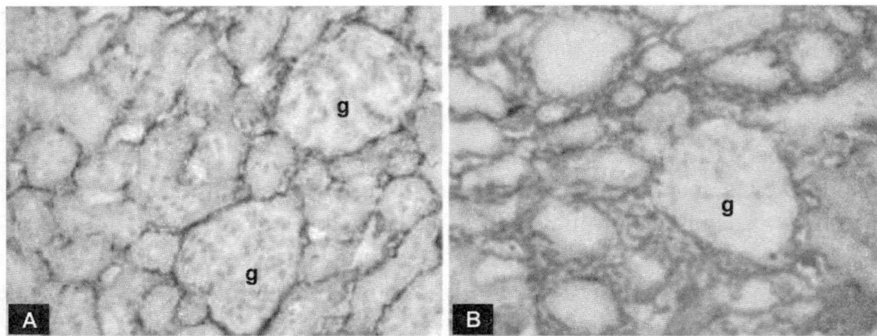

Figure 11.2: Pictures of immunohistochemical staining (red color) for collagen-III in normal kidney (A) and in kidneys with adriamycin-induced nephropathy (B). A single dose of adriamycin (5 mg/kg) was administered in Wistar rats and after 4 weeks staining was performed. Collagen-III deposition in tubulointerstitium was substantially enhanced in adriamycin treatment rats. Sections were counter-stained with hematoxyllin. g = glomerulus. Magnification 20 × 10 (*For color version see Plate 16*)

and renal function. However, a major drawback of this model is that it takes a long time to develop fibrosis and consequently needs long-term treatments.

Protein-overload Rat Model

After many renal insults, plasma proteins filtrate through glomeruli and activate tubular cells, which eventually induce inflammation and fibrosis. To mimic this phenomenon, in the protein-overload model, a large amount of a protein is administered to animals repeatedly which causes excessive protein filtration through glomeruli and eventually leads to tubular damage.[36-38] This model has been studied in mice and rats but rats are used more often. Rats are incised at the flank under anesthesia (isoflurane) and the right kidney is removed. Muscle and skin are stitched layer-by-layer with silk sutures. Animals are treated with postsurgical analgesic buprenorphine (0.05 mg/kg, subcutaneously) after every 12 h for 48 h. After uninephrectomy, rats are administered with daily injections of bovine serum albumin (1 to 2 g) intraperitoneally for several weeks. In this model fibrosis develops slowly and the model has been used to evaluate antifibrotic drugs from 2 to 7 weeks. Similar to the adriamycin-induced nephropathy model, induction of disease can be studied by measuring proteinuria, renal function tests. After sacrificing animals, kidneys are studied for tubular damage, inflammation and fibrosis using immunohistochemical and gene expression analyses.[39,40]

Since, protein overload model develops fibrosis by causing both glomerular and tubular damage, this model is suitable to study antifibrotic effects on both type of tissues. However, daily intraperitoneal injections of protein for several weeks makes this model labor-intensive.

Renal Ischemia/Reperfusion-induced Fibrosis

Ischemia/reperfusion (I/R)-induced renal fibrosis is one of the main factors which leads to the chronic allograft nephropathy, a main cause for allograft failure.[41] I/R injury is well-known to induce tubular damage and inflammation particularly in renal medulla. In I/R injury, renal blood flow is hampered temporarily for 45 to 60 min and then perfused. This process induces hypoxia within kidneys which severely affects medulla, the poorly perfused region in kidney. In addition, I/R injury enhances endothelial cells-leukocyte interaction that leads to leukocyte entrapment in interstitium.[42] Mice and rats have been widely used for this model.

Animals are preferably anesthetized with general anesthesia (2% isoflurane in 2:1 O_2/N_2O, 1 $L.min^{-1}$) and left kidney is exposed via incision in the flank. The renal artery and vein are exposed carefully and clamped individually under microscope. Then a third clamp is placed together at both the renal artery and the vein to completely stop the renal blood flow (see Fig. 11.1). Body temperature is maintained using a heating pad. Saline kept on 37°C is instilled in the peritoneal cavity occasionally. After 45 or 60 min, clamps are removed and reperfusion of the kidney is assessed by the restoration of normal color. Then, the abdominal cavity is closed by stitching muscle and skin layer-by-layer with silk sutures. Animals are treated with postsurgical analgesic buprenorphine (0.05 mg/kg, subcutaneously) after every 12 h for 48 h. In this model, inflammation is prominent in the initial phase of the disease whereas the activation of fibroblasts and the interstitial accumulation of ECM proteins can be detected already after 3-4 days.[43,44] After 3 weeks; the expression of fibrotic markers such as collagens and fibronectin increases significantly. In addition, many studies have used I/R injury with uninephrectomy to mimic the partial condition of an chronic allograft nephropathy.[41]

This model is quite reproducible and is employed often to study the effect of drugs on tubular damage and inflammation after a short time (3-4 days).

Anti-Thy1 Antibody-induced Glomerulosclerosis

Anti-Thy1 antibody-induced glomerulonephritis is an experimental animal model representing immunoglobulin A (IgA) nephropathy in patients. In this model, a monoclonal antibody

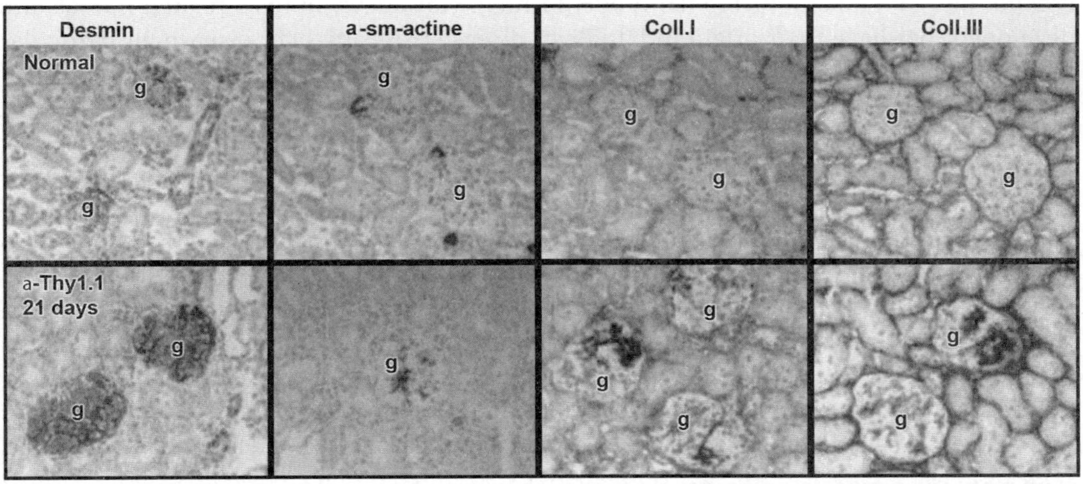

Figure 11.3: Pictures of immunohistochemical stainings (red color) for desmin, alpha-smooth muscle actin collagen type I and collagen type III in normal kidney (upper panel) and in kidneys with anti-Thy1 IgG-induced renal fibrosis (lower panel). A single dose of anti-Thy 1 IgG was administered in Wistar rats and after 21 days staining was performed. The number of fibroblasts (desmin and actin staining) as well as the interstitial matrix deposition (collagens staining) was substantially increased after administration of anti-Thy 1 IgG. Sections were counterstained with hematoxyllin. g = glomerulus. Magnification 20 × 10 (*For color version see Plate 16*)

is administered to animals, which binds to a Thy1-like antigen on the surface of mesangial cells of the kidney.[45] This causes complement-dependent and nitric oxide-dependent lysis of mesangial cells.[46] Since, anti-Thy1-induced glomerulonephritis resolves over 4 weeks in animals if two kidneys are present, uninephrectomy is performed to incite chronic progressive glomerulosclerosis.[47,48]

Male or female Wistar rats (120-180 g) are used commonly in this model. Uninephrectomy is performed as described in the subtotal nephrectomy and unilateral ischemia-reperfusion injury models in this chapter. Three days after surgery, a dose of anti-Thy1 monoclonal antibody (5 mg/kg) is injected intravenously. After 16 weeks, proteinuria is well established and the expression of fibrotic proteins is highly upregulated in tubulointerstitium and glomerulus (Fig. 11.3). In addition, the inflammatory events can be studied in this model, as the infiltration of macrophages and T-lymphocytes is prominent in this model.[48]

The anti-Thy1 model is a reproducible model and can also be used to study the effects on glomerulonephritis in short period of time (< 1 week) as a reversible model, in which anti-Thy1 antibody is injected without performing uninephrectomy.[49]

MODELS OF LIVER FIBROSIS

Several approaches to induce fibrosis in animals are described and these models can be divided according to their stimulus from inciting injury.[18,50] Liver fibrosis models are associated with (1) toxic damage (hepatocytes: CCl4, dimethylnitrosamine (DMN), galactosamine; bile duct epithelial cells: thioacetamide (TAA), (2) immunological-induced damage (heterologous serum and experimental schistosomiasis), (3) biliary damage [common bile duct ligation (BDL) or occlusion] or (4) alcohol-induced damage (baboon ethanol diet or Tsukamoto/French model in rats). Nowadays, fibrosis-related models are developed that have their origin in fatty liver disease (5). Fatty liver disease, in particular the 'malignant' inflammatory form non-alcoholic steatohepatitis (NASH), can progress to liver fibrosis and cirrhosis. It is strongly associated with obesity and diabetes, two modern health problems in Western countries. Of the existing animal models for fatty liver disease, as reviewed by Anstee et al.,[51] the genetic leptin-deficient (ob/ob) or leptin-resistant (db/db) mice and the dietary methionine/choline-deficient models are used in the majority of published research. Progressive fibrosis was reported only in the methionine/choline-deficient models in 100% of the mice.

BDL and CCl_4 are the most widely used rodent models in liver fibrosis research to assess the effectivity of experimental drugs on the pathogenesis, because these models represent features of human pathogenesis. Therefore, these models are the best characterized with respect to histological, biochemical, cell, and molecular changes associated with the development of fibrosis (Fig. 11.4). In the past years, there is a tendency in fibrosis-related research to shift from rat to mice models, and most of the models originally described for rats are now applied in mice. Moreover, new testing models arise due to the development of transgenic or knock-out mice models, which were developed to elucidate the pathogenesis and common pathways in liver fibrosis.[52] Examples of knockouts with spontaneous formation of liver fibrosis are mdr2-/- mice[53,54] lhx2-/- mice,[55] and the mice models for NASH mentioned above.[51]

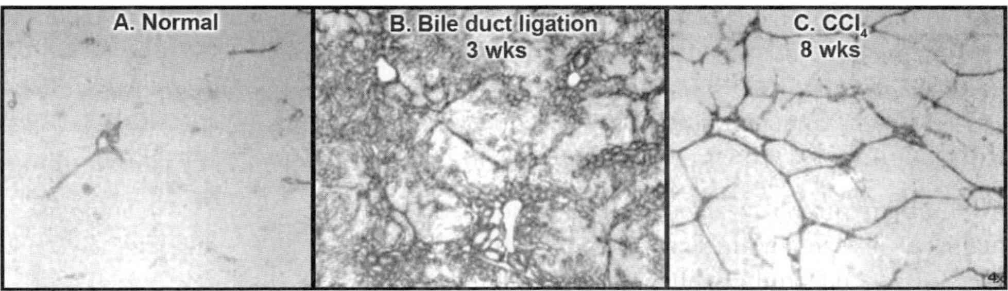

Figure 11.4: Pictures illustrating the enhanced matrix deposition (collagen type III immunostaining) in two important rat models of liver fibrosis as compared to normal livers. (A) normal rat liver (B) rat liver 3 weeks after bile duct ligation, and (C) rat liver 8 weeks after CCl_4 intoxication. Magnification 4 × 10 (*For color version see Plate 16*)

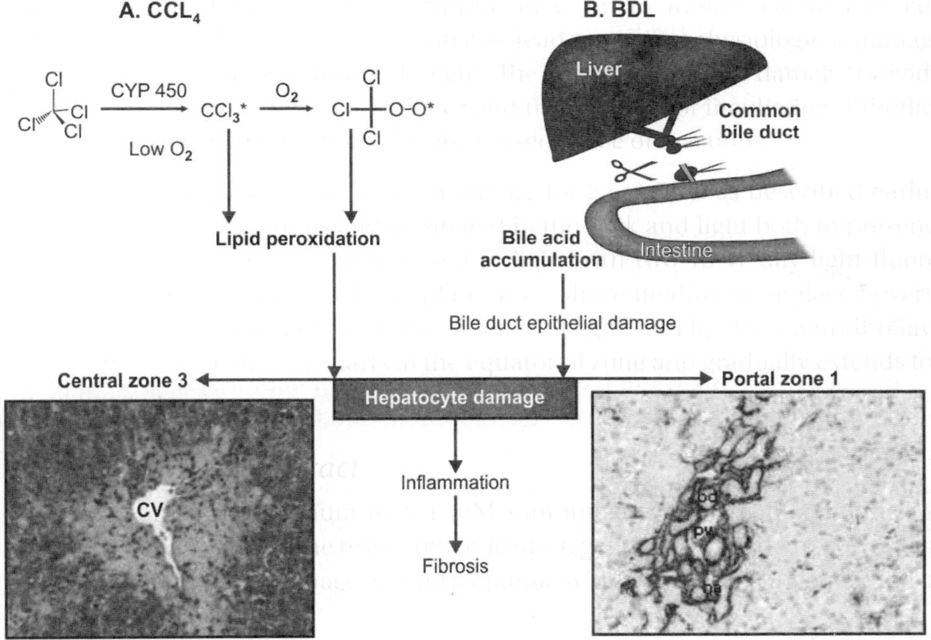

Figure 11.5: Schematic illustration of two different models of liver fibrosis: (A) CCl_4 intoxication and (B) Bile duct ligation (BDL). CCl_4 causes hepatocyte damage predominantly in zone 1 (as illustrated by the PAS stained liver at the left). Ligation of the bile duct causes damage to bile duct epithelial cells and damage is seen in portal area (as illustrated with the collagen I+III stained liver at the right).

Abbreviation: cv=central vein; bd=bile duct; ha=hepatic artery; pv=portal vein. Magnification 20 × 10 (*For color version see Plate 17*)

Acute and Chronic Models with Carbon Tetrachloride (CCl_4)

CCl_4 intoxication results in hepatocyte necrosis and apoptosis with damage predominantly in zone III (around central vein) of the liver. The mechanism behind this hepatocyte damage is the activation of CCl_4 by cytochrome P450, which results in the formation of a trichloromethyl radical in these cells and this free radical initiates lipid peroxidation (Fig. 11.5A).

The damage to hepatocytes by CCl_4 is reflected by high plasma alanine transaminase (ALT) and aspartate transaminase (AST) levels after CCl_4 administration. CCl_4 causes also fatty changes in the hepatocytes. This initial damage is followed by hepatic stellate cell activation and tissue fibrosis.

The CCl_4 model is associated with tremendous inflammation, a feature that is also often seen in livers of patients with liver fibrosis. Disadvantages of this model are the variations obtained in disease induction in the animals and the relatively high rate of mortality after CCl_4 administration (≥ 20%).

In animal models, CCl_4 treatment is used to obtain different stages of the fibrotic process, ranging from early damage and HSC activation until advanced cirrhosis.[50] The fibrotic stage obtained in the rodents depends on the number of injections of CCl_4 that are administered. The models for CCl_4 that are used in liver fibrosis research, as summarized in Table 11.1, represent (1) acute damage (72 hours after a single injection of CCl_4) with HSC activation, (2) early and established fibrosis (4-6 week of twice-weekly CCl_4 dosing), (3) early cirrhosis (8 week of twice-weekly CCl_4 dosing), and (4) advanced micronodular cirrhosis (12 week of twice-weekly CCl_4 dosing). In addition, for each of these models (5) spontaneous recovery from fibrosis can be studied after cessation of dosing of CCl_4.[56,57] This latter model is a valuable model to determine drug induced acceleration of recovery from established fibrosis after removal of the inciting stimulus. This is similar to treatment situations in patients with liver fibrosis in case their inciting stimulus can be eliminated; for instance after alcohol abstinence or after antiviral therapy against hepatitis virus infections.

CCl_4 is administered to the animals via intraperitoneal, subcutaneous, or oral administration, or by inhalation. For intraperitoneal injections, CCl_4 is diluted in olive oil and given in dosages of 0.5-1.0 ml/kg to rats and mice. Often, supplementation of phenobarbital in drinking water (resulting in induction of hepatocyte cytochrome P450) is used to get more reproducible fibrosis development and to accelerate the speed of fibrosis development. Usually, phenobarbital concentrations of 0.3-0.4 g/I in drinking water are used and started 1 week before the initial exposure to CCl_4. In case of inhalation of CCl_4, the animals are placed in an inhalation chamber twice a week with a progressively increasing exposure time (1-5 min). Also with this procedure, supplementary phenobarbital in drinking water is added. To reduce early toxicity and mortality, some research groups vary with the dose of CCl_4 in time. In these cases, gradually increasing dosages in the first weeks are administered to the rats.[58]

Table 11.1: Various rodent models used in liver fibrosis research based on CCl_4 intoxication, that represent different stages of liver fibrogenesis

Model	*CCl_4 injections*	*Time period of injections*	*Stage of disease*
1	1	72 hours	Acute damage, hepatocyte regeneration and HSC activation
2	2x/week	4-6 weeks	Early and established fibrosis
3	2x/week	8 weeks	Early cirrhosis
4	2x/week	12 weeks	Micronodular cirrhosis
5	2x/week	6-12 weeks, cessation for > 4 weeks	Regression models

Bile Duct Ligation (BDL)

The second well-studied experimental animal model of liver fibrosis is the bile duct ligation model.[59,60] This model corresponds with the human pathology of biliary cirrhosis, such as extrahepatic biliary atresia and primary sclerosing cholangitis. Ligation of the bile duct causes acute epithelial damage, and the detergent action of the subsequently released bile salts in the liver is likely associated with the solubilization of plasma membranes and hepatocyte cell death. This latter is visualized by elevated ALT and AST levels in plasma, in particular immediately after ligation (first week). Characteristics of obstruction of the bile is the appearance of bile products, such as bilirubin, into the blood circulation, which causes jaundice in these animals.

The initial damage is followed by a massive expansion of the bile duct epithelial cells and periductal myofibroblasts, which can be referred to as portal expansion (stage I). In total, this results in marked liver enlargement, which can be up to twice the weight as compared to normal. Then, bile duct epithelial cells and myofibroblasts in the portal tract are progressively expanding which results in a gradual remodeling of the liver architecture by linking adjacent portal tracts (biliary cirrhosis stage IV).

To ligate the bile duct, the abdomen of the rat is opened under general anesthesia (preferably N_2O/O_2/halothane inhalation to allow quick recovery from narcosis) to identify the common bile duct. The bile duct runs from the hilum of the liver, where the hepatic ducts meet, through the pancreas, into the lower end of the duodenum. Of note, the rat has no gall bladder in contrast to other rodents. Three ligatures are placed and tied around the bile duct: two close to the liver and one close to the duodenum (Fig. 11.5B). The first ligatures will prevent formation of a reservoir of bile outside the liver. After tight closure, the bile duct is cut between the second and third ligation in order to prevent restoration of the bile flow by bile duct formation around the ligature. Subsequently, the abdomen is closed again and analgesics can be given to the rats. We use a local anesthetic compound (Marcaine® which contains bupivacaine), but also systemic-acting analgesics are sometimes administered (e.g. Temgesic® (containing buprenorphine). For mice, the procedure is a little bit more complicated because a mouse possesses a gall bladder, and attention should be paid to tightly ligate the whole duct, in general, more than three ligatures are needed, to prevent rupture of the bladder and subsequent problems.

Already in the first days after ligation, proliferation of bile duct epithelial cells, activation and proliferation of HSC and myofibroblasts, and deposition of extracellular matrix can be observed microscopically starting in the portal areas of the liver (zone 3). After one week, a fibrous expansion of the portal areas is visible and after about 10-14 days, portal-portal bridging is visible. Three to 4 weeks after ligation, these rats develop advanced cirrhosis characterized by extensive proliferation of the bile ducts, around which the activated and transformed HSC are detectable (markers: a-smooth muscle actin and PDGFbeta receptor) and around which the interstitial collagens (types I and III) are deposited (Fig. 11.6). At this stage, only small islands of hepatocytes are still present (see Fig. 11.4).

A major advantage of the BDL model is the relatively fast development of fibrosis (within 3 weeks) in rats. Furthermore, the model is quite reproducible, and the mortality due to the ligation procedure in rats is low (<10%). Disadvantages of the BDL model are the limited inflammation associated with this type of fibrosis development and the excessive expansion of bile duct epithelial cells. Another drawback with regard to drug screening is that the BDL-induced disease is difficult to reverse with experimental drugs, and a reason for this may be

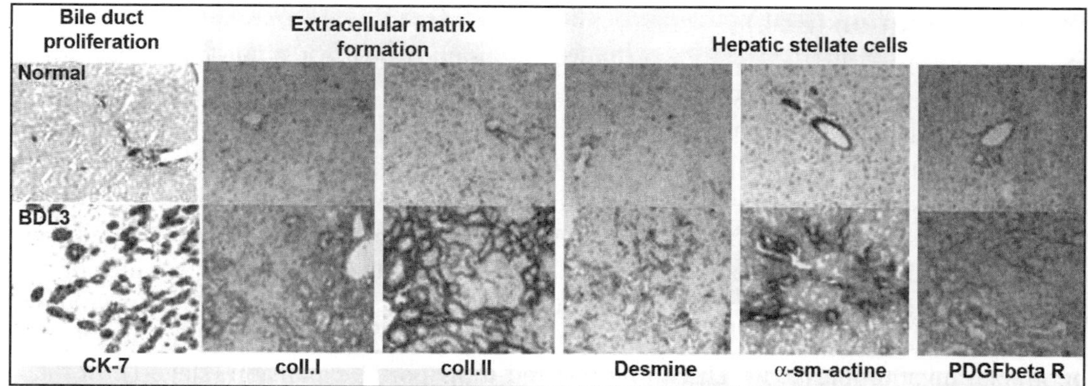

Figure 11.6: Liver fibrosis induced 3 weeks after ligation of the bile duct (BDL3). Pictures of immunohistochemical stainings (red color) for cytokeratin-7 (marker of bile duct epithelial cells), collagen types I and III (matrix formation), desmin (marker for all HSC), and alpha-smooth muscle actin, and PDGFbeta receptor (markers for transformed HSC and myofibroblasts) in normal livers (upper panel) and in BDL3 livers (lower panel). The number of bile duct epithelial cells, myofibroblasts (desmin, actin, and PDGFR staining) as well as the interstitial matrix deposition (collagens staining) was substantially increased after ligation of the bile duct. Sections were counterstained with hematoxyllin. Magnifications 20 × 10 (*For color version see Plate 17*)

because the initiating stimulus (ligation of the bile duct) remains present during treatment periods and causes continuous damage as subsequent fibrosis that troubles the potential treatment effects.

Dimethylnitrosamine (DMN)

DMN induces liver damage leading to fibrosis and cirrhosis. Characteristic for this model is that ongoing administration of this toxic compound finally leads to the development of hepatocellular carcinoma in rodents. DMN induces liver injury by initiating damage to the hepatocyte. It is metabolized primarily in hepatocytes by Cytochroom P450 (isotype 2E1) to more toxic compounds with formation of reactive oxygen species in hepatocytes and subsequently this will lead to lipid peroxidation. In contrast to the hepatotoxin CCl_4, DMN administration does not cause fatty changes, steatosis, in the hepatocytes. To induce the fibrosis, DMN (10 microliter/kg body wt., i.p.) is given 3 days a week for 3 weeks to rats.[61,62]

After administration of DMN, hemorrhagic necrosis is evident in centrolobular part (zone III) of the liver. Incomplete septa appear after 7 days and micronodular cirrhosis is developed after 3 weeks of treatment with DMN. Increased numbers of HSC and myofibroblasts are found in the formed septa. Influx of inflammatory cells, mainly lymphocytes, is noted early in DMN-induced liver injury.

Advantages of this model are that the disease induction is quite reproducible in the animals, and this model is associated with a prominent inflammatory reaction. Furthermore, this model can be used to study the transition from cirrhosis to hepatocellular carcinoma, and the influence of drugs on this process.

HSC in Culture (*In Vitro* System)

HSC are key players in fibrosis and these cells predominantly orchestrate the development of the disease. To assess the antifibrotic efficacy of experimental drugs, these primary cultured cells are useful in assessing specific effects on HSC activities. In particular, the primary isolated HSC are valuable in drug research, because *in vitro* they spontaneously transform into myofibroblasts, and this transformation process is associated with cellular activation, proliferation and matrix production resembling cellular activities that also happen *in vivo*. This transformation does not occur in the various HSC cell lines that are also used in literature.[63] Immediately after isolation they represent a quiescent state, e.g. as present in the normal healthy liver, with vitamin A droplets as their main characteristic. During culture on plastic for about 10-14 days a cell with myofibroblast-like features is obtained (Fig. 11.7).[64] This transformed cell displays different cellular activities as compared to the original isolated one.

The procedure to isolate HSC is well described by various fibrosis research groups.[65-67] Briefly, HSC are isolated from livers of normal rats weighing at least 500 g in order to achieve a good separation from the other hepatic cells. The liver is digested with pronase, collagenase and DNase by *in situ* perfusion. Pronase is essential in the isolation, yet it affects the viability of other hepatic cells (i.e. hepatocytes) and therefore this procedure can only be used to isolate HSC from the liver. After several centrifuge steps, the cell suspension is subjected to a Nycodenz gradient to collect the HSC on top of the Nycodenz layer. The separation is based on the low density of the HSC as compared to other liver cells, as a consequence of their high cellular lipid content. Instead of Nycodenz, also other compounds are used, e.g. Stractan, Metrizamide, or Percoll, to separate the HSC from the other cells by density gradients. The yield of HSC after collagenase/pronase digestion and Nycodenz separation is about 20-40 × 10E6 cells per rat liver. The yield of HSC obtained from a mouse liver is much smaller, and to isolate and purify proper amounts of HSC, about 5 mice have to be used at the same time in one total isolation (Geerts, personal communication).

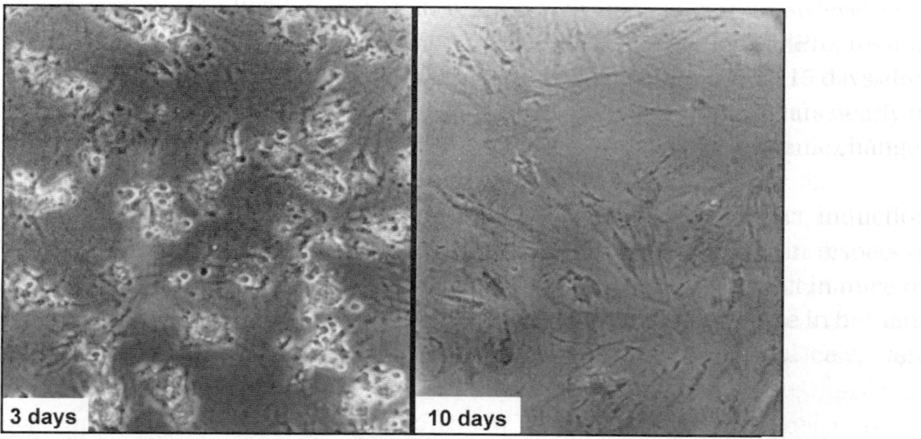

Figure 11.7: Representative photographs of rat hepatic stellate cells at 3 days (quiescent HSC) and 10 days (activated HSC) after isolation from a rat liver. Note the vitamin A droplets in the quiescent HSC and the change in morphology during culture (activated HSC)

Photos are obtained in the lab of Prof. A. Geerts (Brussels, Belgium)

The purity after isolation can be confirmed by phase contrast microscopy or by staining of the cells with markers for hepatic cell types. The isolated cells are cultured in DMEM containing 10% FCS, 100 U/ml penicillin, and 100 µg/ml streptomycin. After 10-14 days in culture, the cells display an activated phenotype as assessed by light microscopy (change in morphology, Fig. 11.7) and acquire the presence of alpha-smooth muscle actin.[64,68]

Additionally, it is also possible to isolate HSC from human livers. Often, (parts of) human livers are used that are unsuitable for transplantation or are derived from tumor-free parts of the human liver and dissected after partial hepatectomy. Roughly, two methods are used to isolate human stellate cells: (i) out-growth of the cells by culturing small pieces of the liver in medium, and (ii) a combined digestion with collagenase/pronase, after which HSC were separated from other liver nonparenchymal cells by centrifugation over density gradients similar to the rat procedure. Of note, the first method will yield a combination of various (myo) fibroblastic cells including HSC and myofibroblasts. These cells are subsequently cultured in DMEM supplemented with 5% Fetal Calf Serum and 5% Human Serum. The myofibroblastic nature of the cells can be microscopically evaluated, and tested for the expression of a-smooth muscle actin.

Liver Slice System

A second *in vitro* test system which was recently developed to assess effects of antifibrotic drugs is the liver slice preparation.[69] Drug studies with tissue slices (8 mm diameter, 250 µm thickness that is about 10-12 cell-layers thick) containing stellate cells in their natural environment that maintain their *in vivo* cellular functional and anatomic relationships, may provide additional information about the hepatocellular specificity of the experimental drug and their effects on all hepatic cells.

Two models have been developed in the past years: one in which CCl_4 induced the activation of quiescent HSC in normal rat liver slices,[70] while in the second model fibrotic rat liver slices were used that were harvested from rats with BDL-induced liver fibrosis and cultured for 1-2 days.[69] In both models, markers of HSC activities were shown to be induced (AB-crystallin, HSP47, alphaSMA and collagen expression). In particular, the slice preparations from fibrotic livers are promising tools for the testing of antifibrotic drugs *in vitro* in their natural multicellular, fibrotic milieu, which cannot be achieved *in vitro* using single cell cultures or co-culture systems.[71]

Liver slices are prepared as follows: Livers are excised from rats and stored in UWsolution (University of Wisconsin transplantation fluid) until the slice procedure starts. Slices were prepared in ice-cold Krebs-Henseleit buffer saturated with carbogen (95% O_2/5% CO_2) and containing 25 mM glucose, 25 mM $NaHCO_3$ and 10 mM Hepes using the Krumdieck tissue slicer. To equilibrate the tissue, slices are pre-incubated for 1 h in Williams Medium E with glutamax-I supplemented with 25 mM d-glucose and 50 µg/ml gentamicin (WEGG) under carbogen-atmosphere at 37°C in six-well culture plates while gently shaken. After that, slices are transferred to six-well culture plates containing fresh medium and incubated under carbogen atmosphere at 37°C for maximally 48 h while gently shaken.

A disadvantage of this system is the limited time period of study. Slices, in particular fibrotic slices, are viable for maximally 48 hours after preparation, which limits the time to study effects of experimental drugs. Another limitation of this method is the absence of blood flow through the slice. Advantages of the slice system is that they can be prepared from normal, fibrotic or cirrhotic tissue, and this *in vitro* system easily allows drug testing in human liver material. Furthermore, the HSC is present in its natural environment including extracellular matrix components and all other resident hepatic cells, which allows testing of multicellular interactions.

CONCLUSION

Animal models are indispensable in the testing of antifibrotic compounds, because of the complex multicellular processes that determine the development of the fibrosis in kidneys as well as in livers. Even the importance of various processes varies during the course of the disease. For both renal and liver fibrosis, various animal models exist, as described in this chapter. Therefore, to evaluate the effects of potential antifibrotic compounds it is essential to choose the proper model and the proper stage of the disease because this will largely determine the outcome of the study. In addition, specific disease markers to describe the fibrotic stage and determine the effects of potential antifibrotic compounds are crucial and therefore additional research searching for new and good discriminating disease markers is needed. The tendency in research seen in the past years to perform efficacy studies in mice instead of rats, is related to the occurrence of specific knock-out mice. However, mice models will also be helpful to assess the effects of for instance biological mediators, such as cytokines and growth factors, on the development of fibrosis, and in particular after chronic administration of these mediators.

REFERENCES

1. Powell DW, Mifflin RC, Valentich JD, et al. Myofibroblasts. I. Paracrine cells important in health and disease. Am J Physiol 1999;277:C1-9.
2. Bonner JC. Regulation of PDGF and its receptors in fibrotic diseases. Cytokine Growth Factor Rev 2004;15:255-73.
3. Eddy AA. Molecular basis of renal fibrosis. Pediatr Nephrol 2000;15:290-301.
4. el Nahas AM, Muchaneta-Kubara EC, Essawy M, et al. Renal fibrosis: insights into pathogenesis and treatment. Int J Biochem Cell Biol 1997;29:55-62.
5. Couser WG. Mediation of immune glomerular injury. Clin Investig 1993;71:808-11.
6. Remuzzi G, Bertani T. Pathophysiology of progressive nephropathies. N Engl J Med 1998;339:1448-56.
7. Zeisberg M, Kalluri R. The role of epithelial-to-mesenchymal transition in renal fibrosis. J Mol Med 2004;82:175-81.
8. Eddy AA. Molecular insights into renal interstitial fibrosis. J Am Soc Nephrol 1996;7:2495-508.
9. Bataller R, Brenner DA. Liver fibrosis. J Clin Invest 2005;115:209-18.
10. Pinzani M, Rombouts K Colagrande S. Fibrosis in chronic liver diseases: diagnosis and management. J Hepatol 2005; 42 Suppl: S22-36.
11. Friedman SL. Mechanisms of disease: mechanisms of hepatic fibrosis and therapeutic implications. Nat Clin Pract Gastroenterol Hepatol 2004;1:98-105.
12. Friedman SL. Molecular regulation of hepatic fibrosis, an integrated cellular response to tissue injury. J Biol Chem 2000;275:2247-50.

13. Fallowfield JA, Iredale JP. Targeted treatments for cirrhosis. Expert Opin Ther Targets 2004;8:423-35.
14. Knittel T, Kobold D, Saile B, et al. Rat liver myofibroblasts and hepatic stellate cells: different cell populations of the fibroblast lineage with fibrogenic potential. Gastroenterology 1999;117:1205-21.
15. Kinnman N, Francoz C, Barbu V, et al. The myofibroblastic conversion of peribiliary fibrogenic cells distinct from hepatic stellate cells is stimulated by platelet-derived growth factor during liver fibrogenesis. Lab Invest 2003;83:163-73.
16. Russo FP, Alison MR, Bigger BW, et al. The bone marrow functionally contributes to liver fibrosis. Gastroenterology 2006;130:1807-21.
17. Sicklick JK, Choi SS, Bustamante M, et al. Evidence for epithelial-mesenchymal transitions in adult liver cells. Am J Physiol Gastrointest Liver Physiol 2006;291:G575-83.
18. Iredale JP. Models of liver fibrosis: exploring the dynamic nature of inflammation and repair in a solid organ. J Clin Invest 2007;117:539-48.
19. Schuppan D, Porov Y. Hepatic fibrosis: from bench to bedside. J Gastroenterol Hepatol 2002;17 (Suppl 3): S300-05.
20. Wu J, Zern MA. Hepatic stellate cells: a target for the treatment of liver fibrosis. J Gastroenterol 2000; 35:665-72.
21. Jovanovic D, Jovovic D, Mihailovic-Stanojevic N, et al. Influence of carvedilol on chronic renal failure progression in spontaneously hypertensive rats with adriamycin nephropathy. Clin Nephrol 2005;63:446-53.
22. Klahr S, Morrissey J. Obstructive nephropathy and renal fibrosis. Am J Physiol Renal Physiol 2002;283:F861-75.
23. Moon JA, Kim HT, Cho IS, et al. IN-1130, a novel transforming growth factor-beta type I receptor kinase (ALK5) inhibitor, suppresses renal fibrosis in obstructive nephropathy. Kidney Int 2006;70:1234-43.
24. Yamate J, Okado A, Kuwamura M, et al. Immunohistochemical analysis of macrophages, myofibroblasts, and transforming growth factor-beta localization during rat renal interstitial fibrosis following long-term unilateral ureteral obstruction. Toxicol Pathol 1998;26:793-801.
25. Muchaneta-Kubara EC, Sayed-Ahmed N, el Nahas AM. Subtotal nephrectomy: a mosaic of growth factors. Nephrol Dial Transplant 1995;10:320-27.
26. Oldroyd SD, Miyamoto Y, Moir A, et al. An IGF-I antagonist does not inhibit renal fibrosis in the rat following subtotal nephrectomy. Am J Physiol Renal Physiol 2006;290:F695-F702.
27. Muchaneta-Kubara EC, el Nahas AM. Myofibroblast phenotypes expression in experimental renal scarring. Nephrol Dial Transplant 1997;12:904-15.
28. Tamaki K, Okuda S, Ando T, et al. TGF-beta 1 in glomerulosclerosis and interstitial fibrosis of adriamycin nephropathy. Kidney Int 1994;45:525-36.
29. Manabe N, Kinoshita A, Yamaguchi M, et al. Changes in quantitative profile of extracellular matrix components in the kidneys of rats with adriamycin-induced nephropathy. J Vet Med Sci 2001;63: 125-33.
30. Vielhauer V, Berning E, Eis V, et al. CCR1 blockade reduces interstitial inflammation and fibrosis in mice with glomerulosclerosis and nephrotic syndrome. Kidney Int 2004;66:2264-78.
31. Ryuzo M, Soares V. Effect of mycophenolate mofetil on the progression of adriamycin nephropathy. Ren Fail 2001;23:611-9.
32. Li J, Campanale NV, Liang RJ, et al. Inhibition of p38 mitogen-activated protein kinase and transforming growth factor-beta1/Smad signaling pathways modulates the development of fibrosis in adriamycininduced nephropathy. Am J Pathol 2006;169:1527-40.

33. Kim HJ, Ryu JH, Han SW, et al. Combined therapy of cilazapril and losartan has no additive effects in ameliorating adriamycin-induced glomerulopathy. Nephron Physiol 2004;97:58-65.
34. Mansour MA, El-Kashef HA, Al-Shabanah OA. Effect of captopril on doxorubicin-induced nephrotoxicity in normal rats. Pharmacol Res 1999;39:233-37.
35. Windt WA, Prakash J, Kok RJ, et al. Renal targeting of captopril using captopril-lysozyme conjugate enhances its antiproteinuric effect in adriamycin-induced nephrosis. J Renin Angiotensin Aldosterone Syst 2004;5:197-202.
36. Eddy AA. Interstitial nephritis induced by protein-overload proteinuria. Am J Pathol 1989;135:719-33.
37. Eddy AA, Giachelli CM. Renal expression of genes that promote interstitial inflammation and fibrosis in rats with protein-overload proteinuria. Kidney Int 1995;47:1546-57.
38. Nagasawa Y, Takenaka M, Kaimori J et al. Rapid and diverse changes of gene expression in the kidneys of protein-overload proteinuria mice detected by microarray analysis. Nephrol Dial Transplant 2001;16:923-31.
39. van Timmeren MM, Bakker SJ, Vaidya VS, et al. Tubular kidney injury molecule-1 in protein-overload nephropathy. Am J Physiol Renal Physiol 2006;291:F456-64.
40. Shimizu H, Maruyama S, Yuzawa Y, et al. Anti-monocyte chemoattractant protein-1 gene therapy attenuates renal injury induced by protein-overload proteinuria. J Am Soc Nephrol 2003;14:1496-1505.
41. Yang B, Jain S, Pawluczyk IZ, et al. Inflammation and caspase activation in long-term renal ischemia/reperfusion injury and immunosuppression in rats. Kidney Int 2005;68:2050-67.
42. Bonventre JV, Zuk A. Ischemic acute renal failure: an inflammatory disease? Kidney Int 2004;66:480-5.
43. Prakash J, Sandovici M, Saluja V, et al. Intracellular delivery of the p38 mitogen-activated protein kinase inhibitor SB202190 [4-(4-fluorophenyl)-2-(4-hydroxyphenyl)-5-(4-pyridyl)1H-imidazole] in renal tubular cells: a novel strategy to treat renal fibrosis. J Pharmacol Exp Ther 2006;319:8-19.
44. Furuichi K, Wada T, Iwata Y, et al. Interleukin-1-dependent sequential chemokine expression and inflammatory cell infiltration in ischemia-reperfusion injury. Crit Care Med 2006;34:2447-55.
45. Bagchus WM, Hoedemaeker PJ, Rozing J, et al. Glomerulonephritis induced by monoclonal anti-Thy 1.1 antibodies. A sequential histological and ultrastructural study in the rat. Lab Invest 1986;55:680-7.
46. van GH, Albrecht EW, Heeringa P, et al. Nitric oxide inhibition enhances platelet aggregation in experimental anti-Thy-1 nephritis. Nitric Oxide 2001;5:525-33.
47. Sakai N, Iseki K, Suzuki S, et al. Uninephrectomy induces progressive glomerulosclerosis and apoptosis in anti-Thy1 glomerulonephritis. Pathol Int 2005;55:19-26.
48. Kramer S, Loof T, Martini S, et al. Mycophenolate mofetil slows progression in anti-thy1-induced chronic renal fibrosis but is not additive to a high dose of enalapril. Am J Physiol Renal Physiol 2005;289:F359-68.
49. Sadlier DM, Ouyang X, McMahon B, et al. Microarray and bioinformatic detection of novel and established genes expressed in experimental anti-Thy1 nephritis. Kidney Int 2005;68:2542-61.
50. Constandinou C, Henderson N Iredale JP. Modeling liver fibrosis in rodents. Methods Mol Med 2005;117:237-50.
51. Anstee QM, Goldin RD. Mouse models in non-alcoholic fatty liver disease and steatohepatitis research. Int J Exp Pathol 2006;87:1-16.
52. Weiler-Normann C, Herkel J Lohse AW. Mouse models of liver fibrosis. Z Gastroenterol 2007;45:43-50.

53. Van Nieuwkerk CM, Elferink RP, Groen AK, et al. Effects of Ursodeoxycholate and cholate feeding on liver disease in FVB mice with a disrupted mdr2 P-glycoprotein gene. Gastroenterology 1996;111:165-71.
54. Popov Y, Patsenker E, Fickert P, et al. Mdr2 (Abcb4)-/- mice spontaneously develop severe biliary fibrosis via massive dysregulation of pro- and antifibrogenic genes. J Hepatol 2005;43:1045-54.
55. Wandzioch E, Kolterud A, Jacobsson M et al. Lhx2-/- mice develop liver fibrosis. Proc Natl Acad Sci U S A 2004;101:16549-54.
56. Iredale JP, Benyon RC, Pickering J, et al. Mechanisms of spontaneous resolution of rat liver fibrosis. Hepatic stellate cell apoptosis and reduced hepatic expression of metalloproteinase inhibitors. J Clin Invest 1998;102:538-49.
57. Issa R, Zhou X, Constandinou CM, et al. Spontaneous recovery from micronodular cirrhosis: evidence for incomplete resolution associated with matrix cross-linking. Gastroenterology 2004;126:1795-808.
58. Zhu J, Wu J, Frizell E, et al. Rapamycin inhibits hepatic stellate cell proliferation in vitro and limits fibrogenesis in an in vivo model of liver fibrosis. Gastroenterology 1999;117:1198-204.
59. Kountouras J, Billing BH, Scheuer PJ. Prolonged bile duct obstruction: a new experimental model for cirrhosis in the rat. Br J Exp Pathol 1984;65:305-11.
60. Hinz S, Franke H, Machnik G, et al. Histological and biochemical changes induced by total bile duct ligation in the rat. Exp Toxicol Pathol 1997;49:281-88.
61. Jezequel AM, Mancini R, Rinaldesi ML, et al. Dimethylnitrosamine-induced cirrhosis. Evidence for an immunological mechanism. J Hepatol 1989;8:42-52.
62. Jezequel AM, Mancini R, Rinaldesi ML, et al. A morphological study of the early stages of hepatic fibrosis induced by low doses of dimethylnitrosamine in the rat. J Hepatol 1987;5:174-81.
63. Gutierrez-Ruiz MC, Gomez-Quiroz LE. Liver fibrosis: searching for cell model answers. Liver Int 2007;27:434-9.
64. Geerts A. History, heterogeneity, developmental biology, and functions of quiescent hepatic stellate cells. Semin Liver Dis 2001;21:311-35.
65. Weiskirchen R, Gressner AM. Isolation and culture of hepatic stellate cells. Methods Mol Med 2005; 117:99-113.
66. Geerts A, Niki T, Hellemans K, et al. Purification of rat hepatic stellate cells by side scatter-activated cell sorting. Hepatology 1998;27:590-8.
67. Friedman SL, Roll FJ, Boyles J, et al. Hepatic lipocytes: the principal collagen-producing cells of normal rat liver. Proc Natl Acad Sci U S A 1985;82:8681-5.
68. Rockey DC, Boyles JK, Gabbiani G, et al. Rat hepatic lipocytes express smooth muscle actin upon activation in vivo and in culture. J Submicrosc Cytol Pathol 1992;24:193-203.
69. van de BM, Groothuis GM, Meijer DK, et al. Precision-cut fibrotic rat liver slices as a new model to test the effects of antifibrotic drugs in vitro. J Hepatol 2006;45:696-703.
70. van de Bovenkamp M, Groothuis GM, Draaisma AL, et al. Precision-cut liver slices as a new model to study toxicity-induced hepatic stellate cell activation in a physiologic milieu. Toxicol Sci 2005;85:632-8.
71. van de Bovenkamp M, Groothuis GM, Meijer DK, et al. Liver fibrosis in vitro: Cell culture models and precision-cut liver slices. Toxicol In Vitro 2007;21:545-57.

CHAPTER

12

Techniques for the Detection of Apoptosis

INTRODUCTION

Apoptosis is naturally occurring cell death. It is physiological in nature, and also known as 'programmed cell death' (PCD). It is an active, genetically controlled process that removes unwanted or damaged cells.[1-3] It is essential for the appropriate development and function of multicellular organisms.

Dysregulated apoptosis results in excessive or insufficient cell death. It is fundamental to the initiation and progression of many human diseases. Diseases associated with increased cell survival/inhibition of apoptosis have been thoroughly reviewed by Thatte and Dahanukar.[4]. It is implicated in neurodegenerative disorders,[5] AIDS,[6] autoimmune disorders,[7] other viral diseases,[8] etc.

The other form of cell death is pathological in nature and is termed as necrosis. Cell death can be distinguished as necrosis and apoptosis, on the basis of morphology and biochemistry.[9] During necrosis there is rapid breakdown of the membrane systems within the cell. In contrast apoptosis is the result of several well-orchestrated events that require RNA and protein synthesis induced by certain stimuli.[10,11] It is characterized by a series of morphological features and biochemical events. The cell breaks up into membrane-bound fragments of various sizes —known as apoptotic bodies in which internal organelles are preserved.[12,13]

As apoptotic bodies are always membrane bound, there is no exposure of intracellular contents. The membrane undergoes changes such as exposure of normally hidden sugar moeities like N-acetyl glucosamine[14] to signal neighboring macrophages to phagocytose these apoptotic bodies. The lack of inflammation is, therefore the hallmark of apoptosis in contrast to necrosis.

PROAPOPTOTIC AND ANTIAPOPTOTIC AGENTS

The manipulation of the apoptotic pathways either by a pharmacological agent or by genetic engineering may be useful in the management of various diseases. The proapoptotic agents are promoters of apoptosis while antiapoptotic agents are inhibitors of apoptosis. The promoters and inhibitors identified are genes and they encode proteins, which either activate or inhibit the apoptotic process.[4,15-18]

The widespread importance of apoptosis in the field of biology and medicine has led to active research in the area. Many different techniques have been developed and are used for the detection of apoptosis. However, none of these are full proof to detect specifically apoptosis and can detect necrosis also. Thus, it is important to use more than one technique to study apoptosis.

CATEGORIES OF CELLULAR CHANGES THAT FORM THE BASIS OF APOPTOSIS ASSAYS

Surface Morphology and Composition

- time-lapse surface morphology
- membrane permeability: impermeable dyes (PI)
- permeable DNA stains (DAPI, Hoechst)
- phospholipid externalization (Annexin V binding).

Nuclear Events and DNA Cleavage

- nuclear morphology: segmentation of chromatin and nuclei DNA cleavage by gels
- large fragments and internucleosomal cleavage DNA cleavage in situ
- detection of strand breaks in situ nick-translation (ISNT)
- TUNEL (terminal transferase)
- anti-single-stranded DNA antibody
- hairpin oligos (double-stranded breaks)
- cell dissolution (pre-GI peak) (apoptotic bodies containing DNA).

Cytoplasmic Biochemical Activation Events

- caspase cleavage products
- caspase activity (caged fluorophores, FRET)
- PARP activity transglutaminase activity
- death antigens.

Mitochondrial Function and Integrity Permeability

- transition (vital dyes)
- mitochondrial antigens (accessibility)
- metabolic activity
- cytochrome c release and alterations.

DETECTION OF APOPTOSIS BASED ON MORPHOLOGY

As described previously, apoptosis is characterized by distinct morphology. During the process of apoptosis the cell shrinks, detaches from the neighboring cells. This is followed by chromatin condensation and nuclear fragmentation into multiple chromatin bodies, leading to the formation of apoptotic bodies, which are phagocytosed, by neighboring cells. These morphological changes can be assessed by light microscopy, fluorescence microscopy or by transmission electron microscopy (TEM).

Light Microscopy

This is one of the most simple, easy and economic method for the quantitation of the apoptotic cell. The tissue sections are stained with routine hematoxylin and eosin stain [19] and observed under an ordinary light microscope. The chromatin condensation characteristic of apoptosis is evident in these cells as "pyknosis", i.e. very dense staining of chromatin by hematoxylin. Giemsa stain can also be used as it differentiates nuclear structures. Preparation of the stains and staining procedure is given in Table 12.1. Periodic acid Schiff-staining is less desirable because its dark, dense coloration fails to distinguish pyknosis and nuclear chromatin condensation. This technique has the advantage of being economic, as it requires a basic microscope and simple reagents. Also, large number of cells from culture and tissue can be examined at the same time. However, the limitation is that the nuclei of quiescent cells might be identified mistakenly as pyknotic nuclei. Apoptosis occurring after administration of certain chemotherapeutic regimens *in vivo* can be readily detected by this technique.[20]

Table 12.1: Preparation of stains and staining procedure

Stains	*Solutions*	*Procedures*
Hematoxylin/ Eosin stain	Hematoxylin (Mayer) 2.0 g/l 0.3% Eosin Y in 70% ethanol	Dip the slide with tissue section in Hematoxylin for 15-30 sec, wash under running tap water for 5 min, then dip in eosin for 5 sec followed by dehydration in 70, 95 and 100% ethanol (The time of dehydration will vary depending upon the tissue and its thickness).
Geimsa	Geimsa: 0.8 g Geimsa, 0.1 g Eosin Y in 100 ml 1:1 v/v glycerol and methanol buffer: 9 ml 0.1 M citric acid in 25% methanol + 11 ml 0.2 M Na_2HPO_4 in 25% methanol + 380 ml DW, pH 6.4 with HCl	Geimsa (after filtration) for 30 sec – 5 min, then washing in Geimsa buffer for 5 min, followed by dehydration in 70, 95 and 100% ethanol (The time of dehydration will vary depending upon the tissue and its thickness).

Fluorescence Microscopy

Apoptosis can also be detected in tissue sections and cultured cells, by examination under fluorescence microscope. The fixed, permeabilized cells are stained with specific DNA stains such as acridine orange, propidium iodide, Hoechst 33258, 4', 6-diamidino-2-phenylindone (DAPI), etc. Nuclear changes such as chromatin condensation and nuclear fragmentation are readily visible by this technique. The advantages and disadvantages are similar to that of light microscopy.

Cells fixed on the glass coverslips are gently rinsed two times with phosphate buffered saline (PBS) and then fixed and permeabilized with methanol: water (4:1) for 15 min. After rinsing with PBS the coverslips are stained with propidium iodide (5 µg/ml) for 5 min in the dark and mounted on glass slides in glycerol: PBS (1:1). Instead of propidium iodide, Hoechst dye 33258 (2.5 µg/ml) can be used to assess apoptosis by nuclear staining (blue) after fixation of cells in 4% paraformaldehyde. The glass slides are preferentially examined under confocal laser scanning microscopy. Apoptotic nuclei are hyper fluorescent, condensed or fragmented, and smaller compared to normal nuclei (Fig. 12.1). The nuclear hyper fluorescence and the

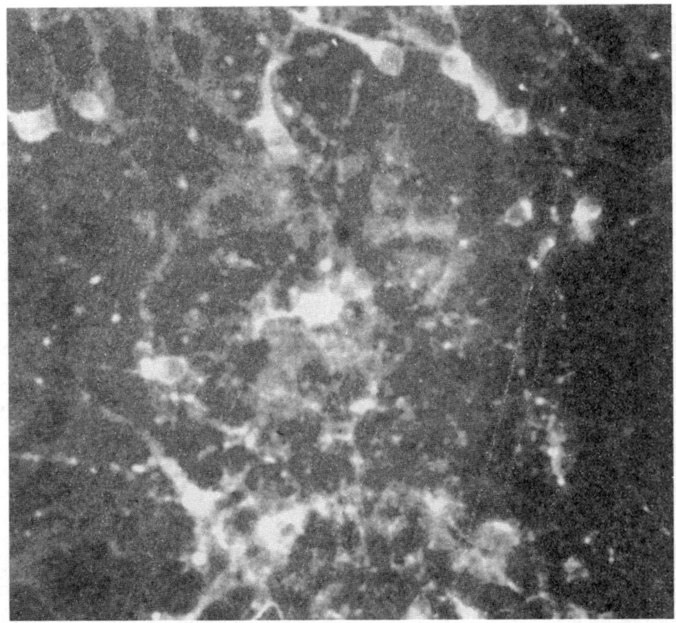

Figure 12.1: Fluorescence microscopy image of 15 weeks gestational age human fetus brain primary cell culture. Cells were stained with Hoechst staining after induction of apoptosis with anti-Fas agonist antibodies. The labeled cells exhibit condensed nuclear fluorescence while viable cells exhibit diffuse nuclear fluorescence. (*Reproduced with permission from J Cell Mol Med 2001; 5: 179-87*) (*For color version see Plate 18*)

nuclear size change can be utilized with appropriate video-image analysis systems to provide a semi-automatic scoring system for apoptotic cells.

Electron Microscopy

Electron microscopy is a reliable qualitative method of characterizing apoptosis both in tissue sections and cell culture. Condensation of nuclei within nuclear margin, blebbing, and shrinkage of the cytoplasm, intact mitochondria and other membranes can be observed in the apoptotic cell under electron microscope.

A mixture of apoptotic and necrotic features are often observed in the sample and therefore the data should be interpreted carefully. Sometimes under tissue culture conditions, secondary necrosis may occur when the ability to remove apoptotic cells by phagocytes is insufficient or compromized. Therefore cells with apoptotic, fragmented nuclei and secondary plasma membrane lysis are frequently observed. Additionally, one should also keep in mind that the same insult can lead to temporally distinct phases of apoptosis and necrosis. For instance Bonfoco and colleagues[21] found that mild insults with glutamate or nitric oxide/superoxide to cerebrocortical neurons *in vitro* led to apoptosis of delayed onset, whereas intense exposure led to more rapid necrosis within a few hours. For cerebellar granule cell neurons in culture, it was found that exposure to glutamate induced a wave of necrosis in a subpopulation of the cells, followed by delayed apoptosis in another subpopulation.[22]

The brief procedure for the preparation of tissue for electron microscopy is: tissue samples or cultures are fixed in 1% glutaraldehyde diluted in 0.1 M phosphate buffer at pH 7.2. The tissue is cut in 1 μm slices and fixed for 5 h at room temperature and then postfixed with 1% osmium tetroxide in PBS for 1 h. After dehydrating samples in acetone and embedding them in epon, thin sections are cut on an ultratome, counterstained with uranyl acetate and examined with an electron microscope.

Electron microscopy is not a suitable technique for quantitation because (i) at a given point of time only few cells are observed, and (ii) the active phase of apoptosis is usually brief.[19]

DETECTION OF DNA FRAGMENTATION

DNA from cells undergoing apoptosis displays a characteristic series of bands known as nucleosomal ladder after agarose gel electrophoresis. This fragmentation pattern results from the preferential cleavage of DNA in the linker regions between nucleosomes double-stranded nuclease that cuts DNA randomly. The nucleases are activated during apoptosis resulting in DNA fragmentation. A variety of techniques described below have been developed based on the detection of fragmented DNA by nucleases.

Conventional Agarose Gel Electrophoresis

DNA can be prepared for agarose gel electrophoresis from whole cells or tissues by a number of treatment protocols. One commonly used protocol involves SDS (Sodium dodecyl sulfate) extraction and protease digestion followed by extraction with phenol to remove peptide fragments. Application of the resulting total cellular DNA to the agarose gel with suitable separation properties, e.g. 1-2% (w/v) agarose, readily demonstrates a ladder of ~180 bp fragments and integer multiples thereof in many models of apoptosis. A brief protocol that can be followed is: Cells (1×10^6) are suspended in 500 μl of TE buffer (10 mM Tris-HCl pH 7.6, 1 mM ethylenediamine tetra acetic acid, pH 8.0) and lysed in 500 ml lysis buffer (3% SDS, 50 mM Tris, pH 12.6) at room temperature for 10 min.[23] Alternatively, cells (1×10^6) can be suspended in 500 μl of extraction buffer (10 mM Tris, pH 8.0; 10 μM EDTA, pH 8.0; 75 mM NaCl; 0.5% SDS and 150 μg/ml proteinase k) and incubated at 50°C for 3 h.[24] After incubation, microfuge the sample for 8 min at room temp. DNA is precipitated from the supernatant by 2 vol. of 100% ethanol with 0.1 M NaCl. The precipitated DNA is washed with 70% ethanol and then treated with DNAse-free RNAse for 60 min. The DNA sample is separated on 2.0% agarose gel electrophoresis and stained by ethidium bromide and photographed under UV illumination. The advantage of this technique is the relatively low cost of the equipment and reagents as well as its simplicity.

In many articles in the literature, agarose gel electrophoresis has often been the single criterion used to detect apoptosis. This is not advisable because it has been shown that DNA laddering is a rather late event in the apoptotic process.[25-27] Therefore, though DNA laddering is typical for apoptosis, its absence cannot be used to exclude apoptosis.[22]

This technique is relatively insensitive and inherently qualitative rather than quantitative. It can distinguish between the nucleosomal ladder of DNA fragments that is characteristic of apoptosis and the random DNA fragmentation that accompanies necrosis, but it is difficult to determine the percentage of the total DNA present in the nucleosomal ladder in a particular lane.[28]

Quantitation of DNA Fragments by Cell Fractionation

Two techniques have been developed to quantify the amount of DNA fragmentation. One of these is based on the observation that double-stranded DNA fragments of less than 10-20 kb can be extracted from nuclei when cells are lysed under nondenaturing conditions in buffer containing EDTA.[29,30] After treatments to initiate apoptosis, cells are suspended in 20 mMTris (pH 7.0 or 8.0) containing EDTA and a neutral detergent. After incubation at 4°C for 10-30 min, the intact chromatin is pelleted at low to moderate speed, leaving the nucleosomal fragments in the supernatant. DNA in the two fractions is then assayed using colorimetric or fluorimetric techniques. Alternatively, if DNA in the cells is uniformly radiolabeled (i.e. greater than one cell cycle) prior to stimulation of apoptosis, DNA in the various fractions is quantitated by scintillation counting.

These approaches allow relatively precise quantitation of the amount of DNA that has been fragmented to oligomers of nucleosome-sized fragments. This information is useful in the time course studies of nuclease activation during apoptosis.[30] Using this simple technique for DNA extraction and assay, large number of samples can be examined. However, these techniques cannot be used to differentiate apoptosis from necrosis as DNA fragments resulting due to necrosis are also extracted. The other drawbacks include: (i) high molecular weight DNA fragments are not extracted under the denaturing conditions and are not detected and (ii) often these results in underestimation of the amount of DNA damage to the cells. For example, if 25% of DNA is extracted, it is not clear whether 25% of the total cells or 25% of DNA in each cell is undergoing apoptosis. The limitations diminish the utility of this approach as a high throughput screening process.

Detection of DNA Fragmentation by Filtration Assays

The rate at which deproteinated DNA flows through the pores of filters is related to the size of the DNA fragments. A variation of this technique has been applied for the quantitation of oligonucleosomal DNA fragmentation.[31] In brief, the DNA in cells is radiolabeled for atleast one generation time. After a suitable postlabeling incubation to chase radiolabeled out of newly synthesized DNA, which has aberrant retention properties on filters, cells are treated with an apoptosis-inducing stimuli. At the desired point(s) in time, cells are then applied to the filters and lysed by addition of an aliquot of deproteinising buffer (e.g. sodium sarkosyl). Low-molecular-weight DNA fragments will flow through the filter with the lysing solution, whereas high-molecular-weight DNA will be retained on the filter unless it is eluted with a large volume of neutral or alkaline buffer pumped through the filter. It is possible to estimate the amount of DNA that has been degraded to low-molecular-weight fragments by quantitating the amount of radiolabel flowing through the filter during cell lysis.

The technique is relatively simple, rapid and the equipment required (a suitable filter manifold and a scintillation counter) is widely available. The approach can also be used for high-throughput screening. However, few precautions should be taken while using this technique. The DNA should be radiolabeled with ^{14}C – labeled nucleotide rather than

^3H-labeled nucleotide because the radiation form ^3H – labeled nucleotide induces apoptosis in some cell types.[32] The labeling step should be followed by sufficient incubation period with radiochemical- free medium to "chase" all the radiolabel into the mature DNA. The limitation is that the technique allows precise quantitation of the amount of DNA that is converted to fragments small enough to pass through the filters during cell lysis; it does not distinguish internucleosomal DNA degradation that accompanies necrosis.

Field-inversion Gel Electrophoresis (FIGE)

Apoptosis is often accompanied by formation of high-molecular-weight DNA fragments (50–200 kb) in addition to nucleosomal ladder[33] by the action of endonuclease on the DNA. The high-molecular-weight DNA fragments are most commonly detected by FIGE. And oligonucleosomal fragmentation is traditionally detected by conventional agarose gel electrophoresis as explained earlier. An elegant combination of these two techniques involving the recovery of small fragments from the plugs used for the FIGE, allows for the simultaneous detection of both high and low-molecular-weight DNA fragments.

To examine DNA by FIGE, cells are treated with an inducing stimulus, encapsulated in agarose (to protect the DNA from shearing during subsequent manipulation), lysed in a deproteinising detergent such as SDS, treated with proteinase k and embedded in the wells of an agarose gel. The DNA is then subjected to an alternating electric field rather than the fixed field utilized in conventional electrophoresis. In this alternating field, larger DNA fragments change migration directions more slowly than smaller fragments. As a consequence, the differences in fragment mobility in pulsed fields, termed "reptation" (reptile like movement through the gel matrix) contribute to separation of high-molecular-weight fragments by size.[34] Molecular weight standards utilized with this technique include oligomers of large viral genomes (e.g. T phage) as well as yeast chromosomes.

The advantage of this technique is its ability to detect the infrequent DNA strand breaks that appear to occur in several models of apoptosis. Because of the widespread and early occurrence of these breaks, it has been suggested that they might be a universal feature of the apoptotic process. However, it is important to note that similar DNA fragmentation has been reported in cells undergoing necrotic cell death as well.[35]

A detailed protocol for the detection of apoptosis in neurons in culture by FIGE as described by Ankarcrona and colleagues[22] is: neurons are gently removed from culture dishes and suspended in a solution containing 0.15 M NaCl, 2 mM KH_2PO_4, pH 6.8, 1 mM EGTA and 5 mM $MgCl_2$. An equal volume of liquefied 1% low melting point agarose gel solution is then added to the suspension, while gently mixing. Next, the mixture is aliquoted into gel plug casting forms and allowed to cool and solidify on ice for 10 min. The resulting agarose blocks are transferred into a solution containing 10 mM NaCl, 10 mM Tris-HCl, pH 9.5, 25 mM EDTA, 1% lauroyl sarcosine and 200 µg/ml proteinase k, and incubated for 24 h at 50°C with continuous agitation. The plugs are then rinsed three times over 24 h at 4°C in 10 mM Tris-HCl, pH 8.0, 1 mM EDTA. Subsequently, the plugs are stored until used for electrophoresis at 4°C in 50 mM EDTA, pH 8.0. FIGE is performed with horizontal or vertical gel chambers equipped with a constant temperature cooling system. The temperature control is very important. Normally, the electrophoresis is run at 180 V in 1% agarose gel in 0.5 TBE (45 mMTris, 1.25 mM EDTA, 45 mM boric acid, pH 8.0) at 12°C. The ramp rate changes from 20-30 sec for the first 6 h, 10-20 sec for the second 6 h and 8–10 sec for the next 12 h applying a forward to reverse ratio of 3:1.

TERMINAL DEOXYRIBONUCLEOTIDYL TRANSFERASE-MEDIATED dUTP NICK END LABELING (TUNEL)

A major disadvantage of all the electrophoretic methods for detecting DNA damage is the inability to determine the number of cells that are affected by the apoptotic process. The limitation has been overcome by the development of *in situ* end-labeling techniques such as TUNEL. It is based on a simple principle. Terminal deoxyribonucleotidyl transferase (TdT) catalyses the addition of nucleosides at a free 3′ OH end of DNA, including the 3′ ends produced by endonuclease action during apoptosis. When the reaction is performed using Co^{+2} as the divalent cation, the enzyme will transfer a nucleoside to a blunt 3′ end, a 3′ protruding end or a 3′ recessed end, albeit with differing efficiencies. A secondary reaction with antibodies or other detection systems is used to detect the nicks. Thus, the TUNEL technique is a method to visualize strand breaks in DNA and can be applied to both tissue sections and cell cultures.[36]

Kits for TUNEL and related assays are commercially available. A detailed procedure to be followed for the assay is supplied with the kit. The precautions to be taken for TUNEL are: the slides should be held in glass slide racks and immersed in glass staining dishes. The solutions should be freshly made. Either superfrost slides or the slides scrubbed with TESPA or poly-L-lysine at least 2 days prior to application should be used to place the tissue sections. 5-10 mm thick paraffin sections of the tissue should be prepared.

A general protocol that can be followed for TUNEL is: Slide-mounted tissue sections are placed on a slide warmer at 45°C for 60 min followed by 15 min each in methanol and 3% hydrogen peroxide respectively. The slide is then incubated for 15 min in 0.3% Triton-X 100 in phosphate buffered saline and rinsed with running de-ionized water. The slide is incubated at 37°C for 1.5-2 h in 100 μl buffer constituted by 20 μl 5 × terminal transferase reaction buffer + 2 μl (40 U) terminal deoxytransferase + 2 μl (2 nmol) biotinylated deoxy UTP and 76 ml sterile distilled water. The slide is then rinsed three times in PBS for 10 min each. Later, the slide is incubated in avidin biotinylated peroxide complex (1:100 dilution) for 2 h at room temperature or alternately for 30 min at 37°C. The slide is rinsed in PBS and incubated for 10 min with 25 mg 3, 3′—diaminobenzidine (Sigma) per 50 ml PBS, with 25 μl 3.0% hydrogen peroxide. The slide is again rinsed with demonized water, dehydrated, defatted and covered with coverslip. The slide is then observed for apoptotic cells under light microscope.

The TUNEL technique has several advantages. The cell morphology and staining intensity can be examined simultaneously; it is therefore possible to compare the time course of DNA fragmentation with morphological changes in individual cells. It can also determine whether DNA degradation is occurring in a small subpopulation of cells as opposed to the entire cell population. However, several groups have reported that cells undergoing necrotic cell death will also be stained by the TUNEL technique.[37,38] Therefore, TUNEL must be considered a sensitive and convenient method for detecting apoptotic cells as long as alternative techniques are also used to confirm that the cells are actually undergoing apoptosis rather than necrosis.

FLOW CYTOMETRY

The flow cytometer measures the amount of fluorescence that is associated with single cells. An aliquot of cell suspension is aspirated into the machine, and the fluid is atomized into droplets so small that the average droplet has 0.05-0.2 probability of containing single cell.

These droplets then flow single file in front of a laser and a series of detectors. As each droplet encounters the laser, photomultiplier tubes detect the light that is scattered as well as the fluorescence emission that results from excitation by the laser.

Several approaches for the study of apoptosis using flow cytometer have been developed. The flow cytometer offers several advantages over microscopic methods. Because of the rapid response of the photomultiplier tubes, it is possible to analyze the fluorescence intensity of hundreds of cells per second. Also, because of the wide dynamic range of photomultipliers, it is possible to precisely quantitate the fluorescence intensity over a 10,000-fold range.

Flow cytometry also has some limitations: it requires relatively expensive and sophisticated equipment that is not easily available; and it is not suitable for the analysis of tissues or even tissue culture cell lines that fail to yield a single-cell suspension.

The flow cytometry techniques that have been developed are described below.

Dye Uptake

The techniques that rely on altered membrane permeability for detection of apoptosis can also be adopted to flow cytometry. The cells can be incubated in dye like Hoechst 33258 or 7-aminoactinomycin D at 4°C and then subjected to flow cytometry. Quantitation of the number of cells that are weakly fluorescent provides an indication of the number of cells undergoing apoptosis.[39]

The principle of the method is that these dyes are excluded from cells at 4°C. Cells that have ruptured readily take up these agents and therefore fluoresce strongly. Whereas, cells undergoing apoptosis take up small amounts of these compounds at 4°C despite the presence of an intact plasma membrane. As a result, cells undergoing apoptosis are weakly fluorescent. It is extremely important to keep cells at 4°C during the entire incubation with the dye because above its phase transition temperature these dyes freely penetrate the plasma membrane.

The advantages of this method are that it is possible to rapidly quantitate the number of cells undergoing apoptosis in a large population of cells. And if these fluorochromes are combined with fluorescently tagged antibodies they permit the precise quantitation of apoptosis in a subset of cells (e.g. CD4—expressing lymphocytes in a larger cell population). The disadvantage of this technique is that the dye uptake is not absolutely specific for apoptosis. Other changes within cells (e.g. ATP depletion) might also allow small amounts of these dyes into the cells. The dye uptake assays appear to offer a rapid and powerful technique for investigating apoptosis in a mixed population of cells as long as this potential limitation is kept in mind.

Decrease in DNA Staining

DNA fragmentation that occurs during apoptosis can also be quantitated by flow cytometry besides cell fractionation technique described previously. For this, the cells treated with an inducing stimulus are fixed with ethanol, extracted with an aqueous buffer lacking divalent cations reacted with propidium iodide or Hoechst 33258, and subjected to flow cytometry.

This technique allows precise determination of the number of cells showing DNA fragmentation. But it does not distinguish between apoptotic and necrotic cells and therefore it can potentially overestimate the number of cells undergoing apoptosis.

Altered Size

Early shrinkage of the cell occurs in apoptosis due to loss of water. Because larger cells scatter light more effectively than smaller cells, cell size can be monitored by changes in light scatter properties. The cells treated with an inducing stimulus are fixed at different time and subjected to flow cytometry. Apoptotic cells are distinguished as those particles that have less forward scatter than control cells.

Although, it is true that apoptotic cells are smaller than nonapoptotic cells, this parameter alone is probably not sufficient as a single discriminator for distinguishing the two populations.[40]

Loss of Mitochondrial Transmembrane Potential (ψ_m)

The predominant localization of Bcl-2 and some of its family members to the mitochondrion indicates a potential role of it in apoptosis. Mitochondria loose transmembrane potential early in the course of apoptosis.

The electrochemical gradient that establishes across the inner mitochondrial membrane during normal oxidative phosphorylation provides energy for concentration of membrane-permeant cationic dyes against concentration gradients. The accumulation ratio of these dyes in mitochondria relative to the extramitochondrial space is directly related to the transmembrane electrochemical gradient. The active concentration of these dyes in mitochondria reflects normal oxidative phosphorylation, and the failure to accumulate these dyes reflects a loss of mitochondrial transmembrane potential.[41] These observations, which were initially made using isolated mitochondria, form the basis for flow cytometry-based methods of assessing mitochondrial transmembrane potential. In these experiments, cells treated with inducers of apoptosis are incubated briefly with membrane-permeant cationic dyes e.g. 5-5',6-6'-tetrachloro-1,1',3-3'—tetraethylbenzimidazolcarbocyanine iodide or 3-3'—dihexyloxacarbocynine iodide, and immediately subjected to flow cytometry. Cells containing normal ψ_m contain larger amounts of these dyes due to their concentration in mitochondria. The appearance of dim staining with this technique reflects a loss of mitochondrial transmembrane potential.

It has been suggested that this change in ψ_m might be the first identifiable biochemical change in cells undergoing apoptosis. However, this change is not universally identifiable and is not specific for apoptosis. Changes in ψ_m have been extensively documented in cells undergoing necrosis and can result from any treatment that alters mitochondrial electron transport or proton transport e.g. metabolic poisons such as cyanide or azide. Accordingly, changes in ψ_m must be interpreted cautiously.

ANNEXIN V STAINING

In healthy cells, sphingomyelin is predominantly present in the outer layer and phosphatidylserine in the inner layer. During the course of apoptosis, this asymmetry is lost. Phosphatidylserine becomes accessible on the surface of cells undergoing apoptosis, and can interact with annexin V, a polypeptide that binds strongly and specifically to phosphatidylserine. These observations form the basis for histochemical and flow cytometry-based methods of detecting cells undergoing apoptosis.[42,43]

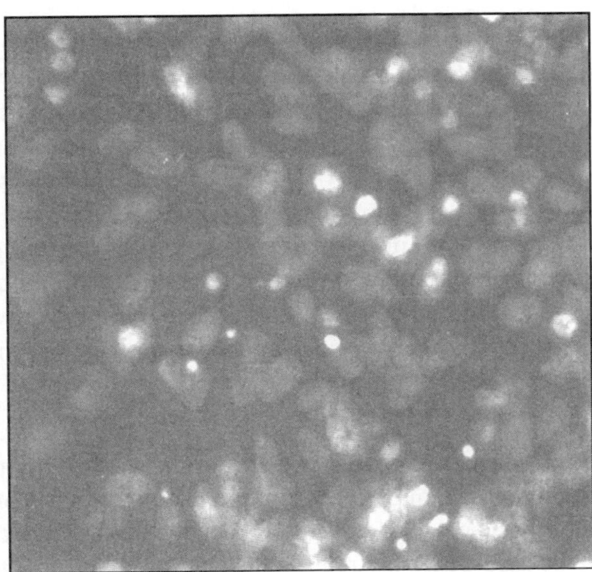

Figure 12.2: Fluorescence microscopy image of 15 weeks gestational age human fetus brain primary cell culture. Cells were stained with annexin V- FITC after induction of apoptosis with anti-Fas agonist antibodies. Labeled cells exhibit condensed nuclear fluorescence while viable cells exhibit diffuse nuclear fluorescence. (Reproduced with permission from J Cell Mol Med 2001; 5: 179-87) (*For color version see Plate 18*)

The cells treated with an inducing stimulus can be fixed using a nonpermeabilizing fixative (e.g. formaldehyde), treated with fluorochrome-coupled annexin V, and examined by fluorescence microscopy or subjected to flow microfluorimetry. Alternatively, cells can be stained without fixation. In either case, cells undergoing apoptosis will be fluorescently labeled (Fig. 12.2), whereas other cells will not.

ALTERATIONS IN PLASMA MEMBRANE PERMEABILITY

Cells that undergo apoptosis are either phagocytosed by neighboring cells or the cells/cell fragments lose membrane integrity. The loss in membrane integrity can be detected by agents that are unable to penetrate viable cells or by the ability to exclude charged dyes such as trypan blue or propidium iodide. Alternatively, it can also be detected as loss of cytoplasmic contents, e.g. ^{15}Cr or lactate dehydrogenase.

The advantages of these methods are that they are quantitative in nature and can be used to examine a large number of cells. However, the disadvantages are: they do not distinguish between apoptosis and necrosis and therefore must be applied only when other techniques have established the apoptotic nature of cell death; also these techniques detect only the change in the later stage of cell death and therefore cannot be used to study earlier changes in the process of cell death; these are not suitable to study changes in individual cells; these techniques are not useful in those apoptotic models that involve phagocytosis of the cells e.g. most *in vivo* models; and lastly these techniques require viable cells.

Vital Dyes

Vital dyes have been one of the most rapid, simple, inexpensive and useful tools for distinguishing between viable and nonviable cells both in tissue culture and in living tissues *in situ*. Trypan blue, erythrosin or nigrosin are unable to enter normal cells but are readily and irreversibly taken up by cells that have lost plasma membrane integrity.[44]

Before applying these dyes, it is important to remember that loss of plasma membrane integrity occur both in apoptosis and necrosis. Besides, because loss of membrane integrity occur relatively late in apoptosis, staining with vital dyes will miss "doomed" cells in the early stages of apoptosis, and will therefore underestimate the number of apoptotic cells. Also dyes such as trypan blue are themselves cytotoxic depending on concentration and/or time.

Release of Sequestered Compounds

The integrity of the plasma membrane can also be assessed by monitoring the release of compounds that are actively sequestered by living cells. Incubation of cells in medium containing diacetyl fluorescein or ^{15}Cr, leads to active uptake and concentration of these compound within cells. Measuring the release of such compounds into culture medium has been used as a means of quantitatively assessing cell death.[45] In a related approach, quantitative information has also been derived by measuring activity of cytoplasmic enzymes (e.g. lactate dehydrogenase or adenylate kinase) released into culture medium by dying cells.[46]

However, these methods are again of little value in understanding the early events of apoptosis. The assays of cytoplasmic enzyme release must be carefully controlled to take into account differences in enzyme activity between cell types or loss of tissue culture sera. Again the method is nonspecific for detection of apoptotic cell death and therefore should be used only in conjunction with the methods that can clearly discriminate between the two forms of cell death.

ENZYME ASSAYS

The identification of morphological and biochemical changes that occur during apoptosis has led to continued efforts to study the enzymatic activities responsible for those changes. Several enzyme activities have been reported to be increased in cells undergoing apoptosis. These include tissue transglutaminases,[47] deoxyribonuclease[48] and ICE family proteases.[49, 50] Studies of these enzymes have generally involved three different approaches: direct assays for activities that are thought to be altered; application of enzyme inhibitors to assess the effect of perturbing enzyme activity; and genetic approaches involving overexpression (transfection) or underexpression (antisense oligoneucleotides or genetic knockouts) to assess the effect of altering enzyme content.

In setting up assays for enzyme activities, several considerations must be kept in mind. First, the assay should be as specific as possible. Second, if assays are being performed to compare relative amounts of enzyme activity present under different conditions, the assays should be performed under conditions in which the product formed is directly related to the amount of enzyme present. Finally, the activity should be investigated under conditions that approximate the intracellular milieu during apoptosis. Adherence to these principles can help eliminate misinterpretations of data.

RECENT ADVANCES

Ribble and colleagues have recently described a simple and rapid technique for quantifying apoptosis in 96-well plates.[51] The authors have modified ethidium bromide and acridine orange staining assay that can be performed entirely in a 96-well plate format. The technique can be used to quantify apoptosis of suspension cells as well as adherent cells. The technique eliminates the detaching and washing steps, which drastically reduces the time needed to perform the test, minimizes damage to adherent cells, and decreases the possibility of losing floating cells.

Lipid Proton MR Spectroscopy

The first MRI technique applied to the detection of apoptosis was lipid proton magnetic resonance spectroscopy.[52] These studies described apoptosis-specific changes, including a selective increase in CH_2 (methylene) relative to CH_3 (methyl) mobile lipid proton signal intensities at 1.3 and 0.9 ppm, respectively. The rise in CH_2 resonance occurred with a wide range of apoptotic drugs as well as apoptosis associated with serum (growth factor) deprivation The CH_2/CH_3 ratio also had a strong linear correlation with other markers of programmed cell death, including fluorescent annexin V cytometry and DNA ladder formation. Although, there was an increase in the methylene resonance, there was no detectable change in total lipid composition or new lipid synthesis, suggesting an increase in membrane mobility as opposed to increased amounts of lipids within cells.[53]

Diffusion Weighed MRI

Diffusion-weighted MRI (DWI) is an alternative MRI modality that can image apoptosis in response to radiation and chemotherapy without the need for a contrast agent.[54] DWI generates image contrast by using the diffusion properties of water within tissues. Diffusion can be predominantly unidirectional (anisotropic) or not (isotropic) and can be restricted or free depending on the amount of water in the extracellular (relatively unrestricted) or intracellular (restricted) compartments. Diffusion-sensitized (weighted) images can be acquired with magnetic gradients of different magnitudes, generating an apparent diffusion coefficient (ADC) map. As increases in cellularity are reflected as restricted motion, DWI has been used in cancer imaging to distinguish between tumor (restricted microenvironment) and peritumoral edema (unrestricted). DWI may also be valuable in monitoring treatment, where changes due to cell swelling and apoptosis are measurable as changes in ADC. The magnitude of changes, however, is small (i.e. < 50% of control), and it may be difficult to separate tumor shrinkage, necrosis, and other processes that can occur with therapy.[55] Therefore, more studies are needed to confirm the validity of DWI as a marker of therapeutic efficacy in the clinic.

Detection of Apoptosis with Ultrasound

High-frequency ultrasound (40 MHz or greater) has been used to detect the unique specular reflections of apoptotic cells *in vitro* and *in vivo*. Backscatter from apoptotic nuclei is up to 6-fold greater than that from nonapoptotic cellular nuclei. The specific nuclear features resolved at 40 MHz include fragmentation of DNA and chromatin condensation, which occur relatively late in the apoptotic cascade. Unfortunately, the significant energy loss with the soft tissues at these higher frequencies currently limits high-frequency ultrasound to the study of the skin and other superficial structures. High-frequency ultrasound, however, could be quite useful for the study of apoptosis in the brain (and possibly other organs) of neonates and young infants. The open fontanels of neonates provide excellent sonographic windows for the high-frequency ultrasonographic study of apoptosis known to be associated with hypoxic ischemic injury.[56] In fact, in the most recent study (2005), Tunis et al. developed statistical methods at a frequency of 20 MHz that enable the monitoring of structural changes within a very low percentage of apoptotic cells in a tissue, raising the possibility of using this technique *in vivo*, particularly in the premature neonatal brain, which is at high risk for periventricular leukomalacia (PVL).[57]

CONCLUSION

It is very important to remember that none of the above techniques are highly specific for the detection of apoptosis. Therefore, it is mandatory to use more than one technique(s) to establish the biochemical nature of cell death as apoptotic. The techniques that can be employed to study apoptosis will depend upon the type of the experiment, expected end result and feasibility to use a particular technique with reference to the tissue under investigation as well as facilities available.

REFERENCES

1. Steller H. Mechanisms and genes of cellular suicide. Science 1995;267:1445-9.
2. Cohen JJ. Apoptosis. Immunol Today 1993;14:126-30.
3. Kerr JFR, Harmon BV. Definition and incidence of apoptosis. An historical perspective. In Tomie LD, Cope FO (Eds): Apoptosis: The Molecular Basis of Cell Death. Cold Spring Harbor: Laboratory Press 1991:5-29.
4. Thatte U, Dahanukar S. Apoptosis: clinical relevance and pharmacological manipulation. Drugs 1997;54:511-32.
5. Martinou I, Frankowski H, Missotten M, et al. Gene tools to study neuronal apoptosis. In Polver I, (Ed). Neuromethods. Vol 29: Apoptosis - techniques and protocols. Humana Press Inc 1997:1-12.
6. Groux H, Torpier G, Monte D, et al. Activation - induced death by apoptosis in $CD4^+$ T cells from human immunodeficiency virus - infected asymptomatic individuals. J Exp Med 1992;175:331-40.
7. Vaux DL. Toward an understanding of the molecular mechanisms of physiological cell death.Proc Natl Acad Sci USA 1993;90:786-9.
8. Akbar AN, Savill J, Gombart W, et al. The specific recognition by macrophages of CD8+, CD45RO+ T cells undergoing apoptosis: a mechanism for T cell clearance during resolution of viral infections. J Exp Med 1994;180:1943-7.
9. Wyllie AH, Kerr JFR, Currie AR. Cell death: the significance of apoptosis. Int Rev Cytol 1980;68:251-306.
10. Cohen JJ, Duke RC. Glucocorticoid activation of calcium dependent endonuclease in thymocyte nuclei leads to cell death. J Immunol 1984;132:38-42.

11. Wyllie AH, Morris RG, Smith AL, et al. Chromatin cleavage in apoptosis: association with condensed chromatin morphology and dependence on macromolecular synthesis. J Pathol 1984;142:67-77.
12. Kontogeorgos G, Kovacs K. Apoptosis in endocrine glands. Endocr Pathol 1995;6:257-65.
13. Schwartzman RA, Cidlowski JA. Apoptosis: the biochemistry and molecular biology of programmed cell death. Endocr Rev 1993;14:133-51.
14. Arends MJ, Wyllie AH. Mechanisms and roles in pathology. Int Rev Exp Pathol 1991;32:223-54.
15. Korsmeyer SJ. Regulators of cell death. Trends Genet 1995;11:101-5.
16. Armstrong RC, Aja T, Xiang J, et al. Fas-induced activation of the cell death related protease CPP 32 is inhibited by Bcl-2 and by ICE family protease. J Biol Chem 1996;271:16850-5.
17. Roquet N, Pages JC, Molina T, et al. ICE inhibitor YVADcmk is a potent therapeutic agent against in vivo liver apoptosis, Curr Biol 1996;6:1192-5.
18. Wang CY, Mayo MW, Korneluk RG, et al. NF - kB antiapoptosis: induction of TRAF 1 and TRAF 2 and c-IAP 1 and CIAP 2 to suppress caspase - 8 activation. Science 1998;281:1680-3.
19. Wyllie AH, Duval E, Cell injury and death. In: McGee IOD, Isaacson PG, Wright NA, Eds. Oxford Text Book of Pathology. Vol. 1. London: Oxford Univ Press 1992:141-79.
20. Martin DS, Stolfi RL, Colofiore JR, et al. Biochemical modulation of tumor cell energy in vivo: II. A lower dose of adriamycin is required and a greater anti tumor activity is induced when cellular energy is depressed. Cancer Invest 1994;12:296-307.
21. Bonfoco E, Krainc D, Ankarcrona M, et al. Apoptosis and nercrosis: two distinct events induced respectively by mild and intense insults with N-methyl-D-aspartate or nitric oxide/superoxide in cortical cell cultures. Proc Natl Acad Sci USA 1995;92:7162-6.
22. Ankarcrona M, Dypbukt JM, Bonfoco E, et al. Glutamate induced neuronal death: A succession of necrosis or apoptosis depending on mitochondrial function. Neuron 1995;15:961-73.
23. Jee SH, Shen SC, Tseng CR, et al. Curcumin induces a p53 - dependent apoptosis in human basal cell carcinoma cells. J Invest Dermatol 1998;111:656-61.
24. Li WC, Kuszak JR, Dunn K, et al. Lens epithelial cell apoptosis appears to be a common cellular basis for non-congenital cataract development in humans and animals. J Cell Biol 1995;130:169-81.
25. Brown DG, Sun XM, Cohen GM. Dexamethasone induced apoptosis involves cleavage of DNA to large fragments prior to internucleosomal fragmentation. J Biol Chem 1993;268:3037-9.
26. Oberhammer F, Wilson JW, Dive C, et al. Apoptotic death in epithelial cells: cleavage of DNA to 300 and/or 50 kb fragments prior to or in the absence of internucleosomal fragmentation. EMBO J 1993;12:3679-84.
27. Zhivotovsky B, Wade D, Gahm A, et al. Formation of 50 kbp chromatin fragments in isolated liver nuclei is mediated by protease and endonuclease activation. FEBS Lett 1994;351:150-4.
28. Tomei LD, Shapiro JP, Cope FO. Apoptosis in C3H/1OT1/2 mouse embryonic cells: evidence for internucleosomal DNA modification in the absence of double - stranded cleavage. Proc Natl Acad Sci USA 1993;90:853-7.
29. Igo - Kemenes T, Greil W, Zachau HG. Preparation of soluble chromatin fractions with restriction nucleases. Nucleic Acids Res 1977;4:3387-400.
30. Kyprianou N, Isaacs JT. Activation of programmed cell death in the rat ventral prostate after castration. Endocrinology 1988;122:552-62.
31. Bertrand R, Kohn KW, Solary E, et al. Detection of apoptosis - associated DNA fragmentation using a rapid and quantitative filter elution assay. Drug Dev Res 1995;34:138-44.
32. Solary E, Bertrand R, Jenkins J, et al. Radiolabeling of DNA can induce its fragmentation in HL-60 human promyelocytic leukemic cells. Exp Cell Res 1992;203:495-8.

33. Dusenbury CE, Davis MA, Lawrence TS, et al. Induction of megabase DNA fragments by 5-fluorodeoxyuridine in human colorectal tumor (HT-29) cells. Mol Pharmacol 1991;39:285-9.
34. de Gennes PB. Reptation of a polymer chain in the presence of fixed obstacles. J Chem Phy 1971;55:572-9.
35. Bicknell GR, Cohen GM. Cleavage of DNA to large kilobase pair fragments occurs in some forms of necrosis as well as apoptosis. Biochem Biophys Res Commun 1995;207:40-7.
36. Gavrieli Y, Sherman Y, Ben-Sasson SA. Identification of programmed cell death in situ via specific labeling of nuclear DNA fragmentation. J Cell Biol 1992;119:493-501.
37. Charriaut-Marlangue C, Ben-Ari Y. A cautionary note on the use of the TUNEL stains to determine apoptosis. Neuroreport 1995;7:61-4.
38. Yasuda M, Umemura S, Osamura RY, et al. Apoptotic cells in the human endometrium and placental villi: Pitfalls in applying the TUNEL method. Arch Histol Cytol 1995;58:185-90.
39. Gong J, Traganos F, Darzynkiewicz Z. A selective procedure for DNA extraction from apoptotic cells applicable for gel electrophoresis and flow cytometry. Anal Biochem 1994;218:314-9.
40. O'Brien MC, Bolton WE. Comparison of cell viability probes compatible with fixation and permeabilisation for combined surface and intracellular staining in flow cytometry. Cytometry1995;19:243-55.
41. Zoratti M, Szabo I. The mitochondrial permeability transition. Biochim Biophys Acta 1995;1241:139-76.
42. Koopman G, Reutelingsperger CPM, Kuijten GAM, et al. Annexin V for flow cytometric detection of phosphatidylserine expression on B cells undergoing apoptosis. Blood 1994;84:1415-20.
43. Martin SJ, Reutelingsperger CPM, McGahon AJ, et al. Early redistribution of plasma membrane phosphatidylserine is a general feature of apoptosis regardless of the initiating stimulus: inhibition by overexpression of Bcl-2 and Abl. Exp Med 1995;182:1545-56.
44. Kaltebach JP, Kaltenbach MH, Lyons WB. Nigrosin as a dye for differentiating live and dead ascites cells. Exp Cell Res 1958;15:112-7.
45. Duke RC, Chervenak R, Cohen JJ. Endogenous endonuclease-induced DNA fragmentation: an early event in cell-mediated cytolysis. Proc Natl Acad Sci USA 1983;80:6361-5.
46. Martin DP, Schmidt RE, DiStefano PS, et al. Inhibitors of protein synthesis and RNA synthesis prevent neuronal death caused by nerve growth factor deprivation. J Cell Biol 1988;106:829-44.
47. Fesus L, Thomazy V. Searching for the function of tissue transglutaminase: its possible involvement in the biochemical pathway of programmed cell death. Adv Exp Med Biol 1988;231:119-34.
48. Schwartzman RA, Cidlowski JA. Internucleosomal deoxyribonucleic acid cleavage activity in apoptotic thymocytes: Detection and endocrine regulation. Endocrinology 1991;128:1190-7.
49. Lazebnik YA, Kaufmann SH, Desnoyers S, et al. Cleavage of poly (ADP-ribose) polymerase by a proteinase with properties like ICE. Nature 1994;371:346-47.
50. Enari M, Talanian RV, Wong WW, et al. Sequential activation of ICE-like and CPP32- like proteases during Fas-mediated apoptosis. Nature 1996;380:723-6.
51. Ribble D, Goldstein NB, Norris DA, et al. A simple technique for quantifying apoptosis in 96-well plates. BMC Biotechnol 2005;5:12-7.
52. Blankenberg FG, Storrs RW, Naumovski L, Goralski T, Spielman D. Detection of apoptotic cell death by proton nuclear magnetic resonance spectroscopy. Blood 1996;87:1951–56.
53. Blankenberg FG, Katsikis PD, Storrs RW, et al. Quantitative analysis of apoptotic cell death using proton nuclear magnetic resonance spectroscopy. Blood 1997;89:3778–86.

54. Charles-Edwards EM, deSouza NM. Diffusion-weighted magnetic resonance imaging and its application to cancer. Cancer Imaging 2006;6:135-43.
55. Deng J, Miller FH, Rhee TK, et al. Diffusion-weighted MR imaging for determination of hepatocellular carcinoma response to yttrium-90 radioembolization. J Vasc Interv Radiol 2006;17:1195-200.
56. Chamnanvanakij S, Margraf LR, Burns D, Perlman JM. Apoptosis and white matter injury in preterm infants. Pediatr Dev Pathol 2002;5:184–89.
57. Tunis AS, Czarnota GJ, Giles A, Sherar MD, Hunt JW, Kolios MC. Monitoring structural changes in cells with high frequency ultrasound signal statistics. Ultrasound Med Biol 2005;31:1041–49.

CHAPTER

13

Anticataract Agents

INTRODUCTION

Cataract is the clouding of lens, now considered to be the inevitable consequence of aging and can only be repaired by surgery. Cataract, responsible for 50% or more of blindness globally, remains the leading cause of visual impairment in all regions of world, despite improvements in surgical outcomes.[1-3] More than 28,000 new cases are reported daily worldwide.[4] Several factors like genes, socioeconomic status, illiteracy, malnutrition, diarrhea, diabetes, myopia, renal failure, hypertension, sunlight exposure, smoking, steroids, etc. are responsible for the development of cataract. Out of 38 million blind persons, 8.9 million are in India and 5.12 million are blind due to cataract.[4] The annual incidence of cataract blindness is about 3.8 million. Annually 2.7 million cataract operations are carried out, yet they are not adequate to clear the backlog.[5] During the last two decades, extensive research inputs have been made to delineate the etiology of cataract. Efforts have been directed to delay the onset and slow down the progression of cataract by a variety of agents. These agents have been classified into different categories; their anticataract properties have been evaluated in different experimental models of cataract.

Cataract, a multifactorial disease, occurs mainly due to the formation of large protein aggregates in the lens. Research has shown that post-translational modifications of lens crystallins such as oxidation, glycation, Schiff's base formation, carbamylation, transamidation, phosphorylation and proteolysis lead to clouding of the lens (Fig. 13.1).[6-8]

Drugs effective in modulating the altered metabolism and lens pathology may delay the progression of protein aggregation and opacification. The agents that are claimed to be effective *in vitro* and *in vivo* models of cataract have been classified as aldose reductase inhibitors, non-steroidal anti-inflammatory drugs, calpain inhibitors, antiglycatics, antioxidants of natural/ synthetic origin and a group of miscellaneous agents having different chemical structure. In this chapter, a few commonly used *in vitro* and *in vivo* experimental models are described.

EXPERIMENTAL MODELS OF CATARACT

Experimental models are indispensable tools for the better understanding of physiology and pathogenesis of cataract. Cataractogenesis can be interrupted in experimental models at intervals to study the intermediate structural changes to establish or determine the causative

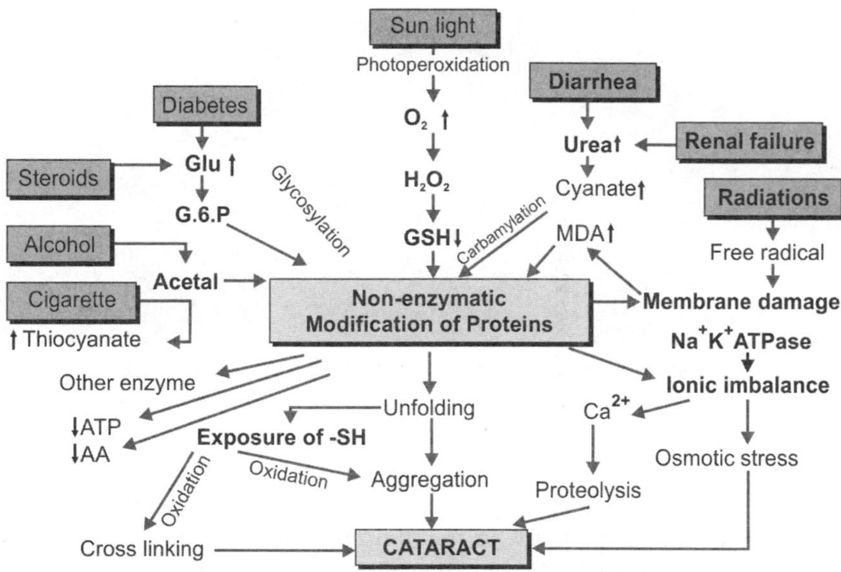

Figure 13.1: Various pathways involved in cataractogenesis

mechanism. Several *in vitro* and *in vivo* models that mimic human senile cataract have been developed indicating crucial targets to intervene and prevent the lens damage. Many of these models however, share few common final steps during the development of cataract.

IN VITRO MODELS

In vitro models include:

- Cell culture
- Organ culture.

Human Lens Epithelial Cell (HLEC) Culture

Most of the studies related to etiology and mechanism of cataract are conducted on animals. In spite of being very closely related to human senile cataract these studies fail to show the exact mechanism. Studies with culture of human lenses are also not possible as enough number of lenses of same age and sex are not easily available. Besides the whole lens is processed for biochemical estimations which results in several fold dilution of the lens epithelial cells. This is the outermost layer and metabolic unit of lens, which is constantly abused by the changing climatic conditions. This layer has various antioxidant enzymes and helps in maintaining the lens homeostasis. Culturing the HLEC makes the studies on etiology and various pathways easier as it offers superior control of physiological environment, accessibility for biochemical monitoring. It is used as a screening model for anticataract agents.[9]

Procedure: Human eyes obtained from the cadaver within 8 h of death are dissected for obtaining the lens epithelium. The anterior capsule with the adhering subcapsular layer of epithelial cells is dissected out and spread on the surface of the culture flask. 4 ml of Dulbecco's

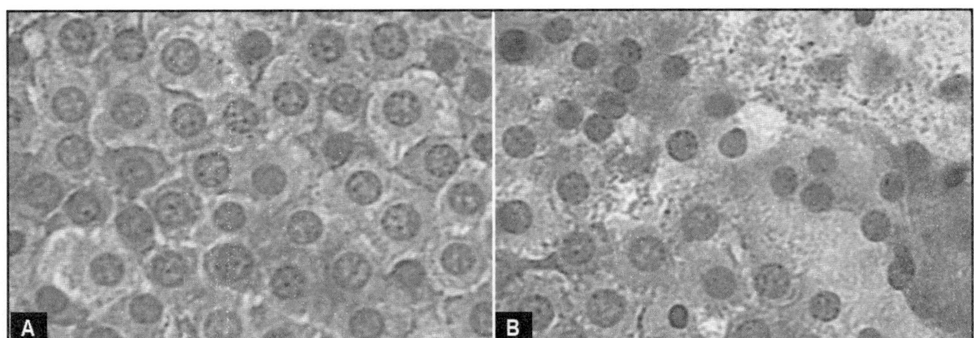

Figure 13.2: Human lens epithelial cells: (A) Normal HLEC cultured in DMEM alone; (B) HLEC cultured in DMEM under oxidative stress (*For color version see Plate 18*)

modified eagle's medium (DMEM), supplemented with 20% fetal calf serum, is added to the flask. The flask is kept in a CO_2 incubator maintaining a temperature of 37°C. The cells are subcultured when they are semiconfluent. To evaluate the potential of anticataract agent the equal number of cells are distributed in different flasks. Cells in one of the flasks are incubated in normal conditions and others are incubated under stress conditions generated by addition of oxidants in the medium. The anticataract agent is added to one of the flasks containing the stress inducer. As per the requirement of the study incubation period may vary. Following incubation morphological and biochemical variations can be evaluated and compared to test the anticataract potential of the agent (Fig. 13.2).[10,11]

Recently the human lens epithelial cell line SRA01/04 is being used for studying various pathways and drug targets involved in opacification of lens.[12] Studies using human lens epithelial cell line have shown that the epithelial mesenchymal transition (EMT) plays a key role in anterior subcapsular cataract (ASC) and posterior capsular opacification (PCO).[13,14] The Jagged/Notch pathway has been reported to be essential in EMT during embryonic development, fibrotic diseases and cancer metastasis. However, the function of Jagged/Notch signaling in LEC EMT is unknown. With the hypothesis that crosstalk between Notch and TGFβ2 signaling could induce EMT in LECs, the studies were conducted and it was shown that inhibition of the Jagged/Notch signaling may have therapeutic value in the prevention and treatment of ASC and PCO.

Human Capsular Bag Model

Posterior capsular opacification is a common complication of cataract surgery. PCO develops a secondary loss of vision in significant number of patients.[15] Modern cataract surgery generates a capsular bag, which consists of a portion of the anterior capsule and the entire posterior capsule. The capsular bag remains *in situ* separating the aqueous and vitreous humors, and, in most cases, houses an IOL. Some of the epithelial cells in spite of the trauma of the surgery remain in the anterior capsule and grow and reach the IOL surface occupy regions of the outer anterior capsule, and colonize the previously cell-free posterior capsule. These cells can finally reach to visual axis hampering the vision if the changes to the matrix and cell organization are severe. This may lead to the need of corrective laser surgery.[16-18] Studies have reported that the rate of PCO can be reduced by improving the design of IOL. These IOLs are manufactured using various range of materials and can affect the progression of PCO because of their contact with the capsule, creating a barrier effect.[19] The IOL designs were tested in rabbit models because of the similarities in lens size, however, the response of injury was more severe in rabbits. Development of human capsular bag model to test the new IOL designs is a valuable tool and reduces the use of animals.

Method: The method for preparing the human capsular bag is an adaptation of the method earlier described by Liu et al.[20] Whole donor eyes are used after ethics committee approval for performing sham cataract surgery with anterior capsulorhexis, nucleus hydroexpression and aspiration of lens fibers.

Sham cataract surgery is done in a laminar flow hood on whole donor eyes obtained within 48 hours of death. The lenses are washed briefly with EMEM. A small rhexis in the anterior surface of the lens capsule is created and central fibrous mass from donor globes is removed. The capsular bag thus obtained can house an IOL when needed. The capsular bag containing an IOL is subsequently removed from the eye separating the zonules with utmost care. It is then transferred to a tissue culture dish with anterior side facing down for better physical interaction between the IOL and capsule. The bag is secured to the dish with entomological pins and maintained in EMEM supplemented with 2% human serum, 10 ng/ml TGF-β_2, and 50 µg/ml gentamicin (Sigma) for a period of four weeks. In the partner capsular bag, no IOL was implanted. Capsular bags are compared using phase-microscopy, immunocytochemistry with fluorescence microscopy.[15, 21, 22]

Organ Culture

Induction of cataract in isolated animal lenses maintained in organ culture has become a convenient, quick and appropriate method for testing the anticataract efficacy of an agent. Opacification of lens is induced by generating oxidative stress/hyperglycemic/hypergalactosemic conditions around the lens by supplementing the culture medium with a variety of exogenous substances.[23, 24]

In general enucleated animal lenses are individually maintained in 2 ml of physiologically competent tissue culture medium (TC-199/MEM) supplemented with 10% fetal calf serum at 37°C and 5% CO_2 atmosphere in a 24 well Falcon plate. The lenses are incubated for 2 to 16 hours prior to the initiation of the cataractogenic insult. Opaque lenses, if any, damaged during the extraction procedure are discarded. Supplementing the medium with different agents causing oxidation of lens proteins/lipids directly/indirectly induces cataractogenesis. Lenses incubated in high sugar containing medium mimic sugar cataract. To carry out the anti-cataract screening process, transparent lenses are divided into different groups as per the requirement of the study. Few lenses are incubated in the plain culture medium, representing normal group and few in culture medium supplemented with stress inducing agent to serve as control. Efficacy of test drug is evaluated by maintaining treated groups, the medium of which as the control is additionally supplemented with different concentration of test drug. Some lenses are also incubated in culture medium containing only the test drug. Lenses belonging to these four groups are further incubated for the period varying from 24 to 72 h depending upon the experimental conditions. Morphological changes and the changes in various biochemical parameters occurring in the different groups are compared to evaluate the efficacy of the test drug. Morphological changes in terms of opacity are categorized as faint peripheral, cortical, dense cortical or nuclear opacities. The biochemical parameters include levels of glutathione (GSH), malondialdehyde (MDA), polyol and enzyme activities such as aldose reductase, sodium potassium ATPase, superoxide dismutase (SOD), catalase (CAT), glutathione peroxidase (GSHPx) and glutathione S-transferase (GST), etc.

Oxidative Stress-induced Experimental Cataract

Oxidative mechanisms play an important role in many biological phenomena including cataract formation. Formation of the superoxide radical in the aqueous humor, lens and its derivatization to other potent oxidants may be responsible for initiating various toxic biochemical reactions leading to the formation of cataract (Fig. 13.3). *In vitro,* such cataracts are induced by agents like selenium, H_2O_2, photosensitizers and enzyme xanthase oxidase. Lenses exposed to 100% oxygen showed optical and structural changes.[25]

Selenite-induced Cataract

Selenium, an essential nutrient but a hazardous element, plays a critical role in maintaining the normal physiological conditions of lens. Selenite-induced cataract models have been used to quantify and characterize events that occur in the lens prior to the formation of nuclear cataract. The critical sulfhydryl (SH) group on Ca^2+ ATPase is oxidized by selenium and opens ion channels in the lens epithelial membrane allowing the influx of calcium from the aqueous humor. Elevated calcium levels activate calpain, a cytosolic calcium activated protease, by autolysis, thereby exposing a buried sulphydryl group in the active site of calpain. Elevated calcium ions translocate calpain to the plasma membrane where phospholipids lower the calcium activation requirement for calpain. The membrane provide localization site for hydrolysis of substrates. High levels of activated cytosolic calpain are also available for proteolysis. The N-terminal extensions on soluble β-crystallin dimer (βL) are cleaved by calpain.

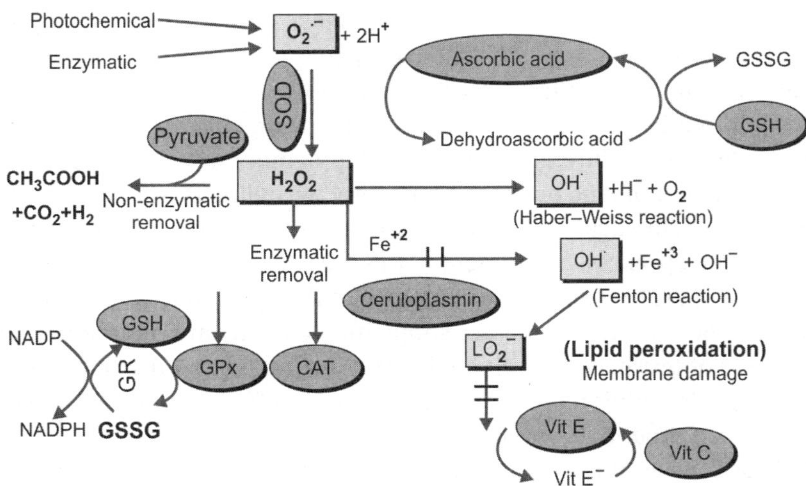

Figure 13.3: Free radical generation in the eye and endogenous defense

This probably exposes charge groups on the βL that interacts to form insoluble aggregates. Hydrophobic interactions may also occur. Hydrolysis of cytoskeleton and membrane proteins by calpain causes further leaking and cell disruption that finally leads to light scattering and opacity.[26,27] Selenium has been used to induce opacity both in isolated lenses and in young rats employing various dosage form and routes of application.[27-29]

Procedure: *In vitro* cataract is produced by supplementing the tissue culture medium with 25 to 100 μM sodium selenite in which freshly enucleated transparent rat lenses are incubated at 37°C. This causes membrane damage and faint cortical opacities within 24 h.

Photochemically-induced Cataract

Photochemically induced oxidative insult is reported by Spector et al.[30] Riboflavin, a photosensitizer is supplemented in the culture medium to induce cataract in cultured lenses. Micro quantities (4-200 μM) of riboflavin lead to severe physiological damage and opacification within 24 h after exposure to light. The initial membrane damage is evidenced by a disturbed cation ratio between lens water and the medium of incubation. Riboflavin on getting photosensitized generates free radicals in a sequence of reactions.

Procedure: Lenses are maintained in organ culture for 24 to 72 h as described earlier. The lenses are divided into four groups and incubated in the dark and light both in presence and absence of riboflavin. The lenses are exposed to light with two 15-W day light fluorescent lamp placed at 8 inches above the cluster plate. The culture medium is replaced every 24 h. Riboflavin shows no effect on the lens in the absence of light, and light without riboflavin has no significant effect. Opacification starts in the equatorial zone and gradually extends towards the center of the lens.[31]

Enzymatically-induced Cataract

Supplementation of culture medium with 1 mM xanthine and 0.1 unit of xanthine oxidase, which acts as substrate and enzyme respectively, leads to generation of superoxide radical. The lenses suffer severe oxidative damage and turn opaque within 24 h when incubated in culture medium at 37°C.[23]

Hydrogen Peroxide-induced Cataract

Incubation of lenses in medium, containing 50-500 μM H_2O_2, produces cataract. Opacification starts in the equatorial region within 24 h. The entire superficial cortex becomes opaque by 96 h. Due to the high instability of H_2O_2 the medium is changed every 2 h during the first eight hours.[31,32]

Sugar-induced Cataract

Diabetes is one of the most important risk factors of cataract. Enzyme aldose reductase (AR) has been implicated to play a pivotal role in sugar cataract formation. AR acts on the sugars like glucose, galactose and xylose and converts them into their respective alcohols. These alcohols (polyols) are not directly involved in the cataractogenic mechanism. If they are found within the lens they accumulate to high levels and produce osmotic effects. Since polyols are not capable of diffusing out easily from the lens nor metabolize rapidly, they accumulate in lens causing hypertonicity. Increase in intralenticular tonicity draws water into the lens fibers causing them to swell. Sugar cataracts have been produced in enucleated lenses *in vitro*.[33,34]

Procedure: Transparent and undamaged lenses are incubated in a basic culture medium with fetal calf serum for 24 to 48 h. The experimental groups are formed as described earlier. In the control group the medium is supplemented with glucose (30 mM), galactose (30 mM) or xylose (20 mM). Lenses develop opacity in the subcapsular region on day 1 and in the central region on day 2. Biochemical analyses reveal raised polyol, malondialdehyde levels and water content, and decreased glutathione levels in these lenses.

Steroid-induced Cataract

Steroid induced experimental cataract is produced *in vitro* by incubating the transparent lenses in the medium containing methyl prednisolone (1.5 mg/ml). To screen anticataract effect of any agent different experimental groups are formed as described earlier. The test agent and methyl prednisolone added alone and together to the medium form drug control, control and treated groups respectively. Early cataract around the equator is produced within 24 h of incubation. Incubation period may be extended to 48 h for dense opacity.[35] Morphological changes and modulation in biochemical parameters between the groups may show the potential of the anticataract agent.

Naphthalene-induced Cataract

Naphthalene is insoluble in the culture medium hence naphthalene metabolites are used for *in vitro* studies of which naphthalene dihydrodiol shows similar morphological and biochemical effect on the cultured lenses as observed in naphthalene fed rats.[36]

Procedure: TC-199 medium modified by Zigler and Hess is used for the pre incubation of lens.[37] Stock solution of naphthalene dihydrodiol is prepared in 20% ethanol at 2.5×10^{-3} M concentration. The stock solution is diluted 1:100 to obtain the final concentration of 2.5×10^{-5} M. The final osmolarity of the solution is 295-300 mOsmol. Rat lenses are incubated in TC-199 medium containing naphthalene metabolite solution. Medium is renewed daily till 72 h. Lenses remain clear during the initial 24 h but form shell like opacity around the nucleus by 48 h. Opacification becomes more peripheral and widespread after 72 h. At 48 h, under such conditions of incubation, development of opacity mimics the *in vivo* naphthalene cataract.[36]

Ca^{++}-induced Cataract

Human and animal cataract lenses contain higher levels of calcium than normal lenses. The homeostasis of ions such as Na^+ and K^+ is affected by the abnormal calcium metabolism. Influx of calcium into the lens activates cysteine proteinase, calpain I and II, which in turn degrades cytoskeleton components and the lens crystallins and eventually causes crystalline aggregation resulting in cataract formation.[38, 39]

Procedure: In this model the control group contains the lenses incubated in the medium enriched with 20 mM Ca^{2+} or 1×10^{-2}mM A23187 calcium ionophore. The treatment group lenses are cultured in the calcium and the test drug-containing medium. Incubation period can range from 24-72 h. Light scattering intensities can be compared as described by Siew and Bettelheim.[40]

Ultraviolet-induced Cataract

Epidemiological studies have shown a link between exposure to UV-B radiation in sunlight and development of cataract. Experimental studies confirm that ultraviolet radiation (UVR) induces cataract. Ultraviolet (UV) light damages the lens by increasing free radicals. Choh et al tested the antioxidant property of a Chinese herb goji berry using *in vitro* model.[41]

Procedure: Bovine lenses are dissected and cultured for 24 hours in the culture medium. Lenses are placed in the medium with or without test drug, then placed into an incubation chamber equipped with UVB light (2.0 J/cm^2) for two hours. Control lenses are placed in lightproof cardboard boxes before being added to the UV irradiation chamber. Optical quality is assessed using a scanning laser monitor. Lenses are scanned prior to UV-irradiation (baseline) and at different intervals post radiation for a period of two weeks. The absorbance of the culture medium with and without test drug is determined at 280- 320 nm UV range.

IN VIVO MODELS

Several animal models of cataract are established for the screening of anticataract agents. These models include sugar, oxidative stress, radiation-induced cataract, etc.

Sugar Cataract Models

Sugar cataract is produced in rats by feeding them high sugar diet such as galactose[28,42,43] or impairing their insulin production using agents like streptozotocin or alloxan. Albino rats (Wistar/Sprague Dawley) are used to evaluate the mechanism of diabetes related cataractogenesis in animals. The eyes of the rats are first examined through a slit lamp to see any abnormality in lens or cornea and if found the rats are discarded. The rats are grouped with a comparable weight distribution. The commonly used sugar cataract models are described below.

Galactose-induced Cataract

Rats of either sex, weighing 50 to 60 g are fed 30% galactose in diet. Diet and water are given ad libitum. The rats are divided into two groups, control and treated. The test agent is administered orally or topically in the treatment group. The eyes of the rats are examined weekly by using a slit lamp to see the cataractogenic changes. The vacuoles start appearing at the periphery of the lens within a week's period, which may be attributed to globular degeneration of the fiber cells. The vacuoles gradually increase in number and size as they extend towards the centre. This takes about 14 days. All these changes are not visible through unaided eye. During the third week opalescence of the lens is visible and it becomes totally opaque in 30 days time (Fig. 13.4). Different stages of cataract are graded as given below.[44]

- Stage 0 — Lenses similar to normal lenses
- Stage I — Lenses showing faint peripheral opacity
- Stage II — Irregular peripheral opacity with slight involvement of the lens in the center

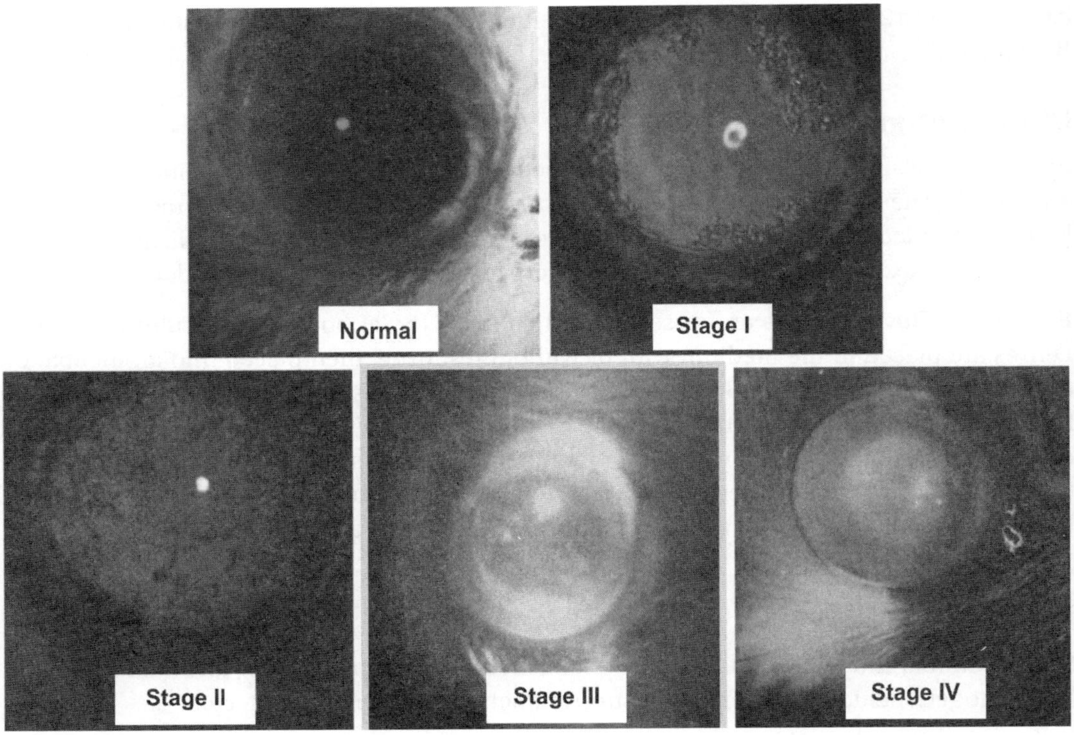

Figure 13.4: Slit lamp photographs of various stages of galactose-induced cataract in rats. Normal: Clear transparent lens; Stage I: Peripheral vacuoles in the lens; Stage II: Vacuoles involving the center of the lens; Stage III: Faint opalescence visible with the naked eye; Stage IV: Mature nuclear cataract. [Reprinted from Nutrition, Vol. 19(9), Suresh Kumar Gupta, Deepa Trivedi, Sushma Srivastava, Sujata Joshi, Nabanita Halder and Shambhu Dayal Verma. 'Lycopene attenuates oxidative stress induced experimental cataract development: An *in vitro* and *in vivo* study', pp 794-9, 2003, with permission from Elsevier] *(For color version see Plate 19)*

- Stage III — Faint opalescence visible with the naked eye
- Stage IV — Mature nuclear cataract
- Stage V — Opacity involving entire lens.

Morphological changes in the lens are compared in all the groups to evaluate the efficacy of the drug. Biochemical changes in lens related to galactose cataract may also be measured at different stages of opacification to support the findings.

A dog model of cataract has also been reported by Sato et al.[45] Nine-month-old beagles are fed a daily diet of 450 g of standard chow containing 30% galactose for 9 months. The dogs developed cataract in 39 months.

Alloxan-induced Cataract

Alloxan is a cyclic urea analog, which produces permanent diabetes in laboratory animals. According to one of the mechanisms proposed it is a highly reactive molecule that is readily reduced to dialuric acid, which is then auto oxidized back to alloxan resulting in the production of H_2O_2, O_2, O_2^-, and hydroxy radical. *In vivo* administration of alloxan induces DNA strand breaks in isolated islets and in islets. However, the other mechanism reveals the ability of alloxan to react with protein sulfhydryl groups on hexokinase, a signal recognition enzyme in the pancreatic β-cell that couples changes in the blood glucose concentration to the rate of insulin secretion. By this mechanism, inhibition of glucokinase and other SH-containing membrane proteins on the β-cell would eventually result in cell necrosis within minutes.

Procedure: Rats of Wistar/Sprague Dawley strain weighing 150 to 200 g are given subcutaneous injection of alloxan @ 100 to 175 mg/kg body weight. After approximately 12 weeks cataractous changes are observed. Alloxan-induced cataract can also be produced in rabbits (2.0 to 3.5 kg) by infusing 150 mg/kg alloxan monohydrate in the ear vein. Morphological examinations of lens of all the animals in age matched normal, control and treated groups for the presence of opacity helps in evaluating the efficacy of the drug.[46-48]

Streptozotocin Cataract

Diabetes related cataractogenic changes are seen in the animals injected with STZ.[49-51] The chemical structure of streptozotocin (STZ) has a glucose molecule with a highly reactive nitrosourea side chain, which supposedly initiates its cytotoxic action. The glucose moiety directs this agent to the pancreatic β-cells. There it binds to the membrane receptor to generate structural damage. At the intracellular level three major phenomena are responsible for β-cell death (i) process of methylation, (ii) frees radical generation and (iii) nitric oxide (NO) production. The damage caused to β-cells alters the sugar metabolism leading to diabetes.

Induction of cataract: Albino rats (Wistar/Sprague Dawley) of 150 to 200 g body weight are used. Diabetes is induced by intraperitoneal injection of streptozotocin 50 to 70 mg/kg body weight. Care should be taken not to puncture the intestine. Streptozotocin is dissolved in 0.02 M sodium citrate buffer. The solution is filtered through a 0.22 μM Millipore filter into a sterilized container placed on ice. The sterile solution thus prepared is used within 10 minutes of preparation. The nondiabetic rats are injected with sterilized buffer alone. Blood glucose levels of each rat are estimated after 3 days. STZ injected rats having blood glucose level <150 mg/dl are reinjected with fresh solution of STZ and tested again for blood glucose.[50] Progression of cataract stages is observed through a slit lamp. The initiation of cataract occurs 15 days after STZ injection. The sutures become prominent and the fully mature cataract appears nearly in 110 days depending upon the age of the rat at the time of injection. The cataractogenic changes can be compared with the age matched buffer injected control rats.

Hegde and Varma (2005) preferred mice to rats for streptozotocin cataract induction because of the reported similarity between the lenses of the mice and humans in respect of AR deficiency and the similarity in morphological changes. They induced cataract in mice by injecting streptozotocin intraperitoneally. Morphological changes similar to those in humans such as shrinkage, elongation, lobulization of the nuclei of the lens epithelial cells were observed.[51]

Care of diabetic rats: Diarrhea often occurs in diabetic rats and they drink large amount of water and produce high urine volume. Bedding is changed frequently to keep the rats dry. The rats should be kept dry or else there is a risk of loosing body heat. Diabetic rats should be provided with plenty of water.

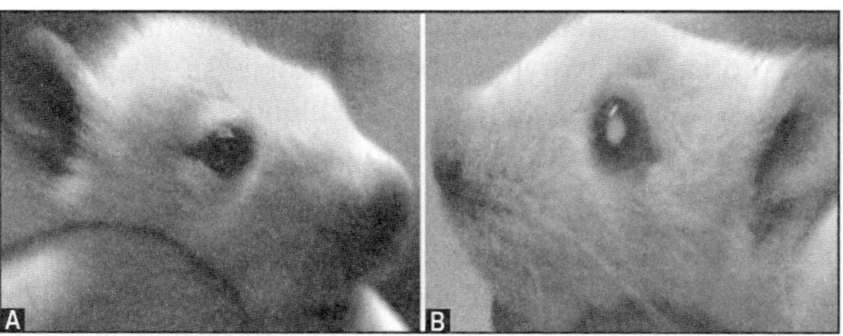

Figure 13.5: Selenite-induced cataract in rat pups: (A) 16-day-old rat pup showing normal eye with clear lens; (B) Rat pup of the same litter injected subcutaneously with sodium selenite showing nuclear cataract (*For color version see Plate 19*)

Selenite-induced Cataract

Selenite cataract is the most reliable and reproducible experimental model for initial screening of potential anti-cataract agents. Selenite cataract resembles human cataract in many ways such as vesicle formation, increased calcium, insoluble protein, decreased water-soluble proteins and reduced glutathione (GSH), etc. However, selenite cataract shows no high molecular weight protein aggregation or increased disulfide formation and is dominated by rapid calpain-induced proteolytic precipitation while senile cataracts may be produced by prolonged oxidative stress.[23,24]

Induction of cataract: Selenite nuclear cataract is usually produced in neonatal albino rats (10 to 14 days) by a single subcutaneous injection of 19 to 30 µmoles/kg body weight of sodium selenite (Na_2SeO_3).[26,27,52-54] Young rats are housed together with their mother. Mother is fed normal diet and water ad libitumand and she suckles the pups. The young rats of same age are grouped into three. One group is left as normal group. Rest of the two groups, control and treated, are given subcutaneous injections of sodium selenite in the scruff of the neck/ abdomen of young rat. Treatment group is given the anticataract agent intraperitoneally four hours prior to the sodium selenite administration. On the 16th day when the eyes of the young rats first open severe bilateral nuclear cataracts are seen (Fig. 13.5). The eyes of the treated group can be compared with the control group to evaluate the efficacy of the drug.[28,52]

Repeated injections of smaller doses of selenite[29] or oral administration are also cataractogenic.[55]

Naphthalene Cataract

Naphthalene cataract model is thought to be a good model for human age related cataract. Van Heyningen and Pirie[56] studied naphthalene cataract in rabbits and proposed the following metabolic pathway. The injected naphthalene is oxidized in the liver first to an epoxide and then is converted into naphthalene dihydrodiol. This stable compound on reaching the eye gets converted enzymatically to dihydroxynaphthalene. Being unstable at physiological pH, 1,2-dihydroxynaphthalene spontaneously autoxidises to 1,2 naphthoquinone and H_2O_2. Rees and Pirie[57] provided further evidence that 1,2 naphthoquinone is a highly reactive compound. It alkylates proteins, glutathione and amino acids, and generates free radicals.

Induction procedure: Albino male rats (125 to 150 g) are used for this model. Naphthalene solution (10%) is prepared in mineral oil by heating at 60°C for 30 min. The rats are dosed with this solution with an 18-gauge needle at 0.5 g per kg per day for three days and 1.0 g per kg per day thereafter. A group of rats is administered with same amount of mineral oil to serve as controls. The drug treatment is given orally by gavage one hour prior to naphthalene administration. Morphological changes in the eyes of the rats are observed through slit lamp examination after dilating the pupil. The lenses are examined and graded twice a week during the first two weeks and thereafter at weekly interval. One week after the administration spoke like opacities in the cortex is seen. By the third week in the deep cortex region an opaque shell is visible which becomes denser and slightly deeper with time.[36]

Hyperbaric Oxygen-induced Cataract

Hyperbaric oxygen (HBO) has been shown to produce cataract in rabbits[58] and guinea pigs.[59-61] Old guinea pigs of 17-18 months age are subjected to 2.5% atmospheres of 100% oxygen for 2.5 h three times per week on alternate days till seven months. This induces high molecular weight aggregate formation in the nucleus resulting in increased nuclear light scattering.

Glucocorticoid-induced Cataract in Developing Chick Embryo

Steroid cataract is reviewed by Urban and Cotlier.[62] Formation of steroid-adduct protein, induction of transglutaminase and reduction of ATPase activity may lead to cataract. Nishigori et al. (1987)[63] suggested that steroid cataract are produced by the activities of glucocorticoids and progressed by way of production of oxidative stress similar to other types of cataract.

Induction of cataract: Fertile white Leghorn eggs are incubated in an incubator at 35.5°C and 68% relative humidity. The onset day of incubation is called day 1. To 15-day-old embryos, hydrocortisone succinate sodium (HC; 0.25 μmol in 0.2 ml sterilized water) is administered through a small hole in the eggshell over the air sac. The puncture is sealed with a cellophane tape and the eggs are incubated for 48 h. Anticataract agent is applied in the same way as HC. For the control embryos same quantity of sterilized water is administered. Lenses are removed from the chick embryo after 48 h of HC administration and the severity of opacity is visually classified according to Nishigori et al. (1983).[64]

L-Buthionine –S, R-Sulfoximine (BSO)-induced Cataract

Glutathione is present in mammalian lens in high concentrations and is involved in the protection of lens against oxidation. In most of the cataracts the decrease in its level is observed.

BSO, a specific inhibitor of GSH, generates cataract in suckling mice when repeatedly injected. Four subcutaneous injections of BSO are administered per day to the mouse pups on postnatal days 7 and 8 at intervals of 2.5 h. The dosage of each injection is 4 μmol per gram body weight (20 ml g^{-1} of a 0.2 M solution of BSO prepared in 0.10 M NaCl). Initiation of opacification occurs on day nine, i.e. within 24 h. The progression of the cataract in 24 h is divided into four stages (i) developing floriform, (ii) mature floriform, (iii) degenerate floriform and (iv) amorphous translucent cataract. Dense cortico-nuclear opacities develop within several days.[65]

N-Methyl-N- Nitrosourea-induced Cataract

Cataract is induced by a single intraperitoneal injection of 100 mg/kg N-methyl-N-nitroso urea (MNU) in 0, 5, 10, 15, or 20-day-old male and female Sprague Dawley rats. In 0, 5, 10 and 15 day old MNU–treated rats, mature cataract develops at 7, 14, 19 and 30 days respectively after dosing. In 20-day-old MNU-treated rats, only subcapsular cataract has been seen 30 days after dosing. Therefore the rats exposed to MNU at an earlier age develop cataract more rapidly and severely. The pathogenesis of MNU-induced cataract is associated with DNA adducts formation in the lens epithelial cell nuclei leading to apoptosis by up regulation of Bax protein, down regulation of BCl-2 protein and activation of caspases-3.[66,67]

Women have a high incidence of cataract and epidemiological data suggests that the increased risk may be caused by a lack of estrogen in postmenopausal year. Effect of estrogen on MNU-induced cataractogenesis is very well documented and serves as a good model for age-related cataractogenesis.

Transforming Growth Factor β (TGF-β)-induced Cataract

Hales, et al produced experimental cataract in nine months old Wistar rats by injecting approximately 60 ng TGF-β into the vitreous.[69] TGF-β stimulates lens epithelial cells to undergo aberrant morphologic and molecular changes that mimic the changes observed in human posterior subcapsular and cortical cataract.

Smoke-induced Cataract

Avunduk et al. induced cataract in Wistar rats by cigarette smoke.[70] Cigarette smoke contains trace and heavy metals.[71,72] The increased metal contents in lens causes lens damage by the mechanism of oxidative stress forming oxygen radicals via metal catalyzed Fenton reaction.[73] In other words cigarette smoke-induced cataractogenesis is associated with the accumulation of iron and calcium in the rat lens.

Procedure: Male Wistar rats of 200 to 350 g weight range are equally divided into control and test groups. The rats are fed with standard rat chow and water ad libitum. The test group rats are exposed to cigarette smoke for 2 h/day continuously for 60 days using an exposure system as described by Chen et al.[74] Control rats are exposed to room air in identical chambers. Morphological and histological changes between the groups are compared; elemental concentration of the lenses of both experimental and control rats can be measured and compared.

UV-induced Cataract

In vivo studies have been conducted to show the effect of UV radiations on eye. There is, however, a lack of data on the age dependence in experimental UVR cataract.

Procedure: Anesthetized albino rats are exposed *in vivo* to UV-B radiation. The UVR source is a mercury lamp with water filter and a double monochromator set to 300 nm and 9 nm full bandwidth at half maximum. The dose ranges between 0.1 and 20 kJ/m^2. The exposure time is 15 minutes. One eye in each rat is irradiated. Before the irradiation the rats receive pupil-dilating eye drops. The animals are kept between 6 h and 32 weeks after exposure. The extracted lenses are photographed. The UVR-induced cataract is produced after one week of the exposure. One or eight weeks after exposure the forward light scattering in the lenses is determined. The lens is placed in a cuvette filled with salt solution. The probing light from the dark-field illumination will in the case of a perfectly transparent lens pass through the lens and not reach the photo detector. If there are scattering centers in the lens, the probing light will scatter and reach the photo detector.[75]

Gamma Rays-induced Cataract

Karslioglu et al.[76] irradiated rats with gamma rays using Cobalt-60 teletherapy unit with a single dose of 5 Gy. Cataract was graded according to Chylack's classification.[77]

Microwave-induced Cataract

Microwave radiation has been reported to produce posterior subcapsular and cortical cataracts in rabbits and dogs within a short span of time at intensities no more than ten folds above safety limits.[78-81] It is believed that microwave radiation have primarily heating effect therefore, there is no need of long-term dosing. Foster, et al conducted single dose experiments in rabbits.[78]

Thermal Cataract

Kramer et al. have produced cataract in rabbits. They circulated hot water intraocularly and maintained the retrolental temperature in the range of 43 to 45°C. Biomicroscopic and light microscopic examination revealed changes similar to microwave-induced cataract. This supports the assumption that microwave-induced cataractogenesis is due to the local production of elevated temperature.[82]

Mechanical Stimulation and Cataract

Mechanical stimulation in the eyes of rabbits (*in vivo*) and in isolated rat lenses (*in vitro*) resulted in high frequency opacification of the lens. The rabbit eyes and the isolated lenses were given vibration from an electric massage machine and tapping. The opacity thus produced was in anterior or posterior subcapsular region.[83]

Hereditary Cataract Model

Hereditary cataract models have been described in many species such as rat, guinea pig, dog, sheep, cattle and birds. Spontaneous hereditary cataract models of dominant trait are found in mouse, such as cataract Fraser mice.[84-86] These models are useful in understanding the physiology of eye lens and the pathogenesis of cataracts. Hereditary dominant cataracts are induced by irradiation or by a chemical mutagen. Representative spontaneous hereditary recessive mutations are Nakano cataract mouse and Deer mouse.[87,88]

Kolosova et al. 2003 have suggested that senescence accelerated OXYS rat strain develop cataract spontaneously with progressive macular degeneration, lenticular changes correspond to human senile cataract.[89]. Deletion of GPR 48 can cause age-related cataracts by decreasing the resistance of lens epithelial cells to oxidative stress, which may be related to altered expression of several antioxidant defense enzymes.[90]

CONCLUSION

The efficacy of an anticataract agent can be tested in the above-mentioned models. The galactose, streptozotocin and alloxan induced models mimic sugar cataracts in humans and are used for evaluating aldose reductase inhibitors. Galactose fed rat model is a popular model as it is easily produced than streptozotocin and alloxan induced models. The rate of mortality is high in streptozotocin and alloxan induced models. The utmost care of the animals has to be taken. Among the models described above selenite model is the widely accepted model for the screening of anticataract agents. It is reproduced easily within a short span of time. It resembles the age-related cataract in humans. Though naphthalene cataract model resembles human cataract still it is not preferred as the rate of mortality is high and reproducibility is less. Hereditary mouse models are more suitable to understand the mechanism of cataractogenesis, however, the cost and maintenance of these mice is high.

REFERENCES

1. WHO. Global data on Visual impairments 2010. WHO/NMH/PBD/12.01, 2012.
2. http://www.iapb.org/vision-2020/global-facts.
3. WHO. Prevention of avoidable blindness and visual impairment. Provisional agenda item 4.9. EB117/35, 117th Session 22 December 2005.
4. Sasikumar S, Mohamed N, Saikumar SJ. Cataract surgical: coverage in Kolenchery, Kerala, India. J Com Eye Health 1998;11:7.
5. Kyselova Z, Stefek M, Bauer V. Pharmacological prevention of diabetic cataract. J Diabetes Complications 2004;18:129-40.
6. Kinoshita JH. Mechanism initiating cataract formation. Invest Ophthalmol 1974;13:713-24.
7. Harding JJ, Rixon KC. Carbamylation of lens proteins: a possible factor in cataractogenesis in some tropical countries. Exp Eye Res 1980;31:567-71.
8. Jernigan HM Jr. Role of hydrogen peroxide in riboflavin sensitized photodynamic damage to cultured rat lenses. Exp Eye Res 1985;41:121-9.
9. Arita T, Lin LR, Reddy VN. Differentiation of human lens epithelial cells in tissue culture. Exp Eye Res 1988;47:905-10.
10. Mohanty I, Joshi S, Trivedi D, et al. Lycopene prevents sugar induced morphological changes and modulates antioxidant status of human lens epithelial cells. Br J Nutrition 2002;88:347-54.
11. Mohanty I, Joshi S, Trivedi D, et al. Pyruvate modulates antioxidant status of cultured human lens epithelial cells under hypergalactosemic conditions. Mol Cell Biochem 2002;238:129-35.
12. Huang S, Liu X, Wu M, Luo L, Liu Z, Zhu L, et al. Inhibition of α-tubulin deacetylase prevents the migration of lens epithelial cells without affecting cell cycle progression. Invest Ophthalmol Vis Sci 2014;55: E-Abstract 1220.
13. Chen X, Ye S, Xiao W, Wang W, Luo L, Liu Y. ERK1/2 pathway mediates epithelial-mesenchymal transition by cross-interacting with TGFβ/Smad and Jagged/Notch signaling pathways in lens epithelial cells. Int J Mol Med. 2014 Jun;33(6):1664-70. doi: 10.3892/ijmm.2014.1723. Epub 2014 Apr 4.
14. Chen X, Xiao W, Ye S , Liu Y. The Jagged/Notch pathway is involved in TGFβ2-mediated epithelial-mesenchymal transition of human lens epithelial cells and rat anterior subcapsular cataract. Invest Ophthalmol Vis Sci 2014;55: E-Abstract 1219.

15. Dawes LJ, Illingworth CD, Wormstone IM. A fully human in vitro capsular bag model to permit intraocular lens evaluation. Invest Ophthalmol Vis Sci. 2012 Jan 3;53(1):23-9. doi: 10.1167/iovs.11-8851.
16. Wormstone IM. Posterior capsule opacification: A cell biological perspective. Exp Eye Res 2002;74:337-47.
17. Moisseiev J, Bartov E, Schochat A, Blumenthal M. Long-term study of the prevalence of capsular opacification following extracapsular cataract extraction. J Cataract Refract Surg 1989;15:531–33.
18. Sundelin K, Sjostrand J. Posterior capsule opacification 5 years after extracapsular cataract extraction. J Cataract Refract Surg. 1999;25:246-50.
19. Nishi O, Nishi K, Wickstrom K. Preventing lens epithelial cell migration using intraocular lenses with sharp rectangular edges. J Cataract Refract Surg. 2000;26:1543–49.
20. Liu CS, Wormstone IM, Duncan G, Marcantonio JM, Webb SF,Davies PD. A study of human lens cell growth in vitro: a model for posterior capsule opacification. Invest Ophthalmol Vis Sci 1996;37:906-14.
21. Dawes Lucy J illingworth CD, Wormstone IM. A fully human in vitro capsular bag model to permit intraocular lens evaluation. Invest Ophthalmol Vis Sci 2012;53 (1):23-9.
22. Wertheimer CM, Siedlecki J, Mueller- Bardorff A, Klingenstein A, Laubichler P, Mackert M, et al. EGF-Receptor Inhibitors Erlotinib and Gefitinib mitigate posterior capsule opacification in the human capsular bag model. Invest Ophthalmol Vis Sci 2014;E-Abstract 1221.
23. Varma SD, Morris SM, Bauer SA, et al. In vitro damage to rat lenses by xanthine–xanthine oxidase; protection by ascorbate. Exp Eye Res 1986;43:1067-76.
24. Ohta Y, Torii H, Okada H, et al. Involvement of oxidative stress in D-xylose induced cataractogenesis in cultured rat lenses. Curr Eye Res 1996;15:1-7.
25. Schaal S, Beiran I, Rozner H, Rubinstein I, Chevion M, Miller B, Dovrat A. Desferrioxamine and zinc–desferrioxamine reduce lens oxidative damage. Exp Eye Res 2007;84:561-8.
26. Shearer TR, David LL, Anderson RS. Selenite cataract. a review. Curr Eye Res 1987;6:289-300.
27. Shearer TR, David LL, Anderson RS, et al. Review of selenite cataract. Curr Eye Res 1992;11:357-69.
28. Gupta SK, Trivedi D, Srivastava S, et al. Lycopene attenuates oxidative stress induced experimental cataract development: An in vivo and in vitro study. Nutrition 2003;19:794-9.
29. Huang LL, Zhang CY, Hess JL, et al. Biochemical changes and cataract formation in lenses from rat receiving multiple low doses of sodium selenite. Exp Eye Res 1992;55:671-8.
30. Spector A, Wang GM, Wang RR, et al. A brief photochemically induced oxidative insult causes irreversible lens damage and cataract 1. Transparency and epithelial cell layer. Exp Eye Res 1995;60:471-81.
31. Cui X-L, Lou MF. The effect and recovery of long-term H_2O_2 exposure on lens morphology and biochemistry. Exp Eye Res 1993;57:157-67.
32. Spector A, Wang G-M, Wang R-R, et al. The prevention of cataract caused by oxidative stress in cultured rat lenses. H_2O_2 and photochemically induced cataract. Curr Eye Res 1993;12:163-79.
33. Kinoshita JH, Merola LU, Dikmak E. The accumulation of dulcitol and water in rabbit lens incubated with galactose. Biochim Biophys Acta 1962;62:176-8.
34. Gupta SK, Agnihotri S, Joshi S. Anticataract action of topical sulindac (1 H-indene-3-acetic acid, 5-fluoro-2-methyl-1-[4-(methylsulfinyl)-phenyl] methylene-(z) in galactosemic rats. Afro Asian J Ophthalmol 1989; VIII:57-61.

35. Ohta Y, Okada H, Majima Y, et al. Anticataract action of Vitamin E: Its estimation using an in vitro steroid cataract model. Ophthalmic Res 1996;28:16-25.
36. Xu GT, Zigler JS Jr., Lou MF. Establishment of a naphthalene cataract model in vitro. Exp Eye Res 1992;54:73-81.
37. Zigler JS, Hess HH. Cataracts in the Royal College of Surgeons rat: evidence for initiation by lipid peroxidation products. Exp Eye Res 1985;41:67-76.
38. Adams DR. The role of calcium in selenite cataract. Biochem J 1929;23:902-12.
39. Li WC, Kuszak JR, Wang GM, et al. Calcium-induced lens epithelial cell apoptosis contributes to cataract formation. Exp Eye Res 1995;61:91-8.
40. Siew EL, Bettelheim FA. Light scattering parameters of rat lenses with calcium induced cataracts. Exp Eye Res 1996;62:265-70.
41. Vivian Choh, Christina Ding, Gah-Jone Won, Adriana Richard. Goji berry effects on cataract development in ultraviolet light irradiated bovine lenses. ARVO 2014 Annual Meeting Abstracts, Program Number: 1212 Poster Board Number: C0300 (accessed from: http://www.arvo.org/webs/am2014/abstract/sessions/162.pdf)
42. Raju TN, Kumar CS, Kanth VR, Ramana BV, Reddy PU, Suryanarayana P, et al. Cumulative antioxidant defense against oxidative challenge in galactose-induced cataractogenesis in Wistar rats. Indian J Exp Biol 2006;44:733-9.
43. Huang R, Shi F, Lei T, Song Y, Hughes CL, Liu G. Effect of the isoflavone genistein against galactose-induced cataracts in rats. Exp Biol Med (Maywood) 2007;232:118-25.
44. Sippel TO. Changes in the water, protein and glutathione contents of the lens in the course of galactose cataract development in rats. Invest Ophthalmol 1966;5:568-75.
45. Sato S, Takahashi Y, Wyman M, et al. Progression of sugar cataract in the dog. Invest Ophthalmol Vis Sci 1991;32:1925-31.
46. Ahmad SS, Tsou KC, Ahmad SI, et al. Studies on cataractogenesis in humans and in rats with alloxan-induced diabetes. Cation transport and sodium potassium dependent ATPase. Ophthalmic Res 1985;17:1-11.
47. Vats V, Yadav SP, Biswas NR, Grover JK. Anti-cataract activity of Pterocarpus marsupium bark and Trigonellafoenum-graecum seeds extract in alloxan diabetic rats. J Ethnopharmacol 2004;93:289-94.
48. Hansen PS, Clark RJ, Buhagiar KA, Hamilton E, Garcia A, White C, et al. Alloxan-induced diabetes reduces sarcolemmal Na+-K+ pump function in rabbit ventricular myocytes. Am J Physiol Cell Physiol 2007;292:C1070-7.
49. Rodrigues B, Poucheret P, Battell ML, et al. Streptozotocin-induced diabetes: Induction and mechanism(s) and dose dependency. In: Mc Neill JH (Ed): Experimental Models of Diabetes. Florida: CRC Press LLC 1999:3-17.
50. Blakytny R, JJ Harding. Prevention of cataract in diabetic rats by aspirin, paracetamol (acetaminophen) and ibuprofen. Exp Eye Res 1992;54:509-18.
51. Hegde KR, Varma SD. Cataracts in experimentally diabetic mouse: morphological and apoptotic changes. Diabetes Obes Metab 2005;7:200-4.
52. Gupta SK, Srivastava S, Trivedi D, Joshi S, Halder N. Ocimum sanctum modulates selenite induced cataractogenic changes and prevents rat lens opacification. Cur Eye Res 2005;30:583-91.
53. Doganay S, Borazan M, Iraz M, Cigremis Y. The effect of resveratrol in experimental cataract model formed by sodium selenite. Curr Eye Res 2006;31:147-53.

54. Yagci R, Aydin B, Erdurmus M, Karadag R, Gurel A, Durmus M, et al. Use of melatonin to prevent selenite-induced cataract formation in rat eyes. Curr Eye Res 2006;31:845-50.
55. Shearer TR, Anderson RS, Britton JL. Influence of selenite and fourteen trace elements on cataractogenesis in the rat. Invest Ophthalmol Vis Sci 1983;24:417-23.
56. van Heyningen R, Pirie A. The metabolism of naphthalene and its toxic effect on the eye. Biochem J 1967;102:842-52.
57. Rees JR, Pirie A. Possible reaction of 1, 2-naphthoquinone in the eye. Biochem J 1967;102:853-63.
58. Padgaonkar V, Giblin FJ, Reddy VN. Disulfide cross-linking of urea-insoluble proteins in rabbit lenses treated with hyperbaric oxygen. Exp Eye Res 1989;49:887–99.
59. Padgaonkar VA, Lin LR, Leverenz VR, et al. Hyperbaric oxygen in vivo accelerates the loss of cytoskeletal proteins and MIP26 in guinea pig lens nucleus. Exp Eye Res 1999;68:493-504.
60. Simpanya MF, Ansari RR, Suh KI, Leverenz VR, Giblin FJ. Aggregation of lens crystallins in an in vivo hyperbaric oxygen guinea pig model of nuclear cataract: dynamic light-scattering and HPLC analysis. Invest Ophthalmol Vis Sci 2005;46:4641-51.
61. Giblin FJ, Padgaonkar VA, Leverenz VR, et al. Nuclear light-scattering, disulfide formation and membrane damage in lenses of older guinea pigs treated with hyperbaric oxygen. Exp Eye Res 1995;60:219–235.
62. Urban RC, Cotlier E. Corticosteroid induced cataracts. Survey Ophthalmol 1986;31:102-10.
63. Nishigori H, Lee JW, Yamamuchi Y, et al. Analysis of glucose levels during glucocorticoid-induced cataract formation in chick embryos. Invest Ophthalmol Vis Sci 1987;28:168-74.
64. Nishigori H, Lee JW, Iwatsuru M. An animal model for cataract research: Cataract formation in developing chick embryo by glucocorticoids. Exp Eye Res 1983;36:617-21.
65. Calvin HI, Patel SA, Zhang JP, et al. Progressive modifications of mouse lens crystallins in cataracts induced by buthioninesulfoximine. Exp Eye Res 1992;54:611-9.
66. Kilichi K, Yoshizawa K, Moriguchi K, Tsubura A. Rapid induction of cataract by a single intraperitoneal administration of N. methyl-N-nitrosourea in 15 days old Sprague Dawley rats. Exp Toxicol Path 2002;54:181-6.
67. Yoshizawa K. Oishi Y, Nambu H, Yamamoto D, Yard J, Senzaki H, et al. Cataractogenesis in neonatal Sprague- Dawley rats by N-methyl-N nitrosourea. Toxicol Pathol 2000;28:555-69.
68. Bigsby RM, Cardenas H, Caperell, Grant A, Grubbsc J. Protective effects of estrogen in a rat model of age related cataract.Proc Natl Acad Sci USA 1999;96:9328-32.
69. Hales AM, Chamberlain CG, Dreher B, et al. Intravitreal injection of TGFβ induces cataract in rats. Invest Ophthalmol Vis Sci 1999;40:3231-6.
70. Avunduk AM, Yardimici S, Avunduk MC, et al. Prevention of lens damage associated with cigarette smoke exposure in rats by a-tocopherol (vitamin E) treatment. Invest Ophthalmol Vis Sci 1999;40:537-41.
71. Mussalo-Rauhamaa H, Leppanen A, Salmela SS, et al. Cigarettes as a source of some trace and heavy metals and pesticides in man. Arch Environ Health 1986;41:49-55.
72. Avunduk AM, Yardimici S, Avunduk MC, et al. Determinations of some trace and heavy metals in rat lenses after tobacco smoke exposure and their relationships to lens injury. Exp Eye Res 1997;65:417-23.
73. Varma SD, Chand D, Sharma YR, et al. Oxidative stress on lens and cataract formation; role of light and oxygen. Curr Eye Res 1984;3:35-7.
74. Chen BT, Weber RE, Yeh HC, et al. Deposition of cigarette smoke particles in the rats. Fundam Appl Toxicol 1989;13:429-38 .

75. Michael R. Development and repair of cataract induced by ultraviolet radiation. Ophthalmic Res 2000; 32-S1:1-44.
76. Karslioglu I, Ertekin MV, Kocer I, Taysi S, Sezen O, Gepdiremen A. Protective role of intramuscularly administered vitamin E on the levels of lipid peroxidation and the activities of antioxidant enzymes in the lens of rats made cataractous with gamma-irradiation. Eur J Ophthalmol 2004;14:478-85.
77. Chylack LT Jr, Leske MC, McCarthy D, Khu P, Kashiwagi T, Sperduto R. Lens opacities classification system II (LOCS II). Arch Ophthalmol 1989;107:991-7.
78. Foster MR, Ferri ES, Hagan GJ. Dosimetric study of microwave cataractogenesis. Bioelectromagnetics 1986;7:129-40.
79. Lipman RM, Tripathi BJ, Tripathi RC. Cataracts induced by microwave and ionizing radiation. Survey Ophthalmol 1988;33:200-10.
80. Jose JG, Pitts DG. Wavelength dependency of cataracts in albino mice following chronic exposure. Exp Eye Res 1985;41:545-63.
81. Harding JJ, Crabbe MJC. The lens: development, protein metabolism and cataract. In. Davson H (ed). The Eye, vol. 18. London: Academic Press. 1984:207.
82. Kramár P, Harris C, Guy AW. Thermal cataract formation in rabbits. Bioelectromagnetics 1987;8: 397-406.
83. Oshita M, Goto H, Yamakawa N, Usui M, Uga S. Experimental cataract models produced by repeated blunt mechanical stimulation and elucidation of the pathogenetic mechanism. Nippon Ganka Gakkai Zasshi 2005;109:197-204.
84. Fraser FC, Schabtach G. 'Shriveled': a hereditary degeneration of the lens in the house mouse. Genet Res 1962;3:383-7.
85. Kador PF, Fukui HN, Fukushi S, et al. Philly mouse: a new model of hereditary cataract. Exp Eye Res 1980;30:59-68.
86. Kuck JFR, Kuwabata T, Kuck KD. The emory mouse cataract: an animal model for human senile cataract. Curr Eye Res 1981-82;1:643-9.
87. Nakano K, Yamamoto S, Kutsukake G, et al. Hereditary cataract in mice. Jpn J Clin Ophthalmol 1960;14:1772-6.
88. Burns RP, Feeney L. Hereditary cataract in Deer mice (Peromyscus maniculatus). Am J Ophthalmol 1975;80:370-8.
89. Kolosova NG, Lebedev PA, FursovaAzh, Moroskova TS, Gusarevich OG. Prematurely aging OXYS rats as an animal model of senile cataract in human. Adv Gerontol 2003;12:143-8.
90. Qiang Hou, Jun Zhu, Lili Tu. Targeted deletion of the murine GPR48 gene decreases lens epithelial cells resistance to oxidative stress and induces age-related cataract formation. ARVO 2014 Annual Meeting Abstracts, Program Number: 1206 Poster Board Number: C0294 (accessed from : http://www.arvo.org/webs/am2014/abstract/sessions/162.pdf).

CHAPTER

14

Evaluation of Pharmacological Activity of Herbal Medicines

INTRODUCTION

Traditional or alternative or complementary systems of medicine are popular not only in developing but also in developed countries. Their popularity can be attributed to various historical and cultural reasons. According to WHO estimates, around 80% of population in developing countries relies on plant derived traditional medicines. Current statistics indicate that the global market for medicinal plants is to the tune of US $62 billion and the demand is growing rapidly. Global resurgence of the interest in herbal drugs has led to the need of their mass production. Consequently, large-scale production has necessitated that standards for their quality, efficacy and safety be clearly defined.

Despite their widespread usage, phytomedicines have not been evaluated scientifically with regard to their safety and efficacy. Moreover, the government policy regarding their registration and regulation remains obscure. With the increasing incidence of metabolic diseases and age-related degenerative disorders that are associated with oxidative processes in the body, the use of herbs has gained much attention; but without careful documentation in well-defined clinical trials, they remain equivocal.[1] It is because of this loophole that spurious, illicit and substandard herbal drugs find their way into the market.[2] International agencies like World Health Organization (WHO), United Nations Industrial Development Organization (UNIDO), International Centre for Science and High Technology (ICS) and Asia Pacific Centre for Transfer of Technology (APCTT) have also emphasized on the need of ensuring quality control of medicinal plant drugs by applying suitable standards employing modern techniques.

Owing to the aforementioned reasons the WHO was requested, to compile a list of medicinal plants and establish their international specifications, during the IVth International Conference of Drug Regulatory Authorities (ICDRA) held in Tokyo in 1986. The guidelines for the assessment of herbal medicines were prepared by WHO and adopted by the VIth ICDRA held in Ottawa, Canada in 1991. The objective of these guidelines was to define basic criteria for the evaluation of quality, safety, and efficacy of herbal medicines and thereby to assist national regulatory authorities, scientific organizations and manufacturers to undertake an assessment of the documentation/submissions/dossiers in respect of such products.

As a general rule in this assessment, traditional experience means that long-term use as well as the medical, historical and ethnological background of these products shall be taken into account. The definition of long-term use may vary according to the country but should be at least several decades. Therefore, the assessment should take into account a description of a herbal medicine in the medical/pharmaceutical literature or similar sources, or a documentation of knowledge on the application of such medicines without a clearly defined time limitation. It may be noted that the traditional description of the herbal preparations are often in vernacular prevalent in those times. Consequently, the description of the plants and their therapeutic uses need to be carefully understood and interpreted, so as to avoid misinterpretation.

WHO defines herbal medicines as finished, labeled medicinal products that contain as active ingredients the aerial or underground parts of plants, or other plant material, or combinations thereof, whether in the crude state or as plant preparations. Plant material includes juices, gums, fatty oils, essential oils and any other substance of this nature. Herbal medicines may contain excipients in addition to the active ingredients. Medicines containing plant material combined with chemically defined, isolated constituents of plants, are not considered to be herbal medicines.

WHO has defined certain related terms to provide consistency and international acceptance for the evaluation and research on herbal medicines.

Definitions

Herbs

Herbs include crude plant material such as leaves, flowers, fruits, seeds, stems, wood, barks, roots, rhizomes or other plant parts, which may be entire, fragmented or powdered.

Herbal Materials

Herbal materials include, in addition to herbs, fresh juices, gums, fixed oils, essential oils, resins, and dry powders of herbs. In some countries, these materials may be processed by various local procedures, such as steaming, roasting, or stir baking with honey, alcoholic beverages or other materials.

Herbal Preparations

Herbal preparations are the basis for finished herbal products and may include comminuted or powdered herbal materials, or extracts, tinctures and fatty oils of herbal materials. They are produced by extraction, fractionation, purification, concentration or other physical or biological processes. They also include preparations made by steeping or heating herbal materials in alcoholic beverages and/or honey, or in other materials.

Traditional Use of Herbal Medicines

Herbal medicines include herbs, herbal materials, herbal preparations, and finished herbal products. Traditional use of herbal medicines refers to their description in ancient literature and long historical use of these medicines. Their use is well established and widely acknowledged to be safe and effective, and may be accepted by national authorities.

Therapeutic Activity

Therapeutic activity refers to the successful prevention, diagnosis and treatment of physical and mental illnesses, improvement of symptoms of illnesses, as well as beneficial alteration or regulation of the physical and mental status of the body.

Active Ingredients

Active ingredients refer to ingredients of herbal medicines with therapeutic activity. In herbal medicines where the active ingredients have been identified, the preparation of these medicines should be standardized to contain a defined amount of the active ingredients, if adequate analytical methods are available. In cases where it is not possible to identify the active ingredients, the whole herbal medicine may be considered as one active ingredient.

Standardization of the presumed active constituents of the drug is perhaps not the best approach, as only in few cases a single component can be held responsible for the pharmacological effect. In majority of the cases, the activity is a synergistic effect of several compounds. In addition, number of factors such as age, origin, time of collection, method of drying, etc. also play a critical role in determining the proportion of the various compounds and ultimately, the effect.

Assessment of Quality

Pharmaceutical Assessment

This should cover all important aspects of the quality assessment of herbal medicines sufficient to make reference to a monograph in pharmacopoeia. The procedures described should be in accordance with good manufacturing practices. The identity and quality of the plant material or preparation must be according to the following headings.

Information for Fresh, Dried, and Processed Plant Materials

i. *Name and characteristics of crude plant materials*
   - Name of the plant material in Latin, native languages, and English.
   - Scientific name and the family to which it belongs.
   - Part and condition (dried, fresh, sliced or decorticated, etc.) of the plant used.
   - Time and method of collection, preliminary preparation, drying, and processing.
   - Description and distribution of plant habitat; growing wild or cultivated (including possible pesticide used). Drawings or photographs of the plants should be provided.
   - Characterizing compounds of the plant materials, which may also be the biologically or therapeutically active principles, should be quantified and described with their structural formulae.
   - Foreign matter (such as stem, rachis fragments in the leaves or leaflets, leaf fragments in the flowers etc.), foreign mineral matter (such as sand and soil adhering to the plant material), impurities and microbial content should be defined or limited.
   - Voucher specimens, representing each lot of plant material processed, should be authenticated by a qualified botanist and should be stored for at least a 10-year-period. A lot number should be assigned and this should appear on the product label.

ii. *Authentication of plant preparations*
Plant preparations include comminuted or powdered plant materials, extracts, tinctures, fatty or essential oils, expressed juices and preparations whose production involves fractionation, purification or concentration. A method for identification and assay of the plant preparation along with a description of the physical and chemical tests for the identification of the plant substances should be provided. If identification of an active principle is not possible, "chromatographic fingerprint" of the mixture is needed to ensure consistent quality of the preparation.

iii. *Packaging, labeling, and storage of finished products*
The manufacturing procedure and formula needs to be described in detail. A method for quantification of the plant material in the finished product should be defined. For imported finished products, confirmation of the regulatory status in the country of origin is needed. The WHO Certification Scheme on the quality of pharmaceutical products moving in international commerce should be applied.

iv. *Product information for the consumer*
Product labels and package inserts should be understandable to the consumer or patient and should include necessary information on the correct use of the product.

v. *Promotion*
Advertisements and other promotional material directed to health personnel and the general public has to be consistent with the approved package information.

vi. *Stability*
The physical and chemical stability of the product should be tested under defined storage conditions and the shelf life has to be established.

Assessment of Safety

Long-term use of a medicine without any evidence of risk may indicate that it is harmless, it is not always definite how far one can rely on it as an assurance of innocuity. Preclinical toxicological studies can be undertaken to study safety of herbal medicines. In addition, side-effects may be documented according to normal pharmacovigilance practices.

Toxicological Studies

Standard methods of nonclinical toxicological studies are indicated below. All tests are not necessarily required for each herbal medicine intended for human use.

Acute Toxicity Test

- Animal species: Some regulatory agencies recommend that at least two species be used, one of them to be selected from rodents and the other from non-rodents.
- Sex: In at least one of the species, males and females should be used.
- Number of animals: In the case of rodents, each group should consist of at least five animals per sex. In the case of non-rodents, each group should consist of at least two animals per sex.

- Route of administration: Ordinarily, the oral route is sufficient as this is the normal route of clinical administration. In cases where it is proposed to administer the herbal preparation to a subject by the parenteral route, it may be sufficient to use this route for animal testing.
- Dose levels: A sufficient number of dose levels should be used in rodents to determine the approximate lethal dose. In non-rodents, sufficient dose levels should be used for the observation of overt toxic signs.
- Frequency of administration: The test substance should be administered in one or more doses during a 24-hour period.
- Observation: Toxic signs and severity, onset, progression and reversibility of the signs should be observed and recorded in relation to dose and time. As a general rule, the animals should be observed for at least 7 to 14 days. Animals dying during the observation period, as well as surviving to the end of the observation period should be autopsied. If necessary, a histopathological examination should be conducted on organs or tissues showing macroscopic changes at autopsy.

Long-term Toxicity Test

- Animal species: At least two species be used, one a rodent and the other a non-rodent.
- Sex: Equal number of males and females should be used.
- Number of animals: In case of rodents, each group should consist of at least ten males and ten females. In case of non-rodents, each group should consist of at least three males and three females.
- Route of administration: Expected clinical route of administration should be used.
- Administration period: The period of administration of the test substance to animals will depend on the expected period of clinical use (Table 14.1). It may vary from country to country, according to its individual regulations.

Table 14.1: Commonly used ranges of administration periods

Expected period of clinical use	*Administration period for the toxicity study*
Single administration or repeated administration for less than one week	2 weeks to 1 month
Repeated administration, between one week to four weeks	4 weeks to 3 months
Repeated administration, between one to six months	3 to 6 months
Long-term repeated administration for more than six months	9 to 12 months

The test substance should be administered seven days a week. Administration periods for the toxicity study must be recorded in each result.

- *Dose levels*: At least three different dose levels should be used. One dose should be a no effect dose, the other should exert-overt toxic effects. Within this range one more dose may be included to observe a dose-response curve for toxic effects.
- *Observations and examinations*: Following points should be considered
  a. General signs, daily body weight, food, and water intake.
  b. Hematological and blood chemistry examination should be done before the start of the drug treatment and compared with that during the administration period and before autopsy values.

c. Renal and hepatic function tests to be performed before, during and after drug administration period.
d. Other function tests include—ECG, visual, and auditory tests.
e. Animals found dead during the examination should be autopsied as soon as possible.

- *Recovery from toxicity*: This is observed in animals that are allowed to live for varying lengths of time after cessation of the period of administration of the test substance.

Local Toxicity Test

This is a sensitization test for dermatological preparations. Usually, guinea pigs are considered the most suitable experimental animals and test methods like patch test, Buehler test, Draize test, Freund's complete adjuvant test, Maximization test, Open epicutaneous test, Optimization test and Split adjuvant test, etc. are usually undertaken.

Special Toxicity Tests

i. *Mutagenicity test*: Reverse mutation test in bacteria, chromosomal aberration test with mammalian cells in culture, micronucleus test with rodents are some of the standard tests which can provide any inkling regarding the toxicity profile of the drug.
ii. *Carcinogenicity test*: Animals are screened in two phases—preliminary and full scale carcinogenicity studies with the same test substance. In preliminary studies, effect of single and repeated doses are observed in a small number of animals and the data from this study is used to determine the dose of the test drug to be used in the full scale carcinogenicity studies. For full-scale carcinogenicity test at least two species of animals are employed. The parameters to be observed are—development of tumor type, frequency of development, onset of development, variety of organs involved, etc.
iii. *Reproductive and developmental toxicity test*: The effect of the test drug is observed on fertility, incidence of spontaneous malformation and susceptibility to substances known to affect reproduction and development.

Assessment of Efficacy

Herbal medicines are currently being used either as first line of medical care or in conjunction with conventional treatment. Citation of existing literature is sufficient to substantiate claims of benefits of herbal medicine being traditionally used. However, in case, any replacement, addition or deletion of traditionally used ingredients from herbal drug product is made, or old product is marketed for new indication, or traditional method of preparation is altered, the "new" herbal product needs to be extensively investigated preclinically and clinically along with post-marketing surveillance.[3]

Activity

The pharmacological and clinical effects of the active ingredients and, if known, their constituents with therapeutic activity should be specified or described.

Evidence Required to Support Indications

According to WHO guidelines the requirements for proof of efficacy of traditional medicines depends on the kind of indication. For treatment of minor and nonspecific indications, some relaxation in requirements for proof of efficacy may be justified, taking into account the extent of traditional use. The relaxation applies to prophylactic use also. Individual experiences of physicians, traditional health practitioners or treated patients should be taken into account.[3]

Combination Products

Many herbal medicines are combination of several active ingredients, and as experience of the use of traditional remedies is often based on combination products, assessment should differentiate between old and new combination products. In the case of traditionally used combination products, the documentation of traditional use (classical texts of Ayurveda, traditional Chinese medicine, Unani, Siddha, etc.) and experience may serve as evidence of efficacy.[3]

An explanation of a new combination of well-known substances, including effective dose ranges and compatibility, should be required in addition to the documentation of traditional knowledge of each single ingredient. Each active ingredient must contribute to the efficacy of the medicine. For study of those herbal medicines, which are used under the principles of traditional medicine, animal models may need to be established according to those principles.[3]

Clinical Trials

The principles of the clinical trials of herbal medicines are similar to those applied to synthetic drugs. Clinical trials of herbal medicines have two objectives—to validate the safety and efficacy claim and to develop new herbal medicines or examine a new indication for an existing herbal medicine. Clinical trial is conducted in a step-wise approach in four phases and the entry point into the phase may be determined by the nature and history of the herbal medicines being studied.[3]

Phase I

New compound or a new formulation is administered for the first time to a small number of healthy volunteers and their tolerance to the herbal medicine is noted. An indication of the intended dose that may be used safely in subsequent phases is decided.

Phase II

Studies are conducted on a limited number of patients to determine clinical efficacy and safety. The dosage schedules established in such studies are then used for a more extensive clinical study.

Phase III

Larger patient groups are usually studied at several centers to validate preliminary evidence of efficacy obtained in earlier studies.

Phase IV

Studies performed after the dosage form is available in the market for general use. This is also known as post-marketing surveillance. Hence, the main purpose of such studies is to detect toxic events that may occur so rarely that they are not detected earlier.

Pharmacovigilance of Herbal Drugs

There is an urgent need to develop pharmacovigilance practices for herbal medicines. The current model of pharmacovigilance and its associated tools are inadequate for monitoring safety of herbal medicines.[4] The matter is further complicated due to the practise of co-administration of herbal and allopathic medicines leading to herb-drug interactions. In such cases, it becomes essential to delineate the mechanism responsible, like activity of metabolic enzymes, active transporters pharmacokinetic profiles etc.[5]

Despite concerted efforts to stimulate reporting of suspected ADRs associated with herbal medicines, such as extending the scheme to unlicensed herbal products, and including community pharmacists as recognized reporters, numbers of herbal ADR reports received remain relatively low. Although, Spontaneous Reporting Schemes form the backbone of pharmacovigilance, it is fraught with an inherent limitation of under-reporting. This limitation is more pronounced for herbal medicines, since users typically do not seek professional advice about their use of such products, or report if they experience adverse effects.

Worldover, herbal medicines are being sold under the garb of neutraceuticals and thereby, circumvent any such targeted monitoring. The herbal sector in the UK has taken the initiative for adverse effect monitoring of herbal drugs by means of spontaneous reporting by the herbal-medicine practitioners. Presently, other tools that are routinely used in pharmacovigilance, such as prescription-event monitoring, computerized health-record databases, offer limited utility in monitoring the safety of herbal medicines, as these drugs are usually sold OTC. Proposed European Union legislation for traditional herbal medicinal products will require manufacturers of products registered under new national schemes to comply with regulatory provisions on pharmacovigilance. In the longer term, other improvements in safety monitoring of herbal medicines may include modifications to existing methodology, patient reporting and greater consideration of pharmacogenetics and pharmacogenomics in optimizing the safety of herbal medicines.[6] Further, it needs to be re-inforced to earnestly take up reporting of adverse events associated with herb use in special population such as pediatric and lactating.[7,8]

REFERENCES

1. Tapsell LC, Hemphill I, Cobiac L, Patch CS, Sullivan DR, Fenech M. Health benefits of herbs and spices: the past, the present, the future. Med J Aust 2006;185(4 Suppl):S4-24.
2. Kinsel JF, Straus SE. Complementary and alternative therapeutics: rigorous research is needed to support claims. Annu Rev Pharmacol Toxicol 2003;43:463-84.
3. Research guidelines for evaluating the safety and efficacy of herbal medicines. World Health Organization, 1993.
4. Shaw D1, Graeme L, Pierre D, Elizabeth W, Kelvin C. Pharmacovigilance of herbal medicine. J Ethnopharmacol 2012; 140(3):513-8.

5. Gouws C, Steyn D, Du Plessis L, Steenekamp J, Hamman JH. Combination therapy of Western drugs and herbal medicines: recent advances in understanding interactions involving metabolism and efflux. Expert Opin Drug Metab Toxicol 2012;8(8):973-84.
6. Barnes J. Pharmacovigilance of herbal medicines: a UK perspective. Drug Saf 2003;26:829-51.
7. Gardiner P, Adams D, Filippelli AC, Nasser H, Saper R, White L. A systematic review of the reporting of adverse events associated with medical herb use among children. Glob Adv Health Med 2013; 2(2):46-55.
8. Budzynska K, Gardner ZE, Low Dog T, Gardiner P. Complementary, holistic, and integrative medicine: advice for clinicians on herbs and breastfeeding. Pediatr Rev 2013;34(8):343-52.

CHAPTER

15

Agents for Immune-based Disorders

INTRODUCTION

The main objective of the human immune system is to discriminate self from non-self (infectious invaders/microbes; dysregulated self/tumors). This requires active and efficient detector and effector mechanisms capable of identifying and destroying the non-self in order to preserve the self. Loss or suppression of immune system functionality can lead to disease conditions like cancer, bacterial, viral or protozoan infections. In contrast, overactive immune system can also cause significant health care problems like autoimmune diseases [rheumatoid arthritis (RA), diabetes mellitus (DM), systemic lupus erythematosus (SLE), multiple sclerosis (MS)], allergic and hypersensitivity conditions. New evidence correlates obese condition with chronic state of low-grade inflammation leading to the pathogenesis of several inflammatory conditions including rheumatic autoimmune and inflammatory diseases.[1]

Immunosuppressive or immuno-stimulant therapies, aiming at immune system mediated diseases have evolved. Antibiotics and antimetabolites have also been successfully used for management of infections and cancer, respectively but not without accompanying side effects. On the other hand, drugs for immunosuppression including glucocorticoids, cyclosporine, tacrolimus and sirolimus have proved to be highly efficacious for management of organ transplant cases, RA and other autoimmune disorders. Unfortunately, these drugs have also proved to be extremely disabling with life threatening side effects like growth retardation, osteopenia, hyperglycemia, nephropathy, hypertension, poor wound healing and increased risk of infection. Consequently, there has been an exponential rise in the need for biological molecules that act specifically to overcome the considerable side effects of non-specifically acting anti-inflammatory and immunosuppressive drugs. Recently, macrophages have been identified for their positive impact upon tissue remodeling following injury. The pivotal role of macrophages can initiate transition from a pro-inflammatory state to a regulated/anti-inflammatory state and reduce scar tissue formation.[2]

Helpful tools in the analysis of drug effects include high-throughput screening techniques such as microarrays, which are used in transcriptomics and pharmacogenomics. Although we are far from using these extensive and costly tests in our daily clinical routine, their application in basic research nevertheless takes us closer to individualized therapeutic strategies, in which the optimal therapeutic regimen is identified for each individual patient.

In Vivo Models

It is imperative to screen novel molecules for management of immune-based disorders and the challenge lies in developing suitable animal models that can help to accurately predict the activity of these agents. Depending on the goal, susceptibility of the animal to the pathogen and innate immune system, various animals like mice, rabbits, goat, sheep and even horse have been used as experimental animals of choice.

Of all the animals, mice have been found to be most useful, as not only they are easy to handle and have a rapid breeding cycle but also because they are genetically well characterized. Genetically identical strains have been developed by inbreeding brother and sister littermates for 20 generations to yield 98% homozygous progeny that are called syngeneic mice. Thus, mice colonies serving as models for cancer types (4T07cg for metastatic breast tumor), diabetes (NOD mice) and other immune-based disorders have been developed to understand underlying pathology of the disease conditions and screen novel drug therapies (Fig. 15.1).[3,4]

Another approach has been to microinject cloned foreign genes (transgenes) into mouse embryos to produce *transgenic mice*. This helps to assess the variation in biological effects induced by the gain of a single gene. Transgenic mice have been of value in studying the immunopathology of human major histocompatibility class II (MHC-II) associated autoimmune diseases like RA, MS and DM by helping to identify the target antigens that are involved in the initiation of these diseases. Many of the mice develop aspects relevant to the human diseases, either spontaneously or following immunization with the relevant antigen, thus providing an *in vivo* disease model, that may be used as a tool for further understanding the disease mechanisms and testing novel immunotherapies.[5,6]

Change in phenotype due to loss of single gene function can also be studied by developing *knockout mice*. In order to develop these mice, the normal gene is replaced with the mutant allele in the cultured embryonic stem (ES) cells. The recombinant ES are then transferred to recipient blastocyst and implanted into foster mother. Finally, the chimeric offsprings that are heterozygous for the disrupted gene are mated to produce homozygous *knockout mice*

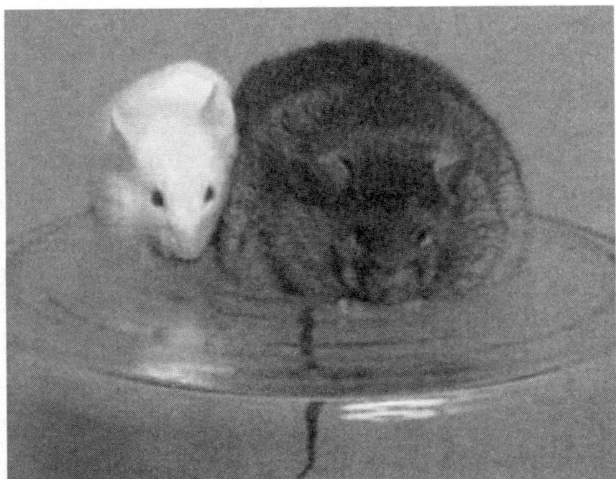

Figure 15.1: Syngeneic mouse-Non-obese diabetic (NOD) mouse as model for screening immune-based disorders *(For color version see Plate 20)*

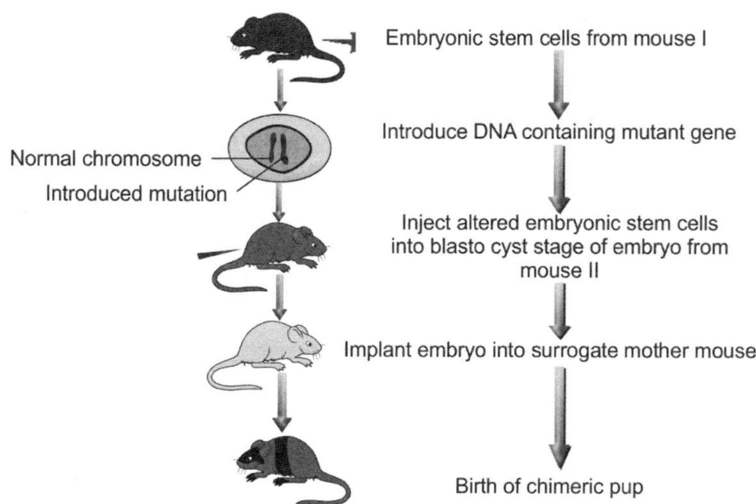

Figure 15.2: Developing knockout mouse (*For color version see Plate 20*)

(Fig. 15.2). These animals have been used to develop novel treatment modalities against cancer, viral infections and autoimmune diseases.[7,8]

An autosomal recessive mutation resulting in severe combined immunodeficiency disease (SCID) developed spontaneously in a strain of mice called CB-17. These CB-17 SCID mice fail to develop mature T and B cells and consequently are severely compromised immunologically. Hence, these animals must be housed in a sterile (germ-free) environment if they are to survive, as they cannot fight off microorganisms of even low pathogenecity. They have proven to be ready recipients of foreign cells and grafts from other strains of mice or even other species. DNA-based vaccine strategies and vectors meant for the treatment of human immunodeficiency virus are being actively developed using this model.[9]

Animal models have been used in the drug development process for the identification of targets for therapeutic intervention and to provide proof of a therapeutic principle. Preclinical animal models for immune-based disorders are briefly described here.

Asthma

One of the major immune disorders is asthma wherein triggering of the immune responses leads to the manifestation of the clinical symptoms. The events leading to clinical manifestation of the disease involve recognition of microbial components (*Chlamydia, Mycoplasma,* bacteria as well as virus and air-borne particles) and their activation through receptors and initiation of the cascade leading to induction of adaptive immune responses. The immune responses and efficacy of therapeutic modalities have been extensively studied using inbred mouse strains like C57BL/6, 129/SvEv.[10]

Six- to eight-weeks old 129/SvEv mice are maintained under sterile laboratory conditions and chow. The mice are immunized with subcutaneous 50 µg of ovalbumin (OVA) alone or in combination with 50 µg of ISS-ODN (TCCATGACGTTCCTGATGCT) or synthetic lipopeptide Pam3Cys (50 µg) on days 0 and 7. The mice are intranasally challenged with 5 µg of OVA 7 days and 1 day before sacrifice. On the 21st day the mice are tested for airway responsiveness to methacholine (3-24 mg/ml) and a bronchoalveolar lavage for the differential lung cell count is performed. Mediastinal lymph nodes are digested with DNAseI/collagenaseVII and restimulated with OVA for T cell ctytokine analysis. ELISA can be used to estimate OVA specific immunoglobulins and interferons in the sera. The modulation of these parameters after drug treatment can evidence the efficacy of the intervention at the cellular and molecular level.[10]

Based on their anatomical similarity and responsiveness of the airway with that of humans, rabbits serve as useful species for screening inflammatory mediators, lung disease pathophysiology and anti-asthmatic agents. Intraperitoneal administration of antigen in combination with adjuvant to neonatal rabbits like soluble bovine serum albumin in conjunction with *Corynebacterium parvum* adjuvant within the first 24 h of life chronically, initiates immune response via production of antigen-specific IgE antibodies. This protocol can be modified, to include other sensitizing agents like ovalbumin, lipopolysaccharide, house dust mite, and ragweed pollen for administration to rabbit neonates and study for various parameters such as comparison of anatomical structures of lung (bronchioles, tracheobronchial capillary bed), lung volume, airway epithelial layer, presence/absence of mucus producing cells, etc.[11]

Immunoinflammatory Disorders of the Central Nervous System (CNS)

Multiple sclerosis is a spectrum of chronic immunoinflammatory diseases of the CNS with multifactorial etiology and a complex pathogenesis. The pathological hallmark of MS is focally demyelinated lesion within the white matter and cortex along with accompanying inflammation, gliosis, axonal pathology and remyelination.[12] While many experimental animal models are available, the use of relevant model that aptly mimics the different forms of the disease is essential. Understanding the cascade can help to identify gene and protein targets for therapy. Experimental autoimmune encephalomyelitis (EAE) in mice and non-human primates shows similar pathogenesis as the clinical disorder.

Experimentally autoreactive T cells alone or T cells plus autoantibodies are used to induce the CNS lesions. For inducing the pathology, emulsion containing Freund's adjuvant in combination with CNS preparations such as brain, spinal cord or myelin antigen are inoculated. EAE is initiated by activation of a pre-existing repertoire of myelin reactive CD^{4+} T cells in peripheral lymphoid organs. The activated cells pass through the blood-brain barrier.

Advances in genetic engineering and the subsequent ease of producing animals with dysfunctional (knock-out/knock-in) genes have helped in probing the disease. Intraperitoneal infection of transgenic mice (C57BL/6, Biozzi ABH) with avirulent A7(74) strain of Semliki-Forest virus or Theiler's virus induces EAE. These protocols have allowed studies on MS-associated immunological responses. Neurovirulent strains of virus induce fatal encephalitis to cause persistent infection and demyelination of the CNS, spinal cord and brainstem.[13]

Non-human primates are attractive models for studying EAE as they share phylogenetic proximity with humans. Based on this, intervention strategies for MS are being actively explored using non-human primate animal models. The common marmoset, a small neotropical primate with significant genetic and immunological similarity to humans provides an excellent model that approximates chronic MS by the clinical and neuropathological presentation.[14] Attempts to evoke MS like syndrome in chimps by inoculation of MS brain material have yielded intriguing results on the viral origin of MS.[15] Macaque also develops neurological deficits associated with CNS inflammation after infection with healthy CNS tissue.[16] Based on these findings, reproducible EAE models have been established for the study of genetic, immunological, pathological features of MS.[17]

Viral Diseases

Non-human primates are complex species including Lemur, Lorisers, Tarsiers, Marmosets, Tamarins and Monkeys. They serve as important models to study human diseases especially of immune origin, as they share a high degree of genetic similarity, susceptibility to pathogens (HIV, HBV, malarial parasite), cascade of pathological events and drug responsiveness. They have proven to be extremely useful for studying mechanisms of immune pathology, exploring interventional therapies and vaccine strategies. However, their use in research requires special ethical permission and dedicated care, attention and housing conditions.[18]

Hepatitis B Virus

Hepatitis B virus (HBV) is infectious to chimps, however, the impact of infection is minimal as compared to humans as they initiate a strong polyclonal cytotoxic T-lymphocyte response immediately.[19] In humans, the response remains restricted and is robust only in chronically infected patients.[17] In the experiment conducted by Bertoni and co-workers, two chimps were inoculated with a terminally redundant copy of the HBV. Both developed acute and self-limited HBV infection. The host interferon-α levels were monitored and associated with decreasing HBV titer. This showed that the chimps could mount an effective response to the infection on the basis of their innate immune response.[20] Further studies exploring the mechanism could provide insight into the cascade of events and management strategies for humans.

Chronic hepatitis B (HBV) infection is one of the most common causes of chronic active hepatitis, and dramatically increases the risk of developing hepatocellular carcinoma (HCC). Because of the narrow host range of this virus, there are very few useful animal models of HBV infection. However, transgenic technology affords the opportunity to produce mouse models of the condition. Moreover, because transgenic technology inevitably involves integration of the donor DNA, this particular characteristic of HBV DNA in HCC can readily be achieved in transgenic mice.[21] Healthy carrier state in hepatitis B virus (HBV) infections, transgenic mice expressing HBV genes were produced according the following protocol. Briefly, fertilized one-cell eggs were microinjected with subgenomic fragments of HBV DNA containing the coding regions for the HBV surface antigen (HBsAg) and pre-S and X antigens. Either the normal (HBV) or metallothionein promoters were used to obtain expression of the HBV genes. There was no evidence of viral replication or tissue pathology. The integrated HBV DNA sequences were inherited in a normal Mendelian fashion. Three of 16 transgenic mice expressed HBV-encoded gene products to which they were immunologically tolerant. Expression was not tissue specific and may be influenced by the genomic integration site and cellular factors. Both HBsAg and pre-S antigen were detectable within the cytoplasm of hepatocytes and renal tubular epithelial cells. High serum concentrations of HBsAg were detectable and the secreted product appeared authentic as judged by mean density, morphology, mean particle diameter, polypeptide composition, and antigenicity.[21]

HBx gene of HBV has also been implicated in HCC and has been introduced under the control of its own promoter into mice, so as to develop a model for HCC.[22] High expression of HBx has been documented in liver, kidney and testis. By 4 months of age focal areas of hepatocyte abnormalities were observed, and definite tumors were diagnosed by 8 to 10 months.

In summary, the species barrier to HBV infection can be overcome in mice by direct microinjection of HBV genes. The genes integrate, and when HBsAg is expressed at high levels, liver cell injury and HCC develop. A serous limitation when working with transgenic mice is that they pose a threat of zoonotic transmission of diseases. It is possible that an animal with the entire genome in every cell could produce mature virions and release them into its serum. In fact, some transgenic mice that carry the entire HBV genome carry core antigens in blood.[23] To date, transmission of disease specific to expression of a transgene from a transgenic animal to man has not been reported. However, it is important to study new proposals involving insertion of human pathogens to determine if risk exists.

Hepatitis C Virus

For the development of effective therapies against hepatitis C virus (HCV), it is essential to develop suitable small animal models. Although the chimpanzee has been a valuable model to study HCV-host interactions but its use is severely hampered by financial and ethical constraints pertaining to large animals. Alternatively, human-liver chimeric mice have been developed as well-characterized tools for the efficacy assessment of antiviral interventions and are widely accepted and used. Transgenic mouse has also been developed immunocompetent mouse model, and is appropriate for the evaluation of both antivirals and murine vaccine responses.[24]

Human Immunodeficiency Virus

Studies indicate that human-immunodeficiency virus (HIV-1 and 2) are products of multiple infections from simian immunodeficiency virus (SIV) infected primates.[25] The difference in response to HIV infection by primates provides clues regarding viral interaction with receptors and co-receptors on the cell surface. Infected chimp in large maintain normal CD^{4+} lymphocytes and do not develop clinical immunodeficiency. The viral-host immune interaction evidences the events leading to AIDS after infection with HIV. It is possible that chimps express favorable homologues that have protective effect.[26]

Chimps deal more effectively with viral infections. The viral load is lower with minimal sequel of events after MHC recognition. Subtle differences in peptide recognition and responses may account for the efficiency of viral clearing. These models are effective for studying cell-cell interactions and mediation of immune response leading to differences in handling of viral challenges.

Rheumatoid Arthritis

Rheumatoid arthritis (RA) is characterized by chronic inflammatory infiltration of the synovium, leading to eventual cartilage and bone destruction. It is a common autoimmune disease, the treatment for which is rarely curative and often tied to major side effects. RA differs from other autoimmune diseases in several aspects, as RA patients often develop extra-articular disease manifestations such as rheumatoid nodules, rheumatic lung disease, and vasculitis, suggesting a more generalized autoimmune process. Genetic susceptibility to RA is associated with human leukocyte antigen (HLA) class II alleles, that share a collection of positively charged amino acids at positions 70–72 of the DRB1 chain, called the 'shared epitope.'[27]

Humanized mouse models of RA have been developed that allow screening of new, less toxic, vaccine-like treatments for RA.[28] Novel screening techniques such as high-throughput screening tools such as microarrays, are also being extensively used. Their application in basic research will takes us closer to individualized therapeutic strategies, in which the optimal therapeutic regimen is identified for each individual patient.

The primary disease phenotype, detected in several different tumor necrosis factor (TNF)-α transgenic mice with constitutive expression of human TNF, is an inflammatory arthritis similar to RA.[29] This phenotype is essentially preserved when these mice are backcrossed to a severe combined immune deficiency background, which lacks the development of B cells and T cells, indicating that arthritis can develop without the participation of lymphocytes.[30-32]

Spontaneous RA-like arthritis was also observed in a murine TCR transgenic model, (KRN×NOD).[33] This TCR is specific for bovine ribonuclease in the context of I-A^k. The transgenic TCRab-positive cells are completely deleted in I-A^k mice. The TCR transgene-positive animals develop arthritis within the first few weeks of life after the first cross to the nonobese diabetic mouse strain (NOD).[33]

Human T cell leukemia virus type-I (HTLV-I) is the etiologic agent of adult T cell leukemia and has also been suggested to be involved in other diseases such as chronic arthritis or myelopathy. To elucidate pathological roles of the virus in disease, transgenic mice were produced that carry the HTLV-I genome. At 2 to 3 months of age, many of the mice developed chronic arthritis resembling rheumatoid arthritis. Synovial and periarticular inflammation with articular erosion caused by invasion of granulation tissues was marked. These observations suggest a possibility that HTLV-I is one of the etiologic agents of chronic arthritis in humans.[34]

T cells have well established diverse role in pathogenesis of RA and mouse models simulating the same have been developed. In SKG mice, point mutation in the gene encoding ZAP70, a tyrosine kinase involved in T-cell receptor signal transduction, results in aberrant TCR signalling. Such self-reactive T cells are understood to lead to the development of spontaneous autoimmune arthritis.[35]

Amyotrophic Lateral Sclerosis

Amyotrophic lateral sclerosis (ALS), also called Lou Gehrigs disease, is an age-related neurodegenerative disorder that primarily involves motor neurons. Although the majority of ALS cases are sporadic, a subset of affected individuals inherits the disease. Rosen and others (1993) observed that a subset of individuals with familial, autosomal dominantly inherited ALS (FALS) harbor mutations of the Cu/Zn superoxide dismutase (SOD-l) gene. These findings indicate a causative relationship between altered SOD-1 activity and motoneuron degeneration. Because humans with ALS are generally not identified until muscle weakness sets in, early medical intervention and prevention is difficult. For these reasons it is highly desirable to develop an animal model of FALS.[36]

Transgenic mouse model of ALS is one of the most important screening model. When a mutation is introduced into the 4th exon of a 15 kb mouse genomic clone, it leads to an alteration in the glycine residue (GGC) at position 86 of the protein, that simulates the mutation found in some families with FALS. The sequence change not only creates a mouse counterpart of a pathogenic human gene sequence, it introduces a recognition sequence for FspI restriction endonuclease. This construct can be microinjected to produce transgenic mice. In mouse lines with high levels of transgene mRNA in the central nervous system (CNS), phenotype that is manifested is development of motor paralysis, degenerative changes of motoneurons within the spinal cord, brainstem, and neocortex. These animals constitute a potentially valuable animal model of ALS.[37]

The transgenic mice produced are of the highly inbred FVB/N strain and are housed under uniform conditions. The appearance and progression of symptoms is very consistent and all mice die between the ages of 94 and 117 days. This is a sensitive model that can be used for testing of potential therapeutic agents or environmental factors involved in the disease.[38]

Recombinant DNA Technology

Recombinant DNA technology is an amalgam of research techniques aimed at gene cloning and DNA sequencing for producing recombinant proteins and providing immunologists with defined components to study structure-function correlation of the immune system at the molecular level.

DNA cloning is a means of amplifying a given DNA fragment and producing unlimited amounts of identical DNA fragments called "cloned DNA". In order to clone DNA, the desired fragment is inserted into an autonomously replicating DNA molecule, called "cloning vector" like bacterial virus (bacteriophage), insect virus and mammalian retrovirus. For producing DNA clones, firstly the vector genes are removed. The desired DNA insert is then incorporated with the remnant vector genome. The expression of the gene is now under the control of the vector promoter region.

Similarly, clones of mRNA can also be produced. First mRNA is isolated from cells and transcribed into complementary DNA or cDNA with the help of reverse transcriptase enzyme. Copies of cDNA are produced by inserting it into an appropriate vector. DNA sequences within vectors representing all the mRNA sequences derived from a cell or tissue is called a cDNA library. The genes from the library are screened to identify, purify and sequence the fragments. Thus, with the advances in technology, it is possible to decipher nucleotide sequences of the corresponding gene if the amino acid sequence is known.

The techniques of protein biochemistry have been very crucial for immunology and have made it possible to elucidate the structure of various immunoglobulins and their functional interactions.[39] Basic techniques like electrophoresis, radio immunoassay, polymerase chain reaction (PCR) and Western blotting have proved to be of central importance and are briefly described here.

Immunoelectrophoresis

Electrophoresis is a separation technique that uses electricity to separate the sample mixture on the basis of size. In gel electrophoresis, the gel acts as a sieve across which the sample moves from the negative to the positive end of the machine. The smaller sized molecules move faster and farther across the sieve than the larger ones. Staining the gel helps to analyze the sample contents quantitatively and qualitatively. Using this technique, DNA, RNA or protein samples can be analyzed. Similarly, antigen mixtures can be separated by electrophoresis and then identified by double immunodiffusion and this qualitative technique is known as immunoelectrophoresis. Here, after the sample components have been separated by electrophoresis, antiserum is added. Consequently, antibody and antigen diffuse towards each other and produce lines of precipitation. The technique is being widely applied to detect the presence or absence of proteins in serum.[40]

Radioimmunoassay

Radioimmunoassay (RIA) is a sensitive technique for detecting antigens and antibodies that was developed by two endocrinologists, S. A. Berson and Rosalyn Yalow in 1960 as an assay for the quantification of insulin in plasma sample. The protocol involves labeling of antigen with ^{125}I or ^{131}I. A mixture of the radioactive antigen and antibodies against that antigen is prepared. Known amounts of unlabeled ("cold") antigen are added to samples of the mixture. These compete for binding sites of the antibodies. At increasing concentrations of unlabeled antigen, an increasing amount of radioactive antigen is displaced from the antibody molecules. The antibody-bound antigen is separated from the free antigen in the supernatant fluid, and the radioactivity of each is measured. From the data, a standard binding curve can be prepared to quantify the test sample. The technique is being applied to detect the presence of marker proteins from the sera and plasma of the patients.[41]

Enzyme-linked Immunosorbent Assay

Enzyme-linked immunosorbent assay or ELISA is similar in principle to RIA but depends on an enzyme rather than a radioactive label. An enzyme conjugated with an antibody reacts with a colorless substrate to generate a colored reaction product. A number of enzymes have been employed for ELISA including alkaline phosphatase, horseradish peroxidase and β-galactosidase. These assays are sensitive, safe and less costly.[42] There are many different types of ELISAs, which can detect the presence of protein in serum or supernatent. One of the most common types of ELISA is the so-called "sandwich ELISA." It is so termed because the antibody that is being detected, gets sandwiched between an antigen and a chromogenically-conjugated antibody. The technique is being experimentally and clinically used to analyse levels of matrix metalloproteinases (MMP), inflammatory and collagen degradation markers, tissue inhibitor of MMPs (TIMP) levels and circulating proteasomes in the systemic circulation and synovial fluid of patients with a variety of autoimmune diseases.[43,44]

Polymerase Chain Reaction (PCR)

PCR is an *in vitro* method for DNA amplification that was invented by Kary Mullis in 1985 for which he was awarded the Nobel Prize in 1993. It is a simplified version of the process that normally occurs during cell division. DNA sample obtained from hospital tissue specimen, single hair strand, or a drop of blood can be amplified and analysed by PCR. The three-step protocol of PCR involves thermal degradation of DNA, followed by primer annealing and lastly, primer extension. The entire procedure can be carried out in specialized equipment called "thermocycler". At the temperature of 94-98°C, within 8 min, the DNA of the sample can be degraded such that the double helical structure opens up into single strands. Now, oligonucleotides of 18-30 bases or "primer" is introduced into the reaction mixture and heated from 5 to 60°C for 1-2 min. The primer is complementary to the DNA template flanks and anneals to the template. The final step involves addition of DNA polymerase or Taq protein, which helps to produce multiple copies of the identified flank. The purity of the product can be determined by electrophoresis, HPLC or direct sequencing. The technique is being used for diagnosing disease condition, polymorphism, developing transgenic animals, gene therapy or quantification of biomarker in disease tissues to provide insights into the mechanisms of action of novel therapeutic agents.[45]

Western Blotting

Western blotting is a technique that helps to identify specific protein from a complex mixture. In contrast, Southern blotting is for identifying DNA fragments and Northern blotting for messenger RNAs (mRNA). Samples are prepared from tissues or cells that are homogenized in a buffer that protects the protein of interest from degradation. The sample is electrophoretically separated using sodium dodecyl sulfate-polyacrylamide gel (SDS-PAGE) and then transferred to a nitrocellulose membrane for detection. The membrane is incubated with a generic protein (such as milk protein) to bind to any remaining sticky places on the membrane. A primary antibody is then added to the solution, which is able to bind to its specific protein. A secondary antibody-enzyme conjugate, which recognizes the primary antibody, is added to find locations where the primary antibody is bound. A number of autoimmune diseases have shown genetic linkage, and Western blotting helps to detect them.[46] For example, SLE is characterized by autoantibody production against different nuclear molecules, including those involved in pre-mRNA processing. The presence of autoantibodies in the sera of patients can be determined using Western blotting and proves to be a crucial diagnostic tool.[47]

REFERENCES

1. Gremese E, Tolusso B, Gigante MR, Ferraccioli G. Obesity as a risk and severity factor in rheumatic diseases (autoimmune chronic inflammatory diseases). Front Immunol 2014;5:576.
2. Brown BN, Sicari BM, Badylak SF. Rethinking regenerative medicine: a macrophage-centered approach. Front Immunol 2014;5:510.
3. Gravekamp C, Sypniewska R, Gauntt S, et al. Behavior of metastatic and nonmetastatic breast tumors in old mice. Exp Biol Med (Maywood) 2004;229:665-75.
4. Ogawa N, List JF, Habener JF, et al. Cure of overt diabetes in NOD mice by transient treatment with anti-lymphocyte serum and exendin-4. Diabetes 2004;53:1700-5.
5. Shibaki A, Sato A, Vogel JC, et al. Induction of GVHD-like skin disease by passively transferred CD8(+) T-cell receptor transgenic T cells into keratin 14-ovalbumin transgenic mice. J Invest Dermatol 2004;123:109-15.
6. Wang Y, Krieg AM. Induction of autoantibody production but not autoimmune disease in HEL transgenic mice vaccinated with HEL in combination with CpG or control oligodeoxynucleotides. Vaccine 2004;22:2641-50.
7. Kerbel RS. Human tumor xenografts as predictive preclinical models for anticancer drug activity in humans: better than commonly perceived-but they can be improved. Cancer Biol Ther 2003;24:S134-9.
8. Stevceva L. Cytokines and their antagonists as therapeutic agents. Curr Med Chem 2002;9:2201-7.
9. Giri M, Ugen KE, Weiner DB. DNA vaccines against human immunodeficiency virus type 1 in the past decade. Clin Microbiol Rev 2004;17:370-89.

10. Redecke V, Hacker H, Data SK, et al. Activation of Toll-like receptor 2 induces a Th2 immune response and promotes experimental asthma. J Immunol 2002;172:2739-43.
11. Kamaruzaman NA, Kardia E, Kamaldin N, Latahir AZ, Yahaya BH. The rabbit as a model for studying lung disease and stem cell therapy. Biomed Res Int 2013;2013:691830.
12. Compston A, Coles A. Multiple sclerosis. Lancet 2002;359:1221-31.
13. Fazakerley JK, Amor S, Webb HE. Reconstitution of Seliki forest virus infected mice, induces immune mediated pathological changes in the CNS. Clin Exp Immunol 1983;52:115-20.
14. 't Hart BA, van Meurs M, Brok HP, et al. A new primate model for multiple sclerosis in the common marmoset. Immunol Today 2000;21:290-7.
15. Brown P, Gajdusek DC. No mouse PMN leukocyte depression after inoculation with brain tissue from multiple sclerosis or spongiform encephalopathies. Nature 1974;247:217-8.
16. Rivers TM, Sprunt DH, Berry GR. Observation of the attempts to produce acute disseminated encephalomyelitis in monkeys. J Exp Med 1933;58:39-53.
17. Rose LM, Richards T, Alvord EC Jr. Experimental allergic encephalomyelitis (EAE) in nonhuman primates: a model of multiple sclerosis. Lab Anim Sci 1994;44:508-12.
18. Bontrop RE. Non-human primates: Essential partners in biomedical research. Immunol Rev 2001;183:5-9.
19. Nayersina R, Fowler P, Guilhot S, et al. HLA A2 restricted cytotoxic T lymphocyte responses to multiple hepatitis B surface antigen epitopes during hepatitis B virus infection. J Immunol 1993;150:4659-71.
20. Bertoni R, Sette A, Sidney J, et al. Human class I supertypes and CTL repertoires extend to chimpanzees. J Immunol 1998;161:4447-55.
21. Chisari FV, Pinkert CA, Milich DR, Filippi P, McLachlan A, Palmiter RD, et al. A transgenic mouse model of the chronic hepatitis B surface antigen carrier state. Science 1985;230:1157-60.
22. Kim CM, Koike K, Saito I, Miyamura T, Jay G. HBx gene of hepatitis B virus induces liver cancer in transgenic mice. Nature 1991;351:317-20.
23. Araki K, Miyazaki J, Hino O, Tomita N, Chisaka O, Matsubara K, et al. Expression and replication of hepatitis B virus genome in transgenic mice. Proc Natl Acad Sci USA 1989;86:207-11.
24. Vercauteren K, de Jong YP, Meuleman P. HCV animal models and liver disease. J Hepatol 2014;61 j:S26–S33.
25. Desrosiers RC, Daniel MD, Li Y. HIV-related lentiviruses of nonhuman primates. AIDS Res Hum Retroviruses 1989;5:465-73.
26. Gao X, Nelson GW, Karacki P, et al. Effect of a single amino acid change in MHC class I molecules on the rate of progression to AIDS. N Engl J Med 2001;344:1668-75.
27. Winchester R. The molecular basis of susceptibility to rheumatoid arthritis. Adv Immunol 1994;56:389-466.
28. Eming R, Visconti K, Hall F. Humanized mice as a model for rheumatoid arthritis. Arthritis Res 2002;4:S133-40.
29. Keffer J, Probert L, Cazlaris H, et al. Transgenic mice expressing human tumour necrosis factor: A predictive genetic model of arthritis. EMBO J 1991;10:4025-31.
30. Feldmann M, Bondeson J, Brennan FM, et al. The rationale for the current boom in anti-TNFalpha treatment. Is there an effective means to define therapeutic targets for drugs that provide all the benefits of anti-TNFalpha and minimise hazards? Ann Rheum Dis 1999;58:I27-32.

31. Feldmann M, Brennan F, Paleolog E, et al. Anti-tumor necrosis factor alpha therapy of rheumatoid arthritis. Mechanism of action. Eur Cytokine Network 1997;8:297-300.
32. Ulfgren AK, Grondal L, Lindblad S, et al. Interindividual and intra-articular variation of proinflammatory cytokines in patients with rheumatoid arthritis: potential implications for treatment. Ann Rheum Dis 2000;59:439-47.
33. Kouskoff V, Korganow AS, Duchatelle V, et al. Organ-specific disease provoked by systemic autoimmunity. Cell 1996;87:811-22.
34. Iwakura Y, Tosu M, Yoshida E, et al. Induction of inflammatory arthropathy resembling rheumatoid arthritis in mice transgenic for HTLV-I. Science 1991;253:1026-8.
35. Kobezda T, Ghassemi-Nejad S, Mikecz K, Glant TT, Szekanecz Z. Of mice and men: how animal models advance our understanding of T-cell function in RA. Nat Rev Rheumatol 2014;10(3):160-70.
36. Rosen DR, Siddique T, Patterson D, Figlewicz DA, et al. Mutations in Cu/Zn superoxide dismutase gene are associated with familial amyotrophic lateral sclerosis. Nature 1993;364:362.
37. Transgenic mice expressing an altered murine superoxide dismutase gene provide an animal model of amyotrophic lateral sclerosis. Ripps ME, Huntley GW, Hof PR, Morrison JH, Goradon JW. Proc Natl Acad Sci 1995;92:689-93.
38. Gurney ME, Pu H, Chiu AY, Dal Canto MC, Polchow CY, Alexander DD, et al. Motor degeneration in mice that express a human Cu, Zn superoxide dismutase mutation. Science 1994;264:1772-75.
39. Nabel GJ. Genetic, cellular and immune approaches to disease therapy: Past and future. Nat Med 2004;10:135-41.
40. Friedman J, Buskirk D, Marino LJ Jr, et al. The detection of brain antigens within the circulating immune complexes of patients with multiple sclerosis. J Neuroimmunol 1987;14:1-17.
41. Lampasona V, Rio J, Franciotta D, et al. Serial immunoprecipitation assays for interferon—(IFN)-beta antibodies in multiple sclerosis patients. Eur Cytokine Netw 2003;14:154-57.
42. Pachner AR. An improved ELISA for screening for neutralizing anti-IFN-beta antibodies in MS patients. Neurology 2003;61:1444-6.
43. Egerer K, Kuckelkorn U, Rudolph PE, et al. Circulating proteasomes are markers of cell damage and immunologic activity in autoimmune diseases. J Rheumatol 2002;29:2045-52.
44. Tchetverikov I, Ronday HK, Van El B, et al. MMP profile in paired serum and synovial fluid samples of patients with rheumatoid arthritis. Ann Rheum Dis 2004;63:881-3.
45. Rioja I, Bush KA, Buckton JB, et al. Joint cytokine quantification in two rodent arthritis models: Kinetics of expression, correlation of mRNA and protein levels and response to prednisolone treatment. Clin Exp Immunol 2004;137:65-73.
46. Vijayakrishnan L, Slavik JM, Illes Z, et al. An autoimmune disease-associated CTLA-4 splice variant lacking the B7 binding domain signals negatively in T cells. Immunity 2004;20:563-75.
47. Vazquez-Talavera J, Ramirez-Sandoval R, Esparza Ibarra E, et al. Autoantibodies against Cajal bodies in systemic lupus erythematosus. Med Sci Monit 2004;10:130-4.

CHAPTER

16

Antihypertensive Agents

INTRODUCTION

Hypertension is a complex multifactorial disease and one of the leading causes of mortality and morbidity due to stroke, heart attack and kidney failure. Because the etiology of essential hypertension is not known and may be multifactorial, the use of experimental animal models may provide valuable information regarding many aspects of the disease, which include etiology, pathophysiology, complications and treatment. As new insights in to the pathogenesis of hypertension are revealed, new models are being developed to produce hypertension in animals. In this chapter, a brief overview of the most widely used animal models, their features and their importance is provided. Nevertheless a cautious approach is mandatory when the experimental findings in these models is extrapoliated to human hypertension.

IN VITRO MODELS

1. Endothelin Receptor Antagonism in Porcine Isolated Hearts

Potent long lasting contractions of isolated blood vessel strips and increase blood pressure *in vivo* is elicited by endothelin peptides. Endothelins have been implicated in the pathophysiology of cardiovascular disorders. In this model, isolated porcine coronary artery is used since the smooth musculature of artery is considered to contain the ET_A receptors.

From porcine hearts left anterior descending coronary arteries are isolated. The endothelium-denuded arteries are cut into spiral strips about 10 mm long and 1 mm wide. The intimal surface of the spiral rings is then rubbed gently with filter paper to remove the vascular endothelium. Each strip is suspended in an organ bath containing Krebs-Henseleit solution bubbled with 95% O_2/5% CO_2 at 37°C. Once the isolated preparation is stabilized reference contraction is isometrically obtained with 50 mM KCl. Concentration-response curves for ET-1 are obtained by cumulative addition of ET-1. Twenty minutes before the addition of ET-1 the endothelin receptor antagonist/test drug is added to the organ bath and concentration response curve is recorded. The pA_2 values and slopes are obtained by analysis of Schild plots.[1]

2. Monocrotaline Induced Pulmonary Hypertension

Monocrotaline is a hepatotoxic and pneumotoxic agent used in rats to induce pulmonary hypertension. It is a pyrrolizidine alkaloid derived from Crotaloria spectabilis and its single injection leads to progressive pulmonary hypertension followed by right ventricular hypertrophy and cardiac failure. Ultrastructural changes such as degeneration and fragmentation of endothelial cells, perivascular edema, extravasation of red blood cells and muscularization of pulmonary arteries and arterioles are also observed. Monocrotaline administration in rats may result in severe right ventricular hypertrophy accompanied by ascitis and pleural effusion.

Sprague Dawley rats (200 to 225 g) are fed with the test drug for one week prior to single subcutaneous injection of 100 mg/kg monocrotaline. The animals are sacrificed 4, 7 or 14 days latter and their hearts and lungs are excised from thoracic cavity. The left ventricle and left lung are weighed. Their pulmonary artery segments, main pulmonary artery, right extra pulmonary and an intra pulmonary artery are also isolated. Each vessel is suspended between stainless steel hooks in tissue baths containing Krebs-Hensleit buffer aerated with 95% O_2 and 5% CO_2 at 37°C. At the end of the experiment vessel segments are blotted, weighed and their dimensions are measured. Cross-sectional area of artery is determined from tissue weight and diameter. After 1 h arteries are made to contract to KCl (6×10^{-2} M). Maximum active force generated by an artery is plotted as a function of applied force and changes in isometric force are monitored using force displacement transducers and recorded on a polygraph. Contractile and relaxant agonist responses are assessed in pulmonary arteries. Cumulative concentration-response curves to KCl, angiotensin II, norepinephrine are plotted. Contractions are expressed as active tension development, force generated per cross-sectional area. Both contractile and relaxation responses are plotted as a function of negative logarithm of agonist concentration.[2] T-test for grouped data is used to compare differences in mean responses.

Rat Models of Hypertension

1. Reno-vascular Hypertension

Experimentally, renal hypertension can be produced by constriction of the renal artery which activates peripheral Renin angiotensin aldosterone system (RAAS) and sympathetic nervous system. In response to decreased blood flow, renin is secreted by kidneys. Renin converts angiotensinogen to angiotensin-I, which is further converted to angiotensin-II by angiotensin converting enzyme (ACE). Angiotensin-II is a potent vasoconstrictor and also causes release of aldosterone leading to salt and water retention resulting in increased blood volume and hypertension . The various methods to produce renal hypertension include:

A. Two-kidney one clip (Goldblatt hypertension, 2K1C)

In the two-kidney one clip method, constriction of only one renal artery is carried out, while the contralateral kidney is left intact. In rats clamping the renal artery for 4 h can induce acute renal hypertension by activation of renin-angiotensin system. After re-opening of the vessel, accumulated renin is released into circulation leading to acute hypertension. This test is used to evaluate antihypertensive activities of drugs.[3,4]

Sprague Dawley rats (300 g) are anesthetized with hexobarbital sodium (100 mg/kg, intraperitoneally). The trachea is cannulated to facilitate spontaneous respiration. Through a pressure transducer connected to carotid artery, blood pressure is measured. Jugular vein is cannulated for administration of test compound. A poly vinyl chloride (PVC) coated clip is placed into the left hilum of the kidney and fixed to the back muscles. The renal artery is occluded for 3.5-4 h. Ganglionic blockade is performed with pentolinium and after obtaining stable reduced blood pressure values, the 'renal arterial clip' is removed. As a consequence of elevated plasma renin level, blood pressure rises. Test compound is administered by intravenous route. Blood pressure is monitored continuously.

Increase in blood pressure after re-opening of renal artery and reduction of blood pressure after administration of test compound is determined. Percent reduction of blood pressure values under drug treatment is calculated as compared to pretreatment values.[5-7]

B. Chronic renal hypertension in rats (1-kidney-1-clip method)

Constriction of the renal artery is done on one side and on the other side the contralateral kidney is removed. As discussed earlier, ischemia of the kidneys induces hypertension. Various modifications of the technique have been described for several animal species. The 1-kidney-1-clip method is one of the most effective modifications in rats in which one kidney is removed.

Sprague Dawley rats (200 to 250 g) are anesthetized with pentobarbitone sodium (50 mg/kg, intraperitoneally). In the left lumbar area, a flank incision is made parallel to the long axis of the rat. The renal artery is dissected, cleaned and a U shaped silver clip is slipped around it near the aorta. The size of the clip is adjusted so that the internal gap ranges from 0.25 to 0.38 nm. The right kidney is removed after tying off the renal pedicel. Four to five weeks after clipping, blood pressure is measured and rats are divided into different groups of different doses. For individual dose each animal is used as its own control. Test compounds are administered for 3 days. Pre-drug and 2 h post-drug blood pressure readings are taken.[8,9] Antihypertensive activity of test drug is determined by comparing treatment blood pressure value with day 1, pre-drug BP Comparisons are made using the paired t-test for evaluation of statistical significance.

C. Chronic renal hypertension in rats [Two kidney two clip (2K2C) method]

In the two kidneys two clip method (2K2C) hypertension; constriction of aorta or both renal arteries is undertaken. When the aorta or both renal arteries are constricted, there is severe renal ischemia caused by renal clipping, occasioning the activation of renin-angiotensin and the sympathetic nervous system and the elevation of serum vasopressin, leading to increased BP. The 2K2C, with a high incidence of spontaneous stroke, can be used as independent of a genetic deficiency. The lesioned small artery or arteriole with thrombotic occlusion is the main cause of cerebral infarction in 2K2C, and this may be similar to lacunar infarction in the human brain. Indeed, one of the most common causes of renal hypertension in human beings is such a patchy ischemic kidney disease.

Sprague Dawley rats (300 g) are anesthetized; trachea, carotid artery and jugular vein are cannulated. The renal arteries are located, U shaped silver clip is slipped around them or near the aorta. Either the renal arteries or the aorta is occluded using renal arterial clips. Test compound are administered by intravenous route via the jugular vein. Blood pressure is monitored continuously. Percent reduction of blood pressure values under drug treatment is calculated as compared to pre-treatment values.[10]

2. Neurogenic Hypertension

Evidence suggests that the central nervous system participates in the genesis of hypertension. Neurogenic hypertension can be defined as a permanent increase in BP resulting from a primarily neural change. One of the most important negative feedback in the control of BP originates from baroreceptors located in the carotid sinus and aortic arch. Denervation of sino-aortic baroreceptors (SAD) is the neurogenic model of hypertension most often used.

A. Blood pressure in pithed rats

The pithed rat model is devoid of neurogenic reflex control that may modulate the primary drug effect; it is frequently used to evaluate drug action on the cardiovascular system.

Male Wistar rats (250 to 350 g) are anesthetized with halothane. The carotid artery is cannulated for monitoring blood pressure and blood sampling. The trachea is cannulated and the animal is maintained on artificial respiration using a ventilation pump (60 cycles/min). The jugular vein is also cannulated for the administration of test drug. Pithing is done by inserting a steel rod, 2.2 mm in diameter and 11 cm in length, through the orbit and foramen magnum down the whole length of the spinal canal. Inspired air is oxygen-enriched by providing a flow of oxygen across a T-piece attached to the air inlet of the ventilation pump. Thirty minutes after pithing, a 0.3 ml blood sample is withdrawn from the carotid cannula and analyzed for pO_2, pCO_2, pH and bicarbonate concentration using blood gas analyzer. Through the carotid artery blood pressure and cardiac frequency is recorded. To measure α_1 and α_2 antagonism, first dose response curves are registered with phenylephrine, a selective α_1 agonist (0.1-30 µg/kg, intravenously) and BHT 920, a selective α_2 agonist (1-1000 µg/kg, intravenously). The test drug is administered intravenously and the agonist dose response curves are repeated 15 min later. The curve of blood pressure response to agonist is obtained. Dose response curves are plotted on a logarithmic probit scale. Potency ratios are calculated from the dose response curves.[11]

3. Dietary Hypertension

It is known that long-term exposure to a special diet (high salt, fat or sugar) results in dietary hypertension in some rats. The presence of oxidative stress and inactivation of Nitric oxide (NO) in rats maintained on the high-fat or high-sugar diet, may contribute to the development of hypertension by enhanced generation of reactive oxygen species (ROS). The reduction in NO availability in the high-fat and high-sugar diet-fed animals was associated with marked salt sensitivity, as evidenced by a significant rise in BP on the high-salt diet. Dietary intake of fats and carbohydrate, particularly the intake of simple sugars and the resultant effects of plasma insulin, adipokine and lipid concentrations, may affect cardiomyocyte size and function, especially with chronic hypertension.[10]

A. Fructose-induced hypertension in rats

Blood pressure increases by intake of either sucrose or glucose and result in the development of spontaneous hypertension or salt hypertension in rats. Fructose feeding also causes insulin resistance, hyperinsulinemia and hypertriglyceridemia in normal rats.

Wistar rats (200 to 250 g) are housed per cage on a 12 h light and dark cycle and fed water and chow diet *ad libitum*. Drinking water consists of 10% fructose solution. Fluid intake, food intake and body weight of each rat are measured every week during the course of drug treatment. Systolic blood pressure and pulse rate is measured using the tail-cuff method. Blood samples are collected before and every second week during treatment and plasma glucose, insulin, triglycerides are measured.[12] One way or two way analysis of variance followed by Newman-Keuls test is used for the statistical analysis.

B. Increased salt induced hypertension in rats

Physiologically, normal kidney has the ability to excrete easily the daily salt load without allowing a marked rise in extracellular volume. However, general epidemiological data have shown that higher the average sodium intake in a given population, the greater will be the prevalence of hypertension. Chronic ingestion of excess salt produces hypertension in rats, which mimics human hypertension morphologically. High salt intake hypertension has been produced in rats by replacing drinking water with 1-2% sodium chloride for 9-12 months.

Wistar rats (200 to 250 g) are fed chow diet *ad libitum*. Drinking water is replaced with 1-2% sodium chloride solution. Fluid intake, food intake and body weight of each rat are measured every week during the course of drug treatment. Systolic blood pressure and pulse rate is measured using the tail-cuff method. Blood samples are collected before and every second week during treatment.[13]

4. Endocrine Hypertension

Mineralocorticoids cause retention of sodium and water in the body until escape diuresis occurs due to increased pressure on the kidneys. No further retention of sodium and water occurs, but general level of body sodium and water is slightly raised. Selye et al. was the first to demonstrate that deoxycorticosterone acetate (DOCA) produces hypertension in rats. There is increased DOCA-induced reabsorption of salt and water leading to increased blood volume and hence increased BP. There is also increased secretion of vasopressin leading to water retention and vasoconstriction. In addition, altered activity of RAAS leads to increased sympathetic activity.

A. DOCA-salt rats

Mineralocorticoid induces hypertension by causing increase in plasma and extracellular volume. Salt loading and unilateral nephrectomy in rats further increases the hypertensive effect. The administration of DOCA, in combination with a high salt diet and unilateral nephrectomy induces a low renin form of hypertension, which can be opposed to the other artificial model, where renin level is high.[14]

Male Sprague Dawley rats (250 to 300 g) are anesthetized with ether. The left kidney is removed through a flank incision. DOCA (20 mg/kg) is dissolved in olive oil and injected subcutaneously to rats, twice weekly for four weeks. Drinking water is replaced with 1% NaCl solution. Blood pressure starts to rise after 1 week and systolic value reaches around 160 to 180 mm Hg after 4 weeks. DOCA pellets or implants in silastic devices can also be used instead of repeated injections. Test drug is administered orally for one month. Blood pressure is measured before and after the administration of the test drug and their values are compared to evaluate the antihypertensive effect.

End organ damage:. The animals are sacrificed and their hearts weighed. Renal changes are seen with proteinuria and glomerulosclerosis. This rat model also demonstrates endothelium dependent relaxations.

5. Psychogenic Hypertension

It has been reported that elevation of BP resulting from repeated exposure to stressful situation may lead to a state of persistent hypertension. Other types of stress that may be applied include emotional stimuli, psychosocial stress, immobilization stress and electric stimuli. However, the degree and stability of hypertension may not be comparable to other types of hypertension. The stress-induced hypertension is associated with either normal or suppressed PRA values, suggesting that the hypertension in these animals is not renin-dependent. As stress plays an important part in development of human hypertension, this model is very frequently used to study the pathophysiology of hypertension.

Air-jet stimulation-induced hypertension

Borderline hypertensive rats (BHR) are useful for psychogenic hypertension. BHRs are exposed to daily sessions of either short (20 min) or long (120 min) duration air-jet stimulation. BP is monitored at regular intervals using tail cuff method. It is generally observed that the BHR develop hypertension within 2 weeks in comparison to home cage controls. Animals exposed to 120 min stress sessions have significantly higher systolic BP relative to the 20 minute group. Its deleterious effects depend on the critical period of exposure, duration and type, as all these factors may alter functions of the basic auto-regulatory stress response components in the hypothalamic-pituitary-adrenal axis, sympathoadrenal medullar system, rennin-angiotensin-aldosterone system (RAAS) and sympathetic nervous system.[15]

6. Genetic Hypertension

A. Salt-sensitive Dahl rats

The salt-sensitive Dahl rats develop severe and fatal hypertension when fed high salt diets, whereas salt resistance Dahl rats do not develop such severe hypertension upon salt loading.[13] Also when fed normal salt diets, the salt sensitive rats become hypertensive, demonstrating that this is a model of genetic hypertension, with the extra feature of salt sensitivity.[14]

Sprague Dawley rats (250 to 300 g) are used for this study. The drinking water is replaced with 8% NaCl saline solution. High Dahl salt diet is prepared in the laboratory by mixing salt with the regular diet. The animals are fed the prepared diet and 8% NaCl solution ad libitum. The test group rats are administered the drug orally for 1 month. Blood pressure changes are recorded. After the completion of the experimental duration, animals of both groups (test and sham control) are sacrificed. Their hearts are removed and total cardiac mass, weight of left and right ventricle is measured and compared. Upon salt feeding (8% NaCl), blood pressure rises steeply, to levels slightly higher than found in spontaneously hypertensive rats (upto 32%). The ability of the test drug to reverse these changes is studied.

End organ damage: Cardiac failure occurs at 4 to 5 months of age in the salt sensitive Dahl rats. Also, renal changes are more severe than spontaneously hypertensive rats, with severe early proteinuria. In this model endothelium dependent relaxations are found to be impaired.

B. Spontaneously hypertensive rats (SHR)
By breeding a strain of spontaneously hypertensive Wistar rats with a female having slightly raised blood pressure, Okamoto and Aoki obtained a strain of rats with spontaneous hypertension, the SHR.[17] Blood pressure rises around 5 to 6 weeks of age and steadily increases to reach systolic blood pressure of 180 to 200 mm Hg. The SHR develop many features of hypertensive end organ damage including cardiac hypertrophy, cardiac failure and renal dysfunction. However, they do not exhibit gross vascular problems. Apart from depressed endothelium dependent relaxations, they have no tendency to develop strokes, and do not develop macroscopic atherosclerosis or vascular thrombosis. The SHR stroke prone (SHR-SP) is a further developed substrain, with even higher levels of blood pressure, and a strong tendency to die from stroke.[18] The SHR have been widely used to evaluate genetic factors in hypertension, yielding a wide variety of genes that seem to co-segregate in various crosses which is not always confirmed.[19]

End organ damage : The untreated SHR exhibit cardiac hypertrophy and develop heart failure between the age of 18 to 24 months. However, not all rats exhibit signs of heart failure after 24 months so that despite the uniformity of the model, individual differences are seen. Impaired endothelium dependent relaxations have been consistently found, although rats until 13 to 15 weeks of age may sometimes have normal endothelium dependent relaxation. Renal damage has also been found in older SHRs. Comparisons between the sham rats (untreated) and treated rats are made on the basis of above-mentioned parameters as well as blood pressure recordings. The ability of the test drug to reverse/delay the changes seen in sham control group is studied and antihypertensive potential of test drug is evaluated.

Methods to measure BP in rats

A. Tail cuff method in rats
The indirect tail cuff method allows the measurement of blood pressure without any surgical procedure. The method is analogous to sphygmomanometry in humans. The indirect tail cuff method is widely used to evaluate the influence of antihypertensive drugs in spontaneously and experimentally induced hypertensive rats.

Charles River Male Spontaneously hypertensive rats (300 to 350 g) are anesthetized with 0.8 ml of 4% chloralhydrate solution. Both kidneys are exposed. A silver clip (0.2 mm diameter) is placed into both renal arteries, kidneys are reposed and wound is closed by suture. After 5 to 6 weeks, operated animals attain renal hypertension with systolic blood pressure of 170 to 200 mm Hg. To measure blood pressure, a tubular inflatable cuff is placed around the base of the tail and a pizoelectric pulse detector is positioned distal to the cuff. The cuff is inflated well above suspected systolic blood pressure until the pulse is obliterated. Thereafter, pressure in the cuff is slowly released and as the pressure reaches the systolic blood pressure, the pulse reappears which is detected and subsequently recorded on a polygraph. The test substance is administered intraperitoneally once a day over a period of 5 days. Blood pressure and heart rate are measured (predose and 2 h post-drug) at days 1, 3 and 5. Percent decrease in systolic blood pressure after administration of the test drug and the duration of effect is determined.[20] Statistical significance is assessed by the Student's t-test. Scores for percentage decrease in systolic blood pressure and for the duration of the effect are allotted.

B. Indwelling catheter for measurement of blood pressure in conscious rats

The method allows direct measurement of blood pressure in conscious rats eliminating the influence of anesthesia on cardiovascular regulation. 7 cm long cannula are prepared by cutting PE 10 and PE 20 tubing respectively. A stylet wire is inserted into the PE 10 tubing and PE 20 tubing is also slipped over the stylet wire. The tube ends are heated in a current of hot air and fused together. Using ridges the cannula is anchored to the animals tissue. In order to make a ridge, the stylet wire is left inside the cannula and the cannula is heated in a jet of hot air. When the polyethylene at the point of heating becomes soft, the cannula is pressed slightly and the ridge is formed.

Male Sprague Dawley rats weighing 300 g are anesthetized with pentobarbitone sodium (45 mg/kg, intraperitoneally). Through a midline incision, the abdominal aorta is exposed, a trocar is passed through the psoas muscles adjacent to the segment of the aorta. Then the cannula is inserted into the trocar and the trocar is withdrawn from the body. The end of the cannula thus comes out from the neck, being anchored by silk sutures to the neck skin and to the psoas muscle. The cannula is filled with heparin solution and the end which is projecting out from the neck skin, is blocked with a tight fitting stainless steel needle. The other end of the cannula is implanted into the aorta. The aorta is wiped with cotton tipped applicator stick over the bifurcation, occluded above this segment and punctured with a bent 27 gauge hypodermic needle. The tip of the PE 10 catheter is inserted through the needle and advanced up the aorta. The intestines are replaced and wounds sutured. The rats are allowed to recover for one week.

After 1 week the occluding stainless steel needle is removed and the cannula is flushed with heparin solution. To restrict the movement of the rat, it is placed in a small cage. The cannula is connected to a Statham P 23 Db pressure transducer and blood pressure is recorded on a polygraph.[21] Test drugs are administered either subcutaneously or orally. Recordings are taken before and after administration of the drug over a period of 1 h. Changes of blood pressure are measured and the maximal changes of each group are averaged and compared with the standard.

Dog Models of Hypertension

1. Chronic renal hypertension

Dogs (8 to 12 kg) are anesthetized intravenously with 15 mg/kg thiopental. Midline abdominal incision is made, one kidney is exposed and wrapped in cellophane and then replaced. The contralateral kidney is exposed and artery, vein and ureter are ligated and kidney is removed. The abdomen is then closed and sutured back. After six weeks of surgery, blood pressure is measured. Blood pressure is recorded either by indirect tail cuff method or by direct measurement through the carotid artery. Test drugs are administered for 5 days. On day 1 readings are taken every 2 h, just before, and 2 and 4 h after oral treatment. On day 3 and 5 blood pressure is recorded before, 2 and 4 h after drug treatment.

The starting value is the average of the 2 readings before application of the drug. Subsequent readings are subtracted from this value and recorded as fall of blood pressure at the various recording times.[22-24]

2. Neurogenic hypertension

Baroreceptors situated in the carotid sinus and aortic arch play an important part in the regulation of blood pressure. Stimulation of the afferent buffer fibers exerts an inhibitory influence on the vasomotor center. A persistent rise in blood pressure is observed on sectioning the baroreceptors. Thus, by this procedure acute neurogenic hypertension is induced in dogs.

Adult dogs (10 to 15 kg) are anesthetized using 15 mg/kg thiopental, 200 mg/kg sodium barbital and 60 mg/kg sodium pentobarbital.[25] Femoral vein is cannulated for the administration of test compounds. Left ventricular pressure and dP/dt are recorded through common carotid artery using Millar microtip pressure transducer. P_{max} and cardiac output are also calculated. The carotid sinus nerves are isolated, ligated and sectioned and a bilateral vagotomy is performed to induce neurogenic hypertension. After 30 min equilibration period, a bolus of test compound is administered by intravenous route. Heart rate, arterial pressure, left ventricular pressure, P_{max} and dP/dt are monitored for 90 min. Changes in cardiovascular parameters are expressed as percentage of the values before and after administration of the drug.[26]

Monkey Model of Hypertension

1. *Renin inhibition in monkeys*

Blood pressure is mainly regulated by the renin angiotensin system and can be influenced by several ways including inhibition of renin. Renin is an aspartyl protease that hydrolyses angiotensinogen to release angiotensin I. Angiotensin I is subsequently converted to angiotensin II by angiotensin converting enzyme. Renin inhibitors developed so far have a high specificity for primate renin and cause only weak inhibition of renin in subprimate species. This suggests that most common laboratory animals such as rats and dogs are not suitable for *in vivo* evaluation of renin inhibitors.

Marmosets (Callithrix jacchus) of 300 to 400 g are fed pellet diet supplemented with fruits. The animals are anesthetized two days prior to the experiment and catheters are implanted in the femoral artery for measurement of blood pressure. Lateral tail vein is cannulated for the administration of test compounds. Furosemide (5 mg/kg) is injected intravenously 30 min before the experiment in order to stimulate renin release. During the experiment, the marmosets are sedated with diazepam (0.3 mg/kg, intraperitoneally) and kept in restraining boxes. Mean blood pressure is recorded continuously, and heart rate is measured at fixed intervals. The test compound and standard drug are injected by intravenous infusion or administered orally. Blood pressure is recorded after 30 min of intravenous infusion. Changes from pretreatment values after various doses of drug are compared. Dose-response curves can be established.[27]

Transgenic Models

1. *Transgenic rats overexpressing the mouse Ren-2 gene {TGR (mRen 2) 27}*

The introduction and overexpression of the mouse Ren-2 gene in the rat leads to severe hypertension, lethal in the homozygous rats. Two important features characterize this rat model: firstly, it is genetic, inherited form of hypertension where the single genetic event is known, and secondly, despite the known genetic alteration, the exact mechanism underlying hypertension remains elusive. In this rat hypertension, is related to an increased renin activity. The severity of hypertension depends partly upon the genetic background of the rats used for breeding the TGR (mRen2) 27. An accelerated and malignant type of hypertension occurs when these rats are bred with Sprague Dawley rats.[28]

End organ damage: 70% of the heterozygous rats survive at least until the age of 5 months. Before that age they develop marked cardiac hypertrophy and impairment of endothelium dependent relaxations.

The ability to specifically introduce genetic constructs and thereby breed transgenic animals, has opened new possibilities for hypertension research.[29] The transgenic rat that was obtained after introduction of the entire mouse Ren2d gene.[30] In this hypertensive model, the hypertension and ensuing end organ damage depends upon increased local angiotensin II formation and is exquisitely sensitive to renin angiotensin system (RAS) inhibition. Other transgenic models have been obtained where the introduction of both renin and human angiotensinogen increases blood pressure in mice and rats.[31]

In the knockout models, genes for ANF and NO-synthase have been knocked out. The ANF knockout rats resulted in salt sensitive hypertension whereas the knockout of the type A receptor for ANF resulted in salt independent hypertension in rats. These models can be used to screen various anti-hypertensive agents.

DISCUSSION AND CONCLUSION

A brief overview of the most widely used animal model strains, and their characteristics has been provided. The most important lesson from a direct comparison of these animal models is that despite the well-known heterogeneity of hypertension, the outcome of hypertension can be similar in some respects: rats from all models exhibit cardiac hypertrophy and all demonstrate impaired endothelin dependent relaxations of isolated arteries. However, the most severe form of end organ damage such as heart failure, stroke and kidney failure occurs in only a subset of hypertensive rats.

Not all classes of antihypertensives are equally effective in all rat models of hypertension: endothelin receptor antagonists are not effective in SHR, but have beneficial effects in DOCA-salt model.

Thus, it seems that rat models of hypertension mainly share high blood pressure, but otherwise display a wide variety of biochemical disturbances, with equally varying course and prognosis. The course and prognosis seem to depend on three main factors:

1. The mechanical stress which is the absolute level of blood pressure, and when above a certain threshold will always cause severe organ damage.
2. The biochemical stress which is an important modifier of the course of hypertension.
3. The ability to recruit coping or adaptive mechanisms.

These models of hypertension provide ample opportunity not only to investigate the mechanisms involved in the pathogenesis of hypertension, but also to learn about the critical balance between stress and coping which eventually determines prognosis.

Summary

In vitro models	*In vivo models*					
	Rat Models					
	Reno-vascular induced	*Neurogenic induced*	*Diet induced*	*Endocrine induced*	*Psychogenic*	*Genetically induced*
Endothelin receptor antagonism in porcine isolated hearts	Two-kidney one clip (Goldblatt hypertension, 2K1C)	Blood pressure in pithed rats	Fructose induced	DOCA-salt rats	Air-jet stimulation induced hypertension	Salt-sensitive Dahl rats
Monocrotaline induced pulmonary hypertension	Chronic renal hypertension in rats (1-kidney-1-clip method)		Increased salt induced			Spontaneously hypertensive rats (SHR)
	Chronic renal hypertension in rats (Two kidney two clip (2K2C) method					
	Dog model of hypertension					
	• Chronic renal hypertension • Neurogenic hypertension					
	Monkey model of hypertension					
	• Renin inhibition in monkeys					
	Transgenic model of hypertension					
	• Transgenic rats overexpressing the mouse Ren-2 gene [TGR (mRen 2) 27]					

REFERENCES

1. Calo G, Gratton JP, Orleans-Juste P, et al. Pharmacology of endothelins: vascular preparations for studying ETA and ETB receptors. Moll Cell Biochem 1996;154:31-7.
2. Altiere RJ, McIntyre MJ, Petrenka J, et al. Altered pulmonary vascular smooth muscle responsiveness in monocrotaline-induced pulmonary hypertension. J Pharmacol Exp Ther 1986;236:390-5.
3. Goldbatt H, Lynch J, Hanzal RF, et al. Studies on experimental hypertension & the production of persistent elevation of systolic blood pressure by means of renal ischemia. J Exp Med 1934;59:347-79.
4. Okakomoto AK. Development of a strain of spontaneously hypertensive rat. Jap Circ J 1963;27:282-93.
5. Baura ALA, Green AF. Antihypertensive agents. In: Laurence DR, Bacharach AL, ed. Evaluation of drug activities: Pharmacometrics. London & New York: Academic Press, 1964:431-6.
6. Cerqua S, Samaan A. Cure of experimental renal hypertension. Clin Sci 1939;40:113-8.
7. Swales JD, Tange JD. The influence of acute sodium depletion on experimental hypertension in the rat. J Lab Clin Med 1971;78:369-79.
8. Brunner HR, Kirshman JD, Sealey JE. Hypertension of renal origin: evidence for two different mechanisms. Science 1971;174:1344-6.
9. Leite R, Salgado MCO. Increased vascular formation of angiotensin II in one kidney one clip hypertension. Hypertension 1992;19:575-81.

10. Badyal DK, Lata H, Dadhich AP. Animal models of hypertension and effect of drugs. Indian J Pharmaco 2003;35:349-62.
11. Curtis MJ, Mc Leod BA, Walker MJA. An improved pithed rat preparation: the actions of the optical enatiomers of verapamil. Asia Pacific J Pharmacol 1986;1:73-8.
12. Brands MW, Hildebrandt DA, Mizelle HL, et al. Sustained hyperinsulinemia increases arterial pressure in conscious rats. Am J Physiol 1991;260:R764-8.
13. Meneely GR, Ball COT. Experimental epidemiology of chronic sodium chloride toxicity and the protective effect of potassium chloride. Am J Med 1958;25:713-25.
14. Rapp JP. Dahl salt susceptible and salt resistant rats. Hypertension 1982;4:753-63.
15. Dornas WC, Silva ME. Animal models for the study of arterial hypertension. J Biosci 2011;36:731-7.
16. Gomez-Sanchez EP, Zhou M, Gomez-Sanchez CE. Mineralocorticoids, salt and high blood pressure. Steroids 1996;61:184-8.
17. Okamoto AK. Development of a strain of spontaneously hypertensive rat. Jap Circ J 1963;27:282-93.
18. Yamori Y. Development of spontaneously hypertensive rat (SHR) the stroke prone hypertensive SHR (SHRSP) and their various substrain models for hypertension related cardiovascular diseases. In: Ganten D, de Jong W, volume eds. Birkenhager WH, Reid JT, series eds. Handbook of Hypertension, Experimental and Genetic models of Hypertension. Amsterdam: Elsevier Press, 1994:26-9.
19. Kreutz R, Struk B, Rubatta S. Role of alpha, beta and gamma subunits of epithelial sodium channels in a model of polygenic hypertension. Hypertension 1997;29:131-6.
20. Bunag RD, Mc Cubbin JW, Page IH. Lack of correlation between direct and indirect measurement of arterial pressure in unanesthetized rats. Cardiovasc Res 1971;5:24-51.
21. Akrawi SH, Wiedlund PJ. Method for chronic portal vein infusion in unrestrained rats. J Pharmacol Meth 1987;17:67-74.
22. Abrams M, Sobin S. Latex rubber capsule for producing hypertension in rats by perinephritis. Proc Soc Exp Biol Med 1947;64:412-6.
23. Gollman A. A simplified procedure for inducing chronic renal hypertension in the mammal. Proc Soc Exp Biol Med 1944;57:102-4.
24. Grimson KS. The sympathetic nervous system in neurogenic and renal hypertension. Arch Surg Chicargo 1941;43:284-305.
25. Angell James JE. Neurogenic hypertension in the rabbit. In De Jong, ed. Handbook of Hypertension: Experimental and Genetic Models of Hypertension. Elsevier Science Press, 1990;4:364-97.
26. Evans DB, Cornette JC, Sawyer TK, et al. Substrate specificity and inhibitor structure-activity relationships of recombinant human renin: implications in the in vivo evaluation of renin inhibitors. Biotechnol Appl Biochem 1990;12:161-75.
27. Franz WM, Muller OJ, Hartong R. Transgenic animal models: new avenues in cardiovascular physiology. J Mol Med 1997;75:115-29.
28. Whitworth CE, Fleming S, Cumming AD. Spontaneous development of malignant phase hypertension in transgenic Ren 2 rats. Kidney Int 1994;46:1528-32.
29. Mullins JJ, Peters J, Ganten D. Fulminant hypertension in transgenic animals harboring the mouse Ren 2 gene. Nature 1990;344:541-4.
30. Okhubo H, Kawakami H, Kakehi Y. Generation of transgenic mice with elevated blood pressure by introduction of the rat renin and angiotensin enzymes. Proc Nat Acad Sci 1990;87:5153-7.
31. Bohlender J, Fukamizu A, Lippoldt A. High human renin hypertension in transgenic rats. Hypertension 1997;29:428-34.

CHAPTER

17

Antiglaucoma Agents

INTRODUCTION

Glaucoma is a progressive optic neuropathy characterized by visual field changes and cupping of optic disc. Elevated intraocular pressure (IOP) is one of the important risk factor. The rise in IOP is due to the increase in aqueous formation, low rate of outflow or a raised pressure in the episcleral veins. An obstruction to the circulation of the aqueous at the pupil or to its drainage through the angle of the anterior chamber causes glaucoma. The normal IOP of an individual ranges from 10-20 mm Hg and can rise up to 60 mm of Hg in glaucoma patients. Raised IOP of this magnitude can result in loss of vision. Optic nerve axons of the eyeball become compressed at the optic disc due to elevated IOP. This compression probably blocks the axonal flow of cytoplasm from the neuronal cell bodies in the retina to the extended optic nerve fibers entering the brain. It results in lack of nutrition of fibers and ultimately causes death of the neurons. Compression of retinal artery may increase the neuronal damage due to reduction in retinal nutrition.[1]

The global estimate of blindness was over 37 million with glaucoma accounting for slightly more than 12% of the blind patients worldwide as per WHO report in 2005.[2] In 2013, the number of people, in the age range of 40–80 years, with glaucoma worldwide was estimated to be 64.3 million, increasing to 76.0 million in 2020 and 111.8 million in 2040.[3] India has a high burden of blind (23.5%) in the world and 13% of the global blindness due to glaucoma is in India. Many population based surveys carried out in the west and in Asia have shown that glaucoma remains undetected in nearly 50% of the cases and hence glaucoma-related blindness and disability is often underestimated.[4,5]

Glaucoma is generally classified as: (i) primary (ii) developmental and (iii) secondary. The commonest form of glaucoma is primary glaucoma; it can be open angle glaucoma or angle closure glaucoma. In primary open angle glaucoma (POAG) the angle of the anterior chamber is always open, at all stages of disease, and aqueous has access to the outflow channels at all times, whether the tension is normal or elevated. There is increased resistance to outflow in the corneoscleral meshwork, whereas in primary angle closure glaucoma no abnormal resistance to outflow in the corneoscleral meshwork is observed. The sole cause of elevated tension is closure of the angle. The iris obstructs the access of aqueous humor to the outflow channels (Fig. 17.1).

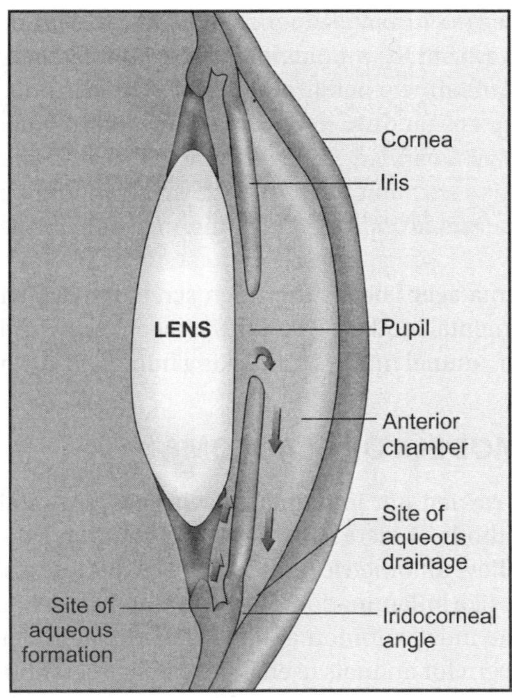

Figure 17.1: Pathway of aqueous flow (*For color version see Plate 21*)

Prompt and effective management of glaucoma is necessary to reduce the incidence of cases of bilateral blindness due to progressive glaucoma. Biological revolution in medicine has provided new avenues for therapeutic intervention. Newer and innovative treatment strategies are being considered for the control of elevated IOP by the use of synthetic and herbal drugs in glaucoma.

The primary goal in the management of glaucoma is to lower IOP below 20 mm Hg in the patients with mild changes in the optic disc and below 15 mm Hg in the patients with more severe changes. Surgical intervention aiming at increasing the aqueous humor outflow is undertaken when IOP remains uncontrolled even with multiple drug therapy.

Tables 17.1 and 17.2 show the groups/drugs widely used in the treatment of glaucoma.

Table 17.1: Topical drugs

Group of drugs	*Formulations*
Cholinergic agonists	Pilocarpine, carbechol, physostigmine
Adrenergic agonists	Forskolin, isoproterenol, salbutamol, epinephrine, brimonidine
Adrenergic antagonists	Timolol, Levobunolol, betaxolol, atenolol, metipranolol
Prostaglandin analogues	Latanoprost, Unoprostone, travoprost, bimatoprost
Carbonic anhydrase inhibitors	Trifluoromethazolamide, aminozolamide, dorzolamide, brinzolamide

Table 17.2: Systemic drugs

Group of drugs	*Formulations*
Carbonic anhydrase inhibitor	Acetazolamide, methazolamide, dichlorphenamide
Hyperosmotic agents	Glycerol, mannitol
Miscellaneous	Cannabinoids, prostaglandins, ACE inhibitors, melatonin, calcium channel blockers, haloperidol, etc.

A potential antiglaucoma agent needs thorough screening, which can be done in various *in vitro* and *in vivo* experimental models. To study the mechanism of glaucoma and the efficacy of the antiglaucoma agent, animal models mimicking human forms of glaucoma are used.

EXPERIMENTAL MODELS OF GLAUCOMA

Studies of glaucoma are carried out in animals having close resemblance of eye structures with human eye. The methods of increasing the IOP should be easy to carry out, produce a reliable increase in IOP, allow tonometric monitoring in experimental animals, and minimize secondary ocular changes like inflammation. Several animal models are used for the screening of IOP lowering drugs. The most common and feasible model under present circumstances, when there is a great concern for animals used in research, is a rabbit model. The surface area and other structures of the eye of a rabbit resemble human eye and they can be housed and handled easily.

Intraocular pressure is measured by tonometery using methods such as:

1. Schiotz method: The eyes are anesthetized and then schiotz tonometer, a small handy instrument is placed on the cornea and pressed lightly to measure the pressure (Fig. 17.2).
2. Applanation method: A flouresein-stained strip is touched to the side of the eye that helps in the examination. The dye is washed out along with the lacrimation. The instrument is fitted on a slit lamp. The probe of the tonometer is made to touch the cornea by moving the instrument forward towards the eye of the patient (Fig. 17.3).
3. Non-contact method: The IOP is measured without any contact of the tonometer to the eye. A puff of air is released when the eye is focused which indents the eye. The force required for indenting the eye is measured (Fig. 17.4).

   The IOP is elevated beyond the limits by the following methods:

   i. Ocular injections
   ii. Reducing the serum osmolarity
   iii. Application of lasers and
   iv. Steroids.

Ocular Injections

There are reports on the production of glaucoma in the experimental animals by injections of a variety of agents like alpha chymotrypsin into the posterior chamber and, methylcellulose, autologous ghost red blood cells, kaolin, prostaglandin, alkali into the anterior chamber of eye which results in elevated IOP.

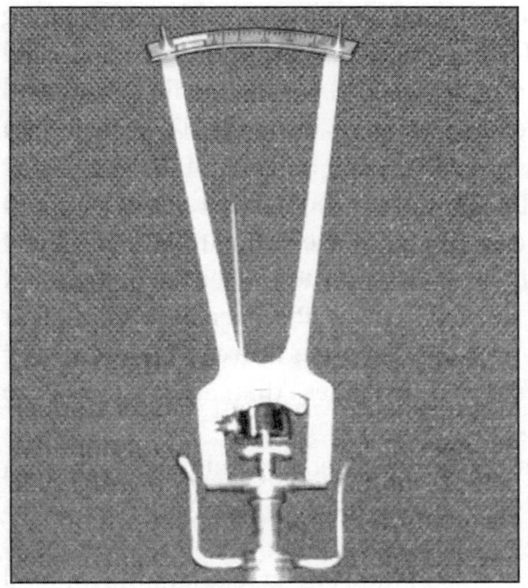

Figure 17.2: Shiotz tonometer
(*For color version see plate 21*)

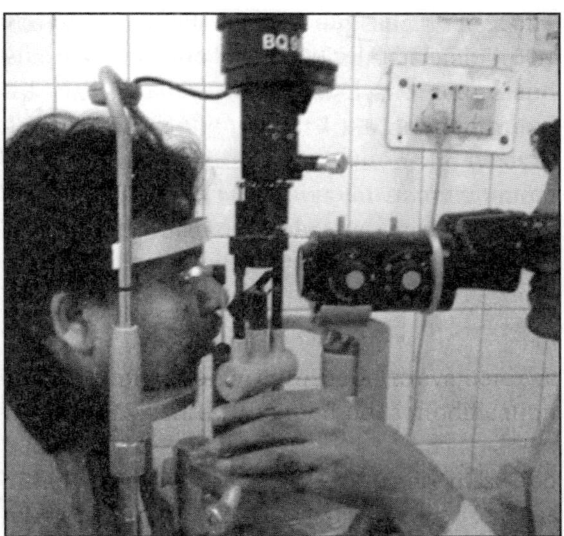

Figure 17.3: Goldman applanation tonometer
(*For color version see Plate 21*)

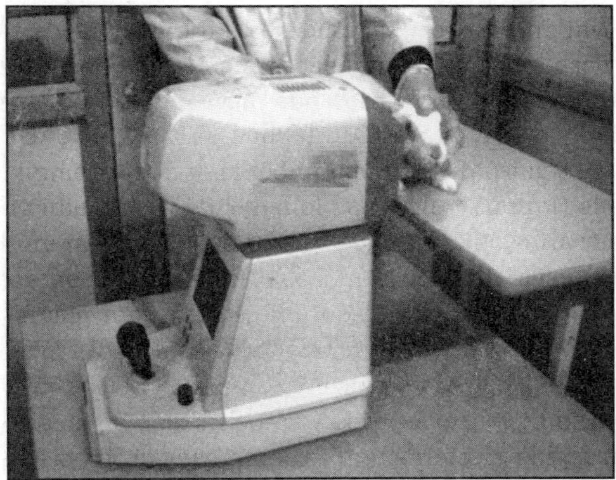

Figure 17.4: Noncontact tonometer
(*For color version see Plate 21*)

Alpha Chymotrypsin-induced Experimental Glaucoma

Alpha chymotrypsin is a proteolytic enzyme secreted by pancreas. It is specific for peptide bonds containing uncharged amino acid residues. Intravitreal injection of alpha chymotrypsin into owl monkeys and rabbits elevates the ocular pressure by 5 to more than 25 mm Hg within 2 to 3 days and suggests that rise in IOP is due to predominant changes in trabecular meshwork caused by α-chymotrypsin. The proteolytic action of α-chymotrypsin on zonular material and the debris of the tissue thus formed blocks the aqueous outflow channels and elevates the IOP. Alpha chymotrypsin induces sustained rise in intraocular pressure for several weeks.[6-8]

Procedure: Sears and Sears established this chronic model of glaucoma.[7] Rabbits of 1.5-2 kg body weight under nembutal anesthesia are used. One of the eyes is anesthetized with local anesthetic 2% xylocaine. The eyeball is fixed by forceps, and a 30 G sterile needle, connected with a tubing to a 1 ml Hamilton syringe, is inserted carefully for intravitreal injection (via limbus). Two minutes after injection, the needle is removed and 2-3 drops of any antibiotic solution are instilled into the eyes to prevent infection. One hundred and fifty units of alpha chymotrypsin dissolved in sterile saline (0.5 ml) are carefully injected into the posterior chamber so that the needle does not damage the lens. Care is taken to prevent the contact of alpha chymotrypsin with the corneal stroma. After two days, the IOP is measured at regular intervals. Stable rise in IOP is achieved within 15 days. A sustained pressure elevation, ranging from 28-45 mm Hg, is observed till 50 weeks. Rabbits showing IOP less than 30 mm of Hg, are excluded from the experiment.

To evaluate antiglaucoma activity, the test agent is administered topically or orally in a suitable formulation once the glaucoma is established (stable IOP). The topical formulations or vehicle are instilled onto the *cul de sac* of one eye (treated eye) and the contralateral eye (control) respectively. The IOP is measured prior to drug instillation and at regular time interval after instilling the eye drops. Change in IOP between the two eyes can be compared to see the potential of the agent. IOP changes can also be calculated.[9]

Chronic Rat Model of Glaucoma

Morrison, et al. have developed a chronic rat model of glaucoma.[10] The aqueous humor escapes the eye through trabecular meshwork, Schlemm's canal and into a vascular plexus circling the limbus. This plexus is connected to the general circulation through several episcleral veins. Injecting mild sclerosants (hypertonic saline) through one of these veins results in the scarring of trabecular meshwork by which decrease in the outflow and increase in the IOP occur.

Procedure: Male Brown Norway rats (*Rattus norvegicus*) of 300 to 400 g weight range are kept in light for minimum 3 days. Rats are anesthetized by intraperitoneal injection of 1.0 ml/kg solution containing 5 ml ketamine (100 mg/ml), 2.5 ml xylazine (20 mg/ml), 1 ml acepromazine (10 mg/ml) and 0.5 ml sterile water. A small propylene ring (5.5 mm diameter) is placed around the globe, covering the equator. The ring has a gap of 1.00 mm in its circumference that is adjusted in such a manner that the passage of one radial aqueous vein in the superior quadrant remains unobstructed. The ring occludes the other aqueous veins and the sclerosing agent (hypertonic saline) is infused to the limbus. The aqueous vein is exposed by incising the conjunctiva. A volume of 50 μl microfiltered 1.75 M hypertonic saline solution is injected into the limbal vascular plexus using a fabricated microneedle assembly. A force sufficient enough to blanch the limbal artery is used for injection. The ring is removed after injecting the saline. Polysporin ointment is applied to the eye and the animals are observed till they recover from anesthesia. Baseline measurements of IOP are taken prior to the injection of saline. Animals have been routinely handled in order to get a reproductive baseline IOP. Following injections of hypertonic saline the IOP is measured twice a week. Elevation of IOP is determined by calculating the difference between the IOP of injected and noninjected eye. Mean IOP elevation ranged from 7-28 mm Hg.[10]

The model is anatomically relevant to the primate model. Prominent globes of the rats and their docile nature helps in measuring the IOP while the animals are awake.

Methylcellulose Induced Glaucoma

Glaucoma can be induced by injecting 0.5-4% methylcellulose in the anterior chamber of animals like minipigs and rabbits.[11-13] Methylcellulose (0.5%) made in 0.9% saline, free of air bubbles is injected into the anterior chamber of rabbit eyes following evacuation of the aqueous humor. The volume of the methylcellulose is equal to the volume of aqueous humor removed (150 µl to 190 µl). Same needle of 0.032 cm diameter is used for both evacuation and refilling along with a three-way stopcock. The needle is inserted into the anterior chamber just above the aperture of iris and aqueous humor is evacuated slowly. In this model the IOP increases from 20 to approximately 30 mm Hg in next 2 hours.[12] Zhu and Cai produced a reliable and about 8 weeks of intraocular hypertension by a series of four intra-anterior chamber injections of 1 or 2% methylcellulose in rabbits.[11]

Autologous Ghost Red Blood Cells Induced Glaucoma

Fixed red blood cells or fixed ghost red blood cells (GBCs) when injected in the anterior chamber of rabbits and monkeys produce chronic glaucoma. GBCs have a relatively rigid membrane and do not possess the flexibility by which the normal red blood cells exit the meshwork. Upon infusion, the GBCs cause trabecular obstruction in eyes with intraocular hemorrhage resulting in secondary glaucoma. IOP elevation lasts in rabbits from 7 to 36 days and in monkeys 2 to 42 days. The model produces increase in IOP easily and without intraocular inflammation.[14]

Hyaluronic Acid Induced Glaucoma

Chronic intracameral administration of hyaluronic acid (HA) in rats induced significant histologic alterations and decreased electroretinographic activity in the retina and optic nerve showing similarity with some characteristics of open angle glaucoma. Injection of hyaluronic acid in the anterior chamber of rabbits and owls monkeys significantly raised the IOP though the effect was short lived being 70 and 24 hours post injection in rabbits and owl monkeys respectively.[15]

Single administration of HA injection induced and maintained the rise in IOP for 8 days. However, injections administered every week induced a sustained elevation of intra ocular pressure for 10 weeks.

Procedure: Male Wistar rats of about 200 $\pm$ 40 g weight are kept in controlled humidity and 21°C temperature, and 12 h day: 12 h night cycle. Rats are anesthetized with intraperitoneally administered mixture of ketamine hydrochloride (50 mg/kg) and xylazine hydrochloride (0.5 mg/kg). Hyaluronic acid (25 µl) is injected into one eye of anesthetized rats and an equal volume of vehicle is injected in the contralateral eye once a week.

Reduced Serum Osmolarity

The animals are subjected to forced ingestion of water or intravenous injections of 5% glucose solution or hypertonic saline.[8,16-18] This reduces the serum osmolarity and a temporary change in the IOP is observed.

Water-loaded Rabbit Model of Glaucoma

This acute model of glaucoma is widely used and established by Sugiyama, et al.[16] Changes in IOP are temporary. This model minimizes the mechanical trauma that can alter the blood aqueous barrier.

Procedure: Albino rabbits of 1.5-2 kg body weight of either sex are required for this model. They are kept fasting overnight and on the day of experiment are anesthetized using 30 mg/kg b.w. of sodium pentobarbitone, 45 minutes before the experiment. Ten minutes before the water loading of the animals, the anesthesia maintenance doses of 4 mg/kg sodium pentobarbitone is administered via the marginal ear vein. The baseline IOP is measured under corneal anesthesia by instilling 2 drops of xylocaine (4%) three times at two minutes interval. Tap water 100 ml/kg is administered orally through an intragastric infant feeding tube within 30 sec. The IOP is measured at baseline 15, 30, 45 and 60 minutes after the water loading till the IOP reaches the baseline values. For evaluating the antiglaucoma activity of an agent, it is administered in the form of eyedrops to one of the eyes of the water-loaded animal, while the vehicle is instilled in the contralateral eye (control). The difference in IOP is observed in the two eyes at various time intervals. Any significant modulation shows the potential of the drug for lowering IOP.

Santafe et al. measured the effect of topical diltiazem in rabbits loaded with 60 ml/kg water.[17]

IOP Recovery Model

This rabbit model for experimental glaucoma has been used by several researchers.[9,19] The intravenous injection of hypertonic saline in the marginal ear vein results in the fall of IOP, which comes back to normal within 2 h. If the drug used is a potential antiglaucoma agent, it will extend the time required for the recovery of normotensive pressure.

Procedure: New Zealand white normotensive rabbits of 2.5-3.0 kg weight range are used for this method. By using an infusion pump, 10% sodium chloride solution (10 ml) is infused through the ear marginal vein, with a flow rate of 1 ml/min. The drug is instilled in the form of eyedrops on to the *cul de sac* of the right eye (treated eye) and vehicle on to the left eye (control eye), immediately after the infusion of hypertonic saline. IOP is measured at 40 and 20 minutes prior to instilling the eyedrops as baseline and then at 0, 20, 40, 60, and 80 minutes thereafter at 20 minutes interval till the baseline values are obtained.

The relative percents of IOP ($IOP_t\%$) can be calculated by the following equations:[9]

$IOP_t\% = (IOP_t/IOP_{-40}) \times 100\%$

$IOP_t\%$: Relative percent of IOP at time t

$\Delta IOP_t\%$: Difference of $IOP_t\%$ between treated and controlled eyes

Perfused Excised Eye Model System

Novel glaucoma therapy includes modulation of cytoskeleton protein actin and tubulin in the trabecular meshwork. Due to induced changes in cell shape and attachment, cytoskeleton of aqueous outflow pathway cells can influence aqueous humor outflow function.

Outflow facility measurement: Freshly excised and chilled porcine eyes are perfused within 4 h. Standard constant pressure perfusion technique is followed using a Grant stainless steel corneal fitting. For the prevention of artificial deepening of the anterior chamber, radial iridotomy is done. Dulbecco's phosphate-buffered saline (DPBS) solution with 0.68 mM $CaCl_2$ supplemented with 5.5 mM D-Glucose is used as perfusion medium. All the solutions are filtered through 0.2 mm filter. The eyes are perfused at 15 mm Hg and 25°C for 1 hour to achieve a steady state flow value and the baseline facility is recorded. The corneal fitting is removed and the anterior chamber is emptied with a cellulose sponge and refilled with the similar perfusion medium containing the test drug. Controls are kept as sham manipulated and receive only the medium for perfusion and drug vehicle. Drug and control solutions are then perfused for the remainder of the experiment.[20] Outflow facilities of experimental and control eyes are measured hourly for 5 hours.[21] Drug effects are expressed as the percentage change in the outflow facility from the baseline value in the experimental eye minus the percentage change in the control eye.

Application of Lasers

Chronic experimental models are produced using laser treatment. Researchers have successfully induced glaucoma in monkeys, rats, mice, etc.

Laser-induced Glaucoma in Monkeys

Normal adult cynomologus monkeys (*Macaca irus*) of 3-4 kg body weight are used for laser-induced glaucoma. Monkeys with normal anterior segments, normal intraocular pressure (15-21 mm Hg) and normal optic nerve heads during baseline examination are selected for the study. The monkeys are anesthetized by intramuscular injection of 9 mg/kg ketamine hydrochloride and intravenous injection of 11 mg/kg sodium pentobarbital. After anesthesia, they are placed in front of the slit lamp of the argon laser delivery system. The eyes are treated with 0.4% oxybuprocaine hydrochloride and approximately 200-400 circumferential laser burns are made with a small gonioscopic lens, aiming at the middle of the trabecular meshwork, with a beam diameter of 50-100 μm for 0.1-0.5 sec at 600-800 mW. The laser treatment is repeated every week for 3-5 weeks. Slit lamp examination, IOP measurement, and fundus photography with a stereofundus camera is performed every 1-2 weeks. The IOP of laser treated eyes increase to 25-45 mm Hg after repeated laser treatment and that of normal eyes remains at 15-21 mm Hg.[22,23] Once the stable IOP is obtained, the antiglaucoma agents are instilled in the test group and the IOPs are compared with the control.

Serle et al. carried out a comparative study of latanoprost (Xylatan) and isopropyl unoprostone (Rescula) in normal and glaucomatous monkeys.[24]

Laser-induced Glaucoma in Rats

WoldeMussie et al. 2001, produced laser induced hypertension in male Wistar rats weighing between 350 to 450 g.[25] Rats are anesthetized with a mixture of ketamine (50 mg/kg), acepromazine (1 mg/kg), and xylazine (25 mg/kg). A blue-green argon laser treatment is given for the elevation of IOP. Laser treatment is performed on the episcleral veins within 0.5 to 0.8 mm from the limbus and on the veins in the limbus. Treatment is given in two parts with a gap of 1 week. The amount of energy used is 1 W for 0.2 seconds for delivering a total of 130 to 150 spots (50–100 μm spot size) with both laser treatments. IOP is measured by tonometer (Tono-Pen) before and after laser treatment. Intramuscular injection of 3.0 mg/kg acepromazine is administered to the rats in order to keep them calm but not to sedate them. Cornea is anesthetized using proparacaine (0.5%) topically. IOP is measured three times for the first 2 weeks and then once a week for the remaining experimental period. IOP values increased twofold from the baseline by the laser treatment, which is maintained for two months. The drug treatment can be given either at the time of or 10 days after IOP elevation.[25]

Unilateral experimental glaucoma in Wistar rats is also induced using a diode laser (532 nm wavelength) aimed at the trabecular meshwork and episcleral veins or only at the trabecular meshwork through the external limbus.[26]

Laser-induced experimental glaucoma is induced in rats after intracameral injection of India ink.[27,28]

Laser-induced Glaucoma in Mouse

Aihara, et al. established this mouse model of laser-induced glaucoma.[29] Laser photocoagulation of the corneal limbus obstructed the outflow of aqueous. They induced mydriasis and flattened the anterior chamber prior to photocoagulation. The procedure used by them is briefly described below.

Thirty minutes before the initiation of laser treatment one eye of each mouse is dilated by topical administration of 4 µl of a mixture of atropine, tropicamide, phenylephrine, and cyclopentolate, 0.25% each. The mouse is anesthetized and placed under a stereomicroscope. In order to prevent the drying of cornea a drop of phosphate-buffered saline is placed on it. A fabricated microneedle is connected to a 1-µl syringe that was mounted on a micromanipulator. The aqueous fluid is aspirated by the microneedle. Once the anterior chamber is flattened, the needle is withdrawn. The anesthetized mouse is kept on the platform of a biomicroscope with a diode laser system. Laser beams of 532 nm wavelengths are then applied to the corneal limbus. The laser power being 100 mW, duration 0.05 second and spot size 200 µm. Laser photocoagulation with flattening of the anterior chamber successfully induces 30% elevation of IOP for at least 6 weeks in mouse eyes without any severe complications.[29]

Steroid Glaucoma

Elevation in intraocular pressure in humans due to the administration of corticosteroids is already reported. Experimental glaucoma induced by steroids is reported in young rabbits and cats.[30,31] An adult feline model is developed by Zhan et al.[31]

Procedure: Adult cats of mixed breeds and of either sex (2.2-4.5 kg) are maintained and trained to accept tonometery. Normal intraocular pressure is in the range of 24 ± 0.5 mm Hg (mean ± SEM). Ocular hypotensive cats show consistently lower IOP 17 ± 0.4 mm Hg for at least 1 month prior to the corticosteroid treatment without any medication.[31] During the baseline period before the first corticosteroid treatment, there is no significant difference between the IOP of the left and right eyes. No signs of ocular irritation or inflammation are present. IOP is measured prior to and during all treatments after corneal anesthesia by topical application of proparacaine hydrochloride 0.5%. IOP is measured preferably at the same time and same interval during the experimental period. During long-term treatments, IOP is measured at 0, 1, 3, and 6 h; thereafter, at least once or twice a week, and daily for a few days after a treatment regimen is started, changed or terminated.

Drug administration: A solution of dexamethasone sodium phosphate (Dex) injection is diluted to the desired concentration of 0.5% or 1% with normal saline. The Dex solution is applied to the corneal surface in a volume of 10 μl (to minimize systemic effect) with an automatic micropipette either unilaterally or bilaterally one, two or three times daily. A gradual intraocular pressure increase is observed which becomes significant within 2 to 3 weeks. Prednisolone acetate 1% solution can also be used instead of dexamethasone.[30]

An ocular hypertension model in rats is generated by instillation of topical dexamethasone to rat eyes 4 times daily for 1, 2, and 4 weeks.[32] Galassi et al. (2006) induced glaucoma by administering dexamethasone phosphate 1% drops topically in rabbit eyes.[33]

Bonomi, et al. administered weekly subconjunctival injections of 4 mg repository betamethasone in rabbits for three weeks.[34] This produced a sustained increase in the intraocular pressure in 96% of the treated rabbits. The steroid treatment was well tolerated and systemic adverse effects were seen in few animals. The rise in IOP was constant, well reproducible and sensitive to antiglaucoma drugs.[34]

Hester, et al. studied the effect of three subconjunctivally injected steroids namely betamethasone, cortisone, and triamcinolone in rabbits. All the three drugs produced elevations in IOP but the most consistent elevation was with triamcinolone.[35]

Gerometta, et al. also produced steroid-induced ocular hypertension in normal cattle using prednisolone acetate topically in one eye 3 times a day for a period of 49 days.[36]

OTHER MODELS

Autoimmune Glaucoma

Glaucoma usually is associated with elevated intraocular pressure, but often occurs or may progress with intraocular pressure in the normal range. It has been suggested that autoimmune response possibly has a role in RGC degeneration in normal pressure glaucoma. Serum samples of glaucoma patients were found to have increased levels of heat shock protein 27 (HSP27) and heat shock protein 60 (HSP60). An *in vivo* rat model was established to elicit the autoimmune response through immunization with HSPs. HSP27 and HSP60 immunization in the Lewis rat induced RGC degeneration and axonal loss 1–4 months later in a pattern similar to human glaucoma. The model is a valuable tool for examining the various roles of immune system in glaucoma. It may assist in finding the treatment strategies to prevent pressure -independent RGC degeneration.[37-40]

Genetic Models

Family history and genetic factors have an important role in glaucoma as it is a progressive disease and affects the elderly. Hereditary models are useful in understanding the genetic and mechanistic basis of the disease.

DBA/2J Mouse Model

This is a genetic mouse model of glaucoma characterized by Chang, et al. (1999) in which IOP increases with age due to pigment dispersion from the iris and obstruction of the trabecular meshwork.[41,42] DBA/2J strain mice spontaneously develop complex ocular abnormalities, such as glaucomatous loss of retinal ganglion cells. Three to 11-month-old DBA/2J mice show retinal degeneration which somewhat resembles human pigment dispersion syndrome and pigmentary glaucoma exhibiting characteristic anterior segment changes and elevated IOP. Neovasculogenesis and myelin-like bodies are observed during aging hence it is recommended that the DBA/2J model requires judicious interpretation as a glaucoma model.[43]

Buphthalmic Rabbits, JWHR bu/bu

Inoue, et al. (2001) evaluated the effect of topical CS-088, an angiotensin AT1 receptor antagonist, on intraocular pressure and aqueous humor dynamics in hereditary ocular hypertensive rabbits (buphthalmic rabbits, JWHR bu/bu).[8]

Human Trabecular Meshwork (HTM) Culture

The trabecular meshwork of the anterior chamber is a circular zone of reticular tissue lying between the Schlemm and the anterior chamber. It is separated into corneoscleral and uveal meshwork. Intertrabecular spaces are present between the trabecular sheets. The aqueous percolates through the trabecular meshwork. Major volume of the aqueous passes through the trabecular spaces into the canal of Schlemm and eventually is emptied into the venous system. Any obstruction in the outflow of aqueous leads to the elevation in IOP. This may be due to the debris of the cells in the intertrabecular spaces, collapse of Schlemm's canal or intrascleral blockade.

Procedure: Human donor eyes enucleated within 48-96 hours of death are used. Whole globe is soaked in DPBS containing 100 U/ml penicillin G sodium, 100 U/ml streptomycin sulfate and 0.25 µg/ml amphotericin B for 15 minutes at room temperature. An incision is made to bifurcate the globes at the equator. The lens, ciliary body, and iris are gently removed from the anterior segment to expose the trabecular meshwork. Preserved anterior segments are rinsed in Dulbecco's modified Eagles Medium with 10% fetal bovine serum, 2 mM L-glutamine, 100 U/ml penicillin, G sodium and 100 µg/ml streptomycin sulfate. Trabecular meshwork is separated from the anterior segment with a 0.5 mm foreign body curette and explanted onto a culture plate. The cells are cultured at 37°C in a 7% CO_2 atmosphere. Upon confluency, the cells are passaged with 25% trypsin 1.0 mM EDTA solution in Hank's balanced salt solution. Subsequent passages are used in the experiments.[20,44]

Drug treatment on cells: Cells are placed onto glass cover slips coated with 2% sterile gelatin solution. On reaching the confluence, the cells are treated with the test drug supposedly interfering with actomyosin function. Sham-treated control samples are performed for each treatment group.[21]

Fixation and cytoskeletal staining: Cells are rinsed to remove the medium and drug after the drug exposure. Cells are washed with buffer. Fixation and cytoskeletal staining is done. Cell viability is assessed by flouresceindiacetate and propidium iodide. The drug effective in inducing a loss of cell-cell attachment and a loss of filamentous actin staining may have a potential in increasing the outflow.

CONCLUSION

Apart from surgery, therapeutic intervention is required for the treatment of glaucoma. A large number of antiglaucoma agents are being discovered; but to screen a potential agent, initially, a suitable animal model is required. Out of the above models, the most commonly used are alpha chymotrypsin-induced, water-loaded and laser-induced models of glaucoma. The alpha chymotrypsin produces irreversible glaucoma. It can permanently damage the eyes of the animal. The changes in the IOP in water-loaded or IOP recovery models are for a short duration. The animal recovers after few hours. Laser-induced glaucoma model in rodents is gradually becoming the most acceptable model. Availability and maintenance of rodents is comparatively easier. In the present circumstances when there is difficulty in the availability of animals one can opt for the *in vitro* models. The cell culture techniques are preferred though they require precision and expertise.

REFERENCES

1. Arthur CG, John EH. The nervous system, the special senses. In Arthur CG, John EH (Eds): Textbook of Medical Physiology (ed. 9), Philadelphia: WB Saunders 1998:633-4.
2. WHO report on Prevention of avoidable blindness and visual impairment. EB117/35 Dec. 2005.
3. Tham YC, Li X, Wong TY, Quigley HA, Aung T, Cheng CY. Global prevalence of glaucoma and projections of glaucoma burden through 2040: a systematic review and meta-analysis. Ophthalmology 2014;121(11):2081-90.
4. Thylefors B, Negrel AD. Global impact of glaucoma. Bull WHO 1994;72:323-6.
5. Thylefors B, Negrel AD, Pararajasegaram R, et al. Global data on blindness. Bull WHO 1995;73:115-21.
6. Hamasaki DI, Ellerman N. Abolition of electroretinogram following injection of alpha chymotrypsin into vitreous and anterior chamber of monkey. Arch Ophthalmol 1965;73:843-50.
7. Sears D, Sears H. Blood aqueous barrier and α-chymotrypsin glaucoma in rabbits. Am J Ophthalmol 1974;77:378-83.
8. Inoue T, Yokoyoma T, Mori Y, Sasaki Y, Hosokawa T, Yanagisawa H, et al. The effect of topical CS-088, an angiotensin AT1 receptor antagonist, on intraocular pressure and aqueous humor dynamics in rabbits. Curr Eye Res 2001;23:133-8.
9. Chiang CH, Chang TJ, Lu DW, Lee AR. Intraocular pressure lowering effects of novel aryl piperazine derivatives. J Ocul Pharmacol Ther 1998;14:313-22.
10. Morrison JC, Moore CG, Deppmeier LMH, et al. A rat model of chronic pressure-induced optic nerve damage. Exp Eye Res 1997;64:85-96.
11. Zhu MD, Cai FY. Development of experimental chronic intraocular hypertension in the rabbit. Aust N Z Ophthalmol 1992;20:225-34.
12. Lorenzetti OJ, Sancilio LF. Procedure for evaluating drug effects on increased intraocular pressure. Arch Ophthalmol 1967;78:624-8.
13. Rosolen SG, Rigaudiere F, Le Gargasson JF. A new model of induced ocular hyperpressure using the minipig. J Fr Ophthalmol 2003;26:259-67.
14. Quigley HA, Addicks EM. Chronic experimental glaucoma in primates. 1. Production of elevated intraocular pressure by anterior chamber injection of autologous ghost red blood cells. Invest Ophthalmol Vis Sci 1980; 19:126-36.

15. Moreno MC, Marcos HJA, Croxatto JO, Sande PH, Campanelli J, Jaliffa CO, et al. A new experimental model of glaucoma in rats through intracameral injections of hyaluronic acid. Exp Eye Res 2005;81:71-80.
16. Sugiyama K, Enya T, Kitazawa Y. Ocular hypotensive effect of 8-hydroxycarteolol, a metabolite of cateolol. Int Ophthalmol 1989;13:85.
17. Santafe J, Martinez de Ibaretta MJ, Segarra J, et al. The effect of topical diltiazem on ocular hypertension-induced by water loading in rabbits. Gen Pharmacol 1999;32:201-5.
18. Shah GB, Sharma S, Mehta AA, et al. Oculohypotensive effect of angiotensin converting enzyme inhibitors in acute and chronic models of glaucoma. J Cardiovasc Pharmacol 2000;36:169-75.
19. Byron HP Li, Chiou GCY. Effects of new clonidine derivatives on rabbit intraocular pressure. Drug Dev Res 1992;26:431-8.
20. Epstein DL, Rowlette LL, Roberts BC. Acto-myocin drug effects and aqueous outflow function. Invest Ophthalmol Vis Sci 1999;40:74-81.
21. Epstein DL, Roberts BC, Skinner LL. Non sulfhydryl reactive phenoxyacetic acids increase aqueous humor outflow facility. Invest Ophthalmol Vis Sci 1997;38:1526-34.
22. Jonas JB, Hayreh SS. Localised retinal nerve fibre layer defects in chronic experimental high-pressure glaucoma in rhesus monkeys. Br J Ophthalmol 1999;83:1291-5.
23. Gherezghiher T, March WF, Nordquist RE, et al. Laser-induced glaucoma in rabbits. Exp Eye Res 1986;43:885-94.
24. Serle JB, Podos SM, Kitazawa Y, et al. A comparative study of latanoprost (xylatan) and isopropyl unoprostone (Rescula) in normal and glaucomatous monkey eyes. Jpn J Ophthalmol 1998;42:95-100.
25. WoldeMussie E, Ruiz G, Wijono M, Wheeler LA. Neuroprotection of retinal ganglion cells by brimonidine in rats with laser-induced chronic ocular hypertension. Invest Ophthalmol Vis Sci 2001;42:2849-55.
26. Levkovitch-Verbin H, Quigley HA, Martin KRG, Valenta D, Baumrind LA, Pease ME. Translimbal laser photocoagulation to the trabecular meshwork as a model of glaucoma in rats. Invest Ophthalmol Vis Sci 2002;43:402-10.
27. Ueda J, Sawaguchi S, Hanyu T, et al. Experimental glaucoma model in rat-induced by laser trabecular photocoagulation after an intracameral injection of India ink. Jpn J Ophthalmol 1998;42:337-44.
28. GuZ, Yamamoto T, Kawase C, et al. Neuroprotective effect of N-methyl-D-aspartate receptor antagonists in an experimental glaucoma model in the rat. Nippon Ganka Gakkai Zasshi 2000;104:11-6.
29. Aihara M, Lindsey JD, Weinreb RN. Experimental Mouse Ocular Hypertension: Establishment of the Model. Invest Ophthalmol Vis Sci 2003;44:4314-20.
30. Knepper PA, Breen M, Weinstein HG, Blacik JL. Intraocular pressure and glycosaminoglycan distribution in the rabbit eye: effect of age and dexamethasone. Exp Eye Res 1978;27:567-75.
31. Zhan GL, Miranda OC, Bito LZ. Steroid glaucoma: corticosteroid-induced ocular hypertension in cats. Exp Eye Res 1992;54:211-8.
32. Sawaguchi Keiko, Nakamura Yoshimi, Nakamura Yuko, Sakai Hiroshi, Sawaguchi Shoichi. Myocilin gene expression in the trabecular meshwork of rats in a steroid-induced ocular hypertension model. Ophthal Res 2005;37:235-42.
33. Galassi F, Masini E, Giambene B, Fabrizi F, Uliva C, Bolla M, et al. A topical nitric oxide-releasing dexamethasone derivative: effects on intraocular pressure and ocular haemodynamics in a rabbit glaucoma model. Br J Ophthalmol 2006;90:1414-9.

34. Bonomi L, Perfetti S, Noya E, Bellucci R, Tomazzoli L. Experimental corticosteroid ocular hypertension in the rabbit. Albrecht Von Graefes Arch Klin Exp Ophthalmol 1978;209:73-82.
35. Hester DE, Trites PN, Peiffer RL, Petrow V. Steroid-induced ocular hypertension in the rabbit: a model using subconjunctival injections. J Ocul Pharmacol 1987;3:185-9.
36. Gerometta R, Podos SM, Candia OA, Wu B, Malgor LA, Mittag T, et al. Steroid-induced ocular hypertension in normal cattle. Arch Ophthalmol 2004;122:1492-7.
37. Bouhenni RA, Dunmire J, Sewell A, Edward DP. Animal models of glaucoma. J Biomed Biotechnol 2012;2012:11 pages. Article ID 692609.
38. Wax MB, Tezel G, Yang J, et al. Induced autoimmunity to heat shock proteins elicits glaucomatous loss of retinal ganglion cell neurons via activated T-cell-derived fas-ligand. J Neurosci 2008;28(46):12085-96.
39. Joachim SC, et al. Complex antibody profile changes in an experimental autoimmune glaucoma animal model. Invest Ophthalmol Vis Sci 2009;50(10):4734-42.
40. Joachim SC, Mondon C, Gramlich OW, Grus FH, Dick HB. Apoptotic retinal ganglion cell death in an autoimmune glaucoma model is accompanied by antibody depositions. J Mol Neurosci 2014; 52(2):216-24.
41. Chang Bo, Smith RS, Hawes NL, Anderson MG, Zabaleta A, Savinova O. Interacting loci cause severe iris atrophy and glaucoma in DBA/2J mice. Nature Genetics 1999;21:405-9.
42. Anderson MG, Libby RT, Gould DB, Smith RS, John SWM. High-dose radiation with bone marrow transfer prevents neurodegeneration in an inherited glaucoma. Proc Natl Acad Sci USA 2005;102:4566-71.
43. Schuettauf F, Rejdak R, Walski M, Frontczak-Baniewicz M, Voelker M, Blatsios G, et al. Acta Neuropathol 2004;107(4):352-8.
44. Stamer WD, Roberts BC, Howell DN, et al. Isolation, culture and characterization of endothelial cells from Schlemm's canal. Invest Ophthalmol Vis Sci 1998;39:1804-12.

CHAPTER

18

Antiarrhythmic Agents

INTRODUCTION

Arrhythmias remain among the most challenging human disorders to diagnose and to treat. The complex pathophysiology of human arrhythmias has proven difficult to model. Direct correlations between the traditional arrhythmia mechanisms, including abnormal excitability, conduction, or repolarization and underlying molecular or cellular biology are poorly defined, as the primary etiologies of many human arrhythmias remain unknown. Since the causes of several arrhythmic syndromes have been identified, genetic models reproducing the mechanisms of these arrhythmias have become feasible. Initial murine modeling has revealed that in many cases the pathophysiology of the respective human disease is more complex than had been suspected. Insights from human genetic studies and animal models strongly suggest that the primary molecular defects may contribute at many stages in the causal chain leading to arrhythmia. The comprehensive analysis of each arrhythmia will require knowledge not only of the membrane effects of the primary defects, but also downstream intracellular signals, the developmental results of these perturbations, and the integration of compensatory responses and environmental factors. Precise modeling will require not only the mutation of specific residues in known disease genes, but also the systematic study of each of the many steps in arrhythmogenesis. Ultimately, such models will enable unbiased screening for disease mechanisms and novel therapies.

Although, no animal model can accurately resemble with human disease condition and species differences also exist, close similarities with humans suffering from or threatened by arrhythmias can be developed by selecting appropriate model and species. Though, an animal is not the same as a human patient, arrhythmogenic mechanisms derived from animal experiments have tremendously helped us to diagnose and adapt therapeutic strategies. Following are the standard models useful for the screening of antiarrythmic drugs:

CELL CULTURE TECHNIQUE

1. Studies on Isolated Ventricular Myocytes

Ventricular arrhythmias, specially torsades de pointes, can be evaluated using isolated ventricular myocytes. Analysis of action potential and patch clamp techniques in isolated ventricular myocytes helps us to clarify the mechanisms underlying the development of torsades de pointes.

Guinea pigs (250–350 g) are sacrificed by decapitation and their hearts are removed and perfused retrogradely through the aorta at a rate of 10 ml/min with oxygenated calcium free HEPES buffered saline at 37°C for 5 min. It is then again perfused with the same solution containing 300U/ml type II collagenase and 0.5 to 1.0 U/ml type XIV protease for 8 min and finally with free HEPES buffered saline containing 0.2 mM calcium chloride for additional 5 min. The heart is digested and cut into small pieces, placed in a 20 ml HEPES buffered saline containing calcium chloride and shaken until single cells are dissociated. The cells are then resuspended in HEPES buffered saline and stored at 24°C. Transmembrane potential is recorded using conventional glass electrodes connected to the headstage of an Axoclamp 2A amplifier. Cells are superfused with HEPES buffered saline at a rate of 2 ml/min at 37°C. Passing brief current pulses (1 ms, 1.2 times threshold), through the recording electrode using an active bridge current, evokes action potentials. Cells are stimulated at a frequency of 1 Hz during the stabilization period and at frequencies of 1 and 3 Hz during control and at 10 min after superfusion with test drugs at cumulatively increasing drug concentration. Four individual action potentials are digitally averaged and measured for each condition. For voltage clamp studies, microelectrodes made from square bore, borosilicate capillary tubing are filled with 0.5 M K^+ gluconate, 25 mM KCl, 5 mM K_2 ATP. A List EPC-7 clamp amplifier is used to voltage clamp the isolated cells. Voltage clamp is performed using whole cell recording mode and cell perfusion is minimized by maintaining constant negative pressure on the electrode using a 1 ml syringe. Outward K^+ currents are measured during superfusion of the cells at a rate of 2 ml/min with calcium free HEPES buffered saline. Concentration response relations are determined by measuring action potentials of currents in each cell during control conditions and during superfusion with two successively increasing concentrations of a given drug.[1]

Action potentials are assessed using a three-way ANOVA to determine significance within treatment variations. Dunett's t test is used to determine significance of individual treatment means compared with control mean values.

IN VITRO MODELS

1. Isolated Guinea Pig Papillary Muscle

A simple and accurate, non-microelectrode method is available to identify and classify potential anti-arrhythmic drugs into class I, II, III and IV. In right ventricular guinea pig papillary muscle developed tension (DT), excitability (EX), and effective refractory period (ERP) are measured. Na^+ channel blockade decreases excitability, K^+ channel blockade lengthens refractory period and Ca^{2+} blockade decreases tension of cardiac muscle.

Guinea pigs (200-400 g) are stunned and their carotid artery is severed. The thoracic cage is opened immediately and the heart is removed. The myocardium is placed into a container filled with pre-oxygenated and pre-warmed physiological solution. The pericardium, atria and other tissues are removed and the heart is pinned to a dissection tray. The right ventricle is opened and tendinous end of papillary muscle is ligated with a silk thread, making sure that the chordae tendinae are freed from the ventricle, while the other end is clamped into a tissue holder, at the end of which is a platinum wire field electrodes. The preparation is transferred to a tissue bath containing physiological salt solution maintained at constant temperature and pressure. The silk thread is used to connect the muscle to a force transducer. Muscles are field stimulated to contract isometrically at stimulus duration of 1 ms, frequency of 1 Hz. Pulses are delivered using a Grass constant voltage stimulator and the developed tension is recorded using a polygraph recorder. The force frequency curve is obtained by measuring developed tension over a range of stimulation frequencies (0.3, 0.5,0.8, 1.0,1.2 Hz). The percent change in post treatment (versus pretreatment) developed tension at 1 Hz is used to quantitate an agent's inotropic effect.[2,3]

The changes in effective refractory period (post treatment minus pretreatment), the degree of shift in the strength duration curve (geometrical area between pre & post treatment curves) and the percent changes in post treatment developed tension at 1 Hz are calculated. The results of this calculation are used to classify the compound as a class I, II, III or IV anti-arrhythmic agent on the basis of its effect on developed tension, excitability and effective refractory period.

2. Action Potential and Refractory Period in Isolated Guinea Pig Papillary Muscle

Following the electrical stimulation, intracellular action potential in the left ventricular guinea pig papillary muscle is recorded. To determine the refractory period, the stimulation frequency is varied. Compounds that affect the duration of the effective refractory period may have anti-arrhythmic or pro-arrhythmic effects. In addition, the inotropic effect of the test compound is determined.

Guinea pigs of Marioth strain (250-300 g) are sacrificed by stunning, carotid artery are severed, thoracic cage is opened, heart is removed and placed on a container of pre-warmed, pre-oxygenated Ringer's solution. The left ventricle is opened and the two strongest papillary muscles removed. A standard micro-electrode technique is applied to measure action potential. The papillary muscle is stimulated with rectangular pulses of 1 V and 1ms duration at an interval of 500 ms. To estimate refractory period, the second stimuli are set in decemental intervals until contraction ceases.[4]

Contractile force and relative refractory period are determined before and after drug administration. ED_{25ms} and ED_{50ms} values are determined. ED_{50} values are calculated from log probit analysis and scored.

3. Langendorff Technique

The basic principle involved is that heart is perfused in a retrograde direction from the aorta either at constant pressure or constant flow with oxygenated saline solutions. Retrograde perfusion closes the aortic valves, just as in the *in-situ* heart during diastole. The perfusate is displaced through the coronary arteries flowing off the coronary sinus and the opened right atrium.

Guinea pigs of either sex weighing 300–500 g are sacrificed by stunning. The heart is removed as quickly as possible and placed in a dish containing Ringer's solution at 37°C. Associated pericardial and lung tissues are removed. The aorta is located and cut below the point of division. A cannula is inserted into the aorta and tied and the heart is perfused with oxygenated Ringer's solution. The heart is transferred to a double wall plexiglass perfusion apparatus maintained at 37°C. Oxygenated Ringer's solution is perfused at a constant pressure of 40 mm Hg at a temperature of 37°C from a reservoir. Ligature is placed around the LAD coronary artery and occlusion is maintained for 10 min followed by reperfusion. Test compound is administered through perfusion medium either before or after occlusion. An epicardial ECG electrode is used for pulsatile stimulation and induction of arrhythmias (rectangular pulses of 0.75 msec duration, usually of 10 V; frequency 400–1800 shocks per min). A small steel hook with a string is attached to the apex of the heart. Contractile force is measured isometrically by a force transducer and recorded on a polygraph. Heart rate is measured through a chronometer coupled to the polygraph. Drugs are injected into the perfusion medium. Incidence and duration of ventricular fibrillation or ventricular tachycardia is recorded in the control as well as test group.[5]

4. Acetylcholine and Potassium-induced Arrhythmia

New Zealand white rabbits of the weight range 0.5–3 kg are used for the study. The animals are sacrificed and hearts removed immediately. The atria are dissected from other tissue in Ringer solution. The atria are attached to an electrode in the lower part of the bath and are suspended. Fibrillation is produced when the atria are exposed to acetylcholine (3×10^{-4} g/ml) or (0.10 g) potassium chloride.[6,7] After 5 min of exposure to acetylcholine or potassium, the atria are stimulated with rectangular pulses of 0.75 ms duration, usually of 10 V (Frequency 400–1800 shocks per min). A mechanical record is taken on kymograph. Control arrhythmias are produced and allowed to continue for upto 6–10 minutes. After a 30 minute rest period, fibrillation is again induced and after allowing the arrhythmia to proceed for 3 minutes, a test compound is added to the bath.

If the atria do not cease to fibrillate within 8–10 minutes following the addition of the test compound, the preparation is washed and allowed to return to normal contraction. Test compound is found to be effective if fibrillation disappears immediately or within 5 min following test drug supplementation to the organ bath.

IN VIVO MODELS

In vivo models used to screen antiarrhythmic drugs can be divided into five groups:

A. Chemically-induced Arrhythmia

A large number of agents alone or in combination are capable of inducing arrhythmias. Administration of anesthetics likes chloroform, ether, halothane (sensitizing agents) followed by a precipitating stimulus, such as intravenous adrenaline, ouabain alkaloids cause arrhythmia. The sensitivity of these arrhythmogenic substances differ among various species.

Aconitine Antagonism in Rats

Aconitine, a plant alkaloid from aconitine root, acts persistently on sodium channels and activates it resulting in ventricular arrhythmias. Drugs considered to have anti-arrhythmic properties can be tested in aconitine intoxicated rats.

Males Ivanovas rats (300–400 g) are anesthetized intraperitoneally with urethane (1.25g/kg). Aconitine (5 μg/kg) is dissolved in 0.1 N HNO_3 and continuously infused into the rat's saphenous vein at a rate of 0.1 ml/min. Lead II ECG is recorded every 30 sec. Test compound is injected orally or intravenously 5 min before the aconitine infusion.

A higher dose of aconitine in the test group compared to untreated group gives an index of antiarrhythmic activity. The antiarrhythmic effect of test compound is measured by the amount of aconitine/100 g animal (infusion duration) and includes ventricular extrasystoles, tachycardia, fibrillation and death.[8,9]

Digoxin-induced Arrhythmia in Guinea Pigs

Digoxin overdose induces ventricular extrasystoles, fibrillation and death. Antiarrhthymic drugs prolong the occurrence of these symptoms.

Male Marioth guinea pigs (350–500 g) are anesthetized with pentobarbitone sodium (35 mg/kg) intraperitoneally. Trachea, jugular vein and one carotid artery are catheterized and the animal is maintained on artificial respiration (45 breaths/min). Through the jugular vein digoxin is infused using a perfusion pump at a rate of 85 µg/kg in 0.266 ml/min until cardiac arrest. ECG is recorded with steel needle electrodes during the whole experiment duration. Blood pressure is recorded through the carotid artery. Test drug is administered either orally 1 hour or intravenously 1 min prior to the infusion. The period until the onset of ventricular extrasystoles, fibrillation and cardiac arrest is recorded.[10]

The total amount of infused digoxin (µg/kg) to induce ventricular fibrillation extrasystoles, ventricular fibrillation, cardiac arrest after treatment with the test drug are compared statistically with controls receiving digoxin only.

Strophanthin/Ouabain-induced Arrhythmia

Ventricular tachycardia and multifocal ventricular arrhythmia are induced with acute intoxication with cardiac glycoside (Strophanthin K).

Dogs (20 kg) of either sex are anesthetized with pentobarbitone sodium (30–40 mg/kg) intraperitoneally. Two peripheral veins are cannulated for administration of the arrhythmia inducing substance (V. brachialis) and the test compound (V. Cephalica antebrachialis). ECG at different time intervals is registered with needle electrodes from lead II. Strophanthin K is infused at a rate of 3µg/kg/min through the brachialis vein. 30–40 min later when ventricular tachycardia or multifocal ventricular arrhythmia occurs, strophanthin infusion is terminated. Test compound is administered after 10 min of stabilization of arrhythmias.[11,12]

A test compound is considered to have antiarrhythmic effect if the extrasystoles disappear immediately after drug administration. If the test compound does not show a positive effect, increasing doses are administered at 15 min intervals. If the test substance does reverse arrhythmias, the next dose is administered after the reappearance of stable arrhythmia.

Adrenaline-induced Arrhythmia

Adrenaline at high dose may precipitate arrhythmia. Dogs (10–11 kg) are anesthetized with pentobarbitone sodium (30–40 mg/kg) intraperitoneally. The femoral vein is cannulated. Adrenaline is infused at a rate of 2–2.5 µg/kg through femoral vein. Lead II ECG and atrial ECG are recorded. Test drug is administered 3 min after adrenaline infusion.[13]

A test compound is considered to have antiarrhythmic effect if the extrasystoles disappear immediately after drug administration.

Calcium-induced Arrhythmia

Wistar albino rats (60–130 g) are anesthetized with Nembutal (60 mg/kg) intraperitoneally. Ventricular flutter and fibrillation are induced by administration of 2 ml/kg 10% aqueous calcium chloride through the femoral vein. During the injection and for 2 min thereafter, the cardiac rhythm and behavior are studied by means of a cardioscope connected to the animal with 2 percutaneous, precordial, clamp electrodes. Test drug is administered two minutes prior to calcium infusion.[14]

Results are graded as isolated ventricular premature systoles, frequent ventricular premature systoles, short and long run of ventricular flutter or fibrillation. The latter two are considered positive. Comparison between test and control is made.

B. Electrically-induced Arrhythmia

Serial electrical stimulation results in flutter and fibrillation and it is possible to reproduce some of the main types of arrhythmias of clinical importance. The flutter threshold or the ventricular multiple response thresholds, may be determined in anesthetized dogs before or after administration of test drug.

Ventricular Fibrillation Electrical Threshold

The maximum frequency at which atria would follow a stimulus can be used to compare antifibrillatory compounds. Several electrical stimulation techniques have been used to measure ventricular threshold such as single pulse stimulation, train of pulse stimulation, continuous 50 Hz stimulation and sequential pulse stimulation.

Dogs (8–12 kg) are anesthetized with sodium pentobarbital (35 mg/kg) intraperitoneally and maintained on artificial respiration. Blood pressure and temperature recordings are monitored, chest opened and the heart is suspended in a pericardial cradle. The SA (sinoatrial) node is crushed and a Ag-AgCl stimulating electrode is embedded in a Teflon disc sutured to the anterior surface of the left ventricle.[15] Anodal constant current (3 ms square) for 400 ms is applied through the driving electrode. Electrical stimulation is programmed through a digital stimulator. A recording electrode is placed on the surface of each ventricle. Lead II of the body surface electrocardiogram is monitored.[16] To determine ventricular fibrillation threshold (VFT), a 0.2 to 1.8 s train of 50 Hz pulses are delivered 100 ms after every 18th basic driving stimulus. The current intensity of pulse train required to induce sustained ventricular fibrillation is defined as the VFT. When ventricular fibrillation occurs heart is immediately defibrillated and allowed to recover to control condition for 15–20 min. Drug is administered through the femoral vein.

VFT is determined before and after administration of test drug and compared using student's t test.

Programmed Electrical Stimulation-induced Arrhythmia

Dogs (8–12 kg) are anesthetized with 30 mg/kg pentobarbital sodium intravenously and maintained on artificial respiration. A cannula is inserted in the left external jugular vein. Left thoracotomy is performed between the 4th and 5th ribs, and the heart is exposed. The left anterior descending coronary artery (LAD) is isolated. After a 20 guage hypodermic needle has been placed on the LAD, a ligature is tied around the artery and the needle. The needle is then removed resulting in critical stenosis of the vessel. LAD is perfused for 5 min. Ischemic injury to the myocardium is achieved by 2 h occlusion of the LAD by a silicon rubber snare. The vessel is then reperfused for 2 h in the presence of the critical stenosis. During the period of LAD reperfusion, an epicardial bipolar electrode is sutured on the interventricular septum, adjacent to the occlusion site. Silver disc electrodes are implanted subcutaneously for ECG monitoring. After 6-9 days, chest is re-opened and programmed electrical stimulation is performed through the electrode implanted on noninfarcted zone. The pacing stimuli is set at 200 ms. After 15 pacing stimulation, an extra stimulus is delivered. Animals with sustained ventricular tachycardia and ventricular fibrillation are used for the study. Heart rate, ECG intervals are determined before programmed electrical stimulation is started. Test drug is administered 30 min after the stimulus.[17]

The minimum current intensity of pulse required to induce sustained ventricular fibrillation is recorded before and after administration of test drugs and mean values of 10 experiments are compared using students t test.

C. Exercise-induced Ventricular Fibrillation

Tests combining coronary constriction with physical exercise, may resemble most closely the situation in coronary patients. This model is suited to evaluate antiarrhythmic drugs for their activity in cardiovascular parameters in an exercise-plus ischemia test.

Mongrel dogs (15–19 kg) are anesthetized with sodium pentobarbitone (10 mg/kg, intravenously), chest cavity is opened, hearts exposed and supported by a pericardial cradle. Around the left circumflex artery, a 20 MHz pulsed Doppler flow transducer and a hydraulic occluder are placed. A pair of insulated silver coated wires are sutured to the epicardial surface of both the left and right ventricular electrogram, from which heart rate is determined using a Gould Biotachometer. A pre-calibrated solid state pressure transducer is inserted into the left ventricle and finally, a two stage occlusion of the left anterior descending coronary artery is performed (partially occluded for 20 min and then tied off). Leads from the cardiovascular instrumentation are tunneled under skin to exist on the back of the animal's neck. Analgesics and antibiotics are administered to the animals to minimize discomfort. Three to four weeks after the production of myocardial ischemia, the animals are walked on a motor driven treadmill and trained to lie quitely without restraint on a laboratory table during this recovery period. Susceptibility to ventricular fibrillation is then tested on the motor driven treadmill. Protocol starts with a 3 min warm up period during which the animals run at 6.4 km/h (0% grade). The grade is increased every 3 min as follows (0%, 4%, 8%, 12% & 16%). During the last minute of exercise, the left circumflex coronary artery is occluded, the treadmill is stopped and the occlusion maintained for one additional min (total occlusion time, 2 min). Electrical defibrillator is used if the animal becomes unconscious. The occlusion is released if ventricular fibrillation occurs. The exercise plus ischemia test is repeated after pretreatment with the test drug and compared to control (saline) group readings. On subsequent day, effective refractory period is determined using Medtronic model 5325 programmable stimulator both at rest and during myocardial ischemia. The effect of test drug on coronary blood flow is also studied using flowmeter.[18]

All hemodynamic data (rate of change of left ventricular pressure) are recorded on to a Gould model 2800 S eight channel recorder. The refractory period data, reactive hyperemia response to each occlusion is averaged and the data analyzed using analysis of variance. The effects of the drug intervention on arrhythmia formation are determined using chi-square test with Yate's correction.

Sudden Coronary Death Model in Dogs

Sudden coronary death is one of the leading causes of death in developed countries. This model in dogs is used to test the protection offered against sudden coronary death. Male mongrel dogs (14–22 kg) are anesthetized with pentobarbital sodium (30 mg/kg) intravenously. The trachea is cannulated and the animals are maintained on artificial respiration. The jugular vein is cannulated for the administration of test drug/saline. The chest cavity is opened and the heart is exposed, then the left anterior descending coronary artery (LAD) is isolated and a 20-guage needle is placed on the LAD. A ligature is then tied across the artery and the needle and subsequently, the needle is removed resulting in critical stenosis of the vessel. The LAD is occluded for 2 h using a silicon rubber snare and then reperfused for 2 h in the presence of critical stenosis. An epicardial bipolar electrode is sutured on the left atrial appendage for artrial pacing and another bipolar plunge stainless steel electrode is sutured on the interventricular septum. Two similar stainless steel electrode are sutured on the left ventricular wall, one at the distribution of the LAD distal to the occlusion and the second in the distribution of the left circumflex coronary artery (LCX). A silver-coated electrode is passed through the wall and into the lumen of the LCX and sutured to the adjacent surface of the heart. For ECG monitoring silver disc electrodes are implanted subcutaneously. Then the surgical incision is closed and animals are allowed to recover. After the animals recover, they are treated with the test drug. A direct anodal 15μA current from a 9-V nickel-cadmium battery is passed through a 250 ohm resistor and applied to the electrode in the lumen of LCX. The cathode of the battery is connected to a subcutaneously implanted disc electrode and lead II ECG is recorded for 30 sec every 15 min on a cardiocasette recorder. The animals are sacrificed after 24 h of constant anodal current or development of ventricular fibrillation. The hearts are removed and the thrombus mass in the LCX is removed and weighed. The heart is sectioned and stained with tetrazolium triphenyl chloride (TTC stain) to study the area of infarction. Time of onset of ventricular ectopy and lethal arrhythmia is studied using recordings of the cardiocassette. Non-sustained and sustained tachyarrhythmias are evaluated.[19]

D. Mechanically-induced Arrhythmia

Arrhythmias can be induced directly by ischemia or by reperfusion. By ischemia induced infarction or by coronary ligation several phases of arrhythmia can be studied. The two stage coronary ligation technique focuses on late arrhythmia. The influence on reperfusion arrhythmia can be tested in various species.

Reperfusion Arrhythmia in Rats

Ligation of the left main coronary artery results in ventricular arrhythmia and myocardial infarction. Electrocardiogram is recorded during ligation and subsequent reperfusion. The amount of infarcted tissue is measured by means of p-nitro-blue-tetrazolium chloride staining in myocardial sections.

Sprague Dawley rats (350–400 g) are anesthetized with pentobarbitone sodium (60 mg/kg) intraperitoneally. The animal is maintained on artificial respiration, jugular vein is cannulated for the administration of test drugs. Blood pressure is recorded from the carotid artery using a pressure transducer connected to a polygraph. Chest is opened and heart is exposed. The left coronary artery is located and ligated for 15–90 min (in case of infarct size studies) and subsequently reperfused for 30 min. Test drug is administered 5 minutes before the ligation. Peripheral blood pressure and ECG lead II are recorded continuously during the whole experiment. The number of ventricular premature beats, ventricular tachycardia and fibrillation are counted in the occlusion and reperfusion periods.[20,21]

At the end of the reperfusion period the animal is sacrificed and TTC (p-nitro blue tetrazolium trichloride) staining is done to quantify the infarct size. The heart is dissected and cut into transverse sections (1 mm thick) and stained with TTC prepared in Sorensen phosphate buffer containing 100 mM, L-maleate in order to visualize the infarct tissue (blue/violet stained healthy tissue, unstained necrotic tissue). Slices are photographed and infarct area is measured by planimetry from projections of all slices. Changes in hemodynamic parameters and infarct size in drug treated animals are compared to control values.

Reperfusion Arrhythmia in Dogs

Coronary artery ligation in dogs may result in increased heart rate, heart contractility, left ventricular end diastolic pressure, blood pressure and ventricular arrhythmias, especially in the reperfusion duration.

Dogs (20–25 kg) are anesthetized with thio-butobarbital sodium (30 mg/kg) intraperitoneally and maintained on intravenous chloralose (20 mg/kg) and 250 mg/kg urethane intravenously followed by subcutaneous administration of 2 mg/kg morphine. Animal is subsequently maintained on artificial respiration. A peripheral vein (saphenous vein) is cannulated for the administration of test compound. ECG is recorded continuously in lead II. Femoral artery is cannulated to measure blood pressure and connected to a pressure transducer. Left ventricular end diastolic pressure and heart rate are determined from the left ventricular pressure curves. Myocardial contractility is measured as a rise of left ventricular pressure. The experimental procedure followed is similar to that in rats. Coronary artery is ligated for 90 minutes. Twenty minutes prior to ligation the test compound is administered. Animal is reperfused for 30 min.[22,23] All the above mentioned parameters are recorded during the whole experiment.
Changes in parameters (mortality, hemodynamic and arrhythmia) in drug treated animals are compared to vehicle controls.

Two Stage Coronary Ligation in Dogs

Mortality in dogs after coronary occlusion with a two stage ligation procedure is lower than one stage ligation method.

Dogs (8–11 kg) are anesthetized by intravenous injection of methohexitone sodium (10 mg/kg) and maintained on artificial respiration. Chest is opened and the heart is exposed. Left coronary artery is located and coronary ligation is performed in two stages. Two ligatures are placed around the artery and a 21 gauge needle. The first ligature is tied around the artery and the needle, which is then removed. Thirty min later, the 2nd ligature is tied tightly around the artery. Chest is closed in layers, 30 min after the 2nd ligature has been tied and the dog is allowed to recover. After 24 and 48 h of ligation, arrhythmias develop and abate within 3–5 days. Lead II ECG, atrial electrogram and mean blood pressure are measured. Test drugs are given as infusion for 10 min after coronary artery ligation.[24] Changes in parameters (mortality, hemodynamics and arrhythmia) in drug treated animals are compared to vehicle controls.

The canine model developed by Boyden and Hoffman, in which right atrial enlargement is produced by banding of the pulmonary artery and by producing tricuspid regurgitation, may also have a clinical counterpart in patients with chronic obstructive pulmonary disease and tricuspid regurgitation.[25] In these dogs, a functional zone of blockade and area of slow conduction sets the stage for reentry, rather than an anatomical obstacle. Functional reentry is also observed in the sterile pericarditis model of canine atrial flutter, first descried by Page et al.[26] This model was developed because of the fact that atrial flutter frequently occurs following cardiac surgery in patients and this may be related to postoperative sterile pericarditis.

E. Genetically-induced Arrhythmia

Genetic Arrhythmia

A colony of German shepherd dogs has been described with inherited ventricular arrhythmias and a predisposition for sudden death that most often occurs during sleep or at rest after exercise or excitement. These dogs can be used to screen potential anti arrhythmic drugs. The electrocardiogram does not show a prolonged QT interval, but frequently there is marked notching of the T wave. The arrhythmias are rapid polymorphic ventricular tachycardia, following long R-R intervals and are most likely due to triggered activity induced by early depolarizations in the Purkinje system. In the epicardial myocytes, the density of the transient outward current (I_o) and the time constant of inactivation are reduced.[27] Deficiencies in cardiac sympathetic denervations also occur. At first glance, this dog model bears resemblance to the congenital long QT syndrome in which bradycardia induced polymorphic ventricular tachycardia and sudden death occurs and in which genetic defects in ion channels regulating repolarization have been described. However, the dogs have no prolonged QT interval. In patients with the long QT syndrome, no deficiencies in I_o have been described.[28,29] Still, this animal model might have a counterpart because patients have been described with polymorphous ventricular tachycardia (*Torsade de pointes*) that has a normal QT interval.

DISCUSSION AND CONCLUSION

Generally speaking, antiarrhythmic drugs exert their effects largely by modulating conduction velocity, or refractory period duration, or both. Conduction velocity on one hand depends, on the passive electrical properties of cardiac tissue, and on the other, the characteristics of the Na^+ and Ca^{2+} channels. In contrast, there are marked differences among species in the K^+ currents that largely determine repolarization, so that action potential duration and duration of refractory period differ widely in various species.

It is clear that species differences do exist with respect to factors that determine arrhythmogenesis and it is also clear that no animal model will accurately mimic the human suffering from or threatened by an arrhythmia. Nevertheless, the knowledge gathered from animal studies, undoubtedly, has been instrumental in devising diagnostic and therapeutic strategies both in supraventricular and ventricular arrhythmias. It is our conviction that in the future, new knowledge will be obtained from experiments performed at many levels: in systems expressing and testing the functions of molecules involved in electrical excitation, in single cells, cell cultures, excised cardiac preparations, isolated whole hearts, whole hearts in anesthetized animals and in conscious animals. It will be the combination of such investigations rather than a single model or experimental technique, which will lead to novel strategies for diagnosis and treatment. Finally, electrophysiological studies should be encouraged in animals with 'naturally' occurring cardiovascular disease.

Animal models have been central to the advances in our understanding of the mechanisms of human arrhythmia, but have also highlighted issues fundamental to all forms of disease modeling. In any complex process, it is preferable to recapitulate as much of the causal pathway as possible, rather than to empirically model individual components. The mechanistic insights that have been gained over the last few decades, emphasize the complexity of the pathogenesis of clinical dysrhythmia.[30] Models capable of integrating the effects of both genetic and epigenetic modifiers will be required to dissect the multi-step pathways involved, which include myocyte heterogeneity, channel processing, and downstream signaling, to name but a few.

Summary

In vitro models	*In vivo models*				
	Chemically induced	*Electrically induced*	*Exercise induced*	*Mechanically induced*	*Genetically induced*
Studies on isolated ventricular myocytes	Aconitine antagonism in rats	Ventricular fibrillation electrical threshold	Sudden coronary death model in dogs	Reperfusion arrhythmia in rats	Genetic arrhythmia
Isolated guinea pig papillary muscle	Digoxin induced arrhythmia in guinea pigs	Programmed electrical stimulation induced arrhythmia		Reperfusion arrhythmia in dogs	
Action potential and refractory period in isolated guinea pig papillary muscle	Strophanthin induced arrhythmia			Two stage coronary ligation in dogs	
Langendorff technique	Adrenaline induced arrhythmia				
Acetylcholine and potassium induced arrhythmia	Calcium induced arrhythmia				

REFERENCES

1. Drolet B, Vincent F, Rail J, Chahine, et al. Thioridazine lengthens repolarization of cardiac ventricular myocytes by blocking the delayed rectifier potassium current. J Pharmacol Exp Ther 1999;288:1261-68.
2. Brown BS. Electrophysiological effects of ACC-9358, a novel class I antiarrhythmic agent, on isolated canine Purkinje fibers and ventricular muscle. J Pharmac Exp Ther 1989;248:552-58.
3. Dawes GS. Synthetic substitutes for quinidine. Br J Pharmacol 1946;1:90-112.
4. Tande PM, Bjornstad T, Refsum H. Dependent class III antiarrhythmic action, negative chronotropic and positive inotropy of a novel I k blocking drug, UK-68, 789: potent in guinea pig but no effect on rat myocardium. J Cardiovasc Pharmacol 1991;16:401-10.
5. Ravelli F, Allessie MA. Effects of atrial dilation on refractory period and vulnerability to atrial fibrillation in the isolated Langendorff-perfused rabbit heart. Circulation 1997;32:52-61.
6. Allessie MA, Lammers WJEP, Bonke FIM, et al. Intraatrial reentry as a mechanism for atrial flutter induced by acetylcholine in rapid pacing in the dog. Circulation 1984;70:123-35.
7. Ten Eick RA, Singer DH. Electrophysiological properties of diseased human atrium. Low diastolic potential and altered cellular response to potassium. Circ Res 1979;44:545-57.
8. Bazzani C, Genedani S, Tagliavini S, et al. Putrescine reverses aconitine induced arrhythmia in rats. J Pharm Pharmacol 1989;41:651-53.
9. Brooks RR, Carpenter JF, Jones SM, et al. Effects of dantrolene sodium in rodent models of cardiac arrhythmia. Eur J Pharmacol 1989;164:521-30.
10. Linz W, Scholkens BA, Kaiser J, et al. Cardiac arrhythmias are ameliorated by local inhibition of angiotensin formation and bradykinin degradation with the converting-enzyme inhibitor ramipril. Cardiovasc Drugs Ther 1989;3:873-82.
11. Brooks RR, Miller KE, Carpenter JF, et al. Broad sensitivity of rodent arrhythmia models to class I, II, III and IV anti arrhythmic agents. Proc Soc Exp Biol Med 1989;191:201-09.
12. Duce BR, Garberg L, Johansson B. The effect of propranolol and the dextro and levo isomers of H 56/28 upon ouabain induced ventricular tachycardia in unanesthetized dogs. Acta Pharmacol Toxicol 1967;25 (2):41-49.
13. Raper C, Wale J. Propranolol, MJ-1999 and Ciba 39089-Ba I ouabain and adrenaline induced cardiac arrhythmias. Eur J Pharmacol 1968;41:119-24.
14. Daoud EG, Knight BP, Weiss R. Effect of verapamil and procainamide on atrial fibrillation induced electrical remodelling in human. Circulation 1997;96:1542-50.
15. Burgess MJ, Williams D, Ershler P. Influence of test site on ventricular fibrillation threshold. Am Heart J 1977;94:55-61.
16. Harumi K, Tsutsumi T, Sato T, et al. Classification of antiarrhythmic drugs based on ventricular fibrillation threshold. Am J Cardiol 1989;64:10J-14J.
17. Wu KM, Hunter TL, Proakis AGI. A dual electrophysiological test for atrial antire-entry and ventricular antifibrillatory studies. J Pharmacol Meth 1990;223:87-95.
18. Belloni FI, Hintze TH. Glibenclamide attenuates adenosine induced bradycardia and vasodilation. Am J Physiol 1991;261:H720-27.
19. Black SC, Chi L, Mu DX, Lucchesi RR. The antifibrillatory actions of UK 68,789, a class III antiarrthythmic agent. J Pharm Exp Ther 1991;258:416-23.
20. Harris S. Delayed development of ventricular ectopic rhythms following experimental coronary occlusion. Circul Res 1950;1:1318-28.

21. Jahnston KM, MacLeod BA, Walker MJA. Responses to ligation of a coronary artery in conscious rats and actions of antiarrhythmics. Can J Physiol Pharmacol 1983;61:1340-53.
22. Black SC, Chi L, Mu DX, et al. The antifibrillatory actions of UK 68,789, a class III antiarrhythmic agent. J Pharm Exp Ther 1991;258:416-23.
23. Cahn PS, Cervoni P. Current concepts and animal models of sudden cardiac death for drug development. Drug Dev Res 1990;19:199-207.
24. Trolese-Mongheal Y, Trolese JF, Lavarenne J. Use of experimental myocardial infarct to demonstrate arrhythmogenic activity of drugs. J Pharmacol Meth. 1991;13:225-34.
25. Boyden PA, Hoffman BF. The effects on atrial electrophysiology and structure of surgically induced right atrial enlargement in dogs. Circ Res 1981;49:1319-31.
26. Page P, Plumb VJ, Okumura K, et al. A new model of atrial flutter. J Am Coll Cardiol 1986;8:872-9.
27. Moise NS, Gilmour RF, Riccio ML. An animal model of spontaneous arrhythmic death. J Cardiovasc Electrophysiol 1997;8:98-103.
28. Freeman LC, Pacioretty LM, Moise NS, et al. Decreased density of Io in left ventricular myocytes from German shepherd dogs. J Am Coll Cardiol 1996;27:1526-33.
29. Doe M, Ursell P, Lee RJ, et al. Heterogeneous sympathetic innervation in German shepherd dogs with inherited ventricular arrhythmias and sudden death. J Am Coll Cardiol 1995; 25:20-25.
30. Milan DJ, MacRae CA. Animal models for arrhythmias. Cardiovascular Research 2005;67:426–37.

CHAPTER

19

Cardiotonic Agents

INTRODUCTION

Congestive heart failure (CHF) is a constellation of symptoms, with hallmarks of fatigue and dyspnea, which continues to be a highly prevalent and morbid clinical syndrome. Because of the growing burden of CHF as the population ages, the need to develop new pharmacological treatments and therapeutic interventions is of paramount importance. Common pathophysiologic features of CHF include changes in left ventricle structure, function, and neurohormonal activation.[1,2]

The progress made in our understanding of the pathophysiology and treatment of CHF would not have been possible without a number of animal models of heart failure and hypertrophy, each having unique advantages as well as disadvantages. The species and interventions used to create CHF depend on such factors as ethical and economical considerations, accessibility and reproducibility of the model.[3,4]

The use of small-animal models to study complex cardiovascular pathophysiology has proven to be invaluable during the past decades. As a direct result of basic and translational studies in murine models, our understanding of pathophysiology of heart failure and its treatment has advanced considerably. Rat models have been used primarily to assess the efficacy of specific pharmacological or molecular therapies. The ability to manipulate the mouse genome has facilitated a particularly elegant approach to identify novel therapeutic targets, offering a "proof of principle" approach to explore the mechanisms underlying heart failure and its progression. Moving forward, these small animal models of heart failure will continue to be critical tools in the identification of new therapeutic targets and evaluation of specific therapies for heart failure.[4]

The recapitulation of the CHF phenotype in large animal models can allow for the translation of basic science discoveries into clinical therapies. Models of myocardial infarction/ischemia, ischemic cardiomyopathy, ventricular pressure and volume overload, and pacing-induced dilated cardiomyopathy have been created in dogs, pigs, and sheep for the investigation of CHF and potential therapies. Large animal models, recapitulating the clinical CHF phenotype and translating basic science to clinical applications, have successfully traveled the journey from bench to bedside. Undoubtedly, large animal models of CHF will continue to play a crucial role in the elucidation of biological pathways involved in CHF and the development and refinement of CHF therapies.[5]

IN VITRO METHOD

1. Isolated Hamster Cardiomyopathic Heart

Isolated Syrian hamster hearts can be used for evaluation of cardiotonic drugs. Hamsters with cardiomyopathy of the age group (50 weeks) are used for the study. Normal Syrian hamsters of the same age are used as controls. The animals are pretreated with heparin (5 mg/kg) intraperitoneally and 20 min later the heart is prepared according to the method of Langendorff and perfused with Ringer's solution and allowed to equilibrate in the isolated state for 60 min at 32°C with a preload of 1.5 g. The force of contractions is recorded isometrically by a force transducer connected to a polygraph. The heart rate is measured using a chronometer. The coronary flow is measured using an electroflowmeter. Test compounds are injected via the aortic cannula into the inflowing heart-Ringer's solution.

The contractile force and coronary flow in hearts of the treated and the sham control group are compared using student's t test. Percentage improvement is calculated and the efficacy of the drug evaluated in increasing the coronary flow and contractile force.[6]

2. Isolated Cat Papillary Muscle

This method using rat capillary muscle has been described by Catell and Gold.[7] Prolonged electrical stimulation of isolated cardiac tissue results in decrease in performance. Cardiac glycosides restore the force of contraction.

Cats (2.5-3 kg) of either sex are anesthetized with ether. Through a left thoracotomy, heart is exposed. Papillary muscle from the right ventricle is isolated and fixed in an organ bath containing Ringer's solution maintained at 37°C. One end of the papillary muscle is tied to a strain guage and other end to the muscle. Electrical stimulus of 4-6 V is applied to the muscle at a rate of 30/min and the contractions are recorded on a polygraph. On electrical stimulation for 1 h, the muscle contractions start diminishing. The cardiac glycosides are added to the bath at this point to restore the contractile force. Ouabain is the standard glycoside that is added at a dose of 300 ng/ml.

Evaluation is based on increase in contractile force on adding the glycoside. Contractile force is calculated as percentage of the predose level and comparisons between different groups are made.

3. Ouabain Binding

The binding kinetics, i.e association process, equilibrium binding and dissociation process on the ouabain receptor, is characteristic of the cardiac glycosides.

Rat hearts are submitted to coronary perfusion and subsequently myocytes are isolated by collagenase digestion. From these isolated membrane fractions, myocyte sarcolemma is obtained. Radioactive ouabain [^{3}H] with specific radioactivity of 20 Ci/mmol is incubated with ligands in 10 ml of binding medium kept at 37°C for 10 min. The composition of binding medium (pH 7.4) is 1 mM inorganic phosphate, 1mM $MgCl_2$ and 50 mM Tris HCl.

Association process: *After* temperature equilibration in the presence of either 10 or 100 nM [3H]ouabain, 200 µg of membrane preparation are added to initiate the reaction. At various times, 4.5 ml are removed and rapidly filtered.

Equilibrium binding: At the end of the temperature equilibration carried out in the presence of increasing concentrations of [3H]ouabain ranging from 10 nM to 3 μM, 40 μg of membranes are added. After 30 min, duplicate aliquots of 4.5 ml are removed and filtered.

Dissociation process: Once equilibrium has been achieved under the experimental conditions used to study association, 10 ml of prewarmed Mg^{2+} plus Pi Tris-HCl solution supplemented with 0.2 mM unlabeled ouabain are added to initiate dissociation of [3H]ouabain. At various times, aliquots of 0.9 ml are removed and rapidly filtered.

The radioactivity bound to the filters and the specific binding measurements are determined. Kinetic parameters for the association and the dissociation process are calculated. The results of equilibrium binding are analyzed by Scatchard plots.

IN VIVO MODELS

Rat Models of Heart Failure

Rat models are relatively inexpensive and because of short gestation period, a large sample size can be produced in a short period of time. Therefore, rat models have been extensively used to study the long-term pharmacological interventions including long term survival studies.[7,8] However, there are several limitations to the use of rat models regarding differences in myocardial function compared to human heart:

1. Rat myocardium exhibits a very short action potential, which normally lacks a plateau phase.
2. Calcium removal from the cytosol is predominated by the activity of sarcoplasmic reticulum calcium pump whereas Na^{+}/Ca^{2+} exchanger activity is less relevant.
3. In normal rat myocardium, α- myosin heavy chain isoform predominates and a shift towards the β-myosin isoform occurs and hemodynamic load or hormonal changes take place.
4. Resting heart rate is five times that of humans and the force-frequency relation is inverse.[9]

1. Rat Coronary Ligation Model

Myocardial infarction following coronary artery ligation in Sprague-Dawley rats is a widely used rat model of heart failure. If the left coronary artery is not completely ligated, heart failure may occur as a consequence of chronic myocardial ischemia.[10] Complete occlusion of the left coronary results in myocardial infarction of variable sizes with occurrence of overt heart failure after 3–6 weeks in a subset of animals with large infarcts. The impairment of left ventricular function is related to the loss of myocardium. Failure is associated with left ventricular dilation, reduced systolic function and increased filling pressures.

Males Sprague Dawley rats (250–300 g) are anesthetized with 200 mg/kg hexobarbital. The trachea is cannulated and the animal is maintained on artificial respiration. The chest cavity is exposed and the left anterior descending carotid artery (LAD) is isolated. A ligature is placed around the LAD and the chest cavity is sutured back and the animal maintained on food and water *ad libitum*. After 4 weeks, the chest cavity is opened and carotid artery as well as jugular vein is cannulated for measurement of blood pressure as well as administration of test compounds. Filling pressure, systolic, diastolic and mean blood pressure are measured. After measuring the hemodynamic parameters, the animals are sacrificed and the isolated hearts are used for studying calcium channel, sarcoplasmic reticulum ATPase and protein levels.

It is observed that in the control group the progression of left ventricular dysfunction and myocardial failure is associated with neurohumoral activation similar to that seen in patients with CHF. Depressed myocardial function is associated with altered calcium transients. The density of L-type calcium channels, SR-Ca^{2+} - ATPase and protein levels decrease continuously with increasing severity of congestive heart failure. Comparison between test group and control group are made on the basis of the above mentioned parameters.

Although a high initial mortality and induction of mild heart failure in most cases may be a disadvantage of this model, it seems to be very useful for long term studies of pharmacological interventions on the neurohormonal activation.[11]

2. Rat Aortic Banding

Restriction of blood flow to the aorta in rats induces not only hypertension but also congestive heart failure within several weeks. After a period of several weeks, ventricular ACE activity may decrease again to normal values, which may be related to normalization of wall stress with increasing cardiac hypertrophy.[12] Furthermore, after several months, a subset of animals goes into cardiac failure.

Sprague-Dawley rats (250–280 g) are fasted for 12 h before surgery. Animals are anesthetized with 200 mg/kg hexobarbitone. The abdomen is shaved, moistened with a disinfectant and opened by a cut parallel to the linea alba. The intestine is moistened with saline and placed in a plastic cover to prevent desiccation. The aorta is prepared free from connective tissue above the left renal artery and underlaid with a silk thread. Then, a cannula no. 1 (0.9 × 40 mm) is placed longitudinally to the aorta and both aorta and cannula are tied. The cannula is removed, leaving the aortic lumen determined by the diameter of the cannula. The intestine is placed back into the abdominal cavity with the application of 5.0 mg rolitetracycline. In sham-operated controls no banding is performed while in the test group animals are administered drugs for 6 weeks. The skin is closed by clipping. It is observed that after 4–6 weeks heart failure develops in these animals.

Total cardiac mass, weight of left and right ventricle of treated rats are compared with operated controls and sham-operated controls. Heart failure is associated with increased myosin heavy chain mRNA and atrial natriuretic factor mRNA. During compensated hypertrophy, while catecholamine levels are normal, there is activation of local myocardial renin-angiotensin system, which may be important for the development of heart failure.[13] The above mentioned parameters are studied in both the test group and the sham control group. At the end of the experiment, blood pressure and heart rate are recorded via the left coronary artery. Moreover, total cardiac mass, weight of left and right ventricle of treated rats is also compared with sham operated controls.

This model seems to be well suited for studying the transition from hypertrophy to failure at the level of myocardium.

3. Dahl Salt Sensitive Rats

This model is well suited to study the transition from compensated hypertrophy to failure.[14] This strain of rats develop systemic hypertension after receiving a high-salt diet.

Sprague-Dawley rats (250–300 g) are selected for this study. Drinking water is replaced with 1% NaCl saline solution. High Dahl salt diet is prepared in the laboratory by mixing salt with the regular diet. Animals are fed the prepared diet and 1% NaCl solution *ad libitum*. The test drug rats are administered the drug orally for 1 month. After the completion of the experimental duration, the animals of both groups (test and sham control) are sacrificed. Their hearts are removed and total cardiac mass, weight of left and right ventricle are weighed and compared. It is observed that the animals in the sham control group develop concentric left ventricular hypertrophy at 8 weeks, followed by marked left ventricular dilation and overt clinical heart failure at 15–20 weeks. Failing heart dies within a short period of time. The ability of the test drug to reverse these changes is studied.[15]

4. Spontaneous Hypertensive Rat

The spontaneous hypertensive rat is a well-established model of genetic hypertension in which cardiac pump function is preserved at 1 year of age.[16] At 18-24 months, cardiac failure develops, which includes reduced myocardial function and increased fibrosis. In this model, although altered calcium cycling is observed, no decrease in mRNA of the sarcoplasmic reticulum calcium pump is found during transition from compensated hypertrophy to failure. The transition to failure is associated with significant alterations in the expression of genes encoding extracellular matrix.[17] Furthermore, an increased number of apoptotic myocytes are observed and it is suggested that apoptosis might be a mechanism involved in the reduction of myocyte mass that accompanies the transition from stable compensation to heart failure.

The animals are divided into two groups. To test group animals, drug is administered orally for 1 month while to sham control group animals, no drug treatment is given. After completion of the experimental protocol, the animals are sacrificed and their hearts are processed for the estimation of number of apoptotic cells, sarcoplasmic reticulum calcium pump mRNA levels and expression of genes encoding for extracellular matrix and results compared.

5. Spontaneous Hypertensive-Heart Failure Rats (SH-HF)

Spontaneous hypertensive rats, which develop failure before 18 months of age, have been selectively bred. Development of heart failure occurs earlier in rats which carry the facp gene (corpulent gene) that encodes a defective leptin receptor (SH-HF/Mcc-facp). In these animals, renin plasma activity, atrial natriuretic peptide (ANP) and aldosterone levels progressively increase with age and renin plasma activity is independently correlated to cardiac hypertrophy. Interestingly, hearts from the SH-HF rats exhibits a more negative force frequency relationship than control rats. In a recent study trial in SH-HF rats, it was observed that calcium current density and function of ryanodine receptors, and sarcoplasmic reticulum calcium uptake were normal. However, it was also observed that the relationship between calcium current density and the probability of evoking a spark was reduced indicating that the calcium influx was less effective at inducing SR calcium release. It was speculated that these changes might be related to spatial remodeling between L-type calcium channels and ryanodine receptors.[18]

Animals are divided into two groups. Group 1 serves as the test drug group (administered drug for one month, orally) while group 2 serves as the sham control group (untreated). After completion of the experiment, comparisons are made between the two groups based on their plamsa renin activity, ANP and aldosterone levels, rynodine receptor density, sarcoplasmic reticulum calcium uptake and endothelial nitric oxide synthase (NOS) activity.

Dog Models of Heart Failure

Generally, dog and other large animal models of heart failure may allow the study of left ventricular function and volumes more accurately than rodent models. In particular, they allow better chronic instrumentation. Furthermore, in dog like human myocardium the β-myosin heavy chain isoform predominates and excitation contraction coupling processes seem to be similar to the human myocardium.[19] The force frequency relationship, the slope of the end-systolic pressure-volume relation, is positive in automatically intact awake dogs as well as during autonomic blockade. On the other hand, dog models are costly and require substantial resources with respect to housing and care.

1. Chronic Rapid Pacing

Chronic rapid pacing at heart rates above 200 beats per minute in previously healthy dogs within several weeks produces the syndrome of CHF.

Adult male dogs (18–25 kg) are anesthetized with pentobarbital (30 mg/kg) intraperitoneally. The animal is maintained on artificial respiration (20–24 strokes/min). The chest cavity is opened through a 3–4 cm long thoracotomy and the heart is exposed. A ventricular pacing lead is attached to the left ventricular apex. The pacemaker is programmed to pace at 240–260 beats/min for 2–4 weeks. After the surgical procedure, the heart is placed back in the chest cavity and the costal ribs closed and the musculus pectoralis placed over the wound. Air from the thorax is removed by applying pressure on both sides of the thorax. After application of an antibiotic emulsion the skin wound is closed. Significant heart failure develops by 4 weeks and continues for upto 10 weeks. In the majority of studies, chronic rapid tachycardia results in progressive biventricular chamber dilatation over a 3–4 week period. The test drugs are administered subcutaneously or intramuscularly over a period of 14 days.

Heart failure is associated with a significant decrease in ejection fraction and diastolic dysfunction, followed by decreased cardiac output and increased systemic vascular resistance.[20] It is important to note that heart failure is reversible with respect to clinical hemodynamic and neurohumoral abnormalities when electrical pacing is stopped. The exact pathogenesis in this model is still unclear. Similar to human heart failure there are time dependent changes in neurohumoral activation and an early sympathetic activation, increase in plasma catecholamine levels and attenuation of parasympathetic tone. In addition, plasma ANP levels are elevated early in the development of left ventricular dysfunction. Systemic activation of renin-angiotensin system is seen with progressive pump failure. Further, more endothelial dysfunction with decreased nitric oxide mediated coronary vasodilation has been observed similar to the patients with heart failure.

Comparison between test group and sham control group is made on the basis of changes in parameter like ejection fraction, cardiac output and systemic vascular resistance. Further, plasma catecholamine, ANP levels and renin acitivty are also evaluated to assess the cardioprotective potential of test drugs.

The technique of tachycardia pacing has also been used in pigs and sheeps, and findings similar to those in dogs have been observed with respect to clinical hemodynamic and neurohumoral changes. This model seems very valuable for studying neurohumoral mechanisms and peripheral circulatory alterations, both of which closely resemble that observed in human heart failure.[21]

In a similar model of CHF, a number of transmyocardial direct current shocks applied through a catheter into the left ventricle chamber in anesthetized dogs, result in left ventricle hypertrophy and dilation, decreased ejection fraction and decreased cardiac output over a 4 months period. This is associated with increased plasma catecholamines but with no change in plasma renin activity.[22]

2. Volume Overload

Prolonged volume overload may lead to development of heart failure. In dogs, volume overload has been produced either by creation of an arteriovenous fistula, where an end to side anastomosis is made between the femoral vein and artery in order to increase venous flow or by destruction of the mitral valve in a closed chest dog by an arterially placed grasping forceps.[23]

Dogs (12–15 kg) are anesthetized with pentobarbital (30 mg/kg) intraperitoneally and maintained on artificial respiration (20–24 strokes/min). Thoracotomy is performed and the heart is exposed. Chronic experimental mitral regurgitation is produced in closed chest dogs by disruption of mitral chordae or leaflets using an arterially placed foreceps. Within 3 months, left ventricular hypertrophy, dilation and development of overt clinical heart failure occurs in this model. After the surgical procedure, the heart is placed back in the chest cavity and the costal ribs closed. By applying pressure on both sides of the thorax, air from the thorax is removed. After application of an antibiotic emulsion the skin wound is closed. Significant heart failure develops by 4 weeks and continues for upto 10 weeks. The test drugs are administered subcutaneously or intramuscularly over a period of 14 days.

Neurohumoral activation including local activation of the Renin Angiotensin System is observed in CHF dogs, which is generally associated with depressed myocardial function. Comparisons between test group and sham control group (untreated animals) are made. The model has been used to study the influence of chronic β-adrenoceptors blockade on myocytes and left ventricular function, both of which significantly improve with treatment.[24]

3. Coronary Artery Ligation and Microembolization

Coronary artery ligation and microembolization have been used to produce myocardial infarction and CHF in dogs.

Dogs of either sex (30 kg) are anesthetized with intravenous bolus injection of 35–40 mg/kg pentobarbitone. Animals are maintained on artificial respiration. A transducer is connected to the right femoral artery for recording peripheral systolic, diastolic and mean blood pressure. A microtip catheter is inserted via the left carotid artery for determination of left ventricular pressure. Systolic, diastolic and mean pulmonary capillary pressure and cardiac output are measured by thermodilution technique using a cardiac index computer. Heart is exposed through a left thoractomy between 4th and 5th intercostal space and pericardium is opened. Polystearyl microsphere is injected through the angiogram catheter into the left atrium. Initially, a 10 ml (1mg/ml) microsphere is injected and later a 5 ml bolus about 5 min apart. The microsphere injection produces stepwise elevation of LVEDP. Embolism is terminated when LVEDP has increased to 16–18 mm Hg or heart rate reaches to 200 beats/min. Intravenous bolus injection or continuous infusion administers the test substance. Recordings are obtained before and after embolization and administration of test compound at various time intervals.[25,26]

The model has several disadvantages. Because of extensive collateral circulation, there are important differences in the pattern of infarction between human and dog. The model is time consuming, technically demanding and expensive. The model is associated with high mortality and a high incidence of arrhythmias.

Rabbit Models of Heart Failure

Rabbit models are less expensive than dog models. In addition, non failing rabbit myocardium exhibits interesting similarities to human heart.

1. The β-myosin heavy chain isoform predominates in adult animals.
2. The sarcoplasmic reticulum contributes by about 70% and the Na^+/Ca^{2+} exchanger contributes by about 30% calcium estimation.
3. The force-frequency relation is positive.

1. Volume and Pressure Overload

Volume overload, pressure overload and the combination of both are used to induce heart failure in rabbits. Chronic severe aortic regurgitation in rabbits, created by aortic valve perforation with a catheter, produces left ventricular hypertrophy, followed by systolic dysfunction and heart failure after a period of months.

Rabbits are anesthetized with pentobarbitone sodium (35 mg/kg) intraperitoneally. Their trachea is cannulated and the animals maintained on artificial respiration. The carotid artery is cannulated. The chest cavity is opened and the heart is exposed. Aortic insufficiency is produced by destroying the aortic valve with the catheter, introduced through the carotid artery. The chest cavity is sutured back and antibiotic is applied to prevent any infection. After 14 days, aortic constriction is performed just below the diaphragm using a PVC clamp. Occurrence of heart failure is more consistent and rapidly observed when aortic regurgitation is combined with aortic constriction. Test drugs are administered for 2 weeks (subcutaneously or intraperitoneally). Heart failure occurs about 4 weeks after the initial procedure. It is associated with alterations in the β-adrenoceptors system similar to those in humans. Furthermore, in this model there is inversion of the force frequency relation and alteration of the post rest potentiation, which closely resembles the situation in the human heart. Interestingly, protein and mRNA levels of the Na^+/Ca^{2+} exchanger are significantly increased in failing compared to nonfailing animals, whereas sarcoplasmic reticulum Ca^{2+} ATPase is not significantly altered. After completion of the experimental protocol, the animals are sacrificed and the above mentioned neurohumoral parameters are studied in the drug treated and sham control groups. The ability of the test group to reverse these changes is studied.[27]

As this model closely mimics alteration of myocardial function observed in the end stage failing human myocardium, this model is well suited to study alteration in excitation contraction coupling during the transition from compensated hypertrophy to failure.

2. Tachycardia Pacing

Recently, chronic rapid pacing at rates between 350–400 beats/min over a period of several weeks in rabbits was shown to produce myocardial depression as well as, hemodynamic and neurohumoral signs of heart failure.[28]

Rabbits are anesthetized with pentobarbitone sodium (35 mg/kg) intraperitoneally. Their trachea is cannulated and the animals maintained on artificial respiration. The chest cavity is opened through a 3–4 cm long thoracotomy and the heart is exposed. A ventricular pacing lead is attached to the left ventricular apex and the pacemaker is programmed to pace at 350–400 beats/min for 2–4 weeks. After the surgical procedure, the heart is placed back in the chest cavity and the intercostal ribs closed and air from the thorax is removed by applying pressure on both sides of the thorax. An antibiotic emulsion is applied and the skin wound is closed. After 4–6 weeks the animals develop heart failure. In one experimental group animals are administered test compound either subcutaneously or intraperitoneally for 2 weeks. After completion of the experimental period, the animals are further subjected to surgery. The carotid artery is cannulated for measuring blood pressure. Hemodynamic parameters like systolic, diastolic, mean blood pressure and heart rate are measured. The animals are then sacrificed and their hearts weighed and processed for estimation of plasma renin activity. Comparisons between test group and sham control group are made on the basis of hemodynamic parameters, plasma renin activity and heart weights.

It is observed that in the sham control group (untreated group) the force frequency relation is severely depressed and inverted at higher stimulation rates. This is similar to the alteration of the force frequency relation observed in failing human hearts. As was observed in the tachycardia-pacing dog failure model, no left ventricular hypertrophy is developed in the rabbit model.

3. Doxorubicin Cardiomyopathy

Doxorubicin exhibits acute and chronic cardiotoxicity and has been used to induce failure in various animal species. Several different mechanisms involved in the pathophysiology of doxorubicin heart failure have been suggested, including free radical generation and lipid peroxidation, reactive sulphydryl groups, binding to channel regulatory sites, or inhibition of mRNA and protein synthesis.[29]

Rabbits (5–6 kg) of both sexes of various strains can be used in this model. Doxorubicin (1 mg/kg intravenously, twice weekly) is given for 6–9 weeks in the sham control group. In the test group the animals are administered test drug for 4–6 weeks either subcutaneously or through the intraperitoneal route. After the experimental duration, the animals are anesthetized with pentobarbitone sodium (35 mg/kg) intraperitoneally and their carotid artery is cannulated for measuring blood pressure. The heart is exposed and cannula is inserted into the left ventricle to measure left ventricular end diastolic pressure (LVEDP) and dP/dt. The animals are sacrificed and the hearts processed for immunohistochemical studies through Western Blot studies. Chronic anthracycline administration to rabbits causes impairment of cardiac contractility and decreased gene expression of the calcium-induced calcium release channel of sarcoplasmic reticulum (SR), the ryanodine receptor (RYR2). The C-13 hydroxy metabolite (doxorubicinol), formed in the heart, has been hypothesized to contribute to anthracycline cardiotoxicity. Left ventricular fractional shortening (LVFS) is decreased by chronic treatment with doxorubicin compared to age-matched pair-fed controls. Doxorubicin, causes a significant reduction in the ratio of RYR2/Ca-Mg ATPase (SERCA2) mRNA levels in the left ventricle. This suggests that doxorubicin may contribute to the downregulation of cardiac RYR2 expression in chronic doxorubicin cardiotoxicity. The above mentioned parameters are also studied in the test drug group and comparisons are made with the sham control group. The ability of the test drug to reverse or reduce these changes is studied. These findings may suggest that this model is suited to study functional consequences of altered ryanodine receptor expression.

Guinea Pig Models

1. Cardiac Insufficiency

CHF in man is characterized by cardiac hypertrophy, peripheral edema, lung and liver congestion, dyspnea, hydrothorax and ascites. Based on these symptoms, CHF has been induced in guinea pigs with symptoms very close to human pathology. Following 8 weeks of banding of the descending thoracic aorta in guinea pigs, overt heart failure develops in a subgroup of animals. Alteration of myocardial function in this guinea pig model has some similarity to end-stage failing human myocardium.

Male guinea pigs (250-400 g) are anesthetized with ether. The chest cavity is opened, pericardium removed and heart is exposed. The beating heart is extruded from the thorax and a ring shaped clamp covered with a thin rubber tube is placed around the basis of the heart, keeping the heart outside of the thorax without closing off the blood circulation. A thread soaked with diluted disinfectant solution is placed as a loop around the heart and tightened so that the apical third of both ventricles is tied off. The degree of tightening of the loop is essential. Complete interruption of blood supply to the apical third resulting in necrosis has to be avoided as well as the loops slipping off. After removal of the clamp, the heart is placed back, the incision between the 4th and 5th costal ribs closed and the musculus pectoralis placed over the wound. Air is removed from the thorax and after application of an antibiotic emulsion, the skin wound is closed. The test drugs are administered subcutaneously or intramuscularly for 14 days.

The animals develop symptoms of CHF with death rate of 80% within 1 day. Lung weight, relative heart weight are significantly increased. Exudate volume in the thorax cavity and ascites is found between 3.5–7.5 ml. Lung edema and liver congestion are found histologically. Peripheral edema, preterminal dyspnoea and tachycardia are observed. The ability of the test drug to reverse these changes is studied. For survival rate ED_{50} of test drug is calculated.

Also a decrease in SR-Ca^{2+} ATPase protein levels and phospholamban protein levels is observed in failing guinea pig heart following 8 weeks of banding of the descending thoracic aorta as compared to an age matched banded group without clinical signs of heart failure. Regarding myosin isoforms, guinea pig myocardium, like the human ventricular myocardium, contains predominantly the β-myosin without any α-myosin heavy chain present in hypertrophied and failing hearts.[30]

The guinea pig model, thus has similarities to human heart failure with respect to calcium cycling, myosin isoforms and myocardial function. This model may be suited to study the transition from cardiac hypertrophy to failure with respect to alterations in excitation-contraction coupling systems.

Syrian Hamster

1. Cardiomyopathic Hamster

Cardiomyopathic strains of the syrian hamsters have been widely used as a model for cardiac hypertrophy and heart failure.[31] The model exhibits an autosomal recessive mode of inheritance, which leads to degenerative lesions in all striated muscles and in particular in the myocardium. The animals develop overt heart failure after 7–10 months. Histologically, necrotic, calcified myocardial lesions are observed initially in the development of the disease. Furthermore, a time dependent change in myosin isoform expression has been observed. The evolution of cardiomyopathic disease is characterized by five distinct phases: A prenecrotic stage, in which no pathology is evident, a phase of fibrosis and calcium deposition, an overlapping period of reactive hypertrophy of the remaining viable myocytes and a final stage of depressed myocardial performance and failure.

The test drugs are administered subcutaneously or intramuscularly for 14 days. The ability of the test drug to reverse or delay the above-mentioned changes is studied.

In summary, the advantages of this model are absence of surgical manipulations, low cost and the ease with which large number of animals can be studied.

It is important to state that there are differences among the strains, in the time course of the pathologic changes, therefore, the time point at which measurements are performed are critically important in this model. Furthermore, sub cellular alterations underlying myocardial failure seem to be different from those in failing human hearts.

Transgenic Mice

Recent developments of techniques to alter specifically the expression of genes have greatly improved the understanding of the pathophysiology of heart failure. Moreover, several genetic models of heart failure by addition or deletion of genes in mice have been developed and miniaturized physiological techniques to evaluate the resulting cardiac phenotypes have been established.[32] These models allow the identification of genes that are causative for heart failure and to evaluate the molecular mechanisms responsible for the development and progression of the disease. Gene targeted disruption of the muscle LIM protein (MLP) in mice is a new model of heart failure. MLP is a regulator of myogenic differentiation. Mice who were homozygous for the MLP knockout develop dilated cardiac myopathy associated with myocardial hypertrophy. Adult mice show clinical and hemodynamic signs of heart failure similar to those in humans.

Development of cardiomyopathy was also observed in mice with knockout of myogenic factor 5. Transgenic mice overexpressing either β-adrenergic receptor kinase or G-protein coupled receptor kinase 5, resulting in uncoupling of the β-adrenergic receptor, also exhibit reduced contractility, but without clinical signs of overt CHF. A recent model of transgenic overexpression of tropomodulin, exhibited dilated cardiomyopathy 2–4 weeks after birth with reduced contractile function and heart failure. This was associated with the loss of myofibrillar organization. One group of animals is administered drug orally, subcutaneously or intraperitoneally for 15 days. At the end of the experimental protocol, the animals in the test drug group are compared to sham control group on the basis of the above mentioned parameters.[33]

DEVELOPING NEW THERAPEUTIC TARGETS IN CHF

Gene Therapy

As the morbidity and cost of CHF have continued to increase, so has the understanding of cellular and molecular derangements which take place in CHF. This increasing knowledge, combined with the urgency to discover and develop novel and improved therapeutic strategies for CHF, has led to targeting molecular entities involved in CHF pathogenesis through gene therapy. Efforts to create CHF therapies targeting molecular causes of myocardial failure have focused on areas such as regulation of cardiomyocyte calcium handling. Kaye et al. used a sheep model of rapid pacing-induced DCM to develop a percutaneous means of myocardial gene delivery of a mutant form of the regulatory protein phospho- lamban, reporting improved cardiac function compared with controls.[34] In a different study, Kawase et al. examined the therapeutic potential of gene delivery in a pig model of volume overload HF. The study observed improved LV contractile performance and myocardial remodeling 2 months after SERCA2a, the cardiac isoform of a family of calcium ATPases, gene delivery administered by antegrade epicardial coronary artery infusion. The first human CHF gene therapy trials have now been initiated on patients with CHF receiving SERCA2a via myocardial gene delivery, providing an example of how large animal models serve a crucial step in the translation of basic science into clinical application.[35,36]

Stem Cells

Advances in the field of cellular therapies have created a new avenue of potential CHF treatments, specifically in area of stem cell research. Stem cells derived from various tissues have been introduced into the post-MI myocardium in efforts to attenuate post-MI LV remodeling. Initial studies using murine models reported dramatic results of stem cells having the ability to localize to the heart and purported to yield new myocardium. These initial small animal studies suggested boundless promises with respect to stem cells and myocardial remodeling. However, more recent clinical studies using mesenchymal stem cells have failed to demonstrate significant effects on post-MI LV remodeling and function.[37] The reasons for the failure of translation from basic stem cell studies to the clinical context are multifactorial, but likely include a lack of consensus regarding optimal stem cell type and preparation, delivery method, delivery location, and cell concentration. Large animal models will play a critical role in defining these factors. For example, the relative efficacy of mesenchymal stem cells has been evaluated in the pig MI model, with reports of improved LV EF after myocardial delivery of mesenchymal stem cells at the time of MI. Other studies have reported decreased MI expansion in pig and sheep MI models with mesenchymal stem cells delivered into the myocardium within 72 hours of MI and attenuation of EF deterioration with delivery 1 month post-MI. Alternatively, intracoronary and systemic delivery of mesenchymal stem cells have also been examined, further exemplifying the utility of large animal models in clarifying variables in stem cell therapies. It is likely that these translational studies in large animal models will be necessary if the tremendous potential suggested by rodent studies is to be realized clinically.[38]

Devices and Mechanical Support

A number of innovative devices aimed at improving LV systolic function and/or cardiac output in patients with HF have been created and refined through large animal models. From comparisons of early LV assist devices with the development of a totally implantable biventricular assist system, large animals have served an integral role in groundbreaking advances in cardiac destination therapies. The adaptation of such devices for neonatal and pediatric use has also been possible through large animal models. The development of minimally invasive devices to unload pressure from the failing LV have also used large animal models. For example, Haithcock et al. used a canine microembolization model of HF to demonstrate the benefits of LV unloading, establishing the basis for a percutaneously placed continuous aortic flow augmentation device, which is now in clinical trial.[39] Other work has been directed toward cardiac restraint devices, which are surgically placed around the heart itself to arrest post-MI LV remodeling. For example, Chakir et al. used a canine rapid-pacing model to demonstrate reduced myocyte apoptosis and improved stress-response molecular signaling with cardiac resynchronization therapy. Further advances and improvements in HF device therapies will surely depend on large animal models to ensure the safety and efficacy of these therapeutic options.[40]

DISCUSSION AND CONCLUSIONS

In the past, a large number of models have been established in animals with overt clinical heart failure to evaluate pathophysiology from the level of the intact instrumented animal to the tissue homogenate. These kind of studies provide a lot of information on hemodynamics, neurohumoral activation, myocardial infarction and sub-cellular and molecular alterations in the failing heart. There are great differences between species and models and only some models mimic human heart failure in some aspects. Such studies seem to be currently less important because with recent invasive and non-invasive technologies, hemodynamics can be studied in-patients. Furthermore, with cardiac transplantation surgery, end stage failing human myocardium became available for functional, biochemical and molecular biology studies allowing the evaluation of alterations, which are present in end-stage failure in the human heart itself. However, it is rather difficult or impossible to study myocardial changes associated during compensated, less severe stages of CHF, during the transition from hypertrophy to failure or during the process of remodeling. Therefore, in order to study transition processes occurring in heart failure, animal models are very important. Furthermore, animal models of heart failure may be relevant to study the effects of new pharmacological strategies on hemodynamics, neurohumoral activation and survival. At present, transgenic animal models of heart failure are critically important to understand the molecular alterations underlying the development of the disease. Addition or deletion of genes in transgenic mice together with miniaturized physiological techniques to evaluate the resulting cardiac phenotypes allow the identification of genes that are causative for heart failure and to evaluate molecular mechanisms responsible for the development and progression of the disease.

In vitro models	*In vivo models*
1. Isolated hamster cardiomyopathic heart 2. Isolated cat papillary muscle 3. Ouabain binding	**Rat models**
	• Rat coronary ligation model
	• Rat aortic banding
	• Dahl salt sensitive rats
	• Spontaneous hypertensive rat
	• Spontaneous hypertensive-heart failure rats (SH-HF)
	Dog models
	• Chronic rapid pacing
	• Volume overload
	• Coronary artery ligation and microembolization
	Rabbit models of heart failure
	• Volume and pressure overload
	• Tachycardia pacing
	• Doxorubicin cardiomyopathy
	Guinea pig model
	• Cardiac insufficiency
	Syrian hamster
	• Cardiomyopathic hamster
	Genetic model
	• Transgenic mice
	New therapeutic targets in CHF
	• Gene therapy
	• Stem cells
	• Devices and mechanical support

REFERENCES

1. American Heart Association. ACC/AHA 2005 guideline update for the diagnosis and management of chronic heart failure in the adult. Circulation. 2005;112:e154-e235.
2. Yamani M, Massie BM. Congestive heart failure: insights from epidemiology, implications for treatment. Mayo Clin Proc 1993;68:1214-18.
3. Ho KKL, Anderson KM, Kannel WB. Survival after the onset of congestive heart failure in Framingham Heart Study subjects. Circulation 1993;88:107-15.
4. Richard D. Patten and Monica R. Hall-Porter. Small animal models of heart failure: Development of novel therapies, past and present. Circ Heart Fail 2009;2:138-44.
5. Dixon JA, Spinale FG, Jennifer A. Large animal models of heart failure: A critical link in the translation of basic science to clinical practice, Circ Heart Fail 2009;2:262-71.
6. Jasmin G, Solymoss B, Proscheck L. Therapeutic trials in hamsters dystrophy, Ann NY Acad Sci 1979;317:338-48.
7. Catell M, Gold H. Influence of digitalis glycoside on the force of contraction of mammalian cardiac muscle. J Pharmacol Exp Ther 1938;62:116-225.

8. Pfeffer MA, Pfeffer JM, Fishbein MC. Myocardial infarct size and ventricular function in rats. Circ Res 1979;44:503-12.
9. Salai S, Miyauchi T, Kobayashi M. Inhibition of myocardial endothelin pathway improves long term survival in heart failure. Nature 1996;384:353-5.
10. Bers DM. Control of cardiac contraction by SR-Ca release and sarcolemmal Ca fluxes. In: Bers DM, ed. Excitation-contraction coupling and cardiac contractile force. Developments in cardiovascular medicine. Boston, London: Kluver Academic Publishers, 1991;122:149-70.
11. Kajstura J, Zhang X, Reiss K. Myocyte cellular hyperplasia and myocyte cellular hypertrophy contribute to chronic ventricular remodelling in coronary artery narrowing-induced cardiomyopathy in rats. Circ Res 1994;74:383-400.
12. Zarain-Herzberg A, Afzal N, Elimban V, et al. Decreased expression of cardiacsarcoplasmic reticulum Ca pump ATPase in congestive heart failure due to myocardial infarction. Mol Cell Biochem 1996; 34:163-4.
13. Holtz J, Studer R, Reinecke H, et al. Modulation of myocardial sarcoplasmic reticulum Ca-ATPase in cardiac hypertrophy by angiotensin converting enzyme. Basic Res Cardiol 1992; 87:191-204.
14. Schunkert H, Lorrel BH. Role of angiotensin II in the translation of left ventricular hypertrophy to cardiac failure. Heart Failure 1994;10:142-9.
15. Dahl LK, Heine M, Tassinari L. Role of genetic factors in susceptibility to experimental hypertension due to chronic excess salt ingestion. Nature 1962;194:480-2.
16. Inoko M, Kihara Y, Morii I, et al. Transition from compensatory hypertrophy to dilated, failing left ventricles in Dahl salt-sensitive rats. Am J Physiol 1994;267:H2482.
17. Okamoto K, Aoki K. Development of a strain of spontaneously hypertensive rats. Jpn Circ J 1963; 27:282-93.
18. Boluyt MO, Neill L, Meredith AL. Alterations in cardiac gene expression during the transition from the stable hypertrophy to heart failure. Marked upregulation of genes encoding extracellular matrix components. Circ Res 1994;75:23-32.
19. Gomez AM, Valdivia HH, Cheng H. Defective excitation-contraction coupling in experimental cardiac hypertrophy and heart failure. Science 1997;276:800-06.
20. Lompre AM, Mercadier JJ, Wisnewsky C. Species and age-dependent changes in the relative amounts of cardiac myosin isozymes in mammal. Dev Biol 1981;84:286-90.
21. Armstrong PW, Stopps TP, Ford Se, et al. Rapid ventricular pacing in the dog: pathophysiologic studies of heart failure. Circulation 1986;74:1075-84.
22. Spinale FG, Mukerjee R. Relation between ventricular and myocyte function with tachycardia induced cardiomyopathy. Circ Res 1992;71:174-87.
23. Mc Danald KM. Francis GS, Carlyle PF. Hemodynamic, left ventricular structural and hormonal changes after discrete myocardial damage in dogs. J Am Coll Cardiol 1992;19:460-7.
24. McCullagh WH, Covell JW, Ross J. Left ventricular dilation and diastolic compliance changes during chronic volume overloading. Circulation 1972;45:943-51.
25. Kleaveland JP, Kussmaul WG, Diters R. Volume overload hypertrophy in a closed chest model of atrial regurgitation. Am J Physiol 1988;254:H1034-41.
26. Sabbah HN, Stein PD, Kono T. A canine model of chronic heart failure produced by multiple sequential coronary microembolizations. Am J Physiol 1991;260:H1379-81.
27. Gengo PJ, Sabbah HN, Steffen RP. Myocardial beta adrenoreceptor and voltage sensitive calcium channel changes in a canine model of chronic heart failure. J Mol Cell Cardiol 1992;24:1361-9.

28. Magid NM, Opio G, Wallerson DC, et al. Heart failure due to chronic experimental aortic regurgitation. Am J Physiol 1990;267:H556-62.
29. Freeman GL, Colston JT. Myocardial depression produced by sustained tachycardia in rabbits. Am J Physiol 1992;262:H63-67.
30. Dodd DA, Atkinson JB, Olson RD. Doxorubicin cardiomyopathy is associated with a decrease in calcium release channel in sarcoplasmic reticulum in a chronic rabbit model. J Clin Invest 1993; 91:1697-705.
31. Malhotra A, Siri FM, Aronson R. Cardiac contractile proteins in hypertrophied and failing guinea pig heart. Cardiovasc Res 1992;26:153-61.
32. Bajusz E. Hereditary cardiomyopathy: a new disease model. Am Heart J 1969;7:686-96.
33. Hoit BD, Khoury SF, Kranais EG et al. In vivo ecocardiographic detection of enhanced left ventricular function in gene targeted mice. Circ Res 1995;77:632-37.
34. Kaye DM, Preovolos A, Marshall T, Byrne M, Hoshijima M, Hajjar R, Mariani JA, Pepe S, Chien KR, Power JM. Percutaneous cardiac recirculation-mediated gene transfer of an inhibitory phospholamban peptide reverses advanced heart failure in large animals. J Am Coll Cardiol 2007;50:253-60.
35. Kawase Y, Ly HQ, Prunier F, Lebeche D, Shi Y, Jin H, Hadri L, Yoneyama R, Hoshino K, Takewa Y, Sakata S, Peluso R, Zsebo K, Gwathmey JK, Tardif JC, Tanguay JF, Hajjar RJ. Reversal of cardiac dysfunction after long-term expression of SERCA2a by gene transfer in a pre-clinical model of heart failure. J Am Coll Cardiol 2008;51:1112-9.
36. Vinge LE, Raake PW, Koch WJ. Gene therapy in heart failure. Circ Res. 2008;102:1458-70.
37. Meyer GP, Wollert KC, Lotz J, Steffens J, Lippolt P, Fichtner S, Hecker H, Schaefer A, Arseniev L, Hertenstein B, Ganser A, Drexler H. Intracoronary bone marrow cell transfer after myocardial infarction: eighteen months' follow-up data from the randomized, controlled BOOST (Bone marrow transfer to enhance ST-elevation infarct regeneration) trial. Circulation 2006;113:1287-94.
38. Lunde K, Solheim S, Aakhus S, Arnesen H, Abdelnoor M, Egeland T, Endresen K, Ilebekk A, Mangschau A, Fjeld JG, Smith HJ, Taraldsrud E, Grøgaard HK, Bjørnerheim R, Brekke M, Müller C, Hopp E, Ragnarsson A, Brinchmann JE, Forfang K. Intracoronary injection of mononuclear bone marrow cells in acute myocardial infarction. N Engl J Med 2006;355:1199-209.
39. Haithcock BE, Morita H, Fanous NH, Suzuki G, Sabbah HN. Hemodynamic unloading of the failing left ventricle using an arterial-to-arterial extracorporeal flow circuit. Ann Thorac Surg 2004;77:158 -63.
40. Chakir K, Daya SK, Tunin RS, Helm RH, Byrne MJ, Dimaano VL, Lardo AC, Abraham TP, Tomaselli GF, Kass DA. Reversal of global apoptosis and regional stress kinase activation by cardiac resynchronization. Circulation 2008;117:1369-77.

CHAPTER

20

Antianginal Agents

Among the cardiovascular pathologies, ischemic heart disease is the leading cause of morbidity, mortality as well as permanent premature disabilities. Ischemic heart disease occurs when coronary blood flow is inadequate to supply the oxygen required by the heart. By far the most frequent cause is atheromatous obstruction of the large coronary vessels (atherosclerosis angina, classical angina). However, transient spasm of localized portions of these vessels, which is usually associated with underlying atheromas, can also cause significant myocardial ischemia and pain (angioplastic or variant angina).

Reperfusion of a previously ischemic heart is a standard clinical procedure. Even if beneficial, reperfusion triggers an inflammatory response that contributes to the acute extension of ischemic injury and later participates in the reparative processes of the damaged myocardium.[1] Occlusion of a major coronary artery in small rodents, followed or not followed by reperfusion, has proven to be a good model to assess the relevance of pathophysiological processes and drug effects in the setting of myocardial ischemia. Models involving reperfusion appear to be particularly suitable to study the inflammatory response, which is much more marked than with permanent ischemia. Ischemia/reperfusion of the myocardium in wild-type and transgenic animals (mostly mice) allows the possibility of testing the vast array of mediators that orchestrate the sequelae of oxidative stress and inflammation. Moreover, the experimental models allow testing of the protective effects of drugs in experimental ischemia and reperfusion injury.

Various animal models are available to screen anti-anginal drugs. Some of the widely used models are discussed in this chapter. These animal models are useful for studying the consequence of a myocardial ischemia and reperfusion on cardiac pathophysiological and physiological functions.

IN VITRO MODELS

1. Langendorff Heart Preparation

Langendorff is a highly reproducible preparation which can be studied quickly in large number at relatively low cost. It allows measurement of broad spectrum of biochemical, physiological and morphological indices. Measurements are made in absence of the confounding effects of the organs. Both global and regional ischemia can be studied using this model. It allows experiments to be continued in face of events (MI, arrhythmias) which would normally jeopardize the survival of an *in vivo* experiment. However, it is a deteriorating preparation though capable of study for several hours. The basic principle involved is that heart is perfused in a retrograde direction from the aorta either at constant pressure or constant flow with oxygenated saline solutions. Retrograde perfusion closes the aortic valves, just as in the *in situ* heart during diastole. The perfusate is displaced through the coronary arteries flowing off the coronary sinus and the opened right atrium. Parameters usually measured are contractile force, coronary flow and cardiac rhythm.

Guinea pigs of either sex weighing 300 to 500 g are used for the study. They are sacrificed by stunning. Diaphragm is assessed by transabdominal incision and cut carefully to expose the thoracic cavity. Thorax is opened by bilateral incision along the lower margins of the last to first ribs. Thoracic cage is reflected over the animal's head exposing the heart. The heart is cradled between fingers and lifted before incising the aorta, vena cava and pulmonary veins. Immediately after excision, heart is dipped in cold perfusion solution (4°C to limit ischemic injury during period between excision and restoration of vascular perfusion). The aorta is located and cut below the point of division. A cannula is inserted into the aorta and tied and the heart is perfused with oxygenated Ringer's solution. The heart is transferred to a double wall plexiglass perfusion apparatus maintained at 37°C.[2] Oxygenated Ringer's solution is perfused at a constant pressure of 40 mmHg at a temperature of 37°C from a reservoir. A small steel hook with a string is attached to the apex of the heart. Contractile force is measured isometrically by a force transducer and recorded on a polygraph. Heart rate is measured through a chronometer coupled to the polygraph. Drugs are injected into the perfusion medium.[3] The anti-anginal effect of the test drug is indicated by an increase in coronary blood flow. The incidence and duration of ventricular fibrillation, coronary flow, inotropic state and K^+ levels after treatment with drug are compared with control.

This method is very useful for testing coronary vasodilator drugs. It has wide applications in the fields of pharmacology and physiology. It is useful to study positive inotropic effects, negative inotropic effects, coronary vasodilatory effect, calcium antagonism, effect on potassium outflow induced by glycosides and determination of hypoxic damage. Metabolic studies, arrhythmogenic, antiarrhythmic and antifibrillatory effects can also be assessed using Langendorff method. Recently this model has been also used to study EDRF release from the coronary vascular bed and electrophysiological evaluation of cardiovascular agents.

2. Isolated Rabbit Aorta Preparation

Aortic rings are used to evaluate the smooth muscle relaxant/contractile activity in this method. Adding potassium chloride or norepinephrine to the organ bath containing slightly modified Kreb's bicarbonate buffer induces contraction of aorta rings.

Using an overdose of pentobarbital sodium, rabbits of either sex weighing 3 to 4 kg are sacrificed. Thorax is opened by bilateral incision. The descending thoracic aorta is rapidly removed and placed in Kreb's bicarbonate buffer maintained at 37°C. Tissue is cleaned, fat and connective tissue is carefully removed. Eight rings of 4-5 mm width are obtained and each is mounted in 20 ml tissue bath containing Kreb's solution. A stabilization period of 2 h is allowed wherein the Kreb's solution is frequently changed followed by stabilization period of 1 h. A tension of 1 g is maintained during these times. A sustained contraction is generated by addition of KCl. Twenty minutes after addition of agonist, the test drug is added. The percent relaxation reading is taken every 30 min after addition of the test drug. There is a 30 min time interval between additions of different test drugs.[4]

Active tension is calculated for the tissue at time point just prior to the addition of the test compound and also at the point 30 min after the addition of each concentration of the test compound. ID_{50} and percentage relaxation caused by the test drug from the precontracted level is calculated.[5] Test drug with calcium channel blocking activity have a relaxing effect and can be evaluated using this method.

3. Calcium Antagonism in Pitched Rat

This model can differentiate calcium entry blockers from other agents that do not directly block entry of calcium.

Sprague Dawley rats (250 to 350 g) are anesthetized intraperitoneally with methohexitone sodium (50 mg/kg). The trachea is cannulated. Thereafter the rats are pitched through one orbit and immediately maintained on artificial respiration. The pithing rod is used as a stimulating electrode and continuous electrical stimulation of the thoracic spinal cord with squarewave pulses at supramaximal voltage (frequency 0.5 Hz and duration 0.5 ms) produces a cardioaccelerator response. Only rats with a resulting tachycardia (100 beats/min) are included for the study. The jugular vein is cannulated for administration of drugs and blood pressure is recorded via carotid artery using a pressure transducer. In the femoral region, an indifferent electrode is inserted subcutaneously.

When cardioaccelerator response is established for 3-5 min, calcium channel blockers and β-blockers are administered. These test compounds dose dependently block tachycardia.[6] The level of tachycardia immediately prior to drug administration is taken as 100% and response to drugs is expressed as percentage of predose tachycardia. ID_{50} is calculated and compared.

4. Relaxation of Bovine Coronary Artery

The relaxation caused by test compounds can be assayed using spiral strips from bovine coronary artery. The tonus of coronary arteries can be regulated by eicosanoids. Prostacyclin induces relaxation whereas thromboxane A_2 causes contraction.

Beef hearts are obtained immediately after slaughtering. They are immersed in cold oxygenated Kreb's solution and immediately transported to the laboratory. The left descending coronary artery is cut into spiral strips and suspended in a 4 ml organ bath under an initial tension of 2 g and immersed in oxygenated Kreb's bicarbonate solution at 37°C. The Kreb's solution contains a mixture of antagonists to inhibit actions from endogenous acetylcholine, 5-hydroxy-tryptamine, histamine or catecholamines. The strips are superfused with a solution of test compound with oxygenated Kreb's solution. Isometric contractions are recorded with force-displacement transducers on a Grass polygraph. The strips are superfused with Kreb's solution three hours prior to the experiment. Standard compounds are 100 ng/ml PGE_2 inducing contraction and 100 ng/ml PGI_2 inducing pronounced relaxation.[7,8]

The maximal response to 100 ng/ml PGE_2 or 100 ng/ml PGI_2 is calculated and the relaxation caused by the test compound is expressed as its percentage.

5. Coronary Artery Ligation in Isolated Rat Heart

Langendorff technique can also be used to produce regional ischemia by clamping the left coronary artery close to its origin. After removal of the clip, changes in the reperfusion period can be observed. Prevention of these symptoms is an indicator of the efficacy of the coronary drugs.

Wistar rats of either sex weighing 280 to 300 g are sacrificed by decapitation. The hearts are removed and dissected free from the epicardium and surrounding connective tissue.[4] A cannula is introduced into the aorta from where the coronary vessels are perfused with the non-circulated perfusion medium according to the Langendorff technique. In the left ventricle a balloon closely fitting the ventricular cavity is placed and connected to an artificial systemic circulation. The balloon is made of silicone material using a Teflon form. The dimensions of the Teflon form are basically derived from casts of left ventricle of K^+ arrested casts by injection of dental cement. During each heart beat the fluid volume pressed from the balloon corresponding to the stroke volume of the heart, can be recorded by means of a flowmeter probe and an integrator connected in series. The preload and afterload are adjusted separately and the perfusate flow is recorded separately. For coronary artery occlusion experiment, the isolated working hearts are perfused for 20 min with Kreb's buffer at 65 mmHg. Acute myocardial ischemia is produced by clamping the left coronary artery close to its origin for 15 min. The clip is then opened and the changes during reperfusion period are monitored for 30 min. Haemodynamic parameters like left ventricular pressure, heart rate, cardiac output and coronary flow are measured.[9] From the coronary effluent, samples are taken for lactate dehydrogenase (LDH), creatine kinase (CK), glycogen, ATP and lactate determinations. The test drug is given into the perfusion medium either before occlusion or 5 min before reperfusion. The incidence and duration of ventricular fibrillation after treatment with test drugs is compared with controls. Left ventricular pressure, left ventricular dP/dt max, coronary flow and myocardial LDH, CPK, glycogen, ATP and lactate are also measured.

6. Isolated Heart-Lung Preparation

The isolated heart-lung preparation of the dog has been used to study various physiological and pharmacological processes. Now this model has also been established in rats.

Wistar rats (300 to 350 g) are anesthetized intraperitoneally with pentobarbitone sodium (50 mg/kg). The trachea is cannulated and the animal is maintained on artificial respiration. The chest cavity is opened and ice-cold saline is injected to arrest the heart. The aorta, superior and inferior vena cava are cannulated. The heart-lung preparation is perfused with Kreb's-Ringer bicarbonate buffer (pH 7.4) containing rat RBC (hematocrit 25%). The perfusate is pumped from the aorta and is passed through the pneumatic resistance and collected in a reservoir maintained at 37°C. It is then returned to the inferior vena cava thus perfusing only the heart and the lung. Test drug is administered into the perfusate 5 min after start of experiment. Cardiac output is recorded with an electromagnetic blood flowmeter and mean arterial pressure from the pneumatic resistance. With the help of a bioelectrical amplifier heart rate is recorded. Hemodynamic data and recovery time of the test drug group and control group (without any treatment) is compared using ANOVA and Kruskal-Wallis test respectively.[10]

7. Plastic Casts Technique in Dogs

Coronary drug when administered for prolonged duration leads to increase in the number and size of interarterial collaterals especially in pigs and dogs. Acute or gradual occlusion of one of the major coronary branches may also stimulate development of collaterals. In order to quantify the collaterals, the arterial coronary bed is filled with plastic. This provides with the possibility to make the collaterals visible.

Dogs (10 to 15 kg) are intravenously anesthetized with pentobarbital sodium (30 mg/kg). They are maintained on artificial respiration, chest cavity is opened and the heart is exposed. The pericardium is removed and Ameroid cuffs are placed around the major coronary branches. The plastic materials gradually swell and occlude the lumen within 3 to 4 weeks. The animals are administered test drugs or placebo for 6 weeks and then sacrificed. After a recovery period of 1 week, their hearts are removed and coronary bed flushed with saline. Liquid araldite is filled in the bulbus aortae, the coronary, arterial and venous tree. Care is taken to maintain the uniformity of the filling pressure, the filling time and viscosity of the filling material. After polymerization is complete, the tissue is digested with 35 % KOH. Plastic casts from the drug treated animals are compared with casts from the sham group (dogs subjected to the same procedure without drug treatment). The ability of the test drug to increase the number and size of collateral's is evaluated.[11]

IN VIVO MODELS

1. Occlusion of Coronary Artery

Compounds that reduce infarct size are studied using this model. Infarct size is studied after proximal occlusion of the left anterior descending coronary artery in open chest dogs. Nitro-blue tetrazolium chloride stain in myocardial sections are used to visualize infarct size in coronary arteriograms made after injection of $BaSO_4$ gelatin mass into the left coronary ostium.

Dogs of either sex (30 kg) are used in this model. The animals are anesthetized with pentobarbitone sodium (35 mg/kg, intraperitoneally) which is followed by its continuous infusion at 4 mg/kg/h. Trachea is cannulated and the animal is maintained on artificial respiration. Peripheral vein (saphenous vein) is cannulated for administration of test compound. ECG is recorded continuously. Femoral vein is cannulated and connected to a pressure transducer for measuring peripheral systolic and diastolic pressure. Left ventricular end diastolic pressure, left ventricular pressure and heart rate are also measured using a Millar microtip catheter (PC 350) inserted via the left coronary artery. Heart is exposed through a left thoracotomy between 4th and 5th intercostal space. The pericardium is opened and the left anterior descending coronary artery is exposed and then ligated for 360 min. Test substance or vehicle is administered by intravenous bolus injection. Haemodynamic parameters are monitored and at the end of the experiment, animals are sacrificed with an overdose of pentobarbital sodium. Area at risk of infarction is measured using coronary arteriograms. The left ventricle is cut into transverse sections. From each slice angiograms are made with X-ray tube at 40 kv to assess the area at risk of infarction by defect opacity : reduction of $BaSO_4$ filled vessels in infarct tissue. The slices are then incubated in p-nitro-blue-tetrazolium

(0.25 g/l) in order to visualize the infarct tissue (blue/violet stained healthy tissue, unstained necrotic tissue). The slices are photographed for determination of infarct area. Mortality, haemodynamic parameters and infarct size are determined. Changes in parameters in drug treated animals are compared to vehicle controls.[12]

2. Microspheres-induced Acute Ischemia

This model can be useful in evaluating the effect of test drugs on myocardial performance during acute ischemic left ventricular failure. Microspheres (50 μm) when injected repeatedly into the left main coronary artery may induce left ventricular failure in anesthetized dogs. Hemodynamic parameters can be recorded and drugs tested on the basis of their improvement of cardiac performance.

Dogs (30 kg) are anesthetized with pentobarbitone sodium intravenously (40 mg/kg) and additionally administered a supplementary dose of 4 mg/kg/h. The trachea is cannulated and the animal maintained on artificial respiration. The brachial vein is cannulated for administration of analgesic and saphenous vein for administration of test compounds. ECG is recorded continuously. The femoral artery is also cannulated and connected to a pressure transducer for the measurement of systolic and diastolic pressure. A Millar microtip catheter is inserted via the left coronary artery for the determination of left ventricular pressure while left ventricular end diastolic pressure (LVEDP) is measured on a high sensitivity scale. From the pressure curve, dP/dt and heart rate are calculated. Mean pulmonary capillary pressure, mean pulmonary artery pressure (PAP) and cardiac output are measured using Cardiac Index Computer and a balloon tip triple lumen catheter with the thermistor positioned in the pulmonary artery via the jugular vein. Through a left thoracotomy, the heart is exposed. Microspheres are injected through the angiogram catheter into the left ostium initially as 10 ml and later as 5 ml boluses about 5 min apart. Embolization is terminated when the LVEDP increases to 16 to 18 mmHg and PAP to 20 mmHg and heart rate 200 beats/min. Test compound is then administered by intravenous route and the above mentioned parameters recorded. In addition to the directly measured hemodynamic parameters, stroke volume, tension index, coronary vascular resistance, total peripheral resistance, pulmonary artery resistance can also be measured. Changes of parameters in drug treated animals are compared to vehicle controls. Also mean embolization time, doses of microspheres and numbers of microspheres are evaluated.[13]

3. Isoproterenol-induced Myocardial Necrosis

Synthetic catecholamines like isoproterenol when injected at high dose produce cardiac necrosis. Rona et al. have studied the infarct like lesions in the rat myocardium.[14] Several drugs such as sympatholytics or calcium antagonists can totally or partially prevent these lesions.

Wistar rats (150 to 200 g) are pretreated with test drug or standard drug orally or subcutaneously for at least a week. These rats are then injected with 85 mg/kg isoproterenol subcutaneously on two consecutive days. Mortality as well as symptoms are recorded in each group and compared to group injected with isoproterenol only. After 48 h of first dose of isoproterenol the animals are sacrificed. The heart is removed, weighed and preserved for histological evaluation or processed for estimation of various biochemical parameters. Before sacrificing, the animal's hemodynamic parameters such as systolic/diastolic blood pressure and heart rate can be recorded by cannulating the carotid artery and connecting it to a pressure transducer. By inserting a cannula in the left ventricle, parameters such as left ventricular end diastolic pressure (LVEDP) and dP/dt can be measured. The degree of histopathological changes can be graded as follows:

Grade 0: No change
Grade 1: Focal areas of necrosis
Grade 2: Focal areas of necrosis and muscle fiber fragmentation
Grade 3: Confluent areas of necrosis, edema and inflammation and muscle fiber fragmentation
Grade 4: Massive areas of necrosis, edema and inflammation and mural thrombi.

Changes of parameters (histological, biochemical and hemodynamic) of drug treated animals are compared to isoproterenol controls.[15]

4. Stenosis-induced Coronary Thrombosis Model

Thrombosis can be induced by stenosis in dogs. This model is characterized by alterations in coronary blood flow with transient platelet aggregation at the site of coronary constriction.

Dogs (15 to 20 kg) are anesthetized with pentobarbitone sodium (30 to 40 mg/kg, intraperitoneally) and then maintained on artificial respiration through a tracheal tube using a positive pressure respirator. Through a left thoracotomy the heart is exposed at the 4th and 5th intercostal space and the pericardium is removed. An electromagnetic flowprobe is placed on the proximal part of the left coronary artery to measure coronary blood flow. Distal to the flowmeter, the vessel is clamped for 5 sec. A small plastic constrictor is placed around the artery at the site of damage. The constrictor is changed several times until the required narrowing of the coronary artery is achieved. In case the artery is occluded, the coronary artery is lifted to induce reflow. Dogs with regular repeated cyclic flow variations of same intensity within a pretreatment phase of 60 min are used for experimental purpose. Hemodynamic parameters are recorded. Test compound is administered intravenously and the cyclic flow variations are registered for 2 to 5 h and compared to pre-treatment values.

In case simple clamping of the coronary artery does not produce cyclic flow variations, additionally adrenaline (0.2 µg/kg) is infused into the peripheral vein, 30 min before and 30 min following drug administration. Also platelet activating factor (PAF; 0.2 nmol/kg/min) when infused for a similar duration as adrenaline into the cannulated lateral branch of the coronary artery may produce cyclic flow variations. Cyclic flow variations are registered and compared to the drug treated group.[16]

5. Electrical Stimulation-induced Coronary Thrombosis

Electrical stimulation can induce thrombosis in the coronary artery in pigs. An alteration in coronary blood flow with transient platelet aggregation at the site of coronary constriction is assessed using this model.

German landrace pigs (20 to 40 kg) are anesthetized with ketamine (2 mg/kg, intramuscularly), metomidate (10 mg/kg intraperitoneally) and xylazine (1-2 mg/kg intramuscularly) and then maintained on artificial respiration through a tracheal tube using a positive pressure respirator. Through a left thoracotomy the heart is exposed at the 4th and 5th intercostal space and the pericardium is removed. A electromagnetic flowmeter is placed on the proximal part of the left coronary artery to measure the coronary blood flow. A vanadium steel electrode is placed in the vessel with the intimal lining and connected with the Teflon coated wire of 9-Volt battery, a potentiometer and an amperometer.[17] To complete the electric circuit, a disc electrode is placed on the thoracic muscle layer. The intima is stimulated with 150 μA for 6 h during which time an occluding thrombosis occurs. The test drug is administered either subcutaneously with the electrical stimulation or 30 min following the electrical stimulation. Hemodynamic parameters - systolic, diastolic, mean blood pressure and heart rate are measured by cannulating the femoral artery and connecting it to a pressure transducer. Left ventricular pressure, left ventricular end diastolic pressure, dP/dt are measured by inserting a micro-tip catheter via the carotid artery retrogradely. ECG is also recorded using lead II. The time interval until the thrombotic occlusion of the vessel occurs and the thrombus size are determined. At the end of the experiment the animals are sacrificed with an overdose of anesthesia. Percent change in mean values for occlusion time and thrombus size in drug treated groups is compared to the control group. Also changes in hemodynamic parameters, cyclic number and cycle area after drug treatment is compared to pre-treatment values.

6. Myocardial Ischemic Preconditioning Model

Myocardial preconditioning (brief duration of ischemia and reperfusion) can reduce the damage produced by prolonged ischemia and reperfusion. Preliminary preconditioning of the myocardium reduces infarct size, reduces leakage of cellular proteins indicative of myocyte death, improves post-ischemic ventricular function, as well as attenuates cardiac arrhythmia associated with frequent ischemia/reperfusion.

Rabbits (New Zealand, weighing 3 to 4 kg) are anesthetized with ketamine (50 mg/ml)/xylazine (10 mg/ml) at a dose of 0.6 ml/kg. The trachea is cannulated and the animal maintained on artificial respiration (30 inflations per min). The right femoral artery and vein are catheterized for measurement of arterial pressure and administration of drugs respectively. Hemodynamic parameters like systolic, diastolic, mean blood pressure, heart rate, left ventricular pressure, left ventricular end diastolic pressure and dP/dt are measured. A 4-0 suture is looped loosely around the marginal branch of left coronary artery to facilitate coronary occlusion during the experiment. Ischemic preconditioning is induced by tightening the loop around the coronary artery for 5 min and then loosening to reperfuse the myocardium for 10 min prior to a subsequent 30 min occlusion. After 30 min ischemia, ligature is released for 120 min of reperfusion. Prior to 30 min of occlusion the rabbits are selected to receive ischemic preconditioning, no preconditioning or preconditioning along with the administration of test compound. The animals are sacrificed after the reperfusion duration. Comparisons between systemic hemodynamic data and infarct size studies are analyzed by ANOVA using statistical software.[18]

7. Models of Coronary Flow Measurement

These models are based on measurement of coronary outflow in open and closed chest animal preparations. Various drugs can be screened for their anti-anginal potential, on the basis of their coronary artery dilating properties.

I. Coronary Inflow Measurement in Anesthetized Dogs

Dogs (15 to 20 kg) are anesthetized with pentobarbitone sodium (30 to 40 mg/kg) intraperitoneally and then maintained on artificial respiration using a positive pressure respirator. Through a left thoracotomy, the heart is exposed at the 4th and 5th intercostal space and the pericardium is removed. Through the jugular vein a catheter is inserted to cannulate the coronary sinus. In the in-vitro studies cannula is inserted through an opening in the atrial appendage into the coronary sinus and drained to measure coronary flow. Haemodynamic parameters - systolic, diastolic, mean blood pressure and heart rate are measured by cannulating the femoral artery and connecting it to a pressure transducer. The test drug is administered through the other jugular vein. Changes in coronary flow and haemodynamic parameters after test drug administration is compared to values before test drug administration.

Advantage of this method is that approximately 95 % of the total coronary venous flow can be measured.[19] Disadvantages of this method are that only 60% of coronary flow returns through coronary sinus. No constant proportion between coronary venous outflow and coronary sinus flow is present.[20] Another method with slight modification in the above mentioned model could also be used to measure coronary blood inflow. In this method blood from superior vena cava is diverted to pulmonary artery and flow from right ventricle is measured.

II. Coronary Outflow Measurement in Anesthetized Dogs

Various devices have been used through ages for measuring coronary flow, of which in-vogue is electromagnetic flowmeter. It is used to measure:

A. Phasic flow: An additional probe is placed around the aorta to record changes in coronary flow with changes in aortic pressure.

B. Mean flow: Average flow through coronary arteries per cardiac cycle.[18]

a. Electromagnetic Flowmeter

Dogs (10 to 12 kg) are anesthetized with pentobarbitone sodium (30 to 40 mg/kg, intraperitoneally). Their trachea is cannulated and animals are maintained on artificial respiration using a positive pressure respirator. Through the left thoracotomy, heart is exposed at the 4th and 5th intercostal space and the pericardium is removed. Two poles of electromagnet are placed in opposite sides of the coronary vessel. Distal to the electromagnets, two chromium-vanadium electrodes are placed adhering to the coronary artery. A magnetic field perpendicular to blood flow generates voltage in the conductor (blood stream). It is picked up by electrodes, amplified and recorded. This method mostly records phasic flow. Mean flow is recorded by electrical damping. Jugular vein is cannulated for the administration of test compound and carotid artery for measurement of blood pressure. Changes in coronary outflow and hemodynamic parameters before and after test drug administration are compared.

To avoid polarization at pickup electrodes, magnetic current is reversed by oscillator either of square wave or sine wave type. Initially probes were big but with advanced technology, nowadays, small sized probes are available. They are used mainly in chronic unanesthetized whole animal experiments by running lead wire through the skin.[21, 22]

III. Other Models to Measure Coronary Flow

The following methods can be employed to measure coronary flow:

a. Inert gas technique

Mainly helium or nitrous oxide is used. A mixture of room air and inert gas is inhaled (known quantity). A series of blood samples are withdrawn simultaneously from a peripheral artery (using needle) and coronary sinus/cardiac vein (using catheter). A-V difference is calculated. A-V difference is the difference between the integrals of arterial and coronary sinus.[20] Blood flow through the organ/time is calculated as:

$$\frac{\text{Amount of substance taken up in unit time}}{\text{A-V difference}}$$

It can measure only mean flow but not regional flow.[23] It takes around 10 min for one determination.

b. Radioactive technique

The radioisotopes mainly used are ^{121}I, ^{3}H and rubidium. Isotopes are inhaled/injected and change in rate over chest wall is measured using giega counter. By appropriate calculations a measure of coronary flow can be determined. It has a close co-relation with the above-described method. It is a fast and simple technique.[24]

c. Radioactive microsphere technique

This method determines regional blood flow including distribution of coronary flow across the ventricular wall. A batch of radioactive microspheres (9-15 μDM) is suspended in a saline detergent solution and injected into the left atrium. Microspheres lodge in only a few capillaries, so no damage/effect on flow is observed.

The number of spheres trapped/unit of myocardial tissue is directly proportional to myocardial blood flow.[25]

d. Thermodilution technique

A catheter having an end hole is passed to the beginning of the coronary sinus. A temperature sensor (thermometer) is placed further down the coronary sinus. Cold saline of known temperature is injected continuously through catheter-diluted by coronary sinus blood flow. Modified temperature is measured by thermometer. The temperature difference obtained is proportional to the blood flow.[26,27]

e. Coronary arteriography

Radio-opaque solutions are injected by a catheter into a coronary artery at the root of aorta. With high speed cinematography clear visualization of coronary circulation before and after drug administration is done. This technique is the most direct, reliable and advanced method.[28] Angina is extremely variable pain syndrome with no anatomical/pathophysiological entity. There is no direct relation between degree of pain and coronary insufficiency. Small areas of ischemia can produce discomfort equal to that of large area ischemia.[29] Also, all antianginal drugs must not be assumed to be coronary vasodilators nor all coronary vasodilators always relieve angina. So, any compound screened positively for angina has to be tested cautiously in a well-planned and controlled clinical trial.

CONCLUSION

In the study of cardiovascular biology, both in healthy and disease conditions, there is a vast spectrum of measurable indices of function and injury. This is particularly so in the case of myocardial ischemia, a disease, which contributes to the majority of deaths in both the developing and developed countries. Each experimental model, each species and each end point has its own inherent advantages and disadvantages and appreciating these will help the investigator select the most appropriate study system for the particular investigation under question.

The key feature of the *in vitro* isolated animal hearts is that global or regional ischemia and reperfusion can be imposed at will and the contractile, biochemical, physiological and morphological consequences can be easily assessed. Furthermore, various degrees of ischemia from zero flow to low flow can be induced and the rate and nature of reperfusion can be manipulated. On the negative side, *in vitro* preparations have a limited laboratory life span that rarely exceeds a few hours; they deteriorate progressively with time and cannot be used for chronic studies. Furthermore, they are deprived of their normal central neural connections; they are isolated from the systemic circulation and are no longer exposed to the host of peripheral neurohormonal factors. The *in vivo* preparations allow measurement of hemodynamic functions such as ECG, ventricular wall motion, and ejection fraction that are of major diagnostic importance. They also provide scope for biochemical, pharmacological, morphological and physiological study. Markers of cardiovascular injury such as lactate, cytokines, catecholamines, creatine kinase or troponin-T from the peripheral circulation can be analyzed.

Nowadays, techniques such as Nuclear Magnetic Resonance (NMR) and Positron Emission Tomography (PET) have increased our ability to study in a non-invasive manner, some aspects of cardiac metabolism, function and coronary flow. However, invasive catheterization procedures will allow the collection of cardiac biopsies, measurement of arteriovenous difference and more sophisticated electrophysiological recording.

Summary

In vitro models	*In vivo models*
1. Langendorff heart preparation	1. Occlusion of coronary artery
2. Isolated rabbit aorta preparation	2. Microspheres induced acute ischemia
3. Calcium antagonism in pitched rat	3. Isoproterenol induced myocardial necrosis
4. Relaxation of bovine coronary artery	4. Stenosis induced coronary thrombosis model
5. Coronary artery ligation in isolated rat heart	5. Electrical stimulation induced coronary thrombosis
6. Isolated heart-lung preparation	6. Myocardial ischemic preconditioning model
7. Plastic casts technique in dogs	7. Models of coronary flow measurement • Coronary inflow measurement in anesthetized dogs • Coronary outflow measurement in anesthetized dogs • Other models to measure coronary flow: – Inert gas technique – Radioactive technique – Radioactive microsphere technique – Thermodilution technique – Coronary arteriography

REFERENCES

1. Chimenti S, Carlo E, Masson S, Bai A, Latini R. Myocardial infarction: animal models. Methods Mol Med 2004;98:217-26.
2. Balderston SM, Johnson KE, Reiter MJ. Electrophysiological evaluation of cardiovascular agents in the isolated intact rabbit heart. J Pharmacol Methods 1991;25:205-13.
3. Burn JH, Hukovic S. Anoxia and ventricular fibrillation: With a summary of evidence on the cause of fibrillation. Br J Pharmacol 1960;15:67-70.
4. Hof RP, Vuorela HJ. Assessing calcium antagonism on vascular smooth muscle: comparison of three methods. J Pharmacol Methods 1983;9:41-52.
5. Matsuo K, Morita S, Uchida MK, et al. Simple and specific assessment of Ca^{2+} entry blocking activities of drugs by measurement of Ca reversal. J Pharmacol Methods 1989;22:265-75.
6. Clapham JC. A method for in vivo assessment of calcium slow channel blocking drugs. J Cardiovasc Pharmacol 1988;11:56-60.
7. Dusting GJ, Moncada S, Vane JR. Prostacyclin (PGX) is the endogenous metabolite responsible for relaxation of coronary arteries induced by arachidonic acid. Prostaglandins 1977;13:3-15.
8. Gilmore N, Vane JR, Wyllie JH. Prostaglandins released by the spleen. Nature 1968;218:1135-40.
9. Linz W, Scholkens BA, Manwen J, et al. The heart as a target for converting enzyme inhibitors: Studies in ischemic isolated working hearts. J Hypertension 1986;4:477-79.
10. Carpi A, Oliverio A. Effect of reserpine on the heart lung preparation of guinea pig. Arch Int Pharmacodyn Ther 1965;157:470-86.
11. Boor PJ, Reynolds ES. A simple planimetric method for determination of left ventricular mass and necrotic myocardial mass in postmortem hearts. Am J Clin Pathol 1977;68:387-92.
12. Gomoll AW, Lekich RF. Use of ferret for a myocardial ischemia/salvage model. J Pharmacol Methods 1990;23:213-23.
13. Smiseth OA, Mjos OD. A reproducible and stable model of acute ischemic left ventricular failure in dogs. Clin Physiol 1982;2:225-39.
14. Rona G, Chappel CI, Balazs T. An infarct like myocardial lesion and other toxic manifestations produced by isoproterenol in rat. Arch Path 1959;67:443-55.
15. Kannengiesser GJ, Lubbe WF, Opie LH. Experimental myocardial infarction with left ventricular failure in the isolated perfused rat heart. Effects of isoproterenol and pacing. J Mol Cell Cardiol 1975;7:135-51.
16. Al-Wathiqui MH, Hartman JC, Brooks HL, et al. Induction of cyclic flow reduction in the coronary, carotid and femoral arteries of conscious, chronically instrumented dogs. A model for investigating the role of platelets in severely constricted arteries. J Pharmacol Methods 1988;20:85-92.
17. Kingaby RO, Lab MJ, Cole AW, et al. Relation between monophasic action potential duration, ST segment elevation and regional myocardial blood flow after coronary occlusion in the pig. Cardiovasc Res 1986;20:740-51.
18. Mickelson JK, Simpson PJ, Lucchesi BR. Streptokinase improves reperfusion blood flow after coronary artery occlusion. Int J Cardiol 1989;23:373-84.
19. Matsuo H, Watanabe S, Kadosaki T, et al. Validation of collateral fractional flow reserve by myocardial perfusion imaging. Circulation 2002;105:1060-65.
20. Antoniucci D, Valenti R, Moschi G, et al. Relation between preintervention angiographic evidence of coronary collateral circulation and clinical and angiographic outcomes after primary angioplasty or stenting for acute myocardial infarction. Am J Cardiol 2002; 89:121-25.

21. Lu TM, Hsu NW, Chen YH, et al. Pulsatility of ascending aorta and restenosis after coronary angioplasty in patients >60 years of age with stable angina pectoris. Am J Cardiol 2001;88:964-68.
22. Carlier SG, Cespedes EI, Li W, et al. Blood flow assessment with intravascular ultrasound catheters: the ideal tool for simultaneous assessment of the coronary haemodynamics and vessel wall? Semin Interv Cardiol 1998;3:21-29.
23. Ohte N, Nakano S, Hashimoto T, et al. Noninvasive evaluation of left ventricular function using new systolic time intervals obtained from continuous-wave Doppler echocardiography. J Cardiol 1990;20:457-64.
24. Bregman D, Kaskel P. Advances in percutaneous intra-aortic balloon pumping. Crit Care Clin 1986;2:221-36.
25. Parker JO, West RO, Di Giorgi S. The effect of nitroglycerine on coronary blood flow and the hemodynamic response to exercise in coronary artery disease. Am J Cardiol 1971;27:59-65.
26. Santomauro M, Cuocolo A, Celentano L, et al. Diagnosis of coronary artery disease with Tc^{99m}-methoxy isobutyl isonitrile and transesophageal pacing. Angiology 1992;43:818-25.
27. Parodi O, Marzullo P, Neglia D, et al. Clinical application of monitoring techniques: radioisotopic methods. Can J Cardiol 1986; Suppl A: 155A-62A.
28. Biagioli B, Borrelli E, Maccherini M, et al. Reduction of oxidative stress does not affect recovery of myocardial function: warm continuous versus cold intermittent blood cardioplegia. Heart 1997;77:465-73.
29. Stewart JT, Gray HH, Calicott C, et al. Heat production by the human left ventricle: measurement by a thermodilution technique. Cardiovasc Res 1990;24:418-22.

CHAPTER

21

Antiplatelet Agents

INTRODUCTION

Platelets were discovered by G. Bizzozero in 1882, but drug industry did not recognize them as viable drug targets till 1960s, after many decades of oblivion. This happened due to the progressive recognition of the role of platelets in physiopathologic and clinical conditions such as inflammation, cancer growth and dissemination, and organ transplant rejection. Initially, the interest of many experts was in the role of platelets in the process of blood coagulation and they were faced with a serious unresolved problem of the normal clotting time even in severe thrombocytopenia. However, during the 1960s, focus shifted to the interaction of platelets with the vascular wall (adhesion) and each other (aggregation). Platelet adhesion and aggregation are central events in hemostasis and the pathophysiology of thrombosis. In 1968, aspirin found that inhibits platelet aggregation and recognized by the FDA (USA) in 1988. Projects for developing antiplatelet drugs are initiated worldwide.

ANTIPLATELET AGENTS

An antiplatelet drug is a member of a class of pharmaceuticals that decreases platelet aggregation and inhibits thrombus formation (Table 21.1). They are effective in the arterial circulation, where anticoagulants have little effect. They are widely used in primary and secondary prevention of thrombotic cerebrovascular or cardiovascular diseases.

Table 21.1: Classification of antiplatelet drugs

Categories	*Drugs*
Cyclooxygenase inhibitors	Aspirin
Adenosine diphosphate (ADP) receptor inhibitor	Clopidogrel, Ticlopidine
Phosphodiesterase inhibitors	Cilostazol
Glycoprotein IIB/IIIA inhibitors	Abciximab, Eptifibatide, Tirofiban
Adenosine reuptake inhibitors	Dipyridamole
Flavonoids	Rutin

IMPORTANCE OF ANTIPLATELET DRUGS

Uncontrolled deposition of platelets on thrombogenic surfaces may lead to the occlusion of vessels, a condition associated with numerous pathophysiological changes, such as acute myocardial infarction and unstable angina, or the ischemic complications of coronary intervention and stroke.[1,2] The contribution of platelets to these disease processes stems from their ability to form aggregates or platelet thrombi, as a consequence of arterial wall injury. Injury of blood vessel walls could occur either acutely or chronically by various pathophysiological processes. Platelets are then activated by a number of activators or agonists that are released from the platelets or from the injured arterial walls, with subsequent adherence, aggregation to the disrupted vessel surface, and resultant formation of an occlusive thrombus in the lumen of the vessel. Platelet aggregation may be stimulated by collagen, thrombin, thromboxane A2, serotonin, adenosine diphosphate (ADP), platelet activating factor (PAF), epinephrine, or most probably by a combination of these factors. These agents are used to induce platelet aggregation in the drug screening methods that are discussed below. Each antiplatelet drug has its own mechanism of antiplatelet action.

Studies have shown that antiplatelet agents can prevent development of thrombotic disorders such as myocardial infarction and peripheral vascular diseases.[3] Inhibitors of aggregation can provide protection against these symptoms that affect millions of people worldwide. Acetylsalicylic acid (aspirin) is one such inhibitor. The chances of a second heart attack can be reduced by as much as 40% by taking aspirin daily.[4] Increasing the level of natural platelet inhibitors in the diet may also reduce the risk of developing cardiovascular disorders mediated by platelet aggregation.

TARGETS FOR NEWER DRUGS

Understanding the mechanisms underlying activation, adhesion and aggregation of platelets, is the key to develop newer antiplatelet drugs. This fact is beautifully illustrated by the widespread clinical use of cyclooxygenase inhibitors, most notably aspirin, as antiplatelet drugs. This was only possible after arachidonic acid metabolism in platelets was fully characterized, which has been shown to be responsible for platelet aggregation. The explosion of cell and molecular biology approaches in the last two decades have led to the discovery and characterization of platelet receptors such as the adenosine diphosphate (ADP) receptor, glycoprotein IIb/IIIa, glycoprotein Ib/IX receptors and prostanoid receptors.[5]

During the last decade, vast information regarding the function of the platelet and about the key role of von Willebrand factor (vWF) interaction with platelet glycoprotein (GP) Ib in the initial contact adhesion of platelets to exposed subendothelium, has been gathered. This interaction leads to the final common pathway for all agonist-induced platelet aggregate formation, initiated by activation of the platelet glycoprotein GP IIb/IIIa and linking of adjacent platelets by fibrinogen bound to the receptor GP IIb/IIIa.[6,7] This binding of fibrinogen is mediated in part by the RGD recognition sequence, which is common to other adhesive proteins that bind to GP IIb/IIIa receptors.[8]

The glycoprotein GP IIb/IIIa belongs to the integrin superfamily of adhesive proteins and is the most abundant platelet cell surface protein. A normal platelet contains approximately

50,000 receptor complexes, which bind like several other integrins to an Arg-Gly-Asp-Ser (RGDS) tetrapeptide recognition sequence.[9] Despite the common motif, integrins are quite specific in their interaction with different adhesive proteins such as fibrinogen, vitronectin, fibronectin, laminin, collagen, or vWF.

Agonist activation causes a morphological change in platelets, placing the GP IIb/IIIa receptors in a conformation having a high affinity for the binding of fibrinogen. The binding of fibrinogen to the activated form of GP IIb/IIIa is both a necessary and sufficient event that can mediate the process of platelet aggregation.[7] vWF is a disulfide-linked multimeric protein composed of identical 275 kDa subunits and mediates the adhesion of platelets to the injured vessel walls by binding both GP Ib and subendotheliums exposed on the injured vessel wall. It is known that some conformational changes in the structure of vWF are necessary for the binding of vWF to GP Ib, and it is likely that *in vivo* these conformational changes are achieved by its binding to exposed subendotheliums, particularly under conditions of high shear stress.[10] Therefore, blocking of GP IIb/IIIa offers a superior approach in effectively preventing arterial thrombosis. Further studies in the platelet signaling pathway and the receptor pathway, coupled with the development of new techniques for studying platelet function, can lead to many new classes of platelet-inhibiting drugs.

Current antiplatelet drugs are mainly effective against one of the many platelet activators. Drugs, such as aspirin and ticlopidine, inhibit only one agonistic pathway and are therefore of limited efficacy. Since, the specific inhibition of a single agonistic pathway leaves alternative routes to platelet activation unaffected and is thus of limited effectiveness in preventing thrombus formation. Antagonism of GP IIb/IIIa with an orally acting agent represents an attractive therapy for chronic treatment of arterial thrombosis. In addition, because no oral GP IIb/IIIa inhibitor exists, there is room for developing oral regimens. Efficacy of new drugs can be screened in various *in vitro* and *in vivo* models of platelet aggregation.

IN VITRO SCREENING METHODS

Selection of Volunteer Blood Donors

It is axiomatic that only normal healthy volunteers should be used for preparing platelets or suspension for drug testing. The healthy volunteers selected should not have clinical signal of von Willebrand's disease or symptoms compatible with primary hemostasis disorders or blood dyscrasias; they are advised not to take aspirin or other nonsteroidal anti-inflammatory drugs (NSAIDs) for 2 weeks before the day of the experiment.

Blood samples are mixed with 1/10 volume of anticoagulant 3.8% sodium citrate during the screening of antiplatelet drugs. Other anticoagulants, such as heparin, EDTA cannot be used as they affect the second wave of aggregation caused by the response to ADP and adrenaline.

Preparation of Platelets and Platelet Aggregation Assays

A typical aggregometer is basically a simple photometer consisting of a light source; usually white light from a low voltage, DC tungsten filament and a photoelectric cell to receive the light beam from passage through the sample. Fresh blood from male rabbit is collected into plastic tubes containing anticoagulant dextrose solution and subsequently centrifuged at 250 g for 10 min to obtain platelet-rich plasma (PRP). PRP samples are stirred at a sufficient speed to maintain platelets in an even suspension and to provide the platelet-to-platelet contact necessary for aggregation to proceed. High speed stirring may traumatize platelets sufficiently to induce release and spontaneous aggregation. Maximal interference with light transmission occurs when platelets are evenly distributed throughout the suspending medium. The levels of light transmission are calibrated as 0% for a platelet suspension and 100% for the Tyrode/HEPES solution. PRP is obtained by plateletpheresis of plasma centrifuged at 120 g for 15 min.

Platelet aggregation is performed according to the turbidometric method of Born.[11] Test drug at concentrations ranging from 1 to 100 μM is incubated with 0.25 ml of PRP for 1 min, followed by activation of the platelet with various agonists. Citrated human PRP is warmed for 5 min at 37°C and then aggregation induced by ADP (100 μM), collagen or thrombin (0.8-6.4 unit/ml). The inhibition of aggregation is expressed as the percentage of the maximal rate of aggregation observed in the absence of antagonists.[10]

Washed Platelets Method

Washed platelets are prepared by the method of Rho, et al.[12] and platelet aggregation is determined by a standard turbidometric method[10] using an aggregometer. Platelets (300 μl) are added to tyrode-BSA (0-35% albumin and apyrase, pH 7.35) in the aggregometer and stirred at 1200 rpm at 37°C for 1 min before addition of the aggregating agents. The platelet count is adjusted to 2×10^8 cells/ml. Platelet aggregation is expressed as an increase in light transmission. Platelet suspension (0.3 ml) in the aggregometer cuvette is preincubated for 5 min at 37°C under continuous stirring at 100 rpm, and then $CaCl_2$ or EDTA is added to a final concentration of 1 mM. After 5 min, aggregating agent (ADP or collagen) was added and platelet aggregation monitored for 10 min. Various concentrations of test drug were preincubated for 5 min before addition of aggregating agent (ADP or collagen) and platelet aggregation was monitored for 20 min.

The effective concentration (EC 100 g/ml) which produces a 100% inhibition of platelet aggregation (rabbit platelet-rich plasma) induced by arachidonic acid is considered as pharmacological response by the test drug.[4] This relatively simple method for determining the platelet aggregation inhibitory activity and compounds giving positive results in this assay also shows interesting properties *ex vivo*.

Whole Blood Aggregometry

In vitro platelet aggregation is measured with a whole blood electrical impedance aggregometer (Chrono-log Corp.). There is a change in the impedance of whole blood, which is proportional to the amount of platelet aggregation occurring in the cuvette. Vascular injury shown necessary for platelet aggregation in the above discussion is achieved by exposing the blood to high shear flow and subendothelial components.

Procedure: Blood is withdrawn from healthy human donors by venipuncture by a 21-gauge needle into a syringe containing the anticoagulant sodium citrate (1 volume of 3.8% sodium citrate to 9 volumes of blood) and is mixed gently. A minimum of two measurements is performed using the blood from the same donor for each condition. An equal volume of Tris-buffered saline (TBS; 10 mM Tris, pH 7.4, and 150 mM NaCl) is added to the blood and mixed by inversion. The blood is stored at 20-22°C during the experiment and used within 4 hr of venipuncture.

One ml of blood/TBS is transferred to cuvettes containing a stirbar. After incubation at 37°C for 3 min, the potential new drug is added (final concentration in whole blood is used). Aspirin is used as positive control. The platelet inhibitory effect of acetylsalicylic acid (aspirin) is measured at 0.36 mM, which is the approximate concentration in the blood of a 70 kg human following a dosage of two 325 mg tablets of aspirin, assuming complete absorption into the circulation. Aspirin is dissolved in 95% ethyl alcohol prior to dilution and then diluted in TBS so that the final level of ethyl alcohol in whole blood is 0.0475%. Platelet aggregation is compared to nonaspirin controls containing an equal amount of ethyl alcohol. Cuvettes are incubated at 37°C for further 4 min. The aggregometer electrodes are then inserted into the blood mixture. Platelet aggregation is induced by adding 5 g/ml collagen. Change in electrical impedance between the electrodes is then recorded over 7 min with stirring. The change in impedance at 6 min is used for all calculations. The test drug and the control drug aspirin both are evaluated four times with each donor's blood.

Preparation of Gel-filtered Platelets

Human blood samples are obtained by venipuncture from drug-free, normal male volunteers and treated with 0.1 ml volume of 3.8% trisodium citrate. PRP is prepared by centrifugation of the blood at 150 g for 10 min at room temperature. Gel-filtered platelets are prepared from PRP by chromatography on a Sepharose 2B (Pharmacia, Sweden) column using modified Tyrode's buffer (138 mM NaCl, 2.7 mM KCl, 0.4 mM NaH_2PO_4, 12 mM $NaHCO_3$, 2 mM $MgCl_2$, 10 mM HEPES, pH 7.4) containing 3.5% bovine serum albumin and 2% glucose for elution. Platelets are counted electronically with a cell counter (CELLTAC MEK-5158, Nihon Kohden, Japan). The final platelet concentration is adjusted to about 3×10^8/ml.

Preparation of Fixed Platelets

Gel-filtered platelets can be stimulated by 20 μM ADP for 10 min. They are then fixed by treatment with 0.8% paraformaldehyde for 30 min at room temperature. The platelets are washed three times with modified Tyrode's buffer.[10]

Platelet Adhesion

Six hundred μl of test drug is added to 2.4 ml of blood. Tris buffer used as control. The drugs are incubated with the blood at room temperature for 5-10 min. After the incubation period, the blood is gently swirled and collected in a 5 ml syringe. The blood is then passed through a bead column at a rate of 1 ml/min. The bead columns are composed of a 2.5 ml disposable plastic syringe filled with 5 g silicone-coated glass beads of diameter 0.45-0.50 mm. Platelet counts are performed in triplicate, after the passage through beads and percent adhesion is calculated by comparing the average of these counts with those performed before bead passage. The results with drugs are compared to those obtained with Tris buffer alone.

Cazenave's group devised a method for evaluating platelet adhesion to glass tubes coated with acid-soluble collagen.[13] The technique utilizes washed, radiolabeled platelets in suspension and a platelet count of 700×10^3/min. 50 μl of drug solution in Tris buffer is added to 1 ml of PRP, mixed, allowed to stand for 5-10 min at 20°C. The tubes are covered with parafilm and rotated end-over-end at 15 rpm for 10 min at room temperature. Adherence is assessed by computing the loss of radioactivity to the collagen surface. If negligible release of labels to the suspending medium occurs, it indicates little or no aggregation.

Platelet Function Analyzer (PFA): Through a 21-gauge cannula inserted into an antecubital vein, a 3 ml blood sample is drawn into a plastic syringe (monovette) containing a buffered citrate solution. Blood samples are stored at room temperature. The PFA-100® (Dade Behring, Düdingen, Switzerland) is composed of a microprocessor-controlled device and single-use test cartridges. An 800 µl sample containing saline or test drug (3 µM) is placed into a test cartridge system for *in vitro* quantitative assessment of platelet function.[11] The test cartridges simulate an injured blood vessel, which consist of a sample reservoir, a capillary and a membrane coated with 2 mg equine type I collagen and either 10 mg epinephrine bitartrate (EPI cartridge) or 50 mg adenosine 5'-diphosphate (ADP cartridge). Blood is pipetted into the reservoir and aspirated through a capillary with a diameter of 200 µm with constant negative pressure thereby simulating high physiological shear forces (5000-6000 s^{-1}). The capillary ends in a membrane aperture with a diameter of 150 µm. Platelets adhere at the aperture where they are activated by the collagen and then aggregate. The two agonist's epinephrine and ADP enhance aggregation. Finally, a platelet plug occludes the aperture and blood flow stops. The time measured in seconds from the beginning of the test until formation of an occluding platelet plug is called closure time (CT), which is a measure of the overall function of the platelets. If an occluding platelet plug does not form after 300 sec, the analysis is stopped.

Microchannel Array Flow Analyzer (MC-FAN)

It is an *in vitro* screening system for platelet aggregation by monitoring aggregation and micro-thrombi formation in the microchannels.[14] In this method, whole blood is collected from the ante-cubital vein of healthy volunteers with no known past medical history including thrombotic disorders or hyperlipidemia. One ml of citrated whole blood is incubated with 10 µl of the indicated concentrations of platelet activation agents or phosphate-buffered saline (PBS) as a control for adjusting the hematocrit. The final concentrations of platelet aggregation triggers in the experiments are as follows: ADP (0–2 µM), collagen (0–100 µg/ml), and ristocetin (0–0.75 mg/ml). Siliconized microchannels are used to evaluate blood coagulation which consists of arrays of microgrooves formed on the surface of a single-crystal silicon substrate and were converted to peak-proof micro-channels by covering them with an optically flat glass plate.

The sample to be tested is transferred into a cylinder graduated in 10 µl units connected to the inlet of the chip holder from which it flowed through the micro-channels when a solenoid valve connecting the outlet of the holder was opened by a negative pressure is 20 cm H_2O.

To determine the effect of anti-platelet agents or anticoagulants on whole blood flow rate in the MC-FAN assay, 1 ml of citrated whole blood was incubated at 37°C and treated with 40 µl of 250 mM $CaCl_2$, platelet activation agent and anti-platelet agent or anticoagulants. Immediately following mixing of 500 µl of the whole blood, a sample is transferred into the cylinder of the MC-FAN. The transit time through the cylinder of successive 10 µl aliquots of the total sample of 100 µl, varying from 30 sec for the control to ~5 min for the highest activated samples is determined. The average transit time through the chamber is used to determine the mean blood flow rate.

To determine the effects of anti-platelet agents and anticoagulants on the blood flow rate of ADP stimulated whole blood, 10 μl of the agents were added to 1 ml of whole blood, incubated for 15 min, stimulated with 2 μM ADP, and the flow rate immediately determined in the MC-FAN. The final concentrations of anti-platelet agents or anticoagulants used in the experiments were as follows: FK633: 0.1–10 ng/ml, cilostazol, dilazep and sarpogrelate: 1–100 μg/ml, heparin and hirudin: 0.1–10 U/ml, APC and sTM: 0.1–1 μg/ml.

A chronolog platelet aggregometer is used to measure the decrease in optical density accompanying aggregation.

After the induction of thrombus formation in the presence or absence of anti-platelet agents or anticoagulants, the siliconized MC-FAN chip was fixed with 2.5% glutaraldehyde in 0.1 M phosphate buffer, pH 7.4. The microchip is washed with phosphate buffer and re-fixed with 1% OsO_4 in 0.1 M phosphate buffer. Adherent cells were dehydrated and dried, mounted on scanning electron microscopy stubs and coated with platinum/palladium. Stubs were stored under desiccation and analyzed with a scanning electron microscope at 15 kV accelerating voltage.

Ex Vivo

Acid soluble collagen (100 μg/kg) is injected into the aortic arch of rabbits via the carotid artery and serial platelet counts performed on blood withdrawn subsequent to collagen administration. The test drug is administered to the animal before the collagen injection.

IN VIVO SCREENING METHODS

Investigation of new drugs in the *in vivo* situation to be used in human disease states, which have a protracted natural history and/or are multifactorial, is more complex and a very frustrating affair. Nowhere is this brutal fact better appreciated than in the search for antiplatelet drugs. Various artificial means are used to induce the platelet activity *in vivo*. It usually involves application to an exposed portion of blood vessels to some form of insult (mechanical, surgical, electrical, photochemical). In all cases, the experiments are either acute or subacute in nature and, therefore, vulnerable to criticism from various fronts. Apart from the obvious species differences, these animal models may not properly reproduce the sequence of events of the disease as it occurs in the clinical situation. Nevertheless, there appears to be sufficient universality in the response of blood platelets to damaged vascular endothelium, which supports these models as useful experimental tools.

Model of Carotid Artery Occlusion in Dogs

A model of electrolytic injury-induced carotid artery occlusive thrombus formation is used.[15] The experimental procedure results in the formation of a platelet-rich intravascular thrombus along with a few erythrocytes and a rough fibrous coating at the site of an endothelial lesion induced by electrolytic injury in proximity to distal arterial stenosis. The carotid artery response to electrolytic injury is similar to that observed in the canine coronary artery. In the case of evaluating intravenous antithrombotic efficacy of a test agent, we can use the right (control) and left (intravenous treatment) carotid arteries or *vice versa* to establish time to occlusion (min) and thrombus weight (milligrams) before and after the intravenous administration of a test agent (i.e., the same animal can serve as control).

Surgical Preparation

Male, mongrel dogs (weight, 15 to 17 kg) are anesthetized (n = 12 for control, n = 5 to 6 for the different oral dose levels of test substance) with sodium pentobarbital (30 mg/kg IV), intubated, and allowed to breathe room air. Both common carotid arteries and the right internal jugular vein are exposed. A catheter is inserted into the jugular vein for blood sampling and administration of the test drug. Arterial blood pressure is monitored from the cannulated femoral artery with the use of a blood pressure transducer. Standard limb lead II of the electrocardiogram is recorded continuously. A Doppler flow probe is placed on each common carotid artery proximal to both the point of insertion of the intra-arterial electrode and the mechanical constrictor. The mechanical constrictor is constructed of stainless steel in a C shape with a polytetrafluoroethylene (Teflon) screw (2-mm diameter) that could be adjusted to control vessel circumference and produce a regional stenosis. The constrictor is adjusted until the pulsatile flow pattern is reduced by 50% without altering the mean blood flow. Blood flow in the carotid vessels is monitored continuously.

Electrolytic injury to the intimal surface of each carotid vessel is accomplished with the use of an intravascular electrode composed of a Teflon-insulated, silver-coated copper wire. Penetration of the vessel wall by the electrode is facilitated by attaching the tip of a 25-gauge hypodermic needle to the uninsulated part of the electrode. Each intra-arterial electrode is connected to the positive pole (anode) of a dual-channel stimulator. The cathode is connected to a distant subcutaneous site. The current delivered to each vessel is monitored continuously on a separate ammeter and maintained at 300 micro A. The anodal electrode is positioned to have the uninsulated portion in intimate contact with the endothelial surface of the vessel. Positioning of the electrodes in each of the carotid arteries is confirmed by visual inspection at the end of each experiment.

Protocol: Prevention of Thrombus Formation

The anodal current is applied for a maximum period of 3 h or is terminated 30 min after blood flow in the involved vessel remains stable at zero flow velocity to verify the formation of a stable occlusive thrombus. Arterial thrombosis and thrombotic occlusion occurs in response to intimal damage, after which the vessel segment is ligated, both proximal and distal to the point of injury, and removed without disturbing the intravascular thrombus. The vessel segment is opened along its length, and the intact thrombus mass is lifted off the intimal surface of the vessel. The weight of the thrombus mass is determined with an analytical balance. Thrombus is formed only at the injury site. Scanning electron micrographic studies demonstrated the presence of a rough surface with fibrous coating containing platelets and a few erythrocytes. Dogs are anesthetized 120 min after ingestion of the capsule, the right carotid artery is cannulated, and electrolytic arterial injury is initiated as discussed before.

Hematological Measurements

Blood is withdrawn for platelet studies from the jugular cannula into a plastic syringe containing 3.2% sodium citrate as the anticoagulant [(1:10 citrate to blood (vol/vol)]. Blood is taken for platelet aggregation and whole blood cell counts at baseline, 60 min, and 240 min after the administration of test drug. Platelet count is determined with an H-10 cell counter. PRP, the supernatant present after centrifugation of anticoagulated whole blood at 1000 rpm for 5 min (140 g), is diluted with platelet-poor plasma (PPP) to achieve a platelet count of 200,000/mm^3. PPP is prepared after the PRP is removed by centrifuging the remaining blood at 12,000 g for 10 min and discarding the bottom cellular layer. *Ex vivo* platelet aggregation is measured by established spectrophotometric methods with a four-channel aggregometer by recording the increase in light transmission through a stirred suspension of PRP maintained at 37°C.[14] Aggregation is induced with ADP (100 μmol/l). Values are expressed as percentages of aggregation, representing the percentage of light transmission standardized to PRP and PPP samples yielding 0% and 100% light transmission, respectively. Bleeding time is measured in anesthetized dogs with a simple device by making incisions on the tongue and blotting the wound with filter paper at 30 sec intervals until blood is no longer transferred to the filter paper.

Inclusion Criteria

Animals included in the final protocol were to satisfy the following pre-established criteria:

1. A circulating platelet count of not less than 1,00,000/mm.^{3}
2. Demonstration of ability of platelets to aggregate in response to arachidonic acid before administration of test compound.
3. Thrombotic occlusion of the right carotid artery (control vessel) within 4 h from the onset of vessel wall injury with a 300 micro A direct anodal current.
4. Absence of heart worms on final postmortem examination.

Photochemically Induced Thrombosis Model in Rats

Male Wistar rats weighing 230-320 g are anesthetized with sodium pentobarbital injected into the femoral muscle (60 mg/kg). The right jugular vein and artery are cannulated for the injection of dye and the monitoring of arterial blood pressure and heart rate, respectively. The small intestine is exteriorized via a midline incision in the abdominal wall into a bath and perfused with saline kept at 37°C. The mesentery around the ileum is spread out carefully on a small circular glass stage and the other parts of the intestine are covered with moistened gauze. Microvessels in the mesentery are observed under transillumination with a halogen lamp for selection of venules of 41-62 μm diameter in which microthrombi are produced. Thrombus formation is induced in microvessels by a filtered light of wavelength 420-490 nm passed through an objective lens.[16] Using a field stop, the area of irradiation around the microvessels is adjusted on the focal plane to a diameter of about 130 μm. The light intensity is controlled at 13.8 mW/mm^2.

Procedure

The test agents are administered by i.v. bolus injection into the jugular vein of a rat. One min after the injection, irradiation with filtered light is started. One min after the start of irradiation, a solution of sodium fluorescein (2.5% w/v) is injected through the jugular vein (1 ml/kg body weight). Whole process is monitored with TV camera after injection of sodium fluorescein. The time when the thrombus begins to form (time of initiation) and the time when blood flow completely stops (time of occlusion) are used as indices of antithrombotic activity. Time is measured by replay of the videotape. If the blood flow does not stop within 30 min, the result is calculated as 30 min. Rats are sacrificed at the end of experiment by overdose of KCl.

Studies of Antiplatelet Efficacy in Rhesus Monkeys

Sixteen rhesus monkeys of either sex, 8-15 years of age, weighing 6-10 kg, are administered test drug as a solution in 0.9% saline (total dosing volume 0.5 ml/kg) at oral doses of 0.1, 0.3, and 1.0 mg/kg. Each dose is given to at least two animals/sex. Oral dosing is achieved by passing a 16 Fr feeding tube through the oral cavity into the stomach. Administration of test drug is followed by a 10-20 ml water flush. Blood sampling at various time points is accomplished by accessing the appropriate sample site (femoral or saphenous vein). The total volume of blood sampled during the study did not exceed 1% of body weight. Blood samples are withdrawn in citrate containing Vacutainer tubes for an assessment of the *ex vivo* inhibition of ADP (100 µM) mediated platelet aggregation.[17]

Antiplatelet Efficacy in Baboons

Six baboons (three per group, each made up of two females and one male) weighing 15-32 kg are fasted overnight, administered atropine (0.04 mg/kg) followed by ketamine (10 mg/kg) and xylazine (2 mg/kg), and restrained on a treatment table. Either the femoral or saphenous vein is cannulated for blood sampling at various time points. Using a nasogastric tube, test drug is administered as a 0.2 or 0.6 mg/ml solution in 5% EtOH-95% saline (0.9%) at oral doses of 0.1, 0.3, 1.0, and 3.0 mg/kg. Blood samples are withdrawn in citrate containing Vacutainer tubes for the assessment of the *ex vivo* inhibition of ADP (100 µM)-mediated platelet aggregation. *In vitro* assessment of platelet function after test drug administration should abolish arachidonic acid-induced platelet aggregation or prolong the lag time between exposure to collagen and aggregation, and decreased plasma thromboxane B_2 levels.[18]

Transgenic Rat Model

The method is developed by Sudo, et al.[19] The genetically modified rat strains are housed at the temperature 23.2°C for two weeks before the experiment. The animals are allowed free access to standard rat chow and water. All rates for platelet aggregation are 12-week-old adult males. Blood (10 ml) is sampled from the inferior vena cava of each rat, under ether anesthesia, with 21G needles into plastic syringes containing 0.1 volume of 3.18% trisodium citrate solution. Platelet, leukocyte and erythrocyte counts in the citrated blood and hematocrit values are obtained with an automatic counter. Blood is stored at room temperature until measurement. Platelet aggregation should be measured within 60-90 min after blood collection.

Examination of PRP Aggregation Using the Turbidimetric Method

Platelet aggregation with PRP, obtained by centrifuging citrated blood, is investigated by using a novel whole blood aggregometer, the WBA analyzer, with a screen filtration pressure

(SFP) method. The measurements for each strain are performed before noon in separate two days. Platelet number is assessed with an automatic counter as described above, and platelets are prepared to 5×10^8 cells/ml with autologous platelet-poor plasma (PPP). To measure changes in the light transmission rate, PRP samples of 200 μl are incubated with stirring for 2 min at 37°C, then with 22.2 ml Adenosine 5′-diphosphate or collagen solution for 5 min at 37°C. The intensity of light transmission over 5 min is then measured using an aggregometer. The baseline is set with PRP and the maximum possible increase in light transmission (Platelet aggregation rate: 100%) is set with PPP. The concentration of ADP and collagen causing a 50% aggregation rate are subsequently calculated as the platelet aggregation threshold index (PATI). Area under the curve of platelet aggregation (AUC) induced by 1μM ADP, 8μg/ml collagen or 50 μM thrombin receptor-activating peptide (TRAP) is calculated (platelet aggregation rate [%] × seconds [sec]). AUC is depending on the lag phase and maximum aggregation rate in collagen, and on maximum aggregation rate and disaggregation in ADP and TRAP.

$FeCl_3$-induced Thrombosis Model

The method of Sudo, et al. and Kurz, et al.[19,20] is applied. Rats are anesthetized with sodium pentobarbital (50 mg/kg ip). The left common carotid artery is surgically exposed and a Doppler flow probe is placed on the surface of the artery. Baseline blood flow is recorded using a Transonic Model flowmeter. Thereafter, filter paper is (± 10 mm) saturated with 40% $FeCl_3$ and applied to the adventitial surface carotid artery, immediately proximal to the probe. Time to thrombotic occlusion after initiation of artery injury is defined as the time required for blood flow to decline to 0.0 ml/min. The times to occlusion beyond 60 min are regarded as 60 min for the purpose of statistical analysis.

REFERENCES

1. Davies MJ, Thomas A. Thrombosis and acute coronary-artery lesions in sudden cardiac ischemic death. N Engl J Med 1984;310:1137-40.
2. Fuster VF, Badimon L, Badimon JJ, et al. The pathogenesis of coronary artery disease and the acute coronary syndromes. N Engl J Med 1992; 326:242-50.
3. Patrono C. Aspirin as an antiplatelet drug. N Engl J Med 1994; 330:1287-94.
4. Dinerman JL, Mehta JL. Endothelial, platelet and leukocyte interactions in ischemic heart disease: insights into potential mechanisms and their clinical relevance. J Am Coll Cardiol 1990;16:207-22.
5. Armstrong RA. Platelet prostanoid receptors. Pharmacol Ther 1996;72:171-91.
6. Vorchheimer DA, Badimon JJ, Fuster V. Platelet glycoprotein IIb/IIIa receptor antagonists in cardiovascular disease. JAMA 1999;281:1407-14.
7. Lefkovits J, Plow EF, Topol EJ. Platelet glycoprotein IIb/IIIa receptors in cardiovascular medicine. N Engl J Med 1995;332:1553-9.
8. Philips DR, Kieffer N. Platelet membrane glycoproteins: function in cellular interactions. In: Palade GE (Ed). Annu Rev Cell Biol 1990;6:329-57.
9. Mousa SA. Antiplatelet therapies: from aspirin to GP IIb/IIIa-receptor antagonists and beyond. Drug Discov Today 1999;4:552-61.

10. Plow EF, Pierschbacher MD, Ruoslahti E, Marguerie GA, Ginsberg MH. The effect of arg-gly-asp-containing peptides on fibrinogen and von Willebrand binding to platelets. Proc Natl Acad Sci USA 1985;82:8057-61.
11. Born GVR. Aggregation of blood platelets by adenosine diphosphate and its reversal. Nature 1962;194:927-9.
12. Rho MC, Nakahata N, Nakamura H, et al. Activation of rabbit platelets by Ca^{2+} influx and thromboxane A_2 release in an external Ca^{2+} dependent manner by Zooxanthellatoxin-A, a novel polyol. Br J Pharmacol 1995;115:433-40.
13. Cazenave JP, Packham MA, Guccione MA, et al. Inhibition of platelet adherence to a collagen-coated surface by nonsteroidal anti-inflammatory drugs, pyrimido-pyrimidine and tricyclic compounds and lidocaine. J Lab Clin Med 1974;83:797-806.
14. Kamada H, Okamoto T, Hayashi T, Suzuki K. An in vitro method for screening anti-platelet agents using a microchannel array flow analyzer. Biorheology 2010;47:153-61.
15. Romson JL, Haack DW, Lucchesi BR. Electrical induction of coronary artery thrombosis in the ambulatory canine: a model for in vivo evaluation of antithrombotic agents. Thromb Res 1980;17:841-53.
16. Sato M, Ohshima N. Platelet thrombus induced in vivo by filtered light and fluorescent dye in mesenteric microvessels of the rat. Thromb Res. 1984;35:319-34.
17. Kaku S, Yano S, Kawasaki T, et al. Comparison of the antiplatelet agent potential of the whole molecule F(ab)2 Fab fragments of humanized anti-GP IIb/IIIa monoclonal antibody in monkeys. Gen Pharmacol 1996;27:435-9.
18. Shoenfeld NA, Yeager A, Connolly R, et al. A new primate model for the study of intravenous thrombotic potential and its modification. J Vasc Surg 1988;8:49-54.
19. Sudo T, Ito H, Hayashi H, Nagamura Y, Toga K, Yamada Y. Genetic strain differences in platelet aggregation and thrombus formation of laboratory rats. Thromb Haemost 2007;97:665-72.
20. Kurz KD, Main BW, Sandusky GE. Rat model of arterial thrombosis induced by ferric chloride. Throm Res 1990;60:269-80.

CHAPTER

22

Drugs Acting on Sympathetic Nervous System

INTRODUCTION

Autonomic nervous system is largely involuntary and is responsible for maintaining the internal homeostasis. Two subdivisions of autonomic nervous system include the sympathetic nervous system and parasympathetic nervous system. Under physiological conditions, stimulation or inhibition of sympathetic activity is in balance with that of parasympathetic activity so as to maintain the internal homeostasis.

Autonomic nervous system consists of two groups of neurons (pre- and postganglionic neurons) to maintain communication between CNS and peripheral organs. The neurotransmitters provide the means of communication between pre and postganglionic neurons.

The neurotransmitter released at the postganglionic sympathetic neurons is noradrenaline. The adrenaline secreted by adrenal medulla provides generalized sympathetic stimulation. The sympathetic neurotransmitters largely act through adrenergic receptors, which are present in heart, bronchi, blood vessels, uterus, gastrointestinal tract, eye, etc. Adrenergic receptors are of two types—α and β, which are further classified into α_1, α_2 and β_1, β_2, β_3 respectively. Stimulation of these adrenergic receptors causes various responses as shown in Table 22.1.

Sympathetic nervous system activation occurs in response to stressful stimuli including physical activity, psychological stress, blood loss, etc. and prepares the body for emergencies. Sympathetic nervous system stimulation leads to increased heart rate and blood pressure, dilatation of pupils, dilatation of trachea and bronchi, stimulation of the conversion of liver glycogen into glucose, shunting of blood away from the skin and viscera to the skeletal muscles, brain, and heart, inhibition of the peristalsis in the gastrointestinal (GI) tract, inhibition of contraction of the bladder and rectum stimulation of uterus and constriction of spleen capsule.

Sympathomimetic drugs are agents with activity that mimics the responses of adrenaline or stimulation of the sympathetic nervous system. The sympatholytic drugs can antagonize the effects of sympathetic stimulation or the effects of sympathomimetic agents. A summary of sympathomimetics and sympatholytics is given in Figure 22.1. The drugs with potential sympathomimetic or sympatholytic activity can be screened using various animal models.

Table 22.1: Adrenergic receptors and their important characteristics

	α_1	α_2	β_1	β_2	β_3
Smooth muscles					
Blood vessels	Constriction			Dilatation	
Bronchi				Dilatation	
GI tract				Relaxation	
GI sphincters	Constriction				
Bladder				Relaxation	
Bladder sphincter	Constriction				
Seminal vesicle	Constriction				
Eye-radial muscle	Constriction				
Ciliary muscle				Relaxation	
Heart rate		Increases			
Force of contraction		Increases			

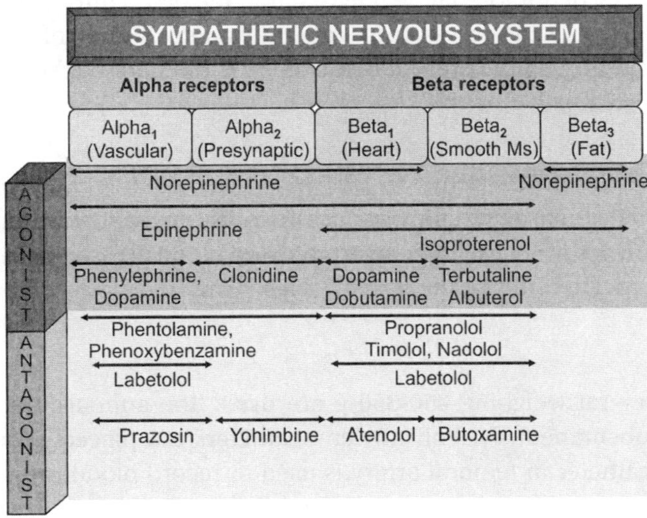

Figure 22.1: Sympathetic agonists and antagonists

IN VIVO METHODS

Cat Spleen Model

This is one of the useful preparations for the evaluation of substances affecting the release and subsequent fate of the adrenergic transmitter from the sympathetic nervous system. After the injection of sympathomimetic amines or electrical stimulation of the pre- and postganglionic sympathetic nerves, spleen contracts. Different doses of the test compound that alter the release of transmitter output of spleen are compared with the known standards.

Released noradrenaline can be measured by collecting spleen venous effluent and analyzing its noradrenaline content. This is achieved after labeling of neuronal stores with radioactive noradrenaline, which is taken up from the splenic arterial circulation and subsequently released after nerve stimulation. The spleen can be used either *in vivo* or *in vitro*.

Procedure

Cats are anesthetized using chloroform. Abdomen is cut open by giving a midline incision and the intestine is removed from the mid-duodenum to the terminal colon. The vascular connections between the spleen and omentum are being cut. The splenic nerves are also cut to avoid liberation of catecholamines from other sites. The adrenal glands are also removed which is helpful to avoid the artifacts due to the release of pressor amines. A ligature is placed around the portal vein just beyond the junction of splenic and superior mesenteric veins and close to the adjoining gastric vein. Heparin is injected intravenously to prevent clotting of blood. The abdominal cavity is filled with warm paraffin and aerated with a mixture of O_2 and CO_2. Venous blood samples are collected by diverting effluent through a cannula by applying increased tension to the ligature placed around the portal vein. Blood is collected in chilled, silicone coated, calibrated centrifuge tubes during the period of stimulation together with a subsequent 20 sec period immediately after cessation of the stimulus. This is enough to capture more than 80% of noradrenaline released into the blood during electrical stimulation and at the same time avoids the excessive loss and unwanted dilution of activity in the plasma. The amount of the noradrenaline present in the blood is estimated by scintillation counter for radioactivity measurement.[1]

The Rat Blood Pressure—Invasive Model

The sympathomimetics like adrenaline induce increase in heart rate and blood pressure while the sympatholytics induce a fall in heart rate and blood pressure. These changes can be recorded in a rat model to evaluate the activity of test drug.[2]

Procedure

The Sprague Dawley rat weighing 250-350 g are used. The animals are anesthetized with urethane 1 g/kg subcutaneously. Polyethylene catheters are placed in femoral artery and femoral vein. The catheter in femoral artery is used to record blood pressure and heart rate while the femoral vein catheter is used for injecting drugs/vehicle. Alternatively, a catheter placed in carotid artery can also be used for recording blood pressure and heart rate. After cannulation the catheters are flushed with 0.2 ml heparinized (20 U/ml) saline solution. The femoral artery catheter is connected with blood pressure transducer and heart rate and blood pressure are recorded. After equilibrium period of 30 min 0.1-0.5 ml of various concentrations of drug or vehicle are injected through the catheter placed in femoral vein and changes in blood pressure and heart rate are recorded to evaluate sympathomimetic/sympatholytic activity. The same volume of adrenaline (2 μg/kg) can be used as standard drug to compare the potential sympathomimetic activity of test drug. To evaluate for the specific receptor agonist activity drug induced changes in BP and HR can be recorded after treatment with specific receptor blockers such as prazosin, an $alpha_1$ blocker (25 μg/kg) or atenolol, a $beta_1$ blocker (1 mg/kg).

The Rat Blood Pressure—Noninvasive Model

Sympathomimetic and sympatholytic drug induced changes in blood pressure and heart rate can also be recorded in a noninvasive model.[3]

Procedure

Adult male Wistar rats (250-300 g) are used. The jugular vein is cannulated in anesthetized rats using a curved polyethylene catheter. The vinyl tubing is led under the skin of neck and exposed on the surface of back to allow for infusion of drugs. The catheter is flushed with heparin (100 units) to prevent clotting. Rats are allowed to recover for at least 24 hours before starting the experiment.

On the day of experiment rats are first placed on heating pads (35-37°C) for 20-30 min. Now the rats are transferred to a restrainer maintained at 37°C. The tail cuff and pulse sensor is placed at the proximal end of the tail and is inflated. The heart rate is determined by manually counting the number of beats per unit time. The systolic blood pressure is indicated at the point where the reappearance of pulsations is detected by pulse sensor. The value for each parameter is taken as average of at least 4 measurements. The measurements are done on three successive days to determine the baseline values. After baseline measurements the drug/vehicle/standard drug are injected through the catheter in jugular vein and changes in heart rate and blood pressure are measured to evaluate for sympathomimetic/sympatholytic activities as in invasive model.

Cat Model of Nictitating Membrane Prolapse

The nictitating membrane of cats relaxes in response to sympatholytic drugs. This activity in cats is used to evaluate sympatholytic activity of a test drug.

Procedure

Unanesthetized cats are used and test compounds are administered orally in the animals. Sympatholytic agents exert relaxant effect on the nictitating membrane of the cat. The extent of relaxation of membrane is measured along the lower lid margin with ruler. Measurement should be done carefully without disturbing the animal. For each dose of the test drug, at least 5-10 animals are used. The relative activity of the different compounds is calculated by dividing the mean duration of the membrane prolapse of a group in hours by the dose in mg/kg.[4,5]

Mouse Eye Model

Norepinephrine, epinephrine and isoproterenol have the property of inducing mydriasis, this effect is blocked by α or β blockers. α-blockers block the mydriatic effect of norepinephrine, β-blockers block the effect of isoproterenol and α and α-blockers block the effect of epinephrine.

Procedure

Mice of weight range 15-20 g are used. Animals are divided into different groups. Vehicle is administered subcutaneously that serves as control. Different doses of test compound are administered subcutaneously. After 30 min, 0.1 mg/kg norepinephrine or 0.05 mg/

kg epinephrine or 20 mg/kg isoproterenol are given intravenously. The pupil diameters are measured before and after vehicle/drug administration. The mean values of pupil diameters are compared between the groups.[6]

Pithed Rat Model

In this model stimulation of the complete sympathetic outflow is performed in the intact animal and agents affecting sympathetic nervous system are evaluated.

Procedure

Rats weighing 250-350 g are used. Animals are anesthetized with either ether or choloroform. The trachea is cannulated. Animals are then pithed by passing a stainless steel rod through the orbit and down the spinal column. Artificial respiration is maintained using respirator. Blood pressure is recorded from the cannulated left carotid artery using a transducer and the arterial pulse is used to trigger a Neilson instantaneous rate meter for the measurement of heart rate. Drugs are administered into the cannulated left femoral vein.

Pithing rod is used as an electrode to stimulate the spinal sympathetic outflow to initiate increase of both the blood pressure and the heart rate. To stimulate thoracolumbar region, rod is insulated with an epoxy resin adhesive except the part in close touch with the thorax and lumbar regions of the spinal cord. Parasympathetic or motor nerve fiber stimulation by spread of the stimulating current is reduced by administration of atropine. The increase in the blood pressure and heart rate can be elicited by the electrical stimulation of supramaximal rectangular pulses of 1.0 ms duration. The magnitudes of the responses are proportional to the frequency of the stimulus usually over the range of 0.5 to 8.0 Hz. Changes in the blood pressure and heart rate are observed after drug (standard/test) administration and dose response curves are plotted for comparison to assess agonistic and antagonistic activity.[7]

To determine α_1 and α_2 antagonismin pithed rats, phenylephrine (selective α_1 antagonist) in the doses of 0.1-30 mg/kg and BHT920 (selective α_2-agonist) in the doses of 1 to 1000 mg/kg are administered intravenously. Their effects on blood pressure and heart rate are observed and dose-response curves are plotted. After that, test drug is administered intravenously and the agonist dose response curves are repeated after 15-30 min to record any shift in the curves of blood pressure response. Finally, potency ratios are calculated using log dose response curves.[8]

Modification

Above method is modified by allowing stimulation of individual pathways of the sympathetic and parasympathetic nerve pathways in pithed rats.[8]

Rat Heart and Uterus Model

β_1 and β_2 receptors are located in the heart and in the uterus respectively. In this method, both heart rate and uterine relaxation are observed in the same animal after drug administration, to determine the β_1 and β_2 activity of the test compound.

Procedure

Female Sprague-Dawley rat is anesthetized with pentobarbital (60 mg/kg ip). After that pithing of the animal is done.[8] Artificial respiration is given to the animal using an animal ventilator. Body temperature of the animal is kept around 36-37°C. For blood pressure monitoring, left carotid artery is cannulated and an instantaneous rate meter is used to monitor heart rate continuously. Drugs are administered intravenously. After that, uterine horns are exposed by giving a midline incision in the abdomen. The ovarian artery is identified and ligated. Uterine horn is dissected free from the ovary. At the free end of the horn a thread is tied and tissue is mounted in an organ bath containing Krebs-Henseleit solution. Temperature is maintained at 37°C and solution is constantly bubbled with 95% O_2 and 5% CO_2.

Isoprenaline (nonselective β-agonist), salbutamol (β_2-agonist) and norepinephrine (β_1 selective agonist) are administered intravenously and their effects on both heart rate and uterine relaxation are recorded. After that, test agent is given intravenously, their effects are observed and compared with the effects of isoprenaline, salbutamol and norepinephrine. A test drug is considered as an agonist when it causes an increase in heart rate and decrease in the height of uterine contractions; whereas if test drug inhibits the effects of isoprenaline on both heart rate and uterine relaxation, it is taken as an antagonist. Dose response curves obtained with isoprenaline in the absence or presence of the β antagonist are compared to assess the antagonistic activity.[9]

IN VITRO METHODS

Cat Spleen Model

The contractile response of splenic capsule in response to norepinephrine can also be determined *in vitro*.

Procedure

The method for the removal of spleen is similar as described above. The removed spleen is placed in a plethysmograph filled with liquid paraffin. The organ is perfused at a rate of 7-16 ml/min with a modified Krebs solution at 37°C gassed with carbogen. Dextran (3%) is added to raise the osmotic pressure of the perfusion fluid. Ascorbic acid at 25 μg/ml is also added to prevent oxidation of noradrenaline. The perfusion is started and samples are collected and estimated for noradrenaline.[1]

Rabbit Pulmonary Artery Model

The pulmonary artery is highly sensitive to sympathomimetic agents. The artery mainly consists of vascular smooth muscle innervated by postganglionic adrenergic sympathetic fibers. The noradrenaline is released in response to the nerve stimulation. The released adrenergic transmitter is measured by labeling the neuronal stores with radioactive noradrenaline and with the use of superfusion technique to reduce the dilution of amines.

Procedure

The rabbit of weight range 1 to 2 kg is sacrificed by exsanguination followed by the removal of main pulmonary artery. The artery is cut transversely and spirally into vertical strip of approximately 4 mm by 30 mm in length. The strip is suspended vertically in an organ bath maintained at 37°C and its lower end is tied to glass support, whereas the other end is connected by thread to an isometric strain gauge transducer. The resting tension is 2 g and the artery is superfused with Krebs bicarbonate solution, which is allowed to flow down the connecting thread and tissue at the rate of 6 ml/min. The tissue is then loaded with ^{3}[H] noradrenaline by submerging it in 20 ml of Krebs bicarbonate solution at 37°C and gassed with 95% O_2 and 5% CO_2. Following incubation of 60 min, the artery strip is superfused with Krebs solution at 37°C for 30 min to wash out extraneuronal ^{3}[H] noradrenaline. During the experiment, superfusates are collected in vials every 2 min. Aliquots of collected samples are then assayed for noradrenaline using scintillation spectrophotometer to count the radioactivity after adding scintillation fluid.

The electrical stimulation is given using bipolar platinum electrodes of 30 mm length and 0.5 mm diameter, placed in parallel or either side of the strip. The gap between the tissue and the electrode allows the strip to develop increased tension without any hindrance. The nerves can be excited by transmural stimulation using strains by supramaximal biphasic pulses of 0.3 ms duration. Responses to successive 2 min period of electrical stimulation are reproducible when applied at 16 min intervals. The tension produced by the tissue increases rapidly after commencement of stimulation and decreases back to original basal value after stimulation has ceased. The response produced is accompanied by increased release of tritium (250% above basal level) onto the superfusate. A further reduction in basal radioactivity in the superfusion fluid occurs after each stimulus period as the tissue gradually loses its stored radioactivity. The total tritium detected in collected superfusates unchanged noradrenaline comprised of approximately 30% during rest period and at least 50% during stimulation.[10,11]

Rat Vas Deferens Model

Vas deferens preparation has exclusive autonomic innervations and it gives constant contractile responses to alpha-adrenergic agonists. It possess both α_1 and α_2 adrenoceptors at post and presynaptic sites, respectively. Norepinephrine gives a contractile response superimposed on the twitch response because of postsynaptic α_1 receptor stimulation.

Procedure

Male Wistar rats weighing 275 to 300 g are used. Animals are killed by stunning. A midline abdominal incision is performed to dissect out vas deferens. Tissue is suspended in an organ bath containing Tyrode solution gassed with O_2 and CO_2 at 35°C. Contractions are recorded using a lever transducer. After 30 min, norepinephrine is administered repeatedly in the concentrations of 0.5, 1.0, 2.0 or 4.0 mg/ml. Test drug is then added into the bath and after 3 min norepinephrine is administered. Phentolamine is used as standard.

To evaluate α antagonistic activity, norepinephrine-induced contractions after test drug administrations are compared with the contractions induced by norepinephrine alone.[12]

Modification

Isolated hypogastric nerve—vas deferens of the guinea pig is also used to evaluate α-sympatholytic activity.[13,14]

Rat Seminal Vesicle Model

Seminal vesicle of rat is used to evaluate a antagonistic activity.

Procedure

Male Wistar rats (40-50 days old) and weighing 125-150 g are used. Animals are killed by stunning. Seminal vesicles are prepared and suspended in an organ bath containing modified Krebs solution, provided as a continuous flow with run rate of 15 ml/min. Resting tension is around 350 mg and solution is bubbled with 5% CO_2 in O_2 at 32°C.

After 30 min of equilibration period norepinephrine is administered repeatedly in the concentrations of 0.5, 1.0, 2.0 or 4.0 mg/ml. Contractions are recorded using lever transducer. Test drug is then added into the bath and norepinephrine is added after 3 min. Phentolamine is used as standard. If a test drug inhibits the contractions induced by norepinephrine, it suggests a sympatholytic activity. To evaluate α antagonistic activity, norepinephrine-induced contractions after test drug administrations are compared with the contractions induced by norepinephrine alone.

The preparation is quite sensitive to a few selected agonists and remains viable for over 4-6 hr. Adrenaline, noradrenaline, dopamine, and acetylcholine all produce concentration-dependent and reproducible contractions. However, histaminergic, serotoninergic, purinergic, and opioid agonists, prostaglandins of the E and F series and the polypeptides angiotensin, vasopressin, and oxytocin are inactive.[15]

Cat Splenic Strip Model

The splenic tissue contracts in response to sympathomimetic agents and therefore can be used for screening of drugs with potential sympathomimtic/sympatholytic activity.

Procedure

Cats of either sex weighing around 1.0-2.8 kg are anesthetized by an intraperitoneal injection of 45 mg/kg sodium pentobarbitone. The spleen is then removed and 25 to 30 mm long and 2 to 3 mm wide strips of the spleen are prepared. The strip is then suspended in an organ bath containing 10 ml of the Krebs-Ringer solution, which at 38°C is aerated with the bubbles of 95% oxygen and 5% carbon dioxide. Isotonic contractions are recorded on a kymograph at 0.5 g tension with magnification 5 to 6 times. To induce contractions, norepinephrine (10^{6} g/ml) or epinephrine (10^{-6} g/ml) is administered after 30 min. Test drug is then added into the bath followed by the administration of α agonists after 3 min. Phentolamine is used as standard. To evaluate α sympatholytic activity, the percent inhibition of epinephrine or norepinephrine induced contractions is determined.[16,17]

Guinea Pig Tracheal Chain Model

Guinea pig tracheal chain preparation contracts in response to muscarinic receptor agonist, carbachol. The carbacholprecontracted tracheal chain preparation when exposed to a beta agonist like isoprenaline shows complete relaxation. Antagonism of relaxant effect of isoprenaline in presence of a beta-blocker can be demonstrated in guinea pig tracheal muscle.

Procedure

Albino guinea pig of either sex weighing 300-550 g is sacrificed by stunning and exsanguination. The trachea is removed and cut into 10-12 rings of the same width. Six rings are connected in series by means of short loops of silk thread and are kept in tyrode solution. The tracheal chain is suspended in an organ bath containing tyrode solution. Solution is aerated with 95% O_2 and 5% CO_2 and temperature is maintained at 37°C. Tension on the lever is around 0.5 g. To block α receptors phentolamine (0.1 mg/ml) and to induce spasm, carbachol (80 ng/ml) are added in the bath. After a period of 30 min, spasm is relieved by adding isoprenaline (β-agonist) in cumulative doses into the bath. After getting complete relaxation with isoprenaline, tissue is washed out at least 2-3 times. Test compound is then added in the bath and isoprenaline is again administered in cumulative doses. Tissue is thoroughly washed out and 10 min later, increased dose of test drug is administered.

β_2 antagonisitic activity would be considered as positive if test drug inhibits the spasmolytic action of isoprenaline.

To evaluate β_2 sympatholytic activity, percent inhibition of isoprenaline-induced relaxation after test drug administration is compared to maximal relaxation induced by isoprenaline.

Above preparation is also used to detect *β_2 agonistic* activity. For this, spasm is induced by carbachol and test drug is added. After 5 min, propranolol (β blocker) is administered in the bath. Spasmolytic effect of the test compound is decreased after propranolol administration. Percent inhibition of spasmolytic effect of the test compound after propranolol administration is measured to assess β_2 sympathomimetic activity.[18,19]

Guinea Pig Isolated Heart Model

The beta adrenergic drugs are potent cardiotonic agents and the effect of these drugs can be evaluated in isolated heart preparation.

Procedure

Guinea pigs of either sex weighing 600-800 g are used. The animals are injected with 100 units of heparin in the marginal ear vein to avoid damage to heart due to clot formation. The animals are now killed by a sharp blow to head, thorax is opened and heart is removed carefully and transferred to a Petridish containing Tyrode's solution. All the blood from the tissue is removed by gently squeezing it. The heart and aorta are dissected free from surrounding fascia and connective tissue. The Lagendroff's method can be used to screen for cardiotonic effects. The aorta is cut just below the point of its division and then the heart is transferred to perfusion apparatus containing Tyrode's solution at 37°C and oxygenated continuously. The aorta is tied to the glass cannula with the precaution that no air bubble enters the aorta. The heart is suspended by a thread through a hook into the ventricle. The thread is connected to spring levers to record contractions. After 20 min stabilization period baseline contractions are recorded to observe for amplitude and frequency of contractions indicating baseline force and rate of heart contractions. Now 0.1 ml of drug/adrenaline (100 µg/ml) is injected into the perfusion fluid and recordings are done to evaluate changes in force and rate of contractions. Beta-adrenergic drugs increase the force and rate of contraction; however they fail to do so in presence of a beta-blocker.[20]

Isolated Rat Aorta Model

The isolated rat aorta model evaluates the aortic smooth muscle contractions in response to $alpha_1$ adrenergic stimulation.[21]

Procedure

Wistar rats weighing 200-250 g are killed by cervical dislocation. The thoracic aorta is separated and gently cleared of fat and connective tissue. The separated aorta is cut into 3 mm ring segments and mounted on steel wires in 20 ml organ bath containing Kreb's solution (NaCl 119 mM; KC1 4.7 mM; $CaCl_2$ 2.5 mM; $MgSO_4$ 1.2 mM; $NaHCO_3$ 25 mM; KH_2PO_4 1.2 mM; D-glucose 11.1 mM) at 37°C and gassed with $O_2 + CO_2$ (95:5). The tissue is placed under 1.5 gram tension and a 60 min period is allowed for equilibrium with repeated washings with Kreb's solution at 15 min interval. Isometric muscle tension can be recorded using forced transducer. After equilibrium period the dose response curve is prepared for phenylephrine (alpha agonist) in the concentration range of 10^{-10} to 10^{-2} M. After washing, the aortic rings are incubated with the test drug and dose response curve (DRC) of phenylephrine is repeated. The shift of DRC to left or right will indicate the agonist or antagonist activity of the test drug. The contractile response to test drug can be repeated after preincubation with prazosin (an alpha blocker) and an inhibitory effect will indicate $alpha_1$ agonistic activity of test drug.

Rat Submaxillary Tissue Model

Adrenergic agonists increase the utilization of glucose in presence of Ca^{2+} by tissues with adrenergic receptors. Since, the rat submaxillary glands contain both the alpha and beta-adrenergic receptors, this property can be utilized for screening of adrenergic agonists.

Procedure

Male Wistar rats weighing 150-200 g are used. The rats are killed by cervical dislocation and submaxillary tissue slices are prepared.[22] The tissue slices (200 mg wet weight) are incubated in 50 ml flasks with 5 ml of Krebs-Henseleit bicarbonate saline containing 5 mM of glucose and gassed with a mixture of $O_2 + CO_2$ (95:5). The estimated quantities of drug/isoproterenol (10 µg/ml) with or without propranolol (20 µg/ml) are added to the flasks. For the control, all additions are made as above except for the tissue. The flasks are sealed and incubated at 37ºC for 1 hour in a shaking water bath. At the end of incubation period the medium is removed and the quantity of glucose is estimated. Glucose removal by the tissue can be calculated from the difference between the amount of glucose in control and that remaining in the experimental flasks. Isoprenaline significantly increases the glucose removal but addition of propranolol significantly inhibits the glucose removal by isoprenaline.[23]

Mice Metabolic Stimulation Model

Exogenous administration as well as endogenous release of catecholamines stimulates the conversion of liver glycogen into glucose and further metabolism of glucose. Alteration in these metabolic parameters in response to catecholamine stimulation can be used for screening of investigational adrenergic drugs.

Procedure

Male mice used in the experiment are anesthetized with sodium pentobarbital (60 mg/kg). The standard treatment group receives intraperitoneal injection of adrenaline (1.25 mg/g) after priming with intravenous adrenaline (0.37 mg/kg). The control animals receive the same volume of saline while the test group receives the test drug. The blood samples are collected from inferior vena cava at 20, 40 and 60 min after injection. Plasma is separated by centrifugation and is used for estimation of glucose, glycerol, nonesterified fatty acids and β-hydroxybutyrate. The plasma concentration of all metabolites increases in response to adrenergic stimulation.[24]

Rat Jejunal Longitudinal Muscle Model

Catecholamines can produce relaxation of non-sphincteric gastrointestinal muscle by an action on either postjunctional α- or β-adrenoceptors or a combination of both. Hence, adrenoreceptor-mediated changes in the contractility by experimental drugs can be demonstrated using this model.[25]

Procedure

Male Wistar rats (200-300 g) are killed by a blow to the head and cervical dislocation. The jejunum is removed and immediately placed in cold and oxygenated Krebs physiological saline solution, at room temperature. Longitudinal muscle strips are dissected from the intestinal segments by gently peeling the muscle in longitudinal direction. Longitudinal smooth muscle strips (3 cm) of jejunum are then suspended in organ baths containing Krebs solution, at 37°C, for isotonic recording. The Krebs solution is gassed with 95% O_2 and 5% CO_2 and consists of (mM): NaCl 118, $CaCl_2$ 2.5, KCl 4.7, $NaHCO_3$ 25, KH_2PO_4 1.2, $MgSO_4$ 1.2 and glucose 11.1. Strips are pre-contracted with potassium chloride (40 mM) before proceeding with cumulative concentration-response curves for agonists and adrenaline can be used as a reference drug. Alternatively, isoprenaline can be used as the intestinal responses are largely β receptor mediated with only a small contribution from α1 receptors. Agonists produce relaxation and the responses are expressed as % relaxation. Response to agonists is repeated in the presence or absence of propranolol (1 μM). Tissues are allowed to equilibrate for 45 min before addition of agonists. The antagonists are added from the beginning of the equilibration period. In the absence of propranolol, agonists produce relaxation of the potassium chloride-contracted strips. Presence of propranolol causes shift of dose-response curve to right by causing β receptor blockade.[25]

Gravid Rat Uterus Model

Stimulation of sympathetic α1 receptors causes uterine contractions and stimulation of β2 receptors causes uterine relaxation. The gravid uterus relaxes in response to epinephrine administration due to β2> α1. Blockade of β receptors abolishes the uterine relaxant effect of epinephrine.

Procedure

Uteri are excised from term pregnant rats. Cross-sectional rings of excised uteri are mounted for isometric force recording. Log dose-response curve is prepared for epinephrine in the concentration range of 10^{-12} to 10^{-6} M. Epinephrine causes dose-dependent reduction in uterine muscle activity. Similarly, agonists produce relaxation and the responses are expressed as % relaxation. Response to agonists is repeated in the presence or absence of propranolol (1 μM). In the absence of propranolol, agonists produce relaxation of the gravid rat uterus muscle. Presence of propranolol causes shift of dose-response curve to right due to β receptor blockade. Careful interpretation is necessary and oxytocin as well as washout of epinephrine also antagonize catecholamine-induced tocolysis.[26]

Murine Macrophage Model

Catecholamines are known to play a protective role during endotoxemia by downregulating the inflammatory response. One of the mechanisms of downregulation of inflammatory response is through suppression of expression of macrophage inducible nitric oxide synthase (iNOS). This model evaluates the effects of catecholamines on lipopolysaccharide (LPS) induced macropahge NO production *in vitro*.[27]

Procedure

The male mice 8-12 week old are used. The peritoneal cavities of mice are lavaged with ice-cold RPMI-1640 medium supplemented with 1% heat inactivated foetal calf serum, 100 U/ml penicillin, 100 μg/ml streptomycin, 25 mMN-2-hydroxyethylpiperazine-N'-2-ethane-sulphonic acid (HEPES) and 10 mM L-glutamine. The fluid now containing resident peritoneal exudates cells is centrifuged at 4° for 7 min at 1100 rpm. The cells are now suspended in the same fluid as above but containing 10% foetal calf serum. The cells in the solution are now counted and viability assessed using trypan blue dye. 100 μl of the cell suspension is now plated on the sterile flat-bottomed culture plates to produce a final concentration of 3×10^5 cells in each well. The plates are incubated at 37° for 2 hr in a 5% CO_2 incubator, followed by removal of non-adherent cell by washing thrice with above medium with 10% calf serum. Cells are further incubated with medium alone, LPS (10 μg/ml) alone, LPS plus drug in presence and absence of propranolol (10^{-2} M) and LPS plus adrenaline (10^{-5} M) in presence and absence of propranolol at 37° for 48 hr. After incubation the supernatant is removed and NO is estimated by Griess reaction. The amount of NO production can be compared among various groups. Adrenergic drugs suppress the NO production by murine macrophages in response to LPS but this suppression is abolished by propranolol. Corticosterone, a steroid hormone known to suppress NO production can be used as negative control in a concentration of 10^5 M.

REFERENCES

1. Brown GL, Gillespie JS. The output of sympathetic transmitter from the spleen of the cat. J Physiol 1957;138:81-102.
2. Keenan D, Romani A, Scarpa A. Differential Regulation of Circulating Mg^{2+} in the Rat by β_1- and β_2-adrenergic receptor stimulation. Cir Res 1995;77:973-83.
3. Zhang YC, Bui JD, Shen L, Phillips MI. Antisense Inhibition of β_1-Adrenergic Receptor mRNA in a single dose produces a profound and prolonged reduction in high blood pressure in spontaneously hypertensive rats. Circulation 2000;101:682.
4. Short JH, Biermacher U, Dunnigan DA, et al. Sympathetic Nervous System Blocking Agents. Derivatives of Guanidine and Related Compounds. J Med Chem 1963;6:275-83.
5. Exley KA. The blocking action of choline 2:6-xylyl ether bromide on adrenergic nerves. Br J Pharmacol chemother 1957;12:297-305.
6. Freundt KJ. Adrenergic α and β receptors in the mouse iris. Nature 1965;206:725-6.
7. Gillespie JS, Muir TC. A method of stimulating the complete sympathetic outflow from the spinal cord to blood vessels in the pithed rat. Br J Pharmacol 1967;30:78-87.
8. Shipley RE, Tilden JH. A pithed rat preparation suitable for assaying pressor substances. Proc Soc Exp Biol Med 1947;64:453-5.
9. Piercy V. Method for assessing the activity of drugs at β_1 and β_2 adrenoceptors in the same animal. J Pharmacol Methods 1988;20:125-33.
10. Su C, Bevan JA. The release of ^{3}H-norepinephrine in arterial strips studied by the technique of superfusion and transmural stimulation. J Pharmacol Exp Ther 1970;172:62-8.
11. McCulloch MW, Bevan JA, Su C. Effects of phenoxybenzamine and norepinephrine on transmitter release in the pulmonary artery of the rabbit. Blood Vessels 1975;12:122-3.
12. Taylor DA, Wiese S, Faison EP, et al. Pharmacological characterization of purinergic receptors in the rat deferens. J Pharmacol ExpTher 1983;224:40-5.
13. Holman M. Nerve muscle preparation of vas deferens. In Daniel EE, Paton DM (Eds): Methods in Pharmacology. New York: Plenum Press, 1975;3:403-17.
14. Hukovic S. Responses of the isolated sympathetic nerve-ductus deferens preparation of the guinea pig. Br J Pharmacol 1961;16:188-94.
15. Sharif SI, Gokhale SD. Pharmacological evaluation of the isolated rat seminal vesicle preparation. J Pharmacol Methods. 1986;15(1):65-75.
16. Innes IR, Kohli JD. An action of 5-hydroxytryptamine on adrenaline receptors. Br J Pharmacol Chemother 1962;19:427-41.
17. De Geus JP, Bernards JA, Verduyn WH. On the rhythmic activity of the cat spleen. Arch Intern PharmacodynTher 1956;106:113-21.
18. Castillo JC, de Beer EJ. The tracheal chain: A preparation for the study of antispasmodics with particular reference to bronchodilator drugs. J Pharmacol ExpTher 1947;90:104-9.
19. Foster RW. The nature of the adrenergic receptors of the trachea of the guinea-pig. J Pharm Pharmacol 1966;18:1-12.
20. Adome RO, Gachihi JW, Onegi B, Tamale J, Apio SO. The cardiotonic effect of the crude ethanolic extract of Nerium oleander in the isolated guinea pig heart. S African Health Sci 2003;3:77-82.
21. Brahmadevara N, Shaw AM, MacDonald. A $alpha_1$ adrenoceptor antagonist properties of CGP 12177A and other beta-adrenoceptor ligands: evidence against $beta_3$ or atypical beta-adrenoceptors in rat aorta. Br J Pharmacol 2004;142:781-7.

22. Thompson MP, Williamson DH. Metabolic effects of α- and β- adrenergic stimulation of rat submaxillary gland in vitro. Biochem J 1975;146:635-44.
23. Thompson MP, Williamson DH. Metabolic effects of α- and β- adrenergic stimulation of rat submaxillary gland in vitro. Biochem J 1976;160:597-601.
24. Tebar F, Grau M, Mena MP, Arnau A, Soley M, RamÍrez I. Epidermal growth factor secreted from submandibular salivary glands interferes with the lipolytic effect of adrenaline in mice. Endocrinology 2000;141:876-82.
25. MacDonald A, Forbes IJ, Gallacher D, Heeps G, McLaughlin DP. Adrenoceptors mediating relaxation to catecholamines in rat isolated jejunum. Br J Pharmacol 1994;112:576-8.
26. Segal S, Csavoy AN, Datta S. The tocolytic effect of catecholamines in the gravid rat uterus. Anesth Analg 1998;87:864-9.
27. Sigola LB, Zinyama RB. Adrenaline inhibits macrophage nitric oxide production through $[beta]_1$ and $[beta]_2$ adrenergic receptors. Immunology 2000;100:359-63.

CHAPTER

23

Drugs Acting on Parasympathetic Nervous System

INTRODUCTION

The parasympathetic nervous system performs maintenance activities and conserves body energy. Acetylcholine is both preganglionic and postganglionic neurotransmitter of parasympathetic nervous system. Acetylcholine, released at the cholinergic synapses and neuroeffector junctions, mediates its pharmacological actions through cholinergic receptors (nicotinic and muscarinic). Nicotinic receptors are found in autonomic ganglion and neuromuscular junction. Muscarinic receptors are found primarily on the autonomic effector cells that are innervated by postganglionic cholinergic nerves and are present in the heart, eyes, glands, smooth muscles and blood vessels. Muscarinic receptors are of five types—M_1, M_2, M_3, M_4, and M_5. Out of these, the first three are functionally well characterized. Stimulation of these receptors gives rise to various responses as shown in Table 23.1.

Table 23.1: Muscarinic receptors and their important characteristics

	M_1	M_2	M_3
Smooth muscles:			
Blood vessels (endothelium)			Dilatation
Bronchi			Constriction
GI tract			Constriction
GI sphincters			Relaxation
Bladder			Constriction
Bladder sphincter			Relaxation
Eye –Circular muscle			Constriction
Ciliary muscle			Constriction
Heart Rate		Decreases	
Force of contraction		Decreases	

Parasympathomimetic/cholinergic agents mimic the effects of acetylcholine. The parasympatholytic/anticholinergic drugs can antagonize the effects of parasympathetic stimulation or the effects of parasympathomimetic agents. A summary of parasymathomimetics (parasympathetic agonists) and parasympatholytics (parasympathetic antagonists) is given in Figure 23.1. The drugs with potential of cholinergic or anticholinergic activity can be screened using various animal models.

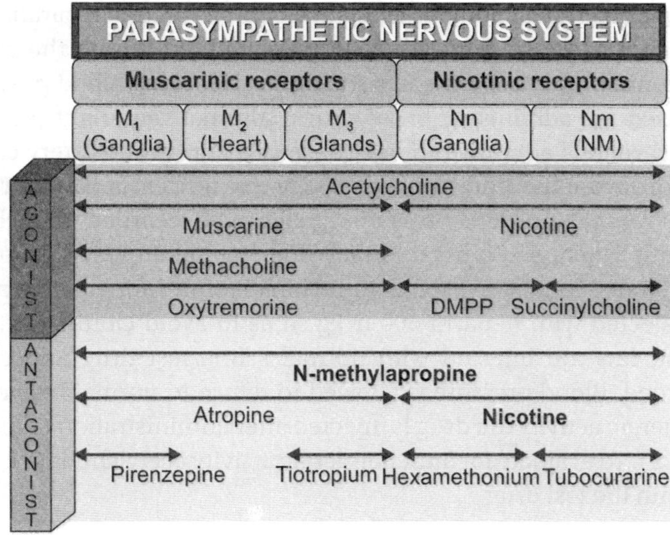

Figure 23.1: Parasympathetic agonists and antagonists

IN VIVO METHODS

Cat Model for Anticholinesterase Activity

Cat is anesthetized using chloralose or pentobarbitone sodium. The common carotid artery is cannulated for recording the blood pressure and the substance to be tested is injected intravenously. The blood pressure and respiration are recorded in the anesthetized animal at different doses of an anticholinesterase agent. For instance, at dose x, no detectable effect is observed. At dose 2x, slight bradycardia followed by fall in blood pressure by 10-20 mm of Hg developed over a period of 5 min. At dose 4x, blood pressure reduces by 50-100 mm of Hg with pronounced bradycardia. Salivary and bronchial secretions are seen with fasciculation of skeletal muscles. Initially, respiration is increased but later on it is depressed. Defecation and urination are also observed. At dose 8x, all effects mentioned are much more prominent as compared to dose 4x. Presence of all these effects indicates that test drug possesses anticholinesterase activity.[1]

Rat Cardiorespiratory Model

The cholinergic and anticholinergic effects of test drug can be evaluated by observing the effects of drug administration on cardiorespiratory functions in rats. Administration of cholinergic drugs produces fall in blood pressure and reduction in heart rate. These cardiac effects are antagonized by muscarinic blocker atropine.[2] Muscarinic receptor stimulation in respiratory tract stimulates secretions and smooth muscle contraction. Atropine in smaller doses causes mild stimulation of medullary centers and in larger doses causes central excitation.

Procedure

Sprague Dawley rats weighing 200-350 g are used. Animals are anesthetized using a 50:50 mixture of 25% urethane and 1% alpha chloralose at a dose 5 ml/kg per body weight. Trachea is cannulated and connected to a pneumotachograph that can record inspiration and expiration. Femoral artery and vein are cannulated using polythene catheters. The catheter placed in femoral artery is connected to pressure transducer for recording blood pressure and femoral vein catheter is used for administration of drugs. Alternatively, right jugular vein may be cannulated for intravenous administration of dose and left carotid artery can be cannulated with a thin polypropylene tube leading to a pressure transducer for blood pressure recording. Heart rate derived from the pulsatile pressure signal can be recorded via tachographic beat to beat conversion with a tachograph preamplifier. Body temperature is monitored with a rectal probe and is maintained at 37.0 ± 0.5°C with heating lamps. Immediately after cannulation, the animals are injected with heparin 600 u/kg so as to avoid clotting. After 30 minutes of equilibrium period rats are injected with normal saline/test drug and changes in blood pressure are recorded. Blood pressure is allowed to return to normal between injections. To evaluate for cholinergic activity the drug is injected after administration of muscarinic blocker atropine (1-6 mg/kg). To evaluate for anticholinergic activity acetylcholine (2 μg/kg) is injected after incubation with the test drug.

Mydriasis Test

Mice of either sex, of weight range 25 to 35 g are used. Test drug and the vehicle are injected intraperitoneally. The pupillary diameters (expressed in mm units) are measured at every 10 minutes interval for the first 60 min of drug administration, and then after 90 and 120 minutes by a dissecting microscope having a graduated scale. If the pupil diameter exceeds 30/25 mm, it is called positive quantalmydriatic effect.[3]

Modification

Rabbits are used instead of mice. At least 3 rabbits per group are taken. The left eyes of the three rabbits are instilled with 2 drops of 0.1% aqueous solution of atropine sulfate, whereas the left eyes of other group of three rabbits are instilled with 2 drops (0.2 ml) of 1% aqueous solution of test compound. The right eye of the used rabbit serves as a control; and after equal intervals, the pupillary diameters of both the eyes are measured. Average mydriasis is expressed as the percent increase of the diameter of the test pupil as compared with that of the control pupil.[4]

Intestinal Spasmolytic Activity in Mice

Fasted Swiss Webster mice of either sex of weight range 25 to 35 g are used. The mice are administered different doses of test drug orally. The aqueous solutions of soluble salts are used for administration and resin complexes are used as suspension in 0.5% carboxymethylcellulose. Test drug solutions are prepared in such a way that the administered dose volume is not allowed to exceed 50 ml/kg of body weight. After 90 min of administration of the soluble salts and 2 h after administration of the resin-complex suspension, the animals are anesthetized by intraperitoneal injection of pentobarbitone. Abdomen is cut open and intestines are exposed. Methacholine (0.25 μg) is applied locally to the intestines and intestines are observed for a period of 3 sec. Data are calculated as points: if methacholine induced contractions are completely prevented, it is scored as 2 points, whereas 1 point is scored if the contractions are only in a limited area or reduced in intensity.[5] The scores obtained are converted to the percent of the ideal mean score and Litchfield and Wilcoxon method is used to calculate the median protective dose.[6]

Continuous Cystometry in Rats

Micturition in rats is mediated mainly by the actions of acetylcholine and ATP, with later controlling the initiation of micturition process and the former maintaining the sustained bladder pressure during micturition. It has been reported that the anticholinergics like atropine reduce the contractility of detrusor and this property can be utilized for evaluation of anticholinergic activity of test drugs in rats.[7]

Procedure

Sprague Dawley rat weighing 230-250 g are used. The animals are anesthetized with pentobarbital sodium (50 mg/kg). A tracheostomy tube is placed to help the respiration and femoral artery is cannulated for administration of drugs. The urinary bladder is exposed after midline incision and a double lumen catheter is inserted at the dome of the bladder. One lumen of catheter is used for infusion while the other is connected to pressure transducer for recording the bladder pressure. At first the bladder is emptied and covered with saline soaked cotton swabs. After an equilibrium period the bladder is emptied and then continuously infused with warm saline (25-30°C) at a rate of 0.1-0.2 ml/min. At least three micturition cycles are recorded to obtain baseline values of urodynamic variables such as basal pressure, micturition pressure (maximum bladder pressure during micturition), bladder capacity (residual volume + volume of infused saline voided) and spontaneous contractile activity (mean amplitude and frequency of bladder contractions before micturition). After the control cystometry, the animal is administered with the test drug and 10 min later the micturition cycles are recoded again to calculate the changes in urodynamic variables. Following administration of muscarinic antagonists like atropine bladder capacity and residual volume increase, the amplitude and frequency of spontaneous bladder contractions decrease and micturition pressure decreases. Atropine can be used as standard in a dose of 1 mg/kg.

Guinea Pig Bronchospasm Model

Parasympatholytic activity of test drug can be evaluated by monitoring the effects on bronchial smooth muscles in guinea pigs.[8]

Procedure

Adult guinea pigs of either sex weighing 400-600 g are used. The animals are placed in a chamber with inbuilt nebuliser and are exposed to acetylcholine chloride (10%) aerosol under a constant pressure of 40 mm Hg. The time interval between the time at exposure and beginning of dyspnea is noted. As soon as the dyspnea appears the animals are removed from the chamber and placed in fresh air. The average time required for dyspnea to appear in response to acetylcholine is calculated.

The experiment is repeated after pretreatment of animals with the vehicle/test drug. Anticholinergic drugs increase the time required for dyspnea to appear following exposure to acetylcholine as they have a relaxant effect on bronchial smooth muscles. Atropine sulfate 2 mg/kg can be used as standard.

Mice Tremor and Salivation Model

Stimulation of central muscarinic receptors elicits several responses including tremors and hence the tremors evoked by intravenous, subcutaneous, intraperitoneal or intraventricular administration of cholinergic agonists have been used to characterize central muscarinic receptor stimulation *in vivo*. Peripheral muscarinic receptor stimulation causes increased salivation and blockade of these receptors results in dry mouth. Therefore, these effects have also been used to investigate cholinergic agonists and antagonists *in vivo*.

Procedure

Mice of either sex weighing 20-25 g are used. Test substances are administered intraperitoneally before subcutaneous injection of oxotremorine (muscarinic agonist; 50-75 μg/kg) at the back of the neck. Tremor intensity and salivation are assessed over a period of 60 min post-oxotremorine injection. Tremor intensity can be scored based on the following scale: 0 = no tremor, 1 = slight tremor (moderate, discontinuous tremor), 2 = strong tremor (intense continuous tremor involving the whole body). Similarly, degree of salivation is scored as follows: 0 = baseline salivation checked by placing an absorbent tissue under the mouth, 1 = slight salivation (weak and continuous salivation), 2 = excessive salivation (profuse and continuous salivation). Alternatively, salivation can be quantified by determining the weight of a preweighed, absorbant foam cube after it has been used to swab the oral cavity. The cholinergic agonists potentiate and cholinergic blockers inhibit the effects of oxotremorine on tremors and salivation.[9]

Modification

Rats weighing 150-200 g may also be used. The procedure used is the same as described for mice, however, the dose of oxotremorine is 150-200 μg/kg. Alternatively, acetylcholine (875 micrograms/kg) may also be used.[9,10]

IN VITRO MODELS

Guinea Pig Ileum

Guinea pig ileum is the most commonly used preparation for screening of parasympatho-mimetic as well as parasympatholytic agents.

Procedure

Guinea pig of either sex (weight range 250 to 550 g) is used. The animal is sacrificed by stunning. The abdomen is cut open by a midline incision. A cord is tied around the intestine just distal to the pylorus. The intestine is gradually removed, mesentery being cut away as necessary. When the colon is reached, the intestine is cut half-way through, so that the glass tube can be inserted. Tyrode solution is passed through the tube and the intestine until the effluent solution becomes clear. Mesentery around the colon is removed. A tissue clamp is attached to the distal end. Pieces of intestine (2-3 cm in length) are cut. One piece is fixed with a tissue clamp, suspended in a 15-20 ml tissue bath and the clamp is tied to a writing lever. Writing lever, which magnifies the contractions 5-10 times, is used. When the spontaneous movements of the muscle subside, acetylcholine (0.01 mg/ml) is added to the bath. Subsequently, doses are increased as per requirement. The procedure is repeated at 10 min interval and 2-3 submaximal contractions are recorded. After getting a response, tissue is washed out every time. When acetylcholine produces a response of 70-90% of maximal, the test substance is added; and if contractions are observed, then it is considered as a stimulant of smooth muscles (parasympathomimetic). If contractions do not occur and addition of acetylcholine produces diminished response of acetylcholine, it is taken as an antagonist of acetylcholine.[11,12]

Modification

Apart from guinea pig ileum, the jejunum of the rat can also be used. Rest of the procedure is same as above. This test has the advantage over the guinea pig ileum as it gives only feeble responses to ganglion stimulants such as nicotine.[13]

Isolated Eye of Rodents

Rats, mice or guinea pigs with pigmented iris are used for this experiment. Immediately after sacrificing the animals, the eyeballs are enucleated. The retrobulbar structures are removed from the eyeball. If corneal removal is necessary, a through-and-through stab incision is given with the help of wheeler knife. The cornea is then cut free along the limbal margin. The eyes are washed in Krebs-Ringer solution and mounted in appropriately sized, hemispherical sockets set in black Lucite trays. The trays are submerged in a bicarbonate buffered Krebs-Ringer solution of approximately 20 ml. The chamber of clear Lucite is designed for this experiment, so that it gets fitted to the standard mechanical stage of a microscope. The pH of the mixture is maintained at 7.4 by continuously bubbling with 95% oxygen and 5% carbon dioxide. The temperature is kept at 37°C by means of a 75 watt heating lamp. The microscope containing ocular micrometer disk with a magnification of approximately 30 times is used to read the pupillary diameter.

The eyes are placed in the chamber and pupillary diameter is measured as control after a period of 30 min. The used Krebs solution is then replaced with fresh Krebs solution, which contains known concentration of the test substance. The pupillary diameter is then measured after 30 min and the response is expressed as a ratio of this diameter to the control diameter.

The above method is also used to determine parasympatholytic activity of a test drug. By antagonism of miosis (induced by cholinomimetic drug), anticholinergic drugs are evaluated.[14]

In Vitro Assay for Anticholinesterase Activity

Acetylcholinesterase activity is detected by the assay described by Ellman et al.[15] This assay is based on measurement of the change in absorbance at 412 nm. In this assay, thiol ester acetylthiocholine was used as a substrate. To detect inhibition of enzyme activity, 2.89 ml phosphate buffer, 0.1 ml of DTNB and 10 ml of sample (serum, plasma, blood or brain homogenate) are mixed and incubated for 10 min. After addition of substrate, absorbance is recorded using spectrophotometer. The rate of change of absorbance is determined and enzyme activity is calculated. Different concentrations of inhibitors of enzymes are used and again rate of reaction is recorded. The percent inhibition as compared to standard activity is calculated.

Isolated Frog Rectus Muscle

The rectus muscle of frog is isolated and suspended in a bath containing 7 ml of frog ringer solution. The fluid is replaced every 5 min by frog ringer solution containing acetylcholine. The effect of acetylcholine is recorded for 90 sec on a kymograph. After that, tissue is washed out. This response is recorded for at least three times. Now to detect the test compound activity, ninety seconds prior to addition of acetylcholine, test drug is added in the bath. Response is observed for 90 seconds. Parasympatholytic drug will decrease the effect of acetylcholine.[3]

Rat Isolated Aorta

The smooth muscles of aorta show a relaxation response when treated with cholinergic drugs. The rat aorta can be used to evaluate this activity.

Procedure

Male Wistar rats of either sex weighing 250-350 g are used. The animals are killed by intraperitoneal sodium pentobarbital and thoracic aorta is dissected clear of the connective tissue and is transferred to a plate containing cold Krebs' solution. Three mm ring segment from the aorta is suspended in a 20 ml organ bath containing Krebs' solution at 37°C and aerated with O_2 + CO_2 (95:5), under 2.0 gram tension with the help of a steel wire. The preparation is allowed to equilibrate for 60 min before starting the experiment. The relaxant response to cholinergic drugs can be observed after precontracting the aortic rings with phenylephrine (10^{-7}-10^{-6} M). Acetylcholine in a concentration range of 10^{-12}-10^{-5} M can be used as standard. The relaxations are expressed as a percentage of the precontraction levels with phenylephrine.[16]

Guinea Pig Trachea

Tracheal smooth muscles contract in response to parasympathomimetic drugs like acetylcholine and relax in response to parasympatholytic drugs. The evaluation of test drugs can be done in guinea pig tracheal smooth muscle preparation.

Procedure

Guinea pigs of either sex weighing 300-350 g are used. The animals are sacrificed by stunning and exsanguination. The trachea is dissected out and transferred to a dish containing Kreb,s solution. The trachea is cut in to 2-3 mm wide rings and 6 such rings are connected to each other with the help of a silk thread. The tracheal ring preparation is now suspended under 1 gram tension in a 10 ml organ bath containing Krebs' solution is 37°C and continuously aerated with O_2 + CO_2 (95:5). The composition of Krebs' solution was as follows (mM): NaCl (118), KCl (4.7), $NaHCO_3$ (25), KH_2PO_4 (1.2), $MgSO_4$ (2.5), $CaCl_2$ (2.5), and glucose (11.1). Carbachol (1 μM) is used as standard. A dose response curve for cumulative concentrations of carbachol is first obtained. The preparation is washed thoroughly with Kreb's solution and the dose response curve for carbachol is repeated after incubation with different doses of the test drug for 10 min. The shift of dose response curve of carbachol to right indicates the parasympatholytic activity of the test drug. [17]

Guinea Pig Isolated Heart

The rate and force of contraction of heart is altered upon exposure to cholinergic and anticholinergic drugs. Guinea pig isolated heart preparation can be used for evaluation of test drugs for cholinergic/anticholinergic activity.[18]

Procedure

Guinea pigs of either sex weighing 600-800 g are used. Guinea pigs are injected with heparin (1000 units) in the ear vein to avoid damage to the heart muscles by clots and then animals are killed by a sharp blow to head. The heart is removed along with the aorta, which is cut at just below the point of its division and is transferred quickly to a dish containing Tyrode's solution. Preparation is gently squeezed to remove all the blood and is then transferred to the perfusion apparatus containing Tyrode's solution at 37°C and continuously aerated with $O_2 + CO_2$ (95:5). The aorta is tied to the glass cannula with the precaution that no air bubble enters the aorta. The heart is suspended by a thread through a hook into the ventricle. The thread is connected to spring levers to record contractions. After 30 min of stabilization the baseline recordings are done for amplitude and rate of contractions. Subsequently, the test drug in various doses is added to the perfusion chamber and changes in amplitude and rate of contractions is recorded. To evaluate for cholinergic activity, the drug is injected after incubation with muscarinic blocker atropine (1-6 mg/kg). To evaluate for anticholinergic activity acetylcholine (2 μg/kg) is injected after incubation with the test drug.

Rabbit Isolated Corpus Cavernosum

Parasympathetic stimulation elicits erection by enhancing the coordinated relaxation of the cavernous vessels and trabecular smooth muscles via the release of ACh and nitric oxide leading to increased blood supply to the sinusoids.[19]

Procedure

Male New Zealand white rabbits weighing 1.5–2.5 kg are used. Animals are anesthetized with pentobarbitone sodium and exsanguinated via the carotid artery. After performing penectomy, corpus cavernosum is dissected in the Krebs solution and cleared of the tunica albuginea and surrounding tissues. Strips of rabbit isolated corpus cavernosum are mounted in an organ bath with warmed (37°C) and oxygenated (95% O_2 + 5% CO_2) Krebs solution at a flow rate of 5 ml/min. Contractions of corpus cavernosum strips are recorded using isotonic or isometric transducer. Tissue strips are, at first, allowed to equilibrate for 90 min and then precontracted with noradrenaline (10^{-6} M). The tissues may also be continuously infused with indomethacin (5.6 mM) to inhibit the generation of cyclo-oxygenase products. Test substance or acetylcholine (0.3–30 nMol) are administered as single bolus injections (10-50 μl). Atropine (1 μM), is infused over the isolated tissues 20 min before and during a bolus injection of the agonists and significantly inhibits the acetylcholine-induced relaxation of rabbit isolated corpus cavernosum tissue.[20]

REFERENCES

1. Hobbiger F. Anticholinesterases. In Laurence DR, Bacharach AL (Eds). Evaluation of Drug Activities: PharmacometricsVol -II. London and New York: Academic Press 1964:467.
2. Salahdeen HM, Yemitan OK, Alada ARA. Effect of aqueous leaf extract of tridaxprocumbens on blood pressure and heart rate in rats. Afr J Biomed Res 2004;7:27- 9.
3. De Elio FJ. Acetylcholine antagonists: a comparison of their action in different tissues. Br J Pharmacol Chemother 1948;3:108-12.
4. Edwards BK, Golberg AA, Wragg AH. Spasmolytic esters of N-sustituted alpha aminophenylacetic acids. J Pharm Pharmacol 1960;12:179-86.
5. Becker BA, McCarthy LE. A comparison of the antispasmodic activities of atropine and scopolamine and their N-methyl derivatives in mice by an in vivo technique. Arch Intern Pharmacodyn Ther 1960;126:307-14.
6. Litchfield JT, Wilcoxon F. A simplified method of evaluation of dose-effect experiments. J Pharmacol Exp Ther 1949;96:99-113.
7. Kwak TI, Lee JG. Inhibitory effects of propiverine, atropine and oxybutynin on bladder instability in rats with infravesical outlet obstruction. Br J Urol 1998;82:272-7.
8. Kumar DA, Ramu P. Effect of methanolic extract of benincasa hispida against histamine and acetylcholine induced bronchospasm in guinea pigs. Indian J Pharmacol 2002;34:365-6.
9. Ogren SO, Carlsson S, Bartfai T. Serotonergic potentiation of muscarinic agonist evoked tremor and salivation in rat and mouse. Psychopharmacology (Berl) 1985;86(3):258-64.
10. Murray CW, Cowan A, Wright DL, Vaught JL, Jacoby HI. Neurokinin-induced salivation in the anesthetized rat: a three receptor hypothesis. J Pharmacol Exp Ther 1987;242(2):500-6.
11. Munro AF. The effect of adrenaline on the guinea pig intestine. J Physiol 1951;112:84-94.
12. Paton WD, Zar MA. The origin of acetylcholine released from guinea pig intestine and longitudinal muscle strips. J Physiol 1968;194:13-33.
13. Van Rossum JM, Ariens EJ. Pharmacodynamics of parasympathetic drugs, structure-action relationships in homologous series of quaternary ammonium salts. Arch Int Pharmacodyn Ther 1959;118:418-44.
14. Beaver WT, Riker WF. The quantitative evaluation of autonomic drugs on the isolated eye. J Pharmacol Exp Ther 1962;138:48-56.
15. Ellman GL, Courtney KD, Andres V Jr, et al. A new and rapid colorimetric determination of acetylcholinesterase activity. Biochem Pharmacol 1961;7:88-95.
16. Brahmadevara N, Shaw AM, MacDonald A. Alpha, 1-adrenoceptor antagonist properties of CGP 12177A and other beta-adrenoceptor ligands: evidence against $beta_3$ or atypical beta-adrenoceptors in rat aorta. Br J Pharmacol 2004;142:781-7.
17. Castillo JC, de Beer EJ. The tracheal chain-I. A preparation for the study of antispasmodics with particular reference to bronchodilator drugs. J Pharmacol Exp Ther 1947;90:104-9.
18. Adome RO, Gachihi JW, Onegi B, Tamale J, Apio SO. The cardiotonic effect of the crude ethanolic extract of Nerium oleander in the isolated guinea pig heart. S African Health Sci 2003;3:77-82.
19. Simonsen U, Garcia-Sacristan A, Prieto D. Penile arteries and erection. J Vasc Res 2002;39: 283-303.
20. Teixeira CE, Bento AC, Lopes-Martins RA, et al. Effect of Tityus serrulatus scorpion venom on the rabbit isolated corpus cavernosum and the involvement of NANC nitrergic nerve fibres.Br J Pharmacol 1998;123(3):435-42.

CHAPTER

24

Neuromuscular Blocking Agents

INTRODUCTION

Neuromuscular blocking drugs act at myoneural junctions to block the neuromuscular transmission causing paralysis of the affected skeletal muscle. The neuromuscular blockers can act presynaptically at receptor sites so as to inhibit the synthesis and release of acetylcholine or postsynaptically at acetylcholine receptors. Although, some drugs like botulinum toxin and tetradotoxin can act presynaptically, the clinically relevant drugs act postsynaptically. The neuromuscular blocking agents fall in two categories:

a. Depolarizing agents, e.g. succinylcholine
b. Nondepolarizing agents, also known as competitive blockers, e.g. tubocurarine.

During evaluation of neuromuscular blocking agents, the following parameters should be studied:[1] (a) potency (initial intravenous mg/kg paralysing dose); (b) time required for development of maximal effect after rapid intravenous administration; (c) duration of action of a single paralysing dose; (d) type of block produced by the initial dose; (e) cumulative effect or tachyphylaxis on repeated administration; (f) change in characteristics of the block after repeated or prolonged administration; (g) effect of tetanic stimulation or exercise on the course of the block; (h) side effects, e.g. autonomic, histamine-releasing and (i) reversibility by antagonists. Numerous experimental methods have been devised to obtain these data; some can be used only in experimental animals; others are suitable for clinical testing in man (Tables 24.1 and 24.2).

Table 24.1: Models used for evaluation of neuromuscular blockers in animals

Unanesthetized	*Anesthetized*	*In vitro*
• Production of contractures in birds • Testing of righting reflex • Inclined screen and inverted grid methods • Rotating drum method • Head drop method • Injection into lymph sac of frog	• Nerve-muscle preparations of lower limbs • Phrenic nerve-diaphragm preparations • Close intra-arterial injection • Determination of dose causing cardiac arrest • Facial nerve stimulation • Reversal of apnea in mouse	• Isolated nerve-muscle preparations • Frog nerve-muscle preparations • Phrenic nerve-diaphragm preparation • Lumbrical nerve-muscle preparation in rabbits • Ionophoretic micro-application technique • Electrical activity of single muscle fiber

Table 24.2: Models used for evaluation of neuromuscular blockers in human

Unanesthetized	*Anesthetized*	*In vitro*
• Test of grip strength • Test of exercise capacity of hand muscles • Measurement of voluntary activity of other muscles • Assessment of twitch response following indirect stimulation • Measurement of respiratory parameters • Electromyographic study • Intra-arterial injection	• Measurement of respiratory parameters • Measurement of twitch response to indirect stimulation	• Fetal phrenic nerve-diaphragm preparation • Intercostal nerve-muscle preparation

Neuromuscular blocking agents show different effects in different species. Variation in effects may also be observed among different members of the same species and even in different muscles of the same individual.[2] Neuromuscular blockers may show different effects in *in vitro* preparations and in intact animals.[3] For this reason, observations made on the neuromuscular effects of an agent in one species in one set of experimental conditions cannot be extrapolated to another species in other experimental conditions. Results obtained from testing in animals cannot be directly applied to man and pharmacologic investigations of each compound in human subjects must be carried out before clinical use.[4]

EVALUATION IN LABORATORY ANIMALS

The marked species differences in sensitivity to neuromuscular blockers[5] emphasize the importance of parallel studies of these compounds in different species.

Intact Unanesthetized Animals

Induction of Contractures in Birds

Administration of a depolarizing blocker in adult fowls, chicks or in pigeons causes a rigid extension of the limbs and retraction of the head.[6] If the dose is lethal, the animal dies in this rigid condition; if the dose is below the lethal level, the recovery is abrupt. Curare, on the other hand, causes flaccid paralysis in birds. The advantage of using this test on avian muscle is the ease with which the difference in the action of these two groups of drugs can be strikingly illustrated.

Testing of Righting Reflex

This reflex may be checked by turning the animal on its back and watching to see if the animal rolls back over onto its sternum. Disappearance of righting reflex in mice, rats and rabbits may be used to determine potency of neuromuscular blocking agents.[7]

Inclined Screen and Inverted Grid Methods

Doses graduated at 0.1 logarithmic intervals are given subcutaneously to groups of 10 mice each. Mice at each dose level are placed on a screen inclined at 50° from the horizontal. Those mice developing typical skeletal muscle paralysis and abruptly sliding off the screen within half an hour after injection are considered positive reactors. This method is used to estimate ED50.[8] Mice or rats can also be tested for their ability to stay on an inverted grid after administration of neuromuscular blocking agents.

Rotating Drum Method

This tests the ability of small laboratory animals to remain upright in a revolving drum after treatment with the drug.[9] In mice the drug is administered subcutaneously. Immediately after injection, the mice are placed in a rotating cylinder and mice falling away from the cylinder during the first twenty minutes are considered as reactors.

Head Drop Method

This method measures the minimal intravenous dose of the drug required to produce head drop. It is applicable to rabbit, mouse, guinea pig, rat, dog and monkey. The end point of the assay, head drop is the precise relaxation state when the animal's head drops forward to the supporting surface and cannot be raised in response to a light tap on the back.[10] Doses graduated at 0.1 logarithmic intervals are given by intravenous injection at the rate of 1 ml/5 seconds to groups of ten rabbits each. After injection, the rabbits are placed in a large enclosure on the floor where they can be observed for the occurrence or absence of head drop. The dose producing head drop in 50% of the rabbits (HD50) is then calculated.

Injection into Lymph Sac of Frog

This method was first described by Bernard.[11] Drugs administered via lateral or dorsal lymph sacs in frogs are rapidly absorbed into the blood. Profound curarisation can be induced in frogs without the need for artificial respiration as respiration occurs primarily through skin.

Anesthetized Animals

Nerve-muscle Preparations of Lower Limbs

Neuromuscular blocking agents can be tested using nerve-muscle preparations of the lower limbs in rats, cats or dogs.[7] Animals are anesthetized and artificially ventilated. The sciatic nerve is isolated and cut. Distal end of the sciatic nerve is stimulated supramaximally and the twitch response of the gastrocnemius, soleus or tibialis muscle is recorded.[12] Diaphragmatic and intercostal respiration is recorded. An induced current is used to stimulate the peripheral end of the sectioned nerve once every 10 sec. After a suitable period, during which a series of contractions of uniform height are obtained, a dose of the test drug is injected rapidly into the femoral vein. Observation is continued until complete recovery occurs. An initial dose of the test drug is selected which produces a partial inhibition of the muscle twitch. When the amplitude of the muscle contractions and respiration return to the preinjection level, subsequent doses of the test drug are increased by 0.1 logarithmic intervals, until complete arrest of nerve impulse transmission is obtained. A crossover comparison may be obtained in the same animal, by administering a graduated series of a second test drug in a similar manner.[8]

Alternatively, the twitch response of tibialis anterior can be observed after stimulation by supramaximal square wave stimuli 0.2 min duration applied to common peroneal nerve at 0.1 Hz. The parameters which can be used to compare the drug treated group with control include the onset time (time interval between the end of injection and maximal block), maximal block (twitch height depression as percentage of control twitch height), recovery time (time between recovery from 25 to 75% of control value) and duration of action (time interval between end of injection and 90% recovery).[12]

Tetanic stimulation of nerve-muscle preparations may be used to differentiate depolarizing and nondepolarizing blocks.

Phrenic Nerve-Diaphragm Preparations

The central stump of the phrenic nerve is isolated in the neck and the nerve action potential is recorded. Simultaneously, electrodes are placed on the ventral surface of the diaphragm to obtain an electromyographic recording.[13]

Facial Nerve Stimulation

New Zealand white rabbits weighing 3.5-4.5 kg are used. Rabbits are sedated by intramuscular injection of ketamine (20 mg/kg) and xylazine (0.05 mg/kg). Rabbits are now intubated and placed under general anesthesia with halothane. The EMG system is set up and subdermal electrode needles are placed in orbicularis oculi and paranasal tissue. The tympanic portion of facial nerve is exposed through middle ear and baseline stimulations are carried out and measured. An induced current (0.05-1.00 mA) is used to stimulate the facial nerve. Once a series of contractions of uniform height is obtained, various doses of the test drug/vehicle are now administered intravenously. These doses are preceded and followed by facial nerve stimulation and monitoring. Vecuronium at a dose of 0.025 mg/kg intravenously can be used as standard to compare the effects of test drug.[14]

Close Intra-arterial Injection

Close intra-arterial injection of neuromuscular blocking agents allows accurate estimation of potency and time required for onset of action and also eliminates the influence of distribution or breakdown en route to the muscle.[15]

Determination of Dose Causing Cardiac Arrest

The dose of neuromuscular blocker producing cardiac arrest is determined in artificially ventilated animals.[8]

Reversal of Apnea in Mouse

Succinylcholine, a depolarizing neuromuscular blocker, has a very short duration of action as it is hydrolyzed by butrylcholinesterase. Patients who carry genetic or acquired deficiency of butyrylcholinesterase are susceptible to succinylcholine-induced apnea. Geyer et al. have shown that a purified recombinant human BChE serves as an ideal antidote for succinylcholine apnea.[16]

Mice are anesthetized with ketamine/xylazine cocktail. Respiratory rate is counted and SpO_2 is recorded in anesthetized animals. Mice are then injected intravenously (tail vein) with 1 mg/kg succinylcholine/experimental drug/vehicle. Respiratory rate and SpO_2 are monitored every 2-3 min. Three minutes after injection, butrylcholine esterase/vehicle is injected to reverse the succinylocholine-induced apnea. Since, this dose of succinylcholine is higher than LD_{50}, all animals injected with succinylcholine and 3 min later with vehicle die of apnea but those receiving butylcholinesterase survive at the end of 15 min. Succinylcholine like experimental drugs with properties of depolarizing neuromuscular blockade show a similar response.[16]

In Vitro Studies

Although, experiments on intact animals may reveal valuable information, *in vitro* experiments allow accurate control of more variables and are likely to be useful in the analysis of the mode of action of drugs. These methods eliminate the influence of circulation, distribution and metabolic transport.

Isolated Nerve-Muscle Preparations

The neuromuscular blocking agent to be studied is added to the bathing fluid into which the amphibian or mammalian muscle is immersed. Electrodes, stimulator and recording system are used. The muscle may be stimulated directly or through the proximal end of the nerve, which is kept outside the bathing fluid. The stimulus rate is 5 per min and working temperature is 40°C. The bathing fluid used is a modified Krebs solution. Glucose is added immediately before use. A gas mixture containing 5% CO_2 and 95% O_2 is equilibrated with the bathing fluid before use. When first set up, the nerve-muscle preparation often shows a partial neuromuscular block, which rapidly recovers in the presence of adequate oxygenation. The twitch tension increases for about an hour and so some time has to be allowed for equilibration of the preparation.

Frog Nerve-Muscle Preparations

Isolated frog gastrocnemius muscle preparation was first used in the classical Claude Bernard[11] experiment in which two nerve-muscle preparations were arranged so that the test drug was applied exclusively to the nerve of one and the muscle of the other. Isolated sartorius and rectus abdominis muscle may be used.[17]

Phrenic Nerve-Diaphragm Preparation

The effects of neuromuscular blocking agents on isolated respiratory muscles may be studied in phrenic nerve-diaphragm preparations from rats[18] and guinea pigs.[19] Rat diaphragm preparation is relatively insensitive to decamethonium and similar agents.[5] Diaphragms from other animals must be from very young animals or from fetuses so that they are thin enough for oxygen diffusion.

A parallel-sided slip of diaphragm is removed with the phrenic nerve. Stimuli are applied alternately to the muscle directly, via electrodes at each end, and to the phrenic nerve. A running control is thus obtained against effects on the muscle as opposed to effects on neuromuscular transmission.

Alternatively, nerve-evoked maximal twitches (T1, T2, T3, T4) of the rat hemidiaphragm to train of four (TOF) stimulation (2 Hz for 2 s every 20 s) can be recorded continuously in the presence and absence of vehicle/test drug. The T1 and T4 response-time profiles can be compared with respect to amplitude depression and the TOF ratio (T4/T1) during the development of and recovery from neuromuscular blockade.[20]

Lumbrical Nerve-Muscle Preparation in Rabbits

The rabbit lumbrical muscle is sensitive to depolarizing blockers. However, it is expensive and difficult to work with; it is vestigial in some rabbits and sometimes has an aberrant nerve supply. Three lumbrical muscles are present in the foot of the rabbit but only the medial of these is generally thin enough to allow adequate oxygen diffusion and at the same time strong enough to operate a lever to record its contractions. The lever bearing and writing tip must be chosen for minimal friction. The lever must be weight-loaded to stretch the muscle optimally and ensure a linear relation between the height of the recording and the work done on the lever by the muscle. Depending upon the time taken during dissection, a partial neuromuscular block may be seen when the preparation is set up. This block is due to anoxia and recovers completely in a few minutes. The preparation is very sensitive to changes in ionic concentration. A fall in the concentration of hydrogen, calcium or magnesium ions, especially calcium, induces spontaneous activity, repetitive response to stimulation and irregularity of behavior, while altering the sensitivity to all types of blocking agents.[21]

Ionophoretic Microapplication Technique using Isolated Tenuissimus Nerve-Muscle Preparation in Cats

The technique has been described by Thesleff.[22] Tenuissimus nerve-muscle has the advantage of being covered by only a thin layer of connective tissue and has generally a number of superficially located end plates, which suit the microapplication of drugs. Furthermore, the tenuissimus muscle can be maintained for a long time in oxygenated Ringer solution without showing signs of deterioration. In these experiments, twin micropipettes with a tip diameter less than 1μ are used. One micropipette contains acetylcholine, while the other contains the drug to be tested. A micromanipulator is used to move the drug pipette to an effective position at a superficial end plate. When the tip of the pipette is close to the receptor structure, a brief positive current pulse applied to the barrel containing acetylcholine releases sufficient amount of drug to produce, in the end plate, a transient depolarization of a few millivolts amplitude and a rapid time course. This potential change is recorded by inserting a microelectrode into the muscle fiber at a distance of about 100 μ from the point of drug application. The position of the drug pipette is adjusted so that stable and maximal responses are obtained when acetylcholine is released by current impulses of constant intensity and duration. With the tip of the pipette in this position, the test drug contained in the second barrel is released in a similar way or by a constant current. Since, the tips of the two drug pipettes are not more than 2 μ apart, both drugs affect the same receptor structure, and it is possible to compare their effects or study their interaction. The current passing through the drug pipette is recorded using an oscilloscope. The advantages of this method are that it is rapid, diffusion times are reduced to a minimum, and much faster events can be studied. Furthermore, the removal of the drug is automatic; there is no need for long periods of washing and many different applications can be made to the same receptor area. The drawback, however, is the uncertainty as to the local drug concentration obtained due to the spatial distribution of drug receptors.

Electrical Activity of Single Muscle Fiber

Frog sartorius muscle is used. The nerve is cut close to its point of entry into the muscle. The muscle is mounted in a bath of Ringer solution on an illuminated stage and observed from above with a binocular microscope. The bath is divided into two compartments by means of a partition and the muscle is drawn through a gap in this partition. Stimulating electrodes are placed in the two compartments. The microelectrode assembly is mounted on the arm of a micromanipulator and attached to a probe. The recording equipment consists of a DC amplifier and oscilloscope. A large amount of information can be obtained in a relatively short time since, the process of mounting and recording from a muscle fiber takes only a few seconds. In this way, average values for a large number of fibers can be determined with reasonable accuracy and the effect of environment can be assessed by comparing the properties of groups of fibers from the same muscle.[23]

EVALUATION IN MAN

In Unanesthetized Subjects

Test of Grip Strength

Onset, duration of action, relative potency and tachyphylactic or cumulative properties of neuromuscular blocking agents can be assessed using this test.[24] Grip strength, measured by a dynamometer, is determined immediately before and after the exercise, consisting of the squeezing of the bulb of an ergograph apparatus for 1 min with the maximum effort of which the subject is capable, before and at 3, 5 and 10 min after the start of the injection of the neuromuscular blockers and at 5 min intervals thereafter. In preliminary studies, the dose of each drug, which produces a 90 to 95% decrease of grip strength, is determined.[25]

Test of Exercise Capacity of Hand Muscles

Information about fatigability of the hand muscles during partial depolarization block can be obtained by this method. Ability of subjects to squeeze the bulb of an ergograph at variable rates is recorded.[25]

Measurement of Voluntary Activity of Other Muscles

Assessment of neuromuscular blockers may be made by recording the muscular strength of finger, foot and abdomen.[26]

Assessment of Twitch Response Following Indirect Stimulation

In the above-mentioned methods, emotional factors may influence the action of neuromuscular blocking agents. To eliminate this, contraction of voluntary muscles caused by indirect stimulation of the corresponding nerves may be made.[27]

Measurement of Respiratory Parameters

Effect of neuromuscular blocking agents on respiratory muscles can be assessed by measuring vital capacity and maximal expiratory pressure.[21] In the preliminary experiments, the dose of each drug which produces a 50-55% decrease of vital capacity is determined.[25]

Electromyographic Study

Response of individual muscles to indirect stimulation during partial depolarization or nondepolarization block can be assessed using this method.[28]

Intra-arterial Injection

Close intra-arterial injections can be given in conscious subjects and the effect of neuromuscular blocking agents on the electromyogram can be studied.

In Anesthetized Subjects

Measurement of Respiratory Parameters

In anesthetized subjects, maximal inspiratory pressure can be measured to assess the degree of paralysis of respiratory muscles.[29] The dose of neuromuscular blocking agent, which causes paralysis of all respiratory muscles, can be measured by monitoring tidal volume.[30]

Measurement of Twitch Response to Indirect Stimulation

In anesthetized subjects, muscle contractions can be measured after indirect stimulation of the corresponding nerve to assess the action of neuromuscular blocking agents.[31]

In Vitro Studies

Fetal Phrenic Nerve-diaphragm Preparation

This isolated nerve-muscle preparation is also used to study the effect of neuromuscular blocking agents *in vitro*.[32]

Intercostal Nerve-Muscle Preparation

This material may be obtained by biopsy under regional anesthesia and may be used to study the effect *in vitro* of neuromuscular blocking agents.[33]

Effect of Anticholinesterases

Neuromuscular blocking agents can be characterized further by assessing the effect of anticholinesterases on their action in conscious and anesthetized human subjects.

Anticholinesterases antagonize the nondepolarizing block and prolong the depolarization block.[34]

CHARACTERIZATIONS OF DEPOLARIZING AND NONDEPOLARIZING BLOCKERS

In laboratory animals, if intra-arterial injection is followed by a spontaneous muscle twitch, tetanus is well maintained during partial neuromuscular block, and there is no post-tetanic stimulation, the compound is a depolarizing agent.[28] On the other hand, absence of a twitch response after intra-arterial injection, poorly maintained tetanus during partial neuromuscular block, and presence of post-tetanic facilitation are characteristics of nondepolarizing agents.[35] In birds depolarizing agents produce contracture, while nondepolarizing agents produce flaccid paralysis.[6]

In human subjects, if intravenous administration of the compound produces relatively less effect on vital capacity as compared to effect on grip strength and produces easy fatigue of the hand muscles after rapid rate of exercise, this indicates that the agent being tested is a nondepolarizing agent. On the other hand, depolarizing compounds affect both vital capacity and grip strength, but exercise at a rapid rate during partial neuromuscular block caused by them does not produce fatigue.[25]

The type of block produced by the compound tested may be determined by intravenous administration of edrophonium chloride, which will rapidly antagonize the nondepolarization block.[36]

DISCUSSION AND CONCLUSION

There is considerable disagreement regarding the applicability of various methods used for testing neuromuscular blocking agents. To obtain complete information about neuromuscular blocking activity of any substance, a variety of *in vitro* and *in vivo* tests must be applied to different species including amphibians, birds and mammals. The species of test animal used and all experimental conditions must be specified when potency, onset, duration of action, etc. are recorded.[1]

Preliminary information of the pharmacological actions of neuromuscular blocking agents can be obtained by relatively simple tests. Depolarizing and nondepolarizing compounds can be differentiated by the production of contracture or paralysis after intravenous injection into birds.[6] The head-drop method can be used to compare relative potency, onset and duration of action of neuromuscular blockers, without elaborate equipment.[10]

For more detailed information, experiments using nerve-muscle preparations in intact animals,[15] isolated nerve-muscle preparations[22] and observations on single muscle fiber with intracellular electrodes[37] should be used. Close intra-arterial injection,[15] observation of the effect of tetanic stimulation on the twitch[13] and electromyogram[28] will provide additional information.

Following testing of a neuromuscular blocking agent in animals, it must be tested in human subjects before it can be introduced into clinical practice.[1] For preliminary testing conscious subjects are used. After intravenous administration, observation of the magnitude and time course of changes produced in grip strength and vital capacity should be made. Unexpected hypersensitivity to both depolarizing and nondepolarizing agents can be seen in apparently normal subjects; and for this reason, during testing on human subjects, equipment and personnel required for respiratory resuscitation must be available.[38] Information regarding cumulation, tachyphylaxis and changes in characteristics of the block can be obtained in anesthetized subjects.[39] Side effects of neuromuscular blocking agents including ganglionic blockade, histamine release and excessive tracheobronchial secretions should also be studied thoroughly before its introduction into clinical practice.[4]

REFERENCES

1. Foldes FF. Animal and clinical techniques for evaluating neuromuscular blocking agents, In Nodine JH, Siegler PE (Eds): Animal and Clinical Techniques in Drug Evaluation. Chicago: Year Book Medical Publishers Inc 1964:383-91.
2. Foldes FF. Factors which alter the effects of muscle relaxants. Anesthesiology 1959;20:464-504.
3. Zaimis EJ. Factors influencing the action of neuromuscular blocking substances. In: Lectures on the scientific basis of medicine. New York: John de Graar 1957:208-18.
4. Foldes FF. The pharmacology of neuromuscular blocking agents in man. Clin Pharmacol Ther 1960;1:345-95.
5. Paton WD, Zaimis E. The methonium compounds. Pharmacol Rev 1952;4:219-53.
6. Buttle GAH, Zaimis EJ. Action of decamethonium iodide in birds. J Pharm Pharmacol 1949; 1: 991-2.
7. Hoppe JO. Observations on potency of neuromuscular blocking agents with particular reference to succinylcholine. Anesthesiology 1955;16:91-124.
8. Hoppe JO. A pharmacological investigation of 2,5-bis-(3-diethyl-aminopropylamino) benzoquinone -bis-benzylchloride (Win 2747): a new curarimimetic drug. J Pharmacol Exp Ther 1950;100:333-45.
9. Collier HO, Hall RA, Fieller EC. Use of rotating drum in assessing activities of paralysant, convulsant and anesthetic drugs. Analyst 1949;74:592-6.
10. Varney RF, Linegar CR, Holaday HA. Assay of curare by rabbit head drop method. J Pharmacol Exp Ther 1949;97:72-83.
11. Bernard C. Lessons on the effects of toxic and medicinal substances: 1857. Cah Anesthesiol 1991;39:55-60.
12. Proost JH, Wierda JM, Houwertjes MC, Roggeveveld J, Meijer DK. Structure-pharmacokinetics relationship of series of aminosteroidal neuromuscular blocking agents in the cat. J Pharmacol Exp Ther 2000;292:861–9.
13. Paton WD, Zaimis EJ. Action of D-tubocurarine and of decamethonium on respiratory and other muscles in the cat. J Physiol 1951;112:311-31.
14. Hester TO, Hasan A, McDonnell F, Valentino J, Jones R. Facial Nerve Monitoring under Neuromuscular Blockade. Skull Base Surgery 1995;5:69-72.
15. Brown GL. Preparation of tibialis anterior (cat) for close intra-arterial injection. J Physiol 1938;92:22P-23P.
16. Geyer BC, Larrimore KE, Kilbourne J, Kannan L, Mor TS. Reversal of succinylcholine induced apnea with an organophosphate scavenging recombinant butyrylcholinesterase. PLoS One. 2013;8(3):e59159.
17. Swanson EE, Gibson WR, Powell CE. Comparative potency of D-tubocurarine chloride USP and dimethyl ether of D-tubocurine iodide. J Am Pharm Assoc 1952;41:487-97.

18. Bulbring E. Observations on the isolated phrenic nerve-diaphragm preparation of the rat. Br J Pharmacol Chemother 1946;1:38-61.
19. Jenden DJ. The effect of drugs upon neuromuscular transmission in the isolated guinea pig diaphragm. J Pharmacol Exp Ther 1955;114:398-408.
20. Cheah LS, Gwee MCE. Train of four fade during neuromuscular blockade induced by tubocurarine, succinylcholine or alpha-bungarotoxin in the rat isolated hemidiaphragm. Clin Exp Pharmacol Physiol 1988;15:937-43.
21. Jenden DJ, Kamijo K, Taylor DB. The action of decamethonium on the isolated rabbit lumbrical muscle. J Pharmacol Exp Ther 1954;111:229-40.
22. Thesleff S. A study of interaction between neuromuscular blocking agents and acetylcholine at mammalian motor endplate. Acta Anaesthesiol Scand 1958;2:69-79.
23. Nastuk WL, Hodgkin AL. Electrical activity of single muscle fiber. J Cell Comp Physiol 1950;35:39-73.
24. Unna KR, Pelikan EW. Evaluation of curarizing drugs in man: VI Critique of experiments on unanesthetized subjects. Ann N Y Acad Sci 1951;54:480-92.
25. Foldes FF, Monte AP, Brunn HM Jr, et al. Studies with muscle relaxants in unanesthetized subjects. Anesthesiology 1961;22:230-6.
26. Poulsen H, Hougs W. Effect of some curarising drugs in unanesthetised man. Acta Anaesthesiol Scand 1957;1:15-39.
27. Botelho SY. Comparison of simultaneously recorded electrical and mechanical activity in myasthenia gravis patients and in partially curarised normal humans. Am J Med 1955;19:693-6.
28. Churchill-Davidson HC, Richardson AT. Decamethonium iodide (C10): some observations on its action using electromyography. Proc R Soc Med 1952;45:179-86.
29. Churchill-Davidson HC, Christie TH. The diagnosis of neuromuscular block in man. Br J Anaesth 1959;31:290-301.
30. Foldes FF, Wolfson MB, Torres KM, et al. The neuromuscular activity of hexamethylene 1, 6-bis carbaminoylcholine bromide (Imbretil) in man. Anesthesiology 1959;20:767-75.
31. Christie TH, Churchill-Davidson HC. The St. Thomas's hospital nerve stimulator in diagnosis of prolonged apnea. Lancet 1958;1:776.
32. Buller AJ, Young IM. Action of D-tubocurarine chloride on foetal neuromuscular transmission and placental transfer of this drug in the rabbit. J Physiol 1949;109:412-20.
33. Dillon J, Fields J, Gumas T, et al. An isolated human voluntary muscle preparation. Proc Soc Exp Biol Med 1955;90:409.
34. Koppanyi T, Vivino AE. Prevention and treatment of D-tubocurarine poisoning. Science 1944;100:474-5.
35. Hutter OF. Post-tetanic restoration of neuromuscular transmission blocked by D-tubocurarine. J Physiol 1952;118:216-27.
36. Randall LO. Anticurare action of phenolic quarternary ammonium salts. J Pharmacol Exp Ther 1950;100:83-93.
37. Graham J, Gerard RW. Membrane potentials and excitation of impaled single muscle fibers. J Cell Physiol 1946;28:99-117.
38. Pelikan EW, Tether JE, Unna KR. Sensitivity of myasthenia gravis patients to D-tubocurarine and decamethonium. Neurology 1953;3:284-96.
39. Artusio JF Jr, Marbury DE, Crews MA. Quantitative study of D-tubocurarine, tri-(diethylamino-ethoxy)-1,2,3-benzene (Flaxedil) and series of trimethyl and dimethylethyl-ammonium compounds in anesthetized man. Ann N Y Acad Sci 1951;54:512-29.

CHAPTER

25

Antiviral Drugs

INTRODUCTION

There are more than hundred viruses known to cause diseases in humans and the need for antiviral drugs is growing rapidly as more and more new viral pathogens are discovered. More than 40 antiviral drugs are approved for clinical use currently and about 20 of them are used for the treatment of HIV infection and the rest for the treatment of other viral diseases.[1] Currently, antiviral drug development strategy is focused to address two main issues: (i) further improvement of existing antiviral therapy such as for hepatitis B (HBV) and C (HCV) viruses, herpes simplex virus (HSV) and influenza viruses. (ii) development of new antiviral drugs for the infections that do not have approved therapy yet, but their prevalence is significantly high and they are associated with considerable morbidity, mortality and high social and economic implications (hemorrhagic fever viruses, human papilloma viruses, severe acute respiratory syndrome (SARS) coronavirus).[2]

Viruses and Viral Life Cycle

Viruses are ultra-microscopic, acellular infectious agents that are obligatory intracellular parasites. Viruses consist of: (i) the genetic material which is either DNA or RNA, (ii) a protein coat (capsid) and in some cases, (iii) an envelope of lipoproteins surrounding the protein coat that is acquired from the host cell membrane. Viruses do not have their own organelles and metabolic processes and hence they can replicate only inside the living host cells.

Virus life cycle depends on the type of virus, but generally includes 6 phases, each of which could be a potential target for new antiviral drugs. The phases in the virus life cycle include the following:

1. Attachment on the surface of host cell
2. Penetration/entry into the host cell
3. Uncoating
4. Gene expression and replication viral DNA or RNA
5. Virion assembly
6. Release of new virions.

Challenges in Development of New Antiviral Drugs

The research in the field of antiviral drug development has dramatically increased over past few decades, however, very few new drugs have been approved for clinical use. Besides high cost, the discovery of new antiviral drugs is associated with some challenges and limitations:

i. Lack of unique targets: As stated above, viruses consist of only the genetic material and protein coat and they completely lack their own metabolic system. It leads to insufficient viral-specific targets for antiviral drugs and hence the possibility of their low efficacy and high toxicity.
ii. Limited availability of *in vitro* and *in vivo* models: Some of viruses do not naturally infect animals and cannot replicate in nonhuman cells. Hence, the availability of animal models and *in vitro* systems is limited making it difficult to investigate newer drugs using multiple models.
iii. High specificity of antiviral drugs. Most of the compounds can target only a single infectious agent and their use for more than one viral infections remains limited.
iv. Emergence of antiviral drug resistance. Viruses are generally characterized by fast replication that results in increased genetic variability and, therefore, greater possibility of development of drug resistance. This further complicates the development of new antiviral drugs.

IN VITRO MODELS

In vitro models are generally used prior to *in vivo* testing for the screening of potential compounds in terms of their cytotoxicity and antiviral efficacy. Usage of *in vitro* models is less time consuming and more cost effective compared to the *in vivo* models. Moreover, for some of the viral infections *in vivo* models are not available or require a particular animal species, for example chimpanzees or other primates, and could be limited by the ethical issues.

Most of the *in vitro* antiviral drug studies are based on virus-induced cytopathic effects and include the detection of median cytotoxic concentration (CC_{50}), median effective concentration (EC_{50}) and selectivity index (SI).

The selection of the type of cells for viral propagation and experimental drug treatment depends on the virus itself. Some viruses, for example HSV, influenza viruses can replicate in different cell lines while for others such as HVB and HVC, replication in cell lines or primary cell cultures is very slow and variable and requires development of the replicon cell culture systems.[3]

Replicon Cell Culture Model for HCV

Discovery of potential therapeutics against HCV was significantly hampered because of lack of the ability of HCV to replicate in cell culture. The situation has been changed by the development of HCV replicon culture system.[4]

Generally, replicon is defined as DNA or RNA molecule that is able to replicate. Subgenomic replicon is derived from the Con1 strain of HCV and recapitulates the intracellular steps of the viral replication in cultured human hepatoma Huh-7 cells.[5] HCV replicon has some advantages compared to wild-type HCV:

i. Subgenomic replicon is able to replicate at high level in cell culture system that allows its easy detection and quantitative analysis.
ii. Subgenomic replicon is avirulent and does not support virus production, thus can be used in a standard cell culture laboratory without particular biosafety concerns.
iii. Persistence of replicon in cell culture causes emergence of drug resistance that could be tested as well.

The HCV replicon system has some disadvantages as well. It is not a complete viral particle and cannot represent entire viral life cycle and some of key steps in the virus life cycle, such as cell entry, uncoating, RNA packaging, virion assembly and release are not represented.[4]

Cell Culture Systems

Vero cells

Vero cells are a continuous cell line originally isolated from kidney epithelial cells of African green monkey (*Cercopithecus aethiops*) by Yasumura and Kawakita. Vero cells are very easily maintained and are extensively used in virology studies as host cells for viral propagation. They are also used for the screening of cytotoxic and therapeutic effects of drugs. One of the most important characteristic of Vero cells making them extremely attractive for virology and screening of antiviral compound is their inability to produce interferon.[6,7] However, Vero cells do have the interferon-alpha/beta receptors and are able to respond to interferon treatment.

Vero cells have been shown to support replication of different viruses including rabies virus, reovirus, Japanese encephalitis virus, dengue fever virus, influenza A and B viruses.[8,9]

There are several lines of Vero cells that are available (*Vero, Vero 76, Vero E6, Vero F6*) but all of them are derived from the same source and follow the same protocol.[10] Vero cells are cultured in Dulbecco's modification of Eagle medium (DMEM), supplemented with 10% heat-inactivated fetal bovine serum (FBS) and 1% penicillin/streptomycin. Cells grow on standard culture plates and should be incubated at 37°C in the presence of 5% CO_2. Vero cells are derived from normal kidney cells so they have not lost their contact inhibition. Actively growing Vero cell culture doubles approximately every 24 hours and when cells reach confluence, they stop growing and die. To avoid that and keep cells in monolayer the cells need to be passaged 2-3 times per week depending on the number of cells seeded and the flask size.[11]

Huh-7 Cells

The classical cell culture system used for HCV is the human hepatoma cell line Huh-7. Huh-7 is a well-differentiated hepatocyte derived cellular carcinoma cell line that was originally obtained from a liver tumor in a 57-year-old Japanese male.

Currently Huh-7 subclones (Huh-7.5, Huh-7.5.1 and Huh-7-Lunet) support more efficient viral replication and production compared to original cell line.[12]

While Huh-7 cells support high level of HCV replication and virus production, they are not normal hepatocytes and have lost some essential properties and characteristics of normal cells. Thus, there are some limitations in the assessment of antiviral effects of the investigational drugs such as their effect on immune response, expression of certain markers etc.[3] However, Huh-7 cells and their subclones are still considered the best available *in vitro* model for HCV.

Other cell culture systems used for HCV

Recently, other non-Huh-7 cell lines (Huh-6, HepG2, IMY-N9, LH86 etc.) and primary human, mouse and chimpanzee hepatocytes have shown the ability to maintain HCV replication. However, viral replication in these cell culture systems was found to be lower compared to that in Huh-7 cells.[3]

Huh-6 cell line is derived from hepatoblastoma and is characterized by low production of Claudin-1, an integral membrane protein responsible for the formation of tight junction strands between cells. Initially, Huh-6 cells were not susceptible for HCV but addition of ectopic Claudin-1 made them support HCV replicon. Huh-6 cells are also highly resistant to interferon-γ treatment making them potentially attractive for antiviral drug screening.[13]

Cell Culture Systems used for HBV

HBV could be reproduced in primary hepatocytes. However, this cell culture model has limitations due to inadequate viral replication, low viral production and poor reproducibility.

HepG2 is an immortal cell line derived from the well-differentiated hepatocellular carcinoma of a 15-year-old Caucasian American male. Since, HepG2 cells are well-differentiated they secrete a large range of plasma proteins, such as albumin, transferrin, and the acute-phase proteins like fibrinogen, alpha 1-antitrypsin, transferrin, plasminogen etc. They have been grown successfully in different cultivation systems and well support the replication of HBV and HCV replicon. [14] HepG2 cells especially 2.2.15 line better support replication of HBV and are widely used to evaluate potential active anti-hepatitis B virus compounds.[15,16]

The other cell culture systems used for HBV include HepAD38, HepAD79, YMDD, PDH.

Cell Culture System used for Influenza Viruses

Influenza viruses A and B are not as demanding as HCV and HBV and may be cultivated in many cell culture systems including Madin Darby canine kidney (MDCK), chick embryo, chick kidney, calf kidney, Vero, mink lung, and human respiratory epithelial cells.[17]

Determination of the Toxicity of the Drug

Assessment of the toxicity of the antiviral drug is based on detection of median cytotoxic concentration (CC_{50}). CC_{50} is the concentration of the drug required to reduce the cell number by 50% compared to untreated control. CC_{50} could be identified using a number of cell viability tests (Fig. 25.1).

There are a number of tests available to assess the cytotoxicity of the investigational compound. The cell viability tests are based on various cell functions such as enzyme activity, cell membrane permeability, ATP production, nucleotide uptake activity, etc. Among the other tests enzyme-based calorimetric tetrazolium salts tests are the most commonly used because of their reproducibility, safety and easy methodology.

MTT assay

The reduction of tetrazolium dyes such as 3-[4,5-dimethylthiazol-2-yl]-2,5-diphenyltetrazolium bromide (MTT) by NAD(P)H-dependent oxidoreductase leads to appearance of formazan

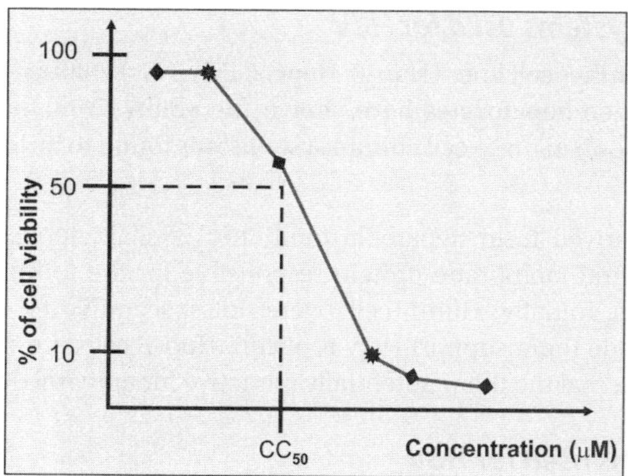

Figure 25.1: Determination of CC_{50}

products that have intense blue or purple color.[18] Oxidoreductase is largely present in the mitochondria and cytoplasm of actively metabolizing cells. Therefore, non-viable or dead cells have low level of oxidoreductase and lose the ability to convert MTT into formazan and hence the color formation. The colored formazan crystals are water insoluble and have to be dissolved in DMSO or any other solubilizer. The absorbance of the dye is measured spectrophotometrically at a certain wavelength (usually 570 nm) using an automated microplate reader. The absorbance corresponding to that of untreated control cells is assumed as 100% cell viability.

The percentage of viable cells in the treated group can be calculated as follows:

$$\% \text{ Cell viability} = \frac{\text{Absorbance of treated cell}}{\text{Absorbance of untreated cells}} \times 100$$

MTS, XTT and WST Assays

More recently developed MTS (3-(4,5-dimethylthiazol-2-yl)-5-(3-carboxymethoxyphenyl)-2-(4-sulfophenyl)-2H-tetrazolium), XTT (2,3-bis-(2-methoxy-4-nitro-5-sulfophenyl)-2H-tetrazolium-5-carboxanilide) and WST (water soluble tetrazolium salts) assays contain tetrazolium reagents that undergoes reduction by viable cells to water soluble formazan products. This improves the assay procedure because a second addition of solubilizing reagent is not required. Measurement of absorbance is usually done at 490 nm.

Determination of Antiviral Activity of the Drug

Antiviral activity of the drug is expressed by the median effective concentration (EC_{50}) which is the concentration of the drug required to inhibit virus replication by 50 percent (Fig. 25.2).

The antiviral activity can be tested by a number of methods, including reduction assays, cytopathic effect inhibition assays, binding and fusion assays, etc.

Some of the most commonly used antiviral assays are based on virus-induced cytopathic effects (CPE), plaque formation or hemagglutination. These methods have disadvantages of

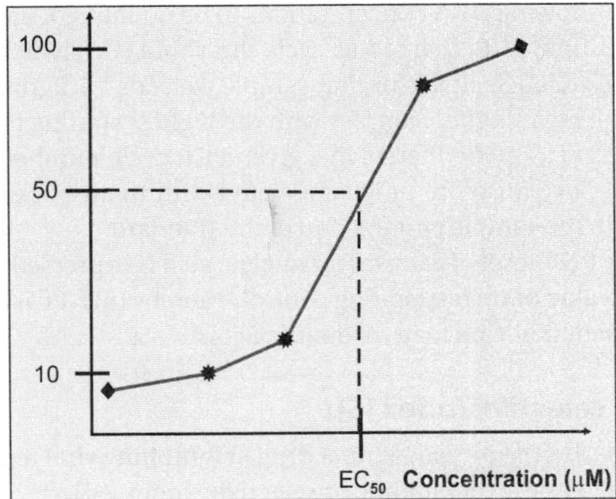

Figure 25.2: Determination of EC_{50}

being time-consuming and labor-intensive, which limit their use for screening. Further more, these methods are less acceptable because different virus strains may differ in their ability to cause cytopathic effects or hemagglutination.

In contrast to cytopathic effect based viral assay, test of polymerase chain reaction (PCR) or quantitative real-time PCR (qRT-PCR) are characterized by much greater sensitivity, specificity and reproducibility. They are currently used for detection of viral DNA or RNA (PCR) and measurement of viral load (qRT-PCR).

PCR

Principle of PCR is based on amplification of a single copy or a few copies of a particular DNA sequence across several cycles and finally generating thousands to millions of copies of primal DNA sequence. Heat-stable DNA polymerase, such as Taq polymerase, is used as an amplifier assembling new DNA strands from single-stranded DNA sample (DNA target). DNA oligonucleotides (DNA primers) that are complementary to the particular DNA template are used for the initiation of DNA synthesis. PCR consists of a series of repeated temperature cycles. Each of them usually includes few steps with different temperature set up as required for initiation and synthesis of new DNA copies. The number, level and time of the temperature steps depend on a wide range of parameters, such as: the type of DNA-polymerase, the concentration of ions, desoxyribonucleotides, etc.

PCR is sensitive, specific and reproducible method however it does not allow quantitation of DNA or RNA and detection of viral load that is essential for determining the efficacy of antiviral drug.

Quantitative Real-Time PCR

qRT-PCR defers from the standard PCR as it allows detection of the amount of DNA or RNA formed after the each cycle with fluorescent dyes or fluorescently-tagged oligonucleotide probes. An increase in DNA/RNA products during PCR, therefore, leads to an increase in fluorescence intensity allowing DNA concentrations to be quantified. Each sample is assigned a specific value in real-time PCR, defined as cycle threshold (Ct), which is the point or cycle number when the fluorescence curve for that sample exceeds background fluorescence and measurements become meaningful. Samples with the highest starting target amount will also have the highest values of amplified target in a given PCR cycle number. The values obtained from qRT-PCR do not have absolute units associated with them but express the amount of measured DNA/RNA in the sample as a fraction of the standard.

The relative DNA or RNA level of each target nucleic acid is expressed as change by number of folds relative to the value of corresponding control. Thereby qRT-PCR allows quantitation of nucleic acids and detection of viral load to identify EC_{50}.

Determination of selective index (SI)

The relative effectiveness of the investigational drug in inhibiting viral replication compared to its cytotoxicity is defined as the therapeutic or selectivity index (SI)

$$SI = \frac{CC_{50}}{EC_{50}}$$

SI allows selecting the compound with highest antiviral activity and minimal cell toxicity.

IN VIVO MODELS

In vivo studies are essential part for antiviral drug discovery. A number of parameters may be used to determine the effectiveness of antiviral drug in animal models. The choice of these parameters depends on the type of viral infection and the animal model used. However, the most commonly used parameters include viral infection associated death, mean time to death, change in water and food intake, change in weight, hyper or hypothermia, blood cell count, coagulation parameters, biochemical parameters, viral titer and histopathological changes in relevant organs and tissues etc.

Unfortunately *in vivo* models available for antiviral drug development studies are very limited (Table 25.1). This can be explained by few reasons: (i) some viruses cannot replicate in nonhuman species or require adaptation by multiple passage through the animal model, (ii) most of the human viruses cannot produce typical clinical picture in nonhuman species, (iii) high cost and ethical issues associated with particular animal models.

All animal models used in the *in vivo* studies could be divided in 3 groups:

1. Chimpanzee and other great apes
2. Nonhuman primates
3. Other animal models.

Chimpanzees (*Pan troglodytes*)

Chimpanzees are the closest living relative to humans sharing more than 98% genetic identity.[19] This explains the greater suitability of chimpanzees compared to all other great apes as an animal model for vaccine development and antiviral drug discovery. Chimpanzees are

Table 25.1: Common animal models for various viral infections

Type of virus	*Animal model*
Cytomegalovirus	Primates, transgenic immunocompromised mice
Dengue virus	Nonhuman primates, transgenic immunocompromised and humanized mice
Ebola and Marburg viruses	Nonhuman primates (rhesus and cynomolgus macaques), mice, guinea pigs, syrian golden hamsters
Hepatitis B and C	Primates, tree shrews, transgenic and humanized mice
HSV	Mice, rabbits
Influenza viruses	Ferrets, guinea pigs, transgenic mice
Japanese encephalitis virus	Syrian golden hamsters
SARS corona virus	Syrian golden hamster, mice
West Nile virus	Syrian golden hamsters

naturally susceptible to most of the human viral photogenes and have the same pathogenic mechanisms, similar clinical symptoms and course of illness as humans. In addition large size of animals provides enough volume of biological materials and facilitates appropriate investigations. Chimpanzees are used as models to study pathogenesis, vaccination and pharmacokinetics and pharmacodynamics of new candidates for the treatment for some viral infections such as norovirus,[20] hepatitis B[21-23] and hepatitis C.[24,25]

However, the use of chimpanzees as an animal model is very limited mostly because of ethical considerations, low availability, and extremely high cost.

Other Nonhuman Primate Models

The genetic proximity of nonhuman primates (NHP) to humans makes them a very attractive animal model for antiviral drug discovery. NHP such as *Cynomolgus macaques, Rhesus macaques, Green monkeys, Chacma Baboons, Cottontop tamarins* and marmosets are more commonly used models for the development of antiviral drugs and vaccines compered to chimpanzees. For example, different macaque species are used as a model for West Nile virus fever, Japanese encephalitis viral infection, avian influenza (H5N1), cytomegalovirus (CMV) infection, dengue, ebola, marburg and some other virus infections.[26-28]

However, the high cost and ethical issues still limit the use of nonhuman primate as an *in vivo* model for antiviral drug development.

Tree Shrews (*Tupaia Belangeri*)

The tree shrews are squirrel-like mammals belonging to Primate order and sharing with them some similarities in anatomy (including the brain anatomy) and phylogenesis. Apparently due to their proximity to primates, they are one of the main animal models used for the studies of various aspects of hepatitis B and C infection including the investigations for efficacy of new antiviral drugs.[15] Many studies have demonstrated that both HBV and HCV enter and replicate in tree shrew primary hepatocytes and infected animals develop hepatitis.[29-32] Closeness to primates, small size and uncommonness make tree shrews currently a very useful model for HBV and HCV research.

Other Animal Models

Mice

Mice and other rodents have traditionally been used as a lab model because of many advantages such as low cost, ease of maintenance and care, small size, which significantly reduces the amount of drugs and other chemicals needed for experiments. Another important advantage of these models is the availability of the large range of reagents, quantification assays, microarray proteome expression and luminex technology-based quantification assays, etc. required for evaluation of disease progression, immune response, histopathological changes and viral titer.

Mice are the most widely used animal model for influenza virus and HSV studies.[33-35] However, most of wild-type of human viruses do not replicate and transmit efficiently and/or do not produce typical clinical signs of viral infections in normal immunocompetent murine lines, requiring to be adopted by the serial passage in suckling, aged or immunocompromised mice to show clinical features and high levels of viral titer.[36] Hence, models currently used for antiviral drug screening studies are mainly transgenic and humanized mice.

Transgenic Mice

Transgenic mice are genetically modified mice with altered genome. Currently, several thousand strains of transgenic mice are available. Usually they are named for the gene which has been disrupted. The genetic engineering technology allows creating the strains of mice with different properties and increases their sensitivity to human viruses.

Knockout mice are lines of genetically modified mice where the activity of a single gene is removed or disrupted. Currently, a large range of knockout mice strains is available for research including pathology, immunology of viral infections and antiviral drug development.

Knockout AG129 mice lacks interferon α, β and γ receptor genes and is more susceptible to virus compared to wild-type mice.[37] This model has been proven useful as a model for dengue virus infection and *in vivo* testing of some antiviral compounds.[38] IKK epsilon mutant mice have loss of the endogenous kinase function in lung, spleen, and embryonic fibroblasts. These mice have increased susceptibility to viral infection due to defective interferon (IFN) signaling and are used as *in vivo* models for influenza virus infection.

UPA mice carry the mouse urokinase-type plasminogen activator (uPA) gene. The overexpression of the uPA gene in the liver results in extensive liver toxicity leading to chronic hepatic insufficiency. It also causes high plasma uPA levels and hypofibrinogenemia, which could result in severe bleeding.

Genetically Humanized Mice

Genetically humanized mice are the mice that express human host factors and usually have inactivation of the production of murine proteins in parallel.

MUP-uPA/SCID/Bg transgenic mice is constructed by the backcross of two murine lines: Severe combined immunodeficiency mice subclone (SCID/Bg) and MUP-uPA. This line expresses the secreted form of human uPA and is used as a model for HCV infection.

Xenotransplantation Mice

Transplantation of human cells or tissues to mice may be very helpful in terms of increasing replication of particular viruses and production of clinical signs of the infection. Immunodeficient mice such as SCID and their subclones are usually used to produce xenotransplantation mice. SCID mice have genetically impaired both the humoral and cellular immunity and thus are able to sustain xenografts.

Human liver-uPA/SCID mice are produced by the cross breeding of uPA and SCID mice followed by intrasplenical injection of human hepatocytes. Transplantation of donor cells should be done within the 2nd week of life. Intrasplenically injected donor cells rapidly migrate through the portal venous system into the liver and support higher level of HCV replication compared to murine hepatocytes.[39]

Hu-PBL-SCID mice are constructed by the injection of peripheral blood lymphocytes to SCID mice and are currently widely used for studies of HIV pathogenesis and anti-HIV drugs. They were first used as a dengue model in 1995.[40]

Rats

Rats are not commonly used as *in vivo* models for antiviral drug research however, some of them such as cotton rats are used for the study of influenza A viruses.[41,42]

Guinea pigs (Cavia Porcellus)

Guinea pigs are very commonly used as an alternative model to mice in viral research. Guinea pigs are susceptible to several viruses and are used as animal models for human viral hemorrhagic fevers, human influenza viruses, HSV, filovirus infection (Ebola and Marburg virus infections) and others. [26,43,44] However, limitations are there due to lack of available reagents and specific assays (ELISA, Western Blot, PCR, qRT-PCR, etc.) to monitor host responses, including immune responses, pathological changes and viral load.

Syrian Golden Hamster (Mesocricetus Auratus)

Syrian golden hamster is widely used as animal model for human infectious diseases caused by bunyaviruses (Crimean-Congo hemorrhagic fever virus), flaviviruses (West Nile virus, dengue virus, Japanese encephalitis virus, yellow fever virus), henipaviruses, and SARS-coronavirus.[45,46] The main drawback of this model is the same as for guinea pig model, i.e. lack of reagents and specific assays.

Ferrets (Mustela Putorius Furo)

The ferrets are attractive and well-established animal model for numerous viruses, such as coronavirus, nipah virus, morbillivirus, influenza viruses and others.[47] Ferrets and humans share similar lung physiology, and human and avian influenza viruses exhibit similar mode of interactions with cellular receptors present in respiratory tract.[47] Moreover, ferrets are very suitable for antiviral drug research because of their relatively small size and ability to exhibit many of the typical clinical signs associated with human disease, especially with regard to influenza virus such as nasal discharge, loss of appetite, congested eyes, otologic manifestations and fever.[48]

CONCLUSION

In conclusion, at the present time, the amount of research for the screening and investigation of new antiviral drugs is increasing due to multiple reasons. Recent advances in the techniques of cultivation and detection of viruses on one hand has contributed to identification of new pathogens and pathogen characteristics while on the other hand there is increasing need for antiviral drugs because of significant outbreaks of well-known viral infections as well as emergence of new viral infections. However, the discovery of new effective antiviral drugs faces enormous limitations due to lack of available *in vitro* and *in vivo* models.

REFERENCES

1. Saxena SK, Saxena S, Saxena R, Swamy MLA, Gupta A, Nair MPN. Emerging trends, challenges and prospects in antiviral therapeutics and drug development for infectious diseases. Electronic J Biol 2010;6(2):26-31.
2. De Clercq E. Recent highlights in the development of new antiviral drugs. Curr Opin Microbiol 2005;8:552-60.
3. Lohmann V, Bartenschlager R. On the history of hepatitis C virus cell culture systems. J Med Chem 2014;57:1627-42.
4. Horscroft N, Lai VCH, Cheney W, Yao N, Wu JZ, Hong Z. Replicon cell culture system as a valuable tool in antiviral drug discovery against hepatitis C virus. Antivir Chem Chemother 2005; 16:1-12.
5. Lohmann V, Korner F, Koch J, Herian U, Theilmann L, Bartenschlager R. Replication of subgenomic hepatitis C virus RNAs in a hepatoma cell line. Science 1999;285:110-3.
6. Desmyter J, Melnick JL, Rawls WE. Defectiveness of interferon production and of rubella virus interference in a line of African green monkey kidney cells (Vero). J Virol 1968;2(10):955-61.
7. Emeny JM, Morgan MJ. Regulation of the interferon system: evidence that Vero cells have a genetic defect in interferon production. J Gen Virol I979;43:247-52.
8. Bente DA, Rico-Hesse R. Models of dengue virus infection. Drug Discov Today Dis Models 2006; 3(1):97-103.
9. Govorkova EA, Murti G, Meignier B, de Taisne C, Webster RG. African green monkey kidney (Vero) cells provide an alternative host cell system for influenza A and B viruses. J Virol 1996; 70(8):5519-24.
10. Ammerman NC, Beier-Sexton M, Azad AF. Growth and maintenance of Vero cell lines. Curr Protoc Microbiol 2008; Ap.4Edoi:10.1002/9780471729259.mca04es11.
11. Nahapetian AT, Thomas JN, Thilly WG. Optimization of environment for high density Vero cell culture: effect of dissolved oxygen and nutrient supply on cell growth and changes in metabolites. J Cell Sci 1986;81:65-103.
12. Duverlie G, Wychowski C. Cell culture systems for the hepatitis C virus. World J Gastroenterol 2007;13(17):2442-5.
13. Windisch MP, Frese M, Kaul A, Trippler M, Lohmann V, Bartenschlager R. Dissecting the interferon-induced inhibition of hepatitis C virus replication by using a novel host cell line. J Virol 2005; 79(21):13778-93.
14. Mabit H, Dubanchet S, Capel F, Dauguet C, Petit MA. In vitro infection of human hepatoma cells (HepG2) with hepatitis B virus (HBV): spontaneous selection of a stable HBV surface antigen-producing HepG2 cell line containing integrated HBV DNA sequences. J Gen Virol 1994:75:2681-9.

15. Schinazi RF, Ilan E, Black PL, Yao X, Dagan S. Cell-based and animal models for hepatitis B and C viruses. Antivir Chem Chemother 1999;10:99-114.
16. Yang L, Shi L, Chen H, Tong X, Wang G, Zhang Y, et al. Isothiafludine, a novel non-nucleoside compound, inhibits hepatitis B virus replication through blocking pregenomic RNA encapsidation. Acta Pharmacol Sin 2014;35:410-8.
17. Sidwell RW, Smee DF. In vitro and in vivo assay systems for study of influenza virus inhibitors. Antiviral Res 2000;48(1):1-16.
18. Berridge MV, Herst PM, Tan AS. Tetrazolium dyes as tools in cell biology: new insights into their cellular reduction. Biotechnol Annu Rev 2005;11:127-52.
19. Watanabe H, Fujiyama A, Hattori M, Taylor TD, Toyoda A, Kuroki Y, et al. DNA sequence and comparative analysis of chimpanzee chromosome 22. Nature 2004;429:382-8.
20. Bok K, Parra GI, Mitra T, Abente E, Shaverb CK, Boon D, et al. Chimpanzees as an animal model for human norovirus infection and vaccine development. Proc Natl Acad Sci USA 2011;108(1):325-30.
21. Carroll SS, Ludmerer S, Handt L, Koeplinger K, Zhang NR, Graham D, et al. Robust antiviral efficacy upon administration of a nucleoside analog to hepatitis C virus-infected chimpanzees. Antimicrob Agents Chemother 2009;53(3):926-34.
22. Gagneux P, Muchmore EA. The chimpanzee model: contributions and considerations for studies of hepatitis B virus. Methods Mol Med 2004;96:289-318.
23. Prince AM, Brotman B. Perspectives on hepatitis B studies with chimpanzees. ILAR J 2001; 42(2):85-8.
24. Bukh J. A critical role for the chimpanzee model in the study of hepatitis C. Hepatology 2004; 39:1469-75.
25. Lanford RE, Bigger C, Bassett S, Klim Pel G. The chimpanzee model of hepatitis C virus infections. ILAR J 2001;42 (2):117-26.
26. Nakayama E, Saijo M. Animal models for Ebola and Marburg virus infections. Front Microbiol 2013;4:267.
27. Rimmelzwaan GF, Kuiken T, van Amerongen G, Bestebroer TM, Fouchier RA, Osterhaus AD. A primate model to study the pathogenesis of influenza A (H5N1) virus infection. Avian Dis 2003;47:931-3.
28. Zompi S, Harris E. Animal models of dengue virus infection. Viruses 2012;4(1):62-82.
29. Amako Y, Tsukiyama-Kohara K, Katsume A, Hirata Y, Sekiguchi S, Tobita Y, et al. Pathogenesis of hepatitis C virus infection in Tupaia belangeri. J Virol 2010;84:303-11.
30. Ruan P, Yang C, Su J, Cao J, Ou C, Luo C, et al. Histopathological changes in the liver of tree shrew (Tupaia belangeri chinensis) persistently infected with hepatitis B virus. Virol J 2013;10:333.
31. Wang Qi, Schwarzenberger P, Yang F, Zhang J, Su J, Yang C, et al. Experimental chronic hepatitis B infection of neonatal tree shrews (Tupaia belangeri chinensis): a model to study molecular causes for susceptibility and disease progression to chronic hepatitis in humans. Virol J 2012;9:170.
32. Bouvier NM, Lowen AC. Animal models for influenza virus pathogenesis and transmission. Viruses 2010;2(8):1530-63.
33. Webre RJM, Hill JM, Nolan NM, Clement C, McFerrin HE, Bhattacharjee PS, et al. Rabbit and mouse models of HSV-1 latency, reactivation, and recurrent eye diseases. J Biomed Biotech 2012;2012:1-18.
34. Zhao X, Tang ZY, Klumpp B, Wolff-Vorbeck G, Barth H, Levy S, et al. Primary hepatocytes of Tupaia belangeri as a potential model for hepatitis C virus infection. J Clin Invest 2002;109:221-32.

35. Crute JJ, Grygon CA, Hargrave KD, Simoneau B, Faucher A, Bolger G, et al. Herpes simplex virus helicase-primase inhibitors are active in animal models of human disease. Nature Medicine 2002;8(4):386-91.
36. Bray M. The role of the Type I interferon response in the resistance of mice to filovirus infection. J Gen Virol 2001;82(Pt 6):1365-73.
37. Johnson AJ, Roehrig JT. New mouse model for dengue virus vaccine testing. J Virol 1999;73(1):783-6.
38. Schul W, Liu W, Xu HY, Flamand M, Vasudevan SG. A dengue fever viremia model in mice shows reduction in viral replication and suppression of the inflammatory response after treatment with antiviral drugs. J Infect Dis 2007;195(5):665-74.
39. Meuleman P, Leroux-Roels G. The human liver-uPA-SCID mouse: a model for the evaluation of antiviral compounds against HBV and HCV. Antiviral Res 2008;80:231-8.
40. Wu SJ, Hayes CG, Dubois DR, Windheuser MG, Kang YH, Watts DM, et al. Evaluation of the severe combined immunodeficient (SCID) mouse as an animal model for dengue viral infection. Am J Trop Med Hyg 1995;52:468-76.
41. Boukhvalova MS, Prince GA, Blanco JC. The cotton rat model of respiratory viral infections pathogenesis and immunity. Biologicals 2009;37(3):152-9.
42. Eichelberger MC. The cotton rat as a model to study influenza pathogenesis and immunity. Viral Immunol 2007;20(2):243-9.
43. Lowen AC, Mubareka S, Tumpey TM, García-Sastre A, Palese P. The guinea pig as a transmission model for human influenza viruses. Proc Natl Acad Sci USA 2006;103(26):9988–92.
44. Van Hoeven N, Belser JA, Szretter KJ, Zeng H, Staeheli P, Swayne DE, et al. Pathogenesis of 1918 pandemic and H5N1 influenza virus infections in a guinea pig model: antiviral potential of exogenous alpha interferon to reduce virus shedding. J Virol 2009;83:2851–61.
45. Zivcec M, Safronetz D, Haddock E, Feldmann H, Ebihara H. Validation of assays to monitor immune responses in the Syrian golden hamster (Mesocricetus auratus). J Immunol Methods 2011;368 (1-2):24-35.
46. Xiao S, Guzman H, Zhang H, Travassos da Rosa APA, Tesh RB. West Nile virus infection in the golden hamster (Mesocricetus auratus): a model for West Nile encephalitis. Emerg Infect Dis 2001; 7(4):714-21.
47. Belser JA, Katz JM, Tumpey TM. The ferret as a model organism to study influenza A virus infection. Dis Model Mech 2011;4:575-79.
48. Sidwell RW, Smee DF. In vitro and in vivo assay systems for study of influenza virus inhibitors. Antiviral Res 2000;48(1):1-16.

CHAPTER

26

Antipsychotic Agents

INTRODUCTION

The word psychosis was first used by Ernst von Feuchtersleben in 1845 and stems from the Greek words psyche (mind) and -osis (diseased or abnormal condition). According to Adolf Meyer (1866–1950), psychosis or schizophrenia is not a discrete disorder with a specific etiology but, rather, as a reaction to a wide variety of biopsychosocial factors. Factors such as gene mutations, brain injury, drug use (cocaine, amphetamine, marijuana, phencyclidine, and steroids), prenatal infection and malnutrition, social isolation and marginalization, have been implicated in the manifestation of the signs and symptoms of schizophrenia. The standardized mortality rate in schizophrenia is about 2.5, with life expectancy between 15 and 20 years. Mortality due to CVD is major contributor and causal factors such as lifestyle, poor diet, lack of physical activity, smoking, and substance abuse, have been identified.[1] The etiopathology of psychosis is complex and genetic basis has been understood to play a definitive role in its genesis with as much as 40-50% risk of developing schizophrenia in population of identical twins. Consequently, pharmacogenetics plays pivotal role in management of schizophrenia, and is known to affect dosage, treatment response, and occurrence of adverse effects.[2]

Overactivity of dopamine neurotransmission and supersensitivity to dopamine has been understood to be the biochemical basis of schizophrenia and the condition is successfully alleviated by drugs that block dopamine D2 receptors.[3] Currently, a number of effective palliative antipsychotic agents including tricyclics, phenothiazenes, thioxanthenes, dibenzepines, butyrophenones and other congeners are available. Besides the lacunae such as delayed onset of action (2 to 3 weeks after initiation of therapy), severe extrapyramidal neurological effects, sedation, hypotension and autonomic side effects, the pharmacological agents used for treating psychotic disorders also have side effects that augment CVD risk.[1] This is owing to their wide array of action which includes not only blockade of D_2 dopamine receptors in forebrain but also D_1 dopaminergic, 5-HT_2 serotonergic and α-adrenergic receptors.

In the past, number of novel antipsychotic drugs were developed with the aim of obtaining agents displaying therapeutic advantages over the first drug generation, often designated “typical” antipsychotic drugs. These include a lower propensity to elicit extrapyramidal side-effects, an improved therapeutic efficacy on negative and affective symptomatology of schizophrenia as well as on refractory forms of the disease. These drugs are designated as "atypical" antipsychotics". Most of the drugs in this new class have been modeled after the prototype drug clozapine. Although, atypical antipsychotic agents possess numerous advantages, they are not devoid of side-effects, creating a need to develop newer agents.

Understanding of underlying neurobiology, neurotransmission anomalies and genetic basis of schizophrenia has made it possible to design and develop animal models which simulate the biological phenomena better. The available models can be divided into three sets, namely, animal models with predictive validity, face validity and construct validity.[1] Most of the currently available models are valid only to make predictions with respect to pharmacotherapy and show pharmacologic isomorphism. These models provide least insight into the processes underlying the disease.[4]

Animal models with face validity are based on symptom similarity and exhibit behavioral isomorphism like catatonia, stereotypy, impaired performance and social withdrawal.[5] These models are few in number and difficult to design, interpret and replicate. Models that mimic the psychopathologic disturbances underlying the disease are classified as animal models with construct validity.[6] Genetic models of schizophrenia fall in this category.

IN VITRO AND *EX VIVO* MODELS

^{3}H-Prazosin Competition Binding for α-1 Adrenoceptors

Direct interaction between a compound and α-1 adrenergic receptor is determined by measuring the inhibition of binding of a radioactive ligand (^{3}H-prazosin) to the receptor. Rats (Male Wistar, 200 to 250 g) are housed in a controlled environment with a 12 h day-night cycle and free access to food and water. The animals are sacrificed; their brains quickly removed, cerebral cortex is taken out and frozen. The tissues are stored at –70°C.

The membrane preparation of rat frontal cortex is prepared and the protein content is measured according to the method of Lowry, et al.[7] Briefly, the tissue is homogenized in 20 volumes of 50 mM Tris-HCl buffer, pH 7.6. The supernatant after centrifugation of the homogenate (1,000 g, 10 min) is recentrifuged at 25,000 g for 30 min and the resulting pellet is stored at –20°C until incubation. Immediately before the assay, the pellet is reconstituted in 50 mM Tris-HCl buffer, pH 7.6 to obtain the final concentration of protein of approximately 1.5 mg/ml. The final incubation mixture contains 450 µl of membrane suspension, 50 µl of the solution of the radioligand and 50 µl of the Tris-HCl buffer or of solution of displacer. Nine concentrations of the test drug are incubated in the presence of one concentration (0.146 nM) of ^{3}H-prazosin. The reference standards used are phentolamine or prazosin. The incubation is carried out at 25°C for 30 min and is terminated by vacuum-assisted filtration through Whatman filters. Filters are washed with ice-cold Tris-HCl buffer and placed in scintillation cocktail. The radioactivity is measured in a liquid scintillation counter and the binding is corrected for the protein content.

Ki [nM] value is calculated from the formula $Ki=IC50/(1+L/KD)$, where L is the concentration of the radioligand and KD is its dissociation constant. Ki value for each compound studied is the mean ± SEM from at least three independent competition-binding studies.

Although, this test is used mostly for *in vitro* studies, it can also be applied for *ex vivo* experiments to determine the effects of a single dose of acutely (or chronically) given test compound on the *in vitro* interaction of reference compound with α-1 adrenergic receptors.

The above-mentioned procedure can be adopted to study the competitive binding between other receptors and their ligands (Table 26.1).

Table 26.1: Radioligand competitive binding with the receptor sub-type

Receptor sub-type	*Radioligand*	*Reference standard*
α-2 adrenoceptors	^{3}H-Clonidine	Clonidine
α-1 adrenoceptors	^{3}H-Prazosin	Phentolamine or Prazosin
β-adrenoceptors	^{3}H-CGP 12177	Propranolol
Benzodiazepine	^{3}H-Flunitrazepam	Clonazepam or Diazepam
D_1 dopamine	^{3}H-SCH 23390	SCH23390
5HT-1A	^{3}H-8-OH-DPAT	8-OH-DPAT
5HT-2	^{3}H-Ketanserin	Ketanserin
μ opioid	^{3}H-Dihydromorphine	Morphine
Ionophore of the NMDA-ionotropic glutamate receptor	^{3}H-MK-801	Phencyclidine
NMDA ionotropic glutamate receptors	^{3}H-CGP39653	L-glutamate
Glycine sites of the NMDA ionotropic glutamate receptors	^{3}H-5,7dichlorokynurenic acid (DCKA)	DCKA
GABA	^{3}H-Muscimol	Muscimol

IN VIVO MODELS

Open Field Test

Automatic recording open field working station is now widely used to record locomotor activities and stereotypic behaviors of the animals. The test field (43 × 43 × 30 cm) is divided into 16 identical squares with a grid of infrared photocells around the arena and illuminated with a dim light (20 lux). On the test day, the animals are individually released into the center of the box and allowed to explore the field freely for 60 min. The general locomotor activities and stereotypic behaviors is recorded by light beam interruptions and data are collected over 30 min by automatic computerized system. Various useful parameters like- ambulatory distance, ambulatory time, resting time, time spent in central area/peripheral area, time spent in stereotypic behaviors (small movements such as scratching, grooming, or digging that repeatedly interrupt only a single optical beam), can be recorded and compared between different groups.[8]

Prepulse Inhibition

Acoustic startle and prepulse response is measured using a startle chamber (ventilate plexiglas cylinder on a plexiglas platform). The mice are subjected to different trial types

i. PULSE ALONE—broadband 120 decibel burst for 40-ms duration
ii. PREPULSE+PULSE—either long 3 decibel for 20 ms duration or long 6 decibel for 120 ms duration or 12 decibel for 20 ms duration prepulse stimuli are given above a 65 decibel background and
iii. NO STIMULUS trial, in which only the background noise is presented.

The animal is allowed to acclimatize in trials presented in a pseudo-random order. Whole-body startle responses of the animal is recorded for each stimulus.[9]

Sucrose Preference Test

Sucrose preference is assessed using a home cage two-bottle choice test. Animals are singly housed with *ad libitum* access to standard chow and two identical water bottles. One bottle is filled with water, while the other bottle contained sucrose solution (up to 15%). The habituation phase (0% sucrose, water only) spans over six days and over next four days sucrose solution is provided. The positions of the bottles are rotated to avoid position preferences. Preference can be calculated as a ratio of the amount consumed from the sucrose bottle to the total liquid volume consumed from both bottles.[10]

Catalepsy in Rodents

Catalepsy in rats is defined as a failure to correct an externally imposed, unusual posture over a prolonged period of time. This is a typical effect of all agents, which inhibit dopaminergic system in the nigrostriatum.

Adult Wistar rats of either sex, weighing between 180 to 220 g each are randomly divided into two groups. One group is dosed with test drug and the other with standard drug (haloperidol 0.5 mg/kg, ip). Catalepsy is evaluated according to the slightly modified method of Delini-Stula and Morpurgo.[11] After an appropriate pretreatment time of the drug, each rat is tested with respect to its right and left front paws, which are first put on columns 3 cm and then 9 cm high. The cataleptic state is scored as 1 and 2, respectively (maximum 6 points for the right and left paws) if a rat maintains an abnormal body posture for more than 10 sec. Catalepsy is scored for 2 or 3 h at 30 min intervals. Three trials are conducted for each animal.

This model tests for the potential of antipsychotic drugs to cause extrapyramidal symptoms in man. Neuroleptics that cause extrapyramidal symptoms in man produce a cataleptic state in rats characterized by immobility, body stiffness and inability to initiate movement.

An increase in catalepsy score predicts that the drug may cause extrapyramidal side effects in humans. If the drug is able to decrease neuroleptic-induced catalepsy, it may have potential antiparkinsonian activity. L-DOPA (+benserazide) or amantadine is used as a reference compound.

Inhibition of Amphetamine-induced Stereotypy in Rats

Amphetamine is an indirect sympathomimetic agent. It induces a characteristic stereotypic behavior (lip smacking, grooming, catalepsy, gnawing) in rats, which can be successfully prevented by classical neuroleptic agents. The test is predictive for antipsychotic drugs with D2-receptor antagonism.

Two groups (n = 6) of adult Wistar rats of either sex, weighing between 180 to 220 g are treated with either test or standard drug and then placed in individual wire cages (21 cm × 21 cm × 23 cm). They are injected with d-amphetamine (5 mg/kg, ip) after 30 min. The onset of stereotypic behavior, its duration and intensity is evaluated at 30 min intervals for 3 hours. An animal is protected if the behavior is reduced or abolished. The intensity of stereotype activity is assessed on an arbitrary rating scale from 0-4 for normal, periodic sniffing, continuous sniffing, licking, gnawing and biting behaviors, respectively. A reduction in mean stereotypy score is indicative for antipsychotic effect.

Inhibition of Apomorphine-induced Stereotypy in Rats

Apomorphine stimulates dopamine autoreceptors and induces stereotypic behavior in rodents like pole climbing, licking, sniffing, gnawing and yawning.[12] Apomorphine-induced climbing behavior can be inhibited by antipsychotic drugs and is predictive for the development of extrapyramidal side effects and tardive dyskinesia. This is a standard test used for the screening of antipsychotic drugs and has good predictive validity for classical as well as atypical neuroleptics.

The mice are placed in individual cylindrical cages (12 cm in diameter, 14 cm in width) with walls made of vertical metal bars (2 mm in diameter, 1 cm apart). After an adaptation period of 30 min, the mice are treated with either test or standard drug (clozapine 10 mg/kg, ip), and, 1 hour later apomorphine (0.75 mg/kg, sc). Immediately afterwards, the behavior is assessed for climbing behavior namely all the paws on the floor, forefeet or all the paws held on the wall, which is rated on an arbitrary scale of 0-2, respectively.

Apomorphine increases the behavioral score by causing climbing behavior in the mice. Antipsychotic drugs can inhibit this behavior.

Phencyclidine-induced Bizarre Pattern of Locomotor Activity and Stereotypy

Phencyclidine (PCP) is a psychotomimetic compound that can induce a schizophrenia-like psychosis in man. In rats, PCP produces locomotor hyperactivity and stereotyped behavior that can be inhibited by antipsychotic drugs.

Male Wistar rats weighing between 200 to 250 g are housed in a controlled environment with a temperature of 22 ± 2°C and a 12 h light/dark cycle. The animals have free access to food and water. Locomotor and stereotypy-like activities of rats are recorded individually for each animal in an activity-monitor. Each cage is equipped with infrared emitters, located on the X and Y-axes, and with an equivalent amount of receivers on the opposite walls of the cage. The locomotor activity is defined as a trespass of three consecutive photo-beams, while other movements observed as repeated interruption of the same photo-beam are regarded as stereotypy-like movements. The PCP-induced locomotor and stereotypy-like activities of rats are measured during a session lasting 150 min. The test may be indicative of possible antipsychotic activity of tested drug.

Phencyclidine-induced Social Withdrawal Measured in the Social Interaction Test

This test helps to show the effectiveness of potential antipsychotic drugs against negative symptoms of schizophrenia. Phencyclidine (PCP) induces stereotyped behavior, hyperactivity and social withdrawal, in rats. All of these behaviors can be evaluated in the social interaction test. The test appears to be specific for antipsychotic drugs and can distinguish between effects on the positive and negative symptoms.[13]

Male Wistar rats of 250 to 280 g are housed in a controlled environment with a temperature of 22 ± 2°C and a 12 h light/dark cycle with free access to food and water. In the PCP-induced social withdrawal test, naive rats are housed in pairs for 10 days prior to the start of the test. During the test one cagemate (familiar rat) is removed and new one—intruder is placed in the cage for 10 min. The amount of the social interaction and locomotor activity both for the resident and intruder is recorded for 10 min. Social interaction is measured as the total amount of time spent on various elements of the interaction, i.e. sniffing, grooming of partner, genital investigation and following the partner. Aggressive behavior is not included (i.e. aggressive posture, sideways threat, biting, boxing, etc.).

Apart from the locomotor stimulant effects, PCP, in a dose of 1-2 mg/kg, decreases the time of social interaction. The doses used in this test are slightly lower than doses, which are required to induce clear locomotor stimulant effects.

Conditioned Avoidance Reflex in Rats

In this model, the rodents are conditioned to avoid a noxious stimuli (electric shock) reflexly, by moving from one chamber to another in response to a cue (light cue or sound buzzer). Antipsychotic drugs decrease the number of conditioned avoidance responses (CAR) in response to cue and prolong the total waiting time (TWT).[14] Adult male Wistar rats weighing 250 to 300 g are housed in a controlled environment with the temperature at 22 ± 2°C and a 12 h light/dark cycle and free access to food and water.

Rats are trained to avoid an electric shock in an automatically controlled, two-compartment shuttle box by moving from one compartment to the other during 3 sec of a light conditional stimulus. If no crossings take place, the light is followed by a 3 sec shock (2 mA during the training and 2.5 mA during the experimental session). The shock is provided through the grid floor of the box. The rats are subjected to daily session of 10 trials for 8 consecutive days (with 30 sec intertrial intervals), which lasts for 5 min. Only rats trained for the criterion (a minimum of 8, out of 10 possible) are used in the experiment. The compounds are administered 30 min before the test on day 9. Two parameters CAR and TWT are recorded.

The standard drugs used in this method are haloperidol (0.2 mg/kg, ip) and clozapine (10 mg/kg, ip). CNS depressants may be delineated from antipsychotics in that the former affects both avoidance and escape but the latter at lower doses affects only avoidance with no effect on escape (i.e. the animal ignores the warning and does not attempt to avoid the noxious stimulus, but escapes once stimulus is applied). At higher doses, due to ataxia and hypnosis both avoidance and escape are affected.

Neurodevelopmental Models

From embryology, it is known that minor physical anomalies and dermatoglyphic deviations are caused by intrauterine disturbances of the first and second trimester, respectively. The second trimester is the critical period for the migration of neural cells to the cortex and of dermal cells to the fingertips.[15] This is the basis of the neurodevelopmental hypothesis of schizophrenia and can explain winter peak of birth, obstetric complications, minor physical anomalies, soft neurologic signs, reduced intelligence, dermatoglyphic differences and structural brain abnormalities. Based on the epidemiological and clinical correlation studies, animal models have been designed to test the etiological theories.

Gestational Malnutrition Model

This is a model of prenatal protein deprivation, which may induce permanent developmental brain deficits. Malnutrition affects neurogenesis, cell migration and differentiation causing disrupted neural circuits and neurotransmitter systems. Thus, deficits in cognition, learning behavior are apparent. However, these are nonspecific, inconsistent and variable and therefore of limited validity.[16]

Viral Infection

Prenatal exposure to virus, like influenza, utero borna disease virus (BDV), and lymphocytic choriomeningitis virus (LCMV), has been implicated in the genesis of schizophrenia. It is hypothesized that these viruses act either by inducing pyramidal cell disarray, defective corticogenesis, hippocampus damage or disruption of the integrity of GABAergic neurons and excitatory amino acid systems. Although, these are attractive models as they simulate the etiology at the cellular level, they do not have concrete relevance to schizophrenia.[17]

Obstetrical and Birth Complications

It is difficult to explore the plausibility of obstetrical and birth complications as a cause for genesis of schizophrenia in animals. However, there are a few reports indicating that in rat models of cesarean section and anoxia at birth, there are changes in limbic dopamine function in adult animals.[18,19] As the trauma and risk factors of C-section in humans are far lesser, obstetrical complications have not been conclusively linked with schizophrenia.

Early Stressful Experience

It has been hypothesized that long-lasting stress in early life affects brain development and shapes adult behavioral responses. In "Two Hit" model of schizophrenia, the rodents are subjected to dual insults, namely, aberrant genetic trait and stressful experience (like maternal separation or social isolation).[20] There are concomitant hormonal, neurochemical and behavioral changes obvious in adult life, which respond to antipsychotic therapy.

Genetic Models

Schizophrenia is a hereditary disorder that involves anomaly of many genes. Targeted gene deletions or gene transfer techniques have been used to set-up the animal models of schizophrenia. These models show construct validity. However, the behavior exhibited in these models does not mimic the disease. These models only serve as tools to study molecular mechanisms underlying the pathogenesis of the disease.[21]

G72/G30 transgenic (Tg) mouse model

Bacterial artificial chromosome (BAC) containing over 117,000 bp of genomic region and encompassing the entire G72/G30 gene complex has to be created. The BAC clone is then microinjected into the fertilized ova of embryos from a female B6CBAF1/J mouse. The male Tg founder mouse is mated with female B6CBAF1/J wild-type (WT) mice to keep the line. The Tg and WT mice of both sexes (2-4 months old) are used in behavioral experiments as test and control group, respectively. The blind experimenter subjects all animals to behavioral tests (viz. open field test, prepulse inhibition, Sucrose preference test, Morris water maze, Forced swimming test etc.) in soundproof behavioral room.[22]

Single Unit Recording of A9 and A10 Midbrain Dopaminergic Neurons

Dopamine D3 receptors are richly located in the limbic areas. D3 receptors are believed to be involved in the pathogenesis of schizophrenia. Therefore, antipsychotic agents are targeted at these sites. *In vivo* electrophysiological recording can be utilized to screen for compounds with potential antipsychotic activity. Briefly, the number of spontaneously active midbrain DA neurons are recorded and studied in anesthetized rats. A decrease in the number of spontaneously active ventral tegmental area (VTA) (A10) and substantia nigra compacta (SNC) (A9) DA neurons produced by the repeated administration of compounds may be correlated with their therapeutic and neurological side effects, respectively.[23] Alternatively, extracellular single unit activity is also recorded to assess the clinical antipsychotic efficacy and side effects of DA receptor blockers on A9 and A10 DA neurons.[24]

Male Albino Sprague Dawley rats (200 to 225 g) are anesthetized (chloral hydrate 400 mg/kg, ip) and mounted in a stereotaxic instrument. A hole is drilled over the A9 and A10 according to the atlas[25] and the dura retracted. Single-barrel microelectrodes are used for recording single-cell activity. Glass micropipettes are pulled with an electrode puller and the tip broken back under a light microscope. They are filled with a solution of NaCl (2 M) saturated with fast green dye (1%). The impedance of the electrodes is usually 0.8 to 1.2 mΩ measured at 135 Hz *in vitro* and 1.5 to 2.0 mΩ *in vivo*. A dopaminergic neuron is identified in the A9-A10 area on the basis of the following criterion: (1) action potential (>2.5 msec, having a distinct initial segment and late positive component; (2) a characteristic low-pitch sound, (3) a slow, regular, or bursting firing pattern; and (4) a spontaneous firing rate of 2 to 9 Hz.[26] The number of spontaneously active DA neurons is determined in 10 different electrode tracks separated from each other by 200 μm, whose sequence is constant in each experiment.[27] Each electrode descent is made in a slow (1-3 μm/sec), uniform speed with a hydraulic microdrive. The number of DA cells encountered in these descents are counted. The DA neuronal spikes obtained after the acute and chronic administration of vehicle, haloperidol, or test drug are analyzed and the following parameters are calculated: spikes per burst, percentage of events in bursts, mean interspike interval (interval between successive spikes), coefficient of variation (ratio of standard deviation and mean interspike interval × 100), and percentage of cells exhibiting burst firing (defined as DA neurons that show two or more bursts of at least three spikes of a series of 500 spikes). These values are determined over a period of 500 intervals between successive DA neuron spikes. The onset of a burst is defined by an interval less than 80 msec and the termination of a burst as an interval exceeding 160 msec.

Extrapyramidal Side Effects Primed Monkey Model

The extrapyramidal side effects (EPS) are one of the most common side effects of anti-psychotic therapy and includes perioral tremors, tardive dyskinesia etc. Monkeys have been used to set up a sensitive model that helps to predict the liability of test drug in generating the side-effect of EPS.[28] The monkeys are sensitized to extrapyramidal side effects (EPS) by prior long-term treatment with classical dopamine D2 antagonists and the EPS observed in these monkeys are very similar to EPS induced by antipsychotics in humans.[29] Other potential side effects, e.g. gastrointestinal side effects, can also be investigated.

Six male Cebus monkeys are used for evaluation. The monkeys were housed in separate cages in a temperature-regulated environment at a 12 h light/dark cycle The monkeys receive haloperidol daily for 2 years and are sensitized to dystonia. The drug is given subcutaneously, in increasing doses until two animals developed dystonia. The EPS can be rated on an arbitrary scale ranging from 0 (not present) to 6 (extreme presence). Other behavioral paradigms that are also recorded are arousal, unrest, stereotypy, locomotion, sedation, bradykinesia and dystonia.

In EPS primed monkey, the test drug is administered behavior paradigms are evaluated at time intervals (t = 30, 60, 120 and 180 min). During each experiment, data recording of the animals can be conducted by videotaping.[30]

This is a useful model to predict whether a new drugs will/will not produce EPS at antipsychotic doses.

COMPUTATIONAL MODELS OF DOPAMINE FUNCTION AND PSYCHOSIS

The temporal difference (TD) algorithm is a prediction method that is gaining attention from neuroscientists for behavioral research. It has been used to study schizophrenia and the consequences of pharmacological manipulations of dopamine on schizophrenia. As in any prediction method, TD takes into account the fact that predictions are often correlated and a pattern can be developed from actually observed value. The firing rate of dopaminergic neurons in brain, dopaminergic receptor manipulation, and the manifested behavior are correlated into a formal framework or algorithm. This algorithm is validated with actually observed data and after validation, TD proves useful as it offers predictive insights into clinical set-up.[31] In context of pre-clinical research, TD has been utilized to explain behavioral phenomena such as the dose-dependent disruption of conditioned avoidance response by anti-psychotic drugs, effect of drugs via receptor modulation and associated behavior paradigms, disruption of latent inhibition by amphetamine, etc.[32]

REFERENCES

1. Ringen PA, Engh JA, Birkenaes AB, Dieset I, Andreassen OA. Increased mortality in schizophrenia due to cardiovascular disease - a non-systematic review of epidemiology, possible causes, and interventions. Front Psychiatry 2014;5:137.
2. Brandl EJ, Kennedy JL, Müller DJ. Pharmacogenetics of antipsychotics. Can J Psychiatry 2014;59(2):76-88.
3. Seeman MV, Seeman P. Is schizophrenia a dopamine supersensitivity psychotic reaction? Prog Neuropsychopharmacol Biol Psychiatry 2014;48:155-60.
4. Ellenbroek BA, Cools AR. Animal models with construct validity for schizophrenia. Behav Pharmacol 1990;1:469-90.
5. Kornetsky C, Markowitz R. Animal models of schizophrenia. In Lipton MA, DiMascio A and Killam KF (Eds): Psychopharmacology: A Generation of Progress. New York Press, 1978;pp 583-93.

6. Matthysse S. Animal models in psychiatric research. Prog Brain Res 1986;65:259-70.
7. Lowry OH, Rosebrough NJ, Farr AL, et al. Protein measurements with the Folin phenol reagent. J Biol Chem 1951;193:265-75.
8. Hall CS, Ballachey EL. A study of the rat's behavior in a field: a contribution to method in comparative psychology. Psychology 1932;6:1-12.
9. Swerdlow NR, Geyer MA. Using an animal model of deficient sensorimotor gating to study the pathophysiology and new treatments of schizophrenia. Schizophr Bull 1998;24(2):285-301.
10. Nielsen CK, Arnt J, Sánchez C. Intracranial self-stimulation and sucrose intake differ as hedonic measures following chronic mild stress: interstrain and interindividual differences. Behav Brain Res 2000;107:21-33.
11. Delini-Stula A, Morpurgo C. Influence of amphetamine and scopolamine on the catalepsy induced by diencephalic lesions in rats. Int J Neuropharmacol 1968;7:391-4.
12. Protais P, Costentin J, Schwartz JC. Climbing behavior induced by apomorphine I in mice: a simple test for the study of dopamine receptors in striatum. Psychopharmacology 1976;50:1-6.
13. Corbett R, Camacho F, Woods, et al. Antipsychotic agents antagonise non-competitive N-methyl-d-aspartate antagonist-induced behaviors. Psychopharmacology 1995;120:67-74.
14. Arnt J. Pharmacological specificity of conditioned avoidance response inhibition in rats: inhibition by neuroleptics and correlation to dopamine receptor blockade. Acta Pharmacol Toxicol 1982;51: 321-9.
15. Bracha HS, Torrey EF, Gottesman II, et al. Second trimester markers of fetal size in schizophrenia: a study of monozygotic twins. Am J Psychiatry 1992;149:1355-61.
16. Cintra L, Granados L, Aguilar A, et al. Effects of prenatal protein malnutrition on mossy fibres of the hippocampal formation in rats of four age groups. Hippocampus 1997;7:184-91.
17. Lipska BK, Weinberger DR. To model a psychiatric disorder in animals: schizophrenia as a reality test. Neuropsychopharmacology 2000;23:223-39.
18. Brake WG, Noel MB, Boksa P, et al. Influence of perinatal factors on the nucleus accumbens dopamine response to repeated stress during adulthood: an electrochemical study in rat. Neuroscience 1997;77:1067-76.
19. Brake WG, Boksa P, Gratton A. Effects of perinatal anoxia on the locomotor response to repeated amphetamine administration in adult rats. Psychopharmacology 1997;133:389-95.
20. Bakshi VP, Swerdlow NR, Braff DL, et al. Reversal of isolation rearing-induced deficits in prepulse inhibition by Seroquel and Olanzapine. Biol Psychiatry 1998;43:436-45.
21. Moises HW. Genetic models of schizophrenia. In Den Boer JA, Westenberg HGM, Van Praag HM (Eds). Advances in Neurobiology of Schizophrenia. John Wiley and Sons Ltd, 1995.
22. Cheng L, Hattori E, Nakajima A, Woehrle NS, Opal MD, Zhang C, et al. Expression of the G72/G30 gene in transgenic mice induces behavioral changes. Mol Psychiatry 2014;19(2):175-83.
23. White FJ, Wang RY. Differential effects of typical and atypical antipsychotic drugs on A9 and A10 dopamine neurons. Science 1983;221:1054-7.
24. Kawashima N, Okuyama S, Omura T, et al. Effects of selective dopamine D4 receptor blockers, NRA0160 and L745,870, on A9 and A10 dopamine neurons in rats. Life Sci 1999;65:2561-71.
25. Paxinos G, Watson C. The rat brain in stereotaxic co-ordinates. Sydney: Academic Press, 1982.
26. Wang RY. Dopaminergic neurons of the rat ventral tegmental area I. Identification and characterization. Brain Res Rev 1981;3:123-40.

27. Chiodo LA. Dopamine-containing neurons in the mammalian central nervous system: electrophysiology and pharmacology. Neurosci Biobehav Rev 1988;12:49-91.
28. Anderson MB, Werge T, Fink-Jensen A. The acetylcholinesterase inhibitor galantamine inhibits d-amphetamine-induced psychotic-like behavior in Cebus monkeys. J Pharmacol Exp Ther 2007;321(3):1179-82.
29. Peacock L, Gerlach J. Effects of several partial dopamine D2 receptor agonists in Cebus apella monkeys previously treated with haloperidol. Eur J Pharmacol 1993;237:329-40.
30. Peacock L, Gerlach J. New and old antipsychotics versus clozapine in a monkey model: adverse effects and amphetamine effects. Psychopharmacol (Berl) 1999;144:189-97.
31. Li W, Li J, Johnson JD. A computational model of sequential movement learning with a signal mimicking dopaminergic neuron activities. Cognitive Sys Res 2005;6:303-11.
32. Smith AJ, Li M, Becker S, Kapur S. Linking animal models of psychosis to computational models of dopamine function. Neuropsychopharmacology 2007;32:54-66.

CHAPTER

27

Antidepressant Agents

INTRODUCTION

Depression is a major affective disorder. It belongs to the heterogeneous group of mental disorders characterized by extreme exaggerations and disturbances of mood, which adversely affect cognition and psychomotor functions. It is a psychobiologic phenomena resulting from abnormal brain mechanisms. An imbalance in the central cholinergic and adrenergic tone is the critical pathophysiologic mechanism in affective disorders. The *Biogenic Amine Hypothesis* proposes an increase in norepinephrine (NE) along with reduction in level of serotonin (5-HT), dopamine (DA) and γ-aminobutyric acid (GABA) as the etiologic mechanism for genesis of depression. Recently, zinc, the essential trace element that is part of regulatory and catalytic protein, has been associated with significant role in the brain development. Imbalance in zinc levels can lead to impaired neuronal activity, initiate neurodegenerative processes leading to depression.[1]

The current therapy includes monoamine oxidase inhibitors (tranylcypromine, clorgiline, moclobemide), tricyclics and related compounds (imipramine, amitryptyline, desipramine, fluoxetine, fluvoxamine). Besides, the limitations of treatment lag, suboptimal efficacy and residual cognitive dysfunction, the typical antidepressants are some of the most toxic psychopharmacological agents and induce sedation, hypotension, and arrhythmias along with anticholinergic symptoms. These factors limit their use. Compounds targeting glutamatergic neurotransmission can be combined with drugs that target 5-HT or inhibit its transport and present new opportunities for antidepressant treatment. Newer multimodal compounds vortioxetine and vilazodone act via such diverse mechanisms in the treatment of depression and associated cognitive dysfunction.[2]

A major problem in the search for new antidepressant drugs is the lack of animal models that resemble depressive illness in humans and are selectively sensitive to simulate effective antidepressant treatments. Most of the available screening methods are based mainly on empirically established relationships between the clinical efficacy of known antidepressants and their effects on various pharmacological test models. In combination with the study of motor activity these tests allow assessment of the specificity of antidepressant activity by establishing a ratio between the "antidepressant" dose and the "stimulant" or "sedative" dose. It can be predicted that a substance will be antidepressant and sedative or stimulant at the same dose if the ratio is close to 1.[3] However, most of classical screening methods are inadequate for detecting novel antidepressant drugs.

IN VIVO METHODS

Chronic Social Defeat Stress (CSDS)

Chronic social defeat can act as stress, especially for adolescents. In order to simulate the condition, the adolescent-age animal is exposed for 2 weeks to daily aggression in agonistic interactions with unfamiliar adult males (hostile environment) and assessed for behavioral changes.

Adult male rodents (potential aggressors) are placed for 5 days into one of the two equal compartments of experimental cages separated by a transparent perforated partition. On the sixth day, single 4-week-old male adolescents are placed into the vacant compartments of common cages. Daily the partitions are removed and it is observed that the adult males demonstrate aggression toward adolescents by way of attacking and chasing the young males, who on the other hand demonstrate defensive behavior. The interaction is allowed for 5 min or for less than 3 min, depending on the intensity of the attack, after which animals are separated. Such exposure is continued for 2 weeks, wherein the adolescent animal faces repeated defeat and social stress. The age-matched animals of the control group are also individually transferred daily to partitioned cage next to an unfamiliar adult but not allowed to communicate physically. At the end of the two weeks, all animals are tested on behavioral and biochemical parameters.[4]

Water Wheel Model

This model demonstrates the antidepressant property of the test drug by use of the '*Behavioral Despair Activity*'. The animal is forced to swim without any escape in a water tank. A rotating wheel in the water tank poses as an option for escape but adds-on to the despair as it turns under the weight of the animal and the animal has to keep rotating the wheel in order to stay afloat. The juncture when the animal is immobile and ceases to struggle and remains floating motionless in the water, making only those movements necessary to keep its head above water is denoted as endpoint. This corresponds to behavioral despair.[5]

The apparatus consists of a plexiglas water tank (20 cm × 8 cm × 18 cm) with a water wheel in its center. The water wheel is made of plexiglas shaft (diameter 3 cm, length 6 cm) on which six paddles (0.5 cm width), move when loads of more than 5 g are attached and the number of rotations of the water wheel are counted. The tank is filled up to a height of 9 cm with water at 25°C, such that paddles just touch the surface of the water. When placed into the apparatus for the first time, the mice swim vigorously to find a way of escaping from the water. On discovering the water wheel, they climb onto it and begin turning it due to their weight. After a few minutes of attempted escape, they cling to the wheel and just float in the water showing complete immobility.

For this method, mice of either sex and in the weight range of 20 to 25 g are selected. The animals are randomly divided into three groups namely control, standard and test groups. First, the animals are put through a preliminary experiment to determine the typical number of rotations of the water wheel prior to the onset of behavioral despair. The animals are treated either with vehicle (control group), standard drug like imipramine (5-20 mg/kg, ip) or test drug in various doses (test group) and rechallenged on the water wheel. A potential antidepressant will increase the number of counts of water wheel turns, indicating increased effort at escape behavior.

The classical tricyclic antidepressants reduce immobility time in this model. However, antidepressants acting selectively on the 5-HT system are inactive in this test and false positive are induced by opiates and antihistaminics.

Lucki and co-workers have enhanced the sensitivity of the traditional Porsolt paradigm and the accuracy of its scoring.[6,7] This enables to better detect selective serotonin reuptake inhibitors (SSRIs) antidepressant activity. The water depth has been increased to 30 cm from the traditional depth of 15-18 cm, and the animal's behavior during consecutive intervals of 5 sec measuring climbing, swimming and immobility activity during each interval has been rated.

Another model on the principles of behavioral despair is the *Forced Swim Test.* The adult male rats are forced to swim in a cylinder (40 cm × 18 cm) with no escape. The animals become immobile after an initial struggling phase. The total duration of immobility is measured throughout the trial. Immobility has been equated to a despair reaction, and when rats are placed back in the water container 24 h later, they remain immobile for a significantly longer time than naïve animals. Antidepressants decrease the immobility time.[8] The forced swimming test is a widely used behavioral model used in rodents. It is both sensitive and selective for clinically effective antidepressant drugs. The test has been validated by most of the current antidepressants. However, the model has the limitation that antidepressant drugs show paradigm shift within 24 hr of treatment initiation, in contrast to weeks required for the recovery from clinical depression. Moreover, high doses of drugs are required to produce effects in most animal tests. [9]

Learned Helplessness Test

In these models, a helpless situation is created for the animal, which results in performance deficits in subsequent learning tasks. The rodents are exposed to chronic stress and not allowed to escape from it. Chronic mild stress is a naturalistic paradigm of a hostile environment, which models anhedonia, a major symptom of depression. This model reproduces a condition of decreased sensitivity to usually pleasurable stimuli, like drinking sucrose, etc.[10] In the classical model "Inescapable Shock Treatment" the chronic stress is provided by foot shock to the animal.[11] Adult Wistar rats of either sex and in the weight range 200 to 250 g are placed in a compartment with steel mesh grid floor. Repeated shocks (15 sec duration, 0.8 mA every min) are applied and this serves as stress to the animals. Rats are exposed for 1 h without any escape route. Control animals are placed in the chamber for 1 h without shocks. This forms the first phase of the model where animal is exposed to 'inescapable shock treatment'.

In the second phase there is 'conditioned avoidance training' where after chronic exposure, the animal is trained. A cue (buzzer or light signal) precedes the shock and simultaneously a door opened for 'safe' chamber, which is unelectrified, and the animal is allowed to escape towards it and avoid the noxious stimulus (electric shock). This is termed as the 'escape response'.

Failure to exhibit escape response by an animal is said to be an indicative of its 'depressive state'.[12] Antidepressants reduce 'escape failure'. This test can be successfully used to screen potential antidepressants and determine their mode of action.[13] This classic paradigm has a variable score of 30-85%, in terms of the percentage of rats, which become hyporeactive after training phase and as a modification, some authors use adrenalectomized rats in order to obtain a consistent high yield.[14]

Isolation-induced Hyperactivity

It is observed that rats when socially deprived for a period of 15 days, exhibit depressive behavior. There is a reduction in spontaneous locomotor activity, exploratory behavior, rearing, and stereotypy.

Adult Wistar rats of either sex weighing 200 to 250 g are housed singly in cages (38 cm × 26 cm × 20 cm) without any visual or auditory contact with their normally housed counter-parts for 10-15 days. The animals are subjected to behavior testing on an arbitrary scale for sleep, reduced response to external stimuli, ambulatory behavior, stereotype and posture.[15]

Both classical and newer antidepressants reduce isolation-induced depressive behavior.

Tail Suspension Test

This model is a modification of the 'behavior despair' test. Mice are rendered immobile by suspending from tail to induce behavioral despair. An animal in that situation alternates between two kinds of behavior: agitation (mobility) and immobility. The cumulative immobility time is a measure of the animal's degree of helplessness ("depression"). Treatment with antidepressant drugs reduces immobility time. It has been observed that mice exhibit better reproducibility of results than rats.[16] In a typical experiment, the mouse (20 to 30 g, either sex, housed under standard laboratory condition with food and water *ad libitum*) is hung on a wire in an upside down posture such that its nostril touches the water surface in a container. Initially, the animal tries to escape by making vigorous movements, but is unable to escape and becomes immobile. The period of immobility during 5 min observation period is noted.

This test is a reliable and rapid screening method for potential antidepressants. Agents acting via the serotonergic pathway can be screened using this method. In contrast, MAO inhibitors fail to answer this test.[16]

A computerized system with 16 channels is available as a single-channel basic configuration for measuring- time of activity, time of immobility, of the animal in real time. The tail suspension monitor is a device for screening antidepressants in mice (Fig. 27.1).

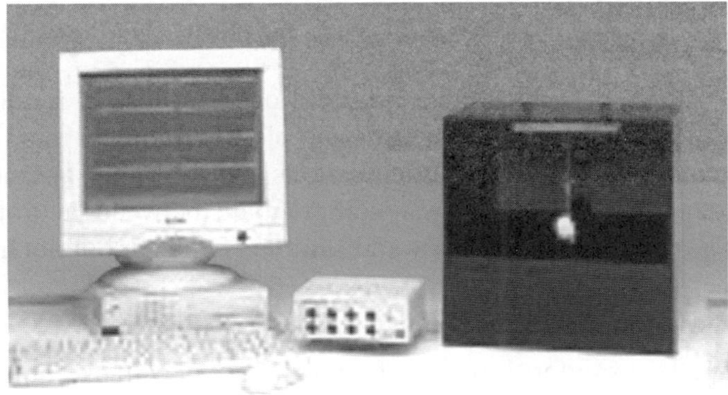

Figure 27.1: Computerized tail suspension monitoring system for screening antidepressant activity in mice

Reserpine-induced Hypothermia

The test measures the ability of compounds to inhibit reserpine-induced hypothermia in mice. The test is used for an early screening of potential antidepressant drugs with the mechanism of action similar to tricyclic antidepressants.

Mice (Male Albino-Swiss, 25 to 30 g) are housed in a controlled environment with a temperature at 22 ± 2°C, 12 h day-night cycle and free access to food and water. Reserpine in a dose of 2.5-5.0 mg/kg, sc induces ptosis, hypothermia, catalepsy. In the experimental model, reserpine (2.5 mg/kg, sc) is given 20 h before the test. Rectal body temperature is measured every 30 min for 3 h after the drug injection. The experiment is preceded by two preliminary measurements and their mean is taken as the initial temperature.[17]

Any pharmacological agent which reverses this typical effect of reserpine may have antidepressant activity. It is a simple and reliable method, which can effectively screen the tricyclics, MAO inhibitors. However, false negatives (mianserin) and false-positives (methyldopa, antihistaminics) are also known to occur.

Amphetamine Potentiation

Amphetamine is a sympathomimetic agent, which promotes neuroexocytosis or displacement of transmitter from axonal terminal. This test is used as a screening method to detect adaptive changes in dopaminergic and noradrenergic systems after repeated treatment with antidepressant drugs. Repeated treatment with antidepressants enhances the amphetamine-induced locomotor hyperactivity.

Rats (male Wistar, 250 to 300 g) are housed in a controlled environment with temperature 22 ± 2°C, 12 h light/dark cycle and free access to food and water. The rats receive the test drug in their home cage usually for two weeks. Ninety minutes after the last dose of test drug, D-amphetamine (5-10 mg/kg, ip) is injected and 30 min later they are placed singly into cages with photocells to record their activity. The locomotor activity of single animal in the activity cage is recorded for 1 hour.

Typical stereotypic effects (sniffing, exploratory activity, body and head movements, gnawing, biting, licking), hyperthermia and increased locomotor activity are seen.[18] Most antidepressants including TCA, MAO inhibitors potentiate amphetamine effects. This model effectively differentiates between neuroleptics and antidepressants.

Apomorphine Antagonism

Apomorphine is a dopamine agonist and in a dose of 16 mg/kg, ip, induces hypothermia, stereotypy and climbing behavior. This method is simple and useful for rapid *in vivo* screening of potential antidepressants. Potential antidepressants antagonize the apomorphine-induced hypothermia in mice. This model helps to differentiate between neuroleptics and antidepressants as the former blocks stereotypy and climbing behavior but not hypothermia.[19]

Resident-intruder Paradigm in Rats

This model is designed to examine the effect of acute treatment with psychotropic drugs on the social behavior of resident rats during encounters with unfamiliar, intruder rat. Antidepressant drugs commonly reduce the level of aggressive behavior exhibited by the resident rats without modifying basal activity levels. This selective effect on rodent agonistic behavior has been observed for all types of antidepressant drugs regardless of their pharmacology.

Male rats are housed under reverse-daylight conditions from weaning, for at least 5 weeks prior to the experiment to allow full entrainment to the phase-shifted light-dark cycle. Standard laboratory chow and water are made available *ad libitum* and all subjects are housed in standard laboratory polypropylene cages (32 cm × 50 cm × 16 cm) throughout each experiment. In all studies, the resident and intruder rats are obtained from different sources to ensure that resident animals have never been in contact with animals in the corresponding intruder group. All age-matched animals within a particular group are housed in closed social groups for at least 3 weeks to allow the development of stable social hierarchies.

Resident rats are treated with test, standard or vehicle and returned to their home cages prior to each social encounter. Resident animals are separated 3 days before each test day and housed individually. All social encounters are performed during the dark phase of the light-dark cycle. At the end of the 10 min encounter, both resident and intruder rats are returned to their respective group cages.

The nonsocial, social and agonistic behavior of the resident rats exhibited during each social encounter is analyzed.[20]

Muricidal Behavior in Rats

Female rats of Holtzman strain exhibit compulsive mouse killing behavior, irrespective of their satiety status. Nonmuricidal rats can be rendered muricidal by pretreatment with pilocarpine (2.5-5.0 mg/kg, ip).[21] It is understood to be a paradigm for depressive state. Agents reducing muricidal behavior exhibit antidepressant action.

Antidepressants attenuate muricidal behavior at doses below that dose which induces motor incoordination while psychotropic agents block at doses inducing motor deficits.[15]

Miscellaneous

Geriatric depression represents an unique set of physiological and biochemical problems due to the regulatory differences in the hypothalamus-pituitary-adrenal (HPA) axis.[22] Male Sprague Dawley rats are obtained when they are 9 weeks or 19 months old and are housed individually with free access to food and water and a 12 h light/dark cycle. After acclimatization, animals are anesthetized and the top of the skull is shaved and a midline frontal incision made in the scalp and the skin retracted bilaterally. Burr holes (2-3 mm) are drilled into the skull 2 mm lateral to the bregma suture, after which the olfactory bulbs are severed from the frontal cortex and aspirated according to established protocols.[23] The cavity is packed with surgical foam, the skin is closed with surgical clips and animal is allowed to recover. Sham-operated animals undergo the same procedure except for excision and aspiration of the olfactory bulbs. After surgery, animals are handled and weighed daily.[24] Aged olfactory bulbectomy (OBX) animals show a loss of passive avoidance. They exhibit locomotor stimulation along with decreased grooming and suppressed feeding.[24] The behavioral changes are visible 2 to 5 weeks after surgery and are attenuated by all classes of antidepressants.

Postpartum depression (PPD) is a form of major depressive disorders that can exert negative effects on both mothers and infants. PPD typically occurs for short durations within the postpartum period and has moderate symptoms. Postpartum adult female cynomolgus monkeys (*Macaca fascicularis*) are observed for typical huddle posture behavior as marker of PPD. The animals are analyzed for locomotive activity, stressful events, hair cortisol levels and for maternal interactive behaviors. This model provides translational efficiency for systematically investigating the etiology, treatment, prevention of PPD.[25]

REFERENCES

1. Tyszka-Czochara M, Grzywacz A, Gdula-Argasinska J, Librowski T, Wiliński B, Opoka W. The role of zinc in the pathogenesis and treatment of central nervous system (CNS) diseases. Implications of zinc homeostasis for proper CNS function. Acta Pol Pharm 2014;71(3):369-77.
2. Pehrson AL, Sanchez C. Serotonergic modulation of glutamate neurotransmission as a strategy for treating depression and cognitive dysfunction. CNS Spectr 2014;19(2):121-33.
3. Bourin M. Is it possible to predict the activity of a new antidepressant in animals with simple psychopharmacological tests? Fundam Clin Pharmacol 1990;4:49-64.
4. Iio W, Takagi H, Ogawa Y, Tsukahara T, Chohnan S, Toyoda A. Effects of chronic social defeat stress on peripheral leptin and its hypothalamic actions. BMC Neurosci 2014;15:72.
5. Porsolt RD, Bertin A, Blavet N, et al. Immobility induced by forced swimming in rats: effects of agents which modify central catecholamine and serotonin activity. Eur J Pharmacol 1979;57:201-10.
6. Detke MJ, Lucki I. Detection of serotonergic and noradrenergic antidepressants in the rat forced swimming test: the effects of water depth. Behav Brain Res 1996;73:43-6.
7. Lucki I. The forced swimming test as a model for core and competent behavioral effects of antidepressant drugs. Behav Pharmacol 1997;8:523-32.
8. Porsolt RD, Anton G, Blavet N, et al. Behavioural despair in rats: a new model sensitive to antidepressant treatments. Eur J Pharmacol 1978;47:379-91.
9. Detke MJ, Johnson J, Lucki I. Acute and chronic antidepressant drug treatment in the rat forced swimming test model of depression. Exp Clin Psychopharmacol 1997;5:107-12.
10. Gambarana C, Scheggi S, Tagliamonte A, et al. Animal models for the study of antidepressant activity. Brain Res Protocol 2001;7:11-20.
11. Overmier JB, Seligman MEP. Effects of inescapable shock upon subsequent escape and avoidance learning. J Comp Physiol Psychol 1967;63:23-33.
12. Martin P, Soubrie P, Simon P. The effect of monoamine oxidase inhibitors compared with classical tricyclic antidepressants on learned helplessness paradigm. Prog Neuropsychopharmacol Biol Psychiatry 1987;11:1-7.
13. Sherman AD, Sacquitne JL, Petty F. Specificity of the learned helplessness model of depression. Pharmacol Biochem Behav 1982;16:449-54.
14. Edwards E, Harkins K, Wright G, et al. Effects of bilateral adrenalectomy on the induction of learned helplessness behavior. Neuropsychopharmacology 1990;3:109-14.
15. Einon D, Morgan MJ, Sahakian BJ. The development of intersession habituation and emergence in socially reared and isolated rats. Dev Psychobiol 1975;8:553-9.
16. Chermat R, Thierry B, Mico JA, et al. Adaptation of the tail suspension test to the rat. J Pharmacol 1986;17:348-50.
17. Willner P. The validity of animal models of depression. Psychopharmacology 1984;83:1-16.
18. Delina-Stula A. Psychotropic agents. In. F Hoffmeister, G Still (Eds): Antipsychotics and Antidepressants: Part I., New York, Springer-Verlag 1980:505.

19. Puech AJ, Chermat R, Poncelet M, et al. Antagonism of hypothermia and behavioral response to apomorphine: a simple, rapid and discriminating test for screening antidepressants and neuroleptics. Psychopharmacology 1981;75:84-91.
20. Grant EC. An analysis of the social behavior of the male laboratory rat. Behavior 1963;21:260-81.
21. Bhattacharya SK, Satayan KS, Ramanathan M. Experimental methods for evaluation of psychotropic agents in rodents:II-Antidepressants. Indian J Exp Biol 1999;37:117-23.
22. Ritchie JC, Scotch RL, Nemeroff CB, et al. The effect of age on DST status and plasma dexamethasone concentration in depressed patients. Bio Psychiatry 1990;27:A45-6.
23. Kelly JP, Wrynn AS, Leonard BE. The olfactory bulbectomized rat as a model of depression: an update. Pharmacol Ther 1997;74:299-316.
24. Slotkin TA, Miller DB, Fumagalli F, et al. Modeling geriatric depression in animals: biochemical and behavioral effects of olfactory bulbectomy in young versus aged rats. J Pharmacol Exp Ther 1999;289:334-45.
25. Xun-Xun CHU, Joshua Dominic Rizak, Shang-Chuan YANG. A natural model of behavioral depression in postpartum adult female cynomolgus monkeys (*Macaca fascicularis*). Zoological Res 2014;35(3):174-81.

CHAPTER

28

Antiepileptics

INTRODUCTION

Epilepsy is a common disorder with an incidence of approximately 0.3-0.5% in different populations throughout the world and a prevalence of 5-10 persons per 1000. The characteristic event in epilepsy is the seizure, which is a paradoxical event due to abnormal, excessive, hypersynchronous discharges from an aggregate of central nervous system neurons.[1] Epilepsy, in contradistinction to seizures, is a chronic disorder characterized by recurrent seizures. Pathophysiology of epilepsy involves alterations in voltage-dependent ion channels: reduction in inhibitory, i.e. GABA-mediated or increase in excitatory, i.e. glutamate-mediated inputs.

Epileptic seizures have been classified [2] into:

- Partial seizures: Begin focally in a cortical site and may or may not generalize. These include simple partial seizures and complex partial seizures.
- Generalized seizures: Involve both the cerebral hemispheres from the onset. Generalized seizures have been classified into absence seizures (Petit mal), generalized tonic-clonic seizures (grand mal), myoclonic seizures and atonic seizures.

Currently available antiepileptic drugs act by modulating GABA or glutamate transmission or by modulating sodium and calcium ion channels. However, drug therapy of epilepsy is empirical therapy and does not address the underlying pathology. Also, inspite of addition of a large number of efficacious antiepileptic drugs during the past decade, they provide relief in only up to 75% patients with absence seizures and in 85% patients with generalized tonic-clonic seizures. Keeping these problems in antiepileptic pharmacotherapy, it has been suggested that the current drug discovery process for antiepileptic drugs should be re-evaluated. In furtherance of the objective of identifying useful models for therapy of pharmacoresistant epilepsy, NIH held a NIH/NINDS/AES models workshop in September 2002.[3] Discovery of newer genetic models of epilepsy and use of models of injury-induced epilepsy based on electrically or chemically induced status epilepticus was recommended at the workshop.

In order to study the antiepileptic effect of drugs and discovering their mechanism of action, various *in vitro* and *in vivo* models of epilepsy have been devised. Some of them, which are used most often, are described below.

IN VITRO METHODS

Hippocampal Slices

In vitro brain slice systems are being increasingly used for study of neurophysiological mechanisms of epilepsies. *In vitro* hippocampal slices have been especially useful due to the involvement of hippocampus in generation of complex partial seizures.[4]

Procedure: A rodent (rat, mouse, guinea pig) is used. The animal is decapitated, its brain is removed and hippocampus is dissected out. Using a vibrotome, slices of about 0.5 mm thickness are made. Cutting approximately perpendicular to the long axis of hippocampus preserves the three-neuron synaptic circuit and associated recurrent circuitry. After cutting, the slices are preincubated for 2 h in a holding chamber in which they are kept moist in 28°C warm saline equilibrated with 95% O_2 and 5% CO_2. Slices can be kept healthy for more than 18 h if handled properly. For recording, the slices are transferred to a Perspex chamber (1.5 × 4 cm) and attached to its bottom. Slices are either kept in 3 mm thick layer of 32°C warm saline or submerged in liquid artificial cerebrospinal fluid. Intracellular recordings from the pyramidal neurons in the slice are done by passing micropipettes (tip diameter <0.5 mm) into the stratum pyramidale under microscopic control.[4-6]

Evaluation: Readings are taken by adding drug to the slice medium and recording the spontaneous or shock evoked repetitive firing of neurons.

In vitro hippocampal slices offer the advantage of mechanical stability, absence of a blood-brain barrier for applied drugs and absence of anesthetics. It is a very useful model for studying the neurophysiological mechanisms of convulsant and antiepileptic drugs and for screening of putative antiepileptic drugs.

Electrical Recording from Isolated Brain Cells

Isolated brain cells are used for testing action of drugs on ion channels in excitable cell membranes using the patch clamp techniques.[7,8] In patch clamp techniques, glass pipettes are directly opposed to membranes in order to record currents through membrane in response to voltage, ionic or chemical change.[9] The isolated brain cells are prepared by either growing cells in tissue culture or by mechanical or enzymatic dissociation of brain slices into Petri dishes.[7] Cells are either obtained from hippocampus or from hypothalamus.

Procedure: The isolated neurons are put in a bath containing 140 mMNaCl, 5 mMKCl, 0.5 mM $CaCl_2$, 1 mM $MgCl_2$, 5 mM HEPES, at pH 7.3. Patch pipettes, filled with same solution as in bath, are attached. Drugs are added to bath solution and recording of capacitative currents is done. Recording is done at room temperature (21-24°C).[6]

Evaluation: Effect of drugs on capacitative component of current Ic is seen.

Ic = C dv/dt

where C = specific membrane capacitance

dv/dt = rate of change of membrane potential

Using this technique, neurophysiologists have explored voltage sensitive calcium and potassium channels, membrane response to neurotransmitters and basic mechanisms of antiepileptic drugs.[5]

In Vitro Assays for GABAergic Compounds

Gamma aminobutyric acid (GABA) is the principal inhibitory neurotransmitter in the central nervous system. It exerts its actions by acting on two distinct types of receptors; $GABA_A$ receptor, which is a ligand-gated Cl^- ion channel or 'ionotropic' receptor and $GABA_B$, which is a member of G-protein-coupled receptor family or 'metabotropic' receptor.[10] Abnormalities in the function of GABA system have been implicated in many diseases of the CNS including epilepsy.

In relation to epilepsy, it has been suggested that enhancing GABA-mediated synaptic inhibition would reduce neuronal excitability and raise the seizure threshold. A number of antiepileptic drugs have been shown to act by enhancing the GABAergic inhibition, e.g. benzodiazepines, barbiturates, vigabatrin and tiagabine.

[^{3}H] GABA Receptor-binding Assay

[^{3}H] GABA-binding assay is a simple and sensitive method to evaluate compounds with GABAergic properties.

Procedure: Rats are used for the experiment. Male rats weighing about 100-150 g are decapitated and their brains removed rapidly. The brains are homogenized in 15 volumes of ice-cold 0.32 M sucrose and centrifuged for 10 min at 1,000 g. The supernatant is then recentrifuged for 20 min at 20,000 g. After discarding the supernatant, the pellet obtained is homogenized in 15 volumes of distilled water and centrifuged for 20 min at 8,000 g. The upper, buffy layer of the pellet is resuspended, by gentle squirling, in the supernatant and then centrifuged for 20 min at 48,000 g. The pellet (synaptic membrane pellet) so obtained is resuspended in 15 volumes of distilled water and centrifuged for 20 min at 48,000 g. After discarding the supernatant, the centrifuge tubes, containing the pellets, are capped with paraffin and stored at –70°C.[6]

Homogenize a frozen membrane pellet in 15 volumes of 0.05 M Tris-maleate buffer (pH 7.1) at 4°C. Add Triton X-100 to a final concentration of 0.05% (enhances the specific GABA receptor binding while lowering the nonspecific binding) and incubate the suspension for 30 min at 37°C. This is now centrifuged for 10 min at 48,000 g. Discard the supernatant and resuspend the pellet by homogenization in 15 volumes of the buffer at 4°C.

The assay tubes are prepared in triplicate. The tissue homogenate is incubated with [^{3}H] GABA (15 nM) in the tris maleate buffer (0.05 M), alone or along with either the test drug or with isoguvacine (0.1 mM) or muscimol (0.1 mM) at 4°C for 5 min and then centrifuged for 15 min at 5,000 rpm. After washing the pellet with the buffer twice, radioactivity is quantified with liquiscint using liquid scintillation photometry.[6]

Evaluation: Specific [^{3}H] GABA binding, i.e. the radioactivity that can be displaced by a high concentration of unlabeled GABA is calculated. Difference between the total bound radioactivity and radioactivity bound in the presence of 0.1 mM of isoguvacine i.e. nonspecific binding gives the specific binding.

Percentage of specifically bound [^{3}H] GABA displaced by a given concentration of the test compound is calculated and its IC_{50} value with 95% confidence limits obtained using computer-derived linear regression analysis.

GABA$_A$ Receptor-binding Assay

GABA$_A$ receptor mediates the bulk of postsynaptic inhibitory actions of GABA. It is a ligand-gated Cl^- channel. It exists as pentamer, composed of 3 different subunits (α, β, γ). The receptor subunits each exist in several subtypes giving heterogeneity to the GABA$_A$ receptors.[11] Muscimol is a powerful GABA$_A$ agonist, whereas bicuculline, picrotoxin and SR 95531 are antagonists. Various centrally acting drugs like benzodiazepines, barbiturates and neurosteroids also modulate GABA$_A$ receptor function. To examine the GABA$_A$ binding sites, [^{3}H] muscimol (agonist) and [^{3}H] SR 95531 (antagonist) are used as radioligands.[12-15]

[^{3}H] Muscimol-binding Assay

[^{3}H] muscimol binding is determined using a concentration of radioligand ranging from 0.5-50 nM. Prior washing of the membrane pellet three times with ice cold buffer followed by centrifugation removes the endogenous GABA from the tissue used for assay. Membrane samples are then incubated with the radioligand in binding buffer (Tris-citrate, pH 7.1) for 60 min at 0-4°C. Nonspecific GABA binding is determined in the presence of 100 mM GABA. The incubation is terminated by centrifugation at 13,000 g for 10 min at 0-4°C. The resulting membrane pellet is rinsed once with 1 ml of ice-cold buffer, and the bottom of the tube containing the pellet is cut into a scintillation vial. Pellet material is dissolved in Protosol (NEN) for 45 min at 40°C and left overnight at room temperature. Scintillation fluid is then added and ligand binding is determined by scintillation counting.

[^{3}H] SR 95531 Binding Assay

The tissue sample is incubated with [^{3}H] SR 95531in buffer (50 mMTris-citrate supplemented with 200 mMNaCl, pH 7.1) for 60 min at 0-4°C. Concentrations of [^{3}H] SR 95531ranging from 1-100 nM are used for the assay and nonspecific binding is determined in the presence of 100 mM of unlabeled compound. The binding assay is terminated by filtration over Whatman GF/B filters on a Brandel filtration manifold. The filters are washed 2 times with ice-cold buffer, dried, and bound radioactivity quantified by liquid scintillation counting.

GABA$_B$ Receptor-binding Assay

GABA$_B$ is a metabotropic receptor, which acts by inhibiting adenylyl cyclase, K^+ channel opening or Ca^{2+} channel blockade.[10] It mediates both presynaptic and postsynaptic inhibition in the central nervous system. Baclofen is an agonist at the GABA$_B$ receptor. GABA$_B$ receptor-binding assay, using [^{3}H] baclofen, allows the screening of drugs with affinity for GABA$_B$ receptors.

Procedure: The tissue homogenate is incubated in buffer along with [^{3}H] baclofen ($1.8\text{-}2 \times 10^{-8}$ M) and either baclofen ($0\text{-}1.2 \times 10^{-6}$ M) or GABA or the test drug for 60 min at 4°C. The binding is terminated by rapid vacuum filtration over glass fiber filters. Filters are washed with ice-cold buffer and radioactivity counted after addition of ethylene glycol monomethyl ether and liquiscint.[6]

Evaluation: Difference of binding of [^{3}H] baclofen in the presence or absence of baclofen gives the specific binding. Dissociation constant (K_i) of the test drug, i.e. the concentration of the test drug at which 50% of the receptors are occupied, is calculated.

[^{3}H] GABA Uptake in Rat Cerebral Cortex

GABA action is terminated by uptake of GABA into neurons and glia via the GAT-1 transporter. Increasing the concentration of GABA by blocking the transporter offers a useful mechanism for anticonvulsant drugs. Tiagabine, a recently introduced antiepileptic drug, acts by inhibition of GAT-1.[16] Various other uptake inhibitors such as nipecotic acid, guvacine and THPO also exhibit anticonvulsant effects. This assay is useful in screening of potential anticonvulsants that act by GABA uptake inhibition.

Procedure: Rats are decapitated and their brains removed rapidly. The cerebral cortices are homogenized in 9 volumes of ice-cold 0.32 M sucrose and centrifuged for 10 min at 1,000 g. The supernatant is recentrifuged for 10 min at 1,000 g. Supernatant is discarded and the pellet is suspended in 9 volumes of 0.32 M sucrose and centrifuged for 10 min at 24,000 g. The pellet is resuspended in 15 volumes of depolarizing Ringer's solution and incubated for 10 min at 25°C. It is then centrifuged for 10 min at 3,000 g. The final pellet is then resuspended in 15 volumes of Ringer's solution.

The assay tubes are prepared in triplicate. The tissue suspension is incubated in Ringer's solution along with either vehicle or the test drug. The nonspecific controls are incubated at 0°C while totals at 25°C for 10 min. Now [^{3}H] GABA is added to each tube and the solution reincubated for 10 min. Centrifuge the tubes for 1 min at 13,000 g. Dissolve the pellet by mixing in Triton X-100+EtOH (1:4, v/v). Incubate for 3 min at 90°C and then recentrifuge for 15 min at 13,000 g. Radioactivity is quantified in 10 ml of liquiscint scintillation cocktail.[6]

Evaluation: Difference between cpm at 25°C and 0°C gives the value for active uptake of [^{3}H] GABA and percentage inhibition of uptake at each drug concentration is calculated. IC_{50} values are calculated using log-probit analysis.

[^{35}S] TBPS-binding Assay

TBPS (t-butylbicyclophosphorothionate) is a convulsant that acts by blocking the GABAergic neurotransmission by interacting with picrotoxin sensitive site of GABA-benzodiazepine-Cl^-channel complex.[17] Inhibition of binding of [^{35}S] TBPS to the rat cortical membranes by test compounds is used for screening of anticonvulsant drugs.

Procedure: Assay tubes are prepared in triplicate. The tissue homogenate is incubated in buffer (0.05 M Tris with 2 M KCl, pH 7.4) and distilled water along with [^{35}S] TBPS (2 nM) and picrotoxin (10^{-5} M) or distilled water or the test compound for 150 min at 25°C, with agitation. The binding is terminated by rapid filtration over Whatman GF/B filters, which are presoaked in buffer. Radioactivity is quantified by counting with 10 ml liquiscint.[6]

Evaluation: Difference between binding in the absence or presence of picrotoxin gives the specific binding which is typically 85-90% of total binding. Percentage inhibition of [^{35}S] TBPS at each drug concentration is measured and IC_{50} value calculated using log-probit analysis.

Excitatory Amino Acid Receptor-binding Assays

Glutamate, and possibly aspartate, function as the principal fast excitatory neurotransmitters in the brain. Glutamate receptors are classified functionally as either ligand-gated ion channels (ionotropic) or G-protein-coupled receptors (metabotropic). The ligand-gated ion channel receptors are further classified, according to the identity of selective agonists, into AMPA, NMDA and kainate receptors.[18] A number of antagonists are now available for these receptors. In case of NMDA receptors, the antagonists may act at various sites on the receptor and antagonize glutamate actions, e.g. phencyclidine, ketamine, MK-801 are open channel blockers, 5,7-dichlorokynurenic acid is an antagonist at the modulatory glycine site, ifenprodil is a closed channel blocker while CPP [3-(2-carboxypirazin-4-yl)-propyl-1-phosphonic acid], AP-7 and AP-5 are competitive antagonists at the glutamate-binding site.[19] Excessive excitatory amino acid neurotransmission has been implicated in the neuropathogenesis of epilepsy, stroke, schizophrenia and various neurodegenerative diseases.[20] Antagonists of NMDA receptors have been shown to act as anticonvulsants and neuroprotective agents.[21]

[^{3}H] CPP-binding Assay

[^{3}H] CPP-binding assay is used to assess the affinity of compounds for the glutamate-binding site on the NMDA receptor complex.

Procedure: Rats are decapitated and their brains removed rapidly. The cerebral cortices are homogenized in 15 volumes of 0.32 M sucrose with a Tissumizer and then centrifuged for 10 min at 1000 g, 4°C temperature. The supernatant is recentrifuged for 20 min at 20,000 g at 4°C. After discarding the supernatant, the pellet obtained is homogenized in 15 volumes of ice-cold distilled water and centrifuged for 20 min at 7,600 g at 4°C. The upper buffy layer of the pellet is resuspended in supernatant and centrifuged for 20 min at 48,000 g at 4°C. The pellet obtained is resuspended in 15 volumes of cold distilled water and centrifuged. Discard the supernatant and store the pellet at –70°C.[6]

Suspend the membrane pellet in 15 volumes of ice-cold 50 mMTris buffer (pH 7.6). Add Triton X-100 to a final concentration of 0.05% and incubate for 15 min at 37°C, with agitation. Now centrifuge it for 20 min at 48,000 g at 4°C. The pellet is washed thrice by resuspending in ice-cold Tris buffer and subsequently centrifuged. Resuspend the final pellet in buffer in a volume 20 times the original wet weight.

Assay tubes are set in triplicate. The tissue homogenate is incubated with [^{3}H] CPP (10 mM) in buffer (0.5 M TrisHCl, pH 7.6), distilled water along with l-glutamic acid (10^{-4} M) or distilled water or the test compound (in appropriate concentration) for 20 min at 25°C with agitation. Tubes are placed in ice bath after incubation. Binding is terminated by centrifugation for 15 min at 7,000 rpm at 4°C. Return the tubes to ice. Discard supernatant and rinse the pellets three times with ice-cold buffer. Radioactivity is quantified by liquid scintillation counting.[6]

Evaluation: Difference of binding in the absence or presence of 10^{-4} M l-glutamic acid gives the specific binding which is typically 60-70% of the total binding. IC_{50} values for the test compound are obtained using log-probit analysis.

[^{3}H] TCP-binding Assay

This assay is used for determining the binding affinity of noncompetitive NMDA receptor antagonists at the phencyclidine (PCP), binding site that lies within or near the NMDA-regulated ion channel. TCP, i.e. 1-[1-(2-thienyl)cyclohexyl]-piperidine is thienyl derivative of PCP.

Procedure: Assay tubes are prepared in triplicate. The tissue homogenate is incubated with [^{3}H] TCP (2.5 nM) in buffer (0.1 M HEPES, pH 7.5) and distilled water along with phencyclidine or vehicle or the test compound and with (for stimulated binding) or without (for basal binding) l-glutamic acid (10^{-4} M) and glyine (10^{-5} M) for 120 min at 25°C with agitation. The binding is terminated by rapid filtration, under reduced pressure, over Whatman GF/B filters, presoaked in 0.05% polyethylene-imine and buffer, using Brandell cell harvesters. Filters are rinsed twice with buffer and then counted for radioactivity with 10 ml of liquiscint.[6]

Evaluation: Difference of [^{3}H] TCP binding in the absence or presence of PCP gives the specific binding. For each test compound, inhibition of [^{3}H] TCP binding is measured both in the absence (basal) and presence (stimulated) of l-glutamic acid and glycine. IC_{50} values for the test compound are obtained using log-probit analysis.

[^{3}H] Glycine-binding Assay

Glycine is a modulator of the NMDA receptor function, which acts at a distinct modulatory site on the NMDA receptor complex. A strychnine insensitive [^{3}H] glycine-binding site is associated with NMDA receptor[22] and has been shown, by autoradiographic studies, to have similar distribution as that of [^{3}H] TCP-binding sites.[23] Binding of both glutamate and glycine is necessary for the NMDA receptor activation. Compounds with affinity for this glycine-binding site provide novel substances for modulation of NMDA receptor function. Such compounds are assayed using the [^{3}H] glycine-binding assay.

Procedure: The assay tubes are prepared in quadruplicate. The tissue homogenate is incubated with [^{3}H] glycine (10 nM) in buffer (0.5 M Tris maleate, pH 7.4) along with glycine (10^{-3} M) or distilled water or the test drug for 20 min in an ice bath at 0-4°C. The binding is terminated by centrifugation for 20 min at 7000 rpm at 4°C. The pellet obtained is rinsed with ice-cold buffer and the radioactivity is quantified by counting with 10 ml of liquiscint.[6]

Evaluation: Difference of binding in the absence or presence of unlabeled glycine gives the specific binding, which is typically 60-70% of the total binding. Inhibition of binding of [^{3}H] glycine by the test compound is measured and IC_{50} value calculated using log-probit analysis.

Disadvantages of *in vitro* models: Although, *in vitro* models provide insight into the mechanism of action of putative antiepileptic drugs and serve as initial screen for drug discovery, they do not give any indication of pharmacokinetics, pharmacodynamics or PK-PD interactions of the compound when introduced into a living animal or human being. Further, it is not possible to study the compensatory changes that occur in body when a drug is given.

IN VIVO METHODS

Electrically Induced Seizures

There are three major types of electrically induced seizure models:[24-26]

1. Threshold models
2. Maximal electroshock seizure (MES) test
3. Focal electrical stimulation such as kindling

These models are used for screening of drugs with efficacy against generalized tonic-clonic and focal seizures.

Threshold for Maximal (Tonic Extension) Electroconvulsions

This test is done to determine the ability of a drug to alter the seizure threshold for tonic limb extension.[26] Drugs effective against generalized tonic-clonic seizures increase this threshold. Used in parallel with MES test, it is a good test for screening of drugs effective against generalized tonic-clonic (grand mal) seizures.

Procedure: Mice are used for the experiment. For each stimulus intensity, male mice (18 to 30 g), in groups of 8-10, are used. Corneal or ear electrodes are used to provide electrical stimulation from a stimulator that either delivers constant current or constant voltage at a frequency of 50-60/sec for 0.2 sec duration. Rectangular pulses are better than sinusoidal pulses in inducing seizures, though either of the two can be used for stimulation.[27] Threshold is usually determined as the current or voltage inducing hind limb extension in 50% of the animals, i.e. CC_{50} and CV_{50} or EV_{50} respectively. Control thresholds in mice are about 6-9 mA (CC_{50}) or 90-140 V (CV_{50} or EV_{50}) depending on strain, age and method of stimulation (thresholds determined via ear electrodes are lower than via corneal electrodes).

Evaluation: Elevation of threshold by the test drug is taken as a measure of its efficacy. Comparison of drug effects requires calculation of dose that elevates the threshold by 20%. Control threshold determination should be undertaken on each day parallel to threshold determinations in drug treated animals. Use of an animal more than once a day is not recommended as post-ictal rise in seizure threshold has been noted.[27]

Maximal Electroshock Seizure (MES) Test

Merritt and Putnam (1938) developed the MES test and discovered the anticonvulsive effect of diphenylhydantoin using this test.[28] This model is useful for screening of drugs effective against primary and secondary generalized tonic-clonic seizures.[29]

Procedure: Groups of 8 to 10 animals (rats or mice) are used per dose of a drug. Electrical stimulation is applied via corneal or ear electrodes with a stimulator that either delivers constant current or constant voltage at a frequency of 50-60/sec. The electrodes are moistened with saline solution before application. All animals are stimulated with the same supra-maximal current strength that is usually 2-5 times the threshold current strength. With constant current stimulators, typical stimulation parameters include 50 mA in mice and 150 mA in rats, 50-60/sec current delivered via corneal electrodes for 0.2 sec.[26,27] With constant voltage stimulators, 250 V is used for mice and 750 V for rats. The resultant seizure passes through various phases: phase of tonic limb flexion of about 1.5 sec duration followed by phase of tonic limb extension lasting about 10 sec and finally followed by a variable short clonic interval which may lead to asphyxial death in some animals.[30]

Evaluation: Suppression of tonic hind limb extension is taken as a measure of efficacy in this test. Anticonvulsant potency is determined by calculation of ED_{50} for suppression of tonic hind limb extension. Drugs effective against generalized tonic-clonic seizures such as phenytoin, carbamazepine, phenobarbitone and primidone are effective while anti-absence seizure drugs like ethosuximide are ineffective in this test.

Disadvantage of electrically induced seizure models: These models, though useful in determining the anti-seizure potential of a compound, do not give any clue regarding the mechanism of action of the compound.

Kindled Rat Seizure Model

Kindling is an animal model of epilepsy that refers to a process whereby repeated administration of an initially subconvulsive electrical stimulus results in progressive intensification of stimulus-induced seizure activity, culminating in a generalized seizure.[31] The effect was discovered by Delgado and colleagues[32] and elaborated by Goddard et al.[24] The kindling phenomenon is a manifestation of the fact that 'epilepsy induces epilepsy'.

Procedure: Adult female Sprague Dawley rats weighing 270 to 400 g are used for the experiment. An electrode is implanted in the right amygdala for electrical stimulation.[6] Although, amygdala is most commonly chosen for the experiment, other regions of the forebrain can also be kindled.[24,33] Animal is allowed to recover from surgery for a minimum of 1-2 weeks, otherwise the sensitivity of the animals to kindling is lowered. Then daily electrical stimulus trains are applied via the electrode using either a fixed current strength (400-500 μA, 1 msec monophasic square wave pulses for 1 sec with 50 or 60/sec frequency) or using the individual threshold current to induce after discharges at the site of stimulation.[27]

During the daily electrical stimulation of amygdala, seizures develop which, as classified by Racine,[34] generally evolve through the following five stages:

Class - 1: Immobility, eye closure, twitching of vibrissae, stereotypic sniffing
Class - 2: Facial clonus and head nodding
Class - 3: Facial clonus, head nodding and forelimb clonus (contralateral to focus)
Class - 4: Rearing, often accompanied by bilateral forelimb clonus
Class - 5: Rearing with loss of balance and falling accompanied by generalized clonic seizures.

Rats are said to be fully kindled when enhanced sensitivity, as evidenced by class five seizures, has developed.[27] If the stimulation is continued for a few weeks, rats develop 'spontaneous' epileptic seizures that persist for as long as 7 months following termination of the stimulation.

Evaluation: The animals to be tested are given the test compound either orally or ip and tested on the day before and after the treatment. Readings obtained after administration of test drug and the control are compared keeping in mind four different measures for drug efficacy which can be recorded in a kindled animal:

1. Seizure latency, i.e. time from stimulation to the first sign of seizure activity.
2. Seizure severity
3. Seizure duration
4. After discharge duration.

Alternatively, drug efficacy can be measured by determining separate ED_{50} values for total suppression of:

1. Generalized seizures (class 4 and 5)
2. Focal seizures (class 1-3)
3. Amygdaloid after discharges.

Kindling model has the merit that the efficacy of a drug against the process of epileptogenesis as well as against the fully kindled state can be measured. Efficacy against generalized seizures provides a valid model for drugs effective in secondary generalized seizures of partial epilepsy, while efficacy against the focal components of kindled seizures provides a valid model for drugs effective in complex partial seizures.[35] Of the anticonvulsant drugs available at present, phenobarbitone, diazepam and valproic acid block the kindled seizures as well as the kindling process while phenytoin and carbamazepine block seizures once kindling has occurred, but do not reliably block the establishment of kindled seizures. Every species so far studied is subject to kindling,[33] from frogs to animals like baboons, rhesus monkeys, cats and dogs.[36-38]

Other Methods of Kindling

1. **Corneal electroshock kindling:** Kindling can be done in rats and mice by giving electroshocks via corneal electrodes. Mice can be kindled by once daily application of 3mA current of 60 Hz frequency for 2 sec while rats can be kindled with twice daily application of 8 mA current of 60 Hz frequency for 4 sec via corneal electrodes. Occurrence of Racine stage 5 seizures (as above) indicates that the animal is kindled. Putative antiepileptic drugs can be tested after the animals have had stage 5 seizures for 10 consecutive times.[39,40]
2. **Kindling by stimulation of other brain areas:** Kindled seizures can also be produced by stimulation of other brain areas like neocortex or hippocampus in rats. Lothman et al. (1985)[41] have described the development of rapidly recurring hippocampal seizure (RRHS) model of kindling in rats. Briefly, bipolar electrodes are implanted stereotactically in either right or left hippocampus of adult albino rats. The animals are allowed to recover for one week. Subsequently via a constant current source stimulator, hippocampus is stimulated with suprathreshold tetanic electrical stimuli in trains of 10 sec, with each stimuli consisting of biphasic square wave pulses of 1ms duration and 10 Hz frequency. The stimulation is repeated every 5 min. Behavioral seizures (Class 1 to class 5 as described above for amygdala kindling) and after discharges on EEG are recorded after every stimulus. Severe limbic seizures (i.e. class 4 or class 5 behavioral seizures) are observed on the first day itself, which intensify on the second day and then remain stable. Effect of putative antiepileptic drugs against the stimulation induced behavioral or EEG seizures and the after discharge duration can be studied. Using the RRHS model of kindling, Lothman et al (1988 a,b)[42,43] have demonstrated that the response pattern of antiepileptic drug against kindling in this model is similar to that with the amygdala kindling.
3. **Chemical induced kindling:** Pentylenetetrazol (PTZ), a proconvulsant chemical acting via antagonism of $GABA_A$ function, can lead to long lasting kindling in rats when given repeatedly in subconvulsive doses. Briefly, adult Sprague Dawley rats are administered 30 mg/kg of PTZ ip 3 times a week for 9 weeks. After every injection, seizures are recorded and scoring done as below:
   0 = no response
   1 = ear and facial twitching
   2 = one to 20 myoclonic jerks in 10 min
   3 = more than 20 body jerks in 10 min
   4 = clonic forelimb convulsions
   5 = generalized clonic convulsions with rearing and falling down episodes
   6 = generalized convulsions with tonic extension episodes and status epilepticus.

Beginning in second week of PTZ administration, the seizure score shows a progressive increase over the period of 9 weeks such that by the end of 9 weeks, about 90% animals are kindled i.e. have seizure score of more than or equal to 3. Efficacy of drugs in preventing the development of PTZ induced kindling can be studied by injecting the putative antiepileptic drug before each PTZ injection.[44,45]

Chemically Induced Convulsions

Numerous chemical compounds can produce seizures. Some, which are used as tools for epilepsy research, include:

1. Chemoconvulsants inducing generalized seizures after systemic administration, e.g. pentylenetetrazol, bicuculline, picrotoxin, penicillin, isoniazid, thiosemicarbazide, allylglycine, DMCM, β-CCM, strychnine, pilocarpine, NMDA, kainic acid, gamma-hydroxybutyric acid, DDT and methionine sulfoximine.
2. Chemoconvulsants inducing focal seizure after central administration, e.g. penicillin, kainic acid, quinolinic acid, and pentylenetetrazol.[27]

Pentylenetetrazol (PTZ) Test

Pentylenetetrazol is a tetrazol derivative with consistent convulsive effect in a large number of animal species like mice, rats, cats, primates, etc. It is believed to act by antagonizing the inhibitory GABAergic neurotransmission.[46] PTZ test is used for screening of drugs effective in petit mal epilepsy or absence seizures.

i. Threshold for Clonic Seizures after IV Infusion of PTZ

Procedure: Eight to 10 mice are used per threshold determination. One percent solution of PTZ is administered by continuous i.v. infusion at the rate of 0.3 ml/min.[27] The animal develops seizures in the following order: one or more isolated jerks (first twitch) followed immediately by a generalized clonic seizure with loss of righting reflexes, followed by maximal tonic clonic seizures after a certain time lag. Dose for the production of generalized clonic seizures with loss of righting reflex is preferably taken as an endpoint. Threshold is calculated as the mean dose (± SD) of PTZ that induces seizures in the group tested and is about 50 mg/kg for clonic seizures and 90 mg/kg for maximal tonic-clonic seizures in mice.

ii. Subcutaneous PTZ Test

Procedure: Mice or rats are used for the experiment. 8 to 10 animals are used per dose of test drug. Prior to drug efficacy experiments, it is better to determine the subcutaneous CD_{97} (convulsive dose in 97% of the animals) of PTZ. CD_{97} is usually about 70 mg/kg in rats and 80-100 mg/kg in mice.[27] Mice are given 1% solution of PTZ, 80-100 mg/kg sc in the scruff of neck. Control mice within 30 min develop a sequence of excitement, myoclonic jerks, clonic seizures, one or more maximal tonic seizures and death.[30] As endpoint, either the first episode of clonic jerking lasting for 5 sec (a threshold seizure) or the first clonic seizure with loss of righting reflex is taken.

Evaluation: Efficacy of a test drug as an anticonvulsant is measured by determining its ED_{50} for suppression of clonic seizure (either threshold seizure or clonic seizure with loss of righting reflex). Drugs effective in petit mal epilepsy like ethosuximide, valproic acid are effective while phenytoin, carbamazepine are not effective in the two models using PTZ.

Systemic Penicillin Test

Cats are used for the experiment. Animals are injected with 3,00,000 units/kg of penicillin G by intramuscular route. Seizure activity begins about 1 h after injection and continues intermittently for 6-8 h and is characterized by recurrent episodes of arrested activity, staring, myoclonus, facial-oral twitching and occasional progression to generalized tonic-clonic seizures.[47] This model is useful for screening of drugs useful in petit mal epilepsy. Ethosuximide and valproate are effective in this model.[48,49]

Modification: Rats can be used for the penicillin model of epilepsy.[50]

Other Chemical Convulsants

Numerous other chemicals have been used systemically to study the anticonvulsant activity of drugs, e.g. bicuculline (a $GABA_A$ antagonist used in a dose of 2.7 mg/kg sc in mice or in a dose of 0.3 mg i.v. in monkeys to induce seizures), picrotoxin, strychnine, NMDA, homocysteine, allylglycine, methionine sulfoximine, fluorothyl (by inhalational route), gamma-hydroxybutyrate and pilocarpine.[29,51-59]

Seizures Induced by Focal Lesions

Topical or intracerebral application of certain metals and chemicals can lead to simple partial seizures. These models are thus useful for screening of potential antiepileptic drugs effective against these seizures.

Cortically Implanted Metals

A state of spontaneously recurrent simple partial seizures can be induced by topical application of certain metals such as alumina cream (aluminium hydroxide), cobalt and tungstic acid onto (or into) the cerebral cortex[60] or by injection of iron into the brain cortex.[61] Aluminium hydroxide gel model is most commonly used.

Aluminium Hydroxide Gel Model

This model was discovered by Kopeloff et al.[62] Four percent aluminium hydroxide is injected into surgically exposed monkey neocortex at few adjacent sites. One to two months after the injection, spontaneous and recurrent seizures begin. These seizures persist for several years. Seizures consist of rhythmic jerking of an extremity or face contralateral to the lesion with occasional progression to secondarily generalized tonic-clonic seizures. Response to standard anticonvulsants parallels that of patients with focal epilepsy.

Miscellaneous Chemicals Used for Producing Focal Lesions

Various other chemicals have been used as convulsants by topical route such as intrahippocampal injections of kainic acid or tetanus toxin, topical application of penicillin, cholinergics, anticholinergics, picrotoxin, bicuculline, strychnine, ganglioside antibody injections, zinc.[63-72]

Focal lesions have also been produced by cryogenic injury to areas of brain using liquid nitrogen probe or ethylchloride, which can lead to highly epileptogenic lesions.[73]

Systemic Focal Epileptogenesis

This model combines the features of focal and generalized epilepsy. Rats are given radiation to a volume of cerebrum equivalent to 0.25 ml. About 3-6 months later, bicuculline methiodide, in a dose of 2 mg/kg, is injected systemically. A seizure focus is produced with recurrent EEG spikes and focal seizures.[74] Seizures last for several weeks after a single injection. Phenytoin, phenobarbital, chlordiazepoxide and valproic acid are effective.

Models of Status Epilepticus

There are a number of animal models that can be used to screen drugs effective in pharmacotherapy of status epilepticus. Some of these are described below in brief:

1. **Pilocarpine-induced status epilepticus:** Pilocarpine, a cholinomimetic agent, can produce behavioral and electroencephalographic seizures suggestive of motor limbic seizures and status epilepticus in rats when given in a dose of 380-400 mg/kg i.p. The seizures can be scored according to the classification of Golarai et al. as follows:
   Stage I - hypoactivity
   Stage II - monoclonic jerks of the head, head bobbing and facial automatism
   Stage III - whole body bilateral activity resembling wet dog shakes
   Stage IV - rearing of forelimbs
   Stage V - generalized clonic-tonic activity and loss of posture.[75-77]
2. **Lithium-pilocarpine induced status epilepticus:** Status epilepticus can be induced in rats by giving pilocarpine (30-40 mg/kg, i.p.) 24 h after pretreating with lithium (3 meq/kg i.p.). Racine classification is used to score the seizures.[78-82]
3. **Lithium-methomyl induced seizures in rats:** Methomyl, a carbamate anticholinesterase, in a dose of 5.2 mg/kg s.c., can induce long lasting status epilepticus in lithium pretreated rats. Diazepam is effective in this model.[83]
4. **Electrical stimulation of hippocampal perforant pathway:** A week after implanting a bipolar stimulating electrode in right angular bundle and a unipolar recording electrode in right hippocampal dentate granule, the perforant pathway is stimulated by 2mA monopolar pulses of 50 microsecond duration and 20 Hz frequency for 2 h. The animals develop self-sustaining limbic status epilepticus when the stimulation is stopped.[84]
5. **D, L-homocysteine induced status epilepticus:** Status epilepticus can be induced by D, L-homocysteinethiolactone in rats with actively epileptogenic cobalt lesions of motor cortex. Diazepam, lorazepam, phenobarbitone and phenytoin are effective against these seizures.[85]
6. **Generalized myoclonic seizures in baboons:** In Papio cynocephalus baboons, generalized myoclonic jerks can be produced by hourly stimulation by stroboscope (15-35 flashes/sec for test periods of upto 5 min), 2-8 h after injecting allylglycine (200 mg/kg i.v.). Phenobarbitone and diazepam are effective against these seizures.[86]

Model of Infantile Spasms

Infantile spasms, which occur in early childhood, are insensitive to most of the available antiepileptic drugs. Velisek et al. (2007)[87] have developed a model of infantile spasms, which includes injecting pregnant Sprague Dawley rats with 2 doses of betamethasone (0.4 mg/

kg i.p.) at 8 AM and 6 PM on gestational day 15. Seizures are produced in the pups on post-natal day 15 by injecting NMDA (15 mg/kg i.p.). The sequence of seizures includes: twisting movements of tail followed by arching for several seconds and finally loss of righting reflex and flexion spasms lasting tens of seconds with multiple recurrences. ACTH, which is the only drug effective against infantile spasms, can delay the onset of NMDA induced seizures in these rats. Betamethasone has been proposed to sensitize the brain to onset of NMDA induced seizures. Although, it is a step forward, this model required validation.

Genetic Animal Models of Epilepsy

Most of the animal models for screening of antiepileptic drugs are basically models of seizures rather than of epilepsy, which is a condition of chronically recurrent spontaneous seizures. Genetic animal models more closely approximate human epilepsy and give opportunity to study genetic and biochemical basis of epilepsy.

Photosensitive Baboons

Baboons, *Papiopapio*, from the Casamance region of Senegal were first reported to suffer from photomyoclonic syndrome by Killiam et al. in 1966.[88] Intermittent light stimulation at frequencies close to 25 flashes per second leads to seizures characterized by eyelid, then face and body clonus and subsequently tonic spasms or full tonic-clonic convulsions.[89] Drugs useful against clinical tonic-clonic and myoclonic epilepsy inhibit photosensitive seizures in Papiopapio. Valproic acid, benzodiazepines and phenobarbital are effective as anticonvulsants in them, while phenytoin, carbamazepine and trimethadione provide less favorable therapeutic effects.[5]

Seizure-prone Mice Strains

Various seizure-prone mice strains have been developed. These include the following:

i. **Audiogenic Seizure Susceptible Mice:** DBA/2J mice, an inbred strain of the house mouse (*Musmusculus*), is the most studied strain of audiogenic seizure susceptible mice and has been known since 1947.[90] Between the ages of 2-4 weeks, these mice exhibit sound-induced seizures, after which susceptibility gradually declines,[91] such that by 8 weeks of age they are totally free of audiogenic seizures.

   Susceptible mice are exposed to sudden, loud sound which contains frequency components in the 12-16 kHz range.[5] The seizure pattern involves a wild running phase, followed by clonic convulsions and a tonic extension ultimately leading to respiratory arrest (in about 60%) or full recovery.[27] Anticonvulsant effect of drugs is evaluated by efficacy against clonic seizures. Audiogenic seizures can be prevented by phenytoin or phenobarbital[92] or valproic acid. Audiogenic seizure susceptible mice are useful as sensitive gross screening model for potential anticonvulsant drugs.

ii. **Totterer Mice**: The homozygous (tg/tg) strain totterer mice are prone to spontaneous epileptic seizures. These mice are recognized by a broad-based ataxic gait. By 3 to 4 weeks of age, they develop frequent partial and absence seizures.[93] Spontaneous focal motor seizures occur a few times a day, manifested as unilateral clonic jerks of limbs with secondary generalization. Ninety-three percent of the seizures last for 15 min or longer.[94] These seizures can be suppressed by diazepam.

Totterer mice also exhibit spontaneous petit mal seizures with synchronous 6-7 per second spike-wave discharges in EEG.[95] These spike-wave discharges last 0.3 to 10 sec and occur hundreds of times per day and are accompanied by a behavioral petit mal seizure. These seizures are blocked by ethosuximide, diazepam and phenobarbital while phenytoin is not effective.[96]

iii. **El Mice**: Imaizumi and colleagues first discovered El mice in 1959.[97] El mice exhibit seizures in response to vestibular stimulation like tossing or spinning. Manifestations of seizure include limb and face automatism like chewing and salivation. There may be secondary generalization to tonic-clonic seizures. EEG recordings indicate onset of electrical discharges in deep limbic structures.[98] Thus, these mice can serve as model for complex partial epilepsy with secondary generalization. Phenytoin and phenobarbitone are effective in this model.

iv. **Quaking Mice**: These are C57BL/6J mutants with myelin defects, tremors, spontaneous or stimulus-induced myoclonic and generalized tonic-clonic seizures. Handling induces seizures in quaking mice. These seizures are blocked by phenytoin, phenobarbitone, carbamazepine and valproic acid. Quaking mice are useful for assessment of potential new anticonvulsant drugs effective against focal motor seizures in humans.[99]

v. **Lethargic (lh/lh) mice**: Hosford et al. (1992) have validated lethargic (lh/lh) mouse model as a genetic model of absence seizures. Lethargic (lh/lh) mice have behavioral, EEG and anticonvulsant drug profiles similar to those in absence seizures in humans. Lethargic mice are recognized by ataxic gate by 3 weeks of age. EEG electrodes are placed intracerebrally in frontal neocortex. Subsequently, 180 min EEG recording sessions consisting of 30 min predrug and 150 min post drug recordings are done to see the effect of drug on frequency of epileptiform bursts. Number of seizures during 150 min period after administration of drug is noted and IC_{50}, i.e. concentration that reduces number of seizures by 50% is calculated. Total duration of seizures during the 150 min recording sessions can give an indication of pro-absence effect of drugs.[100]

vi. **Other mice strains** showing spontaneous seizures (AE mice) or induced seizures (SJL/J strain mice with noise-induced seizures) are also being used for anticonvulsant drug testing.

Seizure-prone Rat Strains

i. **Genetically Epilepsy-prone Rats (GEPRs):** Seizures can be induced in these animals by various stimuli like sound, hyperthermia, chemical and electrical.[101] When stimulated by sound, these GEPRs run about wildly, fall from clonic jerks and may also suffer from tonic extensor convulsions. For anticonvulsant drug evaluation, the tonic-clonic component of the seizure is commonly used.[94] Drugs effective in MES test are effective in this model.

ii. **Rats with Spontaneously Occurring Petit Mal Epilepsy:** About 15-30% of Sprague Dawley and Wistar rats, both males and females, 14 to 18 weeks of age and above exhibit spontaneous spike-wave discharges (7-11/sec) with associated behavioral components like behavioral arrest and myoclonic twitchings mostly limited to the facial musculature.[102] Spontaneous discharges last for 0.5-40 sec and occur hundreds of times a day. Drugs effective in absence seizures in humans suppress these seizures. These rats can serve as a good model for chronic drug efficacy studies.

Mongolian Gerbils

Seizure tendency in Mongolian gerbils was first described by Thiessen et al.[103] in 1968. Seizures in these animals can be precipitated by various stimuli like placing the animal in a new environment, onset of bright light, audiogenic stimuli, vigorous shaking of cage and different handling techniques.[104] Seizures in gerbils can be facial myoclonic (minor) seizures, seen mostly in young animals of 7 to 10 weeks age or generalized myoclonic and tonic-clonic (major) seizures seen in older animals. Young gerbils with minor seizures can serve as model for petit mal epilepsy. Anti-absence seizures drugs are effective in these. While older animals with major seizures can be used to identify drugs with efficacy against generalized tonic-clonic seizures.

Miscellaneous Genetically Seizure-prone Animals

Various other animals can be used for studying the anticonvulsive effect of potential antiepileptic drugs. These include Syrian golden hamsters, photosensitive epileptic chickens and dogs.[105-107]

Morphological Approaches

In many animal SE models, cell necrosis and neurodegeneration are hallmark features. Acute neuronal injury and neurodegeneration are routinely assessed to estimate the extent of protection provided by the test compounds. The following methods are used to determine the neuroprotective potential of test compounds.

Cell Necrosis and Apoptosis

Nissl Staining

Histological assessment is made using Nissl (Cresyl violet, CV) staining techniques, as described previously.[108] CV stains all neurophil components and any changes in cytoarchitecture of the hippocampal cell layers like loss of cells is determined. Cresyl Violet Acetate solution is used to stain Nissl substance in the cytoplasm of neurons. It stains both neurons and glia and is very useful to identify the overall cell loss and neuronal damage.

TUNEL Assay

To measure apoptotic cell death, terminal deoxynucleotidyl transferase and digoxigenin-11-dUTP nick end labeling (TUNEL) staining is mostly widely employed using the Apoptag peroxidase *in situ* apoptosis detection kit.[108] For quantification of cell death, photomicrographs (30-μm) of three sequential sections are taken at dorsal hippocampus level of each animal. The representative sections from different animals ($n = 4$) are permeabilized by treating with 0.25% trypsin solution in 0.01 N HCl for 30 min at 37°C and then washed in PBS, and nonspecific sites are blocked by using 0.1 M Tris buffer containing 3% bovine serum albumin and 20% normal bovine serum for 30 min at 37°C. After this, sections are washed in PBS and incubated in TUNEL reaction mixture for 90 min at 37°C. The TUNEL reaction mixture comprised enzyme solution and fluorescein label solution at a ratio of 1:9. The sections designated as negative controls were incubated in fluorescein label solution only. The nucleus of apoptotic cells in sections treated with the TUNEL mixture exhibits a clear green fluorescence. TUNEL-positive cells within a square millimeter area are counted by an observer blind to the treatment conditions.[109]

Fluoro-Jade B Staining

For detecting degenerating neurons and their processes, Fluoro-Jade B (FJB) staining is commonly performed in brain sections from rodent models. This staining procedure is a sensitive and reliable marker for neuronal degeneration that results from SE or brain injury. The extent of neurodegeneration after the SE is determined with FJB staining in dentate hilus (DH), CA3 and CA1 sub-regions of the hippocampus. The rats are perfused with 4% paraformaldehyde solution and the brains collected and processed in 30% sucrose. Consequently, 30 μm thick sections of these brains are cut with cryostat at the dorsal hippocampus level and collected in phosphate buffer solution (PBS) and later stored at –20°C in cryo-buffer. To visualize neurons undergoing degeneration after SE, three sequential sections each 450 μm apart through the dorsal hippocampi are collected in each animal, mounted on gelatin-coated slides and air dried at room temperature overnight. Slides were then washed sequentially in 100% ethanol, 70% ethanol and deionized water. The slides were then incubated in 0.06% potassium permanganate solution for 15 min (with slow shaking), washed in deionized water, and incubated in 0.004% FJB (Histo-Chem Inc., Jefferson, AK) dissolved in deionized water with 0.1% acetic acid for 30 min. Then slides were washed three times for 1-min in deionized water, dried on a slide warmer at 55°C, briefly immersed in xylene and cover slipped using DPX mounting media. The sections are analyzed by confocal microscope using FITC filter. Cells labeled by FJB were detected as individual green shiny pyramidal shaped spots clearly identifiable from background. The number of FJB positive cells (dying neurons) per image field in the hippocampal DH, CA3 and CA1 are counted in each of the three sections per animal.[116]

Neurodegeneration, Neurogenesis and Mossy Fiber Sprouting

Neurodegeneration

The extent of neurodegeneration after the SE is determined by the immunostaining of sections for NeuN (principal neurons) and parvalbumin- or neuropeptides-Y-positive (interneurons) cells. The neuronal nuclei antigen (NeuN) is a very specific protein that is highly expressed in nucleus and less expressed in cell body in differentiated neurons. NeuN is not expressed in glial cells, oligodendrocytes, astrocytes, or microglial cells, and cerebellar Purkinje cells. Thus, NeuN immunohistochemistry is commonly used to identify neuronal loss and to quantify total number of neurons in various rat brain regions. To analyze the overall neurodegeneration after the SE, the brains are removed, postfixed in 4% paraformaldehyde and cryoprotected in PBS containing 30% sucrose. Cryostat sections are cut at 30-μm coronally through the entire anteroposterior axis of the hippocampus and collected serially in PBS. Every 20th section through the entire hippocampus is selected in each of the animals and processed for Nissl staining. Nissl staining demonstrates the hippocampal cytoarchitecture of principal cell layers and confirmed the presence of bilateral hippocampal injury in rats after SE. The extent of neurodegeneration within different regions of the hippocampus is further assessed by NeuN immunohistochemistry and quantified from 24 to 72 h post-SE. Because the overall neurodegeneration in different regions of the hippocampus appeared mostly symmetrical between the two sides, quantification is performed on only one side. The number of cells in hippocampal subregions such as the dentate hilus (DH), CA3 and CA1 are counted and compared with controls or between various treatment groups. Reduction or lack of neuronal loss is indicative of neuroprotective potential of the test drug.[111]

Neurogenesis

There is strong evidence of dramatic changes in neurogenesis in the hippocampus dentate gyrus subgranular zone following SE and neuronal injury. Quantification of the extent of neurogenesis and type of cells that are born after injury would be helpful to study the pathophysiological role of neurogenesis following SE and acute neuronal injury. Interestingly, hippocampal neurogenesis is very sensitive to physiological and pathological stimuli. Certain pathological stimuli such as seizures alter both the amount and the pattern of neurogenesis. Therefore, it is helpful to identify whether SE-induced changes in neurogenesis contribute to vulnerability to neurological conditions such as cognitive dysfunction, depression and epilepsy. Neurogenesis within the adult central nervous system is demonstrated using an exogenous cell tracer, 5'-bromo-2'-deoxyuridine (BrdU), in combination with endogenous neuronal markers.[111] Specific primary antibodies raised against these markers are widely available and their visualization is possible with the use of fluorescently tagged secondary antibodies. BrdU is a thymidine analog that incorporates into dividing cells during DNA synthesis. Once incorporated into the new DNA, BrdU will remain in place and be passed down to daughter cells following division. Typically, BrdU is injected intraperitoneally. Different survival times required by the desired experimental time-line will yield data on specific phases of neurogenesis: proliferation, differentiation and maturation. One limitation of using BrdU is uncertain penetration of the targeted cells with a uniform concentration of the compound. Thus, for experiments requiring measurements of cell proliferation, Ki67 can be used as an acceptable alternative. The protocol takes 3–5 days, allowing for sectioning and staining.[112]

Mossy Fiber (MF) Sprouting

Sprouting of neuronal axons including MF that contain zinc is generally visualized with Timm staining.[113] In the chronic epilepsy model, MF sprouting is indicative of epileptogenesis and is commonly identified by Timm staining of the brain section at various intervals after induction of SE. There is little or subtle change in Timm staining in acute models of SE; MF sprouting is mostly observed in chronic post-SE models of TLE.

Neuroinflammation Markers

Neuroinflammation is a common consequence of seizures and other neuronal injury events. Acute seizures and SE causes neuroinflammation by activating microglia, astrocytes, and induction and enhancement of inflammatory cytokines such as IL-1β, IL-6 and TNF in key brain regions such as the hippocampus. Further seizure related expression of inflammatory cytokines occurs in brain regions that may undergo neuronal damage A recent report suggests that seizure-induced release of inflammatory cytokines like IL-1β from astrocytes may cause brain inflammation and damage the blood brain barrier. Neuroinflammation and its secondary consequences may partly contribute to generation of recurrence of seizures.[111] Immunohistochemistry of brain sections for specific glial markers such as glial fibrillary acidic protein (GFAP, astrocytes) and Iba-1 (microglia) is helpful to identify the pattern of neuroinflammation and relevant damage. There is a marked increase in the number of astrocytes and microglia and their processes due to inflammation. It is shown that the neurosteroid allopregnanolone can reduce inflammation in traumatic brain injury models. Quantification of biomarkers of neuroinflammation is also very helpful to assess the course of inflammation following seizures and neuronal injury events.

CONCLUSION

A large number of *in vitro* and *in vivo* models for screening of antiepileptic drugs are available. However, there are many more models of seizures than of epilepsies. An ideal model of epilepsy should show the following characteristics:

- Development of spontaneously occurring seizures
- Type of seizure similar to that seen in human epilepsy
- EEG correlates of epileptic-like activity
- Age-dependency in the onset of epilepsy as is seen in many epileptic syndromes

At present, there are no models that satisfy all these criteria. Only the genetic animal models of epilepsy come closest to being called ideal, as they resemble idiopathic epilepsy in humans more closely than any other experimental model. These models can prove to be very valuable for screening of antiepileptic drugs, especially for drug-resistant epilepsies.

The Antiepileptic Drug Development Program of the National Institute of Neurological and Communicative Disorders and Stroke (NINCDS) of the National Institute of Health (NIH), USA is primarily based on two seizure models, the MES test and the s.c. PTZ test,[108] which predict drug efficacy against generalized tonic-clonic and absence seizures, respectively. These models have proved to be very useful for screening of putative antiepileptic drugs.

In vitro models are also very important for gaining insight into the pathophysiology of epilepsies and understanding the mechanism of action of drugs. They are useful in screening of drugs having specific mechanism of action, e.g. the use of [^{3}H] GABA uptake assay for screening of drugs that act by inhibiting GABA uptake.

To conclude, it must be emphasized that use of a single method for screening of antiepileptic drugs cannot predict the full pharmacological profile of the drug. Thus, for successful development of a potential antiepileptic drug, effect of drug in various *in vitro* and *in vivo* models must be studied.

REFERENCES

1. Lowenstein DH. Seizures and epilepsy. In Braunwald E, Fauci AS, Kasper DL, Hauser SL, Longo DL, Jameson JL (Eds). Harrison's Principles of Internal Medicine. New York: McGraw Hill, 2001:2354-69.
2. Commission on Classification and Terminology of the International League Against Epilepsy. Proposal for revised clinical and electroencephalographic classification of epileptic seizures. Epilepsia 1981;22:489-501.
3. Stables JP, Bertram Ed, Dudek FE, Holmes G, Mathern G, Pitkanen, et al. Therapy discovery for pharmacoresistant epilepsy and for disease-modifying therapeutics: summary of the NIH/NINDS/AES models II workshop. Epilesia 2003;44:1472-8.
4. Fisher RS. The hippocampal slice. Am J EEG Tech 1987;27:1-14.
5. Fisher RS. Animal models of epilepsies. Brain Res Rev 1989;14:245-78.
6. Vogel HG. Antiepileptic Activity. In Vogel HG, (Ed): Drug Discovery and Evaluation. Pharmacological Assays. 2nd ed, Berlin: Springer 2002:401-95.

7. Kay AR, Wong RK. Isolation of neurons suitable for patch clamping from adult mammalian central nervous systems. J Neurosci Methods 1986;16:227-38.
8. McLarnon JG. The recording of action potential currents as an assessment for drug actions on excitable cells. J Pharmacol Methods 1991;26:105-11.
9. Lindau M, Neher E. Patch-clamp techniques for time-resolved capacitance measurements in single cells. Pflugers Arch 1988;411:137-46.
10. Brauner-Osborne H, Krogsgaard-Larsen P. Functional pharmacology of cloned heterodimeric $GABA_B$ receptors expressed in mammalian cells. Br J Pharmacol 1999;128:1370-4.
11. Sieghart W. Unraveling the function of $GABA_A$ receptor subtypes. Trends Pharmacol Sci 2000;21:411-3.
12. Edgar PP, Schwartz RD. Functionally relevant γ-aminobutyric acid A receptors: equivalence between receptor affinity (K_d) and potency (EC_{50})? Mol Pharmacol 1992;41:1124-9.
13. Goodnough DB, Hawkinson JE. Neuroactive steroid modulation of [^{3}H] muscimol binding to the $GABA_A$ receptor complex in rat cortex. Eur J Pharmacol 1995;288:157-62.
14. Heaulme M, Chambon JP, Leyris R, et al. Characterization of the binding of [^{3}H] SR 95531, a $GABA_A$ antagonist, to rat brain membranes. J Neurochem 1987;48:1677-86.
15. Sieghart W. Structure and pharmacology of γ-aminobutyric acid A receptor subtypes. Pharmacol Rev 1995;47:181-234.
16. Suzdak PD, Jansen JA. A review of the preclinical pharmacology of tiagabine: apotent and selective anticonvulsant GABA uptake inhibitor. Epilepsia 1995;36:612-26.
17. Im WB, Pregenzer JF, Thomsen DR. Effects of GABA and various allosteric ligands on TBPS binding to cloned rat $GABA_A$ receptor subtypes. Br J Pharmacol 1994;112:1025-30.
18. Dingledine R, Borges K, Bowie D, et al. The glutamate receptor ion channels. Pharmacol Rev 1999;51:7-61.
19. Davies J, Evans RH, Herrling PL, et al. CPP, a new potent and selective NMDA antagonist. Depression of central neuron responses, affinity for [^{3}H] D-AP-5 binding sites on brain membranes and anticonvulsant activity. Brain Res 1986;382:169-73.
20. Parsons CG, Danysz W, Quack G. Glutamate in central nervous system disorders as a target for drug development. Drug News Perspect 1998;11:523-69.
21. Tauboll E, Gjerstad L. Effects of antiepileptic drugs on the activation of glutamate receptors. Prog Brain Res 1998;116:385-93.
22. Kessler M, Terramani T, Lynch B, et al. A glycine site associated with N-Methyl-D-Aspartic acid receptors: characterization and identification of a new class of antagonists. J Neurochem 1989;52:1319-28.
23. Jansen KLR, Dragunow M, Faull RLM. 3H- Glycine-binding sites, NMDA and PCP receptors have similar distribution in the human hippocampus: an autoradiographic study. Brain Res 1989;482:174-8.
24. Goddard GV, McIntyre DC, Leech CK. A permanent change in brain function resulting from daily electrical stimulation. Exp Neurol 1969;25:295-330.
25. Marsan CA. Focal electrical stimulation. In Purpura DP, Penry JK, Tower D, Woodbury DM, Walter R (Eds): Experimental Models of Epilepsy—a Manual for the Laboratory Worker. New York: Raven Press 1972:147-72.
26. Swinyard EA. Electrically induced convulsions. In Purpura DP, Penry JK, Tower D, Woodbury DM, Walter R (Eds): Experimental Models of Epilepsy—a Manual for the Laboratory Worker. New York: Raven Press, 1972:433-58.
27. Loscher W, Schmidt D. Which animal models should be used in the search for new antiepileptic drugs? A proposal based on experimental and clinical considerations. Epilepsy Res 1988;2:145-81.
28. Merritt HH, Putnam TJ. A new series of anticonvulsant drugs tested by experiments on animals. Arch Neurol Psychiatry 1938;39:1003-15.
29. Porter RJ, Cereghino JJ, Gladding GD, et al. Antiepileptic drug development programme. Cleve Clin Q 1984;51:293-305.

30. Toman JEP, Everett GM. Anticonvulsants. In Laurence DR, Bachrach AL (Eds): Evaluation of Drug Activities: Pharmacometrics. London and New York: Academic Press, 1964:287-300.
31. Girgis M. Kindling as a model for limbic epilepsy. Neurosci 1981;6:1695-706.
32. Alonso-DeFlorida F, Delgado JMR. Lasting behavioral and EEG changes in cats induced by prolonged stimulation of amygdala. Am J Physiol 1958;193:223-9.
33. LaSalle GLG. Amygdaloid kindling in the rat: regional differences and general properties. In. Wada JA (Ed). Kindling II. New York: Raven Press, 1981:31-47.
34. Racine RJ. Modification of seizure activity by electrical stimulation. II. Motor Seizure. Electroencephalogr Clin Neurophysiol 1972;32:281-94.
35. Loscher W, Jackel R, Czuczwar SJ. Is amygdala kindling in rats a model for drug-resistant partial epilepsy? Exp Neurol 1986;93:211-26.
36. Wada JA, Osawa T. Spontaneous recurrent seizure state induced by daily amygdaloid stimulation in Senegalese baboon (Papiopapio). Neurology 1976;22:273-86.
37. Wada JA, Mizoguichi T, Osawa T. Secondarily generalized convulsive seizures induced by daily amygdaloid stimulation in rhesus monkeys. Neurology 1978;28:1026-36.
38. McNamara JO. Kindling: an animal model of complex partial epilepsy. Ann Neurol (Suppl.) 1984;16: S72-6.
39. Sangdee P, Turkanis SA, Karler R. Kindling-like effect induced by repeated corneal electroshock in mice. Epilepsia 1982;23:471-9.
40. Matagne A, Klitgaard H. Validation of corneally kindled mice: a sensitive screening model for partial epilepsy in man. Epilepsy Res 1998;31:59-71.
41. Lothman EW, Hatlelid JM, Zorumski CF, Conry JA, Moon PF, Perlin JB. Kindling with rapidly recurring hippocampal seizures. Brain Res 1985;360:83-91.
42. Lothman EW, Perlin JB, Salerno RA. Response properties of rapidly recurring hippocampal seizures in rats. Epilepsy Res 1988;2:356-66.
43. Lothman EW, Salerno RA, Perlin JB, Kaiser DL. Screening and characterization of antiepileptic drugs with rapidly recurring hippocampal seizures in rats. Epilepsy Res1988;2:367-79.
44. Giorgi O, Orlandi M, Lecca D, Corda MG. MK-801 prevents chemical kindling induced by pentylenetetrazol in rats. Eur J Pharmacol 1991;193(3):363-5.
45. Corda MG, Orlandi M, Lecca D, Carboni G, Frau V, Giorgi O. Pentylenetetrazol-induced kindling in rats: effect of GABA function inhibitors. Pharmacol Biochem Behav 1991;40:329-33.
46. Olsen RW. The GABA postsynaptic membrane receptor ionophore complex.Site of action of convulsant and anticonvulsant drugs. Mol Cell Biochem 1981;39:261-79.
47. Taylor CD, Gloor P. Behavioral alterations associated with generalized spike and wave discharges in the EEG of the cat. Exp Neurol 1984;83:167-86.
48. Pellegrini A, Gloor P, Sherwin AL. Effect of valproate sodium on generalized penicillin epilepsy in the cat. Epilepsia 1978;19:351-60.
49. Guberman A, Gloor P, Sherwin AL. Response of generalized penicillin epilepsy in the cat to ethosuximide and diphenylhydantoin. Neurology 1975;25:755-64.
50. Fariello RG. Parenteral penicillin in rats: an experimental model for multifocal epilepsy. Epilepsia 1976;16:217-22.
51. Meldrum BS, Horton RW. Convulsive effects of 4-deoxypyridoxine and of bicuculline in photosensitive baboons (Papiopapio) and in rhesus monkeys (Macaca mulatta). Brain Res 1971;35:419-36.
52. Bigler ED. Comparison of effects of bicuculline, strychnine, and picrotoxin with those of pentylenetetrazol on photically evoked after discharges. Epilepsia 1977;18:465-70.
53. Czuczwar SJ, Frey HH, Loscher W. Antagonism of N-methyl-D, L-aspartic acid-induced convulsions by antiepileptic drugs and other agents. Eur J Pharmacol 1985;108:273-80.
54. Allen IC, Grieve A, Griffiths R. Differential changes in the content of amino acid neurotransmitters in discrete regions of the rat brain prior to the onset and during the course of homocysteine-induced seizures. J Neurochem 1986;46:1582-92.

55. Meldrum BS, Horton RW, Brierley JB. Epileptic brain damage in adolescent baboons following seizures induced by allylglycine. Brain 1974;97:407-18.
56. Harris B. Cortical alterations due to methionine sulfoximine.Ultrastructure during seizure activity. Arch Neurol 1964;11:388-407.
57. Dawson Jr R, Bierkamper G. Fluorothyl seizure thresholds in mice treated neonatally with a single injection of monosodium glutamate (MSG): evaluation of experimental parameters in fluorothyl seizure testing. Pharmacol Biochem Behav 1987;28:165-9.
58. Snead III OC. Gamma-hydroxy butyrate model of generalized absence seizures: further characterization and comparison with other absence models. Epilepsia 1988;29:361-8.
59. Turski WA, Cavalheiro EA, Coimbra C, et al. Only certain antiepileptic drugs prevent seizures induced by pilocarpine. Brain Res Rev 1987;12:281-305.
60. Ward Jr AA. Topical convulsant metals. In Purpura DP, Penry JK, Tower D, Woodbury DM, Walter R (Eds): Experimental Models of Epilepsy—a Manual for the Laboratory Worker. New York: Raven Press, 1972;13-35.
61. Willmore LJ, Sypert GW, Munson JB, et al. Chronic focal epileptiform discharges induced by the injection of iron into rat and cat cortex. Science 1978;200:1501-3.
62. Kopeloff LM, Chusid JG, Kopeloff N. Epilepsy in Macacamulatta after cortical or intracerebral alumina. Arch Neurol Psychiatry 1955;74:523-6.
63. Cavalheiro EA, Riche DA, La Salle GLG. Long-term effects of intrahippocampalkainic acid injection in rats: a method for inducing spontaneous recurrent seizures. Electroencephalogr Clin Neurophysiol 1982; 53:581-9.
64. Mellanby J, Hawkins C, Mellanby H, et al. Tetanus toxin as a tool for studying epilepsy. J Physiol (Paris) 1984;79:207-15.
65. Matsumoto H, Marsan CA. Cortical cellular phenomena in experimental epilepsy: interictal manifestations. Exp Neurol 1964;9:286-304.
66. Turski WA, Czuczwar SJ, Kleinrolk Z, et al. Cholinomimetics produce seizures and brain damage in rats. Experimentia 1983;39:1408-11.
67. Daniels JC, Spehlmann R. The convulsant effect of topically applied atropine. Electroencephalogr Clin Neurophysiol 1973;34:83-7.
68. Usunoff G, Atsev E, Tchavdarov D. On the mechanisms of picrotoxin epileptic seizures (macro- and microelectrode investigations). Electroencephalogr Clin Neurophysiol 1969;27:444.
69. Campbell AM, Holmes O. Bicucullineepileptogenesis in the rat. Brain Res 1984;323:239-46.
70. Knopman DS. Acute strychnine-induced seizures in cats: a Golgi study. Epilepsia 1975;16:791-2.
71. Karpiak SE, Graf L, Rapport MM. Antiserum to brain gangliosides produces recurrent epileptiform activity. Science 1976;194:735-7.
72. Pei Y, Zhao D, Huang J, et al. Zinc induced seizures: a new experimental model of epilepsy. Epilepsia 1983; 24:169-76.
73. Loiseau H, Averet N, Arrigoni, et al. The early phase of cryogenic lesions: an experimental model of seizures updated. Epilepsia 1987;28:251-8.
74. Remler MP, Marcussen WH. Systemic focal epileptogenesis. Epilepsia 1986;27: 35-42.
75. Turski WA, Cavalheiro EA, Coimbra C, et al. Only certain antiepileptic drugs prevent seizures induced by pilocarpine. Brain Res 1987;434:281-305.
76. Biagini G, Avoli M, Marcinkiewicz J, et al. Brain-derived neurotrophic factor superinduction parallels anti-epileptic—neuroprotective treatment in the pilocarpine epilepsy model. J Neurochem 2001;76:1814-22.
77. Golarai G, Cavazos JE, Sutula TP. Activation of the dentate gyrus by pentylenetetrazol evoked seizures induces mossy fibre synaptic re-organisation. Brain Res 1992;593:257-64.
78. Jope RS, Morrisett RA, Snead OC. Characterization of lithium potentiation of pilocarpine-induced status epilepticus in rats. Exp Neurol 1986;91:471-80.

79. Morrisett RA, Jope RS, Snead OC. Effects of drugs on the initiation and maintenance of status epilepticus induced by administration of pilocarpine to lithium-pretreated rats. Exp Neurol 1987;97:193-200.
80. Walton NY, Treiman DM. Response to status epilepticus induced by lithium and pilocarpine to treatment with diazepam. Exp Neurol 1988;101:267-75.
81. Druga R, Kubova H, Suchomelova L, et al. Lithium/pilocarpine status epilepticus-induced neuropathology of piriform cortex and adjoining structures in rats is age-dependent. Physiol Res 2003;52:251-64.
82. Agrawal N, Alonso A, Ragsdale DS. Increased persistent sodium currents in rat entorhinal cortex layer V neurons in a post-status epilepticus model of temporal lobe epilepsy. Epilepsia 2003;44:1601-4.
83. Kaminski RM, Blaszczak P, Dekundy A, et al. Lithium-methomyl induced seizures in rats: a new model of status epilepticus? Toxicol Appl Pharmacol 2007;219:122-7.
84. Gibbs JE, Walker MC, Cock HR. Levetiracetam: antiepileptic properties and protective effects on mitochondrial dysfunction in experimental status epilepticus. Epilepsia 2006;47:469-78.
85. Walton NY, Treiman DM. Experimental secondarily generalized convulsive status epilepticus induced by D,L-homocysteinethiolactone. Epilepsy Res 1988;2:79-86.
86. Meldrum BS, Horton RW, Toseland PA. A primate model for testing anticonvulsant drugs. Arch Neurol 1975;32:289-94.
87. Velisek L, Jehle K, Asche MS, Veliskova MD. Model of infantile spasms induced by N-methyl-D-aspartic acid in prenatally impaired brain. Ann Neurol 2007;61:109-19.
88. Killiam KF, Naquet R, Bert J. Paroxysmal responses to intermittent light stimulation in a population of baboons (Papiopapio). Epilepsia 1966;7:215-19.
89. Naquet R, Meldrum BS. Photogenic seizures in baboon. In Purpura DP, Penry JK, Tower D, Woodbury DM, Walter R (Eds): Experimental Models of Epilepsy—a Manual for the Laboratory Worker. New York: Raven Press, 1972:373-406.
90. Seyfried TN. Audiogenic seizures in mice. Fed Proc 1978;38:2399-404.
91. Seyfried TN, Glaser GH. A review of mouse mutants as genetic models of epilepsy. Epilepsia 1985;26: 143-50.
92. Swinyard EA, Castellion AW, Fink GB, et al. Some neurophysiological and neuropharmacological characteristics of audiogenic seizure susceptible mice. J Pharmacol Exp Ther 1963;140:375-84.
93. Kaplan BJ, Seyfried TN, Glaser GH. Spontaneous poly-spike discharges in an epileptic mutant mouse (tottering). ExpNeurol 1979;66:577-86.
94. Loscher W. Genetic animal models of epilepsy as a unique resource for the evaluation of anticonvulsant drugs: A review. Methods Find Exp Clin Pharmacol 1984;6:531-47.
95. Noebels JL, Sidman RL. Inherited epilepsy: Spike-wave and focal motor seizures in the mutant mouse tottering. Science 1979;204:1334-6.
96. Heller AH, Dichter MA, Sidman RL. Anticonvulsant sensitivity of absence seizures in the tottering mutant mouse. Epilepsia 1983;24:25-34.
97. Imaizumi K, Ito S, Kutsukake G, et al. Epilepsy-like anomaly of mice. ExpAnim (Tokyo) 1959;8:6-10.
98. Suzuki J, Nakamoto Y. Seizure patterns and electroencephalograms of E1 mouse. Electro-encephalogr Clin Neurophysiol 1977;43:299-311.
99. Taylor SM, Bennett GD, Abbott LC, et al. Seizure control following administration of anticonvulsant drugs in the quaking mice. Eur J Pharmacol 1985;118:163-70.
100. Hosford DA, Wang Y. Utility of the lethargic (lh/lh) mouse model of absence seizures in predicting the effects of lamotrigine, vigabatrine, tiagabine, gabapentin, and topiramate against human absence seizures. Epilepsia 1997;38:408-14.
101. Reigel CE, Dailey JW, Jobe PC. The genetically epilepsy-prone rat: an overview of seizure-prone characteristics and responsiveness to anticonvulsant drugs. Life Sci 1986;39:763-74.

102. Van Luijtelaar ELJ, Coenen AM. Two types of electrocortical paroxysms in an inbred strain of rats. Neurosci Lett 1986;70:393-7.
103. Thiessen DD, Lindzey G, Friend HC. Spontaneous seizures in the Mongolian gerbil (Meriones unguiculatus). Psychon Sci 1968;11:227-8.
104. Kaplan H. What triggers seizures in the gerbil, Meriones unguiculatus? Life Sci 1975; 17: 693-8.
105. Yoon CH, Peterson JS, Corrow D. Spontaneous seizures: a new mutation in Syrian golden hamsters. J Hered 1976; 67:115-6.
106. Crawford RD. A new mutant causing epileptic seizures in domestic fowls. Poultry Sci 1969;48:1799.
107. Hegreberg GA, Padgett GA. Inherited progressive epilepsy of the dog with comparison to Lafora's disease of man. Fed Proc 1976;35:1202-5.
108. Gladding GD, Kupferberg HJ, Swinyard EA. Antiepileptic drug development programme. In Frey HH, Janz D (Eds): Antiepileptic Drugs. Handbook of Experimental Pharmacology. Berlin: Springer, 1985;341-7.
109. Rao MS, Hattiangady B, Reddy DS, Shetty AK. Hippocampal neurodegeneration, spontaneous seizures, and mossy fiber sprouting in the F344 rat model of temporal lobe epilepsy. J. Neurosci. Res 2006;83:1088-105.
110. Zeng LH, Rensing NR, Wong M. The mammalian target of rapamycin signaling pathway mediates epileptogenesis in a model of temporal lobe epilepsy. J Neurosci 2009;29:6964–72.
111. Rao MS, Hattiangady B, Reddy DS, Shetty AK. Hippocampal neurodegeneration, spontaneous seizures, and mossy fiber sprouting in the F344 rat model of temporal lobe epilepsy. J Neurosci. Res 2006;83:1088–105.
112. Kuruba R, Shetty AK. Could hippocampal neurogenesis be a future drug target for treating temporal lobe epilepsy? CNS Neurol Disord Drug Targets 2007;6:342–57.
113. Sloviter RS. A simplified Timm stain procedure compatible with formaldehyde fixation and routine paraffin embedding of rat brain. Brain Res Bull 1982;8:771–4.
114. Librizzi L, Noè F, Vezzani A, de Curtis M, Ravizza T. Seizure-induced brain-borne inflammation sustains seizure recurrence and blood-brain barrier damage. Ann Neurol 2012;72:82-90.

CHAPTER

29

Anti-Alzheimer Agents

INTRODUCTION

Alzheimer's disease (AD, the most common form of age-related dementia), is a progressive irreversible neurodegenerative disorder that was first identified and written by Dr. Alois Alzheimer in early 1900s. It occurs gradually affecting the short-term memory at the beginning of the disease, followed by long-term memory loss and results in cognitive impairment, unusual behavior, personality changes, and ultimately death. It is the most common form of adult onset dementia.[1] With the expected aging of the human population, the estimated morbidity of AD suggests a critical upcoming health problem (Juan et al, 2014).[2] Presently, it is the 4th leading cause of death in Western countries, preceded only by heart disease, cancer and stroke.[3] The total number of people with dementia worldwide in 2010 is estimated at 35.6 million and is projected to nearly double every 20 years, to 65.7 million in 2030 and 115.4 million in 2050. The total number of new cases of dementia each year worldwide is nearly 7.7 million, implying one new case every four seconds (Duthey, 2013).[4] Age is by far the main risk factor for AD; its prevalence illustrates an exponential rise with age.[3] Much of the increase is in developing countries, especially India, and their south Asian and western Pacific neighbors (Duthey, 2013).[4]

Approximately 5% of all AD cases have an early onset and are familial, based on mutations of presenilin 1, presenilin 2 or the beta amyloid precursor protein (APP).[5] By contrast, approximately 95% of all AD cases represent the sporadic or late onset form of disease showing no mutations of presenilin 1, presenilin 2 or APP.[6]

AD involves neuronal degeneration with impaired cholinergic transmission in the cerebral cortex and hippocampus in areas of the brain particularly associated with memory and higher intellectual functioning. The primary pathology in AD occurs in the basal forebrain that provides the major cholinergic innervations to the neocortex, hippocampus and amygdala.[7] There is a dramatic loss of neurons and synapses in these areas and are characterized by a number of important pathological changes. The pathophysiology is complex and involves multiple interconnected pathways.[9] It is thought to arise from an interaction of several risk factors, including genetic susceptibility, increased age, female gender, and perhaps a lower premorbid intelligence level.

The cardinal histopathological manifestations of AD are the neurofibrillary tangles (NFT) and amyloid plaques (AP). The NFT is present in the neurons as paired helical filaments and composed of hyperphosphorylated tau and the AP which is composed of a cluster of dystrophic neurites and a few abnormal synapses surrounding a core of beta amyloid are present extracellularly.[8]

The Aβ hypothesis of AD stipulates that increased brain levels of Aβ appear to be a critical event in triggering a wide range of molecular alterations leading to AD (Fig. 29.1). It has been proposed that exposure to sub-toxic concentrations of metals, such as copper, affects secondary structures and acts as a seeding or nucleation core that facilitates Aβ aggregation. Aβ aggregates to form amyloid plaques that are neurotoxic, leading to neurodegeneration accompanied by dementia. The strongest evidence for this hypothesis comes from molecular genetic studies of APP and presenilins in familial AD showing that all mutations increased the propensity for Aβ to aggregate *in vitro*. Studies of the modifier gene product, apolipoprotein E, showing enhanced susceptibility conferred by the E4 allele also found that the E4 isoform increased the rate of Aβ aggregation.

Recently newer hypotheses have been proposed regarding pathogenesis of AD. For one, it is hypothesized that Peroxisome Proliferator-Activated Receptors (PPAR) are nuclear receptors that have potential role in exerting neuroprotective effects in various neurodegenerative disorders, especially AD. This nuclear receptor subgroup is implicated to play a key role in Aβ clearance and shows potential use in AD therapy (Cramer et al, 2012).[10] Another hypothesis proposes that cerebral glucose metabolism is perturbed in the pathogenesis of AD (Fig. 29.2). Abnormality of glucose transportation contributes to intracellular glucose catabolism dysfunction resulting in neuronal degeneration and consequently cognitive deficits in AD patients. Thus, induction of multiple pathogenic factors such as oxidative stress,

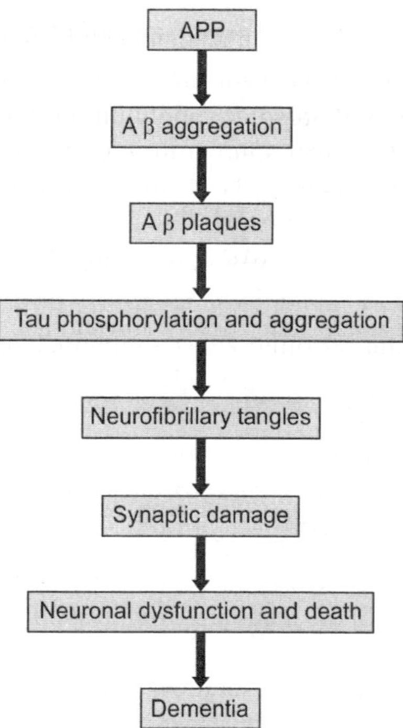

Figure 29.1: Aβ hypothesis of AD

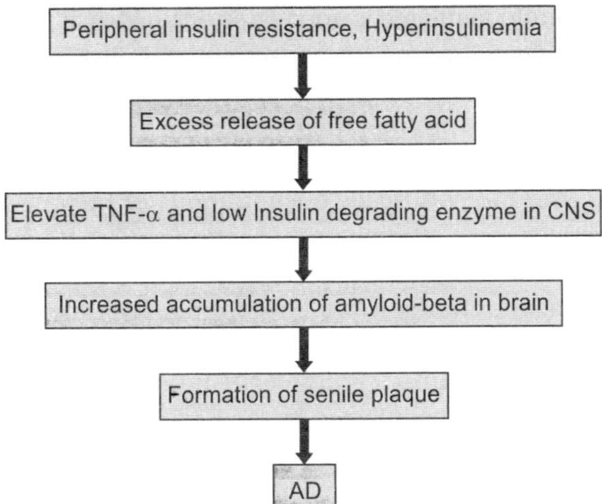

Figure 29.2: Cerebral glucose metabolism hypothesis of AD

mitochondrial dysfunction, and cerebral hypometabolism, etc. are understood to be both causes and consequences of AD (Chen and Zhong, 2013).[11]

Effective treatment and prevention strategies and management of attendant behavioral disturbances are paramount to the management of this illness. The efficacy of any given intervention will ultimately be judged upon its ability to prevent memory loss or restore memory ability. New therapeutic measures against dementia in AD are being aimed at a variety of targets deemed instrumental in the pathogenesis of the disease. The two main targets are amyloid plaques and neurofibrillary tangles and their principal molecular components, Aβ and tau.

The management includes inhibitors of cholinesterase (tacrine, donepezil). However, these drugs are not able to contain the progression of the disease. Moreover, the improvement is modest and a high morbidity exists. Side effects like abdominal cramps, nausea, vomiting and diarrhea are dose limiting. For the development of therapeutic drugs, valid animal models are needed that mimic the pathophysiological change in brain functions and the concomitant behavioral deterioration seen in AD patients.

The ideal model should exhibit the same biochemical, histopathologic and behavioral abnormalities as the human disease state. Behavioral models for studying memory storage, recall and its manipulation by pharmacological agents do not present the typical pathophysiology of AD, i.e. extracellular deposits of beta-amyloid in senile plaques, intracellular accumulations of NFT.[12]

Most of the models currently in use are at best 'Isomorphic Models.' Thus, for the induction and simulation of the pathophysiology underlying AD in experimental animals, amnesia-inducing agents like scopolamine and colchicine are available. Their dosages, mechanisms along with comparative merits and demerits have been tabulated (Table 29.1). The effect of test drug can then be compared to the standard drug in such amnesic animals on the basis of behavioral tests.

The paradigms used for learning and memory can be discussed under two behavioral tasks: behavior in avoidance chambers (active and passive avoidance) and behavior on mazes (elevated plus maze, water maze, etc).

Table 29.1: Comparison of the various amnesic agents

Amnesic agent	*Mechanism of action*	*Dose, route and animal*	*Manifestation*	*Remarks*
Scopolamine	Musacarinic antagonist	0.3-1 mg/kg, ip, mice[33]	Cognitive impairment.	Effect similar to normal elderly but not patients of AD.[32] Unlike the disease the effects are reversible with no compromise of presynaptic cholinergic neurons.[28] Does not produce pathological hallmarks of AD (AP and NFT).
Iboteic acid	Excitotoxicity	Ibotenic acid: 12 g/ml Bilateral lesion in basal forebrain, rats	Cognitive impairment Fall in choline acetyl transferase activity (ChAT).[34]	Kainic acid is also a potent anticonvulsant and can produce distant damage (ibotenic acid is referred).[24] They do not produce the histological characteristics of AD.
Kainic acid		Kainic acid: 1.5-2.5 nM, Nucleus basalis Meynert (nbM)	Decreases ChAT by 70% on 5th day.[35]	Since these excititoxins are not specific to cholinergic cells, they provide limited information on the specific role of cholinergic system in learning and memory deficits.
Streptozotocin	Depletes insulin receptors in brain leading to abnormal glucose metabolism, and cognitive deficit	3 mg/kg, ICV, rat	Damage to myelinated neurons in fornix and corpus callosum, microgliosis),[36] cognitive sporadic impairment, increase in oxidative stress 21st day post-lesion.[37, 39]	Mimics the abnormalities of glucose and energy metabolism found in the brains of patients of AD.[38]
Colchicine	Microtubule inhibitor causing cell death	7.5-14 µg, ICV, rat	Depletion of ACh, ChAT and decrease in muscarinic receptor binding in frontal cortex and hippocampus,[39] produces oxidative stress in brain post-lesion[40]	Selectively lesions cholinergic input into the hippocampus Significant impairment of learning and memory Decrease ChAT activity in the hippocampus Do not produce pathological hallmarks of AD (AP and NFT).
Scopolamine	Musacarinic antagonist	0.3-1 mg/kg, ip, Mice	Cognitive impairment	Effect similar to normal elderly but not patients of AD.[32] Unlike the disease the effects are reversible with no compromise of presynaptic cholinergic neurons.[28] Does not produce pathological hallmarks of AD (AP and NFT).

Contd...

Contd...

Amnesic agent	*Mechanism of action*	*Dose, route and animal*	*Manifestation*	*Remarks*
Iboteic acid	Excitotoxicity	Ibotenic acid: 12 g/ml Bilateral lesion in basal forebrain, rats	Cognitive impairment Fall in choline acetyl transferase activity (ChAT).[34]	Kainic acid is also a potent anticonvulsant and can produce distant damage (ibotenic acid is referred).[24] They do not produce the histological characteristics of AD.
Kainic acid		Kainic acid: 1.5-2.5 nM, Nucleus basalis Meynert (nbM)	Decreases ChAT by 70% on 5th day.[35]	Since these excititoxins are not specific to cholinergic cells, they provide limited information on the specific role of cholinergic system in learning and memory deficits.
Streptozotocin	Depletes insulin receptors in brain leading to abnormal glucose metabolism, and cognitive deficit	3 mg/kg, ICV, rat	Damage to myelinated neurons in fornix and corpus callosum, microgliosis),[36] cognitive sporadic impairment, increase in oxidative stress 21st day post-lesion.[39]	Mimics the abnormalities of glucose and energy metabolism found in the brains of patients of AD.[38]
Colchicine	Microtubule inhibitor causing cell death	7.5-14 μg, ICV, rat	Depletion of ACh, ChAT and decrease in muscarinic receptor binding in frontal cortex and hippocampus,[39] produces oxidative stress in brain post-lesion[40]	Selectively lesions cholinergic input in to the hippocampus hippocampus Significant impairment of learning and memory Decrease ChAT activity in the hippocampus Do not produce pathological hallmarks of AD (AP and NFT).
Ethylcholine mustard aziridinum-AF64A	Structural analogue of choline and selectively cytotoxic against cholinergic-neurons.[21]	1-3 nmol/side, ICV, rat 4 nmol/side/ straitum, rat 2.5 nmol/nbM, rat	Cognitive impairment, fall in Ach[41] and ChAT activity.[42]	Selectively targets cholinergic system and decreases ACh, without altering other neurotransmitters, while AD is multineurotransmitter disease. Does not produce pathological hallmarks of AD (AP and NFT).
192-IgG-saporin	Antineuronal immunotoxin, targets selectively cholinergic nerve terminals in basal forebrain	0.22-1 μg, medial septum, rat[38] 2 μg, ICV, rat[43]	Cognitive impairment, fall in ACh and ChAT activity.[45]	Does not produce pathological hallmarks of AD (AP and NFT).
Intracerebral beta amyloid (Aβ) injections	Beta amyloid is the primary constituent of the amyloid plaques	Aβ[25-35], 20 μg, hippocampus, rat[46] Aβ [1-40], 10-20 μg × 3 days, ICV, rat[47]	Produces behavioral, neurochemical and immunohistochemical changes similar to AD	Throws light on the molecular mechanism of Aβ toxicity and gives support to the pivotal role of Aβ in AD pathogenesis.

Intracerebroventricular (ICV) route is the favored route of drug administration as it allows the drug to be directly injected to the appointed site and bypasses the blood-brain barrier. However, the technique requires good expertise in surgical manipulations and postoperative care of the animals. In contrast, systemic injections are easier to administer, but require higher dose of the test drug, which may inadvertently lead to unwanted side effects. The techniques of brain microdialysis and osmotic minipumps provide a suitable alternative.

IN VITRO AND *EX VIVO* MODELS

Transfected Cell Lines

HEK293 cells are transfected with human APP_{695} and N2a cells with human APP_{695} cDNAs. APP_{695}-HEK293 transfectants are grown in Dulbecco's modified Eagle's medium plus 10% fetal bovine serum, penicillin and streptomycin, whereas, APP_{695}-N2a cells are maintained in Dulbecco's modified Eagle's medium supplemented with 5% fetal bovine serum, penicillin and streptomycin. For drug treatments, cells are treated at confluence as per indicated concentrations and for desired incubation time. Medium is changed regularly, and treatments are continued. For siRNA-directed silencing, 200 pmol of purified siRNA directed against the proteasome subunit β5 are transfected with 10 μl of Lipofectamine 2000 in APP_{695}-HEK293 cells plated in 35 mm dishes. At 48 h post-transfection, cells are incubated in the absence or presence of test drug for another 24 h. Cells and conditioned medium are harvested and analyzed (Marambaud P, Zhao H, Davies P).[13]

Study of Field Excitatory Postsynaptic Potentials

Long-term potentiation (LTP) is a form of synaptic plasticity, which exhibits several features that make it an attractive candidate as the neural basis of vertebrate learning and memory.[14] Study of the amplitude of field excitatory postsynaptic potentials (fEPSPs) evoked in the hippocampal slices, may help to understand the underlying mechanisms involved.

Adult female Wistar rats weighing between 150 g and 200 g are housed under standard laboratory conditions of light, temperature, food and water. The animals are singularly housed in clean cages. On the day of the experiment, they are anesthetized using halothane and decapitated. Transverse hippocampal slices, 400 μm thick, are prepared. The CA3 region is removed before the slices are transferred to a recording chamber at the interface between a warmed (29-31°C) artificial cerebrospinal fluid and oxygen enriched (95% O_2/5% CO_2) humidified atmosphere. The standard perfusion medium comprising of (mM) NaCl 124, KCl 3, $NaHCO_3$ 26, NaH_2PO_4 1.24, $CaCl_2$ 2, $MgSO_4$ 1,D-glucose 10, is bubbled with 95% O_2/5% CO_2 and perfused at a rate of 1 ml/min. Extracellular recordings of fEPSP are obtained from stratum radiatum of the CA1 region using 3 M NaCl filled glass electrodes (resistance 2-10 MΩ). The Schaffer collateral-commissural fibers are stimulated every 30 sec using a bipolar stimulating electrode placed in stratum radiatum towards the fimbrial end of the slice. The stimulus strength is adjusted to evoke a fEPSP half the maximum amplitude and a stable baseline of at least 15-20 min is recorded before any drugs are added. Test drug is administered either by addition to the perfusion fluid for a period of 5 min, or by iontophoresis into the CA1 recording region.

For iontophoretic experiments, triple-barrelled electrodes can be used in which one barrel is used for recording, one contains drug solution and one contains 200 mM NaCl for current balancing. The resistance of the drug and balance barrels is 40-80 MΩ and a holding current of 25-40 nA is applied to the drug barrel to limit leakage.[15]

Cultures of Rat Cerebral Cortical and Hippocampal Neurons

Cultures of rat cerebral cortical and hippocampal neurons have been used to evaluate various intracellular mechanisms involved in synaptic plasticity, neuronal development and learning and memory.[16]

Timed pregnant Sprague-Dawley rats are procured and housed individually in a climate-controlled environment on a 12 h light/dark cycle with free access to food and water. Newborn rat pups are anesthetized with pentobarbitone and their cerebral cortices are dissected and placed in an isotonic salt solution containing 100 units of penicillin G, 100 µg of streptomycin, and 25 µg of amphotericin B per milliliter, pH 7.4. The pia mater and the blood vessels are cleaned from the cortices, which are then chopped into pieces and incubated in 4 ml of an isotonic salt solution containing 0.25% trypsin (w/v) in a shaking water bath at 37°C for 10 min. The reaction is stopped by the addition of 4 ml of 0.016% DNase and further incubation is carried out in a water bath for 5 min. After incubation, regular DMEM (with 10% PDHS) is added and the cells are triturated to dissociate them. The cell suspension is then centrifuged at 600 g for 10 min at 24°C. The supernatant is aspirated and the pellet is resuspended in regular DMEM and plated onto poly-L-lysine-coated culture dishes at a density of 3×10^6 cells/35 mm dish. The dishes are then incubated at 37°C in a 5% CO_2, 95% O_2 atmosphere. On day 3, the media is replaced with fresh DMEM containing 10µ M β-cytosine arabinoside to diminish glial cell proliferation. On day 5, the β-cytosine arabinoside-containing media is aspirated and regular DMEM is added to the cells. The cells are grown for seven more days. The cells express receptors belonging to glutamate family and the cellular mechanism for memory can be studied using these cells in the presence of various agonists and antagonists.[16]

Similarly, hippocampal cultures can be prepared and utilized for determining *in vitro* effects of test drugs. In brief, the hippocampus is dissected, chopped into pieces, and incubated with 2 ml of0.25% trypsin (w/v) in a 37°C water bath for 10 min. The reaction is stopped by addition of 2 ml of 0.016% DNase, followed by four to five times trituration with a fire-polished pipette and a 5 min incubation at 37°C. The supernatant is transferred to a tube containing 20 ml of DMEM/PDHS, and the trypsin treatment is repeated two more times. The procedure for the cortical cultures is then followed and the cells are plated at a density of 1×10^6 cells/35 mm dish. The neurons are maintained similarly to the cortical cultures. The cells are rinsed and incubated for 50 min at 37°C in HEPES buffer (140 mM NaCl, 5.4 mM KCl, 1.8 mM $CaCl_2$, 100 nM glycine, 15 mM glucose, and 25 mM HEPES, pH 7.4) containing 1 µM tetrodotoxin, TTX. Drug treatment is carried out.

Motor-based Intracellular Transport

Motor-based intracellular transport involves directed movement of cargos along microtubules and forms a key component of transport within a cell. Its regulation is crucial to the functioning of a cell, as disruption of transport is linked to Alzheimer's and other neurodegenerative diseases.[17] A model of two-motor arrangement driven cargo transport is one of the simplest case of intracellular motor transport. Motors frequently detach and reattach; so as to transport cargo to the microtubules. Involvement of at least one motor is essential for the transport. In the presence of tau protein, rebinding is suppressed. Therefore, once the first motor disengages from the microtubules, it is unlikely to reattach before the second motor also detaches. The processive motion ceases and is diffused away. Tau protein assumes importance as it reduces cargo travel distances. By blocking rebinding, tau reduces the number of motors that on average drive the cargo. Therefore, tau reduces the total force that the motors can apply to move the cargo as also the force needed to detach the cargoes from microtubules.

This model suggests that it might be possible to regulate the number of engaged motors by controlling motor on rate, i.e. how long it takes motors to bind to the microtubules. The more quickly the motors can reattach to a microtubule, the more time it will spend actively participating in transport. Conversely, if the motors' on rates were lowered, on average fewer of the geometrically available active motors would be bound at any given time. Tau critically controls the number of engaged motors and thereby cargo transport. Thus, this model depicts a potentially important mechanism of local regulation of intracellular transport mechanism.

Hypoxia-induced Memory Deficit

Oxygen homeostasis is essential for the development and physiology of an organism. Hypoxia-inducible factor-1 (HIF-1) (is the principal molecule regulating oxygen homeostasis. The hypoxia) signal transduction pathway plays a major role in vascular development and ischemia, as well as in neurodegeneration.

APP23 transgenic mice carry the human APP751 cDNA with the Swedish double mutation at positions 670/671 (KM→NL) under control of the murine Thy-1.2 expression cassette. Littermates of APP23 mice carrying no human Swedish mutant APP751 cDNA are used as controls. APP23 mice (8 months of age, n = 20, 50% female) are assigned randomly to hypoxia and control groups. The hypoxia group was treated in a hypoxia chamber at 8% O_2 for 16 h/day for 1 month. The oxygen level is regulated by infusing nitrogen into a semisealable chamber controlled by a controller.

This model is useful for evaluating the hypoxia facilitated enzyme cleavage of APP and deposition of Aβ.[18]

Acetylcholinesterase Activity

The procedure was first described by Ellman (1961) and is also known as Ellman Esterase Assay.[19] The method aims to determine the rate of hydrolysis of acetylthiocholine (ATCh) by acetylcholinesterase (AChE) or butyrylcholinesterase (BChE) in tissues taken from the laboratory rat or dog.

This assay is a spectrophotometric method, which involves two linked reactions to produce a colored compound. The production of the compound is monitored by measuring the absorbance of light by the reaction mixture over time. ATCh is hydrolyzed enzymatically to give acetate and thiocholine. Thiocholine reacts with 5,5'-dithiobis-2-nitrobenzoic acid (DTNB) producing the yellow colored 5-thio-2-thionitrobenzoic acid anion (TNB). TNB has absorbance maxima at a wavelength of 412 nm.

Rat striata are homogenized in 10 volumes of 0.1 M phosphate buffer (pH 8.0). Five minutes after the addition of 400 µl of homogenate, 30 µl of test compound solution at various concentrations, and 100 µl of DTNB (10 mM) to 2.45 ml of 0.1 M phosphate buffer (pH 8.0) are added and AChE activity is determined at 25°C over 1 min in a photocell after the addition of 20 µl of acetylthiocholine iodide (75 mM) as substrate.

A substrate blank (i.e., no tissue, only substrate and buffer and DTNB) should be run with each group of assays; this measures nonenzymatic substrate hydrolysis. A tissue blank (i.e., only tissue, buffer and DTNB but no substrate) should be run for each tissue to determine the degree of binding of DTNB to sulfhydryls in the tissue sample. If this is minimal after the preincubation period, then the tissue blank will not be needed on a regular basis for that tissue.

IN VIVO MODELS

The development of animal models mimicking the complex pathogenesis and clinical symptoms of AD still represents a challenge for the preclinical investigators. There is no ideal model of AD, but there are several models, which may help in the screening of potential therapeutic agents so as to accomplish an effective armamentarium to combat AD.

Aging Animals (Rodents and Monkeys)

Impairment of learning and memory in aging animals are severe and consistent with behavioral impairments in the elderly. Since AD is a neurodegenerative disorder associated with aging, aged animals are the most common for investigating drugs potentially active on AD. This model has several advantages namely; (a) old mice and rats are used most frequently since they are easy to obtain and relatively cheap, (b) aged rodents and monkeys show cognitive impairment. Old monkeys have been used as the last preclinical step before clinical trials, and (c) amyloid beta plaques, one of the classical pathological hallmarks, have also been found in aged (23 to 31 years) rhesus monkeys. Therefore, testing in nonhuman primates is an important model.[20,21]

The limitations of this model being: (a) since aging and AD are distinct, aged rodents and monkeys are not ideal animals for this disease, (b) old monkeys are expensive for drug screening, and (c) the poor health of aged animals and individual pharmacokinetic variabilities in drug absorption, metabolism, and distribution may sometimes yield statistically inconclusive data.[22,23]

Transgenic Mice

Identification of AD-related genes (four genes located on chromosomes 21, 19, 14 and 1) has made it possible to rationally design transgenic animal models and test some of the hypothetical mechanisms of amyloidogenesis. The mutations of these genes cause changes in processing of APP, leading to amyloid formation in the brain.[24]

There are now a number of genetically engineered Alzheimer's mouse models. Transgenic mice expressing familial AD mutations or fragments of normal APP: the Minnesota mouse and exemplar/Athena mouse have been developed. Both these models are characterized by accumulation and deposition of amyloid, Minnesota mouse at 7 to 12 months and Athena mouse at 4 to 8 months of age. However, data published for these two models seem to indicate that several key features of AD are established; but in either model, there is no change in the number of neurons in those areas of the brain in which amyloid deposits are found. Moreover, there are no reports showing degeneration of the cholinergic cells of the basal forebrain in APP transgenic mice.[25-27]

Of other transgenic AD animal models exhibiting senile plaques and Abeta-associated neuropathology, different types of transgenic mice expressing human APP, Abeta, the C-terminal fragment of APP and the APP genes carrying familial AD mutations have been created. Transgenic mice over-expressing human APP751, which develop early AD like histopathology with diffuse deposits of Abeta and aberrant tau protein immunoreactivity in some, exhibit age-dependent deficits in spatial learning in a water maze task and in spontaneous alteration behavior in a Y-maze. Transgenic mice models have been reported by number of research groups. The most commonly used models express variants of amyloid precursor protein (APP), presenilin-1 (ps1) or presenilin-2, tau or apolipoprotein E.

The development of transgenic (Tg) mice that over express the Swedish mutation of human APP has been developed. Amyloid plaques in hAPPs mouse brain, like those seen in human AD patients, lead to activated microglia, oxidative stress and alterations in neurotransmitter systems. Distribution of amyloid plaques is not uniform and densely concentrated in the cortex, hippocampus, and amygdala throughout the brains of Tg2576 mice. This is similar to the nature and pattern of the neuropathology seen in human AD patients.

One of the main challenges in cognitive studies of APP transgenic mice has been determining the onset of memory deficits.[28] Although, transgenic mice develop a wide variety of behavioral, biochemical, pathological, and physiological traits, not all traits have been represented within an individual mouse line.

Bigenic Mice

All of the transgenic mice used to evaluate potential therapeutic interventions have been APP transgenic mice or APP/ps1 bigenic mice, because they are the only transgenic mouse models in which both amyloid deposition and progressive memory loss have been shown. The lack of neurofibrillary tangles or significant neuronal loss in app or app/ps1 mice limits the utility of the model. It is possible to produce both amyloid plaques and neurofibrillary tangles within individual mice by crossing APP to tau transgenic mice, the resultant mice are not suitable for learning or memory assessments because they become paralyzed.[29]

Triple Transgenic Mouse Model

3xTg-AD mouse is a Triple Transgenic Mouse Model of AD mouse, which shows etiopathology similar to the progression of the disease in humans. An age-dependent increase in soluble amyloid β (Aβ), its neuronal accumulation and extracellular deposition is recorded by the age of seven months. The relative abundance is seen in the following order: subiculum > amygdale > CA1 region of hippocampus. Concomitantly, changes in behavioral paradigms are recorded from three months onwards. [30]

Femtosecond Laser Ablation for Inducing Vascular Dementia in Transgenic Mice

Vascular dementia (VaD) accounts for roughly 15-20% of all types of dementia making it the second leading cause of dementia behind only Alzheimer's disease. The pathological features commonly associated with VaD include large artery infarctions, small artery subcortical infarctions, cerebral amyloid angiopathy, hippocampal sclerosis, chronic subcortical ischemia leading to selective loss of neurons, glial cells and endothelial cells. Depression, apathy and mood changes leading to personality changes accompany this disease and are an important behavioral component of VaD. The risk factors for vascular dementia are stroke, microbleeds, hypertension, type 2 diabetes and atherosclerosis.

Femtosecond laser ablation can be used to injure the endothelium of a targeted vessel and trigger clotting in transgenic mice that express fluorescent proteins in neurons. Blood flow changes can then be determined by tracking red blood cell motion in 2-photon images. Occlusions in the penetrating arterioles cause a severe drop in flow in the downstream capillaries and lead to a region of neuronal death. Dendrite degeneration, can be observed within minutes of vascular occlusion in real time using. In a stepwise manner, degeneration progresses to cellular death in the ischemic region created due to small vessel occlusions, and lastly measurable behavioral and functional impairment. These lesions are accompanied by activation of inflammatory cells, such as microglia and leukocyte invasion.[31]

BEHAVIORAL PARADIGMS TO ASSESS LEARNING AND MEMORY

Passive Avoidance

Step-down Model

This is a classical model for the assessment of cognitive performance after inducing brain lesions. The term "passive avoidance" is usually employed to describe experiments in which the animal learns to avoid a noxious event by suppressing a particular behavior. The step-down type of passive avoidance task is used to examine the long-term memory based on negative reinforcement.

The apparatus consists of a transparent acrylic cage (30 cm × 30 cm × 40 cm) with a grid floor, inserted in a semi-soundproof outer box (35 cm × 35 cm × 90 cm). The cage is illuminated with a 15 W lamp during the experimental period. A wooden platform (4 cm × 4 cm × 4 cm) is fixed in the center of the grid floor (35 cm above the floor) and electric shocks (1 Hz, 500 msec, 40 V DC) are delivered using an isolated pulse stimulator.

The training is carried out in two sessions. The animal (mouse or rat) is placed on the elevated platform. Due to its innate exploratory behavior, the animal steps down on to the grid. The step-down latency (SDL) is noted. As soon as the animal steps on the grid it is given an electric shock (for duration of 15 sec). SDL, number of flinching reactions and vocalizations are measured.

Animals showing a SDL of 3 to 30 sec during the first training session are selected for second (60 to 90 min after first) and retention trials. Animals staying 60 sec on the platform are considered as remembering the task and do not receive electric shocks any more. The retention test is carried out 24 h after training, in a similar manner, except that the electric shocks are not applied to the grid floor. Each animal is again placed on the platform and SDL is recorded, with an upper cut-off time of 300 sec. Both saline-treated and amnestic-drug treated animals show the same SDL during the first training session. However, amnestic drugs are expected to increase the SDL in the subsequent trials indicating the impairment of learning and retention tasks. The failure should be ameliorated by test drug.[48]

Active Avoidance

Step-through Model

Active avoidance is induced by a sequence of conditioned and unconditioned stimuli to the animal. In response, the animal should actively step through to relocate to an adjoining compartment within a preset time, in order to avert the mild electric shock.[49] The latency from stimuli onset to escape of subject, after the pretraining, is related to the retention of memory task. This model is based on the innate behavior of the animal to seek dark areas and avoid brightly lit area. The trial can be divided into three phases:

1. Familiarization
2. Learning
3. Retention.

After training the animal on this system, it is treated with amnesia-inducing agent and sufficient time is allowed to elapse for the manifestation of the signs and symptoms. The animal is again tested for its step-through latency before and after administering test or standard drug.

A typical shuttle box apparatus consists of two identical opaque dark compartments (31 cm × 18 cm × 29 cm) separated by a wall with a rectangular (7 cm × 10 cm) opening with a sill situated on the grid floor level. Each compartment is illuminated by a 5 W lamp mounted centrally on the top of the apparatus. The floor in each compartment is made of stainless steel bars.

i. Familiarization: The animal is exposed to a conditioned stimulus (darkness). The conditioned stimulus lasts up to 5 sec or until the conditioned reaction emitted, whichever comes first.
ii. Learning: The animal receives a foot shock (Mice—1 mA, 1 sec; Rat—1.5 mA, 2 sec). The animal has 3 to 5 sec to avoid the unconditioned stimulus.
iii. Retention: After learning, the animal takes the cue and avoids step-through thereby increasing latency.

A trained animal is then subjected to scopolamine or colchicine; and after recovery, the animal is again exposed to test. The effect of test drug is compared with standard drug.

Maze

Mazes are traditional tools for assessing learning and memory performance in laboratory animals. Conventionally, maze consists of open and enclosed arms. The rodents have a natural inclination towards enclosed area and spend more time there in comparison to open area. On the basis of this, the transfer latency of the animal is recorded. The animal learns to avoid open arms and shortens transfer latency to enclosed area. Nootropic agents are effectively screened using this paradigm in scopolamine-induced dementia. Elevated Plus Maze, Radial Maze, Y Maze, and Figure 8 Maze are based on this phenomenon.

The plus maze consists of two opposite open arms (50 cm × 10 cm), crossed with two closed arms of the same dimensions with 40 cm high walls. The arms were connected with a central square (10 cm × 10 cm). Rats are placed individually at one end of an open arm, facing away from the central square. Time taken for the rat to move from the open arm and enter into one of the closed arms is recorded and termed as "initial transfer latency" (ITL). Animals are allowed to explore the maze for 30 sec after recording transfer latency. Retention transfer latency (RTL) is recorded by placing the rats similarly on the open arm at specified intervals.[50]

Morris Water Maze

The Morris water maze was developed by Richard Morris in 1984. It is the most popular task in behavioral neuroscience; and in its most basic form, it assesses spatial learning and memory along with nonspatial discrimination learning.[51] Performance in the Morris water maze is acutely sensitive to manipulations of the hippocampus.

The rodents are placed in a large circular pool of water from where they can escape onto a hidden platform to avoid swimming. In this way, the animal learns the spatial location of the platform. The latency to escape from water onto hidden platform is measured. The neuroendocrine mechanisms involved in this case may be responsible for the rapid learning capability of animals. It is useful for studying working and reference memory processes also. Motor, motivational or sensory factors can be easily eliminated. The animals are trained faster, easily and with reliability using water maze in comparison to radial arm maze.

The water maze consists of a large, circular, galvanized steel pool (1.8 m in diameter, 0.6 m in height). A white platform (10 cm in diameter) is placed inside, and the tank is filled with water (22°C) until the top of the platform is submerged 1 cm below the water surface. A sufficient amount of white paint is added to make the water opaque and render the platform virtually invisible. In addition to the visual cues on the walls of the laboratory (shapes), five sheets of paper with black-and-white geometric designs attached to the sides of the tank serve as additional cues. An automated tracking system can be used to analyze the swim path of each subject and calculate escape latencies (the time between being placed in the water and finding the hidden platform), total path lengths, average swim speed and thigmotaxia (percentage of time spent in periphery).

The protocol for reference memory is as follows. Before beginning acquisition training, mice are given a pretraining acclimatization session during which they are allowed to swim in the pool for 5 min without the platform present. On the following day, mice are given seven acquisition sessions that consist of four trials per day with an intertrial interval of 10 min. Throughout the course of this acquisition period, the hidden platform remains in the same fixed position for all mice. Four points along the perimeter of the maze arbitrarily designated as N, S, E, and W, serve as starting points where the mice are released, facing the wall of the tank, at the beginning of each trial (the order of the starting points is determined randomly, except that each starting point is used only once in each session). Once a mouse locates the platform, it is allowed to remain there for 30 sec before being removed from the tank. If a mouse fails to locate the platform within 120 sec, it is manually guided to it. After seven sessions of acquisition training, mice are subjected to a reversal test in which the platform is moved to the opposite side of the tank. Other task parameters remain identical to the acquisition procedures (i.e. 10 min intertrial interval, each trial begins from a different release point).

The training for working memory task is described briefly. The platform is located in one of the 24 possible positions, with the exact platform position on any given day being randomly determined (positions along the perimeter of the tank and in the exact middle are excluded). As in the reference memory procedure, if a mouse fails to locate the platform in 120 sec, it is manually guided to it. The second trial begins after a period of 30 sec on the platform, when the mouse is again released into the water from the same position as the first trial (first trial start positions are still randomly determined). To be eligible for testing with sample or vehicle, the subjects are required to locate the platform in less than 30 sec on two of the three trials subsequent to the first, and are required to meet this criterion on three of their four most recent training sessions.

Sample tests are conducted once or twice per week, with at least 72 h and one training session between tests to ensure sample clearance. In addition, the tests are conducted identically to training sessions except that only two trials are run.

Experiments using a cued procedure can also be conducted. The location of the platform is made known to the mice by placing a black rubber stopper (height, 3 cm; radius, 1.5 cm) on the platform that extends about 2 cm above the surface of the water. The platform, which remains submerged 1 cm below the surface of the water, is moved to a new location each day in the same manner as in the working memory procedure. Test sessions consist of four trials, each starting from one of the four release points. Mice are allowed to rest on the platform for 30 sec in between trials.[52]

Conditioned Avoidance Response (CAR)

This test characterizes the influence of the compound on both learning ability and memory (retention of the avoidance behavior after extinction period, i.e. the rest period without training and drug treatment). The method is valid and considered as essential *in vivo* procedure for testing the cognition-enhancers, nootropics and neuroprotective agents (e.g. piracetam, nimodipine, bilobalide, memantine). This test shows particularly convincing results in neurodeficit-animal models in which memory processing is impaired by scopolamine, lesions or aging. The test is also often used to identify drugs with antipsychotic activity where antipsychotics disrupt learning.

Test is carried out in a shuttle-box, which is divided into two equal compartments, which are connected. The floor of each compartment contains a steel grid with the help of which the unconditioned stimulus, a foot-shock of 2.0 mA is delivered. The protocol for the experiment is described in the chapter "Antipsychotics".

A shortening of avoidance latency and an increase in the number of correct responses relative to the vehicle-treated group indicate that the test drug improves avoidance behavior and enhances memory processing.[53]

Microdialysis of Acetylcholine Release

In vivo microdialysis techniques can be used to estimate the cholinergic neuronal activity in the hippocampus of freely moving rats.

Adult Wistar rats (200 to 250 g, either sex) are anesthetized with ketamine (100 mg/kg, ip) and a 3 mm concentric guide cannula stereotaxically implanted into the hippocampus (5.08 mm posterior, 4.8 mm lateral to the bregma, 4.0 mm ventral to the dura). Two days after surgery, a dialysis probe is inserted through the guide cannula and perfused at a flow rate of 1 µl/min with Ringer's solution (KCl 2.7, NaCl 147, $CaCl_2$ 2.3 mM) containing 10 µM physostigmine. Perfusion is performed to obtain the stable baseline for 120 to 180 min, and successive 20 µl samples are collected at 20 min intervals.

Test samples can be administered into the hippocampus via the dialysis probe. The extracellular levels of ACh are measured using high performance liquid chromatography

(HPLC) with an electrochemical detector. ACh and choline are separated using an AC-Gel column attached to enzyme reactor containing acetyl cholinesterase and choline oxidase. ACh can be assayed using the HPLC-electrochemical detector following its conversion to hydrogen peroxide, which is electrochemically detected with a platinum working electrode at 450 mV versus the Ag/AgCl reference electrode. The mobile phase contains 0.1 M sodium phosphate buffer (pH 8.5), 0.6 mM tetramethylammonium chloride and 0.8 mM sodium 1-decanesulfonate. The HPLC separation and enzymatic reactions are to be performed at 33°C.[54]

REFERENCES

1. Clegg A, Bryant J, Nicholson T, et al. Clinical and cost-effectiveness of donepezil, rivastigmine and galantamine for Alzheimer's disease: a rapid and systematic review. Health Technol Assess 2001;5:1-137.
2. Zolezzi JM, Candia SB, Santos MJ, Inestrosa NC. Alzheimer's disease: relevant molecular and physiopathological events affecting amyloid-β brain balance and the putative role of PPAR. Front Aging Neurosci 2014;6:176.
3. Bush TL, Miller SR, Criqui MH, et al. Risk factors for morbidity and mortality in older population: An epidemiological approach. In: Hazard WR, Beirman EL, Blass JP, et al (Eds): Principles of Geriatric Medicines and Gerontology. New York: McGraw Hill, 1994:153-66.
4. Duthey B. Update on 2004 Background Paper, BP 6.11 Alzheimer Disease and other Dementias. February 2013;1-74.
5. Selkoe DJ. Physiological production of the b-amyloid protein and the mechanism of Alzheimer's disease. Trends Neurosci 1993;16:403-9.
6. Cummings JL, Cole G. Alzheimer's disease. JAMA 2002;287:2335-8.
7. Lewis AJ, Tierney MC, Fisher RH, et al. Pathologic diagnosis of Alzheimer's disease. Neurology 1988;38:1660.
8. Carr DB, Goate A, Phil D, et al. Current concepts in the pathogenesis of Alzheimer's disease. Am J Med 1997;103:3S-10S.
9. Doraiswamy PM. Non-cholinergic strategies for treating and preventing Alzheimer's disease. CNS Drugs 2002;16:811-24.
10. Cramer PE, Cirrito JR, Wesson DW, Lee CY, Karlo JC, Zinn AE. ApoE-directed therapeutics rapidly clear β-amyloid and reverse deficits in AD mouse models. Science 2012;335:1503-6.
11. Chen Z, Zhong C. Decoding Alzheimer's disease from perturbed cerebral glucose metabolism: implications for diagnostic and therapeutic strategies. Prog Neurobiol. 2013;108:21-43.
12. Reddy DS. Assessment of nootropic and amnestic activity of centrally acting agents. Indian J Pharmacol 1997;29:208-21.
13. Marambaud P, Zhao H, Davies P. Resveratrol promotes clearance of Alzheimer's disease amyloid-beta peptides. J Biol Chem. 2005; 280(45):37377-82.
14. Bliss TVP, Collingridge GL. A synaptic model of memory: long-term potentiation in the hippocampus. Nature 1993;361:31-9.
15. Collins DR, Davies SN. Potentiation of synaptic transmission in the rat hippocampal slice by exogenous L-glutamate and selective L-glutamate receptor subtype agonists. Neuropharmacology 1994;33:1055-63.

16. Chetkovich DM, Sweatt JD. NMDA receptor activation increases cyclic AMP in area CA1 of the hippocampus via calcium/calmodulin stimulation of adenylyl cyclase. J Neurochem 1993;61:1933-42.
17. Vershinin M, Carter BC, Razafsky DS, King SJ, Gross SP. Multiple-motor based transport and its regulation by Tau. Proc Natl Acad Sci 2007;104:87-92.
18. Sun X, He G, Qing H, Zhou W, Dobie F, Cai F, et al. Hypoxia facilitates Alzheimer's disease pathogenesis by up-regulating BACE1 gene expression. Proc Natl Acad Sci 2006;103:18727-32.
19. Ellman GL, Courtney KD, Andres V, Jr, et al. A new and rapid colorimetric determination of acetyl cholinesterase activity. Biochem Pharmacol 1961;7:88-95.
20. Fisher A, Hanin I. Potential animal models for senile dementia of Alzheimer's type, with emphasis on AF64A-induced cholinotoxicity. Annu Rev Pharmacol Toxicol 1986;26:61-181.
21. Pepeu G. Overview and perspective on the therapy of Alzheimer's disease from a preclinical viewpoint. Prog Neuropsychopharmacol Biol Psychiatry 2001;25:193-209.
22. Price DL, Martin LJ, Sisodia SS, et al. Aged non-human primates: an animal model of age-associated neurodegenerative disease. Brain Pathol 1991;1:287-96.
23. Bartus RT. The need for common perspectives in the development and use of animal models for age-related cognitive and neurodegenerative disorders. Neurobiol Aging 1988;9:445-51.
24. Loring JF, Paszty C, Rose A, et al. Rational design of an animal model for Alzheimer's disease: introduction of multiple human genomic transgenes to reproduce AD pathology in a rodent. Neurobiol Aging 1996;17:173-82.
25. Hsiao K. Transgenic mice expressing Alzheimer amyloid precursor proteins. Exp Gerontol 1998; 33:883-9.
26. Quon D, Wang Y, Catalano R, et al. Formation of beta-amyloid protein deposits in brains of transgenic mice. Nature 1991;352:239-41.
27. Moran PM, Higgins LS, Cordell B, et al. Age-related learning deficits in transgenic mice expressing the 751-amino acid isoform of human beta-amyloid precursor protein. Proc Natl Acad Sci U S A 1995;92:5341-5.
28. Ashe KH. Learning and memory in Transgenic mice modeling Alzheimer's Disease. Learn Mem 2001;8:301-8.
29. Lewis J, Dickson DW, Lin WL, Chisholm L, Corral A, Jones G, et al. Enhanced neurofibrillary degeneration in transgenic mice expressing mutant tau and APP. Science 2001;293:1487-91.
30. Rosario ER, Carroll JC, Oddo S, LaFerla FM, Pike CJ. Androgens regulate the development of neuropathology in a triple transgenic mouse model of Alzheimer's disease. J Neurosci 2006;26:13384-9.
31. Nishimura N, Schaffer CB. Big effects from tiny vessels: imaging the impact of microvascular clots and hemorrhages on the brain. Stroke 2013;44:S90-S92.
32. Ebert U, Kirch W. Scopolamine model of dementia: Electroencephalogram findings and cognitive performance. Eur J Clin Invest 1998;28:944-9.
33. Ridley RM, Barratt NG, Baker HF. Cholinergic learning deficit in the marmoset produced by scopolamine and ICV hemicholinium. Psychopharmacologia 1984;83:340-5.
34. Saporito MS, Brown ER, Carswell S, et al. Preservation of cholinergic activity and prevention of neuron death by CEP-1347/KT-7515 following excitotoxic injury of the nucleus basalis magnocellularis. Neuroscience 1998;86:461-72.
35. Li L, An X, Qiao J. Pathological characteristic of Alzheimer's disease by lesion in nucleus basalis of Meynert in rats. Chin Med J 1998;111:638-40.

36. Prickaerts J, Fahrig T, Blokland A. Cognitive performance and biochemical markers in septum, hippocampus and striatum of rats after an ICV injection of streptozotocin: a correlation analysis. Behav Brain Res 1999;102:73-88.
37. Sharma M, Gupta YK. Intracerebroventricular injection of streptozotocin in rats produces both oxidative stress in the brain and cognitive impairment. Life Sci 2001;68:1021-9.
38. Lannert H, Hoyer S. Intracerebroventricular administration of streptozotocin causes long-term diminutions in learning and memory abilities and in cerebral energy metabolism. Ann N Y Acad Sci 2000; 920:256-8.
39. Bhattacharya SK, Kumar A. Effect of Trasina, an ayurvedic herbal formulation, on experimental models of Alzheimer's disease and central cholinergic marker in rats. J Altern Complement Med 1997;3:327-36.
40. Veerendra Kumar MH, Gupta YK. Intracerebroventricular administration of colchicine produces cognitive impairment associated with oxidative stress in rats. Pharmacol Biochem Behav 2002;73:565-71.
41. Hiramatsu M, Yamatsu T, Kameyama T, et al. Effects of repeated administration of (-) nicotine on AF64A- induced learning and impairment in rats. J Neural Transm 2002;109:361-75.
42. Liu J, Ho W, Lee NT, et al. Bis(7)-tacrine, a novel acetyl cholinesterase inhibitor, reverses AF64A-induced deficits in navigational memory in rats. Neurosci Lett 2000;282:165-8.
43. Johnson DA, Zambon NJ, Gibbs RB. Selective lesion of cholinergic neurons in the medial septum by 192 IgG-saporin impairs learning in a delayed matching to position T-maze paradigm. Brain Res 2002;943:132-41.
44. Galani R, Jeltsch H, Lehmann O, et al. Effects of 192 IgG-saporin on acetyl cholinesterase histochemistry in male and female rats. Brain Res Bull 2002;58:179-86.
45. Rossner S. Cholinergic immunolesions by 192IgG-saporin—useful tool to simulate pathogenic aspects of Alzheimer's disease. Int J Dev Neurosci 1997;15:835-50.
46. Shen YX, Xu SY, Wei W, et al. The protective effects of melatonin from oxidative damage induced by amyloid beta-peptide 25-35 in middle-aged rats. J Pineal Res 2002;32:85-9.
47. Nakamura S, Murayama N, Noshita T, et al. Progressive brain dysfunction following intracerebroventricular infusion of beta (1-42)-amyloid peptide. Brain Res 2001;912:128-36.
48. Sahgal A. Passive avoidance procedures. In Sahgal A (Ed): Behavioral Neuroscience: A Practical Approach. Oxford Univ Press 1993:49-56.
49. Bartus RT, Flicker C, Dean RL. Logical principles for the development of animal models of age-related memory impairments. In Crook T, Ferris SH, Bartus RT (Eds). Assessment in Geriatric Psychopharmacology. New Canaan (CT): Mark Powley Assoc 1983:263-99.
50. Sharma AC, Kulkarni SK. Evaluation of learning and memory mechanisms employing elevated plus-maze in rats and mice. Prog Neuropsychopharmacol Biol Psychiatry 1992;16:117-25.
51. Morris R. Developments of a water maze procedure for studying spatial learning in the rat. J Neurosci Methods 1984;11:47-60.
52. Varvel SA, Lichtman AH. Evaluation of CB1 receptor knockout mice in the morris water maze. J Pharmacol Exp Ther 2002;301:915-24.
53. Francis PT, Palmer AM, Sims NR, et al. Neurochemical studies of early onset Alzheimer's disease. Possible influence on treatment. N Engl J Med 1985;313:7-11.
54. Matsumoto M, Togashi H, Mori K, et al. Evidence for the involvement of central 5-HT (4) receptors in cholinergic function associated with cognitive processes: Behavioral, electrophysiological, and neurochemical studies. J Pharmacol Exp Ther 2001;296:676-82.

CHAPTER

30

Antiparkinsonian Agents

INTRODUCTION

Parkinson's disease (PD), a neurological syndrome is characterized by bradykinesia, postural instability, rigidity and involuntary tremors. These motor symptoms result from progressive neurodegeneration marked by selective and extensive loss of dopaminergic neurons of substantia nigra. It is understood that interplay of genetic and environmental factors may disrupt normal intrinsic physiology and contribute to neuronal death along with possible initiation of repair mechanisms. Biochemically, there is depletion of dopamine (DA) and increment of acetylcholine (Ach) in the affected area.

In India, with an aging population and increased life expectancy, it is expected that the disease burden due to PD will be enormous, but there is no prospective study to estimate its incidence and mortality. The incidence rates (IRs) in different countries vary from 1.5 to 20 per 100,000 per year.[1]

Recently, manganese has also been held responsible for neurotoxicity in the central nervous system and the basal ganglia, and produces neurological symptoms that are similar to that of Parkinson's disease.[2] Chronic exposure to manganese initiates a cascade of events that leads to selective dopaminergic dysfunction, neuronal loss, gliosis in basal ganglia structures, astrocytic changes ultimately leading to a disruption of oxidative phosphorylation. In addition, manganese causes a number of other functional changes in astrocytes that lead to compromised energy metabolism and neurotoxicity.

Advances in understanding of pathogenesis of PD indicate role of Renin-angiotensin system (RAS). Angiotensin, via type 1 receptors, activates NADPH-oxidase complex, to mediate key events leading to oxidative stress. Hyperactivation of RAS and its components in the basal ganglia and nigrostriatal system exacerbates OS and the microglial inflammatory response and contributes to progression of dopaminergic degeneration. In addition counter-regulatory interactions between angiotensin and dopamine have also been observed in several peripheral tissues.[3]

Belladonna alkaloids, antispasmodics and antihistaminics are some of the class of drugs, which have been traditionally used for the management of parkinsonism. However, their introduction into the physician's itinerary has been incidental and not as a result of systematic search. Recent studies using adenosine receptor agonists have also shown neuroprotective effect in PD through the reduction of excitatory neurotransmitter release, apoptosis and inflammatory responses.[4] The current drug therapy includes dopamine precursor (l-dopa), dopamine agonists and anticholinergics. L-dopa is decarboxylated to dopamine in the dopaminergic neurons which helps to maintain adequate motor functions. L-dopa provides therapeutic benefit for most early-stage PD patients. However, from the available line of drugs, no single agent is capable of controlling neuronal degeneration. They only provide symptomatic relief. In addition, there are reports that l-dopa is itself neurotoxic and an active participant in the oxidative stress cascade.[5,6] Further debilitating conditions like neurogenic orthostatic hypotension are part of PD and no pharmacotherapy exists. Recently, short-term clinical trials have shown the potential of Droxidopa, an oral prodrug converted by decarboxylation to norepinephrine, for symptomatic relief of neurogenic orthostatic hypotension in PD. Improvement in daily activities, falls, and standing systolic blood pressure has been reported.[7] It is, therefore, essential to have an alternative line of therapy, which not only provides symptomatic relief but also has a neuroprotective activity. Since to date no such wonder drug is available, it is imperative that the research in this field be intensified.

The molecular players in genesis of PD have been identified as inflammatory cytokines (tumor necrosis factor-α, interleukin [IL]-6, and IL-1 β), nitric oxide, prostaglandin E2, and reactive oxygen and nitrogen species (Fig. 30.1). Uncontrolled activation of microglia, the resident innate immune cells, affects neurons by releasing the molecular mediators of neuroinflammation leading to PD.[8] Addressing these lacunae may prove useful strategy for development of future preventive and therapeutic agents for this neurodegenerative disorder. Appropriately designed models, which allow such investigations are essential.

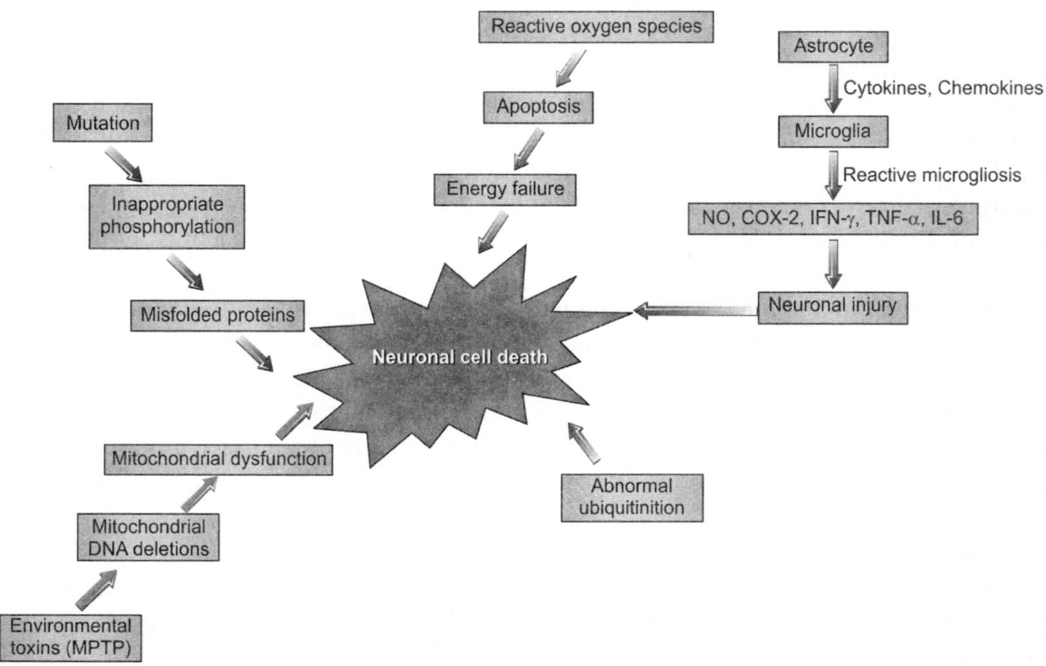

Figure 30.1: Etiopathology of Parkinson's disease

The patients suffering from idiopathic PD exhibit the three cardinal symptoms of muscular rigidity, resting tremors and hypokinesia. The rodents or primates *per se* do not exhibit these signs and symptoms. Hence, to induce the underlying pathologic changes and mimic the condition of parkinsonism in experimental animals, certain chemical agents are available. Compounds, which were reported to produce adverse effects resembling parkinsonism in patients, were tested in laboratory animals for the induction of extrapyramidal disorders. Major tranquilizers, reserpine and phenothiazine derivatives have been successfully used to set-up models of parkinsonism in animals. The protective effect of the test drugs can then be compared to that of standard in these animals by assessing them on various behavioral paradigms.

IN VITRO AND *EX VIVO* MODELS

In Vitro Primary Microglial Cultures

Primary rat microglial-enriched cultures are obtained from cerebral cortices of two-day-old rat pups. After removing the meninges, cortices are sectioned and washed in Hank's Balanced Salt Solution supplemented with Hepes/Na pH 7.4 (10 mM), $MgSO_4$ (12 mM), 50 U/ml penicillin and 50 μg/ml streptomycin and dissociated with 2.5 mg/ml trypsin type IX in the presence of 1 mg/ml deoxyribonuclease for 10 min at 37°C. The cell suspension obtained is diluted in medium containing 10% horse serum and centrifuged (50 g for 15 min). The cells are cultured in Minimum Essential Medium Eagle supplemented with 10% horse serum, 33 mM glucose, 2 mM Glutamax, 50 U/ml penicillin, 50 μg/ml streptomycin and 20 ng/ml GM-CSF and maintained in flasks at 37°C in a humidified 5% CO_2 incubator. Microglia cells are obtained by gentle manual shaking of the flasks two to three days after dissection. Detached cells (about 75 to 85% microglia with a 15 to 25% astrocytic contamination) are plated with fresh medium containing GM-CSF on 12-well plates coated with poly-l-lysine (100 μg/ml). Purity of highly-enriched microglial cells is assessed.

Stimuli (LPS, IL-1β, TNF-α and INF-γ) are administered to the culture medium and assessed for activation of inflammatory and neurodegenerative processes in microglia.[9]

Experiments Using Rat Striatal Slices

Striatum is the brain region, which is primarily affected in parkinsonism. The release of the neurotransmitters like dopamine and acetylcholine in response to test agent serves as a good *in vitro* marker of its activity.

Male Sprague Dawley rats (150 to 250 g) are decapitated; the skull is opened and the right and left striata are removed and placed in ice-cold Krebs' solution of the following composition (in mM): NaCl 118, KCl 4.85, $CaCl_2$ 1.3, KH_2PO_4 1.15, $NaHCO_3$25 and $C_6H_{12}O_6$ 11.1. The striata is cut into 0.4 mm thick slices using a tissue chopper. The slices are kept floating for 30 min in Krebs solution continuously gassed with 95% O_2 and 5% CO_2 at room temperature. The slices are labeled by incubating for 30 min at 37°C with [^{3}H] dopamine (5 mCi/ml) and [^{14}C] choline (2 mCi/ml) in the presence of 0.15 mM pargyline chloride and 0.1 mM ascorbic acid. Labeled slices are transferred to superfusion chambers and perfused with Krebs solution at 37°C at a flow rate of 0.5 ml/min. After washing and stabilization, 5 min fractions of superfusate are collected. The perfusion buffer contains 1 mM nomifensine to inhibit dopamine reuptake and

10 mM hemicholinium to inhibit choline uptake. The slices are subjected to field stimulation with rectangular pulses of alternating polarity, with a current strength of 10-15 mA/cm^2 and a pulse duration of 2 msec at a stimulation frequency of 3 Hz for 5 min. Drugs to be tested are present in the superfusion fluid. The radioactivity in the superfusate samples and in the tissue is determined by liquid scintillation counting.[10]

The radiolabelled choline method makes it possible to study ACh release *in vitro* without inhibiting cholinesterase, thus minimizing auto inhibition of transmitter release caused by an accumulation of unhydrolysed ACh.

Dopamine-stimulated Adenylyl Cyclase Activity

Male Sprague Dawley rats (150 to 250 g) are decapitated and the right and left striata are removed. Striatal tissue is homogenized by teflon glass homogenizer in chilled buffer containing 10 mM imidazole, 2 mM EGTA, and 10% sucrose, pH 7.3. The homogenate is centrifuged at 1,000 g for 10 min, and the supernatant that is obtained is re-centrifuged at 27,000 g for 20 min. The pellet obtained is washed twice and suspended in 10 mM imidazole, pH 7.3. Membrane protein is determined by Bradford's method using bovine serum albumin as standard. Adenylyl cyclase activity is measured by calculating the conversion rate of [^{32}P] ATP to [^{32}P] cAMP. The assay is performed in 250 µl of solution containing 10 mM imidazole, pH 7.3, 2 mM $MgCl_2$, 0.1 mM papaverine, 0.2 mM EGTA, 1 mM dithiothreitol, 1 µM GTP, 0.1 mM ATP, 2 mM phosphocreatine, 5 units of creatine phosphokinase, and 1 µCi of [a-^{32}P] ATP. The reaction mixture is preincubated at 30°C for 5 min, and the reaction is initiated by adding 50 to 60 µg of membrane proteins and incubated for an additional 10 min. The reaction is terminated by the addition of 300 µl of stopping solution (2% SDS, 25 mM ATP, and 1.3 mM cAMP). Formed [^{32}P] cAMP is separated from [^{32}P] ATP by chromatography.[11]

Radioligand Binding Studies for D_1 and D_2 Dopamine Receptors

Male Sprague Dawley rats (150 to 250 g) are decapitated and the right and left striata removed. Striatal tissue is homogenized with teflon glass homogenizer in 20 volumes of ice-cold buffer containing 50 mM Tris-HCl, pH 7.4, 2 mM EGTA, and 10% sucrose. The homogenate is centrifuged for 5 min at 800 g, and the supernatant is centrifuged for 20 min at 49,000 g. The pellet is washed and suspended in 50 mM Tris-HCl buffer, pH 7.4. Reaction mixtures containing 50 mM Tris-HCl buffer, pH 7.4, 120 mM NaCl, 5 mM KCl, 2 mM $CaCl_2$, 1 mM $MgCl_2$ and [^{3}H] SCH23390 (0.1-6.4 nM) or [^{3}H] raclopride (0.25-16 nM), in a total volume of 250 µl is incubated at 37°C for 30 min and terminated by vacuum filtration through Whatman filter. Further, washing with cold 50 mM Tris-HCl buffer, pH 7.4 may be given. Nonspecific binding is defined as binding in the presence of 10 µM cis-flupenthixol for D_1 dopamine receptor binding or 1 µM haloperidol for D_2 dopamine receptor binding. In addition, 10 µM of mesulergine is added into the D_1 dopamine receptor-binding assay to prevent binding of SCH23390 to serotonin receptors. The receptor densities and affinities are calculated by scatchard analysis.[11]

Dopamine Release from Synaptosomes

Mice are bred in pathogen-free colony and maintained on a 12 h light/dark cycle and housed five in a cage with same-sex littermates, free access to food and water. Each mouse is sacrificed by cervical dislocation and the brain removed and immediately placed on ice and chilled for 5 min. One millimeter coronal slices are taken and nucleus accumbens (NA) dissected from slices in which the anterior commissure is visible using a 1.2 mm glass capillary tube. Frontal cortex (FC), olfactory tubercle (OT), and striatum (ST) are dissected from the slices using forceps. Tissue is homogenized in 0.5 ml of 0.32 M sucrose buffered with 5 mM HEPES, pH 7.5. P2 synaptosomal pellets are then prepared from each region by centrifugation at 1000 g for 10 min, followed by centrifugation of the resulting supernatant at 12,000 g for 20 min. The P2 pellets are resuspended in perfusion buffer (in mM): NaCl 128, KCl 2.4, $CaCl_2$ 3.2, KH_2PO_4 1.2, $MgSO_4$ 1.2, HEPES 25, glucose 10, ascorbic acid 1, and pargyline 0.01, pH 7.5). Synaptosomes are diluted 5- to 15-fold with perfusion buffer to maintain uptake in a linear range (below 10% of input counts per minute). Test and standard drugs are dissolved directly into perfusion buffer. Aliquots of synaptosomes (90 μl) are added to appropriate concentrations of drugs (10 μl) and incubated at 37°C for 5 min before addition of 0.5 μCi of [^{3}H] dopamine (final concentration 0.1 μM). After an additional 5 min of incubation at 37°C, each sample is diluted with 0.5 ml of cold buffer and filtered. Radioactivity is determined by scintillation counting.[11]

In Vitro Neuroprotective Efficacy

Human Neuroblastoma cells, SH-SY5Y are cultured and maintained in Dulbecco's modified Eagle's medium supplemented with 10% (v/v) fetal calf serum and a 1% (v/v) penicillin/streptomycin antibiotics mixture. Cells were grown in an atmosphere of 95% air and 5% CO_2 at 37°C for 24 h. SHSY5Y cells are seeded at a density of 4×10^4 cells/well in 96-well culture plates and allowed to attach overnight. The cells are subjected to stress by incubating with or without hydrogen peroxide (100 or 300 μM) for 6 h. Appropriate concentration of test drug is added to culture plate 0.5 h before H_2O_2, so as to evaluate its efficacy as neuroprotective agent.

The cell survival is evaluated, by performing the MTT. Briefly, MTT is added to the cultures at a final concentration of 0.2 mg/ml, and after incubation at 37°C for 2 h, the media is removed carefully and the reaction is stopped by addition of isopropanol containing 0.04 N HCl. The absorbance of each well is measured at 590 nm by using a microplate reader.

Increase in viability of the cells in test wells may indicate the efficacy of the test drug as neuroprotective agent against a stress of H_2O_2.[12]

BEHAVIORAL MODELS OF PARKINSONISM

Reserpine-induced Parkinsonism

Reserpine is an alkaloid extracted from the dried roots of *Rauwolfia serpentina* belonging to the family, Apocynaceae. The pharmacological activity of this herb is well documented in the ancient literature and was used for the management of hypertension and psychosis. It acts by interfering with vesicular uptake and storage of Nor-epinephrine (NE), DA and serotonin (5-HT), both centrally and peripherally. Depletion of biogenic amines impairs the sympathetic activity, which takes about weeks to restore after discontinuation of the drug. However, owing to its CNS side effects, the drug has been discontinued for therapeutic use. Currently, it finds use as an agent for inducing extrapyramidal symptoms in laboratory animals.

Both intravenous (5 mg/kg) and intraperitoneal (2.5 mg/kg) injections of reserpine in rats produce the signs and symptoms of parkinsonism. After 20-30 min of drug administration, motor disorders are apparent. The animals are sedated and markedly hypokinetic with poor movement coordination. Hind limb rigidity, arched body position, fixed facial expression and ptosis are the other typical effects of reserpine. The effects peak at 1-2 h postadministration and subsides within 24 h. The animals may be divided into three groups, namely, test, standard and vehicle control. About 30 min after reserpine administration, the test or standard drug may be administered and percentage inhibition of the peak reserpine effect may be evaluated. Various behavioral paradigms are established to quantitatively score the effect of the test drug.

Assessment of Hypokinesia

A wooden box of 88 cm × 88 cm × 60 cm is constructed and the floor is divided into 16 equal squares. For a total duration of 120 min, the number of squares entered per 2 min by the rat is counted. In a hypokinetic animal, the score reduces significantly.

Assessment of Muscular Rigidity

A simple grasping test helps to assess the muscular rigidity of the animal. A metal rod (id 0.5 cm) is held at a height of 50 cm above table. The animal is made to grasp the rod with its forelimbs and the total time for which it remains on bar is noted.

Assessment of Catatonia

Appearance of catalepsy is the most obvious behavioral consequence of acute injection of a dopamine antagonist. It is hypothesized that catatonia may be equated with Parkinson's disease as it also originates as a dysfunction at the level of cortico-cortical and cortico-subcortical connectivity. Clinical similarities between Parkinson's disease and catatonia with respect to akinesia may be related with involvement of the basal ganglia in both disorders.[13] The ability of antiparkinson drugs to counteract this manifestation is an often studied behavioral paradigm. An arbitrary scale is used to grade the degree of catatonia by challenging each paw to different heights (0-9 cm).

The advantage of using reserpine model is that it helps to simulate the symptoms of parkinsonism effectively. Thus, it helps to predict the *in vivo* pharmacological activity of the test agent. However, as reserpine produces sudden depletion of biogenic amines without producing neurodegeneration of neurons, this model cannot be used to screen potential neuroprotective agents.

Neuroleptics-induced Parkinsonism

Neuroleptics act by blocking striatal dopamine receptors and are useful for the management of psychosis in patients. However, phenothiazine derivatives with piperazine side chain like trifluoperazine, thioproperazine and chlorpromazine produce typical extrapyramidal side effects and are used as a pharmacological tool to mimic parkinsonism in laboratory animals.

Chlorpromazine in a single dose of 4 mg/kg, ip, in rats produces marked catatonia, muscular rigidity and bradykinesia. The reversal of neuroleptic effect by test and standard drugs may be quantitated using various behavior scoring systems (described in the previous model). Hypokinesia may also be accompanied with tremors and rigidity, when rats are administered chlorpromazine chronically (2 mg/kg, ip, daily for 7 days). Chlorpromazine also diminishes exploratory behavior and conditioned avoidance response (Method for assessment described in the chapter "Antipsychotics").

Assessment of Tremors

The animal is lifted by tail such that its hindquarters are suspended approximately 8 cm above table. The forelimbs are maintained in this position for 10 sec and observed for body/hindleg tremors and scored on the basis of degree of tremors on an arbitrary scale from 0-4.

Cumulative scores of 30-60 min are analyzed in vehicle control, standard and test groups. Test agent with antiparkinsonism effect will significantly reduce the scores. Instruments, which allow digital recording of the tremors, have also been devised.[13] There are many pitfalls of this model. Catalepsy is the primary symptom observed in this model of parkinsonism. L-dopa, which is the choice of drug for management of parkinsonism in humans, partially antagonizes this symptom in rodents.[14] On the other hand, anticholinergic agents, which provide symptomatic relief to patients of parkinsonism, are quite effective in ameliorating the signs and symptoms of neuroleptics-induced parkinsonism in rodents.[15] Moreover, the neurobehavioral symptoms produced by neuroleptics are due to temporary blockade of dopamine neurotransmission and not owing to degeneration of dopaminergic neurons. Thus, this model does not accurately simulate the underlying pathogenesis of the disease.

Cholinomimetics-induced Parkinsonism

In PD loss of nigrostriatal dopaminergic inhibitory neurons results in cholinergic hyperactivity. In accordance with this hypothesis, anticholinergic agents are used for management of parkinsonism in patients and cholinomimetics used to set-up experimental models of parkinsonism.

Cholinomimetics like ACh, arecoline, tremorine and its potent derivative oxotremorine, carbachol, physostigmine, nicotine, harmine and harmaline have been traditionally used, both centrally (0.5-1.5 mg, intrastriatally) and peripherally (1 mg/kg, ip), to produce cholinergic symptoms like tremors, excitement, limb rigidity, salivation, lacrimation, defecation, urination and stereotypy and convulsions at higher doses (1 mg/kg, iv) in rodents. Tremorine is also known to produce rage in cats. These are observational symptoms. The ability of the test agent to ameliorate these symptoms indicates its anticholinergic activity.

Oxotremorine-induced tremors in mice is a sensitive, useful and convenient method for finding antiparkinsonian drug. This model serves as a simple, precisely defined, observational method for screening drugs with anticholinergic activity.

However, neuroleptics, antidepressants and antihistaminics can also give false positive results in this model. In such case, the test drug may be subjected to further tests to clearly delineate its mechanism of action:

i. *In vitro* antagonism of the effect of ACh on isolated tissue preparation—frog rectus abdominus, guinea pig ileum.
ii. Peripheral *in vivo* effect on mouse pupil—atropine-like drugs produce dilatation, whereas acetylcholine produces constriction.
iii. Directly testing anticholinergic effect in central nervous system—ability to antagonize physostigmine-induced sinistrotorsion in guinea pigs.

Certain precautions ought to be taken when any drug is being centrally administered. Firstly, its pH should be correctly balanced to avoid any drug-induced lesion in brain. Secondly, the osmolarity of the drug solution should be checked. It is advisable to prepare all solutions in CSF buffer. Thirdly, the volume of the drug injection should be kept to minimum (0.5-2 ml) as large volumes can displace brain tissue. All injections should be made slowly so as to avoid diffusion of solution into a large area.[16]

Surgical Induction

Direct lesion of the nigrostriatal dopaminergic neurons by injecting 6-OH-dopamine (6-OH-DA), 1-methyl,4-phenyl,1,2,3,6 tetrahydro pyridine (MPTP) or electrolesion are selective and reproducible ways to simulate the clinical condition in animals.

Unilateral Administration of 6-OH-DA

Unilateral administration of 6–OH-DA in the substantia nigra, ventral tegmentum or medial forebrain bundle in rats produces degeneration of the nigrostriatal pathway.

Adult male Wistar rats weighing between 200 to 250 g are housed under standard laboratory conditions of 12 h day/night cycle, with food and water *ad libitum*. The animals are anesthetized with ketamine hydrochloride (80 mg/kg, ip) and the head region between eye and ear of the animal is shaved. The rat is positioned on the stereotaxic apparatus with the incisor bar at 5° below the interaural line. The animal is held in position with the help of ear-bars. A longitudinal midline incision is made and the skin retracted. A point is marked at the appropriate stereotaxic coordinate and a burr hole is made.[17] A prefilled probe drive with a microliter syringe mounted on top is lowered to appropriate height and a slow infusion made. The test group is administered with 8 mg of 6-OH-DA and the control rats receive equivalent volume of the vehicle. Minimum volume of vehicle (normal saline) is used to dissolve the drug. Ascorbic acid (0.2 mg/ml) is added to prevent auto-oxidation. After 5 min of injection, the infusion probe is slowly withdrawn and the wound sutured. The animal is allowed to recuperate for 10-15 days before challenging it to battery of tests.

The neurotoxin 6-OH-DA induces permanent and selective damage of the neuronal region where it is injected. The altered levels of cerebral monoamines, i.e. norepinephrine, 5HT and DA induce behavioral deficits.[18] In rats, inhibition of spontaneous locomotor activity, hypokinesia, adypsia, aphagia and increase in pain sensitivity are some of the typical effects of central administration of 6-OH-DA. Ipsilateral and contralateral turning of lesioned rats in response to psychomotor stimulant administration is a critical behavior paradigm used to assess the activity of test drug.

a. *Spontaneous locomotor activity*: A well-illuminated, sound attenuated chamber (45 cm × 50 cm × 35 cm) containing a transparent acrylic cage (37 cm × 24 cm × 30 cm) is fabricated. It is fitted with a photocell beam system (described in chapter "Antipsychotics"). This system can be used to record the spontaneous locomotor activity and rearing behavior in a variety of animals such as rats, mice and marmosets. The animal is introduced into the acrylic cage and allowed to acclimatize for 5-10 min. The total counts of the interruptions of the photocell beam, for a predecided duration are made. The numbers of events of rearing behavior are also counted.

Motor activity is a good index for studying the effects of pharmacological agents. Traditionally, investigations center around counting the number of times an animal interrupts a photocell beam, but novel methods also use interruption of magnetic field as a paradigm. The interruptions are significantly reduced in a hypokinetic rat. Novel sensor systems with provision for multichannel measurements (body heat measurement, online cannulation and monitoring) are also available.[19]

b. *Rotational behavior in rats*: The neurotoxin 6-OH-DA depends upon DA transporter for selective presynaptic uptake, where it exerts neurotoxicity. Unilateral lesion of nigrostriatum by 6-OH-DA in rats, induces a selective presynaptic terminal loss of dopaminergic neurons along with postsynaptic hypersensitivity in the lesioned hemisphere.[20] The rotational behavior model, as proposed by Ungerstedt, is an important model. Systemic or central injection of apomorphine stimulates the intact but hypersensitive postsynaptic dopamine D_2 receptors and induces contralateral rotations in rat. On the other hand, amphetamine acts on the intact presynaptic terminals in the hemisphere contralateral to the lesion, and induces release of DA. Thus, the rat rotates in a direction ipsilateral to the lesioned hemisphere.

In unilaterally lesioned rats, a clear cut rotational behavior is observed in response to very low doses of apomorphine (0.05 mg/kg, ip). The onset is within 5 min of drug administration and lasts for 30-40 min. The total number of rotations is recorded for this duration and its modulation by the test drug reveals the nature of activity of the test drug. Concomitant stereotypy (gnawing, sniffing, rearing, ptosis) and cholinergic (defecation, salivation, urination) behavior are also observed. Comparable effects of apomorphine in normal rats are observed at a dose 10-20 times of the magnitude. Implantation of chronic cortical and neck muscle electrodes helps to record EEG and EMG in lesioned rats and study disease progression along with chronic effects of drug administration.[21]

L-dopa induces similar rotational behavior at a threshold dose of 10 mg/kg. The cholinergic and stereotypy behavior is less pronounced. Doses between 200 and 1000 mg/kg are required to induce rotations in normal rats.[22] Dexamphetamine is an indirect dopaminergic agent which at a dose of 5 mg/kg, ip induces ipsilateral rotations.[23]

Unilaterally lesioned animal model is at best a representation of hemiparkinsonism. In contrast, both the brain hemispheres are affected in humans. Moreover, these animals do not exhibit the triad symptoms like rigidity, akinesia and tremors.

Bilateral Administration of 6-OH-DA

Bilateral administration of 6-OH-DA in the medial forebrain bundle at the level of the lateral hypothalamic area results in a widespread depletion of regional brain catecholamine content and are accompanied with severe neurobehavioral disturbances.[24]

Adult Wistar male rats weighing between 200 to 250 g are housed under standard laboratory conditions of 12 h day/night cycle, with food and water *ad libitum*. They are fixed on the stereotaxic instrument as described earlier. A bilateral infusion of 6-OH-DA (2 × 5 mg) is made to the lateral hypothalamic site. The neurochemical and behavioral deficits are evident 48 h later. Prominent hypokinesia, muscular rigidity, and resting tremors are accompanied with severe adypsia, aphagia and weight loss.[25] Modulation of behavior by test drug is evaluated using paradigms described earlier.

MPTP Model

1-methyl-4-phenyl-1, 2,3,6-tetrahydropyridine (MPTP) is an environmental toxin, which produces a parkinsonian syndrome after its conversion to 1-methyl-4-phenylpyridine (MPP^+) by B-form monoamine oxidase (MAO) in the brain. MPP^+ perfusion into the striatum increases extracellular DA levels. This increase may concomitantly induce the formation of reactive free oxygen radicals (.OH), which induce lipid peroxidation of striatum membranes, as detected by increased nonenzymatic formation of 2,3-dihydroxybenzoic acid (DHBA).[26] MPTP treatment has provided best animal model of PD primarily in primates and later in mice. It produces the same syndrome as in clinical situation and the animals respond to the same therapeutic modalities as their human counterparts. The side effects (dyskinesia etc.) to the drugs administered are also the same.

All primate species are sensitive to MPTP, though most studies have been conducted on cynomolgus monkeys (*Macaca fascicularis*). The MPTP salt should be handled with due precaution as it is a very potent neurotoxin. Monkeys weighing between 2 to 4 kg are used for the experiment. For the injection, they are placed in a chair and MPTP solution is administered intravenously in the leg vein or subcutaneously. The dosage schedule is fixed as 0.3 mg/kg/d for 5 days. Immediately after each injection, the animals exhibit a syndrome for 10-30 min characterized by agitation, ataxia, myoclonus, hallucinations, linguinal dyskinesia and vomiting. The animals become akinetic progressively followed by stooped posture, adypsia and aphagia, to an extent that it has to be intubated. After 6 to 8 weeks, the syndrome stabilizes and experiments to test antiparkinsonian agents can be initiated. The response to test agent has to be evaluated in terms of motor parameters. Tremors, rigidity by electromyography, and akinesia by photocells fixed within cages. Disability scoring systems, inspired from the scoring system of human patients, have been employed to assess the degree of disability amongst the animals.

Common marmosets (*Callithrix jacchus*; 300–350 g) may also be used as animals to study parkinsonism. The animals are kept in controlled housing conditions, with constant temperature (25°C), relative humidity (50%), and 12 h light/dark cycles and free access to food and water. Marmosets are rendered parkinsonian by administration of MPTP-hydrochloride (2 mg/kg s.c. for 5 consecutive days). Following stabilization of the parkinsonian state, the animals are treated with standard (12 mg/kg L-DOPA and 3 mg/kg benserazide) or test drug and observed for behavioral paradigm as described above.

C57 BL/6 mice are also sensitive to systemic administration of MPTP. MPTP (2 × 40 mg/kg, s.c., separated by a 24 h interval) is administered. After 4 to 6 weeks, the symptoms stabilize and behavioral testing can be conducted.[27] Striatal dopamine levels fall by 90%.[28] There is reduction of all three behavior parameters of spontaneous motor activity, i.e. locomotion, rearing and total activity, during both the initial, exploratory stage (first 90 min), and later stages of the 3 or 4 h test periods.[29]

Primate model is an expensive and tedious method. Despite the disadvantages, it serves as an excellent platform to test new drugs before initiating them for patients. The effect on the various components of Parkinson's syndrome is established along with potential to induce side effects.

A modification in the protocol has been described by Jackson-Lewis et al. (1995) to induce severe and mild parkinsonism in mice. In severe model, the mice receive four-dose of MPTP (20 mg/kg, ip × 4) at 2 h intervals. Two doses of the same protocol induce milder cell injury.

$FeCl_3$-induced Model of Parkinsonism

The cause of degeneration of nigrostriatal dopaminergic neurons in idiopathic PD is unknown. The "oxidative stress" hypothesis suggests that there is an imbalance between the formation of cellular oxidants and the antioxidative processes.[30] Abnormalities in the metabolism of the transition metals, iron and copper, have been demonstrated to play a crucial role in its pathogenesis.[31] Iron is central in the initiation of fenton reaction mediated cascade of events, which ultimately ends in neuronal death.[32] Based on this hypothesis *in vivo* rat model of parkinsonism has been established.

Adult Wistar rats of either sex, weighing between 200 to 250 g are housed under standard laboratory conditions of light, temperature, food and water. After acclimatization the animals are prepared for stereotactic lesion. The animals are anesthetized using ketamine (80 mg/kg, ip) and fixed on the stereotaxy instrument as described above. According to the coordinates for substantia nigra the prefilled probe is lowered through the burr hole. The test group receives 50 mg of $FeCl_3$ dissolved in 5 ml of normal saline, whereas the control group receives equivalent volume of vehicle. After 5 min of infusion, the probe drive is slowly withdrawn to avoid spreading of chemical. The wound is sutured and the animal allowed recuperating for 15 to 20 days. On 21st day postlesion, the animal is subjected to apomorphine (1 mg/kg, ip) challenge. The animals suffering from nigral lesion exhibit ipsilateral rotations. The number of rotations executed for duration of 40 min is counted and its modulation by test and standard drug indicates their interaction with the dopaminergic system.

In $FeCl_3$-induced unilateral lesion of substantia nigra there is free radical mediated injury to which both pre- and postsynaptic neurons are equally susceptible. Hence, when apomorphine is systemically administered, it acts on the intact neurons in the contralateral hemisphere and induces ipsilateral rotations.[33]

In concordance with the human patients, this model also induces permanent damage from which the system cannot recover. In contrast, studies indicate that there are signs of recovery from toxicity of 6-OH-DA.[34]

Alternatively, unilateral destruction of nigrostriatal dopaminergic neuron can also be conducted using Ferrous citrate (2 mM in 0.9% NaCl). Rats are anesthetized (Tiletamine hydrochloride, 125 mg/kg,ip + Zolazepam hydrochloride, 125 mg/kg, ip) and positioned on stereotaxic instrument. The 4.0 μL of ferrous citrate solution (2 mM) is infused through microdialysis probe with glued outlet and tear off membrane at the flow rate of 0.8 μL/min to the right SNC using stereotaxic coordinates; AP: 3.2 mm, L: 2.1 mm and DV: 2.0 mm relative to bregma. The injections were delivered over the period of 5 min and probes were kept *in situ* for an additional 5 min after each injection to avoid the reflux along the injection tract. The sham controls were injected with 4.0 μL of 0.9% NaCl. After surgery, animals are observed for behavior paradigms and sacrificed at different time intervals and brain sections assessed histologically and biochemically for DA levels.[35]

Ultrafine Particle Air Pollution Model of Parkinson's Disease

Exposure to components of air pollution and agricultural pesticides has been associated with lesions of neurons in substantia nigra and striatum and increased risk of PD in humans. Based on this, mice are exposed to concentrated ambient ultrafine particles (CAPS; <100 nm diameter) during the first two weeks, postnatal. Parkinson-like pathology can be further induced during adulthood using agricultural pesticides (paraquat+maneb, 10+30 mg/kg, ip, 2 × per week × 6 weeks). Symptoms of loss in locomotor activity along with alterations in striatal GABA inhibitory function, nigrostriatal dopamine, dopamine-glutamate function in midbrain and excitotoxicity can be recorded.[36]

Monitoring Dopamine Concentration Using Microdialysis

Microdialysis has become a widely used method for the analysis of the extracellular fluid composition in anesthetized and moving animals.

Male Wistar rats weighing between 220 to 240 g are housed individually at ambient temperature, 12 h light/dark cycle and food and water *ad libitum*. The animals are allowed to acclimatize for 4 days before initiating experiment. The animals are anesthetized using pentobarbitone (70 to 80 mg/kg, ip) and placed on stereotaxic apparatus. The head is shaved and the skin retracted. The exposed skull bone is cleaned and allowed to dry. A guide cannula with a stainless steel obturator is implanted with its tip at the upper limit of the striatum.[37] The cannula is fixed into place using screws and dental cement. One week post-surgery the animal is subjected to repeated dialysis after treating with test or standard drug. To perform dialysis, the obturator is removed and dialysis probe inserted into the guide cannula and connected to microinjection pump. It is perfused with artificial CSF (in mM: NaCl 147, KCl 4, $CaCl_2$ 3.4) at a flow rate of 1 ml/min. After 30 min equilibration, 20 ml samples are collected in microtubes containing 0.5 M perchloric acid and refrigerated at –80°C. At the end of dialysis, the probe is gently removed and the obturator reinserted. The dialysate is separated by HPLC (flow rate- 0.3 ml/min, C_{18} reverse phase column, mobile phase: 100 mM KH_2PO_4, 0.1 mM EDTA, 0.28 ml triethylamine, 1 mM octanesulfonic acid, 10% methanol/acetonitrile, 2/1 v/v, pH 4.4 adjusted with citric acid).[31] This model helps to measure DA levels and concentrations repeatedly up to 4 months. It can be successfully used for kinetic monitoring of a given neurotransmitter during chronic drug treatment.

Monitoring Dopamine Concentration Using LC-MS/MS

Liquid chromatography with triple quadrupole tandem mass spectrometer (LC-MS/MS) can be used to detect DA in brain samples. Briefly, striatum is accurately weighed and mixed with acetronitrile containing 200 μg/ml dithiothreitol and 2 μg/ml cimetidine (internal standard). The homogenized mixture is vortexed and centrifuged (8,000 rpm) and supernatant is collected, dried under nitrogen, and reconstituted in methanol (containing 0.1% formic acid). The sample is injected into LC-MS/MS system with ESI operated in the positive ion mode and analyzed under the multiple reaction monitoring (MRM) mode: DA (m/z 154 → 177, CE = 10 eV), BH_4 (m/z 242.2 → 166.0, CE = 17 eV), cimetidine (m/z 253.1 → 159.0, CE=14 eV). For chromatographic separation hydrophilic interaction chromatography column can be used. The recommended mobile phase is of 0.1% formic acid-acetonitrile/water (75:25, *v*/*v*).[35]

Effect of Dopamine Receptor Stimulation on Electrophysiological Output from Rat Basal Ganglia

The basal ganglia functional model predicts that DA, by stimulating the striatonigral pathway via D_1 receptors and inhibiting the striatopallidal pathway via D_2 receptors, should inhibit output from the substantia nigra pars reticulata and internal pallidal segment (SNpr/GPi). Inhibition of output from the SNpr/GPi should in turn disinhibit the thalamus to facilitate movement.[38]

Male rats (250 to 275 g) are implanted bilaterally with 23-gauge stainless steel guide cannulae into the VLS just before electrophysiological experiments. Activities of SNpr neurons are recorded in rats anesthetized with chloral hydrate (400 mg/kg ip). SNpr neurons are located within the pars reticulata region of the substantia nigra, within the following stereotaxic coordinates: L, 2.0 to 2.4 mm; A, 2.8 to 3.2 mm; V, >7.0 mm. These neurons are distinguished electrophysiologically by their sharp, biphasic extracellular waveforms, duration (<1 msec), firing rates (10-40 spikes/sec), and location just ventral to the pars compacta dopamine neurons.[37] Electrodes are glass micropipettes filled with 1% pontamine sky blue dye in 2 M NaCl. Standard methods are used for amplifying, displaying, and discriminating the single unit activities of SNpr neurons.[38] At the end of recording periods, a small amount of the blue dye is iontophoretically deposited in the brain at the recording site. The animal is sacrificed and the brain is removed, sectioned, and mounted on slides to verify location of the blue spot within the pars reticulata. The effects of striatal drug infusions on SNpr firing are evaluated by first obtaining a stable 3 to 5 min period of baseline firing then infusing bilaterally into the VLS over 2 min test or standard drugs or saline (1 μl/side). SNpr neuronal firing is monitored for 30 min after infusions. Firing rates are averaged over 5 sec intervals and plotted as a percentage of the preinfusion baseline firing rate of the cell. For each drug treatment, the average percentage of change in firing of all SNpr neurons after the infusions is compared with their preinfusion (baseline) rates.[35,36]

REFERENCES

1. Das SK, Misra AK, Ray BK, Hazra A, Ghosal MK, Chaudhuri A, et al. Epidemiology of Parkinson disease in the city of Kolkata, India: a community-based study. Neurology 2010;75(15):1362–9.
2. Normandin L, Hazell AS. Manganese neurotoxicity: an update of pathophysiologic mechanisms. Metab Brain Dis 2002;12:375-87.
3. Labandeira-García JL, Garrido-Gil P, Rodriguez-Pallares J, Valenzuela R, Borrajo A, Rodríguez-Perez AI. Brain renin-angiotensin system and dopaminergic cell vulnerability. Front Neuroanat 2014;8:67.
4. Rivera-Oliver M, Díaz-Ríos M. Using caffeine and other adenosine receptor antagonists and agonists as therapeutic tools against neurodegenerative diseases: a review. Life Sci 2014;101(1-2):1-9.
5. Isaacson SH, Skettini J. Neurogenic orthostatic hypotension in Parkinson's disease: evaluation, management, and emerging role of droxidopa. Vasc Health Risk Manag 2014;10:169-76.
6. More SV, Kumar H, Kim IS, Song SY, Choi DK. Cellular and molecular mediators of neuroinflammation in the pathogenesis of Parkinson's disease. Mediators Inflamm 2013;2013:952375.
7. Rascol O, Fabre N. Dyskinesia: L-dopa-induced and tardive dyskinesia. Clin Neuropharmacol 2001;24: 313-23.
8. Fahn S. Is levodopa toxic? Neurology 1996;47:S184-95.

9. Lazzaro M, Bettegazzi B, Barbariga M, Codazzi F, Zacchetti D, Alessio M. Ceruloplasmin potentiates nitric oxide synthase activity and cytokine secretion in activated microglia. J Neuroinflammation 2014;11:164.
10. Jin S, Fredholm BB. Role of NMDA, AMPA and Kainate receptors in mediating glutamate and 4-AP induced dopamine and acetylcholine release from rat striatal slices. Neuropharmacology 1994;33:1039-48.
11. Grady SR, Murphy KL, Cao J, et al. Characterization of nicotinic agonist-induced [3H] dopamine release from synaptosomes prepared from four mouse brain regions. J Pharmacol Exp Ther 2002;301:651-60.
12. Northoff G. What catatonia can tell us about "top-down modulation": a neuropsyhiatric hypothesis. Behav Brain Sci 2002;25:555-77.
13. Iwashita A, Yamazaki S, Mihara K, Hattori K, Yamamoto H, Ishida J, et al. Neuroprotective effects of a Novel Poly(ADP-Ribose) Polymerase-1 Inhibitor, 2-{3-[4-(4-Chlorophenyl)-1-piperazinyl] propyl}-4(3H)-quinazolinone (FR255595), in an in vitro Model of Cell Death and in Mouse 1-Methyl-4-phenyl - 1,2,3,6-tetrahydropyridine Model of Parkinson's Disease. J Pharmacol Exp Ther 2004;309:1067-78.
14. Dill RE, Dorman HL, Nickey WM. A simple method for recording tremors in small animals. J Appl Physiol 1968;24:598-9.
15. Derkach P, Larochelle L, Bieger D. L-Dopa-chlorpromazine antagonism on running activity in mice. Can J Physiol Pharmacol 1974;52:114-8.
16. Arnt J, Christensen AV, Hyttel J. Differential reversal by scopolamine of effects of neuroleptics in rats: relevance for evaluation of therapeutic and extrapyramidal side effect potential. Neuropharmacology 1981; 20:1331-4.
17. Matthews RT, Chiou CY. Cholinergic stimulation of the caudate nucleus in rats: a model of Parkinson's disease. Neuropharmacology 1978;17:879-82.
18. Paxinos G, Watson C. The rat brain in stereotaxic coordinates. Sydney: Academic Press, 1982.
19. Butterworth RF, Belanger F, Barbeau A. Hypokinesia produced by anterolateral hypothalamic 6-hydroxydopamine lesions and its reversal by some antiparkinson drugs. Pharmacol Biochem Behav 1978;8:41-5.
20. Masuo Y, Matsumoto Y, Morita S, et al. A novel method for counting spontaneous motor activity in the rat. Brain Res Protocol 1997;1: 321-6.
21. Ungerstedt U, Arbuthnott G. Quantitative recording of rotational behaviour on rat after 6-OHDA lesions of the nigrostriatal dopamine system. Brain Res 1970;24:485-93.
22. Buonamici M, Maj R, Pagani AC, et al. Tremor at rest episodes in unilaterally 6-OHDA induced substantia nigra lesioned rats: EEG-EMG and behavior. Neuropharmacology 1986;25: 323-5.
23. Ernst AM. Mode of action of apomorphine and dexamphetamine on gnawing compulsion in rats. Psychopharmacologia 1967;10: 316-23.
24. Boules M, Warrington L, Fauq A, et al. Antiparkinson-like effects of a novel neurotensin analog in unilaterally 6-hydroxydopamine lesioned rats. Eur J Pharmacol 2001;428:227-33.
25. Ervin GN, Fink JS, Young RC, et al. Different behavioral responses to L-DOPA after anterolateral or posterolateral hypothalamic injections of 6-hydroxydopamine. Brain Res 1977;132:507-20.
26. Vos PE, Steinbusch HW, Ronken E, et al. Short-and long-term plasticity after lesioning of the cell body or terminal field area of the dopaminergic mesocorticolimbic system in the rat. Brain Res 1999;831:237-47.

27. Obata T. Dopamine efflux by MPTP and hydroxyl radical generation. J Neural Transm 2002;109: 1159-80.
28. Fredriksson A, Palomo T, Archer T. Effects of co-administration of anticonvulsant and putative anticonvulsive agents and sub/suprathreshold doses of L-dopa upon motor behaviour of MPTP-treated mice. J Neural Transm 1999;106:889-909.
29. Fredriksson A, Palomo T, Chase T, et al. Tolerance to a suprathreshold dose of L-Dopa in MPTP mice: effects of glutamate antagonists. J Neural Transm 1999;106:283-300.
30. Fredriksson A, Plaznik A, Sundstrom E, et al. MPTP-induced hypoactivity in mice: reversal by L-dopa. Pharmacol Toxicol 1990;67:295-301.
31. Sherer TB, Betarbet R, Greenamyre JT. Pathogenesis of Parkinson's disease. Curr Opin Investig Drugs 2001;2:657-62.
32. Perry G, Sayre LM, Atwood CS, et al. The role of iron and copper in the aetiology of neurodegenerative disorders: therapeutic implications. CNS Drugs 2002;16:339-52.
33. Hirsch EC, Faucheux BA. Iron metabolism and Parkinson's disease. Mov Disord 1998;13:39-45.
34. Mathur R, Gupta YK. Adenosinergic and dopaminergic interaction in nigrostriatum in FeCl3-induced model of parkinsonism in rats. Methods Find Exp Clin Pharmacol 1999;21:435-9.
35. Aryal B, Lee JK, Kim HR, Kim HG. Alteration of striatal tetrahydrobiopterin in iron-induced unilateral model of Parkinson's disease. Korean J Physiol Pharmacol 2014;18(2):129-34.
36. Allen JL, Liu X, Weston D, Conrad K, Oberdörster G, Cory-Slechta DA. Consequences of developmental exposure to concentrated ambient ultrafine particle air pollution combined with the adult paraquat and maneb model of the Parkinson's disease phenotype in male mice. Neurotoxicology 2014;41:80-8.
37. Sengstock GJ, Olanow CW, Dunn AJ, et al. Progressive changes in striatal dopaminergic markers, nigral volume and rotational behaviour following iron infusion into rat substantia nigra. Exp Neurol 1994;130:82-94.
38. Martin-Fardon R, Sandillon F, Thibault J, et al. Long-term monitoring of extracellular dopamine concentration in the rat striatum by a repeated microdialysis procedure. J Neuorsci Methods 1997;72:123-35.

CHAPTER

31

Antimigraine Agents

INTRODUCTION

Migraine is a neurovascular disorder characterized by episodes of severe, throbbing headache that is frequently unilateral, usually associated with nausea, vomiting or sensitivity to light, sound or movement. When untreated, these attacks typically last for 4–72 h.[1] In about one-third of the patients, migraine attacks are usually preceded or accompanied by transient focal neurological symptoms, which are usually visual; such patients have migraine with aura (previously known as classical migraine),[2] while majority of patients do not present with such symptoms of aura (migraine without aura or common migraine).[3] Migraine is a very common disorder with a prevalence of 15–18% in females and 6% in males.[4]

The exact pathophysiology of migraine is still not known. Neurovascular hypothesis has been proposed to explain the pathophysiology of migraine.[3,5] The initiating trigger, which remains unknown, is followed by a wave of cortical spreading depression.[6] There is subsequent decrease in regional cerebral blood flow leading to aura symptoms. This phase of oligemia is followed by vasodilatation of cranial extracerebral large arteries and arteriovenous anastomoses in the dura mater, base of skull and scalp during the headache phase. The pathophysiology of this vasodilatation involves changes in the activity of the neurons innervating these blood vessels. These neurons may release various vasodilating neurotransmitters like 5-HT, substance P, calcitonin gene-related peptide (CGRP), vasoactive intestinal peptide (VIP)[7] and nitric oxide.[8] This vasodilatation leads to stimulation of 'stretch' receptors in the vessel wall leading to increase in perivascular (trigeminal) sensory nerve activity that provokes headache and other associated symptoms. These trigeminal nerve fibers may also release neuropeptides, which reinforce vasodilatation and perivascular sensory nerve activity.[9]

The mechanisms by which various antimigraine drugs are proposed to act include: constriction of the dilated extracerebral blood vessels,[10,11] reduction of neuropeptide release and plasma protein extravasation across dural vessels[12] and inhibition of impulse transmission centrally within the trigeminovascular system.[13]

At present, there are no true animal models that can reproduce a complete clinical picture of migraine. However, the constituent parts of migraine can be explored to a large extent in experimental animals, both *in vivo* and *in vitro*. Some of the models used in the screening of potential antimigraine drugs are described below.

IN VITRO MODELS

[^{3}H]5-HT-binding Assay

[^{3}H]5-HT-binding assay is done for screening of potential antimigraine drugs, acting as 5-$HT_{1B/1D}$ agonists. The assay is performed using rat or bovine brain tissues in the presence of spiroperidol, which inhibits the binding of 5-HT to 5-HT_{1A} and 5-HT_2 receptors.

Procedure: Male Wistar rats are used for the assay. The rats are sacrificed, decapitated and their striata removed and weighed. These are homogenized in 20 volumes of 0.05 M Tris buffer, pH 7.7 and subsequently centrifuged at 48,000 g for 10 min. The supernatant is discarded and the pellet suspended in same volume of 0.05 M Tris buffer and incubated at 37°C for 10 min. This is again centrifuged at 48,000 g for 10 min. The final pellet is suspended in 0.05 M Tris buffer containing 10 mM pargyline, 4 mM calcium chloride and 0.1% ascorbic acid.

The binding assay consists of 50 μl [^{3}H]5-HT, 50 μl of spiroperidol (final concentration 1 mM), 800 μl of tissue preparation, 80 μl of 0.05 M Tris buffer with calcium chloride, pargyline and ascorbic acid and 20 μl of vehicle/5-HT (final concentration of 10^{-5} M)/the test drug. Following incubation at 25°C for 15 min, the binding is terminated by vacuum filtration through Whatman GF/B filters. The filters are then washed twice using 5 ml of ice-cold 0.05 M Tris buffer. Radioactivity is determined in 10 ml of liquiscint scintillation cocktail.[14]

Evaluation: Specific binding is determined in the presence or absence of 10^{-5} M 5-HT. IC_{50} values are calculated from the percent specific binding at each drug concentration. The K_i value is determined by Cheng Prusoff equation.[14]

Contraction of Isolated Blood Vessels

A number of isolated blood vessels from various species including the canine basilar and coronary arteries, canine and rabbit saphenous vein and human middle meningeal artery[15-18] contract in response to acutely acting antimigraine drugs. These are used for studying the action of potential antimigraine drugs on the 5 $HT_{1B/1D}$ receptors.

Contraction of Dog Isolated Saphenous Vein

Procedure: Beagle dogs of either sex, body weight 7–12 kg are used. The animals are anaesthetized and their lateral saphenous veins removed and cut spirally into strips. Four preparations are obtained from each vein. The strips are suspended in organ bath containing modified Krebs solution, under resting tension of 0.5 g and continuously aerated with 95% O_2 and 5% CO_2 at 37°C. All tissues are equilibrated for at least 1 hour and then primed with KCl (final bath concentration of 30 mM). Test drugs are given at least 30 min following washout of KCl. To exclude the actions of 5-HT and the test drug on other receptor sites, blockers of various receptors are used viz. atropine (1 μM), ketanserine (1 μM) and mepyramine (1 μM). Cumulative concentration response curves to 5-HT are obtained on all tissues. One hour later, a cumulative concentration response curve of the test drug is determined in one preparation and of 5-HT in another preparation (to monitor any spontaneous changes in sensitivity to 5-HT).

To find out the effect of antagonist on the contractile effect of the test drug, concentration response curves to the test drug are established in the presence of a single fixed antagonist concentration in the bath, allowing 30 min of antagonist contact time.[19-21]

Evaluation: EC_{50} is calculated for 5-HT and the test drug by log concentration response curves. Relative potency is determined by dividing EC_{50} for the test compound with EC_{50} value of 5-HT in the same preparation. This value is then corrected for spontaneous changes in sensitivity to 5-HT by dividing it with the ratio of EC_{50} values for 5-HT in the control strip.[21]

Contraction of Rabbit Isolated Saphenous Vein

Procedure: Right and left lateral saphenous veins of male New Zealand white rabbits (2.5–3.0 kg) are cleaned of surrounding adipose and connective tissue *in situ* under a binocular microscope. The veins are then cut off and placed in cold oxygenated Krebs-bicarbonate buffer solution, and cut into 4 rings of approximately 5 mm in length. The tissue is suspended with wire hooks and mounted in an organ bath filled with 10 ml Krebs-bicarbonate solution maintained at 37°C and continuously gassed with 95% O_2 and 5% CO_2 at 7.4 pH. Initial optimal resting force of 4 g is applied and tissues are equilibrated for 60-90 min before the concentration responses with repeated washings at every 15 min. Isometric contractions are recorded on a physiological recorder with isometric force displacement transducers. The response of the test drug is obtained in the presence of standard agonist and antagonist. [22-24]

Contraction of Human Isolated Middle Meningeal Artery

Procedure: Pieces of dura mater containing segment of middle meningeal arteries are obtained, as from the neurosurgery department. The arteries are dissected free from the dura mater and ring segments (2–3 mm in length) are prepared. These are mounted in organ baths containing standard physiological salt solution, under a resting tension of 4 g and aerated with 95% O_2 and 5% CO_2 at 37°C. Contractile response to the reference agonist, KCl (45 mM) is taken. After a 30 min wash-off period, cumulative concentration-effect curves to 5-HT, 5-carboxamidotryptamine (5-CT) and the test drug are obtained. Concentration-response curves to the test drug are also obtained in the absence or presence of $5HT_{1B/1D}$ antagonists like GR125,743 or GR 127,935 (10 nM), equilibration time 30 min.[18]

Evaluation: The concentration-effect curves to the agonist are calculated as a percentage of KCl evoked contractions. For the antagonist experiment, the responses are expressed relative to the maximum response obtained in the control (in the absence of antagonist) curve (=100%). The data are analyzed using weighted least square nonlinear regression analysis and the equation:

$$E = E_{max}/[1 + \{EC_{50}/(\text{agonist})^{nH}\}]$$

Where E_{max} is the maximum contraction evoked by the agonist, EC_{50} is the molar concentration of an agonist eliciting half maximal response and nH is the Hill coefficient.[18]

Contraction of Isolated Human Coronary Artery

This model is used for screening the antimigraine compounds for their coronary side effect potential.

Procedure: Hearts of patients who die of noncardiac causes like cerebrovascular accidents, trauma, hypoxia, etc. are obtained. The right epicardial coronary artery is removed and cut into rings approximately 4 mm long. These are suspended in organ baths containing Krebs bicarbonate solution, maintained at 37°C and aerated with 95% O_2 and 5% CO_2. Vessel segments containing macroscopically visible atherosclerotic lesions are discarded. Segments are allowed to equilibrate for at least 30 min with 2–3 washings in between and then K^+ (30 mM) is added twice. To verify the functional integrity of the endothelium, relaxation in response to substance P (1 nM) after precontraction with prostaglandin $F_2\alpha$(1 μM) is observed. Any segment that does not relax to substance P is discarded. After washout, the maximal contractile response to K^+ is determined by exposing the tissue to 100 mM of K^+. The tissue is then equilibrated in Krebs solution for 30 min.

After equilibration, cumulative concentration response curves to the test and standard drugs are obtained. Responses are expressed as a percentage of K^+ (100 mM)-induced contractions. All curves are obtained in a paired, parallel experimental set up. The averaged data per artery are used for further analysis.[25,26]

Evaluation: pD_2 values [-log of molar concentration of an agonist needed to reach half of its maximal effect (E_{max}), i.e. -log EC_{50}] are obtained and averaged for the agonist. Data are analyzed using multiple analysis of variance (MANOVA) followed by paired t-test.[25]

IN VIVO MODELS

Constriction of Carotid Arteriovenous Anastomoses in Anesthetized Animals

Dilatation of carotid arteriovenous anastomoses has been implicated in the pathogenesis of migraine.[27] It has been postulated that selective constriction of carotid arteriovenous anastomoses is responsible for the antimigraine effect of a number of drugs including the ergot alkaloid and the triptans.[28-30] This screening method is thus useful for screening of potential antimigraine drugs acting by constriction of carotid arteriovenous anastomoses.

Procedure: Domestic pigs (Yorkshire X Landrace; 10–15 kg) are used. After an overnight fast, the pigs are anesthetized, intubated and connected to a respirator for intermittent positive pressure ventilation. Arterial blood gases and pH are maintained within physiological limits (pH 7.35–7.48, pCO_2 35–48 mm Hg, pO_2 100–120 mm Hg) by adjusting the respiratory rate, tidal volume and oxygen supply. Body temperature is kept at about 37°C and continuous infusion of saline is given to maintain fluid and electrolyte balance. Inferior vena cava is catheterized via the left femoral vein for administration of drugs and aortic arch is catheterized via the left femoral artery for measurement of arterial blood pressure and withdrawal of arterial blood for determining blood gases.

After cutting both vagi and the accompanying cervical sympathetic nerves, a catheter is placed in the right external jugular vein for withdrawal of venous blood samples and a needle is inserted into the right common carotid artery against the blood flow for the administration of radioactive microspheres. Right carotid blood flow and heart rate are measured using a flow probe (internal diameter: 2.5 mm) and tachograph, respectively. After a stabilization period of 1 hour, baseline heart rate, mean arterial blood pressure, carotid blood flow and its distribution are measured. Arterial and jugular venous blood gases are monitored continuously. The test drug is then given and its effect on the hemodynamic variables is seen at different time-points.

For determining the distribution of common carotid blood flow, a suspension of about 2,00,000 microspheres [15 ± 0.1 (SD) μm diameter labeled with either ^{141}Ce, ^{113}Sn, ^{95}Nb, ^{103}Ru or ^{46}Sc] is injected into the carotid artery. At the end of the experiment, the animal is sacrificed. Heart, kidneys, lungs and the different cranial tissues are dissected, weighed, put in vials and radioactivity counted in these vials for 5–10 min in a gamma-scintillation counter.[26,31]

Evaluation: Effect of the test drug on the arterial and jugular venous O_2 saturation (A-V O_2 difference), systemic hemodynamics (mean arterial blood pressure, heart rate, changes in distribution of blood to other organs) and on carotid hemodynamics (total carotid blood flow and its arteriovenous anastomotic fraction, capillary fraction of blood flow) is seen. Data are evaluated statistically using Duncan's new multiple range test and paired t-test.

For calculating the distribution of carotid blood flow to different tissues (by the use of microspheres), the ratio of tissue and total radioactivities is multiplied by the total common carotid blood flow at the time of injection of microspheres. The amount of radioactivity in the lungs is an index of the arteriovenous anastomotic fraction of the carotid blood flow.[26]

Neurogenic Plasma Extravasation Model

This screening method is used for studying the ability of potential antimigraine drugs to block the release of vasodilating peptides from trigeminal sensory nerve endings.

Procedure: Male Sprague-Dawley rats (380–450 g) are used for experiment. After anesthetizing the animal, femoral vein is cannulated for intravenous injections. Animals are placed in a stereotaxic frame with the incisor bar set at –1.5 mm. Burr holes are drilled symmetrically 4 mm lateral and 4 mm posterior to the bregma. Paired nonconcentric bipolar electrodes are lowered bilaterally into the trigeminal ganglia, which are located 9.5 mm from the dura mater. The animals are now injected with ^{125}I radiolabeled human serum albumin (50 μCi/kg) and Evan's blue (20 mg/kg). Drug or vehicle is administered 5 min later. The left or right trigeminal ganglion is stimulated electrically (5 Hz, 2 ms, 2.2 mA, 3 min duration) 10 min after drug administration. To wash the blood from the head region, animals are perfused with 0.9% saline via the left cardiac ventricle for 5 min at a constant pressure of 120 mm Hg immediately after stimulation. The dura mater is then dissected, weighed and counted for radioactivity. Samples of extracranial tissues innervated by the trigeminal nerve (eyelid, conjunctiva and lower lip) are also removed, weighed and counted for radioactivity.[32]

Evaluation: ^{125}I human serum albumin extravasation ratio is expressed as the ratio of cpm/mg wet weight (stimulated side) to cpm/mg wet weight (unstimulated side). Maximum inhibition for a drug is achieved when the ratio of radioactivity on the stimulated versus the unstimulated side does not differ from 1.[33] Data are analyzed using student's unpaired t-test.

Inhibition of Neurogenic Dural Vasodilatation in Anesthetized Animals

This procedure is used for testing the ability of test drug to block the release of vasoactive peptides like CGRP from the trigeminal sensory nerve endings and thereby inhibit the vasodilatation of dural vessels.

Procedure: Male Sprague-Dawley rats (300–400 g) or male Dunkin Hartley guinea pigs (300–450 g) are used. After anesthesia, the trachea is cannulated for artificial respiration. The left carotid artery and jugular vein or the femoral artery and vein are cannulated for measurement of mean arterial blood pressure (MABP) and i.v. injections of drugs. The animals are now placed in a stereotaxic frame and their skull exposed. Using a saline cooled drill, the right parietal bone is thinned until the dural blood vessels are clearly visible through the intact skull. Using an intravital microscope, a branch of middle meningeal artery is viewed and a video dimensions analyzer continuously measures dural blood vessel diameter. A bipolar stimulating electrode is placed on the surface of the cranial window close to the vessel of interest. To evoke dilatation of dural blood vessels, the cranial window is electrically stimulated (5 Hz, 1 ms, 250–300 μA for 10 sec). Test drugs are administered 15 min before the electrical stimulation. In guinea pigs, the dural vessels are observed to be fully dilated following introduction of cranial window. Therefore, it is necessary to preconstrict the vessels by giving intravenous endothelin-1 (ET-1, 3 μg/kg) 3 min before electrical stimulation.[34,35]

Evaluation: Ability of the test drug to constrict the dilated blood vessels is taken as a measure of efficacy. The effect of electrical stimulation is calculated as a percentage increase from the prestimulation baseline diameter. The control responses are compared to the responses obtained after drug administration. The data obtained are analyzed using ANOVA and paired student's t-test.[35]

Activation of CB2 Receptors: Potential Therapeutic Target for Migraine[36]

Existence of interactions between the endocannabinoid system and pain mediation in migraine have been suggested by experimental animal models. Role of cannabinoid-1 (CB1) receptor in antinociception has been demonstrated and it has been suggested that CB2 receptors, located outside the central nervous system, play a role in the perception of pain. Systemic administration of nitroglycerin (NTG) consistently induces spontaneous-like headache attacks in migraneurs; in the rat, systemic NTG induces hyperalgesia, probably through the activation of cerebral/spinal structures involved in nociceptive transmission. Greco et al. 2014 evaluated the role of CB2 receptors in animal models of pain that may be relevant for migraine.[36]

Knockin Mouse Models[37]

A group of researchers generated a knockin mouse model carrying the human pure FHM-1 R192Q mutation and observed multiple gain-of-function effects. These include increased $Ca_v2.1$ current density in cerebellar neurons, enhanced neurotransmission at the neuromuscular junction, and in the intact animal, a reduced threshold and increased velocity of cortical spreading depression (CSD; the likely mechanism for the migraine aura). They showed that the increased susceptibility for CSD and aura in migraine may be due to cortical hyperexcitability. The R192Q FHM-1 mouse is a promising animal model for testing novel therapeutic strategies for migraine aimed at decreasing neuronal hyperexcitability and/or preventing CSD.[37]

REFERENCES

1. Headache Classification Committee of the International Headache Society. Classification and diagnostic criteria for headache disorders, cranial neuralgias and facial pain. Cephalalgia 1988; 8:1-96.
2. Rasmussen BK, Olesen J. Migraine with aura and migraine without aura: An epidemiological study. Cephalalgia 1992;12:221-8.
3. Ferrari MD. Migraine. Lancet 1998;351:1043-51.
4. Lipton RB, Stewart WF. Prevalence and impact of migraine. Neurol Clin 1997;15:1-13.
5. Goadsby PJ, Lipton RB, Ferrari MD. Migraine-current understanding and treatment. N Engl J Med 2002;346:257-70.
6. Read SJ, Parsons PA. Cortical spreading depression and migraine. In Edvinsson L (Ed): Migraine and Headache Pathophysiology. London: Martin Dunitz, 1999:81-92.
7. Gulbenkian S, Cunha e Sa M, Barosso PC, et al. Innervation of intracranial blood vessels. In Edvinsson L (Ed): Migraine and Headache Pathophysiology. London: Martin Dunitz, 1999:17-30.
8. Olesen J, Thomsen LL, Iversen H. Nitric oxide is a key molecule in migraine and other vascular headaches. Trends Pharmacol Sci 1994;15:149-53.
9. Saxena PR. The pathogenesis and pharmacology of migraine. Rev Contemp Pharmacother 1994;5:259-69.
10. Saxena PR, Ferrari MD. 5-HT1-like receptor agonists and the pathophysiology of migraine. Trends Pharmacol Sci 1989;10:200-4.
11. Humphrey PPA, Feniuk W. Mode of action of the antimigraine drug sumatriptan. Trends Pharmacol Sci 1991;12:444-6.
12. Moskowitz MA. Neurogenic versus vascular mechanisms of sumatriptan and ergot alkaloids in migraine. Trends Pharmacol Sci 1992;13:307-11.
13. Goadsby PJ. Current concepts of the pathophysiology of migraine. Neurol Clin 1997;15:27-42.
14. Vogel GH. Serotonin receptor binding. In Vogel GH (Ed): Drug Discovery and Evaluation. 2nd edition. New York: Springer, 2002:417-8.
15. Skingle M, Beattie DT, Scopes DIT, et al. GR127935: A potent and selective 5-HT1D receptor antagonist. Behav Brain Res 1996;73:157-61.
16. Terron JA. GR127935 is a potent antagonist of the HT1-like receptor mediating contraction of the canine coronary artery. Eur J Pharmacol 1996;300:109-12.
17. Razzaque Z, Longmore J, Hill RG. Differences in the effects of ketanserin and GR127935 on 5-HT receptor mediated responses in rabbit saphenous vein and guinea pig jugular vein. Eur J Pharmacol 1995;283:199-206.
18. Razzaque Z, Heald MA, Pickard JD, et al. Vasoconstriction in human isolated middle meningeal arteries: Determining the contribution of 5-HT1 B-and 5-HT1F-receptor activation. Br J Clin Pharmacol 1999;47:75-82.
19. Apperley E, Feniuk W, Humphrey PPA, et al. Evidence for two types of excitatory receptor for 5-hydroxytryptamine in dog isolated vasculature. Br J Pharmacol 1980;68:215-24.
20. Feniuk W, Humphrey PPA, Watts AD. Presynaptic inhibitory action of 5-hydroxytryptamine in dog isolated saphenous vein. Br J Pharmacol 1979;67:247-54.
21. Humphrey PPA, Feniuk W, Perren MJ, et al. GR43175, a selective agonist for the 5-HT1-like receptor in dog isolated saphenous vein. Br J Pharmacol 1988;94:1123-32.

22. Bhandare A, Vyawahare N, Kshirsagar A, et al. In vivo and in vitro screening of antimigraine drugs: studies in animal model of migraine. IJPRD 2010;2 (9):11-21.
23. Valentin JP, Bonnafous R, John GW. Influence of the endothelium and nitric oxide on the contractile responses evoked by 5-HTID receptor agonists in the rabbit isolated saphenous vein. Br J Pharmacol 1996;119:35-42.
24. Arulmozhi DK, Sridhar N, Bodhankar SL, et al. In vitro pharmacological investigations of Sapindus trifoliatus in various migraine targets. J Ethnopharmacol 2004; 95:239-45.
25. Bax WA, Renzenbrink GJ, van Heuven-Nolsen D, et al. 5-HTreceptors mediating contractions of the isolated human coronary artery. Eur J Pharmacol 1993;239:203-10.
26. Saxena PR, De Vries P, Heiligers JPC, et al. BMS-181885, a HT1B/1D receptor ligand, in experimental models predictive of antimigraine activity and coronary side-effect potential. Eur J Pharmacol 1998; 351:329-39.
27. Heyck H. Pathogenesis of migraine. Res Clin Stu Headache 1969;2:1-28.
28. Johnston BM, Saxena PR. The effect of ergotamine on tissue blood flow and the arteriovenous shunting of radioactive microspheres in the head. Br J Pharmacol 1978;63:541-9.
29. Den Boer MO, Villalon CM, Heiligers JP, et al. Role of 5-HT1-like receptors in the reduction of porcine cranial arteriovenous anastomotic shunting by sumatriptan. Br J Pharmacol 1991;102:323-30.
30. Martin GR. Pre-clinical pharmacology of zolmitriptan (Zomig™; formerly 311C90), a centrally and peripherally acting 5-HT1B/1D agonist for migraine. Cephalalgia 1997;17:4-14.
31. De Vries P, Willems EW, Heiligers JPC, et al. Investigation of the role of HT1B and HT1D receptors in the sumatriptan-induced constriction of porcine carotid arteriovenous anastomoses. Br J Pharmacol 1999;127:405-12.
32. Gupta P, Brown D, Butler P, et al. The in vivo pharmacological profile of a HT1 receptor agonist, CP-122,288, a selective inhibitor of neurogenic inflammation. Br J Pharmacol 1995;116:2385-90.
33. Lee WS, Moskowitz MA. Conformationally restricted sumatriptan analogues, CP-122,288 and CP-122,638 exhibit enhanced potency against neurogenic inflammation in dura mater. Brain Res 1993;626:303-5.
34. Williamson DJ, Hill RG, Shepheard SL, et al. The antimigraine HT1B/1D agonist rizatriptan inhibits neurogenic dural vasodilation in anaesthetized guinea pigs. Br J Pharmacol 2001;133:1029-34.
35. Akerman S, Williamson DJ, Kaube H, et al. The effect of antimigraine compounds on nitric oxide-induced dilation of dural meningeal vessels. Eur J Pharmacol 2002;452:223-8.
36. Greco R, Mangione AS, Sandrini G, et al. Activation of CB2 receptors as a potential therapeutic target for migraine: evaluation in an animal model. J Headache Pain 2014;15:14.
37. van den Maagdenberg AM, Pietrobon D, Pizzorusso T, et al. A Cacna1a knockin migraine mouse model with increased susceptibility to cortical spreading depression. Neuron 2004;41(5):701-10.

CHAPTER

32

Analgesic Agents

INTRODUCTION

Pain is an unpleasant sensory and emotional experience associated with actual and potential tissue damage. Various types of pain are seen in humans, e.g. somatic pain (arising from the skin, muscles, joints, ligaments and bones), visceral pain, referred pain, neuropathic pain, cancer pain, etc.

Chemical mediators of pain are numerous. These mediators come from sources intrinsic to the neuron, including various neurotransmitters such as 5-HT and substance-P, and extrinsic to the nervous system, including substances from inflammatory/immune cells and red blood cells such as prostaglandins, kinins, cytokines, chemokines and ATP that are released following injury to the tissue.

Pain is produced by the excitation of particular receptors, the nociceptors or of their afferent fibers. These remarkable cells respond to a broad spectrum of physical (heat, cold and pressure) or chemical noxious stimuli. In general, perception of noxious stimuli is termed as nociception. Nociception is not exactly same as pain, pain is a subjective experience and includes a strong affective component, whereas nociception lacks affective component. Most of the afferent fibers that are excited by noxious stimuli are non-myelinated C-fibers with low conduction velocities (< 1 m/s), known as C-polymodalnociceptors (PMN) other fibers are fine myelinated (Aδ) fibers with rapid conduction.

Pain can be classified as acute or chronic. The distinction between acute and chronic pain is not based on its duration of sensation, but rather the nature of the pain itself. Acute pain, which has as its source soft tissue damage, infection and/or inflammation, will be short in duration. The primary distinction is: acute pain serves to protect one after an injury, whereas chronic pain does not serve this or any other purpose. Acute pain is the symptom of pain. Chronic pain was originally defined as pain that lasts 6 months or longer. It is now defined as, "the disease of pain". The most common causes of chronic pain include cancer pain, neuropathic pain and arthritic pain.

MECHANISM AND MODULATION OF PAIN/NOCICEPTION

Nociception is the mechanism whereby noxious peripheral stimuli are transmitted to the central nervous system. Nociceptive fibers terminate in the superficial layers of the dorsal horn, forming synaptic connections with transmission neurons running to the thalamus. PMN neurons release glutamate, substance P, etc. contributing to neurogenic inflammation. Transmission in the dorsal horn is subjected to various modulations constituting the gate control theory. Descending inhibitory pathways from the midbrain (Periaqueductal gray area) and brainstem (nucleus raphe magnus) exert a strong inhibitory effect on dorsal horn transmission. Main transmitters in this pathway are enkephalin, 5-HT and noradrenaline.

Drugs in clinical use as analgesics belong to two main groups—narcotic or morphine group and analgesic-antipyretic (nonsteroidal anti-inflammatory drugs) group. Morphine-like drugs produce analgesia by acting on the central nervous system, while analgesic-antipyretic drugs act by both central and peripheral mechanisms.

ANIMAL MODELS OF ACUTE PAIN

Animal tests used in the search for new analgesics are designed as models for the treatment of pathological pain in man; but they usually differ from the original in that the drug is given before the noxious stimulus (thermal, electrical, chemical, and mechanical types of stimuli). Hence, these tests only measure the power of a drug to increase the minimal stimulus required to elicit pain or nociceptive response. The methodology to perform these tests using above stimuli is described below.

MODELS USING THERMAL STIMULUS

Hot Plate Method

Hot plate method has been widely used to evaluate opioid analgesics.

Procedure

Mice weighing 18–22 g are used. Animals are placed on the hot plate, which consists of electrically heated surface. Temperature of the hot plate is maintained at 55–56°C. Responses such as jumping, withdrawal of the paws and licking of the paws are seen. The time period

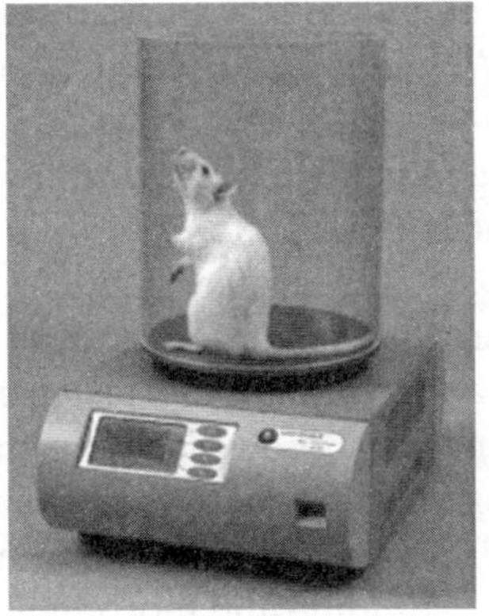

Figure 32.1: Hot plate

(latency period), when animals are placed and until responses occur, is recorded by a stopwatch.

Test compounds are administered orally or subcutaneously and latency or latency period is recorded after 20, 60 and 90 min. These values are compared with the values before administration of the test drug by using t-test.[1,2]

The Tail-Flick Test

The tail-flick test is a widely and reliably used test for revealing the potency of opioid analgesics. In this also heat is used as the noxious stimulus. The stimulus causes a simple nociceptive spinal reflex response in which the rat or mouse flicks its tail away from the heat source. The dependent variable in this test is the time taken by the animal to flick its tail. It is a very useful test for discrimination between centrally acting morphine like analgesics and non-opioid analgesics. Another advantage of the method lies in the fact that there is minimal interanimal variation.

There are two variants of the tail-flick test. One consists of applying radiant heat to a small surface of the tail and the other involves immersing the tail in water at a predetermined temperature.

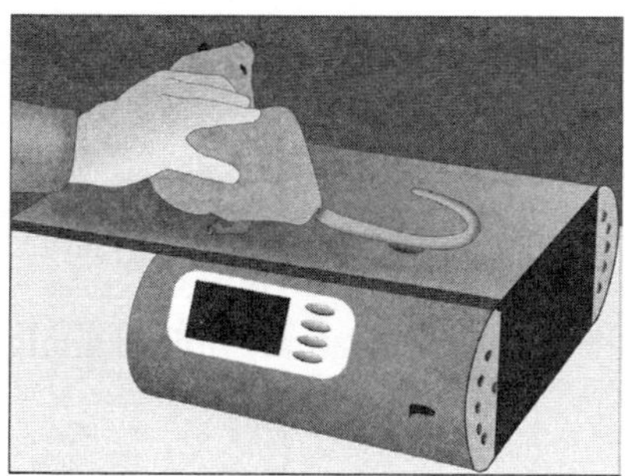

Figure 32.2: Tail-Flick apparatus

The Tail-Flick Test Using Radiant Heat

Procedure

Mice weighing 18–22 g are used and placed into small cages, leaving the tail exposed. Mouse-tail is held gently by the observer. A light beam is focused (exerting radiant heat) to the proximal third of the tail. The mouse tries to pull the tail away and rotates the head, this reaction is known as escape reaction. The reaction time of this movement is recorded. The reaction time varies with the surface area stimulated.

The test drug and standard are administered either orally or subcutaneously. Same procedure is repeated and reaction time is noted after 30, 60 and 120 min. A lengthening of the reaction time is interpreted as an analgesic action of test drug.

At each time interval those animals that show higher reaction time than the time before drug administration are regarded as positive. Percentages of positive animals are counted for each time interval and each dose and ED_{50} values of test compounds can be calculated according to Litchfield and Wilcoxon. Codeine, pethidine and morphine are used as standard.[3,4]

The Tail-Flick Test Using Immersion of the Tail

Young female Wistar rats weighing 170–210 g are used. Rats are placed into separate cages in such a way that their tail hangs out freely. The distal 5 cm part of the tail is marked, which is immersed (maximum upto 15 sec) in a cup filled with warm water (temperature 55°C). A tail withdrawal reflex is seen within a few seconds. This reaction time is noted by stopwatch. Normal reaction time is 1–5.5 sec. The test substances are given orally or subcutaneously and reaction time is recorded after 0.5, 1, 2, 3, 4 and 6 h.

Centrally acting analgesic drugs are capable of causing prolongation of tail withdrawal reflex, and hence, a withdrawal time of more than 6 sec in test animals denotes positive analgesic response of the test drug.[5]

Modifications

Cold Tail-Flick Test

In the test, 1–2 cm of the tails of rats are immersed in a cold 1:1 mixture of water and ethylene glycol at –10°C. The reaction time is measured as the time taken by the rats to deflect their tails. The first reading is discarded and the reaction time is taken as the mean of the last two readings. A test drug having potential of analgesic (centrally acting) would increase the reaction time.[6]

Cold Ethanol Tail-Flick Test (CET)

Cold ethanol tail-flick test can also be used for evaluating opioid analgesics. In the test –20°C is selected as the noxious cold stimulus. Male Sprague-Dawley rats weighing between 175 and 225 g are used and their tails submerged, approximately, halfway into the bath containing a bath solution of water or 75% ethanol (temp –20°C). The nociceptive threshold is taken as the latency until the rat removes or flicks its tail from the bath. The time from immersion to tail removal is measured to the nearest tenth of a second with a timer.[7]

MODELS USING ELECTRICAL STIMULUS

Tooth Pulp Test

In the test electrical stimulus is given in rabbits tooth pulp.

Procedure

Rabbits weighing 2–3 kg are used and anesthesia is given with thiopental in the doses of 15 mg/kg intravenously. Using dental drill, tooth pulp chambers are exposed close to the two front upper incisors. Clamping electrodes are placed into the drilled holes. After 30 min, electrical stimulus is applied by rectangular current (frequency 50 Hz) upto 1 sec. Current is started with 0.2 mA and increased until animal starts licking. After that, a threshold is determined at least 3 times in each animal. Animal serves as its own control. Test compound is administered orally or intravenously. After 15, 30, 60 and 120 min, threshold current is measured and compared with the threshold current prior to drug administration.[8]

Modifications

Electrical Stimulation of the Tail

Electrical stimuli of gradually increasing intensities can be delivered by subcutaneous electrodes in the tail of the rat or the mouse. When such gradually increasing intensities of electrical stimuli are applied, a reflex movement of the tail can be observed. The threshold for this response is determined before (relative ratio: 1, 1.5, and 3, approximately) and 45 min after the administration of test drug. The results are expressed as percentages of these thresholds on a semilogarithmic chart. Over the range of doses used, if test drug increases the threshold for the responses, it would have analgesic potential.[9-11]

Monkey Shock Titration Test

The monkey shock titration test is used for final evaluation of a new compound having analgesic potential.

Procedure

The monkeys are seated in restraining chairs. By a Coulbourn Instrument Programmable Shocker electrical current is delivered through electrodes, which are coupled to two test tube clamps attached to a shaved portion of tail. The current ranges from 0–4 mA through 29 progressive steps. The monkey presses a bar to interrupt the shock. For each monkey, a stable baseline shock level is recorded. After 24 h, drug is administered and shock titration activity is measured according to a change in maximum level of median shock intensity for drug as compared to control levels.[12,13]

MODELS USING CHEMICAL STIMULUS

The chemical tests involve administration of an irritant, algogenic chemical agent as the nociceptive stimulus. Chemical stimulation induces a slow form of stimulation. The characteristic features of chemical stimuli are that they are progressive and persist for a longer duration.

Hence, chemical tests can be distinguished clearly from those mentioned above, in terms of their physical nature, duration, and measurement of a behavioral score in units of time. Without doubt, these experimental models are the closest in nature to clinical pain. Tests where chemical stimulus is applied are:

Formalin Test

The formalin test uses a 10% formalin solution as a chemical noxious stimulus. By injecting the formalin solution into the paw of a rat or a mouse, a model of persistent (chronic) pain caused by peripheral tissue injuries and inflammation is created. This model is highly sensitive for opioids like drugs. In formalin test, animals show two phases (biphasic) of nociceptive behavior involving two different stimuli. The first (early) phase starts immediately after injection of formalin and last for 3–5 min. This occurs due to chemical stimulation of nociceptors causing C-fiber activation. Second (late) phase starts after 10–15 min of formalin injection and lasts for 20–40 min. This phase appears due to combination of an inflammatory reaction in the peripheral tissue and functional changes in the dorsal horn of the spinal cord. The C-fiber barrage initiates functional changes during the early phase. Opioid analgesics are antinociceptive for both phases, although the second is more sensitive to these substances. Non-steroidal antinflammatory drugs are effective in second phase, while the first phase remains unaffected.[14,15]

Procedure

Male Wistar rats weighing 180–300 g are used. In the dorsum of front paw of the animal 0.05 ml of 10% formalin is injected subcutaneously. Each animal is placed into separate cage for observation of pain responses in early and late phases. These responses are elevation or favoring of the paw or excessive licking and biting of the paw. Scoring of these pain responses is done according to a pain scale. After administration of the test drug, again scoring is done after 30, 60 min for comparison. If both paws of the animal are allowed to rest on the floor with no obvious favoring of the injected paw, this is taken as a positive analgesic response.[16]

Writhing Test

This is a model of visceral or peritoneal pain in animals, which also involves the administration of algogenic agents. This test is used to detect peripheral analgesic activity of a test compound. In this test, pain is induced by intraperitoneal administration of chemicals that irritate serous membranes and provoke a stereotyped behavior in the mouse or rat known as writhing. These behaviors are considered reflexive, and are evidence of peritoneovisceral or visceral pain associated with visceral chemoreceptors.[17]

Procedure

Mice of either sex approximately 20–25 g are used. Rats can also be used in this test. Phenylquinone (0.02%) is suspended in 1% suspension of carboxy methylcellulose. An aliquot of 0.25 ml of this suspension is injected intraperitoneally in each animal. The animal reacts with a characteristic stretching behavior, i.e. a series of constrictions occur that travel along the abdominal wall, sometimes accompanied by turning movements of the body and extension of the hind limbs. This response is called as writhing.

A group of animals (n=6) is used as test group in which prior to phenylquinone administration, test drugs are administered orally or subcutaneously. The mice are placed individually into glass chambers and number of writhes are recorded for 10 min in each animal.

For scoring, a writhe is indicated by stretching of the abdomen with simultaneous stretching of at least one hind limb. Formula for computing percent inhibition is: average writhes in the control group minus writhes in the test group divided by writhes in the control group times 100%. The time period with the greatest percent of inhibition is considered the peak time.[18]

Other Chemical Compounds that can Elicit Writhing

Several other chemicals can give rise to writhing behavior. For example: acetic acid, acetylcholine, bradykinin, prostaglandin E_1, aconitine, 4% NaCl, ethacrynic acid. [19-23]

Distension of Hollow Organs Using Chemical Stimulus

Such tests involve injecting chemical substances directly into hollow organs and they represent as models for true visceral pain such as:

Rat Sigmoid Colon Model

This model is a true visceral pain model.

In this model, formalin (50 µl, 5%) is administered into the rat sigmoid colon, which produces a complex biphasic pain behavior involving an initial phase of body stretching and contraction of either the flanks or the whole body followed by a second phase, showing abdominal licking and nibbling. A pain score can be calculated after analysis of the formalin-induced behaviors. The score can be dose-dependently reduced by test drug with analgesic activity.[24]

Inflammatory Uterine Pain Model

This model resembles closely a state of inflammatory uterine pain and also provides further insight into the neural processes contributing to visceral nociception.

Procedure

Mustard oil is injected into one uterine horn in the rat to produce chemical inflammation. Control rats are sham-operated. Rat behavior is observed using non-stop video-tape recording for 7 days. Rats with uterine inflammation show abnormal behavior during the first 4 days (hunching, hump-backed position, licking of the lower abdomen, repeated waves of contraction of the ipsilateral oblique musculature with inward turning of the ipsilateral hind limb, stretching, squashing of the lower abdomen against the floor) suggestive of visceral pain and evidence of flank muscle hyperalgesia over 7 days indicative of referred visceral pain.[25]

MODELS USING MECHANICAL STIMULUS

Haffner's Tail Clip Method

In this method, mechanical stimulus is applied. The preferred sites for applying nociceptive mechanical stimuli are the hind paw and the tail. This method is highly sensitive for centrally acting drugs. Tests using constant pressure have been abandoned progressively for those applying gradually increasing pressures.

Procedure

Male mice weighing 18–25 g are used. An artery clip is placed at the root of the tail of the mice to apply noxious stimulus. A quick response of the animal is seen as biting the clip or tail, where clip has been placed. The time (reaction time) between application of the clip and response is noted by a stopwatch. For testing analgesic activity, test compounds are administered subcutaneously or orally. After 15, 30 or 60 min, same procedure is repeated and reaction time is measured. For evaluation of analgesic drugs cut off time is determined, i.e. average reaction time plus 3 times the standard deviation of the combined latencies of the control mice at all time periods.

Reaction time of the test animals, greater than the cut off time denotes a positive response indicating analgesic activity.[26,27]

Randall Selitto Test

The principle of the test is that inflammation increases the sensitivity to pain, and thus, decreases pain threshold. In Randall Sellito test, inflammation is induced by subcutaneous administration of Brewer's yeast and then pressure is applied, which increases the intensity of pain. This test is used to detect peripheral analgesic activity of a test compound.

Procedure

Male Wistar rats are divided into two groups—test and control. In the test group, test agents are administered and vehicle is administered in control group animals. After 15–30 min, 0.1 ml of Brewer's yeast (20% suspension) in distilled water is injected subcutaneously into the plantar surface of the left hind paw of the rat. After 3 h, using a special apparatus (Randall Selitto apparatus) pressure is applied to the plantar surface of the rat's foot at a constant rate until animal struggles or squeals. In both the groups each animal is tested for its control pain threshold and then comparison is made between the groups. Animal, which is showing control pain threshold greater than 80 g, is eliminated.[28]

Colburn et al. evaluated a mechanical visceral pain model, where chronic intermittent intestinal distension (repeatable and reversible) is produced in the rat using a chronic indwelling intraduodenal balloon catheter.[29,30]

Commonly used animal models of acute pain, according to types of stimuli are shown in Table 32.1.

Table 32.1: Common animal models of acute pain according to types of stimuli

Thermal	*Mechanical*	*Chemical*	*Electrical*
Tail-flick test	Haffner's tail clip method	Formalin test (intradermal injections)	Tail stimulation
Hot-plate test	Randall and Selitto test	Writhing test (intraperitoneal injections)	Tooth pulp test
		Chemical stimulation of visceral organs	

ANIMAL MODELS OF CHRONIC PAIN

Neuropathic Pain Models

Partial somatosensory nerve injury is the cause of causalgiform pain disorders in man. Causalgia is characterized by spontaneous burning pain combined with hyperalgesia and allodynia. The presence of pain in the inflammation models is inferred by an increased response to a noxious stimulus (hyperalgesia) or a nocifensive behavior in response to an innocuous stimulus, normally not perceived as painful allodynia. This model represents disorders of neuropathic pain sensation like those seen in man.

Procedure

Male Sprague-Dawley rats are used and anesthetized with 4% halothane. A local incision is given and sciatic nerves of both legs are exposed at the level of mid thigh. Four (4-0) chromic gut sutures are tied loosely with a square knot around the right sciatic nerve. Left sciatic nerve is just mobilized. Incisions are closed layer to layer. During the next days animals show a mild aversion of the affected paw and foot drop.[31] The thermal nociceptive threshold of hind paws is measured in each animal. For this, rats are placed beneath a transparent plastic cage upon a raised glass plate, such that a halogen projector lamp could be placed below it. Lamp (source of radiant heat) is focused at the planter area of one hind paw. As soon as heat is applied a withdrawal response of hind paw is seen. The time interval between the exposure of heat and withdrawal response is measured in each animal.[32] After 7–8 days, test drug and vehicle are injected intrathecally in test and control group, respectively. Paw withdrawal latency (PWL) of hind paws is recorded before and after 5, 15, 30, 60 and 90 min of drug and vehicle administration. PWL, which was the maximum during the first 30 min after drug or vehicle injection is called as maximum PWL. To evaluate hyperesthesia, the difference score (DS) is calculated by subtracting the maximum PWL of the control side (left side) from the maximum PWL of the affected side (right side). For evaluation of drug effects in hyperesthetic rats, the dose is plotted against the change in DS (post- drug difference score minus pre-drug difference score).

Modifications

A rat model of partial sciatic nerve injury has also been produced.[33] This model produces reproducible tactile allodynia and thermal hyperalgesia. Unilateral tight ligation of about half of the sciatic nerve in rats rapidly produces sympathetically dependent neuropathic pain that lasts many months and resembles causalgia in humans.

An animal model of persistent peripheral neuropathic pain has also been produced involving spared nerve injury. This involves a lesion of two of the three terminal branches of the sciatic nerve (tibial and common peroneal nerves) leaving the remaining sural nerve intact. Co-mingling of distal intact axons with degenerating axons is restricted, and it permits behavioral testing of the non-injured skin territories adjacent to the denervated areas. The spared nerve injury model results in early (< 24 h), prolonged (> 6 months), robust (all animals are responders) behavioral modifications.[34]

Vincristine-induced Neuropathy Model

Hyperalgesia induced by vincristine in the rat provides a good model for the experimental study of painful peripheral neuropathies in patients receiving vincristine as a chemotherapeutic agent.

Procedure

Vincristine (100 μg/kg) is administered daily for 2 weeks in rats. A decrease in mechanical nociceptive threshold and hyperalgesia occurs after the second day of administration. Chronic lowered threshold and increased response to stimuli (determined 24 h after each injection) is seen during the second week of vincristine administration. Responses gradually return to baseline following discontinuation of treatment. Thermal hyperalgesia is also produced with vincristine in this model.[35]

Diabetic Neuropathy Model

Painful diabetic neuropathy is one of the most common complications of insulin-dependent diabetes in man. The streptozotocin-induced diabetic rat has been put forward as a model of chronic pain with signs of hyperalgesia and allodynia that may reflect signs observed in diabetic humans.

Procedure

Streptozotocin (STZ) (75 mg/kg, ip) is administered in rats so that they develop diabetes (hyperglycemia > or = 14 mM). The animals are subjected to various pain stimuli: mechanical, thermal (warm and cold) and chemical. The time course of the scores was followed for 4 weeks simultaneously with the clinical symptoms (weight, body and skin temperature, motility) and hyperglycemia. A decrease in reaction thresholds to noxious heat stimuli and to non-painful thermal (cold: 10°C, and warm: 38–42°C) and mechanical stimulation (paw pressure) is observed. This serves as evidence for hyperalgesia and allodynia, respectively. These troubles appear after 2 weeks of establishment of diabetes. Four weeks after the induction of diabetes, the scores can be obtained in diabetic rats injected with formalin (chemical stimuli). If score is greater than those in normal rats, it indicates hyperalgesia.[36]

Kiguchi S et al. evaluated the antinociceptive effect of oxcarbazepine (OCBZ), a keto derivative of carbamazepine in diabetic neuropathy rat model and suggested that OCBZ has an analgesic action and is a possible therapeutic agent for the treatment of painful diabetic neuropathic pain.[37]

Persistent Post-thoracotomy Pain Model

Chronic post-thoracotomy pain (CPTP) recurs or persists after a thoracotomy incision at least 2 months following the surgical procedure.[38] This pain is described as a continuous dysesthesia with burning and aching in the general area of the thoracotomy incision.

This type of pain is chronic and persistent in nature and commonly seen after thoracotomy, although its basis and therapy have not been well characterized. In this model, the allodynic responses (mechanical and cold) as well as the histopathologic changes after thoracotomy and rib retraction in rats are observed to evaluate the antinociceptive potential of test drug.

Procedure

Male Sprague-Dawley rats are anesthetized and the right 4th and 5th ribs surgically exposed. The pleura is opened between the ribs and a retractor placed under both ribs and opened 8 mm. Retraction is maintained for 5, 30, or 60 min. Control animals are given pleural incision only.

After two days post-surgery, animals are tested for mechanical allodynia using calibrated von Frey filaments and cold allodynia using acetone applied to the incision site. Two weeks after surgery, animals are tested for reduction of allodynia with administration of test drugs. In 50% of the animals with 60 min retraction, allodynia develops and when the retraction time was 5 and 30 min allodynia is seen in 11% and 10% of animals, respectively. Control animals do not develop allodynia. Allodynic animals show extensive axon loss in the intercostal nerves of the retracted ribs. If a test drug reduces allodynia, it would have analgesic potential. This model is useful for quantifying the efficacy of techniques to reduce the frequency and severity of long-term post-thoracotomy pain.[39]

Rat Model of Incisional Pain

This model helps to understand mechanisms of sensitization caused by surgery and investigate new therapies for postoperative pain in humans. In the model, it is revealed that both the sural and tibial nerves are responsible for transmitting input from the incision that produces hyperalgesia.

A longitudinal incision of 1 cm is given through skin, fascia and muscle of the plantar surface of the hind paw in halothane-anesthetized rats. Withdrawal responses are measured using von Frey filaments at different areas around the wound before surgery and for the next 6 days. The results of tests for withdrawal responses suggest that a surgical incision of the rat foot causes mechanical hyperalgesia lasting for several days after surgery.[40]

Pharmacological Characterization of Rat Model of Incisional Pain

Whiteside et al. assessed the validity and reliability of rat model of postincisional pain and evaluated the effects of different classes of clinically effective analgesic drugs against multiple behavioral end points, the time course of mechanical hyperalgesia, tactile allodynia using the Randall-Selitto (paw pressure) assay and electronic von Frey, respectively. Behavioral evaluations began 24 h following surgery, and continued for 9–14 days.[41]

MODELS OF CANCER PAIN

Rat Model of Bone Cancer Pain

Bone metastasis is one of the major causes of cancer-related pain, and not all bone cancer pain can be effectively treated.

In this model, bone cancer is induced in the rat by the syngeneic MRMT-1 mammary tumor cell line. Model is characterized by mechanical hyperalgesia and allodynia along with the progression of the tumor in the bone marrow cavity, while the general condition of the animal remains satisfactory.

Procedure

Sprague-Dawley rats are given intra-tibial injections of syngeneic MRMT-1 rat mammary gland carcinoma cells. Control rats receive heat-killed cells or vehicle. Sprague-Dawley rats, given intratibial injections of syngeneic MRMT-1 rat mammary gland carcinoma cells, develop behavioral signs indicative of pain, including: mechanical allodynia, difference of weight bearing between hind paws and mechanical hyperalgesia. The development of the bone tumor and structural damage to the bone was monitored. Intra-tibial injections of $3 \times 10^{(3)}$ or $3 \times 10^{(4)}$ syngeneic MRMT-1 cells produced a rapidly expanding tumor within the boundaries of the tibia, causing severe remodeling of the bone. Damage to the cortical bone and the trabeculae by day 10–14 after inoculation of $3 \times 10^{(3)}$ MRMT-1 cells, and by day 20, the damage was threatening the integrity of the tibial bone. A large number of polykariotic cells, resembling those of osteoclasts within the tumor are observed with tartarate-resistant acid phosphatase staining.

No tumor growth was observed after the injection of heat-killed MRMT-1 cells. No changes in body weight and core temperature occurs after intra-tibial injections of $3 \times 10^{(3)}$ or $3 \times 10^{(4)}$ MRMT-1 cells, heat-killed cells or vehicle. The general activity of animals after injection with live or heat-killed MRMT-1 cells was higher than that of the control group, however, the activity of the MRMT-1 treated group declined during the progress of the disease.

Rats receiving intra-tibial injections of MRMT-1 cells show development of mechanical allodynia and mechanical hyperalgesia/reduced weight bearing on the affected limb, beginning on day 12–14 or 10–12 following injection of $3 \times 10^{(3)}$ or $3 \times 10^{(4)}$ cells, respectively. Rats receiving heat-killed cells or vehicle do not show these symptoms.[42]

Modifications

In modified model, syngeneic Walker 256 mammary gland carcinoma cells are injected into the tibia medullary cavity via intercondylar eminence in rats. The rats inoculated with carcinoma cells show significant ambulatory pain, mechanical allodynia, and reduction in weight bearing, as well as increased incidence of spontaneous activity in Abeta fibers in affected limb, whereas PBS (vehicle) or heat-killed cells (sham) injected rats showed no significant difference in comparison to normal rats.[43]

Zhao C et al. used sarcoma cells (NCTC 2472) that were injected into the medullary cavity of the humerus, femur, or calcaneus.[44]

Lee BH et al. developed another mouse model of cancer pain, in which Murine hepatocarcinoma cells, HCa-1, were inoculated unilaterally into the thigh or the dorsum of the foot of male C3H/HeJ mice. Four weeks after inoculation, behavioral signs were observed for mechanical allodynia, cold allodynia, and hyperalgesia using a von Frey filament, acetone, and radiant heat, respectively. Bone invasion by the tumor commenced from 7 days after inoculation of tumor cells and was evident from 14 days after inoculation. Cold allodynia, but neither mechanical allodynia nor hyperalgesia, was observed in mice that received an inoculation into the thigh. On the contrary, mechanical allodynia and cold allodynia, but not hyperalgesia, were developed in mice with an inoculation into the foot. Sometimes, mirror-image pain was developed in these animals.[45]

IN VITRO METHODS

Identification of several types of opioid receptors in the brain has allowed to perform *in vitro* binding tests to study the action of central analgesics. Various new receptors have been identified by using *in vitro* methods as therapeutic targets for the treatment of pain, especially neuropathic and cancer pain, such as receptors for nociceptin, vasoactive intestinal peptide, cannabinoids and vanilloid receptors. Agonists and antagonists for these receptors are being evaluated.[46-49]

^{3}H-Naloxone Binding Assay

Opiate agonists and antagonists have ability to displace radiolabeled naloxone that is a potent narcotic antagonist. ^{3}H-Naloxone binding assay is developed to classify opioid analgesics as agonists, mixed agonist-antagonists and antagonists. The basic principle of this assay is to determine IC_{50} values for ^{3}H-Naloxone in the presence or absence of Na^+.

Reagents that are used in the assay are: ^{3}H Naloxone (38–58 Ci/mmol): concentration is 5 nM in 3 test tubes.

Levorphanol tartrate: 1 mM stock solution of levorphanol is diluted 1:200 in distilled water and in 3 tubes 20 μl is added to yield a final concentration of 0.1 μM in the assay.

Dextrorphan tartrate: 1 mM stock solution is diluted 1:200 in distilled water and in 3 tubes 20 μl is added to get a final concentration of 0.1 μM in the assay.

Test compounds: 1 mM stock solution is made in an appropriate solvents and diluted serially to get the final concentration in between 10^{-5} and 10^{-8} M.

Procedure

Male Wistar rats are decapitated and their brains are removed. Whole brains without cerebella are homogenized in 50 volumes of ice-cold 0.05 M tris buffer with a tissue homogenizer. Centrifugation of homogenate is done at 40,000 g for 15 min. Pellet is resuspended in buffer and recentrifuged at 40,000 g. After this, the final pellet is resuspended in freshly prepared 0.05 M tris buffer. Finally, tissue concentration in the assay becomes 10 mg/ml.

In test tubes a mixture is prepared, which consist of 310 μl H_2O, 20 μl 5 μM dextrorphan (total binding) or 5 μM levorphanol (non specific binding), 50 μl 2 M NaCl or H_2O, 50 μl 0.05 M Tris buffer, pH 7.7, 20 μl drug or vehicle, 50 μl ^{3}H-Naloxone and 500 μl tissue suspension. The tubes are incubated for 30 min at 37°C. Vacuum filtration through Whatman GF/B filters is done to stop the assay and washing is performed at least 3 times with ice-cold 0.05 M Tris buffer, pH 7.7. The filters are then counted in 10 ml of Liquiscint liquid scintillation cocktail. Difference between binding in the presence of 0.1 μM dextrorphan and 0.1 μM levorphanol is known as stereospecific binding.

Specific binding is around 1% of the total added ligand and 50% of the total bound ligand in the absence of Na^+ and 2% of the total added ligand and 65% of the total bound ligand in the presence of Na^+ (100 mM). An increase in specific binding denotes an increase in binding.

To evaluate analgesic activity, data are converted into % stereospecific ^{3}H-naloxone binding displaced by the test drug. Determination of IC_{50} is done by using computer-derived log-probit analysis. IC_{50} is used to calculate sodium shift. Opioids agonists show high sodium shifts, antagonists show low shift and mixed opioids agonists-antagonists show medium shift. Data are analyzed by a computer program.[50,51]

μ Opiate Receptor Binding Assay

Opioids drugs exert their analgesic effects mainly through μ opioid receptors. ^{3}H-Dihydromorphine is highly selective for μ receptors. The compounds that inhibit binding of ^{3}H-dihydromorphine in a synaptic membrane preparation from rat brain can be identified by this assay.[52]

Reagents that are used in the assay are—20 nM stock solution of ^{3}H-dihydromorphine, 0.1 mM stock solution of levallorphan tartrate and 1 mM stock solution of test compounds. All compounds are taken in 3 test tubes. 50 μl of ^{3}H-dihydromorphine and 20 μl of levollarphan tartrate are added to each tube. In the assay final concentration of ^{3}H-dihydromorphine and levollarphan tartrate are 0.5 nM and 0.1 μM, respectively and concentration of test compounds ranges from 10^{-6}–10^{-9} M. Total volume of assay mixture is 2 ml.

Procedure

Male Wistar rats are used. Animals are sacrificed by decapitation. Whole brains without cerebella are removed, weighed and homogenized in 30 volumes of ice-cold 0.05 M Tris buffer, pH 7.7. Centrifugation of homogenate is performed at 48,000 g for 15 min and pellet is resuspended in the same volume of buffer. This homogenate is incubated to remove the endogenous opiate peptides and centrifuged again. The final pellet is resuspended in 50 volumes of 0.05 M Tris buffer.

In test tubes, a mixture consisting of 1850 µl tissue suspension, 80 µl distilled water, 20 µl vehicle or levallorphan or appropriate concentration of drug and 50 µl ^{3}H-dihydromorphine is prepared. Then incubation is performed for 30 min at 25°C. The assay is stopped by vacuum filtration through Whatman GF/B filters, which are washed twice with 5 ml of 0.05 M tris buffer. Filters are placed into scintillation vials with 10 ml liquiscient scintillation cocktail and counted. Specific binding is the difference between total binding and binding in the presence of 0.1 mM levollarphan. At each drug concentration IC_{50} values are calculated from the percent specific binding.[53,54]

Assay to Study Cannabinoids Activity

Cannabinoids such as 9-THC (tetrahydrocannabiol) are capable of inhibiting nociception, i.e. pain transmission. Cannabinoids exert their effects by cannabinoid receptors CB_1 & CB_2, that are localized in the brain. These receptors have been well characterized and cloned. Cannabinoids produce analgesia without respiratory depression that is associated with opioids analgesics.

Procedure

Male Sprague-Dawley rats of around 150–200 g are decapitated and brains are removed immediately. The cortex is dissected free and immersed in 30 ml of ice-cold centrifugation solution (320 mM sucrose, 2 mM Tris EDTA, 5 mM $MgCl_2$). The process is repeated until the cortices of five rats are combined. The cortical material is homogenized with a Potter-Elvehjem glass-Teflon grinding system, which is then centrifuged for 15 min at 1,600 g. The supernatant is combined with the two subsequent supernatant obtained from washing and 1,600 g centrifugation of the P_1 pellet. The combined supernatants are centrifuged at 39,000 g for 15 min. The P_2 pellet resuspended in 50 ml buffer (50 mM Tris HCL, 2 mM Tris EDTA, 5 mM $MgCl_2$, pH 7.0) and incubated for 10 min at 37°C. Then centrifuged again at 23,000 g for 10 min. The P_2 membrane is resuspended in 50 ml of buffer A, incubated again and centrifuged at 11,000 g for 15 min. Finally, obtained and wash treated P_2 pellet is resuspended in assay buffer B, (50 mM Tris HCL, 3 mM Tris EDTA, 3 mM $MgCl_2$, pH 7.4) to a protein concentration of approximately 2 mg/ml. Four aliquots are prepared from the preparation and freezed in dry ice solution and 2 methylbutane and stored at –80°C.

150 mg of P_2 membrane is added to test tubes that contain [^{3}H] CP-55,940 (79 Ci/mmol), a cannabinoid analog (for displacement studies) and a sufficient quantity of buffer C (50 mM Tris-HCI, 1 mM Tris EDTA, 3 mM $MgCl_2$, 5 mg/ml BSA) to get the total incubation volume to 1 ml. In displacement studies, the concentration of [^{3}H] CP-55,940 is 400 pM and in saturation studies it varies from 25 to 2500 pM. Nonspecific binding is measured by the addition of 1 mM unlabeled CP-55,940. The standard CP-55,940 and other cannabinoid analogs are prepared in suspension buffer C from a 1 mg/ml ethanolic stock, without evaporation of the alcohol.

After this, incubation is performed for 1 h at 30°C, binding is terminated by addition of 2 ml ice-cold buffer D (50 mM Tris-HCl, 1 mg/ml BSA) and vacuum filtration. Reaction vessels are washed once with 2 ml of ice-cold buffer D, and the filters washed twice with 4 ml of ice-cold Buffer D. Filters are placed into 20 ml plastic scintillation vials with 1ml of distilled water and 10 ml of Budjet-Solve. After shaking for 1 h, the radioactivity is determined by liquid scintillation photometry.[55,56]

ROLE OF VASOACTIVE INTESTINAL POLYPEPTIDE (VIP) AND PITUITARY ADENYLATE CYCLASE- ACTIVATING PEPTIDE (PACAP) AND NOCICEPTIN IN ANALGESIA

Vasoactive intestinal polypeptide and pituitary adenylate cyclase-activating peptide (PACAP), play a role in the altered transmission of sensory information in neuropathic pain (arising from trauma or compression injury of peripheral nerves). Both of these peptides act through G-protein coupled receptors, named VPAC (VIP_1), $VPAC_2$ (VIP_2), PAC_1 (PACAP type 1) receptors. These receptors would be used as new therapeutic targets for the treatment of neuropathic analgesia. Various agonists and antagonists for VIP have been evaluated.

To study properties of these receptors, CHO cell lines are used, which stably express VIP-PACAP type I & type II receptors.[57,58]

Nociceptin or orphanin FQ is a heptadekapeptide, which acts through a specific receptor that has been cloned and well characterized in man and animals and named as opioid receptor like (ORL_1) receptor. Nociceptin receptor (ORL_1) and opioid receptors show structural and transductional similarities. Hence, nociceptin receptor has been included into the opioids receptor family with the name of $OP_{4.}$ Nociceptin induces analgesia when given intrathecally in rats.[59-60]

CONCLUSION

The word pain is applied to a wide variety of subjective phenomenon ranging from the perception of an experimental noxious stimulus to the most severe and excruciating pain in humans suffering from cancer, trigeminal neuralgia, etc. Animal models have been used extensively in basic pain research based on the premise that animal models can serve as surrogate assays that can reliably predict the potency and efficacy of the pharmacologic action of, and, in some cases, the molecular response to, agents that work in human pain states. But in contrast to the polymorphic nature of pain in humans, pain in animals can be estimated only by examining their reactions to various chemical, thermal, and mechanical stimuli, with the latency or nature of response altered in the pain state. Most commonly used methods for evaluation of analgesic drugs are tail-flick test and hot plate test. However, formalin test has also been widely used.

Although different pain models based on use of nociceptive stimuli (electrical, thermal, mechanical, or chemical) have been used, none is ideal. However, test using chemical stimuli probably most closely mimic acute clinical pain. The monitored reactions are almost always motor responses ranging from spinal reflexes to complex behaviors. Most have the weakness that they may be associated with, or modulated by, other physiological functions. The weaknesses of the tests, include (i) in most tests responses are monitored around a nociceptive threshold,whereas clinical pain is almost always more severe; (ii) differences in the fashion, whereby responses are evoked from healthy and inflamed tissues; and (iii) problems in assessing threshold responses to stimuli, which continue to increase in intensity.

In summary, animal models have contributed much to the understanding of the mechanisms of pain in humans, and current clinical treatments are based, in part, on those studies. But the future of effective strategies that go beyond palliative care will also use these models to screen novel, safe, and useful approaches in a preclinical setting. Much resource effort and expense can be conserved by testing novel methodologies in multiple animal models—not relying on a single animal model, strain, or species—before clinical testing begins. As pain in humans is chronic in nature, there is a critical need for development of such models that could provide knowledge about mechanisms involved in chronic pain in humans. As far as neuropathic pain is concerned, it is difficult to design this type of model in animals for both technical and ethical reasons and much more difficult is to devise tests that could measure affective component of pain.

REFERENCES

1. Woolfe G, MacDonald. The evaluation of the analgesic action of pethidine hydrochloride (DEMEROL). J Pharmacol Exp Ther 1944;80:300-7.
2. Kitchen I, Gowder M. Assessment of the hot plate antinociceptive test in mice: A new method for the statistical treatment of graded data. J Pharmacol Meth 1985;13:1-7.
3. Geller I, Axelor LR. Methods for evaluating analgesics in laboratory animals. In Soulairac A, Cahn J, Charpentier J (Eds): Pain. London, New York: Acad Press, 1968;153-63.
4. Howes JF, Harris LS, Dewey WL, et al. Brain acetycholine levels and inhibition of tail-flick reflex in mice. J Pharmacol Exp Ther 1969;169:23-8.
5. Sewell RDE, Spencer PSJ. Antinociceptive activity of narcotic agonist and partial agonist analgesics and other agents in the tail-immersion test in mice and rats. Neuropharmacol 1976;15:683-8.
6. Pizziketti RJ, Pressman NS, Geller EB, et al. Rat old water tail flick: a novel analgesic test that distinguishes opioid agonists from mixed agonist-antagonists. Eur J Pharmacol 1985;119:23-9.
7. Wang JJ, Ho ST, Hu OY, et al. An innovative cold tail-flick test: the cold ethanol tail-flick test. Anesth Analg 1995;80:102-7.
8. Piercy MF, Schroedor LA. A quantitative analgesic assay in the rabbit based on response to tooth pulp stimulation. Arch Int Pharmacodyn Ther 1980;248:294-304.
9. Nilsen PL. Studies on algesimetry by electrical stimulation of the mouse-tail. Acta Pharmacol Toxicol 1961;18:10-22.
10. Paalzow L. An electrical method for estimation of analgesic activity in mice. II. Application of the method in investigations of some analgesic drugs. Acta Pharm Suec 1969;6:207–26.
11. Carroll MN, Lim RK. Observations of the neuropharmacology of morphine like analgesia. Arch Int Pharmacodyn Ther 1960;125:383-403.
12. Weiss B, Laties VG. Analgesic effects in monkeys of morphine, nalorphine and a benzomorphan narcotic antagonist. J Pharmacol Exp Ther 1964;143:169-73.
13. Romer D. A sensitive method for measuring analgesic effects in the monkey. In Soulaireac A, Cahn J, Charpentier J, eds. Pain. London, New York: Acad Press, 1968:165-70.

14. Abbot FV, Franklin KBJ, Westbrook RF. The formalin test: scoring properties of the first and second phases of the pain response in rats. Pain 1995;60:91-102.
15. Dubuission D, Dennis SG. The formalin test: A quantitative study of the analgesic effects of morphine, meperidine and brain stem stimulation in rats and cats. Pain 1977;4:161-74.
16. Hunskaar S, Hole K. The formalin test in mice: dissociation between inflammatory and non-inflammatory pain. Pain 1987;30:103-14.
17. Hammond DL. Inference of pain and its modulation from simple behaviors. In Chapaman CR, Loeser JD, (Eds): Issues in pain management: advances in pain research and therapy. New York: Raven Press; 1989;69-91.
18. Hendershot LC, Forsaith J. Antagonism of the frequency of phenylquinone- induced writhing in the mouse by weak analgesics and non-analgesics. J Pharmacol Exp Ther 1959;125:237-40.
19. Amanuma F, Wakaumi C, Tanaka M, et al. The analgesic effects of non-steroidal anti-inflammatory drugs on acetylcholine-induced writhing in mice. Folia Pharmacol Japon 1984;84:543-51.
20. Koster R, Anderson M, de Beer EJ. Acetic acid for analgesic screening. Fed Proc 1959;18:412.
21. Emele JF, Shanaman J. Bradykinin writhing: A method for measuring analgesia. Proc Soc Exp Biol Med 1963;114:680-2.
22. Sancillo LF, Nolan JC, Wagner LE, et al. The analgesic and anti-inflammatory activity and pharmacologic properties of bromfenac. Arzneim Forsch/Drug Res 1987;37:513-9.
23. Bjorkman RL, Headner T, Hallman KM, et al. Localization of central antinociceptive effects of diclofenac in the rat. Brain Res. 1992;590:66-73.
24. Miampamba M, Chéry-Croze S, Gorry F, et al. Inflammation of the colonic wall induced by formalin as a model of acute visceral pain. Pain 1994;57:327-34.
25. Wesselmann U, Czakanski PP, Affaitati G, et al. Uterine inflammation as a noxious visceral stimulus: behavioral characterization in the rat. Neurosci Lett 1998;246:73-6.
26. Haffner F. Experimental Prufungs chimerzstillender Mittel. Dtsch Med Wschr 1929;55:731-3.
27. Bianchi C, Franceschini J. Experimental observations on Haffnerés method for testing analgesics. Br J Pharmacol 1954;9:280-4.
28. Randal LO, Selitto J J. A method for measurement of analgesic activity on inflamed tissue. Arch Int Pharmacodyn 1957;111:409-19.
29. Colburn RW, Coombs DW, Degnan CC, et al. Mechanical visceral pain model: chronic intermittent intestinal distension in the rat. Physiol Behav 1989;45:191-7.
30. deLeo JA, Colburn RW, Coombs DW, et al. The differentiation of NSAIDS and prostaglandin action using a mechanical visceral pain model in the rat. Pharmacol Biochem Behav 1989;33:253-5.
31. Bennet GJ, Xie Y K. A peripheral neuropathy in the rat that produces disorders of pain sensation like those seen in man. Pain 1988;33:87-108.
32. Hargaeves K, Dubner R, Brown F, et al. A new and sensitive method for measuring thermal nociception in cutaneous hyperalgesia. Pain 1988;32:77-88.
33. Seltzer Z, Dubner R, Shir Y. A novel behavioral model of neuropathic pain disorders has also been produced in rats by partial sciatic nerve injury. Pain 1990;43:205-18.
34. Decosterd I, Woolf CJ. Spared nerve injury: an animal model of persistent peripheral neuropathic pain. Pain 2000;87:149-58.
35. Aley KO, Reichling DB, Levine JD. Vincristine hyperalgesia in the rat: a model of painful vincristine neuropathy in humans. Neurosci 1996;73:259-65.

36. Courteix C, Eschalier A, Lavarenne J. Streptozocin-induced diabetic rats: behavioural evidence for a model of chronic pain. Pain 1993;53:81-8.
37. Kiguchi S, Imamura T, Ichikawa K, et al. Oxcarbazepine antinociception in animals with inflammatory pain or painful diabetic neuropathy. Clin Exp Pharmacol Physiol 2004;31:57-64.
38. Merskey H. Classification of chronic pain: description of chronic pain syndromes and definitions of pain terms. Pain 1986;3:S138-9.
39. Buvanendran A, Kroin JS, Kerns JM, et al. Characterization of a new animal model for evaluation of persistent post-thoracotomy pain. Anesth Analg 2004;99:1453-60.
40. Brennan TJ, Vandermeulen EP, Gebhart GF. Characterization of a rat model of incisional pain. Pain 1996; 64:493-501.
41. Whiteside GT, Harrison J, Boulet J, et al. Pharmacological characterisation of a rat model of incisional pain. Br J Pharmacol 2004;141:85-91. Epub 2003 Nov 3.
42. Medhurst SJ, Walker K, Bowes M, et al. A rat model of bone cancer pain. Pain 2002;96:129-40.
43. Mao-Ying QL, Zhao J, Dong ZQ, et al. A rat model of bone cancer pain induced by intra-tibia inoculation of Walker 256 mammary gland carcinoma cells. Biochem Biophys Res Commun 2006;345:1292-8. Epub 2006 May15.
44. Zhao C, Wacnik PW, Tall JM, et al. Analgesic effects of a soy-containing diet in three murine bone cancer pain models. J Pain 2004;5:104-10.
45. Lee BH, Seong J, Kim UJ, et al. Behavioral characteristics of a mouse model of cancer pain. Yonsei Med J 2005;46:252-9.
46. Xu X-J, Hao J-X, Wiesenfield-Hallin Z. Nociceptin or antinociceptin: potent spinal anti nociceptive effect of orphanin FQ/nociceptin in the rat. Neuro Report 1996;7:2092-4.
47. Dickinson T, Fleetwood-Walker SM. VIP and PACAP: very important in pain. Trends Pharmacol Sci 1999;20:324-9.
48. Devane WA, Dysarz FA, Johnson MR, et al. Determination and characterization of a cannabinoid receptor in rat brain. Mol Pharmacol 1988;34:605-13.
49. Szallasi A, Blumberg PM. Vanilloid receptor: new insights enhance potential as a therapeutic target. Pain 1996;68:195-208.
50. Pert CB, Synder SH. Opiate receptor binding of agonists and antagonists affected differentially by sodium. Mol Pharm 1974;10:868-73.
51. McPherson GA. Analysis of radioligand binding experiments. A collection of computer programs for the IBMPC. J Pharmacol Meth 1985;14:213-28.
52. Mansour A, Lewis ME, Khachaturia H, et al. Pharmacological and anatomical evidence of selective μ, δ and κ opioid receptor binding in the rat brain. Brain Res 1986;399:69-79.
53. Pasternak GW. Opioid receptors. In Meltzer HY, ed. Psychopharmacology: The third generation of progress. New York: Raven Press, 1997;281-8.
54. Childers S, Creese I, Snowman AM, et al. Opiate receptor binding affected differentially by opiates and opioid peptides. Eur J Pharmacol 1979;55:11-8.
55. Felder CC, Glass M. Cannabinoid receptors and their endogenous agonists. Ann Rev Pharmacol Toxicol 1998;38:179-200.
56. Compton DR, Rice KC, de Costa BK, et al. Cannabinoid structure-activity relationships: correlation of receptor binding and in vivo activities. J Pharmacol Exp Ther 1993;265:218-26.
57. Ciccarelli E, Vilardaga JP, de Neef P, et al. Properties of the VIP-PACAP type II receptor stably expressed in CHO cells. Regul Pept 1994;54:397-407.

58. Gourlet P, Vardermeers A, Vertongen P, et al. Development of high affinity selective VIP1 receptor agonists. Peptides 1997b;18:1539-45.
59. Civelli O, Nothacker HP, Reinschied R. Reverse physiology: discovery of the novel neuropeptide, orphanin FQ/nociceptin. Crit Rev Neurobiol 1998;12:163-76.
60. Hamon M. The new approach to opioid receptors. Naunyn-Schmiedeberg's Arch Pharmacol 1998;358(suppl 2):SA 5.3.

CHAPTER

33

Anti-inflammatory Agents

INTRODUCTION

Inflammatory diseases cover a broad spectrum of conditions including autoimmune diseases (e.g. rheumatoid arthritis), osteoarthritis, asthma, chronic obstructive pulmonary disease, interstitial cystitis, prostatitis, inflammatory bowel disease, multiple sclerosis, allergic rhinitis, infectious diseases, various types of cancers and cardiovascular diseases, etc.[1] Therefore, inflammation can be described as a universal host defense process involving complex cell-cell, cell-mediator and tissue interactions. These events involved in inflammation may appear common across various inflammatory diseases, but there are underlying differences in paracrine signaling mechanisms which are orchestrated by differences in chemokines, cytokines and growth factors, lipids and genetic influences.[2,3]

Although, inflammation is the unifying factor across a host of diseases but the treatment approach is often unique for each of the inflammatory disease. Each disease population has distinct therapeutic needs that are inadequately served by current prevention and treatment strategies. Therefore, there is need for improved method to search for new drugs. Inflammation most commonly occurs when microbial invasion or tissue injury overcomes the body's non-specific defense mechanisms.[4] Subsequent to infection, immune system gets activated, communication and coordination occurs between different classes as well as actions of immune cell to produce inflammation. Normally, inflammation is tightly regulated by the body and is the starting point of the body's self repair process initiated by body's defense system to thwart pathologic assaults but occasionally it runs amok, leading to physiological chaos and death.[5]

Inflammation occurs in response to a variety of harmful exogenous and endogenous stimuli. Exogenous stimuli can be of physical, chemical, mechanical, nutritional and biological origin, whereas endogenous stimuli can be of immunological, neurological and genetic origin. The inflammation could be acute, subacute or chronic in nature. The acute inflammation is short lasting, whereas chronic inflammation may persist for weeks, months or years. The classic triad of acute inflammation is: (a) pain, fever and swelling, which is caused by increased blood flow, (b) increased capillary permeability and (c) increased migration of leukocytes of which neutrophils are first to ingress into the affected tissue area. Acute inflammatory response often transitions into chronic inflammation, which is defined by tissue proliferation, granuloma, and repair. The cardinal features of inflammation are shown in Figure 33.1.

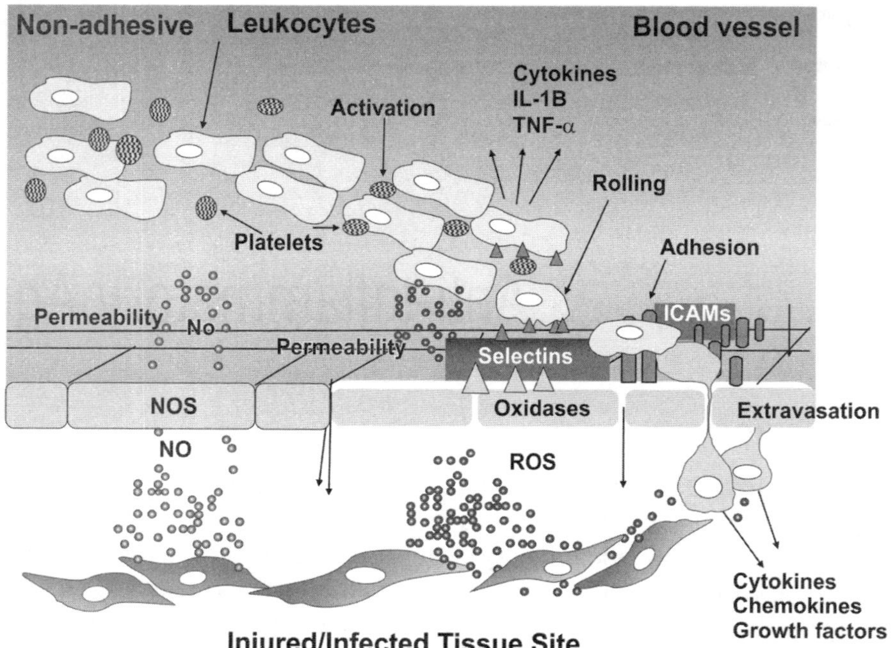

Figure 33.1: Inflammation is a characteristic response of tissue to injury or microbial invasion. Classic triad of inflammation at injury site is initiated by vasodilation following release of Nitric oxide (NO) from endothelium, then increased capillary permeability facilitates extravasation (increased migration) of leukocytes especially neutrophils towards the affected tissue area. Release of chemokines by injured cells drives the chemoattraction of other leukocytes such as monocytes, neutrophils and lymphocytes from blood. Extravasation of leukocytes to injured tissue requires expression of molecules, such as selectins, which supports rolling and stable arrest of leukocytes bound to platelets on activated vascular endothelium. Adhesion molecules, such as ICAM-1 associates with receptors of the integrin family to induce a reversible adhesion interaction

In the recent years, there has been increased focus on leukocyte migration. The first steps in leukocyte recruitment include rolling of the leukocytes on the vessel wall mediated by selectins and glycoproteins bearing the sialyl Lewis^x moiety[6] (Fig. 33.1). Adhesion between the activated platelets and neutrophils is mediated by one of the selectins, P-selectin. Drug screen methods based on adhesion assays evaluate the binding of thrombin-activated human platelets to neutrophils. Adhesion molecules, vascular cell adhesion protein 1 (VCAM-1), intracellular cell adhesion molecule (ICAM-1) also play a major role in the development and persistence of inflammatory diseases.[7]

Accumulating research evidence has proven that inflammation is an orchestra involving many players including histamine, prostaglandins (PGE2 and prostacyclins), leukotrienes (LTB4), serotonin, bradykinin, cytokines (IL-1, IL-6, IL-8, TNF-α), growth factors,[6] lysosomal contents of neutrophils, adipokines (leptin, adiponectin, resistin), reactive oxygen species (ROS), etc.[6] Reactive oxygen species (ROS) generated in endoplasmic reticulum and mitochondria contribute to the inflammation by participating in the process of autophagy, which is a highly conserved housekeeping pathway that plays a critical role in the removal of aged or damaged intracellular organelles. ROS include Superoxide (O_2.-), Hydrogen peroxide (H_2O_2), Hydroxyl radical (OH.), singlet oxygen. Gasotransmitters like Hydrogen sulfide (H_2S)

together with Nitric oxide (NO)[8] and carbon monoxide CO, are also emerging as a regulators of inflammation.[9] Efforts to develop new, safer and more effective anti-inflammatory drugs are based on the improved understanding of the role of key mediators and the processes involved in triad of inflammation (Fig. 33.1).

Advent of genomic era has emphasized on the role of altered gene expression as fundamental to the etiology of inflammation and immune disorders.[10] Many genes for proinflammatory enzymes (e.g. COX-2, iNOS,)[8] acute phase proteins and cytokines (e.g. TNF-α) contain binding sites for multiple transcription factors in their regulatory elements, which are activated by a variety of exogenous stimuli like bacterial lipopolysaccharide (LPS) and endogenous stimuli, cytokines (IFN-γ, IL-6) and growth factors. Consensus sequences for the transcription factors NF-κB, AP-1 and STAT1 have been found, e.g. in the promoters of COX-2[11] and iNOS.[9] Proinflammatory agents like TNF-α and LPS activate the mitogen-activated protein (MAP) kinase pathways resulting in the stimulation of ERK1/2, c-Jun, N-terminal kinases and p38 kinases which in turn activate transcription factors AP-1, NF-κB which participate in the regulation of expression of immediate early genes involved in immune, acute phase and inflammatory responses.

Cytokines have been shown to play central roles in inflammatory diseases[12] such as psoriasis, rheumatoid arthritis and septic shock, and inhibition of their action or their activation is a proven approach to modulation of these diseases. The secretion of these diffusible growth factors and heparin- binding chemokines by resident tissue is further amplified by immune cells during inflammation.[13] It has been demonstrated that chemokine expression temporally precedes the inflammatory cell infiltration.[14] Certain hyper inflammatory states are linked to inflammasome activation, which facilitates caspase-1 and interleukin IL-1β processing by autophagy, leading to amplified inflammatory response.[15-17] During autophagy, cell size increase and the presence of increased numbers of membrane vacuoles termed autophagosomes is noticeable. Autophagy can limit inflammasome activity by lysosome mediated destruction of inflammasomes. Autophagy can therefore be described as a double-edged sword as destruction of inflammatory cells like macrophages and inflammasome by autophagy is desirable in control of inflammation,[18] but unchecked autophagy of differentiated cells could have serious implications[19] in aging and degenerative diseases.

Until a few years ago, inflammatory disorders were treated primarily with relatively nonselective anti-inflammatory drugs such as corticosteroids and various nonsteroidal anti-inflammatory drugs, however, nowadays specific mediator antagonists alone or in combination and gene therapy are also being tried. Inhibitors, which specifically interfere with components of different intracellular signaling pathways or inhibit the activation of transcription factors responsible for the expression of disease, related genes might have applications as novel therapeutic agents in inflammation.[11,20-22] In order to search new inhibitors of signaling involved in inflammation, inducible reporter gene vectors are constructed containing the natural promoters of inflammatory genes (COX-2, iNOS, TNF-α)[11,20-22] or using binding sites for defined transcription factors (NF-κB, AP-1, glucocorticoid receptor, STATs). Present day anti-inflammatory drug discovery is based on preliminary *in vitro* observations in a number of standard anti-inflammatory assays, in which the test compound produces unusually potent antagonism of inflammatory pathways. The effective candidate drug in *in vitro* tests is later tested in whole animal models of acute, subacute and chronic inflammation.

IN VITRO METHODS

Measurement of NO Production in LPS/ IFN-γ- costimulated and unstimulated murine macrophage RAW264.7 cell line

In this *in vitro* screening method, ability of test drug to inhibit NO, which is one of the early mediators of inflammation through increased vasodilation (Fig. 33.1), is evaluated. Murine macrophage cell line RAW264.7 is maintained at 37° C in Dulbecco's modified eagle medium (DMEM) containing 10% fetal bovine serum (FBS), penicillin (100 units per ml) and streptomycin sulfate (100 μg/ml) in a humidified atmosphere of 5% CO_2.[23] The cells are stimulated with either 1 μg/ml of LPS for 4 h or 20 ng/ml IFN-γ and then test compounds, Griess reagent (100 μl) is added to 100 μl of each supernatant from LPS or IFN-γ stimulated cells in triplicate. Inhibitory test compounds are dissolved in DMSO before addition to cell line; final concentrations of DMSO is kept at 0.1% or less than that. Controls with DMSO alone are also run alongside the test drugs. The protein determination is performed by Bradford protein assay. The plates are read at 550 nm against a standard curve of sodium nitrite. Nitrite accumulation is used as an indicator of NO production in the medium and is assayed by the Griess reaction. Hydrocortisone, a well-known steroidal anti-inflammatory drug, is used as a positive control for such experiments and potential candidates are compared against hydrocortisone for efficacy measurement.

Inhibition of Oxidative Stress by Reducing Reactive Oxygen Species (ROS) Generation

Generation of excessive ROS has been implicated in a number of diseases including inflammatory diseases (Fig. 33.1). Cells of murine macrophage cell line RAW264.7 grown overnight are treated with the test drugs in different concentration for 24 h, and then incubated with fluorescent marker 5 μM carboxy-2',7'-dichlorodihydrofluorescein diacetate at 37°C for 30 min. Drug treated cells are compared to positive control cells exposed to hydrogen peroxide H_2O_2 (0.03%) for 1h prior to being stained with 5 μM of carboxy-2',7'-dichlorodihydrofluorescein diacetate. Treated cells are washed with PBS, and fluorescent cells are counted by flow cytometry. Decrease in percentage of fluorescent cells relative to positive control is index of ROS generation. Another *in vitro* model of superoxide (O_2^-) generation by polymorphonuclear cells PMNs has been used by Dianzani et al. 2006 for drug screening.[24] These investigators have cultured the PMNs and challenged them with a concentration of 10^{-7}M n-FMLP (N-formylmethionyl-leucyl-phenylalanine) to optimally generate O_2^-. Superoxide production was determined spectrophotometrically by measuring the superoxide dismutase inhibit able reduction of cytochrome C reduced/10^6 PMNs/min.

Blocking Inflammasome Activation

Inflammasome are cytoplasmic and multimolecular protein complexes, which activate Caspase-1, enzyme present in an inactive pro-form in the cytoplasm.[15-17] Isolated macrophages/ mast cells from mouse peritoneum or cell lines such as RAW264.7 and HMC-1 plated overnight can be used for this assay. Cultured cells are pretreated with test drugs (0.1, 1, and 10 μg/ml) for 1 h before stimulation with LPS (100 ng/mL)[25] or proinflammatory cytokine (interleukin-1beta, IL1β, 5 ng/ml) for 24 h. Afterwards, the cells and supernatants are harvested for analysis.

Caspase-1 activity is quantitatively measured by Western blot of pro- and processed caspase-1 in drug treated tissue homogenates.[26] Efficacy of drugs in blocking inflammasome activation is measured by reduction in the active form of caspase-1 and the increased level of pro caspase-1 form relative to active drug comparator.

Induction of Autophagy

Recent studies on autophagy frequently use RAW264.7 macrophage cells that stably or transiently express a green fluorescent protein (GFP)-tagged LC3 protein (microtubule-associated protein 1 light chain 3). RAW264.7 macrophage cells stably expressing GFP-LC3 are grown in multi-well plates and exposed to test drugs and positive controls. Drugs capable of inducing autophagy cause characteristic redistribution of GFP-LC3, which leads to a change from diffuse fluorescence throughout the cytosol to numerous punctate with concentrated fluorescent signal in vesicles due to vacuole formation.[18] Effect of potential anti-inflammatory drugs in causing redistribution of fluorescence is measured by confocal microscope.[27] The differences in expression levels of LC3-II and LC3-I in immunoblots can serve as a quantitative measure of autophagy induction.[18]

Autophagy occurs in a stepwise fashion as cells gain in size with increase in numbers of membrane vacuoles termed autophagosomes. The final step of autophagy involves the fusion of the autophagosome with the lysosome to form the autophagolysosome, in which the gathered cargo is degraded by lysosomal hydrolases. In the drug screen for autophagy, GFP-LC3 is recruited from the cytosol to become part of the autophagosome and there it undergoes site specific proteolysis and lipidation near the C terminus to form LC3-II. Effect of test drugs on the expression of autophagy-related proteins such as light chain 3B (LC3B), autophagy protein 5 ATG5, beclin 1, LAMP-2, can be used as measure of efficacy.[28]

Mast Cell Degranulation

Mast cells play a key part in allergic inflammation as their degranulation releases cytokines, chemokines, proteases, and histamine after re-exposure to an allergen.[29] Previous drug screen methods relied on harvesting peritoneal mast cells to evaluate ability of test drugs to inhibit mast cell degranulation. Recent studies used phorbol 12-myristate 13-acetate (PMA) plus A23187-stimulated mast cell line, HMC-1[29] for this purpose. Cultured mast cell line is exposed to test drugs for 30 min prior to stimulation with PMACI (20 nM of PMA plus 1 μM of A23187) and incubated at 37°C for 6 h. The cells are separated from the released histamine by centrifugation at 400 rpm for 5 min at 4°C. Histamine levels are then measured in supernatant by measuring fluorescent intensity at 460 nm (excitation at 355 nm) using a spectrofluorometer. The total content is measured after treatment of the cell suspension with Triton X-100. The percentage release determined is considered the index of anti-inflammatory activity.

Measurement of Cytokine Expression in Murine Macrophages

Macrophages are the crucial agents for chronic inflammation and therefore serve as ideal platform for screening agents against chronic inflammation. To obtain primary macrophages, female CD-1 mice, 5 to 10 weeks of age are injected intraperitoneally with 2 ml of 4% thioglycollate broth. Four days after injection, peritoneal macrophages are harvested and processed according to Ding's procedure.[30] Cells are seeded in 96-well plates at 2×10^5 cells/

well and incubated for 48 h with 20 ng/ml IFN-γ in the presence or absence of test drugs. Following treatment, cytokines levels in medium from drug treated and untreated cells can be measured by ELISA or by multiplex.[31] Besides protein, the effect of tested agents on the mRNA expression of proinflammatory mediators can be assessed by harvesting the cells and processing for semiquantitative reverse transcription polymerase chain reaction (RT-PCR) or quantitative PCR (qPCR).[23,32]

Measurement of Inflammatory Gene Expression

Murine peritoneal macrophages are isolated[26] as described above and treated with test drugs in the presence or absence of LPS (5μg/mL) for 18 h. Effect of test drugs on inducible NOS (iNOS), COX-2[33] and microsomal PGE synthase-1 protein, and p38 MAPK phosphorylation[34] is evaluated by Western Blot analysis. Effect of drugs on NF-κB nuclear translocation can be visualized using the technique of immunofluorescence.

Adhesion Assays

The vascular proteins VCAM-1, ICAM-1, and E-selectin, are investigated in primary cells derived from umbilical vein (HUVEC) and a microvascular cell line (HMEC-1) owing to their prominent roles in regulating leukocyte extravasation. Adhesion assays using cultured (HUVECs) or human dermal microvascular endothelial cells (HDMECs) are used to recapitulate the *in vivo* setting.[35] Confluent monolayers of endothelial cells are cultured overnight in 96 well plates and then incubated with test drug at concentrations from 10^{-6} to 2×10^{-5} M for 20 min prior to stimulation with TNF-α 20 ng/ml for 24 h. TNF-α upregulates intercellular adhesion molecule (ICAM)-1 expression and 24 h stimulation with TNF-α can be replaced in this assay with another noxious stimulus of LPS 4 mg/L for 6 h.[36] Neurophills intravitally labeled with 2′, 7′- bis-(carboxyethyl)-5-(and-6)-carboxyfluorescein (BCECF) are overlaid (2×10^5 cells/well) and allowed to adhere for 20 min to TNF-α stimulated endothelial cells at 37°C. Fluorescently labelled cells of human monocytic leukemia cell line THP-1 can also be used instead of neutrophils. Adherent cells are rinsed with PBS and adherence is then evaluated by lysing adherent cells with 0.5% CTAB (cetyl-trimethyl-ammonium bromide), and measuring fluorescence at 485 nm in an ELISA reader which is a quantitative measure of the activity present in test drug.

FMLP-induced Adhesion of PMN to HUVEC

The bacterial peptide FMLP only activates the PMN adhesive machinery, therefore this stimulus was selected by Dianzani et al. 2006 to evaluate the anti-inflammatory activity of various compounds on PMN adhesion to HUVEC.[24] The near maximal concentration of FMLP (10^{-7}M) produced maximal activation of PMNs. PMNs and HUVEC can also be challenged with other inflammatory stimuli like platelet activating factor (PAF), IL-1β, TNF-α and phorbol myristate acetate (PMA) to observe adhesion phenomenon in inflammation. PAF (10^{-7}) induced stronger inhibition of PMN adhesion than other stimuli at the concentration used.

Platelet-neutrophil adhesion: Thrombin-activated human platelets are incubated with drug (10^{7}–10^{-4} M) at 20°C for 10 min, and mixed with neutrophils at a ratio of 10:1. Neutrophils with two or more (number positives) and one or no adherent platelets (number negatives) are counted as index of activity. The test drug blocks the adhesion with respect to controls.

Neutrophil adhesion to hypoxia-stimulated porcine aortae: Fresh porcine aortae are stimulated by placing them into PBS gassed with N_2, and fixed between a Teflon block and a stainless steel plate with drilled holes. Neutrophils and the test drug (10^{-5} to 10^{-7} M) are added onto the luminal side for 90 min. Adhesion is blocked by test drug, and the adherent cells are lysed to assess the (MPO activity photometrically.

Interleukin 1beta-stimulated human articular chondrocytes

Human chondrocytes (CHs) isolated from osteoarthritic patients[37] can serve as ideal screen to test potential drugs for arthritis. Isolated cells are stimulated with a proinflammatory cytokine (interleukin-1beta, IL1beta, 5 ng/ml) and the effect on NO and cytokine expression is measured as described for macrophages in above sections.

Cyclooxygenase (COX) Assays

The enzyme COX catalyses the conversion of arachidonic acid to prostaglandins. COX is now known to exist in two isoforms COX-1 and COX-2, which are constitutive and inducible in nature, respectively. Thus, constitutive form is associated with physiological function whereas inducible form plays a pathological role (major role in inflammation). The *in vitro* assays for these enzymes may be carried out as under.

COX-1 assay: Briefly, purified recombinant human COX-1 (50 µl of 1 µg ml^{-1} in 100 mm Tris-HCl, pH 8.0, 5 mm EDTA, 1 mm phenol, 1 µm hematin)[38] is preincubated with 2 µl of test drug solution for 15 min. The reaction is then initiated by the addition of 5 µl of 1 µM arachidonic acid to obtain a final concentration of 0.1 µM. After a 7 min incubation at room temperature, the reaction is stopped by the addition of 5 µl 1M HCl and 50 µl acetonitrile. Aliquots of 50 µl of each reaction mixture are analyzed for substrate conversion into PGE_2 by a PGE_2 enzyme immunoassay.

COX-2 assay: Drugs can be tested for COX-2 inhibitory activity spectrophotometrically by measuring the velocity of oxidation of N, N, N', N'-tetramethyl-p-phenylenediamine (TMPD).[39] TMPD is oxidized during the reduction of PGG_2 to PGH_2. The assay mixture consists of 100 mM sodium phosphate, 1 µM of hematine, 1 mg/ml gelatin, 2-5 µg/ml of purified COX-2 and 4 µl of test compound in DMSO. The total volume of assay mixture is 180 µl. This is then preincubated for 15 min at 22°C and then 20 µl of a solution of 1 mM arachidonic acid and 1mM TMPD in the assay buffer is added. The assay buffer contains the assay solution except hematin and enzyme. The absorbance at 610 nm is measured over the first 36 sec and percentage inhibition calculated. The nonenzymatic oxidation of TMPD in the absence of COX-2 is also observed and subtracted from the activity in the presence of COX-2.

IN VIVO METHODS

Animal models are the way in which the results from simpler *in vitro* research can be tested in "intact" biological systems. The logical link of animal modeling to the clinical context can help build a confidence in a new drug before clinical trial. Animal studies can be viewed as hierarchical in nature as studies using rodents and small laboratory animals are relatively simpler to perform and maintain than studies done using larger animals. Research done with small mammals is less expensive, more accessible and less time-consuming to carry out.

However, none of the models currently employed using variety of phlogistic agents inducing varying degree and duration of inflammation; adequately mimic the chain of events underlying inflammation in patients. Various models that have been used to date have different strengths and weaknesses and findings should ideally be reproduced in more than one mammalian species before extrapolating data to human subjects. A recent PNAS paper reported that mouse models of inflammatory diseases correlate poorly with the human conditions,[40] which makes clinical translation of findings from certain mouse models less certain. The revised chapter lay greater emphasis on rat models over mouse models. The use of rats also affords superior pain behavior modeling, and their comparatively larger size facilitates surgical manipulation. It is important that these aspects are taken into account for identifying experimental findings that constitute general principles that are predictive of clinical efficacy from those that are unique to a model.

It is recommended to concomitantly use several *in vivo* methods, which together can mimic a broad spectrum of acute, subacute and chronic inflammatory events such as redness, heat, plasma exudation, edema, pain, leukocyte migration, tissue proliferation and partial necrosis. Whole animal like guinea pig, rat, mouse, rabbits or dog may be used for this purpose. Most prominent *in vivo* models of inflammation are croton oil-induced mouse ear edema, carrageenan induced edema,[41] carrageenan-induced rat pleurisy,[42] and cotton pellet induced rat granuloma.[43] The models inducing edema screen drugs for their ability to halt vasodilation and edema formation, whereas models inducing pleurisy and granuloma evaluate test compounds against exudative phases and proliferative phases of inflammation, respectively. Various *in vivo* models of inflammation have been given in Table 33.1. Preliminary anti-inflammatory mechanisms, is determined in the animal models by measuring the levels of myeloperoxidase (MPO) for assessing neutrophil migration and levels of free radical damage by measuring superoxide dismutase (SOD) and malondialdehyde (MDA) in tissue.

Table 33.1: Various *in vivo* models of inflammation

S. No	*Model of inflammation*	*Animal species*	*Site of application/ injection of inflammogen*	*Reference(s)*
1.	UV-β-induced erythema	Guinea pig	Depilated skin	44,45
2	Ear edema	Mice	Topical application on ear	41, 43
3.	Carrageenan-induced paw edema	Rats, mice	Subplantar region	44, 46, 47, 48
4.	Pleural exudation	Rats	Pleural space	42
5.	Cotton pellet-induced granuloma	Rats, mice	Subcutaneously through the skin incision, groin region, flanks	43
6.	Freund's adjuvant arthritis	Rats	Subplantar region	53
7.	Papaya latex-induced arthritis	Rats	Subplantar region	54
8.	Collagen/LPS-induced accelerated arthritis	Mice	Intradermal injection at the base of the tail	55, 56
9.	Air pouch	Rats, mice	Dorsal surface	51, 52
10.	Cyclophosphamide-induced cystitis	Rats, mice	Systemic injection	8, 57
11.	Prostatitis	Rats, mice	Intraprostatic application	33, 46
12.	TNBS-induced colitis	Rats, mice	Rectal application	64

UV-B-induced Erythema in Guinea Pigs

Erythema (redness) is the earliest sign of inflammation, not yet accompanied by plasma exudation and edema. Guinea pigs are the frequently used animals to study the anti-inflammatory activity of drugs in this model.[44] In albino guinea pigs, the pure erythema reaction appears 2 h after exposure of the depilated skin to ultraviolet irradiation.[28] Guinea pigs are pretreated with the test drugs half an hour before UV-exposure from a UV lamp that emits radiation in the wavelength of 180-200 nm. This model can be used as a pure measure of the vasodilatory phase in the inflammatory reaction. However, the test suffers from the drawback that shaving of skin is required before application of irritant. The test also depends on the skin thickness and the intensity of erythema. It is difficult to quantify and requires a skilled investigator. However, the method is easily translatable in clinic and in recent studies it has been applied to Human volunteers.[45]

Ear Edema Model

Croton oil is obtained from the expression of the seeds of *Croton tiglium*. Apart from its role as a promoting agent in chemical carcinogenesis, it is widely used agent to induce ear edema in mice. Croton oil ear edema (induced by topical application) is a predictable model to detect the activity of topical anti-inflammatory drugs. In this test, the inflammatory response is quantified by measuring the increase in earplug weight at single time interval (peak at 6 h) after croton oil application.[41] The method can be used to test both steroidal and nonsteroidal anti-inflammatory drugs. Both the rats and mice can be used for this test.

A total of 15 μl of an acetonic solution containing 75 μg of croton oil is applied to the outer and inner surface of the right ear of each mouse (about 1 cm^2 area). The left ear remains untreated. Control animals receive only the irritant while indomethacin (100 μg/ear) serves as the reference. Varying dose levels of the test drug are applied to the inner surface of the right ear of each mouse either 1 h before drug administration or by dissolving the drug in croton oil solution. The animals are sacrificed by cervical dislocation 6 h later and a plug (6 mm in diameter) is removed from both the treated and untreated ear. The difference in weight between the two plugs is taken as a measure of edematous response.[43] The inhibition percentage was calculated by the following equation:

$$\text{Inhibition (\%)} = (E_{control} - E_{treated}) \div E_{control} \times 100$$

where $E_{control}$ and $E_{treated}$ is the extent of edema from the control group and treated groups. Possible mechanism of action is determined by measuring MPO activity in harvested tissue.

Carrageenan-induced Paw Edema Model

To study the acute and subacute phases of inflammation in rodents (rats and mice), carrageenan is a widely used irritant or inflammogen or a phlogistic agent.[41] Chemically, it is a sulfated polysaccharide from seaweeds. The experimental tissue injury caused by this irritant initiates a cascade of events leading to formation of exudates. The inflammation induced by it is biphasic in nature.[46] Injection of carrageenan induces inflammatory cell infiltration and increased COX-2 expression, which facilitates inflammatory processes. COX-2 derived prostaglandins, particularly prostaglandin E2, is the primary pathogenic factor of symptoms, representing the classic triad of inflammation.[11,20-22] The well recognized method of Winter et al. 1962[47] is followed. A 1% w/v suspension of carrageenan is prepared freshly in normal saline and injected into subplantar region of left hind paw (usually 0.1 ml in rats and 0.025-0.05 ml in mice).[48] In control animals, only vehicle is injected. Test drug is usually administered orally or intraperitoneally, according to body weight immediately or half an hour or one hour before (depending on the expected peak effect) carrageenan challenge.[49] A mark is made at the ankle joint of each rodent. Paw volume up to the ankle joint is measured in drug treated and untreated groups before and 3 h after carrageenan challenge using a plethysmograph filled with mercury.[50] However, paw edema in rats has also been measured beyond 3 h also after carrageenan challenge.

The sophisticated electronic devices are also being used nowadays to record the paw volume or rodents. The % reduction in edema is calculated using the following formula:

$$\%\text{ Reduction in edema} = \frac{\text{Mean edema in untreated control group} - \text{mean edema in drug treated group}}{\text{Mean edema in control group}} \times 100$$

The method is simple, easy and short lasting as well as reproducible. However, it is non-specific and difficult to quantify. It is also difficult to examine cells and their modification by anti-inflammatory drugs. One must avoid injecting the irritant in both the hind paws of the animal on account of severe pain. The carrageenan causes unalleviated pain and deformity.

Carrageenan in this model can be replaced by other irritants such as formalin, mustard oil, snake venom, dextran and polyvinylpyrollidone, etc., which produce varying degree of inflammation.

Carrageenan-induced Rat Pleurisy

Various irritants produce nonimmune acute inflammation when injected into natural cavities (pleural and peritoneal cavities, knee joints). The pleural cavity of rats and guinea pigs has been successfully utilized for screening of anti-inflammatory drugs. In this model, it is easy to measure the volume of exudates and to determine the amounts of protein, mediators and leukocytes in the exudates. Pleurisy can be induced in rats by an intrapleural injection of carrageenan,[42] turpentine, Evan's blue, Arabic gum, glycogen and dextran, enzymes, antigens, microbes, mast cell degranulators, etc. This model not only allows quantitation of the anti-inflammatory activity, but also allows for investigating the mechanism underlying the action of new test drugs. The method is suitable for detection of both steroidal and nonsteroidal anti-inflammatory drugs.

Experimental pleurisy is produced by injecting 0.1 ml of turpentine oil into right pleural space in rats under light anesthesia as described by Spector. The test drugs are injected intraperitoneally in graded doses 1 h before turpentine injection. The rats are decapitated and pleural exudate is collected half an hour after turpentine treatment. The exudate is removed, preferably by washing the pleural cavity with a known volume of Hank's solution to ensure complete recovery of the exudate and integrity of the cells. Volume of the exudate is measured as an index of activity of the test drug.

Cotton Pellet-induced Granuloma

This method is widely used to study the exudative and proliferative phases of inflammation. Sterile cotton pellets (5 mg), each impregnated with 0.4 ml of 5% aqueous solution of ampicillin, are used.[43] Under ether anesthesia, pellets are inserted subcutaneously through skin incision in the back of the animal (rats and mice). Drug treatment is started 2 h after cotton pellet implantation and continued for 5 consecutive days. Vehicle treated animal receive normal saline for the same duration as the test group receives drug. On 5th day, animals are sacrificed, granulomas are removed, dried for 24 h at 60°C and the dry weights determined. The weight of granulomatous tissue formed is calculated by subtracting initial weight from the final dry weight of cotton pellets and % protection by the drug can be calculated. Cotton pellets of larger size (30 mg) introduced subcutaneously into the groin region have also been used. The proinflammatory effect of cotton pellets can be enhanced by soaking the pellets in turpentine, carrageenan or some other irritants.

Air Pouch Model

The air pouch model of acute inflammation has been used over the last 30 years for screening anti-inflammatory drugs as well as for other applications.[51,52] Injection of air into dorsal surface of rat or mouse followed by a suitable irritant provides a useful model of non-immune subacute exudative inflammation. The air pouch model was originally devised by Selye, 1953 and later on modified by several investigators. Subcutaneous dorsal pouches are created in anesthetized mice by injecting 5 ml of air. [51,52] After 3 days, the pouches are re-injected and on day 6, 1 ml of 1% w/v carrageenan in sterile saline is injected. Control animals receive saline alone. Twenty-four hours after carrageenan, mice are anesthetized and killed. The anti-inflammatory effect of different doses of test compound is investigated by giving them orally 30 min before, 8 and 20 h after carrageenan. Controls receive drug vehicle. Indomethacin (5 mg/kg) orally is kept as standard and fed according to the above schedule. The pouches are washed with 1ml of saline, exudates are immediately cooled on ice and the volume is recorded. The total number of leukocytes migrated into the pouch are evaluated after staining with erythrosine B and the remaining exudate is centrifuged at 3,000 rpm for 10 min at 4°C and supernatant stored at -20°C until use. The chemical mediators involved in this inflammation remain unknown, protein synthesis and kinin formation are necessary for this granuloma formation.

Adjuvant Arthritis

Adjuvant arthritis in rats is considered to be an immunologically mediated and most frequently investigated model of chronic inflammation. This model depicts the very close similarity with the clinical rheumatoid arthritis. The strain of rat, preparation (emulsion or suspension) of the adjuvant (emulsion induces both primary and secondary lesions in greater% of animals), site of injection and the time of measurement of primary and secondary lesions affects the results obtained.[53] The arthritis is induced by s/c injection of either Freund's complete adjuvant FCA or mycobacteria suspended in oil. The subplantar injection of 50-100 μl of this suspension results in a primary, non-immune, localized inflammatory response in the paw followed by the secondary immune systemic disease. Mycobacterial constituents in FCA are recognized by toll like receptors and activate Th1 immune response leading to production of TNF-α and IL-12 and arthritic changes. The local swelling begins in the injected paw within 24 h, reaches a peak on day 4 or 5 and becomes stabilized on day 6 to 11. The systemic disease usually starts on day 7 and is characterized by the swelling of the contralateral non-injected limb. Foot thickness and body weight changes can be monitored in the drug treatment group and compared with that of untreated control. This model allows evaluation of chronically administered drug against inflammation. Drug administration is done daily starting a day before injection of adjuvant. There is delayed systemic response to the Freund's adjuvant, which makes this model superior to other models in assessing the efficacy of all types of potential anti-rheumatic drugs.

Papaya Latex-induced Arthritis

The slow reacting antirheumatic drugs (SARDs) such as gold, chloroquine, levamisole and penicillamine etc. have failed to show significant activity in the conventional experimental models. It has now been demonstrated that lysosomal enzymes play an important role in adjuvant induced arthritis. These enzymes are known to cause tissue damage. Keeping in view the disease etiology, papaya latex induced model of experimental rheumatoid arthritis has been developed to test the anti-inflammatory activity of SARDs. Cartilage destruction in this model is caused by cysteine protease called caricain found in the latex of papaya. 0.1 ml of 0.25% solution of papaya latex (prepared in 0.05 M sodium acetate buffer, pH 4.5 containing 0.01% thymol) is injected into the rat hind paw.[54] The peak effect occurs at 3 h and lasts for more than 5 h. The method is sensitive for evaluating NSAIDs like aspirin, ibuprofen and steroidal anti-inflammatory drugs (particularly SARDs), which do not show appreciable activity in adjuvant induced arthritis and other models of inflammation.

Collagen-induced Arthritis (CIA)

This mouse model of arthritis is induced by immunization with type II collagen in FCA, which induces an autoimmune disease directed against the cartilage in the joints.[55,56] Unlike other models, CIA is characterized by inflammation and destruction of the joints in a T cell- and B cell-specific manner. The model successfully predicted the clinical efficacy of (TNF-α) antibodies in rheumatoid arthritis.

Chicken collagen type II[55,56] is solubilized overnight at 10°C in 0.05 N acetic acid at a concentration of 1 mg/ml and emulsified in FCA at a ratio of 1:1 (v/v). Using 0.1 ml emulsion each adult female DBA/1 Lac J mice (age 12-14 weeks, weighing 22-26 g) are immunized by an intradermal injection at the base of the tail with 100 μg of chicken type II collagen. Seventeen days later, the immune response to collagen is boosted by a subcutaneous injection in the back of the neck with 200 μg of LPS solubilized in 0.2 ml PBS. The thickness of each affected hind paw is measured daily with microcalipers. Clinical severity of inflammation (redness, swelling, joint deformity) is scored periodically on a scale of 0-3 in all 4 extremities as follows: 0 = normal, 1 = slight swelling and/or erythema, 2 = pronounced edematous swelling, and 3 = joint rigidity. Each limb is graded, thus allowing a maximum score of 12 per mouse. This experiment was repeated on 3 separate occasions. The incidence and frequency of arthritis is calculated as follows:

Incidence was the number of mice having at least one affected paw divided by the number of mice per group.

$$\text{Frequency} = \frac{\text{Number of affected paws}}{\text{Total number of paws per group}}$$

The advantages of this method are:

i. This model is specifically well suited for high throughput screening to identify novel inhibitors of integrin VLA-4, the very late antigen-4.
ii. The end point of the model is reached within 21 days whereas in other models it takes weeks to months.
iii. Inflammation is not self-limiting as with other models and therefore mimics clinical arthritis.
iv. It limits the amount of test compound required for the study by administration of the test compound at appropriate time (these investigators have administered antibody to VLA-4 on day 16-22 (effector phase of the response). Therefore, the animals do not need to be treated from the time of collagen immunization.
v. Administration of LPS causes a highly synchronous response with reduced variability.

Cyclophosphamide-induced Cystitis in Rodents

Systemic chronic administration of cyclophosphamide (CYP) in rodents has been proposed as a relevant preclinical model of urinary bladder inflammation or cystitis.[8,57] Single or repeat systemic injections of CYP in mice or rats can induce acute or chronic model of bladder inflammation. Cyclophosphamide is metabolized in liver and kidney into acrolein, which is the actual agents that cause bladder injury leading to bladder inflammation. Acute cystitis is induced by a single intraperitoneal (ip) injection of CYP at the dose of 100-150 mg/kg. Inflammation in bladder tissue is characterized by submucosal edema (Fig. 33.2), infiltration of inflammatory cells, telangiectasia (prominent dilated blood vessels engorged with red blood cells) increase in proinflammatory cytokine gene expression. Increased bladder weight and wall thickness were associated with edema and hemorrhage. Bladder tissue levels of IL-1β, IL-6, MCP-1 and VCAM-1, and urinary levels of PGE2 were increased. Oral administration of anti-inflammatory agents aspirin and ibuprofen reversed the increased bladder wall thickness, macroscopic damage and levels of cytokines IL-1β, IL-6 and PGE2.[58] Therefore, the model of bladder inflammation allows noninvasive repeat assessment of the drug effect from the same animal without the need of animal sacrifice. The two genders respond differently to CYP and females perform better in this model.[8,57] Model allows evaluation of both local[59] and systemic treatments.

Rat model of Prostatitis: Compared to cystitis which is typically observed in females, prostatits is a quintessential male disorder as it is the inflammation of prostate. Several animal models have been reported in last 30 years including chemical induced prostatitis, bacterial infection-induced prostatitis models, hormone-associated prostatitis models and other miscellaneous prostatitis models. For chemically induced prostatitis, irritant chemicals are directly injected into the surgically exposed prostate of male rat. Chemicals used in studies so far include, capsaicin, 5% formalin[33] and 3% carrageenan[46] in saline.

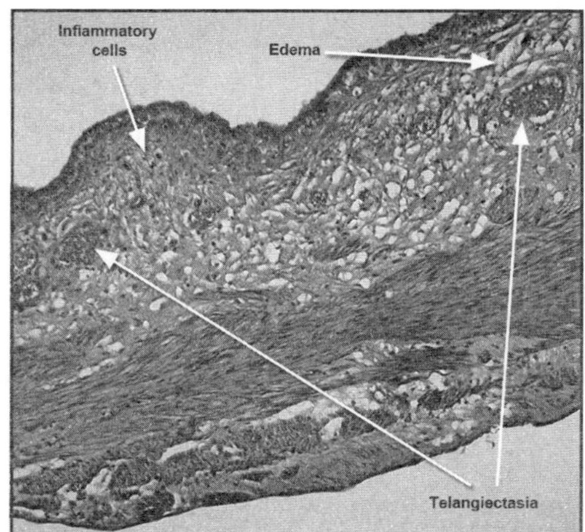

Figure 33.2: Cyclophosphamide induced inflammation in rat bladder. Bladder tissue harvested 24 h after injection showing interstitial edema and infiltration of inflammatory cells and telangiectasia (prominent dilated blood vessels engorged with red blood cells). Hematoxylin and eosin stain, original magnification 4x

For intraprostatic injection, rats are anesthetized with isoflurane (5% for induction and 3% for maintenance) and lower abdomen above the penis is shaved and the skin in this area sterilized using 3 applications of 10% povidone-iodine solution. A small midline incision is made in the sterile area to expose the bladder and the adjacent prostate at the bladder outlet. With a 30-gauge needle, 50 ul injection of irritant chemical is made into both right and left ventral lobes of the prostate gland. For the control group, commensurable sterile normal saline is injected in similar sites. After the injection, surgical site is sutured back and animals allowed to recover from anesthesia. At different time points (after 24 h, 7 days, 14 days and 30 days of injection), rats are sacrificed and the prostate is harvested. For histological analysis, one part of the prostate is fixed in buffered 10% formaldehyde for 24 h, embedded in paraffin, cut with a microtome, and stained with hematoxylin-eosin. Under a low-power microscopy field, each slide is evaluated randomly in 4 different areas containing inflammatory cells (Fig. 33.3).

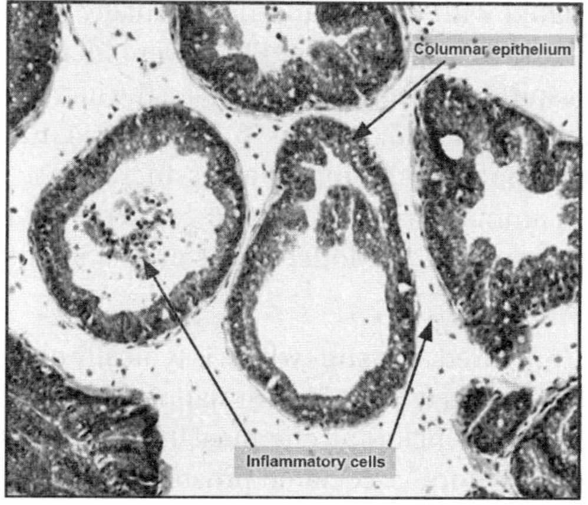

Figure 33.3: Intraprostatic injection of 5% formalin induces a model of prostatic inflammation (prostatitis) marked by a host of inflammatory changes including hyperplastic acini lined by tall columnar epithelium and infiltration shown by arrows. Hematoxylin and eosin stain, image is magnified 20x

Compared to saline injected prostate, intraprostatic injection of chemicals causes prostatic edema and increased inflammatory cell accumulation. There is inflammation of prostate with minimal tissue necrosis and damage without any bacterial infection. Compared to capsaicin induced prostatitis[60] that lasts only for a week, the formalin induced prostatitis lasts up to a month to test interventions.

Bacterial prostatitis in male rats is induced by injecting 10^5 -10^8 colony-forming units (CFU)/ml of *E. coli* in to the urinary tract.[61] Frozen bacterial isolate is cultured in tris-buffered saline (TBS) immediately prior to the injection to a concentration of 10^8 CFU. Male rats are anesthetized and a sterile polyethylene tube (0.9 mm outer diameter, 2.5 cm length) is inserted to the urethra, and 0.2 ml of *E. coli* suspension instilled into prostatic urethra using insulin syringes. Sufficient time for the bacteria to infiltrate to the inside of the prostate is maintained by preventing excretion of urine through maintenance of anesthesia for 1 h. Model can be validated 4 weeks after the injection of *E. coli* by performing McConkey culture test on collected urine or prostate biopsy to detect bacteria. This model is suitable for assessing the effect of drugs with chronic action.

A mice model of experimental autoimmune prostatitis also exists, which is developed by subcutaneous injection of prostate antigen[62] or spermine binding protein (p25) peptide[63] which induces immune mediated prostatic inflammation. However, these immune mediated models of prostatitis in mouse frequently develop diabetes and other organ-specific autoimmune diseases that may interfere in the study of drugs targeting prostatic inflammation.

Trinitrobenzene Sulfonic Acid (TNBS)-induced Experimental Colitis

Under normal conditions the intestinal mucosa functions within a delicate balance of inflammatory cells where cytokine synthesis and cytokine-induced signal transduction pathways are tightly regulated by intricate feedback mechanisms and regulatory T-cells. Colitis leads to a dramatic shift/imbalance in the cytokine production profile at different stages of the disease process. TNBS induces inflammation of the rat colon called colitis. Intracolonic administration of 2, 4, 6-trinitrobenzene sulfonic acid (50 mg/ml) dissolved in 50% ethanol (v/v) is administered via a transanal approach (total volume 0.5 ml) using a PE-90 catheter whose tip will be placed approximately 6 cm proximal to the anal verge.[64] Sham animals receive 0.5 ml of normal saline. Inflammation is examined in 8 cm distal part of rat colon 14 days later. Cytokines are principal mediators of the innate and adaptive arms of the immune responses in mucosal inflammation and TNBS induces drastic increase. TNBS instilled rats show colonic damage, weight and adhesions (macroscopic and microscopic), diarrhea, body weight and increased colonic levels of free radicals (nitric oxide and lipid peroxidation).

CONCLUSION

From the searched literature, it is evident that numerous experimental methods for evaluation of anti-inflammatory drugs have been developed over the last few years. The lead compounds may be identified using *in vitro* assays and may be subjected to further testing *in vivo*. These methods help in understanding of inflammation process as well as in identifying a potential drug. The findings they generate may drive medical advances and understanding, but the information gained must be interpreted within the limitations of the model. Irrespective of the type of animal model used, findings should be carefully validated before extrapolation to humans. How closely the chosen model reproduces the disease in question will dictate the extent of validation necessary for translation.

Most of the currently available antirheumatic drugs have shown anti-inflammatory activity in carrageenan-induced edema, which utilize the transudative and exudative phases of inflammation. One of the key steroidal anti-inflammatory drug hydrocortisone failed to show anti-inflammatory activity in pleural exudation method. So, this method is not the most recommended one for testing inflammatory activity. Therefore, for detecting anti-inflammatory activity in a new compound, one may rely either on the inhibition of the proliferative phase of inflammatory reaction viz. inhibition of granulation tissue formation or in the reduction of exudative phase of inflammation viz. carrageenan induced edema. The former methods are more-time consuming and require larger quantities of drugs. Carrageenan-induced edema seems most suitable for screening anti-inflammatory drugs because it is convenient, less time-consuming and detects activity in all the clinically useful drugs. Collagen-induced arthritis is suitable model for new biotechnology based drugs for arthritis, considering the successful prediction the clinical efficacy of TNF-α antibodies this model.

REFERENCES

1. Bostanci Y, Kazzazi A, Momtahen S, Laze J, Djavan B. Correlation between benign prostatic hyperplasia and inflammation. Curr Opin Urol 2013;23:5.
2. Nathan C. Points of control in inflammation. Nature 2002;420:846.
3. Luster AD. Chemokines--chemotactic cytokines that mediate inflammation. N Engl J Med, 1998; 338:436-45.
4. Lenz A, Franklin GA, Cheadle WG. Systemic inflammation after trauma. Injury, 2007;38:336.
5. Borges Lda S, Bortolon JR, Santos VC, de Moura NR, Dermargos A, Cury-Boaventura MF, et al. Chronic inflammation and neutrophil activation as possible causes of joint diseases in ballet dancers. Mediators Inflamm 2014:846021.
6. Kashyap M, Kawamorita N, Tyagi V, Sugino Y, Chancellor M, Yoshimura N, et al. Down-regulation of nerve growth factor expression in the bladder by antisense oligonucleotides as new treatment for overactive bladder. J Urol 2013;190:757.
7. Corcoran AT, Yoshimura N, Tyagi V, Jacobs B, Leng W, Tyagi P. Mapping the cytokine profile of painful bladder syndrome/interstitial cystitis in human bladder and urine specimens. World J Urol 2013;31:241.
8. Tyagi P, Tyagi V, Yoshimura N, Witteemer E, Barclay D, Loughran PA, et al. Gender-based reciprocal expression of transforming growth factor-beta1 and the inducible nitric oxide synthase in a rat model of cyclophosphamide-induced cystitis. J Inflamm (Lond) 2009;6:23.
9. Lo Faro ML, Fox B, Whatmore JL, Winyard PG, Whiteman M. Hydrogen sulfide and nitric oxide interactions in inflammation. Nitric Oxide 2014;41:38.
10. Tyagi P, Tyagi V, Qu X, Lin H, Kuo H, Chuang Y, et al. Association of inflammaging (inflammation + aging) with higher prevalence of OAB in elderly population. Int Urol Nephrol 2014;46:871.
11. Aoki T, Narumiya S. Prostaglandins and chronic inflammation. Trends Pharmacol Sci 2012;33:304-11.
12. Tyagi P, Killinger K, Tyagi V, Nirmal J, Chancellor M, Peters KM. Urinary chemokines as noninvasive predictors of ulcerative interstitial cystitis. J Urol 2012;187:2243.

13. Bouchelouche K, Alvarez S, Horn T, Nordling J, Bouchelouche P. Human detrusor smooth muscle cells release interleukin-6, interleukin-8, and RANTES in response to proinflammatory cytokines interleukin-1beta and tumor necrosis factor-alpha. Urology 2006;67:214.
14. Pérez de Lema G, Maier H, Nieto E, Vielhauer V, Luckow B, Mampaso F, et al. Chemokine expression precedes inflammatory cell infiltration and chemokine receptor and cytokine expression during the initiation of murine lupus nephritis. J Am Soc Nephrol 2001;12:1369.
15. Yang SJ, Lim Y. Resveratrol ameliorates hepatic metaflammation and inhibits NLRP3 inflammasome activation. Metabolism 2014;63:693.
16. Weber K, Schilling JD. Lysosomes integrate metabolic-inflammatory cross-talk in primary macrophage inflammasome activation. J Biol Chem 2014;289:9158.
17. Ma Q, Chen S, Hu Q, Feng H, Zhang JH, Tang J. NLRP3 inflammasome contributes to inflammation after intracerebral hemorrhage. Ann Neurol 2014;75:209.
18. Williams-Bey Y, Boularan C, Vural A, Huang NN, Hwang IY, Shan-Shi C, et al. Omega-3 free fatty acids suppress macrophage inflammasome activation by inhibiting NF-kappaB activation and enhancing autophagy. PLoS One 2014;9:e97957.
19. Zang QS, Wolf SE, Minei JP. Sepsis-induced Cardiac Mitochondrial Damage and Potential Therapeutic Interventions in the Elderly. Aging Dis 2014;5:137.
20. Prado FC, Araldi D, Vieira AS, Oliveira-Fusaro MC, Tambeli CH, Parada CA. Neuronal P2X3 receptor activation is essential to the hyperalgesia induced by prostaglandins and sympathomimetic amines released during inflammation. Neuropharmacology 2013;67:252.
21. Peeraully MR, Sievert H, Bullo M, Wang B, Trayhurn P. Prostaglandin D2 and J2-series (PGJ2, Delta12-PGJ2) prostaglandins stimulate IL-6 and MCP-1, but inhibit leptin, expression and secretion by 3T3-L1 adipocytes. Pflugers Arch 2006;453:177.
22. Griffin EW, Skelly DT, Murray CL, Cunningham C. Cyclooxygenase-1-dependent prostaglandins mediate susceptibility to systemic inflammation-induced acute cognitive dysfunction. J Neurosci 2013;33:15248.
23. Huang BP, Lin CH, Chen YC, Kao SH. Antiinflammatory effects of Perilla frutescens leaf extract on lipopolysaccharide stimulated RAW264.7 cells. Mol Med Rep 2014;10:1077.
24. Dianzani C, Collino M, Gallicchio M, Di Braccio M, Roma G, Fantozzi R. Effects of anti-inflammatory [1, 2, 4]triazolo[4, 3-a] [1, 8]naphthyridine derivatives on human stimulated PMN and endothelial cells: an in vitro study. J Inflamm (Lond) 2006;3:4.
25. Shim H, Moon JS, Lee S, Yim D, Kang TJ. Polyacetylene Compound from Cirsium japonicum var. ussuriense Inhibited Caspase-1-mediated IL-1beta Expression. Immune Netw 2012; 12:213.
26. de Luca A, Smeekens SP, Casagrande A, Iannitti R, Conway KL, Gresnigt MS, et al. IL-1 receptor blockade restores autophagy and reduces inflammation in chronic granulomatous disease in mice and in humans. Proc Natl Acad Sci USA 2014;111:3526.
27. Sims K, Haynes CA, Kelly S, Allegood JC, Wang E, Momin A, et al. Kdo2-lipid A, a TLR4-specific agonist, induces de novo sphingolipid biosynthesis in RAW264.7 macrophages, which is essential for induction of autophagy. J Biol Chem 2010;285:38568.
28. Park EJ, Zahari NE, Kang MS, Lee SJ, Lee K, Lee BS, et al. Toxic response of single-walled carbon nanotubes synthesized by HIPCO method in mice and RAW264.7 macrophage cells. Toxicol Lett 2014;229:167.
29. Nam SY, Kim MH, Seo Y, Choi Y, Jang JB, Kang IC, et al. The (2'S,7'S)-O-(2-methylbutanoyl)-columbianetin as a novel allergic rhinitis-control agent. Life Sci 2014;98:103.

30. Naik SK, Mohanty S, Padhi A, Pati R, Sonawane A. Evaluation of antibacterial and cytotoxic activity of Artemisia nilagirica and Murraya koenigii leaf extracts against mycobacteria and macrophages. BMC Complement Altern Med 2014;14:87.
31. Nirmal J, Wolf-Johnston AS, Chancellor MB, Tyagi P, Anthony M, Kaufman J, et al. Liposomal inhibition of acrolein-induced injury in rat cultured urothelial cells. Int Urol Nephrol 2014;46:1947.
32. Petrera E, Coto CE. Effect of the potent antiviral 1-cinnamoyl-3,11-dihydroxymeliacarpin on cytokine production by murine macrophages stimulated with HSV-2. Phytother Res 2014;28:104.
33. Funahashi Y, O'Malley KJ, Kawamorita N, Tyagi P, DeFranco DB, Takahashi R, et al. Upregulation of androgen-responsive genes and transforming growth factor-beta1 cascade genes in a rat model of non-bacterial prostatic inflammation. Prostate 2014;74:337.
34. Aparicio-Soto M, Alarcon-de-la-Lastra C, Cardeno A, Sanchez-Fidalgo S, Sanchez-Hidalgo M. Melatonin modulates microsomal PGE synthase 1 and NF-E2-related factor-2-regulated antioxidant enzyme expression in LPS-induced murine peritoneal macrophages. Br J Pharmacol 2014;171:134.
35. Ku SK, Kwak S, Bae JS. Orientin inhibits high glucose-induced vascular inflammation in vitro and in vivo. Inflammation 2014;37:2164.
36. Zhao Y, Feng Q, Huang Z, Li W, Chen B, Jiang L, et al. Simvastatin inhibits inflammation in ischemia-reperfusion injury. Inflammation 2014;37:1865.
37. Burguera EF, Vela-Anero A, Magalhaes J, Meijide-Failde, R, Blanco FJ. Effect of hydrogen sulfide sources on inflammation and catabolic markers on interleukin 1beta-stimulated human articular chondrocytes. Osteoarthritis Cartilage 2014;22:1026.
38. Riendeau D, Percival MD, Boyce S, Brideau C, Charleson S, et al. Biochemical and pharmacological profile of a tetrasubstituted furanone as a highly selective COX-2 inhibitor. Br J Pharmacol 1997;121:105.
39. Pang YY, Yeo WK, Loh KY, Go ML, Ho HK. Structure-toxicity relationship and structure-activity relationship study of 2-phenylaminophenylacetic acid derived compounds. Food Chem Toxicol 2014;71:207.
40. Seok J, Warren HS, Cuenca AG, Mindrinos MN, Baker HV, Xu W, et al. Inflammation and Host Response to Injury, L. S. C. R. P.: Genomic responses in mouse models poorly mimic human inflammatory diseases. Proc Natl Acad Sci USA 2013;110:3507.
41. Sakat SS, Mani K, Demidchenko YO, Gorbunov EA, Tarasov SA, Mathur A, E, et al. Release-active dilutions of diclofenac enhance anti-inflammatory effect of diclofenac in carrageenan-induced rat paw edema model. Inflammation 2014;37:1.
42. Allegra M, Ianaro A, Tersigni M, Panza E, Tesoriere L, Livrea MA. Indicaxanthin from cactus pear fruit exerts anti-inflammatory effects in carrageenin-induced rat pleurisy. J Nutr 2014;144:185.
43. Cai C, Chen Y, Zhong S, Ji B, Wang J, Bai X, Shi G. Anti-inflammatory activity of N-butanol extract from Ipomoea stolonifera in vivo and in vitro. PLoS One 2014;9:e95931.
44. Okumura Y, Yamauchi H, Takayama S, Kato H, Kokubu M. Phototoxicity study of a ketoprofen poultice in guinea pigs. J Toxicol Sci 2005;30:19.
45. Mandalari G, Arcoraci T, Martorana M, Bisignano C, Rizza L, Bonina FP. Antioxidant and photoprotective effects of blanch water, a byproduct of the almond processing industry. Molecules 2013;18:12426.
46. Zeng F, Chen H, Yang J, Wang L, Cui Y, Guan X, et al. Development and validation of an animal model of prostate inflammation-induced chronic pelvic pain: evaluating from inflammation of the prostate to pain behavioral modifications. PLoS One 2014;9:e96824.

47. Winter CA, Risley EA, Silber RH. Carrageenan-induced edema in hind paw of the rat as an assay for anti-inflammatory drugs. Proc Soc Exp Biol Med 1962;111:544.
48. Boonyarikpunchai W, Sukrong S, Towiwat P. Antinociceptive and anti-inflammatory effects of rosmarinic acid isolated from Thunbergia laurifolia Lindl. Pharmacol Biochem Behav 2014;124C:67.
49. Soares DG, Godin AM, Menezes RR, Nogueira RD, Brito AM, Melo I S, et al. Anti-inflammatory and antinociceptive activities of azadirachtin in mice. Planta Med 2014;80:630.
50. Gupta SK, Bhardwaj RK, Tyagi P, Sengupta S, Velpandian T. Anti-inflammatory activity and pharmacokinetic profile of a new parenteral formulation of nimesulide. Pharmacol Res 1999;39:137.
51. Huang Z, Zhao C, Chen Y, Cowell JA, Wei G, Kultti A, et al. Recombinant human hyaluronidase PH20 does not stimulate an acute inflammatory response and inhibits lipopolysaccharide-induced neutrophil recruitment in the air pouch model of inflammation. J Immunol 2014;192:5285.
52. Hassan HM, Al-Gayyar MM, El-Gayar AM, Ibrahim TM. Effect of simvastatin on inflammatory cytokines balance in air pouch granuloma model. Inflamm Allergy Drug Targets 2014;13:74.
53. Shabbir A, Shahzad M, Ali A, Zia-Ur-Rehman M. Anti-arthritic activity of N'-[(2,4-dihydroxyphenyl) methylidene]-2-(3,4-dimethyl-5,5-dioxidopyrazolo[4,3-c][1,2]benzothiazin-1(4H)-yl) acetohydrazide. Eur J Pharmacol 2014.
54. Gupta OP, Sing S, Bani S, Sharma N, Malhotra S, Gupta BD, et al. Anti-inflammatory and anti-arthritic activities of silymarin acting through inhibition of 5-lipoxygenase. Phytomedicine 2000;7:21.
55. Hou Y, Lin H, Zhu L, Liu Z, Hu F, Shi J, et al. The inhibitory effect of IFN-gamma on protease HTRA1 expression in rheumatoid arthritis. J Immunol 2014;193:130.
56. Inglis JJ, Notley CA, Essex D, Wilson AW, Feldmann M, Anand P, et al. Collagen-induced arthritis as a model of hyperalgesia: functional and cellular analysis of the analgesic actions of tumor necrosis factor blockade. Arthritis Rheum 2007;56:4015.
57. Smaldone MC, Vodovotz Y, Tyagi V, Barclay D, Philips BJ, Yoshimura N, Tyagi P. Multiplex analysis of urinary cytokine levels in rat model of cyclophosphamide-induced cystitis. Urology 2009;73:421.
58. Auge C, Chene G, Dubourdeau M, Desoubzdanne D, Corman B, Palea S, et al. Relevance of the cyclophosphamide-induced cystitis model for pharmacological studies targeting inflammation and pain of the bladder. Eur J Pharmacol 2013;707:32.
59. Tyagi P, Banerjee R, Basu S, Yoshimura N, Chancellor M, et al. Intravesical antisense therapy for cystitis using TAT-peptide nucleic acid conjugates. Mol Pharm 2006;3:398.
60. Chuang YC, Yoshimura N, Wu M, Huang CC, Chiang PH, Tyagi P. Chancellor MB. Intraprostatic Capsaicin injection as a novel model for nonbacterial prostatitis and effects of botulinum toxin A. Eur Urol 2007;51(4):1119-27.
61. Wu J, Yuan Q, Zhang D, Zhang X, Zhao L, Zhang X, Ruan J. Evaluation of Chinese medicine Qian-Yu for chronic bacterial prostatitis in rats. Indian J Pharmacol, 2011;43:532.
62. Rudick CN, Schaeffer AJ, Thumbikat P. Experimental autoimmune prostatitis induces chronic pelvic pain. Am J Physiol Regul Integr Comp Physiol 2008;294:R1268.
63. Altuntas CZ, Daneshgari F, Veizi E, Izgi K, Bicer F, Ozer A, et al. A novel murine model of chronic prostatitis/chronic pelvic pain syndrome (CP/CPPS) induced by immunization with a spermine binding protein (p25) peptide. Am J Physiol Regul Integr Comp Physiol 2013;304:R415.
64. Yoshizawa S, Kawamorita N, Oguchi T, Funahashi Y, Tyagi P, Chancellor MB, Yoshimura N. Pelvic organ cross-sensitization to enhance bladder and urethral pain behaviors in rats with experimental colitis. Neuroscience 2015;284:422-9.

CHAPTER

34

Ocular Inflammation

INTRODUCTION

Ocular inflammation is responsible for a number of eye ailments. Ocular inflammation can cause number of ocular disorders like blepharitis (lids), conjunctivitis (inflammation of conjunctiva), keratitis (inflammation of cornea), scleritis (inflammation of sclera), uveitis (inflammation of uvea), etc. These inflammations commonly occur due to bacterial or viral infections and hypersensitivity. Surgical procedures and physical injury to the eye are important causes of ocular inflammation.

Any type of ocular inflammation can affect the vision of an individual. The recurrent inflammation requires immediate attention as several internal structures get adversely affected and vision is hampered. Gram-negative bacterial infections cause severe ocular surface inflammations. Lipopolysaccharide (LPS), a component of gram-negative bacterial membrane has potent proinflammatory and proapoptotic effect, which is mediated through membrane receptors expressed on host cells. Inflamed cells or tissues release inflammation mediators (histamine, bradykinin, prostaglandin, leucotrienes, cytokines etc.) in case of acute or chronic inflammation. The concentration of mediators suggests the degree of inflammation. The efficacy of the anti-inflammatory drug can be evaluated by determining the levels of these mediators.

One of the common forms of ocular inflammation is uveitis, which is the inflammation of uveal tract comprising iris, ciliary body and choroid. Uveitis is responsible for over 2.8% of blindness in the United States. Each year, 17.6% of active uveitis patients experience a transient or permanent loss of vision.[1]

It can be categorized into:

1. Anterior uveitis: Inflammation of the anterior part of the uvea causing iritis and iridocyclitis.
2. Intermediate uveitis: Inflammation of the middle part of the uvea affecting the ciliary muscles.
3. Posterior uveitis: Inflammation of the posterior portion of the choroid.
4. Pan uveitis: All anterior, middle and posterior zones are affected.

Ocular inflammation can be treated by corticosteroids. Instillation of steroids and pupil dialators help in reducing the inflammation and pain. Systemic medications are supplemented for treating appropriate cases. If the treatment gets delayed it may lead to several complications like glaucoma, cataract and development of new blood vessels ultimately resulting in visual loss.

The ethical and practical limitations prevent the availability of human ocular tissues with active inflammation at different time intervals. Therefore, the studies on animal models remain the main source of the information. Various animal models have been established to evaluate the anti-inflammatory activity of new therapeutic interventions. The models are mainly categorized into non-immunogenic model and immunogenic model, besides inflammation can be produced experimentally by inflicting injury to the cornea.

EXPERIMENTAL MODELS FOR OCULAR INFLAMMATION

Guinea Pig Model of Giant Papillary Conjunctivitis

Chronic exposure to foreign bodies like contact lenses, leads to giant papillary conjunctivitis (GPC). Increased incidence is seen during the spring season although it is not related to any allergan. Levels of IL-3, IL-4, and IL-5; IgG, IgE, and IgM have been found increased in tears.[2]

Procedure: Contact lens associated GPC, is mimicked in guinea pigs. A sterile needle is inserted directly into the conjunctiva of unsensitized animal. Pricking results in high number of neutrophil infiltration in the traumatized tissues.[3] This model does not represent the true histopathological picture found in human GPC.

Rat Models of Allergic Conjunctivitis

Ovalbumin Induced

Ovalbumin induced allergic conjunctivitis model is a generally used experimental model for studying the inflammatory responses and effect of various therapeutic approaches.[4]

Procedure: Brown Norway rats, of 8-10 weeks age, are injected subcutaneously in the hind footpad with 100 μg of ovalbumin emulsified with 100 μl Complete Freund's Adjuvant (CFA). Then, the intraperitoneal injection of the test compound or phosphate buffered saline (PBS) treatment is given for 13 days. On 13th day all the rats are instilled with ovalbumin eye drops (250 μg in 50 μl of PBS). After 24 h the rats are sacrificed and the eyes, blood and lymph nodes are used for histologic studies and other related parameters.[4, 5]

Pollen Induced

Ragweed pollen (RW): RW has been used as an allergan for inducing conjunctivitis. Iwamoto et al. (2000) has compared the effects of immunization with ragweed pollen in two different adjuvants.

Procedure: Lewis or Brown Norway rats are immunized with 100 μg of RW in emulsion with aluminum hydroxide or CFA. The rats are instilled with ragweed pollen eye drops in phosphate buffer saline (PBS) after three weeks. Inflammatory parameters are observed after 24 h of drug instillation in eyes, blood and lymph. The response to ragweed pollen is similar to that of ovalbumin.[6]

Fukushima et al. (2006) induced allergic conjunctivitis in mice using ragweed pollen as per the method described below:

Procedure: BALB/c mice are actively immunized with ragweed pollen. The ragweed pollen, which is adsorbed on alum, is injected in the hind footpad and the tail base. Each injection contains 50 μg of RW and 2 mg of alum. The test drug is administered intraperitoneally on alternate days till day 8. RW in a dose of 2 mg in 10 μl of PBS per eye is instilled in the eyes of mice on the tenth day. After the 24 h of ragweed challenge the conjunctivae are processed for the evaluation of histological changes and other parameters as needed in the study.[7]

An experimental model of allergic conjunctivitis to ragweed was produced in guinea pigs by Merayo-Lloves et al. in 1995.[8] The model mimics human hay fever conjunctivitis and helps in evaluating the reponse of conjunctivitis to various therapeutic approaches.[8] Merayo-Lloves et al. in 1996 exposed SWR/J mice to ragweed by topical contact with the conjunctival and nasal mucosas. Serum IgE levels and histopathological changes, infiltration of conjunctival eosinophils, change in number of mast cells, cytokine release is evaluated.[9]

Japanese cedar pollen: It has been used by Yasuda et al. (2004) for developing allergic conjunctivitis in guinea pigs.[10] The method is useful in analyzing the mechanism of allergic conjunctivitis.

Procedure: Small gelatin sponge pieces containing pollen extracts and aluminum hydroxide are inserted into the palpebra superior and/inferior sulci of both eyes of Male Hartley guinea pigs for 8 h/day for 6 days. Three pieces are inserted in each eye. After six days the guinea pigs are challenged once a week by instilling pollen suspension in each eye.[10]

Rabbit Model of *Staphylococcus aureus* Keratitis

Oguz et al. (2005) tested a broad-spectrum nonantibiotic antimicrobial agent against bacterial keratitis.[11] They used rabbit model of *Staphylococcus aureus* keratitis for the study and compared the efficacy of the test compound with topical ciprofloxacin, ofloxacin, and 5% cefazolin.

Procedure: One of the corneas of the rabbits is intrastromally injected with 100 colony-forming units of *Staphylococcus aureus* ATCC strain 25923. The animals are divided into different group as per the need of the experiment. The eyes are instilled with the test drug every 30 min from 4 to 9 h post injection. At 10 h post injection signs of inflammation are scored by slit-lamp examination. Then, the corneas are processed for further evaluation. The number of colony-forming units per cornea in all eyes is also calculated.[11]

Endotoxin-induced Uveitis (EIU)

This is a model for acute anterior uveitis in human beings. Lipopolysaccharide (LPS) is a glycolipid component of the outer membrane of Gram-negative bacteria. It induces a generalized proinflammatory response during infection. Systemic administration of sublethal dose of LPS produces bilateral acute ocular inflammationin rats and mice. Maximum effect of EIU is seen in 24 h of LPS injection and wanes out in the next 48 h. Percolation of proteins from the serum and infiltration with macrophages and neutrophils into the eye is the characteristic feature of EIU.[12]

In Rabbits

LPS induced uveitis in rabbits has been used by several workers for testing anti-inflammatory response of the drugs (Fig. 34.1).[12-17] The mechanism of EIU is not clearly known, but the role of cytokines has been clearly mentioned.[18,19] Cytokines are signaling proteins released by cells

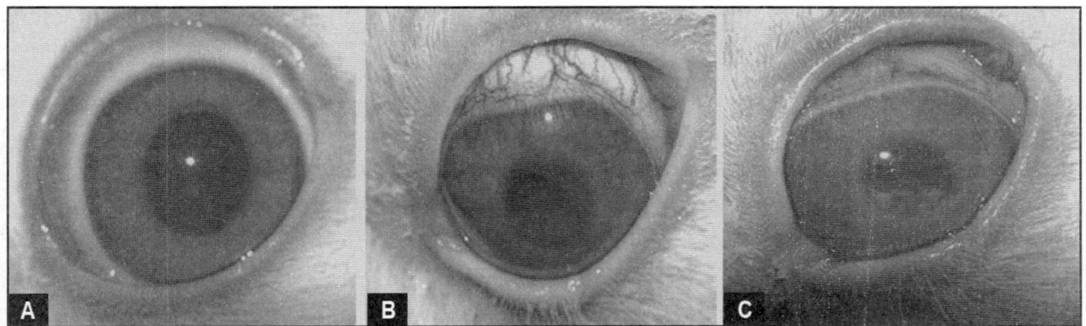

Figure 34.1: Clinical signs of anterior uveitis in control group: (A) Just before intravitreal endotoxin injection; (B) 24 hours post intravitreal endotoxin injection; (C) 72 hours post-intravitreal endotoxin injection.

[*Courtesy*: Researchers of Ocular Pharmacology Laboratory, Delhi Institute of Pharmaceutical Sciences and Research, New Delhi. (*For color version see Plate 22)]*

and act as important mediators. The upregulation of cytokines such as tumor necrosis factor (TNF)-α, interleukin (IL)-6, monocyte chemoattractant protein (MCP)-1, and macrophage inflammatory protein (MIP)-2 has been reported in rabbits, rat and mice models of EIU.[12]

Procedure: New Zealand male rabbits weighing between 1.5 and 2.0 kg are used for inducing uveitis. Rabbits are anesthetized using proparacaine HCl topically. *E. coli* endotoxin (LPS) is dissolved in sterile physiological saline solution at a concentration of 10 ng/μl. Intravitreal injection of 10 μl (100 ng) of the LPS is given into both eyes of each rabbit using a 30 G needle attached to a Hamilton constant range syringe. The severity of the inflammation is compared in the treated group with their own vehicle treated control group, as the grade of uveitis is known to vary from one experiment to another. The test drug is administered to rabbits one h before intravitreal injection of endotoxin. Within 24 h time maximal inflammation occurs and wanes out in 48 h. The rabbits are euthanized 24 h after the LPS injection with an overdose of pentobarbital sodium and immediately aqueous humor is withdrawn by paracentesis using 30 G needle. To dissect the ciliary body the eyes are enucleated and dissected around the equator. Various parameters can be evaluated in aqueous humor and ciliary body.[13]

Burgundy Fawn rabbits of 2.5 to 3.9 kg weight range are also used using ketamine and same dose of LPS as mentioned above.[14]

Liang et al. (2006) used two new tools to assess the ocular inflammation induced by LPS.[16] They used Confocal Microscopy for the evaluation of inflammatory infiltrates and conjunctival impression cytology for assessing TNF alpha and TNF receptor-1 expression.

In Rats

In endotoxin induced uveitis in Lewis rats mainly anterior segment (iridocyclitis) is inflamed and the inflammatory cells get into the vitreous humor and retina.[12,20] Lewis eight-week-old rats weighing between 180 to 220 g are used. LPS from Salmonella typhimurium is diluted in sterile saline and 200 μg/0.1 ml is injected in one of the footpads of the rats to induce the uveitis. Test drug is given immediately after LPS injection in the test group whereas vehicle is administered in the control group.

Satofuka et al. (2006) produced EIU in Long Evans rats by a single intraperitoneal injection of 100 μg LPS.[21]

In Mice

In order to induce EIU Ohta et al. injected 200 μg LPS from *Salmonella typhimurium* in PBS in footpads of C3H/HeN mice of 8-10 weeks. An acute intraocular inflammation is induced that peaks within 24 h and dissipates by 48 h.[15]

Autoimmune Uveitis

Experimental autoimmune uveitis (EAU) is a model of idiopathic human uveitis.[1] EAU is produced against S-antigen, a major protein on retinal photoreceptor cell, interphotoreceptor retinoid binding protein (IRBP) like retinal proteins in susceptible strains of rats, mice and subhuman primates.[15, 22-25]

Interphotoreceptor Retinoid-Binding Protein-induced Uveitis

A method for inducing experimental autoimmune uveitis by Ohta et al. is described briefly.

Procedure: B10.A mice are immunized (s.c) with 50 μg interphotoreceptor retinoid-binding protein (IRBP) in 0.2 ml emulsion mixed in a ratio of 1:1 with complete Freund's adjuvant supplemented with *Mycobacterium tuberculosis* to a final concentration of 2.5 mg/ml. Simultaneously, 500 ng of pertussis toxin is injected intraperitoneally to the mice as an additional adjuvant. Aqueous humor is collected at different time points and assayed for leukocyte content and the ability to suppress or enhance T-cell proliferation. Inflammation in the anterior segment is detected after 10 days.[15]

Fox et al. (1987) compared the inflammatory response produced by IRBP and S-antigen. They immunized Lewis rats with IRBP and found that the response was more compared to S-antigen in lower doses (less than or equal to 4 μg/rat) however, uveitis produced by S-antigen at higher doses (greater than or equal to 20 μg/rat) was more severe in comparison to the inflammation produced by same dose of IRBP. They also observed that the rats differ in susceptibility when immunized with these two proteins.[22]

Ke et al. (2007) induced autoimmune uveitis in C57BL/6 mice by transfer of activated T-cells specific for the IRBP 1-20 peptide. Disease onset occurs at 10 days. The test compound can be given at 0 or 10th day. Clinical signs, ocular histology and infiltrated inflammatory cells in the eye are compared.[26]

Bovine Serum Albumin-induced Uveitis in Guinea Pigs

Ultrastructural changes and leptin expressions in the guinea pig eyes were studied by Kükner, et al. in 2006.[27] Retinas of uveitis induced group when observed under light and electron microscope showed oedematous ganglion cells and increased thickness of inner plexiform layer. They reported that leptin expressions are closely related to ocular inflammation. They also observed the effect of intraperitoneal vitamin E, melatonin and aprotinin on leptin expression.

Procedure: Male guinea pigs are divided into control and treated groups and are injected intravitreally with bovine serum albumin (BSA) to produce experimental uveitis. On the third day, the test group is given the test drugs and on the sixth day, the clinical scoring of the inflammation produced and histopathological examination is done. Leptin expressions are evaluated in retina, choroids, sclera and episclera.[27]

Melanin-induced Uveitis

A number of researchers have used Experimental melanin-protein-induced uveitis (EMIU) also known as experimental autoimmune anterior uveitis (EAAU) model induced by melanin granules extracted from bovine choroids, iris, hair and skin, and from human, monkey and rabbit choroids.[28-32]

Procedure: Susceptible strains of rats (Lewis, Fischer 34, Porton rats) of 10 weeks are housed at 21°C and 50% humidity in a 12 h light and 12 h dark cycle, and fed water and dried feed. Melanin is extracted from bovine choroids as per the procedure of Broekhuyse et al. (1993).[29] Susceptible Lewis rats are immunized with bovine ocular melanin with a dose of 250 μg, which induced maximally severe disease in all injected animals in about 10 days of treatment. Rats are given 125 μg of bovine ocular melanin in a 1:1 emulsion of sterile, non-pyrogenic normal saline and Hunter's TitreMax adjuvant by right hind footpad injection (60 μl). Immediately afterwards, they are injected intraperitoneally with the same quantity of melanin mixed with 1 μg of pertussis toxin in normal saline (40 μl). Animals are examined daily through slit-lamp biomicroscope for clinical signs of uveitis, and are scored using a clinical scoring system.[33] Inflammatory cellular infiltrates into the iris, ciliary body, and the anterior chamber show predominance of CD4+ T-cells, monocytes/macrophages, and neutrophils.[34]

Myelin Basic Protein-induced Anterior Uveitis

Adamus et al. (1998) induced experimental autoimmune encephalomyelitis (EAE) with myelin basic proteins (MBP). EAE is an acute CD4+ T-cell mediated inflammatory disease of the central nervous system. It is an animal model for multiple sclerosis (MS) and is induced in susceptible animals by a number of myelin antigens including MBP.[34-35] Lewis rats are immunized with MBP or certain peptides of MBP with adjuvant and develop a self-limited form of AAU along with EAE. MBP-induced EAU persists for more than 11 days post immunization even after clinical signs of EAE subsides, with spontaneous AAU remission occurring about 30 days after immunization. The inflammatory cellular infiltrates accumulate around anterior surface of iris, trabecular meshwork and in some cases within the ciliary body and aqueous humor.[34-36]

Kuchroo et al. (1991) inducted experimental allergic encephalomyelitis by myelin proteolipid-protein-(PLP) specific T-cell clones and synthetic peptides in SJL(H-2s) mice.[37]

T-Helper Lymphocytes Type 2-induced Ocular Inflammation

Ocular inflammation is often mediated by T-helper (Th) lymphocytes. These are divided into two Th1 and Th2, and differ in their cytokine production and biological activities. Kim et al. (2002) induced inflammation using T-helper lymphocytes Type 2. They examined the capacity of Th1 and Th2 cells to induce ocular inflammation.[38]

Procedure: Transgenic (Tg) mice are used for induction of ocular inflammation. These mice express hen egg lysozyme (HEL) in their lens, by adoptively transferring Th cells, which transgenically express HEL-specific receptor. Th1 and Th2 populations are polarized *in vitro*, and their selective cytokine production is checked by RT-PCR. Conventional histological methods are used for monitoring the inflammation.[38]

Inflammation-induced by Topical Irritants

Topical irritants like carageenan, nitrogenized mustard, Freund's adjuvant, croton oil, etc. have been used in establishing a model of ocular inflammation. The model fulfills most of the criteria sought by the researchers such as the induction of pathological inflammatory changes in the eyes to study inflammatory activity that can be quantified using standard methods such as estimation of edema, inflammation, mediators, inflammatory cells, etc. The model is easily standardized and reproduced.[37]

Croton Oil-induced Uveitis

Rabbits are instilled with 3% croton oil. Croton oil is dissolved in 2-ethoxyethanol and 40 µl (single drop) is instilled in the cornea. The model probably involves the activation of arachidonic acid pathway and breakdown of blood-aqueous barrier and permits the entry of high molecular weight proteins in aqueous humor.[39]

Villena et al. also induced inflammation by applying 80 µl (40 µl at the interval of 5 min) of 0.1 and 0.2% carageenan using 1% carboxymethyl cellulose and 1% between 80 and; 120 µl (40 µl at 5 min interval) Freund's adjuvant.[39]

Schistosoma mansoni Model of Ocular Inflammation

The model has an important role in screening of the chemotherapeutic agents for suppressing the granulomatous uveitis and understanding the cellular interaction in the formation of granuloma. The role of immunologic factors in ocular defense mechanism can also be understood.[40]

Procedure: Golden Syrian hamsters are injected with 200 cercariae of *Schistosoma mansoni*. After 8 weeks the eggs are recovered from the livers by trypsin digestion and sieving. Eggs are counted and transferred to the tuberculin syringes. New Zealand rabbits of 2.0 kg weight are anesthetized. *S. mansoni* eggs are injected in the eye through pars plana carefully so that the lens and retina is not damaged. The eggs are injected in various concentrations. After 5 days an inflammatory response involving vitreous, choroids, retina, and optic nerve is seen which depends on the number of eggs injected.[40]

Laser-induced Ocular Inflammation

Several workers have induced ocular inflammation in rabbits, rats, mice, primates using laser. Apart from changes in the IOP the injury due to laser produces ocular inflammation. Laser-induced ocular hypertension model can also be used as ocular inflammation model.[41] Laser treatment to the iris of rabbits causes miosis, a rise in intraocular pressure and an increase in the protein content of the aqueous humor. These effects on IOP and the blood-

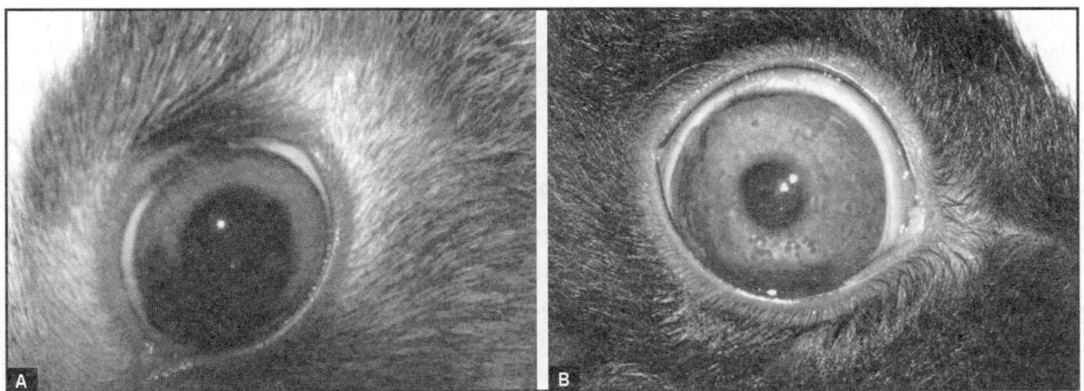

Figure 34.2: Laser treatment in pigmented rabbit eyes: (A) Normal eye (B) post-laser with hyphema (*Courtesy*: Researchers of Ocular Pharmacology Laboratory, Delhi Institute of Pharmaceutical Sciences and Research, New Delhi) (*For color version see Plate 22*)

aqueous barrier are to some extent due to the release of prostaglandins of the E type and are reduced by pretreatment with prostaglandin synthetase inhibitors. The miosis and part of the rise in intraocular pressure and breakdown of the blood-aqueous barrier may also be due to antidromic stimulation of sensory nerves. A combination of indomethacin and local anesthetic helps to block the miosis and elevation in IOP and greatly reduces the increased protein content of the aqueous humor. The human eye may react in a similar way to laser irradiation of the iris.[42]

Gherezghiher and Koss (1989) applied argon laser of 0.75 watts, 0.5 sec duration and 8 spots of 500-micron size to the iris of pigmented rabbits. This resulted in acute rise in IOP and miosis together with an increase in aqueous protein concentration. The response lasted for three days.[41]

Neodymium-yttrium aluminum garnet (Nd-YAG) laser was used by Joo and Kim (1992) to induce ocular changes like prostaglandin E, protein, pupil diameter, and intraocular pressure by photo disruption of pigmented rabbit iris.[43] Figure 34.2 shows post laser hyphema in pigmented rabbits treated with the Nd-Yag laser for producing hypertension.

Zhou et al. (2005) induced choroidal neovascularization by laser photocoagulation in adult male C57BL/6J mice. A brief procedure used by them is given below.[44]

C57BL/6 male mice between 6 to 8 weeks old are fed standard laboratory chow and maintained in a 12 h light 12 h dark environment. The mice are anesthetized with ketamine (80 mg/kg) and xylazine (8 mg/kg), and pupils are dilated with topical 1% tropicamide. Both eyes of mice are photocoagulated by Diode laser (75 µm spot size, 0.1 s duration, 140 mW). They evaluated neutrophil infiltration and showed that post-laser treatment neutrophils infiltrated the sites of laser injury on the day 1 and peaked at day 3.[44]

Endophthalmitis

Inflammation of the ocular cavities and their adjacent structures is defined as endophthalmitis. It may occur as a complication of intraocular surgeries and can lead to loss of vision or sometimes enucleation of the eye. One of the most common causes of this disease is bacterial or fungal infection. Trauma and foreign bodies may also result in endophthalmitis. The symptoms usually are pain; redness of conjunctiva and episclera and sometimes hypopyon is also present. Some of the fungi and bacteria induced experimental models, used by researchers for evaluating the therapeutic potential of the drugs or understanding the mechanism, are described here.

Candida albicans Induced Endophthalmitis

With candida endophthalmitis becoming common Demant and Easterbrook (1977) produced an experimental rabbit model of endophthalmitis to understand whether a clinical lesion can be related to the number of organisms present in it as the drugs required to treat this condition are very toxic and need to be stopped as early as possible. The model produced by them gave reproducible results making it a convenient model for experimental endophthalmitis.[45]

Procedure: A suspension of *Candida albicans* is injected in rabbits intravenously, which produced typical ocular lesions in all of them. The rabbit fundus is examined by indirect ophthalmoscopy. As per the requirement the rabbits are killed to prepare quantitative cultures of their eyes.[45]

In a recent study, Kusbeci et al. (2007) injected New Zealand white rabbits by inoculation of 1 × 104 colony forming units (CFU)/ml of *C. albicans*. The test drug is injected in the vitreous after seventy-two h of inoculation. Differences in the clinical scores and histopathological scores and mean CFU/ml between the control and test group are evaluated.[46]

Fusarium solani-induced Endophthalmitis

Mayayo et al. (1998) induced inflammation in immunocompetent mice by Fusarium solani to produce an experimental model, which can be used for evaluating the efficacy of various treatments and can establish the pathogenecity of the fungus in eye.[47]

Procedure: Isolates of *F. solani* are injected in the lateral tail vein of immunocompetent mice to produce systemic infection along with ocular infection. Each mouse is injected with 5×10^6 conidia.

The study of Mayayo et al. showed that out of the 20 *F. solani* injected mice 16 developed panophthalmitis, four had bilateral infection and 34% showed presence of fungal infection.[47]

Bacteria-induced Endophthalmitis

Bacterial infections lead to endophthalmitis with tissue destruction and also produce host inflammatory response. Inflammatory cells infiltrate to the site of infection mediated by adhesion molecules expressed on the surface of endothelial and inflammatory cells. In order to understand the mechanism of infiltration of the inflammatory cells, the model is produced and described by Giese et al.[48-50]

Procedure: Female Lewis rats of 8-10 weeks are used. One of the eyes of rats is intravitreally injected with 25 µl of *S. aureus*. Controls can be given normal saline. To confirm the number of *S. aureus* injected into the eye 25 µl of *S. aureus* suspension is added to rabbit and sheep blood agar plates and kept under incubation at 37°C for 24 h. The maximum inflammatory response occurs at 24 to 48 h after injection and then reduces.[49]

Kowalaski et al. (2005) and Deng et al. (2006) induced inflammation using *Staphylococcus* species in rabbits. The inflammation thus produced was reproducible.[51,52]

Meyers-Elliott and Dethlefs (1982) injected *Klebsiella oxytoca* in the vitreous of rabbits to produce a model of endophthalmitis with anterior segment inflammation. They observed polymorphonuclear leucocytes at corneal limbus, adjacent to endothelium, in iris and ciliary body, vitreous and optic nerve within 24 h. Within 48 h retinal photoreceptor degeneration was seen. Mononuclear cells were observed in the vitreous in 72 h.[53] Davey et al. 1987 also induced endophthalmitis in rabbits using a different species of *Klebsiella*, i.e. *K. pneumoniae* and *Pseudomonas aeruginosa*. Rabbits were injected intravitreally with either of the organisms. The injection containing 500 colony-forming units of organisms in 0.1 ml of saline were given to produce unilateral inflammation.[54]

Experimental animal models of ocular inflammation are contributing a lot in understanding the mechanism of the ocular inflammations in humans and the efficacy of newer therapeutic agents though researches in this direction are still going on. There are numerous models of inflammation of which only few have been described here. Models using different fungal or bacterial strains have been produced to evaluate antibacterial or antifungal agents for treating the particular disease condition. Corneal transplant models and several other eye irritants or allergens are also used for producing the inflammatory responses in the experimental animals.[55]

REFERENCES

1. Bora NS, Kaplan HJ. Intraocular diseases - anterior uveitis. Chem Immunol Allergy 2007;2:213-20.
2. Groneberg DA, Bielory L, Fischer A, Bonini S, Wahn U. Animal models of allergic and inflammatory conjunctivitis. Allergy 2003;58:1101-13.
3. Hann LE, Cornell-Bell AH, Marten-Ellis C, Allansmith MR. Conjunctival basophil hypersensitivity lesions in guinea pigs. Analysis of upper tarsal epithelium. Invest Ophthalmol Vis Sci 1986;27:1255-60.
4. Fukushima A, Fukata K, Ozaki A, Takata M, Kuroda N, Enzan H, et al. Exertion of the suppressive effects of IFN-g on experimental immune mediated blepharoconjunctivitis in Brown Norway rats during the induction phase but not the effector phase. Br J Ophthalmol 2002;86:1166-71.
5. Nishino K, Fukushima A, Okamoto S, Ohashi Y, Fukata K, Ozaki A, et al. Suppression of experimental immune-mediated blepharoconjunctivitis in Brown Norway rats by topical application of FK 506. Graefes Arch Clin Exp Ophthalmol 2002;240:137-43.
6. Iwamoto H, Nishino K, Magone TM, Whitcup SM, Yoshida O, Yoshida H, et al. Experimental immune-mediated blepharoconjunctivitis in rats induced by immunization with ragweed pollen. Graefes Arch Clin Exp Ophthalmol 2000;238:346-51.
7. Fukushima A, Yamaguchi T, Ishida W, Fukata K, Ueno H. Role of VLA-4 in the development of allergic conjunctivitis in mice. Molecular Vision 2006;12:310-7.
8. Merayo-Lloves J, Calonge M, Foster CS. Experimental model of allergic conjunctivitis to ragweed in guinea pig. Curr Eye Res 1995;14:487-94.
9. Merayo-Lloves J, Zhao TZ, Dutt JE, Foster CS. A new murine model of allergic conjunctivitis and effectiveness of Nedocronil Sodium. J Allergy Clin Immunol 1996;97:1129-40.

10. Yasuda M, Kato M, Nabe T, Nakata K, Kohno S. An experimental allergic conjunctivitis induced by topical and repetitive application of Japanese cedar pollens in guinea pigs. Inflammation Research 2004;48:325-36.
11. Oguz H, Ozbilge H, Oguz E, Gurkan T. Effectiveness of topical taurolidine versus ciprofloxacin, ofloxacin, and fortified cefazolin in a rabbit Staphylococcus aureus keratitis model. Curr Eye Res 2005;30:155-61.
12. Ohgami K, Ilieva IB, Shiratori K, Emiko I, Yoshida K, Kotake S, et al. Effect of human cationic antimicrobial protein 8 peptide on endotoxin-induced uveitis in rats. Invest Ophthalmol Vis Sci 2003;44:4412-8.
13. Kulkarni P, Srinivasan BD. Ocular Inflammation: A pharmacological model. Trends Pharmacological Sciences 1987;8:375-7.
14. Goldblum D, Rohrer K, Frueh BE, Theurillat R, Thormann W, Zimmerli S. Ocular distribution of intravenously administered lipid formulations of amphotericin B in a rabbit model. Antimicrob Agents Chemother 2002;46:3719-23.
15. Ohta K, Wiggert B, Taylor AW, Streilein JW. Effects of experimental ocular inflammation on ocular immune privilege. Invest Ophthalmol Vis Sci 1999;40:2010-8.
16. Liang H, Baudouin C, Labbé A, Pauly A, Martin C, Warnet JM, et al. In vivo confocal microscopy and ex vivo flow cytometery: new tools for assessing ocular inflammation applied to rabbit lipopolysaccharide-induced conjunctivitis. Mol Vis 2006;12:1392-402.
17. Adibkia K, Shadbad MR, Nokhodchi A, Javadzedeh A, BarzegarJalali M, Barar J, et al. Piroxicam nanoparticles for ocular delivery: physiochemical characterization and implementation in endotoxin induced uveitis. J Drug Target 2007;15:407-16.
18. de Vos AF, van Haren MA, Verhagen C, Hoekzema R, Kijlstra A. Kinetics of intraocular tumor necrosis factor and interleukin-6 in endotoxin-induced uveitis in the rat. Invest Ophthalmol Vis Sci 1994;35:1100-6.
19. Yoshida M, Yoshimura N, Hangai M, Tanihara H, Honda Y. Interleukin-1 alpha, interleukin-1 beta, and tumor necrosis factor gene expression in endotoxin-induced uveitis. Invest Ophthalmol Vis Sci 1994;35:1107-13.
20. Tuaillon N, Shen de F, Berger RB, Lu B, Rollins BJ, Chan CC. MCP-1 expression in endotoxin-induced uveitis. Invest Ophthalmol Vis Sci 2002;43:1493-8.
21. Satofuka S, Ichihara A, Nagai N, Yamashiro K, Koto T, Shinoda H, et al. Suppression of ocular inflammation in endotoxin-induced uveitis by inhibiting nonproteolytic activation of prorenin. Invest Ophthalmol Vis Sci 2006;47:2686-92.
22. Fox GM, Kuwabara T, Wiggert B, Redmond TM, Hess HH, Chader GJ, et al. Experimental autoimmune uveoretinitis (EAU) induced by retinal interphotoreceptor retinoid-binding protein (IRBP): differences between EAU induced by IRBP and by S-antigen. Clin Immunol Immunopathol 1987;43:256-64.
23. Iwase K, Fujii Y, Nakashima I, Kato N, Fujino Y, Kawashima H, et al. Experimental autoimmune uveoretinitis (EAU) in mice. Curr Eye Res 1990;9:207-16.
24. Singh VK, Biswas S, Anand R, Agarwal SS. Experimental autoimmune uveitis as animal model for human posterior uveitis. Indian J Med Res 1998;107:53-67.
25. Gasparin F, Takahashi BS, Scolari MR, Gasparin F, Pedral LS, Damico FM. Experimental models of autoimmune inflammatory ocular diseases. Arq Bras Oftalmol 2012;75(2):143-7.

26. Ke Y, Sun D, Zhang P, Jiang G, Kaplan HJ, Shao H. Suppression of established experimental autoimmune uveitis by anti-LFA-1alpha Ab. Invest Ophthalmol Vis Sci 2007;48:2667-75.
27. Kü. Kükner A, Colakoðlu N, Serin D, Alagöz G, Celebi S, Kükner AS. Effects of intraperitoneal vitamin E, melatonin and aprotinin on leptin expression in the guinea pig eye during experimental uveitis. Acta Ophthalmol Scand 2006;84:54-61.
28. Broekhuyse RM, Kuhlmann ED, Winkens HJ. Experimental autoimmune anterior uveitis (EAAU). II. Dose-dependent induction and adoptive transfer using a melanin-bound antigen of the retinal pigment epithelium. Exp Eye Res 1992;55:401-11.
29. Broekhuyse RM, Kuhlmann ED, Winkens HJ. Experimental autoimmune anterior uveitis (EAAU): induction by melanin antigen and suppression by various treatments. Pigment Cell Res 1993;6:1-6.
30. Broekhuyse RM, Kuhlmann ED, Winkens HJ. Experimental melanin-protein induced uveitis (EMIU) is the sole type of uveitis evoked by a diversity of ocular melanin preparations and melanin -derived soluble peptides. Jpn J Ophthalmol 1996;40:459-68.
31. Bora NS, Kim MC, Kabeer NH, Simpson SC, Tandhasetti MT, Cirrito TP, et al. Experimental autoimmune anterior uveitis. Induction with melanin-associated antigen from the iris and ciliary body. Invest Ophthalmol Vis Sci 1995;36:1056-66.
32. Fang I-Mo, Yang CH, Yang CM. Chitosan oligosaccharides attenuate ocular inflammation in rats with experimental autoimmune anterior uveitis. Mediators Inflamm 2014;2014:827847.doi.org/10.1155/2014/827847.
33. Smith JR, Hart PH, Parish CR, Standfield SD, Coster DJ, Williams KA. Experimental melanin-induced uveitis in the Fischer 344 rat is inhibited by anti-CD4 monoclonal antibody, but not by mannose-6-phosphate. Clin Exp Immunol 1999;115:64-71.
34. Chang JH, McCluskey PJ, Wakefield D. Acute Anterior Uveitis and HLA-B27. Surv Ophthalmol 2005; 50:364-88.
35. Adamus G, Amundson D, Vainiene. Ariail K, Machnicki M, Weinberg A, et al. Myelin basic protein specific T-helper cells induce experimental anterior uveitis. J Neurosci Res 1998;44:513-8.
36. Constantinescu CS, Lavi E. Anterior uveitis in murine relapsing experimental autoimmune encephalomyelitis (EAE), a mouse model of multiple sclerosis (MS). Curr Eye Res 2000;20:71-6.
37. Kuchroo VK, Sobel RA, Yamamura T, Greenfield E, Dorf ME, Lees MB. Induction of experimental allergic encephalomyelitis by myelin proteolipid-protein-specific T cell clones and synthetic peptides. Pathobiology 1991;59:305-12.
38. Kim SJ, Zhang M, Vistica BP, Chan C-C, Shen De-Fen, Wawrousek EF, et al. Induction of Ocular Inflammation by T-Helper Lymphocytes Type 2. Invest Ophthalmol Vis Sci 2002;43:758-65.
39. Villena C, Vivas JM, Villar AM. Ocular inflammation models by topical application: Croton oil induced uveitis. Curr Eye Res 1999;18:3-9.
40. Stein PC, Char DH. Intraocular granuloma: a Schistosoma mansoni model of ocular inflammation. Invest Ophthalmol Vis Sci 1982;23:479-88.
41. Gherezghiher T, Koss MC. Argon laser-induced ocular hypertension: animal model of ocular inflammation. J Ocul Pharmacol 1989;5:7-17.
42. Perkins ES. Prostaglandins and ocular trauma. Adv Ophthalmol 1977;34:149-52.
43. Joo CK, Kim JH. Prostaglandin E in rabbit aqueous humor after Nd-YAG laser photodisruption of iris and the effect of topical indomethacin pretreatment. Invest Ophthalmol Vis Sci 1992;33:1685-9.
44. Zhou J, Pham L, Zhang N, He S, Gamulescu M-A, Spee C, Ryan SJ, Hinton DR. Neutrophils promote experimental choroidal neovascularization. Mol Vis 2005;11:414-24.

45. Demant E, Easterbrook M. An experimental model of Candida endophthalmitis. Can J Ophthalmol 1977;12:304-7.
46. Kusbeci T, Avci B, Cetinkaya Z, Ozturk F, Yavas G, Ermis SS, et al. The effects of caspofungin and voriconazole in experimental Candida endophthalmitis. Curr Eye Res 2007;32:57-64.
47. Mayayo E, Guarro J, Pujol I. Endogenous endophthalmitis by Fusarium solani: an animal experimental model. Med Mycol 1998;36:249-53.
48. Giese MJ, Berliner JA, Riesner A, Wagar EA, Mondino BJ. A comparison of the early inflammatory effects of an agr-/sar- versus a wild type strain of Staphylococcus aureus in a rat model of endophthalmitis. Curr Eye Res 1999;18:177-85.
49. Giese MJ, Shum DC, Rayner SA, Mondino BJ, Berliner JA. Adhesion molecule expression in a rat model of Staphylococcus aureaus endophthalmitis. Invest Ophthalmol Vis Sci 2000;41:145-53.
50. Giese MJ, Rayner SA, Fardin B, Sumner HL, Rozengurt N, Mondino BJ, Gordon LK. Mitigation of neutrophils infiltration in a rat model of early Staphylococcus aureus endophthalmitis. Invest Ophthalmol Vis Sci 2003;44:3077-82.
51. Kowalaski RP, Romanowski MS, Mah FS, Yates KA, Gordon YJ. Intracameral VigamoxR (Moxifloxacin 0.5%) is non toxic and effective in preventing staphylococcal endophthalmitis. Am J Ophthomol 2005;140:497-504.
52. Deng SX, Penland S, Gupta S, Fiscella R, Edward DP, Tessler HH, et al. Methotrexate reduces the complications of endophthalmitis resulting from intravitreal injection compared with dexamethasone in a rabbit model. Invest Ophthalmol Vis Sci 2006;47:1516-21.
53. Meyers-Elliott RH, Dethlefs BA. Experimental Klebsiella-induced endophthalmitis in the rabbit. Arch Ophthalmol 1982;100:1959-63.
54. Davey P, Barza M, Peckman C. Spontaneous inhibition of bacterial growth in experimental gram-negative endophthalmitis. Invest Ophthalmol Vis Sci 1987;28:867-73.
55. Horai R, Silver PB, Chen J, Agarwal RK, Chong WP, Jittayasothorn Y, et al. Breakdown of immune privilege and spontaneous autoimmunity in mice expressing a transgenic T cell receptor specific for a retinal autoantigen. J Autoimmun 2013;44:21-33. doi: 10.1016/j.jaut.2013.06.003. Epub 2013 Jun 28.

CHAPTER

35

Antiulcer Agents

INTRODUCTION

The term peptic ulcer refers to a spectrum of disorders that includes gastric ulcers, duodenal ulcers and postoperative ulcers at or near the site of surgical gastrointestinal anastomosis. There are two types of duodenal ulcers - acute and chronic duodenal ulcers. Pathogenesis of peptic ulcers involves disturbances in the acid-pepsin status of the gastric contents and infection with *H. pylori*. Neutralization of gastric acid by antacids or inhibition of acid secretion by drugs like H_2 receptor blockers, proton pump (H^+ K^+-ATPase) inhibitors, cytoprotective prostaglandin analogs and various other drugs are the main modes of pharmacological treatment of peptic ulcers. Due to the high morbidity associated with this disease, there is a continuous need for newer anti-ulcer drugs. Screening models of antiulcer agents have been reviewed recently by many investigators.[1,2] This chapter further updates various methods used for the screening of potential anti-ulcer agents. Before the selection of experimental ulcer model, it is desirable that the following requirements are met.[1]

1. They should be simple, reproducible and allow for easy quantification of results.
2. They should make use of a variety of animal species.
3. They should induce characteristic ulceration in specific locations (stomach and duodenum).
4. They should involve different mechanism by which ulceration is produced.
5. The ulcers induced should not spontaneously heal during the observation period.

Apart from above requirements the selected model

6. Should also be cost effective and
7. Model should not be time consuming.

IN VITRO METHODS

[^{125}I] Gastrin Binding Assay

Gastrin is one of the major stimuli for gastric acid secretion. Its release is also triggered by partially digested proteins, peptides, blood borne factors and by vagal stimulation.[3] After release from gastric antrum, it stimulates acid secretion by binding to its receptors on parietal cells as well as by releasing histamine from enterochromaffin-like cells. Compounds with gastrin receptor antagonistic activity can prove to be useful antiulcer drugs. [^{125}I] Gastrin is used for radioligand binding assay for gastrin receptors. Proglumide like drugs, which are a CCKR antagonists, may also be screened using this assay.[4]

Procedure: The assay is done using fundic gland suspension obtained from guinea pig stomach. For the binding and competition assays, the gland suspension is incubated with 50 μl of [^{125}I] gastrin in the presence of either buffer alone (for total binding) or in the presence of unlabeled gastrin (for non-specific binding) or in the presence of test compound for 90 min at 37°C. Subsequently, ice cold buffer, in microcentrifuge tubes, is layered with incubated mixture and centrifuged for 5 min at 10,000 g. Radioactivity is quantified in pellet after discarding the supernatant.

Evaluation: Total binding, non-specific binding and specific binding are determined. Percentage of specifically bound [^{125}I] gastrin displaced by a given concentration of the test compound is calculated and its IC_{50} and dissociation constant (Ki) values are calculated.[5-7]

[^{3}H] Tiotidine Binding Assay for Histamine H_2 Receptors

Histamine H_2 receptor blockers have been the mainstay of anti-ulcer therapy since the early 1970s due to their potent acid-suppressing properties. Tiotidine is an H_2 receptor blocker that is used for H_2 receptor binding assay.

Procedure: The assay is done using cerebral cortex homogenate obtained from male White leghorn chicks or from guinea pigs. The cerebral cortex homogenate is incubated with [^{3}H] tiotidine for 90 min at 4°C in the presence of Na_2HPO_4/KH_2PO_4 buffer (pH 7.4) alone to determine total binding or in the presence of unlabeled ranitidine and buffer to determine non-specific binding or in the presence of test compound in buffer for competition assay. 5 ml of ice-cold phosphate buffer is added to terminate the incubation. Subsequently the reaction mixture is filtered under vacuum through glass fiber filters that are pre-soaked with buffer. Filters are then washed with 5 ml of ice-cold buffer twice and radioactivity measured by liquid scintillation counting.[8,9]

Evaluation: Specific binding, i.e. total binding minus non-specific binding and IC_{50} are determined.

In another study, the [^{3}H]-tiotidine has also been used as a specific ligand for H_2 receptors in dispersed mucosal cells from guinea pig stomach and it was found to have limited binding to H_2 receptors and as such [^{3}H]-tiotidine was not a suitable ligand for labelling the H_2-receptor on gastric mucosal cells.[10]

H^+/K^+- ATPase Inhibition Assay

H^+/K^+- ATPase or proton pump is the final step in the synthesis of acid by parietal cells. It exchanges intracellular H^+ with extracellular K^+ in the canaliculi of parietal cells in response to stimulation by all gastric acid secretagogues, i.e. histamine, acetylcholine and gastrin. Proton pump inhibitors like omeprazole, lansoprazole, etc. are now established antiulcer drugs.

Procedure: The assay is carried out using homogenates of microsomal gastric H^+/K^+-ATPase obtained from pig gastric mucosa.[11] For inhibition assay, 80 ng microsomal H^+/K^+-ATPase is incubated with 100 μl buffer (pH 7.4), 1 mM ATP and test compound in microtitre plate for 30 min at 37°C. After 30 min of incubation, the reaction is stopped by adding malachite green colorimetric reagent and then after 10 sec 15% sodium citrate is added for 45 min. Release of orthophosphate from ATP is quantified by colorimeter at 570 nm. For study of omeprazole and other proton pump inhibitors available at present, which produce active metabolite at acidic pH, the microsomal homogenate is initially suspended in buffer at pH 6.1 along with the drug and incubated for 30 min. This homogenate is then transferred to buffer at 7.4 and the procedure described above is followed. Percentage inhibition of H^+/K^+- ATPase is calculated.[12]

Percentage of enzyme inhibition is calculated using the formula:

$$\% \text{ Inhibition} = \frac{[\text{Activity (control)} - \text{Activity (test)}]}{\text{Activity (control)}} \times 100$$

IN VIVO METHODS

Pylorus Ligation in Rats

This procedure was described by Shay et al.[13] The basis for this model is that accumulation of unbuffered gastric juice over a certain length of time leads to peptic ulceration in rats whose pylorus has been ligated.

Procedure: Wistar rats (150 to 180 g) are used for the experiment. The animals are fasted for 48 hours before the operative procedure. However they are given free access to water ad libitum. To prevent cannibalism and coprophagy, the animals are housed singly in cages with raised bottoms of wide wire mesh. Under ether anesthesia, a one-inch midline abdominal incision is given below the xiphoid process. The pylorus is carefully lifted out with minimal handling and traction and ligated without damaging its blood supply. The stomach is now replaced and the abdominal wall closed with sutures. The test compound is administered either orally or subcutaneously and the animals are placed in plastic cylinders. About 17-19 h after pyloric ligation, the animals are sacrificed and the stomach dissected out. The contents of the stomach are drained into a graduated centrifuge tube and their acidity determined by titration with 0.1 N NaOH. The stomach is opened along its greater curvature, pinned on a cork plate and inner surface examined for ulceration with a binocular microscope. The ulcer index is calculated and the ulcer severity graded as mentioned below.

Ulcer severity is graded as:

0—No ulcer, 1—Superficial ulcer, 2—Deep ulcer and 3—Perforation

The ulcer index (U_I) is calculated by the following equation:

$$U_I = U_N + U_S + U_P \times 10^{-1}$$

where, U_N = Average of number of ulcers/animal; U_S = Average of severity scores; U_P = Percentage of animals with ulcers.

Ulcer index and acidity of the gastric content of the treated animals are compared with the control.

Aspirin alone at a dose of 150 mg/kg p.o. can induce ulcers in rats.[14] Aspirin plus pylorus ligation induced gastric ulcers in rats have also been successful to study the antiulcerogenic effects of drugs.[15]

Stress Ulcer Models

Stress plays a significant role in the pathogenesis of gastric ulcers in human being. However, the recent studies suggest no harmful effect of chronic stress on gastric ulceration.[16] Selye (1936), for the first time, described the use of restraint for the production of gastric ulcers.[17] Various models involving various types of stress have since been developed. The involvement of psychogenic factors and the ease of production of gastric ulcers using these models is a real advantage over the pyloric ligation method of gastric ulcer production.

Restraint-induced Ulcers

Procedure: Albino rats, of either sex, weighing 150 to 200 g, are used for the study. After 36 hours of fasting, the test drug is administered. Thirty minutes later, the animals are subjected to restraint by molding a special galvanized steel window screen around the animal and tying the limbs of the animal in pair so that the animal cannot move. The animals are kept under restraint for 24 h. The animals are then sacrificed and their stomachs dissected out. The stomachs are opened along greater curvature and fixed to cork plate.[18] Ulcer index and ulcer severity are determined as described in the pyloric ligation method.

Cold Water Immersion-induced Ulcers

It has been observed that when the restrained animals are subjected to additional cold water immersion, the occurrence of gastric ulcers is accelerated and this also shortens the immobilization time.[19,20]

Procedure: Wistar rats (150 to 200 g) are used for the experiments. After fasting the animal for 16 hours, the test compound is administered orally. The animals are placed individually in restraint cages vertically and then immersed in water at 22°C for 1 h. Azovan blue (Evan's blue), in a dose of 30 mg/kg, is injected intravenously via the tail vein after removal of the rats from the cage. They are sacrificed 10 min later. The stomach is removed and ligated at both ends. It is filled with formol saline and kept overnight. On the next day, the stomach is opened along the greater curvature, washed in warm water and examined for ulcerative lesions. Evan's blue helps in evaluation of the lesion score, which is calculated by adding the lengths of the longest diameters of the lesions.[20] Gastric mucosal lesions can also be induced by 2 h of cold restraint stress in rats.[21]

Abdel-Sater KA et al,[22] 2012 have used acute cold restraint stress by fixing the four limbs of the rat and placing it in a refrigerator at 4°C for 3 h to study the gender difference of selective serotonin reuptake inhibitors, fluoxetine. Stressed male rats were found to be more responsive to the antiulcer effect of fluoxetine more than stressed females.

Stress and NSAIDs-induced Ulcers

Procedure: Wistar rats (150 to 200 g) are used for the experiment. The animals are fasted for 24-36 h and then given the test agent (in 1% carboxymethyl cellulose) via gastric intubation and an NSAID such as aspirin, indomethacin or diclofenac intraperitoneally. After placing the rats in stress cages, they are immersed in water up to the level of xiphoid process at 23°C for 7 h. The animals are then sacrificed, their stomach removed and evaluated for ulcer index.

The dose of NSAID required to increase gastric erosion by 100% relative to immobilization is compared with that of NSAID required to produce 100% increase in gastric erosion under the protective effect of test drug.[23]

Swimming Stress Ulcers

Procedure: Albino rats of either sex are fasted for 24 h with free access to water. The rats are forced to swim in a deep concrete tube filled with water at 23°C for 5 h. The animals are removed from the tube after five hours, sacrificed and their stomachs removed. The stomachs are opened along the greater curvature and severity grading is done and ulcer index calculated. Severity of the ulcerative lesions is graded as follow:

0—no lesions, 1—lesions with diameter less than 1 mm, 2—lesions with diameter 1-2 mm, 3—lesions with diameter 2-4 mm, and 4—lesions with diameter more than 4 mm.

Ulcer index is calculated by summation of scores for individual erosions and ulcers.[24]

Histamine-induced Gastric Ulcers

Histamine has been used widely for the production of gastric ulcers. Enhanced gastric acid secretion has been implicated in the production of ulcers due to histamine.[25]

Procedure: Male guinea pigs, weighing 300 to 400 g, are used for the experiment. The animals are fasted for 36 h with water available *ad libitum*. Histamine acid sulphate is injected in a dose of 50 mg intraperitoneally. To prevent histamine toxicity, promethazine hydrochloride is injected intraperitoneally 15 min before and 15 min after the histamine injection in a dose of 5 mg. The test drug is administered 30-45 min before the histamine injection. Four hours after the histamine injection, the animals are sacrificed and their stomachs dissected out. The degree of ulceration grading is done as follows:

- Type 0: No visible ulceration on gross examination
- Type 1: 1-3 mm ulcers, ten or less in number
- Type 2: 1-3 mm ulcers, eleven or more in number
- Type 3: 4-6 mm ulcers, one or more in number
- Type 4: 7 mm or bigger ulcers, one or more in number
- Type 5: Gastric or esophageal wall perforation.[26]

Other routes of administration of histamine such as intraperitoneal/intramuscular have also been found useful.[27] Repeated administration of histamine by intraperitoneal route (0.09 mg/kg) or intramuscular route 0.09 mg/kg × 8 doses) has been found to selectively induce gastric or duodenal ulcers demonstrating differential of histamine in ulcer induction.

Modification: Duodenal ulcers were also induced by repeated ip administration of histamine acid phosphate at a dose of 0.25 mg/kg at every 30 min interval for 4 h after 45 min of test drug administration.[28]

Apart from guinea pig, other animals such as rats can also be used to induce histamine gastric ulcers. Histamine, intraperitoneal injection at a dose of 300 mg/kg induces gastric lesions.[29]

Methylene Blue-induced Ulcers

Methylene blue (MB), a synthetic drug has been used for the induction of duodenal and gastric ulcers in rats. Methylene blue uncouples the ATPase enzyme and also possesses the affinity for muscarinic receptors. The model is used for the screening of antiulcer agents involving H^+/K^+ ATPase system or via anticholinergic action exerted via muscarinic receptors.

Procedure: Methylene blue produces ulceration of gastric mucosa by reduction in blood supply to gastric mucosal region that causes oxidative stress. Rats are fasted for 24 h before the administration of MB. Animals are administered MB at a dosage of 5-125 mg/kg body weight p.o. followed by the administration of the test drug. After 4 h the animals are sacrificed and ulcer index is determined.[30]

Serotonin-induced Gastric Ulcers

Adinortey et al. 2013 have reviewed the serotonin (5-HT)-induced gastric ulcer model. Serotonin produced local vasoconstriction and thus reduced the gastric mucosal blood supply, resulting in local mucosal injury.[2]

Procedure: Rats were administered with a single dose of serotonin creatinine sulfate (0.5 ml of 50 mg/kg subcutaneous injection) for the induction of glandular lesions after fasting for 24–36 h and water deprivation for 2 h before the experiments. They are housed in wide mesh wire bottom to prevent coprophagy. Serotonin was administered by intragastric intubation with the aid of an orogastric cannula. Six hours later, the animals are sacrificed by cervical dislocation for examination.

Endogenous serotonin is also reported to play a dual role in the pathogenesis of indomethacin induced small intestinal ulceration in mice - proulcerogenic action via 5-HT_3 receptor and antiulcerogenic action via 5-HT_4 receptors.[31]

Ethanol-induced Mucosal Damage

Ethanol (absolute)-induced gastric lesion is a reproducible method in experimental animal.[32] Using a transmission densitometer, it is possible to quantify the extent of gastric lesions induced by ethanol, by measuring the optical density of photographic negatives of gastric mucosa.[33]

Procedure: Wistar rats, weighing 250 to 300 g, are used for the experiment. The animals are placed individually in cylindrical stainless steel cages with flat bottoms to limit their mobility and prevent coprophagy. They are fasted for 18 h but given water ad libitum. Now the test drug or the vehicle is given to the animals orally. Thirty minutes later, 1 ml of absolute ethanol is given orally. The animals are sacrificed 1 hour later and their stomachs dissected out. The stomachs are opened along the greater curvature, washed with tap water and ulcer severity grading done. Using a cork borer, 13 mm, full thickness circular patches are cut from each lobe of the fundus below the ridge dividing glandular from non-glandular portion of the stomach and placed into holes of a special template. Photographs of the tissues are taken and the negatives examined under light transmission densitometer. Damaged areas have lower optical density values.[32,33]

Absolute ethanol has also been used at higher dose of 5 ml/kg to induce gastric lesions in rats. Animals were sacrified after 1 h and stomach opened to observe gastric lesions.[34]

Khazaei and Salehi,[35] 2006 have induced gastric ulcers in male albino rats by administering ethanol 50% (in distilled water) at a dose of 10 ml/kg. One h after ethanol administration, rats were killed and lesions produced in glandular part of stomach were measured/counted with a graticules under stereo microscope and effects of test drug observed. Ethanol induced severe gastric hemorrhagic erosions. It induced both long ulcers and petechial lesions. Decrease in gasric mucus and increased lipid peroxidation are the mechanisms suggested for ethanol induced gastric ulcers.

Acetic Acid-induced Gastric Ulcers

This model produces chronic ulcers that resemble human ulcers and is used to screen drugs for their gastroprotective effect in chronic gastric and duodenal ulcers. Spontaneous relapse of healed ulcers > 100 days after ulceration is the characteristic feature of this model.[36]

Procedure: Albino rats are used for the experiment. A volume of 0.05 ml of acetic acid (1-30%) is injected into the submucosal layer of the stomach, which results in the formation of penetrating peptic ulcers that are confined by adhesions to contiguous organs like liver. They are typically chronic ulcers with repeated healing and re-aggravation. 100% acetic acid can also be applied to the serosal surface of stomach or duodenum for production of ulcers. Effect of test drug given twice daily for 10-15 days is noted.[37]

Rabbit gastric ulcer models namely acetic acid induced and mucosal resection-induced models are more clinically relevant models in terms of round, deep ulcers with clear-cut margin and well-defined healing stages that are difficult to define in rat models.[38]

Qin and Chen,[39] 2005 have used modified method for induction of gastric ulcers. Gastric ulcers were produced in male Sprague-Dawley rats by application of round filter paper (diameter 5 mm) immersed in a 100% acetic acid on the serosal surface of the anterior wall of the stomach approximately at the center of the corpus for 30 sec and the process was repeated twice. Immediate production of necrosis of the entire mucosa and submucosa (but not serosa) within the area (20 mm^2) where the acetic acid applied, was observed. Excess of acetic acid was then removed and serosa was gently washed with saline. The abdomen was then sutured and the animals were allowed to recover and returned to their cages with free access to food and water. The above method was found useful to study the synergistic action of famotidine and chlorpheniramine on acetic acid-induced gastric ulcer in rats.

Indomethacin-induced Gastric Ulcers

Gastric ulcers may be induced by oral administration of indomethacin (25 mg/kg) after 24 h fasting male albino rats. Indomethacin is dissolved in sodium bicarbonate to form a clear solution. Gastric ulcer can be examined after 4 h of indomethacin administration by opening the stomach along the greater curvature, washed in normal saline to remove debris and pinned on a cork mat for ulcer screening. This can be done by locating the wounds in the glandular region under a simple microscope. The length (mm) of all the elongated black-red lines parallel to long axis of the stomach in the mucosa is measured. Ulcer index is calculated by adding the lengths of all the lesions in the glandular region of the stomach. NSAIDs are believed to cause inhibition of COX and thereby inhibiting the production of cytoprotective prostaglandins and causing gastrointestinal side effects. Indomethacin has shown to cause oxidative stress also leading to formation of gastric ulcers.[40]

Reserpine-induced Chronic Ulcers

Histamine liberation from the mast cells in stomach wall with subsequent increase in gastric acid secretion has been implicated in reserpine-induced gastric glandular ulcer formation in rats.[41]

Procedure: Female Sprague-Dawley rats, weighing 130 to 180 g, are used. The animals are fasted for 48 hours with free access to 0.8% sucrose in 0.2% NaCl w/v. They are housed in wide mesh wire bottom cages to prevent coprophagy. One h before starting the experiment, the liquid diet is also withdrawn. Now the animals are injected with the test drug intraperitoneally and half an hour later reserpine (5 mg/kg) or vehicle is injected intraperitoneally. Four h later, the animal is sacrificed and stomach removed and examined for mucosal lesions.[42] Reserpine dose (5 mg/kg intraperitoneally, 18 h before sacrifice) has also been used by other investigators,[43] and it induced marked glandular ulceration with release of free β-glucuronidase.

Cysteamine-induced Duodenal Ulcers

Selye and Szabo[44] first described the production of duodenal ulcers in rats by cysteamine HCl (β-mercaptoethylamine HCl). The pathogenesis of cysteamine-induced duodenal ulcers involves: inhibition of alkaline mucus production, increased gastric acid secretion, increased serum gastrin levels and delayed gastric emptying. This model is widely used to evaluate the anti-ulcer activity of anticholinergics, antacids, prostaglandins and H_2 receptor antagonists.

Procedure: Female Sprague-Dawley rats are used. Cysteamine (10% in normal saline) is administered in dose of 28 mg/100 g body weight, 3 times at intervals of 3.5 h orally or 20 mg/100 g body weight, twice at an interval of 4 h subcutaneously. The animals are sacrificed 28 hours after the first dose in case of orally administered cysteamine and 40 h after subcutaneous administration of cysteamine. Perforating duodenal ulcers are produced that are located 2-4 mm from the pylorus, mainly on the anterior wall of the duodenum. Presence of necrotic material and acute inflammatory response on the luminal layers of the crater are characteristics of active ulcers. The ulcer and its features in test group are compared to those in control group.

Acute duodenal ulcers can be induced in rats by administration of a single dose of cysteamine hydrochloride (400 mg/kg p.o.). For induction of chronic type duodenal ulcers, rats are administered with cysteamine (400 mg/kg p.o.) twice at an interval of 4 h followed by addition of cysteamine hydrochloride to drinking water.[45]

Dimaprit-induced Duodenal Ulcers

Dimaprit, an H_2 receptor agonist, has been shown to induce gastric erosions in rats after a single intravenous dose and duodenal ulcers in guinea pigs after repeated subcutaneous doses.[46] This model is especially useful for screening of H_2-blockers.

Procedure: Female Sprague-Dawley rats (150 to 180 g) or female guinea pigs (250 to 300 g) are used for the experiments. The animals are fasted for 24 h before the experiment but allowed free access to water. In rats, dimaprit is given in a dose of 100 mg/kg intravenously, single dose. The animal is sacrificed one hour later and the stomach dissected out and examined for gastric erosions. The test drug or vehicle is given orally 60 min before injecting dimaprit.

In case of guinea pigs, the animals are given multiple subcutaneous injections of dimaprit (2 mg/kg every hour for 6 h). The test drug is given either 30 min before the first dose of dimaprit or 30 min before and then hourly along with dimaprit. The animals are sacrificed one hour after the last dimaprit injection and stomach and duodenum are examined for lesions.[46]

Other routes of administration of dimaprit such as intramuscular injection at a dose of 0.09 or 0.18 mg/kg body weight and intraperitoneal injection at a dose of 1.81 or 3.62 mg/kg have also been used in guinea pigs for induction of duodenal ulcers. The intramuscular injection produced particularly severe ulcers.[27]

Mepirizole-induced Duodenal Ulcers

Okabe et al. (1982) have described the production of duodenal ulcers in rats by mepirizole, a non-steroidal anti-inflammatory drug. This model is a useful model for screening of antiulcer drugs like antacids, anticholinergics and H_2 receptor antagonists as mepirizole-induced gastric secretions are inhibited by these drugs thereby important in study of pathogenesis of duodenal ulcers.[47]

Procedure: Male Sprague-Dawley rats, 200-220 g in weight, are administered 200 mg/kg of mepirizole suspended in 1% carboxymethyl cellulose solution via gastric intubation. Subsequently rats are kept in cages with raised mesh bottom and deprived of food and water for 24 h. This leads to ulceration in proximal duodenum and erosions in antrum. Antiulcer drug therapy is started after 24 h of mepirizole administration. On the 11th day, the animals are sacrificed and their duodenum and stomach evaluated for ulcer area under microscope. Ulcer or erosion indices are calculated from the sum of area of ulcers and erosions, respectively.[48]

Duodenal ulcers can also be induced by subcutaneous administration of mepirizole at doses of 60 and 200 mg/kg to increase acid secretion in a dose dependent manner within 8 hours.[49]

Gastric Mucosal Injury by Local Ischemia-Reperfusion in Rats

Gastric ischemia-reperfusion is an important model for studying acute gastric mucosal injury.

Procedure: Wistar rats, 180-200 g weight, are deprived of food for 24 h before experiments, but allowed free access to tap water. The animals are anesthetized and their abdomen opened by a midline incision. Celiac artery is identified and clamped by a microvascular clamp, 0.5 cm from its origin, for 30 min to induce ischemia and then reperfusion for 60 min is performed by removal of clamp. After completion of reperfusion, the animals are sacrificed by exsanguination and stomach removed and lesions examined macroscopically and microscopically. Ulcer index is then calculated.[50-53]

Modifications: Hassan et al. (1997) produced ischemia by clamping left gastric artery for 15 min and then reperfusion for 30 min before sacrificing the animals by cervical dislocation. The stomachs were removed and opened along the greater curvature and photographed for assessment of macroscopic mucosal injury planimetrically. Microscopic injury was also assessed by staining a sample of corpus with hematoxylin and eosin, and examining under a microscope.[54]

Mojzis et al.[55] 2000 induced gastric ischemia in male Wistar rats by 30 min clamping of the coelic artery followed by 30 min of reperfusion and the mucus content, extent of gastric lesions and length of lesions was determined at the end of ischemia/reperfusion. The method has been used to evaluate the effects of sucralfate, malotilate, 0.5% methylcellulose and N-acetylcysteine.

In Silico Model Based Approach for the Development of Antiulcer Antibiotics

Mandal and Das,[56] 2014 have developed an *in silico* based approach for the development of antiulcer antibiotics. They targeted bacterial lysine biosynthetic pathway for antibacterial drug development using inhibitors of *H. pylori* DapE-encoded N-succinyl-L,L-diaminopimetic acid desuccinylase, an essential enzyme responsible for lysine synthesis in bacterial cell wall.

Procedure: The study used 3D structured model of DapE-encoded *H. pylori* having two domains, one catalytic domain and other dimerization domain developed by MODELLER software. After conformation of the stability of the model by GROMACS, the identification of inhibitors of DapE, drug-like small molecule screening library was developed by Tanimoto based Pubchem Database with DapE substrate L, L- SDAP as a query molecule followed by docking approach by using GLIDE XP to identify the potential inhibitors of DapE which can be used further in the development of novel antibacterial antiulcer drugs.

REFERENCES

1. Lahiri S, Palit G. An overview of the current methodologies used for evaluation of gastric and duodenal antiulcer agents. Pharmacologia 2012;3(8):1-8.
2. Adinortey MB, Ansah C, Galyuon I, Nyarko A. In vivo models used for evaluation of potential antigastroduodenal ulcer agents. Hindawi 2013:1-12.
3. Regulation of gastrointestinal function. In: Review of Medical Physiology, 20th International Ed 2002 (Editor - Ganong WF), Mc Graw Hill: pp 467-67.
4. The gastrointestinal tract. In: Elsevier's Pharmacology, 5th Ed 2005 (Rang et al), Churchill Livingstone, International Print-O-Pac Limited, Noida.
5. Praissman M, Walden M, Pellechia C. Identification and characterization of a specific receptor for cholecystokinin on isolated fundic glands from guinea pig gastric mucosa using a biological active 125I-CCK-8 probe. J Recept Res 1983;3:647-65.
6. Berglindh T, Obrink KJ. A method for preparing isolated glands from the rabbit gastric mucosa. Acta Physiol Scand 1976;96:150-9.
7. Gully D, Frehel D, Marcy C, et al. Peripheral biological activity of SR 27897: a new potent non-peptide antagonist of CCKA receptors. Eur J Pharmacol 1993;232:13-9.
8. Zawilaska JB, Wolden-Tambor A, Nowak JZ. Histamine H2-like receptors in chick cerebral cortex: effects of cyclic AMP synthesis and characterization by [3H] tiotidine binding. J Neurochem 2002;81:935-46.
9. Gajtkowski GA, Norris DB, Rising TJ, et al. Specific binding of [3H]tiotidine to histamine H2-receptors in guinea-pig cerebral cortex. Nature 1983;304:65–7.
10. Betzri S, Harmon JW. Is [3H]-tiotidine a specific ligand for the H2-receptor? Pharmacology 1986;32(5):241-7.
11. Rabon EC, Im WB, Sachs G. Preparation of gastric H,K-ATPase. Methods Enzymol 1988;157:649-54.
12. Smolka AJ, Goldenring JR, Gupta S, et al. Inhibition of gastric H,K-ATPase activity and gastric epithelial cell IL-8 secretion by the pyrrolizine derivative ML 3000. BMC Gastroenterology 2004;4. Article accessed from http://www.biomedcentral .com/1471-230X/4/4.
13. Shay H, Komarov SA, Fels SS, et al. A simple method for the uniform production of gastric ulceration in the rat. Gastroenterology 1945;5:43-61.

14. Onasanwo SA, Singh N, Olaleye SB, Mishra V, Palit G. Anti-ulcer and antioxidant activities of Hedranthera barteri {(Hook F) Pichon} with possible involvement of H+K+ ATPase inhibitory activity. Indian J Med Res 2010;132:442-9.
15. Sen S, Ashok Kumar K, Umamaheshwari M, Sivashanmugam AT, Subhadradevi V. Antiulcerogenic effect of gallic acid in rats and its effect on oxidant and antioxidant parameters in stomach tissue. Indian J Pharm Sci 2013;75(2):149-55.
16. Filaretova L, Morozova O, Laszlo F, Morschl E, Zelena D. Does chronic stress enhance the risk of diseases? Endocr Regul 2013;47(4):177-88.
17. Selye H. A syndrome produced by various noxious agents. Nature 1936;138:32-5.
18. Brodie DA, Hanson HM. A study of the factors involved in the production of gastric ulcers by the restraint technique. Gastroenterology 1960;38:353-60.
19. Takagi K, Kasuya Y, Watanabe K. Studies on the drugs for peptic ulcers: A reliable method for producing stress ulcer in rats. Chem Pharm Bull 1964;12:465-72.
20. West GB. Testing for drugs inhibiting the formation of gastric ulcers. J Pharmacol Methods 1982;8:33-7.
21. Zhu D, Tong Q, Liu W, Tian M, Xie W, Ji L, Shi J. Angiotensin (1-7) protects against stress-induced gastric lesions in rats. Biochem Pharmacol 2014;87(3):467-76.
22. Abdel-Daiem WM, SayyedBakheet M. The gender difference of selective serotonin reuptake inhibitor, fluoxetine in adult rats with stressed induced gastric ulcer. Eur J Pharmacol 2012;688 (1-3):42-8.
23. Leitold M, Fleissig W, Merk A. Antiulcer and secretion-inhibitory properties of the tricyclic derivative doxepin in rats and dogs. Arzneimittelforschung 1984;34:468-73.
24. Nagy L, Fiegler M, Mozsik GY, et al. Some metabolic and biochemical alterations during the development of stress ulcers in rats forced to swim. Int J Tiss Reac 1983;5:363-71.
25. Djahanguiri B, Sadeghi D, Pousti A, et al. Effect of a single dose of phentolamine, MJ 1999 and isoproterenol on histmaine-induced gastric ulcer in guinea pigs. Eur J Pharmacol 1968;2:315-6.
26. Barrett WE, Rutledge R, Plummer AJ, et al. Inhibition of ulcer formation in the shay rat and reduction of gastric acidity in dogs by antrenyl (oxyphenonium) (BA5473) diethyl (2-hydroxyethyl) methylammonium bromide ◎-phenyl-cyclohexaneglycolate, an anticholinergic agent. J Pharmacol Exp Ther 1953;108:305-16.
27. Cho CH, Pfeiffer CJ. Gastrointestinal ulceration in the guinea pig in response to dimaprit, histamine, and H1 and H2 blocking agents. Digest Dis Sci 1981;26(4):306-7.
28. Parmar NS, Desai JK. A review of the current methodology for the evaluation of gastric and duodenal antiulcer agents. Indian J Pharmacol 1993;25:120-35.
29. Sirmaqul B, Killic FS, Batu O, Erol K. The effects of verapamil on stress and histamine–induced gastric lesions in rats. Methods Find Exp Clin Pharmacol 2004;26(10):763-7.
30. Shah DI, Santani DD, Goswami SS. A novel use of methylene blue as a pharmacological tool. J Pharmacol Toxicol Methods 2006;54(3):273-7.
31. Kato S, Matsuda N, Matsumato K, Wada M, Onimaru N, Yausda M, et al. Dual role of serotonin in the pathogenesis of indomethacin induced small intestinal ulceration: proulcerogenic action via 5-HT3 receptor and antiulcerogenic action via 5-HT4 receptors. Pharmacol Res 2012;66(3):226-34.
32. Robert A, Nezamis JE, Lancaster C, et al. Cytoprotection by prostaglandins in rats: Prevention of gastric necrosis produced by alcohol, HCl, NaOH, hypertonic NaCl, and thermal injury. Gastroenterology 1979;77:433-43.

33. Witt CG, Will PC, Gaginella TS. Quantification of ethanol induced gastric mucosal injury by transmission densitometery. J Pharmacol Methods 1985;3:109-16.
34. Arumugam S, Selvaraj SV, Velayutham S, Natesan SK, Palaniswamy K. Evaluation of anti-ulcer activity of Samanea saman(Jacq)merr bark on ethanol and stress induced gastric lesions in albino rats. Indian J Pharmacol 2011;43(5):586-90.
35. Khazaei M, Salehi H. Protective effect of Falcaria vulgaris extract on ethanol-induced gastric ulcer in rat. Iranian J Pharmacol Ther 2006;5:43-6.
36. Okabe S, Amagase K. An overview of acetic acid ulcer models - the history and state of the art of peptic ulcer research. Biol Pharmaceutical Bull 2005;28(8):1321-41.
37. Kimura M, Saziki R, Arai I, et al. Effect of 2'- carboxy-methoxy-4,4'-bis(3-methyl-2-butenyloxy) chalcone (sofalcone) on chronic gastric ulcers in rats. Jpn J Pharmacol 1984;35:389-96.
38. Maeng JH, Lee E, Lee DH, Yan SG. Rabbit gastric ulcer models: Comparison and evaluation of acetic acid-induced ulcer and mucosectomy-induced ulcer. Lab Anim Res 2013;29(2):96-102.
39. Qin Z, Chen C. Synergistic action of famotidine and chlorpheniramine on acetic acid induced chronic gastric ulcer in rats. World J Gastroenterol 2005;11(45):7203-7.
40. Ajeigbe KO, Olaleye SB, Oladejo EO, Olayanju AO. Effect of folic acid supplementation on oxidative gastric mucosa damage and acid secretory response in the rat. Indian J Pharmacol 2011;43(5): 578-81.
41. Lau HK, Ogle CW. The influence of cimetidine, a histamine H2-receptor antagonist, on the gastric effects of reserpine in rats. Eur J Pharmacol 1981;70:139-48.
42. Kim KS, Shore PA. Mechanism of action of reserpine and insulin on gastric amines and gastric acid secretion and the effect of monoamine oxidase inhibition. J Pharmacol Exp Ther 1963;141:321-5.
43. Pfeiffer CJ, Cho CH, Cheema A, Saltman D. Reserpine induced gastric ulcers: Protection by lysosomal stabilization due to zinc. Eur J Pharmacol 1980;61(4):347-53.
44. Selye H, Szabo S. Experimental model for production of perforating duodenal ulcers by cysteamine in the rat. Nature 1973;244:458-9.
45. Szabo S. Animal model of human disease. Duodenal ulcer disease : Cysteamine induced acute and chronic duodenal ulcer in the rat. Am J Pathol 1978;73(1):273-76.
46. Del Soldato P, Ghiorzi A, Cereda E, et al. Cimetidine, ranitidine and mifentidine in specific gastric and duodenal ulcer models. Pharmacology 1985;30:45-51.
47. Okabe S, Ishihara Y, Inoo H, et al. Mepirizole-induced duodenal ulcers in rats and their pathogenesis. Dig Dis Sci 1982;27:242-9.
48. Ishihara Y, Okabe S. Effects of antiulcer agents on healing of mepirizole-induced duodenal ulcers in rats. Digestion 1983;27:29-35.
49. Ueshima K, Takeuchi K, Ohuchi T, Okabe S. Acid secretory and duodenal ulcerogenic responses induced by mepirizole in anaetetized rats. Digest Dis Sci 1994;39(8):1625-32.
50. Brzozowski T, Konturek PCh, Konturek SJ, et al. The role of melatonin and L-tryptophan in prevention of acute gastic lesions induced by stress, ethanol, ischemia and aspirin. J Pineal Res 1997;23:79-89.
51. Ueda S, Yoshikawa T, Takahashi S, et al. Role of free radical and lipid peroxidation in gastric mucosal injury induced by ischemia-reperfusion in rats. Scand J Gastroenterol Suppl 1989;162:55-8.
52. De La Lastra CA, Cabeza J, Motilva V, et al. Melatonin protects against gastric ischemia-reperfusion injury in rats. J Pineal Res 1997;23:47-52.
53. Wada K, Kamisaki Y, Kitano M, et al. Protective effect of cystathionine on acute gastric mucosal injury induced by ischemia-reperfusion in rats. Eur J Pharmacol 1995;294:377-82.

54. Hassan M, Kashimura H, Matsumaru K, et al. Gastric mucosal injury induced by local ischemia-reperfusion in rats. Role of endogenous endothelin-1 and free radicals. Dig Dis Sci 1997;42:1375-80.
55. Mojzis J, Hegedusova R, Mirossay L. Role of mucus in ischemia/reperfusion-induced gastric mucosal injury in rats. Physiol Res 2000;49:441-6.
56. Mandal RS, Das S. In silico approach towards identification of potential inhibitors of Helicobacter pylori DapE. J Biomol Struct Dyn 2014;9:1-14.

CHAPTER

36

Agents Affecting Gut Motility

INTRODUCTION

The change in absorptive, secretory and motor functions of the gut can undermine human well-being. Appropriate motility along the gut plays a significant role in the absorption of nutrients and water across the gastrointestinal tract. Drugs can stimulate or reduce intestinal motility and thus alter the transit time of compounds across intestine and thereby hinder or stimulate absorption. Following are some of the models most commonly employed to study the effect of drugs on intestinal motility.

IN VITRO MODELS

[^{125}I]CCK Receptor Binding Assay

Cholecystokinin (CCK) is an important hormone regulating gastric emptying, intestinal motility and biliary and pancreatic secretions. Dexloxiglumide, a CCK-A receptor antagonist, is in clinical development phase for the therapy of gastroparesis and constipation-dominant irritable bowel syndrome.

Procedure: [^{125}I]CCK receptor binding assay is performed using rat pancreatic membrane suspension.[1,2] The membrane suspension is incubated with 40 pM of [^{125}I]CCK in presence of buffer alone (for total binding) or in presence of CCK (for non specific binding) or in presence of test compound (for competitive assay) for 40 min at 25°C. Subsequently, ice cold buffer supplemented with 0.5% bovine serum albumin, in microcentrifuge tubes, is layered with the incubated mixture and centrifuged for 5 min at 10,000 g. Radioactivity is determined in γ–scintillation counter.

Evaluation: Specific binding, i.e. radioactivity that can be displaced by a high concentration of unlabelled CCK is calculated by taking difference between the total binding and nonspecific binding. IC_{50} value is further calculated by computer-derived linear regression analysis.

[^{3}H]GR-113808 Binding Assay for 5-HT_4 Receptors

5-HT is one of the major transmitters affecting gut motility. It acts via 5-HT_4 receptors to stimulate gut motility. Thus, 5-HT_4 agonists will have motility stimulating activity in the gastrointestinal (GIT). Tegaserod, a partial agonist at 5-HT_4 receptors, is approved for use in constipation-dominant irritable bowel syndrome. Prokinetic drugs like cisapride, mosapride and metoclopramide act as agonists at these receptors. GR-113808 is a 5-HT_4 receptor antagonist used for radioligand studies.

Procedure: Guinea pig striatal or hippocampal brain tissue homogenates are obtained as described by Grossman et al.[3] For binding and competition studies, 400 μl of [^{3}H]GR-113808 in HEPES buffer is incubated for 30 min at 37°C in presence of either buffer alone (for total binding) or 5-HT (for non-specific binding) or the test compound. Reaction is terminated by rapid vacuum filtration and washing with ice-cold buffer. Radioactivity is counted by scintillation counter after placing the filters in scintillation cocktail overnight.

Evaluation: Specific binding (total binding minus non-specific binding) and IC_{50} are calculated.

[^{3}H]Zacopride Binding Assay for 5-HT_3 Receptors

5-HT, acting via 5-HT_3 receptors, contributes to relaxation of gut. Thus 5-HT_3 antagonistic activity can stimulate the gut motility. Cisapride, a prokinetic drug, has weak 5-HT_3 antagonistic activity in addition to its 5-HT_4 agonistic activity. Zacopride is a 5-HT_3 receptor antagonist used for radioligand binding studies.

Procedure: Assays are performed using homogenates of tissue from entorhinal cortex of male Hooded-Lister rats.[4] For binding studies, 50 μl of [^{3}H]zacopride is incubated in presence of buffer alone for 20 min at 37°C (for total binding) or in presence of 5HT (for non-specific binding) or test compound for 15 min at 37°C. Reaction is terminated by rapid filtration and the filters are washed with ice-cold buffer. Radioactivity is quantified by liquid scintillation counting.

Evaluation: Specific binding (total binding minus non-specific binding) and IC_{50} are determined.

Guinea Pig Ileum

Magnus for the first time described this method.[5] It is one of the most commonly used models to study the effect of drugs on gut motility, like screening of drugs for spasmolytic activity. Other parts of the gut, such as duodenum and colon, can also be used as isolated preparations for gut motility studies.

Procedure: Guinea pigs of either sex are used for the experiment. The animal is sacrificed by stunning. The abdomen is cut opened. After tying a ligature around the intestine just distal to the pylorus, the intestine is cut above the ligature and carefully dissected free up to colon after cutting the mesentery. The intestine is severed near the ileocolic junction. Now, a nick is made in the intestine near the cord at the upper end. A glass tube is inserted through the cut and the intestine is flushed thoroughly with Tyrode's solution until the solution coming out of the other end is clear. The intestine, preferably the lower part (more sensitive), is cut into 2.5-3.0 cm long pieces and kept in Tyrode's solution. A piece of intestine is selected and suspended in an organ bath containing Tyrode's solution, under a preload of 1 g and aerated with 95% O_2 and 5% CO_2 at 37°C. After a 30 min incubation period, concentration-response curve to the standard drug is obtained. Subsequently, the concentration-response curve of the test drug (agonist) or of the standard in the presence of test drug (antagonist) is established. The contractions can be recorded on a kymograph under a magnification of 5-10 times. Alternatively, the contractions can be recorded on a polygraph using isometric force transducer. Drugs acting as agonists or antagonists on various receptors like muscarinic, nicotinic, serotonergic, histaminergic, prostaglandin receptors as well as directly acting agents like $BaCl_2$ and papaverine can be assayed using guinea pig ileum. The agonists (acetylcholine, carbachol, histamine, $BaCl_2$, serotonin, PGE_2) and antagonists (atropine, scopolamine, papaverine) can be used as standards for the experiments.

Cascade Superfusion Technique

The technique was developed by Gaddum.[6] Using rat stomach strip, guinea pig ileum, guinea pig vas deferens and various other isolated tissues, Vane (1964) has extended the technique to multiple tissue superfusion for identification and assay of circulating hormones in the blood of animals.[7]

Procedure: Depending on the activity to be tested, tissues of various origins like guinea pig ileum and vas deferens, rat fundus, rat duodenum, rat colon, rat bladder, and rabbit stomach strip, etc. can be used for the cascade superfusion. Up to 5 tissues can be simultaneously used. The tissues are suspended one above the other, on plastic platforms attached to a vertical rectangular rod inside an organ bath consisting of double-wall glass container (20-25 cm in height and 7-8 cm inner diameter). The plastic platforms are placed in such a way that the effluent from the donor tissue above bathes the tissue below and so on. Depending on the tissue used, various physiological salt solutions can be used as superfusion fluid. The tissues are aerated with 95% O_2 and 5% CO_2. Warm water is circulated through the outer jacket of the organ bath to maintain a temperature of 38°C.

For recording, the threads from various organs, separated from each other by about 5 mm, are connected over isotonic levers to isometric tension transducers. The superfusate is passed down the cascade of tissues at uniform flow rate and tension from each tissue is recorded on a polygraph.

Isolated Rat Thoracic Esophageal Muscularis Mucosae

This method is useful for study of drugs acting on $5\text{-}HT_4$ receptors as this tissue is rich in these receptors.

Procedure: Sprague-Dawley rats, 180-300 g weight, are used. The animal is sacrificed and its esophagus removed. External muscularis propria is carefully separated from the tunica muscularis mucosae of lower 2 cm of esophagus. The tissue is suspended in organ bath containing Krebs' Henseleit solution, under an initial tension of 1g and aerated with 95% O_2 and 5% CO_2. The tissue is allowed to equilibrate at 37°C for 60 min. Tissue is washed every 15 min. After 60 min equilibration, 3 μM of carbachol is added to the organ bath for contracting the tissue and then a cumulative concentration-response curve to 5-HT is obtained. 5-HT will relax the precontracted tissue. Tissue is then washed and allowed 60 min recovery period. Subsequently, the antagonistic test compound is added for 45 min and again concentration-response curve is obtained or for agonist drug, a concentration-response curve to the agonist is obtained on the precontracted tissue. All responses are recorded isometrically.[8,9]

IN VIVO MODELS

Charcoal Passage Test

After administration of a test compound, the distance traveled by charcoal meal can be used to determine the effect of the compound on gut motility.

Procedure: Rats or mice can be used. The animals are fasted for 18 h, but with free access to water, before experiment. After varying time intervals of oral or subcutaneous administration of the test drug, the animals are administered a charcoal meal consisting of 10% charcoal powder, 5% gum Arabic with or without 1% carboxymethylcellulose suspension in distilled water. The dose of charcoal meal is 0.3 ml/mouse or 1 ml/100 g/rat. The animals are sacrificed by cervical dislocation or asphyxiation with CO_2 at various time intervals after the meal depending on the goal of study, e.g. for gastric emptying studies, the animals are sacrificed after 5 min while for intestinal transit, the animals can be sacrificed after 20, 40, 60 or 120 min. Immediately after sacrifice, the GI tract is removed and distance traveled by charcoal meal through the intestine is measured and expressed as percentage of total length of intestine from pylorus to cecum.[2,10-12]

In Vivo Evaluation of Spasmolytic Activity

To assess organ selectivity of spasmolytics, Maggi and Meli (1982) devised an *in vivo* procedure for determining the comparative potencies of spasmolytics against smooth muscle contractions induced by topically applied acetylcholine on rat colon, rectum and urinary bladder.[13]

Procedure: Male albino rats, weighing 350 to 400 g are used. After anesthetizing the animal, the left jugular vein is cannulated for injecting the test drugs. The abdomen is opened and colon and rectum isolated. Pocket-like spaces are made in them by applying occluding silk ligatures at a distance of 2 cm from each other; and into these spaces, flanged tips of polyethylene tubing (internal diameter 1 mm and outer diameter 1.5 mm) are inserted via a small incision. Similarly, a polyethylene tube is inserted into the urinary bladder via a small uretheral incision. The free ends of the tubes are connected to pressure transducer and the whole system is filled with saline. Warm saline, at 37°C, is filled into the organs so as to obtain a resting pressure of 4-12 mm of Hg and warm saline soaked cotton-wool swabs are used to maintain the temperature and moisture of the exteriorized organs. The organs are allowed to stabilize for 15 min and then concentration-response curve to acetylcholine is obtained by bathing the outer surface of organs with 0.5 ml of acetylcholine solution. After 3 or more comparable control curves are obtained at 10 min interval from each other, antagonist is injected intravenously and dose-response curve to acetylcholine obtained. ED_{50} values are calculated, and from them, DR_{10} values (dose of antagonist required to produce an acetylcholine dose ratio of 10) are calculated according to the method of Daly et al.[14]

Colonic Motility Studies in Rats

The anesthetized rat is used as one of the experimental models to study the influence of spasmolytic drugs on colon motility induced by carbachol. Bickel (1983) used this model to study the stimulant property of an enkephalin analogue pentapeptide.[15]

Procedure: Male Sprague-Dawley rats, weighing 350 to 500 g are used. The animals are fasted for 18 h with free access to water. After anesthetizing the animal, the abdomen is opened and a latex balloon inserted into colon ascendens and recording of intraluminal pressure changes done.[15] Duration and height of colonic contractions in response to carbachol in the absence or presence of the test drug are noted.

Gut Motility Studies in Dogs

This method includes the study of intraluminal pressure and motility of the small intestine in unanesthetized dogs with balloon catheter systems via a duodenal Mann-Bollman fistula.

Procedure: Male beagle dogs, weighing 15 to 20 kg, are used. After anesthetizing the animal, the abdomen is opened by a midline incision. Terminal ileum and the portion of the intestinal tract, where the fistula is desired, are exposed and carefully packed off. A 15-20 cm loop of ileum is isolated, clamped at both ends and cut so that the two cut ends are left in clamps. The remaining ileum is anastomosed end-to-end or side-to-side. Without stretching the mesentery of the isolated loop, it is anastomosed end-to-side with the intestine at the desired site of fistula. The free end of the loop is brought to the surface through a stab wound and sutured to the skin. The abdomen is closed in layers.[16,17]

Gut motility experiments are carried out in these animals after they have been fasted for 18 h. For measurement of intraluminal pressure of intestines, air filled latex balloons attached to air filled polyethylene catheters are placed in intestine through the fistula and filled with air at a pressure of 10 mm of Hg. Recording is done on a polygraph after connecting the catheters to a pressure transducer. Frequency and amplitude of pressure waves are recorded over 10 min and comparison of predrug and postdrug readings is made.

Gastrointestinal Motor Activity in Conscious Dogs

Beagle dogs of either sex, weighing 9-13 kg, are used. The animal is anesthetized and abdominal cavity is opened. Force transducers are implanted extraluminally in gastric antrum (3 cm proximal to pyloric antrum) and in colon (10 and 20 cm distal to the ileo-caecal valve). Through an incision between the scapulae, the lead wires are brought out at the back of animal and sutured to the skin. A 6.5 F catheter is placed in superior vena cava of the animal (for intravenous injection of drugs) and the outer end sutured to the skin. The animal is covered with a protective jacket and allowed to recover for 2 weeks. For gut motility experiments, the test drug is given intravenously, 2-3 hr after food and GI motor activity recorded by connecting lead wires to polygraph system. Motor index is calculated from the amplitude of contraction and the time for which the contraction remains in an area over a fixed time period (30 min period is taken). Motor index with and without the drug are compared.[9,18]

REFERENCES

1. Steigerwalt RW, Williams JA. Characterization of cholecystokinin receptors on rat pancreatic membranes. Endocrinology 1981;109:1746-53.
2. Gully D, Frehel D, Marcy C, et al. Peripheral biological activity of SR 27897: a new potent non-peptide antagonist of CCKA receptors. Eur J Pharmacol 1993;232:13-9.
3. Grossman CJ, Kilpatrick GJ, Bunce KT. Development of a radioligand binding assay for 5HT4 receptors in guinea-pig and rat brain. Br J Pharmacol 1993;109:618-29.
4. Barnes NM, Costall B, Naylor J. [3H]zacopride: ligand for the identification of 5HT3 recognition sites. J Pharm Pharmacol 1988;40:548-51.
5. Magnus R. Versuche am uberlebenden Dunndarm von Saugethieren. Pflugers Arch 1904;102:123-51.
6. Gaddum JH. The technique of superfusion. Br J Pharmacol 1953;8:321-6.
7. Vane JR. The use of isolated organs for detecting active substances in the circulating blood. Br J Pharmacol 1964;23:360-73.
8. Baxter GS, Craig DA, Clarke D. 5-Hydroxytryptamine4 receptors mediate relaxation of the rat oesophageal tunica muscularis mucosae. Naunyn-Schmiedeberg's Arch Pharmacol 1991;343:439-46.
9. Mine Y, Yoshikawa T, Oku S, et al. Comparison of effect of mosapride citrate and existing 5-HT4 agonists on gastrointestinal motility in vivo and in vitro. J Pharmacol Exp Ther 1997;283:1000-08.
10. Vischer P, Casals-stenzel J Influence of prostacyclin and indomethacin on castor oil-induced gastrointestinal effects in rats. J Pharm Pharmacol 1983;35:152-6.
11. Mascolo N, Izzo AA, Barbato F, et al. Inhibitors of nitric oxide synthetase prevent castor oil-induced diarrhea in the rat. Br J Pharmacol 1993;108:861-4.
12. Izzo AA, Mascolo N, Pinto L, et al. The role of cannabinoid receptors in intestinal motility, defaecation and diarrhea in rats. Eur J Pharmacol 1999;384:37-42.
13. Maggi CA, Meli A. An in vivo procedure for estimating spasmolytic activity in the rat by measuring smooth muscle contractions to topically applied acetylcholine. J Pharmacol Methods 1982;8:39-46.
14. Daly MJ, Flook JJ, Levy GP. The selectivity of β-adrenoceptor antagonists on cardiovascular and bronchodilator responses to isoprenaline in the anaesthetized dog. Br J Pharmacol 1975;53:173-81.
15. Bickel M. Stimulation of colonic motility in dogs and rats by an enkephalin analogue pentapeptide. Life Sci 1983; 33:469-72.
16. Tasaka K, Farrar JT. Intraluminal pressure of the small intestine of the unanaesthetized dog. Pflugers Arch 1976;364:35-44.
17. Mann FC, Bollman JL. A method for making a satisfactory fistula at any level of the gastrointestinal tract. Ann Surg 1931;93:794-7.
18. Itoh Z, Honda R, Takeuchi S, et al. An extraluminal force transducer for recording contractile activity of the gastrointestinal smooth muscle in conscious dogs: Its construction and implantation. Gastroenterol Jpn 1977;12:275-83.

CHAPTER

37

Antiemetic Agents

INTRODUCTION

Nausea and vomiting are amongst the most common and distressing symptoms observed in a variety of conditions such as pregnancy, peptic ulcer, gastrointestinal infections, gastrointestinal obstruction, renal disorders, hepatitis, motion sickness, following anesthesia and surgery and as adverse effect of treatment with a wide range of drugs especially the cancer chemotherapeutic agents. Nausea and vomiting are also an important component of defense mechanism of the body against accidental ingestion of toxins. Nausea is a nonobservable subjective feeling of having an urge to vomit. The unpleasant sensation is experienced at the back of throat and epigastrium that may or may not culminate into emesis.[1] The emesis consists of retching and vomiting. The retching is characterized by attempt to vomit without expulsion of the contents of upper gastrointestinal tract. During retching muscles of diaphragm and abdomen contract and relax simultaneously. The vomiting consists of more sustained abdominal contraction in coordination with intercostal muscles and muscles of larynx and pharynx. The glottis is closed, the soft palate elevated, the gastric fundus relaxes and contents of stomach, both solid and liquid, are forcefully expelled out through the nose or mouth. The occurrence and frequency of retching and vomiting can be measured objectively.

Acute emesis usually occurs within a few minutes to several hours of exposure to emetogen. It usually resolves within 24 h. Emesis that occurs before the person receives the emetic stimuli such as the cancer chemotherapy is known as the anticipatory emesis. It is a conditioned response due to negative past experiences. Emesis occurring despite the prophylactic antiemetic treatment and requiring rescue antiemetic therapy is known as the breakthrough emesis. Delayed emesis is observed more than 24 h after the institution of cancer chemotherapy. It usually peaks at 48-72 h and can continue for 6-7 days.

Integration of the complex interplay of physiological events ultimately leading to emesis takes place in the vomiting center located in medulla oblongata. Output neurons that control the muscles involved in emesis are scattered throughout the medulla oblongata. Afferent inputs to the vomiting center originate from four sources that include (Fig. 37.1):

1. Cerebrocortical pathways, stimulated by learned associations.
2. Chemoreceptor trigger zone (CTZ) in area postrema of cortex, stimulated by chemical stimuli from blood and cerebrospinal fluid.
3. Vestibular pathway, stimulated by positional changes of the body.
4. Peripheral pathways, stimulated by neurotransmitter receptors in gastrointestinal tract.

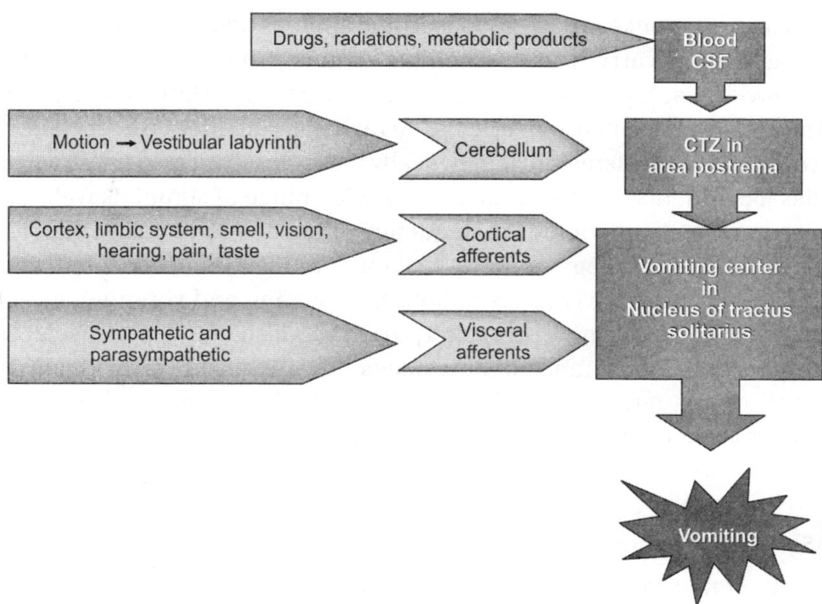

Figure 37.1: Pathophysiology of nausea and vomiting

To further elaborate the understanding of the pathways involved in generation of the sensation of nausea and reflex vomiting, to identify pharmacological approaches for development of new antiemetics and to understand the underlying problems in diseases with nausea and vomiting as the cardinal features, use of appropriate animal models is required.

IN VIVO MODELS

Choice of Animal Models

Animals

For research in nausea, emesis and antiemetics, selection of appropriate animal species is extremely important. In general, the vomiting reflex, although not essential for survival, is an important defense mechanism, which helps body to get rid of ingested toxins. Many animal species used in laboratory research such as rat, mouse, rabbit, guinea pig and hamster appear to lack the vomiting reflex as is seen in human. There are isolated reports suggesting presence of a degenerate vomiting reflex in rodents[2,3] and presence of a neophobic character to avoid ingestion of toxins.[4] Vomiting reflex is present in other mammalian species such as dogs, monkey, cat, ferret, pigs and vertebrates like birds, reptiles, fishes and amphibians.[5-9] However, it should be noted that all species with vomiting reflex are not sensitive to all emetic stimuli and function of vomiting reflex in some species is to get rid of undigested material and not the defense against the toxins.

Animal species commonly used to evaluate antiemetic activity of test drugs include dogs, cat, monkeys, ferret, house musk shrew (*Suncus murinus*), least shrew (*Cryptotis parva*), gerbils and pigeons. Rodents do not possess the emetic reflex, however exposure to emetic stimuli can lead to significant increase in the intake of non-food substances, a response known as pica. Dogs, cats and monkeys have good learning abilities and therefore cannot be used for repeated testing. Pigeons carry viruses infectious to human and therefore they are not widely used. Ferret is a widely accepted animal model and the emesis in ferret closely resembles that in human. The disadvantage in using ferret is the high maintenance cost. The *Suncus murinus* is an insectivore and is considered phylogenetically more closely related to primates than other animal species like rodents. Emetic response to a wide range of stimuli is well-known in this animal species however, sometimes the frequency of retches can be very high as compared to other species such as cat, dog and ferret making it difficult to observe individual retches. Therefore, the emetic response consists of both the retching and vomiting and is measured as emetic episodes. The least shrew (*Cryptotis parva*) was also found to be useful as it showed the emetic response to a wide range of emetogens.[10,11] Animals are individually housed and maintained in standard environmental conditions with free access to food and water. The observation cages are kept in a quite room. A wide range of emetogens can be used to evaluate antiemetic properties of test drugs.

Emetogens

The commonly employed emetic stimuli in animals include drugs such as cancer chemotherapeutic drugs like cisplatin and methotrexate, apomorphine and copper sulfate. The cancer chemotherapeutic drugs act by directly stimulating the enterochromaffin cells in small intestinal mucosa to secrete serotonin. Serotonin is thought to stimulate vagal afferent fibers through 5-HT_3 receptors located at the vagal afferent terminals. Sensory signals reach the area postrema to initiate nausea and emesis. Apomorphine is a derivative of morphine and induces vomiting by stimulating central dopamine receptors. Copper sulfate is an irritant to gastrointestinal mucosa and its oral administration initiates emesis by stimulating the vagal afferents. Other drugs used as emetogens include cyclophosphamide, doxorubicin, morphine, nicotine, etc.

Other useful emetogens used in experimental studies include motion stimulus, which induces emesis through vestibular pathways and radiations acting through early peripheral and late central serotonergic pathways.

Parameters

Emetic episodes are easy to study and can be overtly measured in laboratory animals showing vomiting reflex. Observations are made for latency to first retching and vomiting and number of vomiting episodes are counted for each animal. An interval of at least 1 min is needed to separate one emetic episode from the next. Episodes of retching and vomiting are considered separate when animal changes position in the observation cage or when the interval between the retches and/or vomiting is more than 5 seconds. Exposure to emetogens can also induce behavioral changes in animals, which are considered analogous to nausea. These behavioral changes include increases in the incidence of swallowing, lip licking, backward walking, burrowing, curling up, rearing or decreases in locomotor activity. It is considered relatively straightforward to assess if a compound has an activity to reduce retching and vomiting, but more problematic to determine a reduction of nausea, since animals are unable to communicate directly their emotional status.

Animals with absent vomiting reflex such as rats are also used to study behaviors associated with nausea and vomiting. These specific behaviors include conditioned flavor avoidance (CFA) or pica. Mitchell et al (1976, 1977) suggested that pica, i.e. eating of nonnutritive substances such as kaolin, is an illness-response behavior in rats.[12,13] These behavior responses are often measured as indicators of emesis in rats. Kaolin is prepared using the pharmacological grade kaolin (or hydrated aluminum silicate) and acacia mixed in a ratio of 99:1. A thick paste is prepared by mixing with distilled water. The paste is rolled and cut into pieces resembling regular rat chow pellets, which are then dried at room temperature for 72 h.[14] Rats expressing pica behavior show increase in the wet weight of stomach, which can be measured at the end of the experiment. An incision is made proximal to the gastroesophageal junction and distal to the pyloric sphincter to isolate the stomach. After isolation, the stomach is blotted dry, and the wet weight is recorded.[15]

Emesis is associated with delayed gastric emptying due to reduced gastric motility. Increase in the rate of gastric emptying in response to administration of test drugs may also indicate their antiemetic efficacy.[16] To determine the rate of gastric emptying, 200-250 g rats are orally administered with a 1.5 ml of test meal consisting of 0.05% phenol red in a 1.5% aqueous methylcellulose solution. Rats are sacrificed 45 min after the meal. Stomach is removed and homogenized in 100 mL of NaOH 0.1 M. Stomach tissue proteins are precipitated with 20% trichloroacetic acid (0.5 ml of trichloroacetic acid in 5 ml homogenate) and centrifuged. The supernatant is mixed with 4 ml of NaOH 0.5 M and absorbance of the sample is read at a wavelength of 560 nm. Phenol red recovered from the stomach of rats sacrificed immediately after administration of methylcellulose meal serves as standard. The percentage gastric emptying of each rat is calculated as follows:

$$\text{Gastric emptying (\%)} = 1\text{-}C_{\text{phenol red (test stomach)}}/C_{\text{phenol red (standard stomach)}} \times 100$$

Drug-induced Emesis Models

Cisplatin-induced Emesis Model

Cancer chemotherapy based on cisplatinum is known to be associated with the adverse effects of nausea and vomiting. Emesis occurring within first 24 h of the institution of therapy is the early phase acute vomiting and can be effectively antagonized by 5-HT_3 receptor antagonists. The emesis occurring 24-120 h after the start of therapy is delayed emesis and does not respond well to 5-HT_3 receptor antagonists.[17,18] Cisplatin is popularly used as an emetogen in animal models to evaluate antiemetic drugs especially for early phase emesis and is usually prepared in normal saline at 70°C followed by slow cooling to 40°C. Dogs are most sensitive to cisplatin followed by ferret, cat and *Suncus murinus*.

Cisplatin-induced Dog Model

Cisplatin-induced emesis in dogs has previously been described by Gylys et al. (1979)[19] and can be used to evaluate antiemetic properties of 5-HT_3 receptor antagonists. Animals are divided into test and control groups. Test group receives the test drug and control group receives the vehicle. Ten minutes later cisplatin is administered intravenously at a dose of 3.2 mg/kg/ml. Animals are then observed continuously for next 5 h for emetic episodes. Dogs with no obvious toxicity are retested after an interval of 4 weeks.

Cisplatin-induced Cat Model

John et al. (2000) have described the use of Cisplatin-induced cat model.[20] Cats of either sex weighing 2-6 kg are used. On the day of experiment animals are fed with 200 g of cat food. Light anesthesia is administered using 5% halothane. A cannula is then inserted into the cephalic vein through which cisplatin (3-7.5 mg/kg) is infused slowly over a period of 4 min. Cisplatin administration is immediately followed by administration of drug/vehicle. Cannula can now be removed and animals transferred back to cages for observation of emesis as in case of dogs. A video-monitoring system can also be used to monitor behavioral changes during prolonged observation period if drug is being tested for effects on delayed emesis.

Cisplatin-induced Ferret Model

Ferrets weighing 1-1.5 kg are used. After overnight fasting each ferret is administered simultaneously with the test drug/vehicle and cisplatin (10 mg/kg) intravenously. If the test drug is administered orally, cisplatin can be administered 30 minutes after the test drug administration. Following cisplatin administration the animals are observed for emesis for next four hours.[21]

Cisplatin-induced Pigeon Model

Adult pigeons weighing 350-550 g are used. Cisplatin 4 mg/kg is administered intravenously via the brachial wing vein. Test drug/vehicle is administered prior to cisplatin administration and time interval between the drug and cisplatin administration depends upon the expected time required for the drug to act. Following cisplatin administration animals are kept under observation for emesis.[22]

Cisplatin-induced Suncus murinus Model

Adult *Suncus murinus* of either sex weighing 30-80 g are maintained under standard laboratory conditions are allowed to acclimatize in transparent cages to make the observations easier. Test drug/vehicle is administered usually by subcutaneous route and 30 min later the emetic stimulus cisplatin (20 mg/kg) is administered intraperitoneally. Animals are individually observed for next two hours for the behavioral effects to characterize nausea status, latency to emetic episodes and frequency of emesis.[23]

Cisplatin-induced Rat Model

Administration of cisplatin in rats induces significant kaolin intake, which can be used as the measure analogous to emesis in other species. Rats pretreated with drug/vehicle are administered with cisplatin (3-10 mg/kg, intraperitoneal) 30 minutes later. Kaolin intake, food intake, and body weight were measured every 24 h for 120 h.[24]

Methotrexate-induced Delayed Emesis Model

Cisplatin induced emesis in animals may fail to demonstrate delayed emesis, which occurs 24 h after the start of chemotherapy. To evaluate the antiemetic activity against delayed emesis during chemotherapy, methotrexate (MTX) is a useful emetogen.[25] It can be used in dogs, cats, ferrets and *Suncus murinus*. MTX is prepared by dissolving in 5% dextrose. Test drug/vehicle is administered at 24, 36, 48 and 60 after MTX. Animals are kept under observation soon after MTX administration till 72 h. It is preferable to use a video camera with automatic night photographic system so as to provide with a continuous record of animal behavior for 72 h post MTX treatment. Animals can be retested with MTX at least 6 weeks later.

Apomorphine-induced Emesis Model

Apomorphine is an opiate that acts as a potent central dopamine agonist directly at the area postrema via dopamine receptors.[26,27] As the vestibular pathways are also involved in apomorphine-induced emesis the active animals develop emesis readily as compared to animals that are sedate and motionless. Dogs are the most sensitive to apomorphine followed by ferret while *Suncus murinus* is unresponsive. Use of apomorphine in cat is controversial as the administration of apomorphine can cause excitation in cats.

Apomorphine-induced Dog Model

Dogs are very sensitive to emetic response to apomorphine. Apomorphine hydrochloride is prepared as solution in saline. Each animal receives the test drug/vehicle subcutaneously or orally. Apomorphine is administered at a dose of 0.3 mg/kg subcutaneously. The interval between the administration of drug and emetogen can be modified depending upon the expected time required for drug action.[20] Subsequently, animals are observed for emetic episodes.

Apomorphine-induced Ferret Model

Ferrets have been used successfully to evaluate antiemetic drugs against apomorphine-induced emesis. Animals are allowed to habituate in the observation cages 2 h every day for 4-5 days. On the day of experiment the animals are kept in the observation boxes for at least 30 min prior to the start of experiment. Animals are then administered with the test drug/vehicle and 30 min later apomorphine hydrochloride (0.25 mg/kg) is injected subcutaneously. The animals are now observed for further 60 min for behavioral changes as well as emetic episodes.[28]

Apomorphine-induced Rat Model

Administration of apomorphine in rats induces pica (ingestion of non-food substances e.g. kaolin). The antiemetic activity of test drug can be determined by observing this behavior in animals (pretreated with drug/vehicle) before and after challenge with apomorphine (10 mg/kg, intraperitoneal).[29]

Copper Sulfate-induced Emesis Model

Copper sulfate is a powerful oxidizing agent and an irritant to mucous membranes. If administered orally causes irritation of gastric mucous membrane and leads to nausea and vomiting. It has conveniently being used as an emetogen in experimental studies.

Copper Sulfate-induced Dog Model

After overnight fasting dogs receive the test drug or the vehicle depending upon the group they belong to. Copper sulfate solution prepared by dissolving copper sulfate pentahydrate in distilled water is rapidly administered at a dose of 100 mg/kg through an orogastric tube. Animals are observed for next one hour for episodes of emesis and those showing no toxicity can be retested two weeks later.[30]

Copper Sulfate-induced Cat Model

Evaluation of antiemetics can be done in adult cats after administering copper sulfate in a dose of 40 mg/kg orally. Alternatively, the threshold dose is determined by once a week administration of copper sulfate orally in a dose of 20, 30 and 40 mg/head. The cats with a threshold of more than 40 mg or latency of less than 5 min or of more than 45 min should be excluded. Cats included in the experiment are administered with the test drug/vehicle followed by oral administration of the threshold dose of copper sulfate. The efficacy of test drug can now be evaluated by observations for the emetic episodes.[31]

Copper Sulfate-induced Ferret Model

Copper sulfate-induced emesis can also be induced in ferrets. After overnight fasting and pretreatment with drug/vehicle ferrets are administered with the solution of copper sulfate 40 mg/kg orally. Subsequently, animals are observed for latency and frequency of emetic episodes.[32]

Copper Sulfate-induced Suncus murinus Model

Suncus murinus can also be used to investigate antiemetic effects against copper sulfate induced emesis. Copper sulfate is administered 40 mg/kg (intragastric) 30 min after the administration of test drug/vehicle. The animal is observed for further 60 min for emetic episode.[23]

Copper Sulfate-induced Chick Model

Antiemetic activity of experimental drugs may also be evaluated using chick emesis model. 4-day old chicks are administered with experimental drug or vehicle orally. Subsequently, after 10 min, copper sulfate is administered orally at a dose of 50 mg/kg body weight and animals are observed for latency and frequency of emetic episodes.[33]

Motion-induced Emesis Model

Dog is probably as sensitive to motion-induced emesis as man. Motion-induced emesis can also be established in cats, *Suncus murinus* and rats.

Motion-induced Cat Model

Cats weighing 1.5-3 kg are placed in a Plexiglas chamber on a circular platform having holes at the base so as to reduce air resistance during oscillations. Chambers are suspended from the ceiling by springs. A gentle push is applied to initiate and maintain the vertical oscillations at ~0.3 Hz through a distance of ~75 cm. The motion sickness is characterized by repetitive licking, salivation often dripping out of the mouth, or vomiting. The increased latency and/or decreased frequency of motion-induced emesis in cats pretreated with the test drug indicates antiemetic property of the test drug.[34]

Motion-induced Suncus murinus Model

Suncus murinus after receiving the test drug/vehicle are placed individually in transparent cages, which are then kept on a reciprocal shaker. This is followed by a period of 5 min for acclimatization. Shaker is then started to give a horizontal oscillation of 4 cm at a frequency of 1 Hz for 10 min. The emetic episodes are noted during motion as well as after the motion ceases. Individual animals can be exposed only twice at an interval of 1 week as more exposures lead to adaptation to motion stimulus.[35]

Motion-induced Rat Model

In rats, 60 min double rotation can induce increased kaolin intake indicating motion-induced emesis. Pretreatment with the test drug if found to decrease the kaolin intake, indicates antiemetic activity of the test drug.[29]

Radiation-induced Emesis Model

Ferrets are most sensitive to radiations followed by dogs. Cats are considerably resistant to radiations.

Radiation-induced Dog Model

A radiation-induced emesis can be induced in dogs by using ^{60}Co and 8 Gy administered to total body surface. An irradiated control group is established which is given no medication or vehicle while the other similarly irradiated groups receive the test drug. Latency to retching/vomiting and number of vomiting episodes are observed in each animal and a comparison can be made to evaluate efficacy of the antiemetic drug. Alternatively, drug/vehicle pretreated dogs are exposed to 8 Gy ^{60}Co gamma mid-abdominal irradiation. Subsequently, animals are observed for latency and frequency of emetic episodes in two groups.[36]

Radiation-induced Ferret Model

The radiation-induced model can also be induced in ferret. The ferrets are irrradiated with bilateral ^{60}Co gamma radiation at 201 cGy. An emesis incidence of 100% is reported at 201 cGy in ferret.[37] Increased latency and/or reduced frequency of emetic episodes indicates antiemetic property of test drug.

Radiation-induced Rat Model

Exposure to radiation can induce pica in rats. Pica is a behavior characterized by ingestion of non-nutritive substances such as kaolin and can be used as an index of radiation-induced vomiting. Rats pretreated with drug/vehicle are exposed to 4 Gy of total-body irradiation. The 4 Gy of abdominal irradiation is reported to be more effective to induce pica than that of head irradiation.[38] Inhibition of kaolin intake in drug treated group as compared to control is considered a measure of antiemetic properties of test drug.

Suncus murinus Model for Anticipatory Nausea and Vomiting

Anticipatory nausea and vomiting, often associated with cancer chemotherapy, is described as the conditioned response to cues present at the time of exposure to toxins as a result of pairing. Conditioned retching in *Suncus murinus* was found to provide an effective model to evaluate efficacy of drugs against anticipatory nausea and vomiting by Parker et al. 2006.[39] The emetic stimuli, which can be effectively used in this model, include horizontal motion (1 Hz, 4 cm, 10 min), nicotine, 4 mg/kg sc and lithium chloride 100 mg/kg ip.

Shrews of either sex weighing 20-50 g are used. All animals included in the study are weaned at the age of 20 days. They are individually housed and maintained under standard laboratory conditions. Animals are housed in transparent cages with a mirror fitted at the bottom so as to allow the observation of the ventral surface of the shrews. Observation chambers are kept in a well-illuminated room with a video camera fitted to record the activities of shrews. Animals are then divided into test and control groups. All animals now receive three conditioning trials 72 h apart. Within each group (study, control) half the animals receive of lithium chloride while the other half will receive the vehicle intraperitoneally just before they are put in the observation chambers. The episodes of vomiting and retching are observed over next 45 minutes. Lithium treated animals develop retching and vomiting during these conditioning trials. Six days after completing the three conditioning trials the animals receive two test trials 72 hours apart. On the day of trial the animals are first injected with the test drug/vehicle and returned to their home cages. Thirty minutes later all animals are injected with 60 ml/kg of physiological saline just before putting them in observation chambers. The shrews are then observed and behavior is video recorded for next 45 minutes. Finally four groups of animals i.e. test drug-lithium conditioned, test drug-saline conditioned, vehicle-lithium conditioned and vehicle-saline conditioned are compared to evaluate efficacy of test drug. The shrews display conditioned retching upon exposure to a context associated with drug-induced vomiting in vehicle treated lithium conditioned group.[40] The frequency of retching can be more than that during the last conditioning trial. Decreased frequency of retching episodes in drug treated lithium conditioned group indicates efficacy of drug against anticipatory vomiting. The cannabinoids have been found to be effective against anticipatory nausea and vomiting however, 5-HT_3 antagonists are not as effective.

Rat Model for Anticipatory Nausea and Vomiting

Effectiveness of the test drugs against anticipatory nausea and vomiting can also be evaluated in rats.[41] The animals undergo 4 conditioning trials 72 h apart as described for *Suncus murinus*. Seventy two hours after 4th conditioning trial, all rats are surgically implanted with intraoral cannulae. For implantation of cannulae, first a thin-walled 15-gauge stainless steel needle is inserted at the back of the neck, directed subcutaneously around the ear and is brought out behind the first molar inside the mouth. A length of thin plastic tubing with an inner diameter of 0.86 mm and an outer diameter of 1.27 mm is then passed through the needle and then the needle is removed. Two circular elastic discs are placed over the tubing and drawn to the exposed skin at the back of the neck to stabilize the cannulae. The tubing is secured in the oral cavity by a ring, which is sealed behind the tubing prior to cannulation surgery. This indwelling cannulae is connected with an infusion pump through a plastic tube for delivery of 0.1% saccharin solution. Cannulae are flushed daily with chlorhexidine solution to prevent infection.

All animals are subjected to test trials after receiving drug/vehicle as described for *Suncus murinus*, 72 h after implantation of cannulae. During the 30 min trial in observation chamber, rats receive an intraoral infusion of 0.1% saccharin solution every 5 min for 1 min (at a rate of 1 ml/min), resulting in a total of 6 infusions in 30 min. During the intraoral infusions, the rat's somatic and orofacial responses are video-recorded. Grading is done for gaping, rearing and active locomotion. Gaping is rapid, large-amplitude opening of the mandible expressed while rats are infused with 0.1% saccharin. Frequency of gaping is recorded separately for the duration of saccharine infusion (6 min) and for inter-infusion interval (24 min). The rearing activity is obtained by recording the frequency when both front forepaws of rat are lifted off the floor and not touch the wall of the chamber. An overall activity duration score is obtained by summing the frequency of instances of forward locomotion i.e. movement of the rat's forepaws along the floor of the chamber. These scores are converted to an activity/min score and a comparison is made among groups.

Rats display the characteristic response of gaping when intraorally infused with a flavor previously paired with lithium chloride. The gaping response of the taste reactivity test appears to be a selective marker of nausea in rats. Only drugs that produce emesis in species capable of vomiting produce conditioned gaping.

IN VITRO MODELS

The *in vitro* models can be used to demonstrate the pharmacological activity of the newer drugs indicating their potential use as antiemetics. A large number of antiemetics belonging to different classes of drugs are in therapeutic use. These include selective H-1 receptor antagonists, anticholinergics, antidopaminergics, corticosteroids and cannabinoids. Among all, 5-HT_3 receptor antagonists are considered potent antiemetics. The experimental drugs with possible antiemetic activity can be evaluated for 5-HT_3 receptor antagonist activity using *in vitro* methods.

5-HT_3-Receptor Antagonists

Selective 5-HT_3 receptor antagonists such as ondansetron are extremely potent antiemetics especially in the treatment of emesis associated with cancer chemotherapy. The possible 5-HT_3 receptor antagonist activity indicative of antiemetic activity can be evaluated using isolated guinea pig colon preparation.

Male guinea pig is killed by blow on the head, abdomen opened and distal part of colon is removed and placed in a dish containing Krebs-Henseleit solution (pH 7.3–7.5) consisting of NaCl 118 mM, KCl 4.7 mM, $CaCl_2$ 2.5 mM, KH_2PO_4 1.2 mM, $NaHCO_3$ 25 mM, $MgSO_4$ 1.2 mM and glucose 10 mM. A 20 mm piece of colon (in relaxed condition) is washed with Krebs-Henseleit solution. The piece of colon is now suspended in 10 ml organ bath containing Krebs-Henseleit solution at 37°C and bubbled through with oxygen/carbon dioxide (95% O_2 + 5% CO_2). The preparation is fixed with an isotonic transducer loaded with 1-gram weight. After 60 min to achieve equilibrium, a selective 5-HT_3 receptor agonist 2-methyl-5-HT (initial concentration10^{-5} M) is used to elicit the concentration-response curve. The preparation is washed with bath solution every 5 min until the baseline is achieved. The test compound is now pipetted into the organ bath and 30 min time is allowed to equilibrate before challenging with the agonist again. Selective 5-HT_3 receptor antagonist competitively inhibits the contractile responses to 2-methyl-5-HT or it can enhance the inhibitory activity of another selective 5-HT_3 antagonist like tropisetron (0.1 mmol.l^{-1}). 5-HT_3 receptor antagonist will fail to affect the contractile response evoked by acetylcholine receptor agonist carbachol (1 mmol/l^{-1}).[42]

REFERENCES

1. Rhodes VA, Watson PM, Johnson MH. Development of reliable and valid measures of nausea and vomiting. Cancer Nurs 1984;7:33-41.
2. Andrew BL, The nervous control of the cervical oesophagus of the rat during swallowing. J Physiol 1956;134:729-40.
3. Furukawa T, Yamada K. The alpha-naphthoxyacetic acid-elicited retching involves dopaminergic inhibition in mice. Pharmacol Biochem Behav 1980;12:735-8.
4. Mitchell D. Experiments on neophobia in wild and laboratory rats: a revaluation. J Comp Physiol Psychol 1976;90:190-7.
5. Andrews PL, Davis CJ, Bingham S, Davidson HI, Hawthorn J, Maskell L. The abdominal visceral innervation and the emetic reflex: pathways, pharmacology, and plasticity. Can J Physiol Pharm 1990;68:325-45.
6. Andrews PL, Axelsson M, Franklin C, Holmgren S. The emetic reflex in a reptile (Crocodylus porosus). J Exp Biol 2000;203:1625-32.
7. King GL. Animal models in the study of vomiting. Can J Physiol Pharm 1990;68:260-8.
8. Sims DW, Andrews PL, Young JZ. Stomach rinsing in rays. Nature 2000;404:566.
9. Tanihata S, Oda S, Nakai S, Uchiyama T. Antiemetic effect of dexamethasone on cisplatin-induced early and delayed emesis in the pigeon. Eur J Pharmacol 2004;484:311-21.
10. Darmani NA. Serotonin 5-HT_3 receptor antagonists prevent cisplatin-induced emesis in Cryptotis parva: a new experimental model of emesis. J Neural Transm 1998;105:1143-54.
11. Darmani NA, Zhao W, Ahmad B. The role of D2 and D3 dopamine recptors in the mediation of emesis in Cryptotis parva (the least shew). J Neural Transm 1999;106:1045-61.
12. Mitchell D, Wells C, Hoch N, Lind K, Woods SC, Mitchell LK. Poison induced pica in rats. Physiol Behav 1976;17:691-7.
13. Mitchell D, Krusemark ML, Hafner D. Pica: a species relevant behavioural assay of motion sickness in the rat. Physiol Behav 1977;18:125-30.
14. Aung HH, Dey L, Mehendale S, Xie JT, Wu JA, Yuan CS. Scutellaria baicalensis extract decreases cisplatin-induced pica in rats. Cancer Chemother Pharmacol 2003;52:453-8.
15. Malik NM, Liu YL, Cole N, Sanger GJ, Andrews PL. Differential effects of dexamethasone, ondansetron and a tachykinin NK1 receptor antagonist (GR205171) on cisplatin-induced changes in behaviour, food intake, pica and gastric function in rats. Eur J Pharmacol 2007;555:164-73.
16. Scarpignato C, Capovilla T, Bertaccini G. Action of cerulin on gastric emptying of conscious rats. Arch Int Pharmacodyn Ther 1980;246:286-94.
17. Kris MG, Gralla RJ, Clark RA, Tyson LB, O'Connell JP, Wertheim, et al. Incidence, course, and severity of delayed nausea and vomiting following the administration of high-dose cisplatin. J Clin Oncol 1985;3:1379-84.

18. Kris MG, Pisters KM, Hinkley L. Delayed emesis following anticancer chemotherapy. Support Care Cancer 1994;2:297-300.
19. Gylys JA, Doran KM, Buyniski JP. Antagonism of cisplatin-induced vomiting in dogs. Commun Chem Pathol Pharmacol 1979;23:61-8.
20. Rudd JA, Tse HYH, Wai MK. Cisplatin-induced emesis in the cat: effect of granisetron and dexamethasone. Eup J Pharmacol 2000;391:145-50.
21. Yoshikawa T, Yoshida N, Oka M. The broad-spectrum anti-emetic activity of AS-8112, a novel dopamine D_2, D_3 and 5-HT_3 receptors antagonist. British J Pharmacol 2001;133:253-60.
22. Tanihata S, Hiroaki I, Masami S, Toshimitsu U. Cisplatin-induced early and delayed emesis in the pigeon. British J Pharmacol 2000;130:132-8.
23. Andrews PLR, Okada F, Woods AJ, Hagiwara H, Kakaimoto S, et al. The emetic and anti-emetic effects of the capsaicin analogue resiniferatoxin in Suncus murinus, the house musk shrew. British J Pharmacol 2000;130:1247-54.
24. Mehendale S, Han A, Anbao W, Jun-Jie Y, Chong-Zhi W, Jing-Tian X, et al. American ginseng berry extract and ginsenoside Re attenuate cisplatin-induced kaolin intake in rats. Cancer Chemoth Pharmacol 2005;56:63-9.
25. Hisashi Y, Hiroe S, Yasue M, Katsunori I, Hiroyuki S, Masahiko M, et al. Probable involvement of the 5-hydroxytryptamine4 receptor in methotrexate-induced delayed emesis in dogs. Pharmacol Exp Ther 2000;292:1002-7.
26. Andrews PLR, Davis CJ, Maskell L. The abdominal visceral innervation and the emetic reflex: pathways, pharmacology, and plasticity. Can J Physiol Pharm1990; 68:325-45.
27. Andrews PLR, Kovacs M, Watson JW. The anti-emetic action of the neurokinin(1) receptor antagonist CP-99,994 does not require the presence of the area postrema in the dog. Neurosci Lett 2001;314:102-4.
28. Lau AH, Ngan MP, Rudd JA, Yew DT. Differential action of domperidone to modify emesis and behaviour induced by apomorphine in the ferret. Eur J Pharmacol 2005;516:247-52.
29. Takeda N, Hasegawa S, Morita M, Horii A, Uno A, Yamatodani A, et al. Neuropharmacological mechanisms of emesis. I. Effects of antiemetic drugs on motion- and apomorphine-induced pica in rats. Methods Find Exp Clin Pharmacol 1995;17:589-90.
30. Fukui H. Yamamoto M, Sasaki S, Sato S. Possible involvement of peripheral 5-HT4 receptors in copper sulfate-induced vomiting in dogs. Eur J Pharmacol 1994;257:47-52.
31. Kayashima N, Hyama T. Reproducibility of emesis by orally administrated copper sulfate in cats. Nippon Yakurigaku Zasshi 1976;72:287-91.
32. Nakayama H, Hisashi Y, Mika H, Hirofumi I, Katsunori I, Masahiko M, et al. Antiemetic Activity of FK1052, a 5-HT_3- and 5-HT_4-Receptor Antagonist, in Suncus murinus and Ferrets. J Pharmacol Sci 2005;98:396-403.
33. Akita Y, Yang Y, Kawai T, Kinoshita K, Koyama K, Takahashi K, et al. New assay method for surveying anti-emetic compounds from natural sources. Natural Product Sciences 1998;4:72-77.
34. Ivan ML, Sarna SK, Shaker R. Gastrointestinal motor and myoelectric correlates of motion sickness. Am J Physiol Gastrointest Liver Physiol 1999;277:G642-52.
35. Ueno S, Matsuki N, Saito H. Suncus murinus as a new experimental model for motion sickness. Life Sci 1988;43:413-20.
36. Ignacio A, Gomez-de-Segura, Antonio G, Grande, Enrique DM. Antiemetic effects of lerisetron in radiation-induced emesis in the dog. Acta Oncologica 1998;37:759-63.

37. King GL. Characterization of radiation-induced emesis in the ferret. Radiat Res 1988;114:599-612.
38. Yamamoto K, Noriaki T, Atsushi Y. Establishment of an animal model for radiation-induced vomiting in rats using pica. J Radiat Res 2002;43:135-41.
39. Parker LA, Magdalena K, Raphael M. Delta-9-tetrahydrocannabinol and cannabidiol, but not ondansetron, interfere with conditioned retching reactions elicited by a lithium-paired context in Suncus murinus: an animal model of anticipatory nausea and vomiting. Physiol Behav 2006;87:66-71.
40. Parker LA, Kemp SWP. Tetrahydrocannabinol (THC) interferes with conditioned retching in Suncus murinus: an animal model of anticipatory nausea and vomiting (ANV). Neuro Report 2001;12:749-51.
41. Limebeer CL1, Hall G, Parker LA. Exposure to a lithium-paired context elicits gaping in rats: a model of anticipatory nausea. Physiol Behav 2006;88(4-5):398-403.
42. Yuan Y, Xu D, Hu G. Pinacidil suppression on 5-HT_3 receptor contraction. Acta Pharmacologica Sinica 1998;19:31-5.

CHAPTER

38

Absorption and Metabolism

INTRODUCTION

Absorption and metabolism are important pharmacokinetic parameters for effective drug therapy. Many drugs are absorbed by the small intestine. Drug absorption is affected by multiple factors such as physiochemical factors—solubility of the drug, particle size, routes of administration, gastrointestinal motility, permeability area of absorbing surface, etc. The small intestinal epithelium acts as a primary barrier to control the absorption of orally administered xenobiotics and nutrients. Apart from its absorptive property, it is also involved in the first pass metabolism of the drugs, involving both phase I and phase II reactions. The outcome of an orally administered drug depends on both physicochemical properties of the drug and physiological factors like gastric emptying rate, intestinal motility, intestinal mucosal cells and composition of the intestinal juice. Sufficient intestinal absorption of orally administered drugs from gastrointestinal tract is one of the essential requirements for the success of oral drug therapy.

Further, after absorption of drug from any route, it undergoes distribution and metabolism in the body before being excreted. Liver is the main site of metabolism of most of the xenobiotics. CYP450 superfamily of enzymes catalyzes most of the metabolism reactions. Drug metabolism studies are very important both from the industrial perspective, where they are used to study drugs in discovery and development as well as in the pursuit of basic research. Importance of metabolic studies can be gauged from the recent banning of terfenadine, astemizole and cisapride, due to their propensity to cause serious ventricular arrhythmias when given in conjunction with CYP450 inhibitors like erythromycin, ketoconazole, etc. Some of the commonly used methods for the screening of drugs for absorption and metabolism are described below.

ABSORPTION STUDIES

IN VITRO MODELS

Everted Gut Sac Model

Wilson and Wiseman in 1954[1] first introduced everted intestinal gut sac model to study nutrient transport. The technique was later modified to study drug transport across the intestine.[2]

Male Sprague-Dawley rats of 250–300 g weight range are used. Small intestine is quickly removed from the decapitated animal and placed in Krebs-Henseleit bicarbonate buffer solution. Using a glass rod, the intestine is inverted and tied at both the ends to prepare an intestinal sac. The sac is then filled with the physiological solution using blunt needle syringe. A small air bubble is also injected to oxygenate the serosal side of the intestinal segment. The everted sac is then placed in a beaker containing the compound of interest dissolved in well-oxygenated physiological salt solution. The amount of drug permeated through the intestine layers to the serosal side is measured.[3]

This model can be used for measuring absorption of test compounds at different sites in the intestine.[4] The model is also used to study pro-drug conversion in different intestinal sites and also to investigate efflux transporters, like 'p' glycoprotein mediated efflux of [^{3}H] vinblastine, [^{14}C] doxorubicin and veraparmil. Thus, can be prove as an important tool for study of p-glycoprotein mediated transport and potential p-glycoprotein substrate modifiers.[5] It is also useful for estimating the first-pass metabolism of drugs in intestinal epithelial cells. A potential disadvantage of this approach is limited tissue viability[6] and the presence of the muscularis mucosa, which is not usually removed from everted sac preparations. Thus, the compound has to cross all the layers (including muscles) of the small intestine. Apart from this, as the volume of fluid on the serosal side, i.e. inside the sac is limited; there may be possibility of saturation of transport due to accumulation of compound. This model has recently been reviewed by Alam et al. 2011.[7] This model is affected by the age of the animal, sex and species, pathological conditions, chronic therapy and intestinal selectivity. Many experimental factors such as pH, media, temperature, substrate related factors (time lapse in the harvesting of the intestine and animal state—live or dead) affect active transport in the duodenal segments of the animal. This model is very useful to study product conversion in different intestinal sites, drug interaction and mechanism of transport, screening of excipients and formulation in transport modulation and to study permeability of drugs in various experimental settings.

Tissue Mounted in Ussing Chamber

The technique of performing drug absorption studies, using intestinal tissue mounted in Ussing chamber, was first introduced by Ussing and Zerahn[8] for studying active transport of sodium as a source of short circuit current in isolated frog skin. Later on, it was modified to study the transport of drugs. In this system, the drug can be exposed at either the mucosal side (apical side of enterocytes) or the serosal side (basolateral side of enterocytes). The procedure for carrying out the intestinal Ussing chamber studies is described by Jezyk et al.[9]

Albino rats, weighing 225–275 g, are used. After an overnight fast, the animal is decapitated. The small intestine is removed and small sections, 2.5–3 cm in length, are made. These are opened along the mesenteric border. The tissue is mounted in Ussing chamber, which is then placed in a 37°C heating block, aerated with 95% O_2/5% CO_2 and filled with 5 ml buffer at 37°C and pH 7.4. After 15 minutes of equilibration period, the original buffer is replaced with warm fresh buffer solution. The transport studies are initiated by the addition of labeled and unlabeled drug to either the apical or the basolateral chamber. Samples of 500 μl are taken from the receiver chamber every 30 min for up to 120 min and replaced with fresh warm buffer of same pH. Sample activity is then measured by liquid scintillation counter. Some researchers have used a stirring rotor system instead of gas lift, to avoid excess foaming when surfactants or proteins are used in buffer solution preparations.[10]

The usefulness of Ussing chambers for intestinal transport studies has long been recognized, and they have also been used to study the intestinal metabolism of xenobiotics.[11] When properly equipped with electrodes, Ussing chambers are useful for studying the effects of compounds on electrophysiological parameters of the intestinal barrier.[3] However, to study this effect, integrity and viability of intestinal segments is very important and this is ensured by electrophysiological parameters, like transepithelial resistance (TEER) responsible for tissue integrity and short circuit current (SSC) reflects the ionic flux across the membrane epithelium.[12] Molecules like mannitol and PEG 400 can be used as marker to check the integrity of cell layers of intestinal segment.

Porcine Intestinal Tissue System

Healthy porcine intestinal tissue mounted in an Intestine™ system to predict human intestinal absorption of compounds with different chemical characteristics and within bio relevant matrices has been a new approach used. Feasibility of this new approach to study regional differences (duodenum, jejunum and item) in permeability of compounds and to study the effects of luminal factors on permeability was also investigated. The authors concluded that this system can be applied as a reliable tool for the assessment of intestinal permeability in the absence and presence of bio relevant samples.[13]

Cell Culture Models

Cell culture models are based on the assumption that intestinal epithelium, in the form of monolayer of cells, is the main barrier for the drug molecules to reach the systemic circulation. These models are used to perform rapid screening of compounds for their absorption across the intestine. As enterocytes present in the intestinal epithelium play a major role in the absorptive functions, various immortalized tumor cells having intestinal epithelial cells are used to investigate the transport of drugs across the intestinal epithelium. One of the most commonly used cell lines for studying the drug absorption is Caco-2 cell line.

Caco-2 Cells

Caco-2 cells are derived from human colon carcinoma cells and have similarity to the intestinal enterocytes. Drug transport studies can be carried out, as recently described by Kim et al.[14] and Pauli-Magnus et al.[15] Caco-2 cells are grown as polarized monolayers on semiporous filters.

During this period, P-glycoprotein is expressed on their apical surface. These cells allow study of vectorial transcellular transport, i.e. basal to apical and apical to basal. Cells of passage number 33–50 are plated on polycarbonate transwell cell culture insert plates with a cell count of 2×10^5 cells/well. Transport experiments are performed on day 7 after plating. About 1 hour prior to the start of the experiment, the medium in each compartment is replaced by transport medium. Test drug is then added for the transport experiments either in the apical or the basolateral compartment and the amount of drug appearing in the opposite compartment (basal or apical) after 1, 2, 3 and 4 h is measured in 25 µl aliquots. Net basal to apical transport is calculated after 4 hours by substracting the apical to basal from the basal to apical transport rate. Permeability coefficient (P_{app}) is determined according to the equation:

$$P_{app} = dQ/dt * 1/(A * C_o) \text{ [cm/sec]}$$

Where, dQ/dt (μmol/sec) is the transport rate, C_o (μmol/cm^3) is the initial concentration in the donor chamber and A (cm^2) is the surface area of the monolayer.[16] Inhibition of P-glycoprotein-mediated transport across confluent Caco-2 cell monolayers is determined in a similar manner after addition of the putative inhibitor to both compartments. Experiments are conducted only in those wells that show transepithelial electrical resistance (TEER) of more than 350 ohms. TEER is verified after each transport experiment in all the wells to determine the effect of test substance on the monolayer integrity.

Apart from expression of P-glycoproteins, they also express transporter protein and phase II conjugation enzymes to model a variety of transcellular pathways as well as metabolic transformation of test substances. Caco-2 cells, in contrast to normal cells, lack expression of cytochrome P450 isozyme particularly CYP 3A4, however, drug treatment of Caco-2 cells with vitamin D3 can induce this enzyme.

Caco-2 cell permeability assays may be used employing LCMS and LC-MS–MS for simultaneous measurement of multiple compounds. Caco-2 cells are useful in studying more than one pharmacokinetic parameter.[17]

Permeability characteristics of HT29-18-C1 colonic epithelial cell line with Caco-2 have been compared. It was concluded that HT29-18-C1 monolayers can be used to study drug permeability at transepithelial electrical resistance (Rt) values similar to human intestine without the need for Ca^{2+} chelation and as such they offer a useful alternative to Caco-2 for modeling intestinal drug absorption.[18]

Other Cell Lines

Various other cell lines like Madin Darby Canine Kidney (MDCK) cells isolated from a dog kidney by Madin and Darby,[19] Intestinal Epithelial Cell line (IEC)[20] and Rat Intestinal Epithelial (RIE) cell line[21] are also being used for drug intestinal absorption studies.

Advantages and Disadvantages of Cell Culture Models

Cell lines offer a variety of advantages:

- Easy to work with once cell culture conditions are established
- Less amount of test drug needed than in other systems
- Importance of different cell populations in absorption and metabolism of drugs can be studied by culturing specific cell types like enterocytes, crypt cells, etc.

Some of the disadvantages associated with the use of cell culture models include:

- Some are cancerous in origin, and thus, may not mimic the exact physiological features of normal intestinal cells
- Are not necessarily phenotypically stable and properties may differ with passage number
- Great expertise is needed in handling cell culture systems
- Molds, bacteria and fungi can infect the cultured cells and lead to erroneous results.

IN SITU MODEL

In Situ Rat Gut Perfusion

In situ rat gut perfusion technique is an important model for the investigation of intestinal transport, since *in situ* perfusion of the intestinal segments in anesthetized rats more closely mimics the *in vivo* absorption studies. A significant advantage of the model is that biliary excretion and enterohepatic circulation are eliminated, thus allowing the study of intestinal events in isolation.

Male Wistar rats, weighing 225–275 g, are used. Overnight fasted animals are anesthetized with urethane 30 min before surgery. The small intestine is exposed through a midline longitudinal abdominal incision. A silicon cannula is then inserted into the duodenum and an outlet cannula is inserted just proximal to the ileocecal junction. The intestine is then flushed using isotonic saline followed by infusion of air to remove the remaining solution. The drug solution with or without inhibitor is then infused and the effluent samples are estimated for drug content. The amount of the drug measured in the inlet and the outlet cannula is used to calculate the permeability coefficient of the drug across the small intestinal epithelium.[22,23]

In-silico Model

For *in-silico* predictions of gastrointestinal drug absorption in pharmaceutical products development, SjÖrgen E et al. 2013[24] successfully developed a mechanistic absorption model. The GI-Sim deployed a compartmental gastrointestinal absorption and transit model as well as algorithms describing permeability, dissolution rate, salt effects, partitioning into micelles, particle and micelle drifting in aqueous boundary layer particle growth and amorphous or crystalline precipitation. The model's overall predictive performance was good in screening the selected APIs.

METABOLISM STUDIES

An overview of different *in vitro* models such as supersomes, microsomes, cytosol, S9 fraction cell lines, transgenic cell lines, primary hepatocytes, liver slices, isolated perfused liver with advantages, disadvantages and future prospectives is given by Brandon et al. 2003.[25] For successful screening of drug candidate's selection of proper models and data interpretation are crucial. Methodologies for investigating drug metabolism at the early drug discovery stage and prediction of hepatic drug clearance and P450 contribution are reviewed by Emoto C et al. 2010.[26] Recently, different *in vitro* and *in vivo* preclinical experimental models of drug metabolism and drug disposition in drug discovery and development are described in detail by Donglu et al. 2012.[27]

IN VITRO MODELS

For drug metabolism studies, various *in vitro* models are used. These models involve the use of liver slices and hepatocytes in evaluating the metabolism of the test compound. The advantages offered by these models are the presence of drug metabolizing enzymes like CYP450s, other microsomal and cytosolic enzymes and also cofactors that contribute to metabolism. However, interindividual genetic variations in enzyme expression lead to differences in variable rate of drug metabolism. Such genetic variations, leading to variable human CYP 3A-mediated metabolism are covered by Lamba et al. 2002.[28] These models can also be used for studying the hepatotoxic potential of the compounds. However, these cellular systems also have some inherent disadvantages, like the cells and slices cannot be easily frozen and subsequently thawed for use in assays, cell culture of hepatocytes are primary and cannot be passaged and these cellular systems cannot be prepared from liver tissue that has previously been frozen. There is also an alternative approach of using a complete mixture of enzymes that involves working with simple homogenates of liver or other tissues. Although all of the enzymes are present in the system containing homogenates, but their cofactors are diluted.

Hepatocytes

Hepatocytes are the functional units of liver, the major site responsible for xenobiotic and drug metabolism. Hepatocytes isolated from a large number of laboratory animal species, such as rat, mouse, dog, monkey as well as human liver tissue, have been used. Hepatocytes can be used to study several aspects of drug metabolism, such as metabolite profiling, biotransformation pathway reaction phenotyping, metabolic drug-drug interactions comparison of metabolism of xenobiotics and drugs and the detoxification of toxicants of xenobiotics derived from metabolism. The collagenase perfusion method, first developed using rat liver, is now used for preparation of hepatocytes using various species of animals. Collagenase perfusion is used because the extracellular matrix of the liver comprises largely of collagen (1 mg/g of wet weight in rats and 5 mg/g in humans), thus yielding the highest viable hepatocytes.

To carry out the isolation of hepatocytes from rat liver, liver is obtained and portal vein is cannulated. To remove blood from the liver, it is perfused with calcium free oxygenated buffer (Krebs-Ringer bicarbonate buffer, Hanks balanced salt solution or Dulbecco's phosphate buffered saline) at a flow rate of 20–40 ml/min under a hydrostatic pressure of 20–25 cm of H_2O for 5–10 min. Too high or too low perfusion rates can damage the liver tissue by causing shearing and anoxia, respectively. EGTA (ethylene glycol bis β-aminoethyl ether N, N, N, N tetra-acetic acid), a calcium-chelating agent, can be added to the perfusion buffer to favor cleavage of hepatocytes. Collagenase is then added to the reservoir and the liver perfused for an additional 10-15 min or until visible softening is evident. Subsequently, disruption or removal of liver capsule and gentle stroking of the cell mass leads to dissociation of liver cells. The resulting cell suspension is filtered through a double layer of sterile cotton gauze or nylon mesh of 50-250 μm. The cells are washed twice by centrifugation and the cloudy supernatant, which contains residual collagenase, nonparenchymal cells, erythrocytes, nonviable hepatocytes and cell debris, is discarded. The hepatocytes are then centrifuged again through a density gradient of porcell to obtain hepatocytes of the highest viability.[29] Using trypan blue exclusion assay; the hepatocytes are then tested for their viability. More than 90% viability is desirable. The cells are then cultured in collagen-coated (95–98% type I collagen), 100-mm diameter plates at a density of 10^7 cells/7 ml of culture medium. Hepatocytes are cultured for the first 4 h in 1:1 (v/v) Ham's F12/William's medium E supplemented with fetal calf serum, sodium bicarbonate, penicillin, streptomycin, ethanolamine, transferin, insulin, dexamethasone, glucagon, linoleic acid, glucose, sodium pyruvate, ascorbic acid and trace elements and subsequently cultured in serum free medium[30] in a humidified atmosphere of 5% CO_2/95% air at 37°C. The drug with and without inhibitor is put in the different wells of the plate to study the metabolism of the drug.

In vitro human hepatocyte-based experimental systems for the evaluation of human drug metabolism, drug-drug interactions, and drug toxicity are recently described by Shahi J et al. 2010[31] and Li, 2014.[32]

Precision-cut Liver Slices

Precision-cut liver slices are used frequently for *in vitro* metabolism studies. Liver slices from a large variety of laboratory animals, including human beings, can be used for metabolism studies. The liver samples are obtained and stored in ice-cold culture medium consisting of Earle's Balanced Salt Solution (EBSS) containing 25 mM of D-glucose, 50 µg/ml of gentamicin and 2.5 µg/ml of fungizone till the initiation of slicing procedure. The medium is pregassed with 95% O_2 and 5% CO_2. Tissue is prepared for slicing in tissue cylinders with the help of a motor driver tissue coring tool. Using a Krumdieck tissue slicer, 200-300 µm tissue slices are prepared in well-oxygenated culture medium. The tissue slices are now floated onto steel mesh inserts and incubated in culture medium in polystyrene vials for 30 min at 37°C in an atmosphere of 95% air and 5% CO_2, using a roller system rotated at 9 rpm. Pre-incubation enables the liver slices to restore their ATP levels. Subsequently, the tissue is incubated with culture medium containing the test drug and the medium is analyzed for metabolites.[33]

Precision-cut tissue slices from various organs and different species can provide excellent *in vitro* models for biotransformation and chemical-induced organ specific toxicity. They offer the advantage of maintaining tissue architecture and avoiding damage to the cells as may occur during cell isolation procedures. Further, the technique for preparing tissue slices is relatively easy and can be employed for preparing tissue slices from different organs from different species.

Microsomes

Majority of drugs administered by the human beings are metabolized in the liver by CYP3A4 enzymes. It is important to choose a proper experimental system to study the drug metabolism. Microsomes of varied origin are used *in vitro*. The experimental approaches using cytochrome P450 are reviewed by Zuber et al. 2002,[34] based on drug metabolising system. Briefly, for CYP1A mediated pathways all the commonly used experimental models are appropriate except probably the dog; on the contrary the dogs are suggested to be suitable for modeling of processes depending on the CYP2D. With CYP2C, which is possibly the most large and complicated subfamily, the system based on monkey (*Maccacus rhesus*) is suggested to be a good representative. The CYP3A is suggested to be well modeled by pig or minipig CYP3A29.

The use of microsomes is another *in vitro* approach to study the metabolism of test compound and patterns of biotransformation. For the preparation of liver microsomes, the organs from the sacrificed animals are immediately removed and placed in ice. Using a mechanical meat grinder, these are grounded and then homogenized in 2 volumes of 0.25 M sucrose, 0.05 M HEPES (pH 7.4) using a potter Elvehjem homogenizer coupled with a motor driven Teflon pestle (2,500 rpm). The homogenate is then diluted by adding 25% w/v buffered sucrose and centrifuged at 10,000 g for 20 min to remove the cell debris, nuclei and mitochondria. The mitochondrial supernatant is again centrifuged for 45 min at 1,00,000 g. The microsomal pellet so obtained is suspended in 0.15 M KCl containing 0.02 M HEPES (pH 7.4) and centrifuged at

1,92,000 g for 45 min. The washed pellet is resuspended in buffered KCl.[35] The protein content of the microsomal preparation is estimated by the method of Lowry et al.[36]

To perform metabolism studies, substrate is preincubated with 50 μg of microsomal protein, 30 mM $MgCl_2$, and 50 mM KH_2PO_4, pH 7.4 for 2 min in a shaking water bath at 37°C. The reaction is started by the addition of 4.8 mM NADPH and incubated for another 5 min. The reaction is terminated after 5 min with the addition of 1.7 ml of ice-cold ethanol. The incubation performed in presence of different concentration of inhibitors is used to determine the nature of the inhibition.[37]

The microsomal preparations can be stored in liquid N_2 or at –80°C for long duration. Human liver microsomes can be availed from industries or from other sources. The disadvantage with human liver microsomes is the presence of different subfamilies of CYP450. Normally, liver is considered as a main enzyme source, although depending on the specific enzyme and xenobiotic, other organs may also play an important role in drug metabolism.[38]

Recombinant Systems

Due to the technical difficulties in purification of specific CYP450 enzymes from human liver and the unavailability of tissues, various recombinant systems expressing CYP450s have been developed for drug metabolism studies. Several cell lines expressing individual human CYP450s, including V79 Chinese hamster[39] and human lymphoblastoid cell lines, have been developed and are commercially available. High level of CYP450 expression has also been achieved in yeast,[40] insect cells using recombinant baculovirus[41] and bacteria.[42] For toxicological studies, expression of P450 in mammalian cells is most appropriate as exemplified by activation and inactivation of chemotherapeutic drugs.[43] The advantage of recombinant systems is the availability of large amount of purified enzymes for drug metabolism studies, but the cost of these systems has limited their use.

ACKNOWLEDGMENTS

The encouragement from Dr GN Singh, Secretary-cum-Scientific Director, Indian Pharmacopoeia Commission, Ghaziabad and Professor SK Gupta, Delhi Institute of Pharmaceutical Sciences and Research, Pushp Vihar, New Delhi-110017, during the revision of this chapter is gratefully acknowledged. Typing assistance provided by Ms Reena Tripathi is also acknowledged.

REFERENCES

1. Wilson TH, Wiseman G. The use of sacs of everted small intestine for the study of the transference of substances from the mucosal to the serosal surface. J Physiol 1954;123:116-25.
2. Leppert PS, Fix JA. Use of everted intestinal rings for in vitro examination of oral absorption potential. J Pharm Sci 1994;83:976-81.
3. Hillgren KM, Kato A, Borchardt RT. In vitro systems for studying intestinal drug absorption. Med Res Rev 1995;15: 83-109.
4. Chowhan ZT, Amaro AA. Everted rat intestinal sacs as an in vitro model for assessing absorptivity of new drugs. J Pharm Sci 1977;66:1249-53.

5. Carrreno Gomez B, Duncan R. Everted rat intestinal sacs : a new model for the quantification of P-glycoprotein mediated efflux of anticancer agents. Anticancer Res 2000;20:3157-61.
6. Barthe L, et al 1998. An improved everted gut sac as a simple and accurate technique to measure paracellular transport across the small intestine. Eur J Drug Metab Pharmacokinet 1998;23(2):313-23.
7. Alam MA , Al-Jenoobi FI, Abdullah MA. Everted gut sac model as a tool in pharmaceutical research: limitations and applications. J Pharm Pharmacol 2011;64:326-36.
8. Ussing HH, Zerahn K. Active transport of sodium as the source of electric current in the short-circuited isolated frog skin. Acta Physiol Scand 1951;23:110-27.
9. Jezyk N, Li C, Stewart BH, et al. Transport of pregabalin in rat intestine and Caco-2 monolayers. Pharm Res 1999;16:519-26.
10. Ungell AL, Andreason A, Lundin K, Utter L. Effects of enzymatic inhibition and increased paracellular shunting on transport of vasopressin analogues in the rat J. Pharma Sci 1992;81:640-5.
11. Soderholm JD, Hedman L, Artursson P, et al. Integrity and metabolism of human ileal mucosa in vitro in the Ussing chamber. Acta Physiol Scand 1998;162:47-56.
12. Polentarutti Bl, Peterson AL, Sjoberg AK, Anderberg EKL, Utter LM, Ungell AL. Evaluation of viability of excised rat intestinal segments in the Ussing chamber:investigation of morphology, electrical parameters and permeability characteristics. Pharma Res 1999;16(3):446-54.
13. Westerhout J, van de Steeq E, Grossouw D, et al. A new approach to predict human intestinal absorption using porcine intestinal tissue and biorelevant matrices. Eur J Pharm Sci 2014;63:167-77.
14. Kim RB, Fromm MF, Wandel C, et al. The drug transporter P-glycoprotein limits oral absorption and brain entry of HIV-1 protease inhibitors. J Clin Invest 1998;101:289-94.
15. Pauli-Magnus C, von Richter O, Burk O, et al. Characterization of the major metabolites of verapamil as substrates and inhibitors of P-glycoprotein. J Pharmacol Exp Ther 2000;293:376-82.
16. Artursson P, Karlsson J. Correlation between oral absorption in humans and apparent drug permeability coefficients in human intestinal epithelial (Caco-2) cells. Biochem Biophys Res Commun 1991;175:880-5.
17. van Breemen RB, Li Y. Caco-2 cell permeability assays to measure drug absorption. Expert Opin Drug Metab Toxicol 2005;1(2);175-85.
18. Collet A, Sims E, Walker D, et al. Comparison of HT 29-18-C1 and Caco-2 cell lines as models for intestinal paracellular drug absorption. Pharm Res 1996;13(2):216-21.
19. Gaush CR, Hard WL, Smith TF. Characterization of an established line of canine kidney cells (MDCK). Proc Soc Exp Biol Med 1966;122:931-5.
20. Quaroni A, Beaulieu JF. Cell dynamics and differentiation of conditionally immortalized human intestinal epithelial cells. Gastroenterology 1997;113:1198-213.
21. Blay J, Brown KD. Characterization of an epithelioid cell line derived from rat small intestine: demonstration of cytokeratin filaments. Cell Biol Int Rep 1984;8:551-60.
22. Komiya I, Park JY, Kamani A, et al. Quantitative mechanistic studies in simultaneously fluid flow and intestinal absorption using steroids as model solutes. Int J Pharm 1979;4:249-62.
23. Doluisio JT, Billups NF, Dittert LW, et al. Drug absorption. I. An in situ rat gut technique yielding realistic absorption rates. J Pharm Sci 1969;58:1196-200.
24. Sjogren E, Westergren J, Grant I, et al. In silico predictions of gastrointestinal drug absorption in pharmaceutical product development: application of the mechanistic absorption model GI-Sim. Eur J Pharm Sci 2013;49(4):679-98.

25. Brandon Esther FA, Raap Christiaan D, Meijerman I, et al. An update on in vitro test methods in human hepatic drug biotransformation research:pros and cons. Toxicol Applied Pharmacol 2003;189:233-46.
26. Emoto C, Murayama N, Rostami-Hodjegan A, et al. Methodologies for investigating drug metabolism at the early drug discovery stage: prediction of hepatic drug clearance and P450 contribution. Current Drug Metab 2010;11(8):678-85.
27. Zhang D, Luo G, Ding X, et al. Preclinical experimental models of drug metabolism and disposition in drug discovery and development. Acta Pharmaceutica Sinica B 2012;2(6):549-61.
28. Lamba JK, Lin YS, Schuetz EG, et al. Genetic contribution to variable human CYP3A-mediated metabolism. Adv Drug Deliv Rev 2002;54(10):1271-4.
29. Bissell DM, Hammaker LE, Meyer UA. Parenchymal cells from adult rat liver in nonproliferating monolayer culture I Functional Studies. J Cell Biol 1973;59:722-34.
30. Hutchings SE, Sato GH. Growth and maintenance of HeLa cells in serum-free medium supplemented with hormones. Proc Natl Acad Sci USA 1978;75:901-4.
31. Sahi J, Grepper S, Smith C. Hepatocytes as a tool in drug metabolism, transport and safety evaluations in drug discovery. Curr Drug Discov Technol 2010;7(3):188-98.
32. Li AP. In vitro human hepatocyte-based experimental systems for the evaluation of human drug metabolism, drug-drug interactions, and drug toxicity in drug development. Curr Top Med Chem 2014;14(11):1325-38.
33. Steensma A, Beamand JA, Walters DG, et al. Metabolism of coumarin and 7-ethoxycoumarin by rat, mouse, guinea pig, cynomolgus monkey and human precision-cut liver slices. Xenobiotica 1994;24:893-907.
34. Zuber R, Anzenbacherova, Anzenbacher P. Cytochromes P450 and experimental models of drug metabolism. J Cell Mol Med 2002;6(2):189-98.
35. Bend JR, Hook GE, Easterling RE, et al. A comparative study of the hepatic and pulmonary microsomal mixed-function oxidase systems in the rabbit. J Pharmacol Exp Ther 1972;183:206-17.
36. Lowry OH, Rosebrough NJ, Farr AL, et al. Protein measurement and folin phenol reagent. J Biol Chem 1951;93:265-75.
37. Kroemer HK, Echizen H, Heidemann H, et al. Predictability of the in vivo metabolism of verapamil from in vitro data: contribution of individual metabolic pathways and stereoselective aspects. J Pharmacol Exp Ther 1992;260:1052-7.
38. Birkett DJ, Mackenize PI, Veronese ME, et al. In vitro approaches can predict human drug metabolism. Trends Pharmacol Sci 1993;4:292.
39. Doehmer J, Oesch F. V79 Chinese hamster cells genetically engineered for stable expression of cytochrome P450. Methods Enzymol 1991;206:117-23.
40. Gautier JC, Urban P, Beaune P, et al. Engineered yeast cells as model to study coupling between human xenobiotic metabolizing enzymes. Simulation of the two first steps on benzo[a]pyrene activation. Eur J Biochem 1993;211:63-72.
41. Lee CA, Kadwell SH, Kost TA, et al. CYP3A4 expressed by insect cells infected with a recombinant baculovirus containing both CYP3A4 and human NADPH-cytochrome P450 reductase is catalytically similar to human liver microsomal CYP3A4. Arch Biochem Biophys 1995;319:157-67.
42. Guengerich FP, Martin MV, Guo Z, et al. Purification of functional recombinant P450s from bacteria. Methods Enzymol 1996;272:35-44.
43. Friedberg T, Tritchard MP, Bandera M, et al. Merits and limitations of recombinant models for the study of human P 450 mediated drug metabolism and toxicity:an interlaboratory comparison. Drug Metab Rev 1999;31(2):523-44.

CHAPTER

39

Hormones of Pituitary, Thyroid, Parathyroid, Adrenal Cortex, Ovary and Testes

INTRODUCTION

Functions of the body are mainly regulated by two control systems, the nervous system and the endocrinal system. The endocrine system is a collection of glands that secrete chemical messengers known as hormones. A hormone is a specialized molecule that is synthesized, stored and secreted by a group of specialized cells known as the endocrine gland. These glands are ductless gland and secret hormones directly into the blood stream to reach the target organ possessing cells with appropriate receptors. The hormones deliver the message through receptors to bring about changes in cellular functions.

The neural center for the control of endocrinal secretions is located in the hypothalamus. The hypothalamus secretes releasing or inhibitory hormones and sends them to pituitary via hypothalamic-hypophyseal portal veins. The pituitary gland often known as the 'master gland' is responsible for secretion of a battery of hormones that collectively influence virtually all physiological processes of the body (Figs 39.1 and 39.2).

An integrated feedback regulation mediated by complex interactions among the hypothalamus, pituitary and peripheral endocrine glands is present, and better understanding of the mechanisms responsible for the interactions provides the rationale to diagnose and to treat the endocrine disorder. Various endocrine disorders mostly arise from the endocrine gland dysfunction, which may result in excessive or scanty secretion of hormones resulting in clinical symptoms.

The elucidation of the structures of various hormones of different origin with the advancement of the protein chemistry made it possible to produce synthetic peptide agonists and antagonists that play very important role in diagnostic as well as therapeutic application. To evaluate these drugs, various *in vitro* and *in vivo* experimental models have been developed. This chapter deals with the different biological screening models of hormones, which are useful to evaluate various natural and synthetic derivatives of hormones for their pharmacological activity.

GROWTH HORMONE

Growth hormone (GH) is the most abundant anterior pituitary hormone. It produces growth at open epiphyses via stimulation of insulin-like growth factor I (IGF-I, somatomedin C). It also

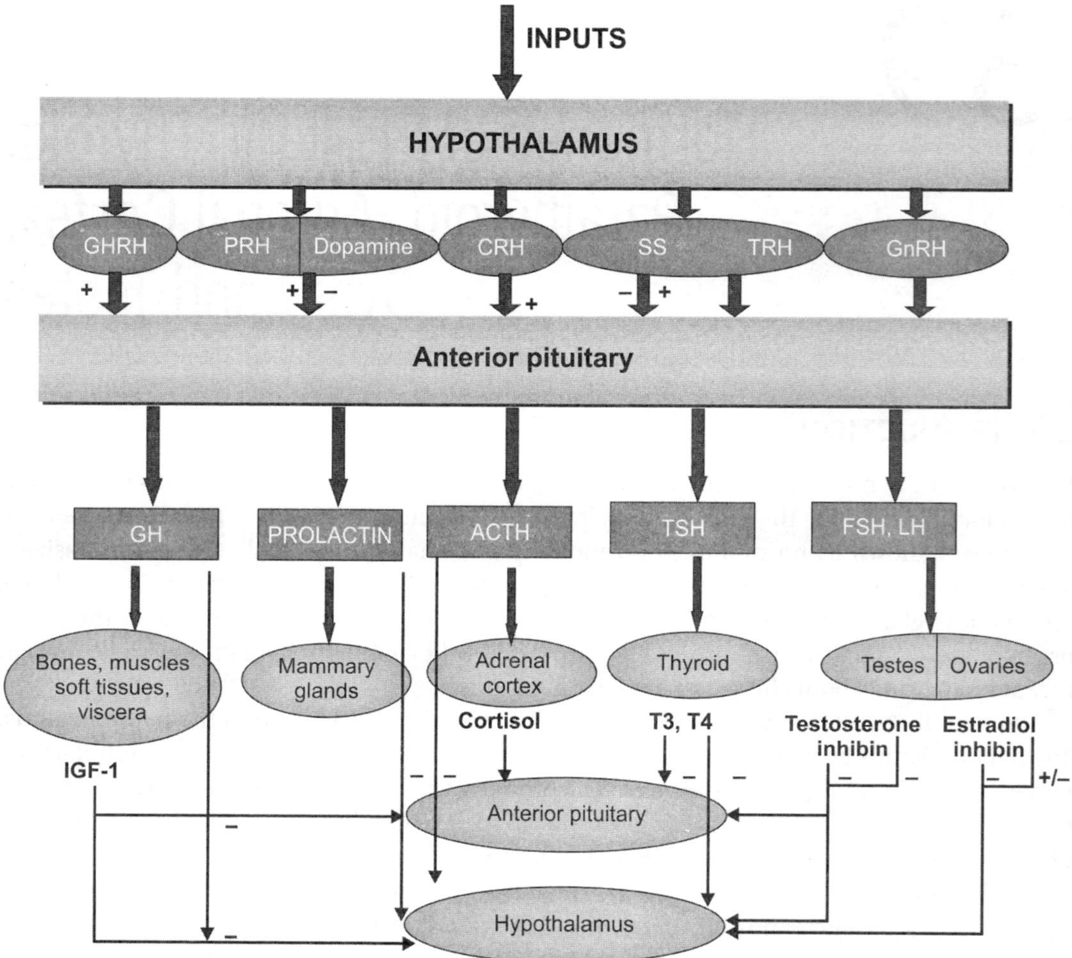

Figure 39.1: Hormones of hypothalamus and anterior pituitary

causes lipolysis in adipose tissue and growth of skeletal muscle. *In vitro* and *in vivo* bioassays used for screening GH analogues include the following models.

IN VITRO STUDIES

Glucose Uptake Inhibition

The conversion of glucose to lipid in murine adipocytes is inhibited by human growth hormone (hGH) in a dose-dependent manner. This is a very sensitive *in vitro* method developed by Foster et al.[1] and is used to screen growth hormone analogues for their biological activity.

Procedure

Murine fibroblasts cells are grown in Dulbecco's Modified Eagle's Medium (DMEM) containing antibiotics. These cells are plated in 60 to 100 mm plastic culture dishes at a

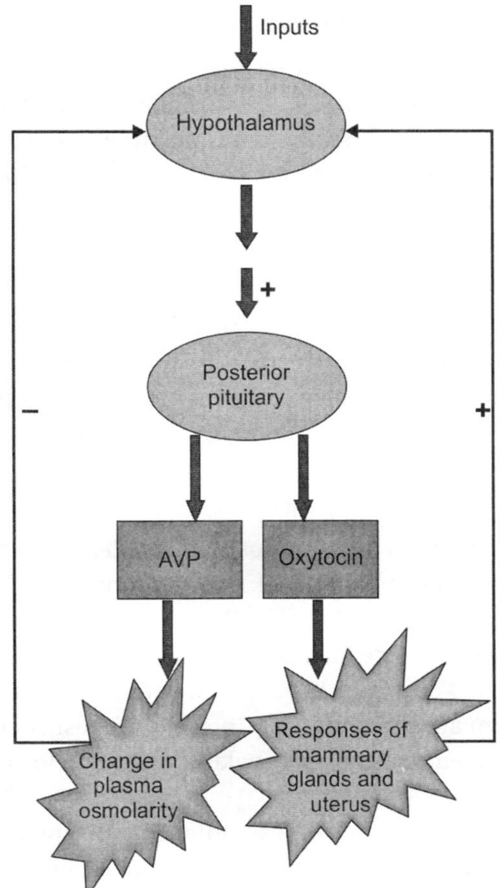

Figure 39.2: Hormones of hypothalamus and posterior pituitary

density of 200 cells/cm^2 and are allowed to be confluent in 25 mM galactose and 10% fetal calf serum supplemented media with 90% air and 10% CO_2 at 37°C. Medium is replaced every 2 to 3 days; and once fibroblasts are confluent, they are converted to characteristic adipocytes by incubation for 48 h in a medium supplemented with 25 mM glucose, 10% FCS, 0.5 mM methylisobutylxanthine, 2 µg/ml insulin and 250 nM dexamethasone. The medium is then replaced by the medium which contains 10% fetal bovine serum and 2 µg/ml of insulin every 2 days for 5 to 8 days until at least 70% of the cells have characteristics of adipocytes as assessed by phase contrast microscopy.

For the evaluation of growth hormone activity, the DMEM medium is uniformly radiolabeled with [^{14}C] D-glucose. Cultures are incubated with increasing concentrations of standard and test preparations or with medium alone for 24. The cells are treated with Doles reagent followed by the scraping of cells and finally the contents are transferred to glass tube. Lipids are extracted and the radioactivity is determined by the scintillation counter. Lipid accumulation in the control cells is considered to be 100%. Decrease in lipid accumulation is directly proportional to the increase in dose range. From dose response curve, activity of the unknown can be calculated.

Human Growth Hormone (hGH) Bioassays

Bioassay of hGH can be assessed either by evaluating biological interaction of hGH with its receptor through Ligand binding assay or its intracellular activity that it evokes on particular cell. Based on affinities of binding on receptor it is possible to screen the agents having hGH activity. hGH bioassays include radioreceptor assays, receptor modulation assays and cell proliferation assays.

Radioreceptor Assays

The biological potency of hGH is determined by employing competitive binding between unlabeled and radiolabelled hGH to its receptor. It has been known that radiolabeled agent that is bound to the receptor can be replaced by the unlabeled agent in direct proportion to their biological activity.

Procedure

The method of radioimmunoassay was proposed by Nederman and Sjodin et al.[2] Human lymphocytes cells (IM-9) are cultured in RPMI 1640 medium complemented with FCS (10%), L-glutamine (2 mM), streptomycin (100 mg/ml) and penicillin (100 IU/ml). These cells in the late log or early plateau phase are harvested and washed in assay buffer (100 mM Hepes, 120 mM NaCl, 1.2 mM $MgSO_4$, 2.5 mM KCI, 15 mM sodium acetate, 10 mM glucose, 1 mM EDTA and 1% bovine serum albumin, pH 7.0). The cells are resuspended in assay buffer and preincubated at the desired temperature in a shaking waterbath for 1 h before incubation was started.

The cells (400 ul) are added to the tubes containing purified tracer [^{125}I] hGH (about 1.0 ng/ml) and serial concentrations of unlabeled hGH or other samples to be assayed. The incubation is carried out for 90 min at 30°C in a constant temperature water bath. To determine binding, duplicate aliquots of the incubation mixture are layered over iced assay buffer in polypropylene microfuge tubes. The samples are centrifuged at 90,00 g for 1min. The resulting pellets are washed three additional times with iced assay buffer. The radioactivity in the duplicate washed pellets and in corresponding duplicate medium samples is counted in a gamma counter.

Total binding is calculated as percentage of radioactivity in the medium samples. Non-specific binding, defined as the binding of [^{125}I] hGH in the presence of unlabeled hGH, is subtracted from the total binding to obtain the specific binding.

Cell Proliferation Bioassays

The bioactivity of hGH can be evaluated by cell proliferation assays utilizing human cell lines or other cell types. The cell proliferation assays are based on the somatotrophic response produced by hGH in dose dependent manner as described by Ishikawa et al.[3] This assay reflects not only receptor binding of hGH but also mimic signal induction at the intracellular level.

Procedure

Establishment of Ba/F3-hGHR

Mouse pro-B cell lymphoma cells expressing hGH receptors are developed as described by Wada et al.[4] The Ba/F3-cells are cultured in RPMI-1640 supplemented with 10% FCS, 50 mM 2-mercaptoethanol, 50 mg/ml streptomycin sulfate, 50 U/ml penicillin G, and 1 ng/ml recombinant mouse IL-3. Fifty micrograms of mammalian plasmid pCXN2-hGHR are transfected into 1×10^7 Ba/F3 cells. Cells expressing hGHR are cultured in selection medium (RPMI-1640 medium containing 1 mg/ml G418, 10% FCS, 50 mM 2-mercaptoethanol, 10 nM 22K-hGH, and antibiotics). Resultant hGH-responsive cells are examined for hGHR expression by binding assay to [^{125}I] 22K-hGH.

Bioassay with Ba/F3-hGHR cell line

The procedure for the bioassay was explained by Ishikawa et al.[3] Approximately, 4h before the start of experiment, cells are washed twice with assay medium (RPMI 1680, supplemented with 5% FCS, 50 mM 2-mercaptoethanol, and antibiotics, without hGH) and are transferred to the assay medium and incubated for 4-6 h to slow down the rate of cell replication. The cells are collected by centrifugation (3 min at 1000 rpm) and resuspended in the assay medium at a concentration of 1×105 cells/mL of which an aliquots (200 µl) distributed in each well of 96-well microplate. Standards hGH are diluted with 0.01 M PBS supplemented with 0.1% BSA. Samples are incubated at 56°C for 40 min to inactivate the serum. Standards or samples (25 µl) are added to each well. The cultures are incubated in a CO_2 incubator (5% CO_2, 95% air) for 48 h at 37°C. At the end of the incubation, the colorimetric end point is determined by an eluted stain bioassay (ESTA). Briefly, 20 µl MTT solution (3-[4, 5-dimethylthiazol-2-yl]-2,5-diphenyltetrazolium bromide) (5 mg/ml in 0.01 M PBS) is added to each well and incubated at 37°C for 4 h in a CO_2 incubator. During this time, activated cells reduce the yellow MTT salt to purple formazan. The plate is centrifuged at 800 rpm for 10 min, and the stain is eluted into dimethyl sulfoxide (100 µl). Bioactive responses are determined with a kinetic microplate reader reading optical densities at the test wavelength of 550 nm and a reference wavelength of 650 nm to correct for differential scattering. A control serum with known bioactivity was used at every assay for the quality control.

The bioactivity of hGH is evaluated on the basis of cell proliferation in the dose dependent manner which serve as a standard curve for quantification of unknown sample.

IMMUNOASSAYS

These tests are the widely used, sensitive proficiencies for the determination of hGH in biological fluids with high degree of accuracy and reproducibility. These are based on detection of immunological epitopes present on the polypeptide human growth hormone. Antibodies are being developed on the basis of detection of these epitopes such as monoclonal and polyclonal antibodies. However, these techniques are having shortcomings viz. it do not reflect the biological activity of hGH. Immunoassays include radioimmunoassays (RIAs), immunoradiometric assays (IRMAs), enzyme-linked immunoassays (ELISAs) and immunofunctional assays (IFAs).

IMMUNOFUNCTIONAL ASSAY (IFA)

hGH has been known to contain two receptor binding epitopes and induces dimerization of receptor as an initial step of signal transduction mechanism in target cells. Immunofunctional assay is developed to combine the speed of immunoassay and merit of bioassay. The IFA is based on the interaction of hGH with an immobilized mAb specific for binding site 2 epitope of the hormone and with biotin-labeled recombinant hGH (rhGH)-binding protein (hGHBP), which represents the full length hGH receptor ecto domain (Strasburger et al.).[5]

Procedure

The method of IFA was demonstrated by Strasburger et al.[5] Anti-hGH mAb 7B11, which binds to an epitope largely overlapping with binding site 2 of the hGH molecule, is adsorbed to flat bottom 96 well microtiter plates by incubation of 500 ng mAb 7811 in 200 μl 50 mmol/l sodium phosphate buffer, pH 9.6. The plates are sealed with a self-adhesive cover film and stored at 4°C for 12 h to 1 month. After aspiration of the coating solution, the plates are washed three times with washing solution. Twenty-five microliters of standard or sample are pipetted into the wells, followed by 175 μl assay buffer. The plates are incubated at ambient temperature for 3 h on a horizontal shaker. After a 3-fold wash step, 50 ng/well biotinylated rhGHBP are added in 200 μl assay buffer, and the plates are sealed and incubated overnight (12-16 h) at 4°C. After a 3-fold wash step, the plates are incubated with streptavidin-europium and processed as described above. The calibration curve is produced by plotting the hGH concentration of standards and the signal from the time-resolved fluorometric end point. Concentrations of unknown samples are read by interpolation of the signal obtained on the standard curve.

IN VIVO METHODS

Weight Gain Model

After attaining maturity at six months of age, female rats continue to grow at a very slow rate and they almost reach the plateau of weight gain process. However, they can be induced to grow and gain weight by the administration of growth hormone. Though this method needs a large amount of test materials, it is highly specific for the evaluation of growth hormone activity.

Procedure

Ten female Wistar rats weighing between 250 to 280 g who fails to gain more than 10 g in 20 days period are used. Various doses of unknown growth hormone preparations and standard dissolved in saline are injected subcutaneously for 20 consecutive days. During this period, weight gain between 10 to 40 g is expected. A relationship exists between the logarithm of the daily dose level and the increase in body weight of the rats in grams.

The mean values of the weight gain are calculated after administration of 2 doses of standard and 2 doses of test preparations used for 2+2 point assay.[6]

Rat Model of Suboptimal Nutrition

In the regulation of secretion of GH and insulin like growth factor I (IGF), nutritional status and energy intake play a critical role. Poor nutritional status and energy intake reduce the serum GH and IGF levels leading to retarded growth. In animals with suboptimal nutrition, growth can be stimulated by administration of growth hormone.

Procedure

The procedure was described by Carrillo et al. (1998).[7] Four-month-old Sprague Dawley rats are maintained under standard laboratory conditions with *ad libitum* access to water. Daily record of body weight and estimation of food intake is obtained for each animal. Various doses of unknown growth hormone preparation and standard dissolved in saline are injected subcutaneously in the back. Control animals are treated with same volume of normal saline. Within each group the rats are fed with balanced purified 1:1 carbohydrate to fat diet at three energy levels, i.e. *ad libitum* and 80 and 60% of ad libitum. Protein and micronutrient levels are maintained at constant level. Each rat from ad libitum group is paired with one rat each from 80 and 60% diet restriction groups. The amount of food to be fed to the diet restricted groups is calculated from the amount of food intake by corresponding rat of ad libitum group according to the following formula:

Food consumed by the ad libitum fed rat in the previous day/weight of this rat in the previous day) × (0.8 or 0.6, depending on the restriction level) × (the current weight of the rat for which the food is calculated).

Body weight is recorded daily and tail length measured from hairline to the tip of the tail. For each rat weekly average is determined for body weight gain, increase in tail length, calorie intake and food sufficiency. Calorie intake is calculated by multiplying the amount of food intake by calorie density of diet. Food efficiency is calculated by multiplying the ration of amount of food intake and body weight gain by 100. In addition at the end of the experiment the rats can be sacrificed and blood is collected for estimation of insulin and insulin growth factor using radioimmunoassay. The growth hormone treated rats in restricted diet groups show higher growth as compared to vehicle treated groups.

Tibia Test

Cessation of epiphyseal growth occurs after hypophysectomy. Following hypophysectomy, width of the epiphyseal cartilage is markedly reduced. Remarkable increase in the width of the epiphyseal cartilage plate can take place by administration of the growth hormone to hypophysectomized rats.

Procedure

Hypophysectomy is done in female Sprague Dawley rats at the age of 26 to 28 day. They are used for the experiment 12 to 14 days after the operation. Animals are randomly divided into different groups of standard and test preparations, each comprising of 6 to 8 animals. The drugs are administered (i.p.) twice daily for 4 days. On fifth day, animals are sacrificed and both tibias are dissected out and freed from soft tissue. The bones are split into half with a sharp knife. The halves are washed in water, then immersed in acetone and again washed in water; and thereafter, they are placed in 2% silver nitrate solution and rinsed with water. While rinsing with water, bones are exposed to a strong light so that calcified portions of the bone turn dark brown. The stained tibia are then processed to a microscopic stage and the width of the uncalcified cartilage plate, which does not take stain, is measured under low power with a calibrated micrometer eyepiece. Ten individual readings are taken across the epiphysis.

Mean values are obtained and average is calculated for the each dose group. The potency ratio of the test preparations is calculated using 2+2 point assay.[8]

Uptake of ^{35}S

In hypophysectomized animal, radiolabeled sulfur uptake into the cartilage is greatly reduced and is found to be restored following growth hormone application. This phenomenon can be utilized to evaluate the growth hormone activity in the compounds.

Procedure

Hypophysectomized female Sprague Dawley rats (21 day old) are used for this experiment. Three weeks after hypophysectomy, animals are given growth hormone together with radiolabeled sulfur (i.p.) once daily for 4 days. Eight to ten animals are used for various doses for standard and test preparations. The rats are sacrificed 24 h after the last injection and the amount of radiosulfur present in seventh rib cartilage is determined. The radiosulfur uptake is directly proportional to the dose of the growth hormone.

Mean value of each group is calculated and potency ratios of the test preparations compared to the standard are calculated with the help of 2+2 assay.[9]

PROLACTIN

Prolactin is a 198 amino acid peptide hormone produced in the anterior pituitary. It is the principal hormone responsible for lactation. A deficiency of prolactin, which can occur in states of pituitary deficiency, is manifested by failure to lactate or by a luteal phase defect. Hyperprolactinemia can produce galactorrhea and hypogonadism and may be associated with symptoms of a pituitary mass. No preparation is available for the use in prolactin deficient patient. For patients with symptomatic hyperprolactinemia, inhibition of prolactin secretion can be achieved with bromocriptine and other dopamine agonists.

Radioimmunoassay

Prolactin is a glycoprotein hormone with specific activity. For evaluation of gonadotropin-releasing activity or prolactin inhibiting factor activity, radioimmunoassay is necessary.

Procedure

Standards or samples are incubated with antiserum (rabbit-anti-rat-prolactin) for 24 h at 4°C. Now ^{125}I-rat-prolactin is added and incubated for another 48 h. The secondary antibody (1:50), 200 ml/tube is added and incubated for 48 h at 4°C. Separation is done with 1 ml ice-cold phosphate-buffered saline, pH 7.4. The vials are centrifuged at 13,000 g for 15 min. Thereafter, the supernatant is discarded and the residue is counted for 1 min in a gamma counter.[10]

Pigeon Crop Method

Pigeons are very sensitive to lactogenic hormone. Suitable assay method has been developed on the basis of this phenomenon.

Procedure

Pigeons of 2-3 months old of either sex are injected with various doses of standard and test preparations once daily for 4 days intraperitoneally. On the 5th day, the birds are euthanized. A midventral incision is made through the skin and crop wall from keel to head. The contents of the crop and the adherent crop milk are removed. The two lateral pouches are removed, cleaned and wet weight is recorded.

Mean values of various doses of standard and test preparations are calculated and plotted against log dose of the corresponding group. Potency ratios with confidence limits are also calculated.[11]

Lactation in Rabbits

For mammalian assays of lactogenic hormone, only rabbits and guinea pigs have shown satisfactory results so far. There is an induction of mammary growth and milk secretion of pseudopregnant animal following prolactin administration. This is useful to evaluate compounds having prolactin-like activity.

Procedure

Pseudopregnancy is induced in mature estrus rabbits by 50 IU of human chorionic gonadotropin given intravenously. On the 14th day, animals are examined for the presence of well-developed mammary gland, which is characteristic of pregnancy. Various doses of standard and test preparations are injected (s.c.) once daily for 6 days. Animals are euthanized on the 7th day and the abdominal skin is incised in the midline and separated from the mammary gland underneath. The degree of glands enlargement with secretion is rated as the following:

- No response

+ All ducts are filled with milk

++ All ducts and most of the lobules are filled with milk

+++ Entire gland is filled with milk

++++ Mammary glands are greatly extended with milk

Mean values of 6 animals in each group of test are compared with the standard mean.[12]

CORTICOTROPIN

Adrenocorticotropin is a peptide hormone produced by anterior pituitary. Its primary endocrine function is to stimulate synthesis and release of cortisol by the adrenal cortex. Corticotropin can be used therapeutically, but a synthetic derivative, e.g. cosyntropin is more commonly and almost exclusively used to assess adrenocortical responsiveness.

IN VITRO STUDIES

Receptor-binding Assay

Adrenocorticotropin hormone (ACTH) was one of the first hormones that were shown to cause an increase in intracellular cAMP and one of the first peptides shown to bind specifically and reversibly to a cell surface receptor.[13] This receptor is primarily expressed in the adrenal cortex and the role of ACTH is to stimulate steroid production by target cells.

Demonstration of specific-binding of ACTH to receptors is extremely difficult. Cloning of the human ACTH receptor in 1992[14] permitted a detailed investigation of the ligand-binding and agonist properties of ACTH and its analogues.

Procedure

Stable Transfection of HeLa Cells

Human HeLa cells are cultured in DMEM with 10% FBS. The mouse ACTH receptor expression vector, in which the coding region of the gene is inserted into the pcDNA1 vector, is co-transfected with the pTK and neomycin resistance expression vector. Cells are selected in G418 (final conc. 800 µg/ml) and several resistant colonies are picked by ringing after 2 weeks. These cells are further cultured and are characterized for cAMP generation response to ACTH.

Stimulation of Cells with ACTH and Analogues

HeLa cells (5×10^5) are seeded into 6 well tissue culture dishes 24 h before stimulation. On the day of the experiment, cells are incubated in DMEM that include 1 mM 3-isobutyl-1-methylxanthine and incubated for 20 min at 37°C with increasing concentrations (10^{-12} to 10^7 M) of ACTH and various analogues. After incubation, the cells and the media are placed into Eppendorf tubes and boiled for 10 min, centrifuged at 10,000 rpm to discard the cell debris and stored at –20°C until aliquots are assayed to determine levels of cAMP, which is measured by a specific protein-binding assay.[15]

Ligand-binding Assay

The-binding assay is done by the method described by Penhoat et al.[16] HeLa cells are seeded into 12 well culture plates at a density of 10^6 cells/well. On the second day of the culture, the cells are washed and incubated for 60 min at 20°C with increasing concentrations of nonradioactive ACTH or various ACTH analogues and the reaction initiated on the addition of (^{125}I-iodotyrosyl) ACTH (2000 Ci/mmol, final concentration 0.1 pmol/l) in DMEM. Post incubation, the medium is removed and the cells washed for three times with 0.9% NaCl and then dissolved in 0.5 M NaOH/0.4% sodium deoxycholate (w/v). Each point is determined in triplicate and radioactivity is measured using a gamma counter. Specific-binding is determined by subtracting from the total-binding. Binding parameters are determined using the LIGAND programme.[17]

IN VIVO MODELS

Thymus Involution

Corticotropin can reduce thymus weight in a dose dependent manner. Young Wistar rats are sensitive to this effect of corticotropin.

Procedure

Sprague Dawley or Wistar rats of either sex of 7 to 10 days of age (10 to 15 g) are used and animals from the same litter are preferred for this experiment. The rat pups are randomly distributed into different groups of standard and test compounds. Drugs (both standard and test agents) are injected subcutaneously at different doses in oily suspension once daily for 3 days. Animals are sacrificed after 24 h of the last injection. Thymus glands are immediately dissected out and weighed. The response is expressed as the average of the individual weight for each dose of standard and test drug.[18]

Dose response curve of average weight is plotted against log dose of the drugs and the potency ratios are calculated by using 3+3 point assay.

Modifications

The sensitivity of the method can be enhanced by using the quotient between increase of the weight of the adrenals and decrease of the weight of the thymus gland.

Depletion of Adrenal Ascorbic Acid

Temporary reduction in adrenal ascorbic acid is observed after the administration of pituitary ACTH. The depletion of ascorbic acid is dose dependent. This relationship has been used for the quantitative assay of ACTH.

Procedure

Hypophysectomy is done in male Wistar rat (100 to 200 g) one day prior to the experiment. Three doses of test and standard are used. Test and standard preparations are dissolved in 0.5% phenol solution and diluted with gelatin solution. The hypophysectomized rats are randomly divided into 6 groups, each comprising of 6 to 8 animals. Each animal is injected (s.c.) with various doses of test compounds and standard. Post-treatment animals are anesthetized and both adrenal glands are removed, freed from external tissues, and finally their weight is recorded. The glands are homogenized in 4% trichloroacetic acid and the ascorbic acid determination is done according to the method of Roe and Kuether.[19]

Ascorbic Acid Determination

Trichloroacetic acid (4%) is added to 0.0, 0.5, 1, 2, 3, 4, 6, 8 ml of the 0.02% (w/v) ascorbic acid solution and 1, 1.5 and 2 ml of the 0.2% ascorbic acid solution to reach final volume of 8 ml. About 100 mg charcoal is added to each sample and is mixed by shaking for 1 min. The solutions are filtered after 5 min and an aliquot of 0.1 ml of the 6% thiourea solution is added to 2.0 ml of the filtrate followed by 0.5 ml dinitrophenylhydrazine solution. The whole mixture is shaken and heated at 57°C for 45 min in a water bath. The solutions are then placed in ice-cold water bath; and with further cooling, 2.5 ml of 85% sulfuric acid is added. At the wavelength of 540 nm, the calibration curve is established using the solution without ascorbic acid as a blank.

Preparations of the Adrenal Glands

The dissected adrenal glands are homogenized in 200 mg purified sand and 8 ml of 4% TCA. The reagents are added in a similar way for the calibration curve. The potency including the confidence limits is calculated by 3+3 assay.

Modifications

This ascorbic acid depletion test can also be performed in dexamethasone blocked rats. However, the potency ratios of various synthetic corticotropins have been found to be different in hypophysectomized rats.

Increased Corticosterone Level in Blood

In hypophysectomized or dexamethasone blocked rats, ACTH activity can be measured by the increase in corticosterone level in venous blood. This phenomenon is useful to measure the corticotropin activity of the corticotropin analogues.

Procedure

Male Sprague Dawley rats (150 to 200 g) are injected ACTH preparation or the standard dexamethasone (5 mg/kg) subcutaneously 24 h and 1 h prior to the experiment. Eight animals are taken for the each dose of test and standard. Rats are anesthetized with pentobarbital (60 mg/kg, i.p.) at various time intervals after ACTH injection and blood is withdrawn by cardiac puncture. One ml plasma is diluted with 2 ml distilled water and extracted with 5 ml petrol ether in order to remove the lipids. The petrol ether is discarded and 2 ml of water layer is extracted twice with 5 ml of methylene chloride by vigorous shaking for 15 minutes. The methylene chloride phase is separated by centrifugation. Both methylene chloride extracts are unified and shaken with 1 ml ice-cold 0.1 N NaOH. The water phase is immediately removed and the methylene chloride extracts dried by addition of sodium sulfate. Five ml of methylene chloride aliquot is mixed with 5 ml of fluorescence reagent. After vigorous shaking, the methylene chloride phase is removed and fluorescence is measured with primary filters of 436 mμ and secondary filters of 530 to 545 mμ. To establish a calibration curve, concentrations of 0, 20, 50, 100 and 250 μg/ml corticosterones are treated identically and measured in each assay.[20]

Using 3 doses of test compounds and standard, activity ratios with confidence limit can be determined with the help of 3+3 point assay.

Modifications

Corticosteroid can also be determined fluorimetrically in guinea pigs.[21]

GONADOTROPINS

Hypophysectomized Female Mice Model

Effect of FSH like activity can be evaluated by studying ovarian follicular development in adult hypophysectomized mice.

Procedure

Adult female mice undergo hypophysectomy and 12 days later the animals start receiving various doses of drug, subcutaneously daily for 4 day. The control group receives the same volume of vehicle subcutaneously. Ovine FSH subcutaneously (4 μg/day) can be used as standard to compare the FSH like activity of test drugs. After 4 days of treatment the ovaries are examined for follicular development. The FSH activity leads to increased number of preantral follicles (stage 1-3) as compared to control. The number of antral follicle, i.e. stage 4 and 5 starts increasing after 1 day of treatment with concomitant decrease in the number of atretic follicles. After 2 days of FSH treatment the follicles reach the stage 6 or the preovulatory size. The serum levels of progesterone and androstenedione also increase in the drug treated groups if the test drug possesses FSH like activity.[22]

Immature and Mature Male Rat Model

The male sex hormone, testosterone is secreted by the Leydig cells located in the interstitium of testes. The functions of Leydig cells are regulated by Luteinizing Hormone (LH) however the studies have revealed that FSH can modulate the LH response of Leydig cells indirectly through Sertoli cells.

Procedure

Twenty-eight day old immature or 90 day old adult male rats are used. The test group of rats receives different doses of drug by intraperitoneal route for 6 days. The control group receives the same volume of vehicle by same route. Another group of animals treated with recombinant human FSH (rFSH) (100 ng/day for immature rats and 300 ng/day for adult rats in 100 μl of gelatin phosphate buffered saline (GPBS) by intraperitoneal route for 6 days is added to compare the efficacy of test drugs. On the 7th day the animals are sacrificed and the testicular tissue from different groups is used to isolate Leydig cells and estimate *in vitro* testosterone production. The Leydig cells are isolated by collagenase dispersion of the testis and Percoll density gradient fractionation as described by Hardy et al. (1990)[23] and Sriraman et al. (2000).[24] As described by Sriraman and Rao (2004)[25] the Leydig cells (1×10^5) are cultured in 1 ml of medium containing 0.1% BSA at 34°C for 4 h in shaking water bath with or without 100 ng of hCG or 22-R-hydroxycholesterol (20 μM). The testosterone secreted in to the medium is estimated by radioimmunoassay. There is a significant increase in the amount of testosterone production in FSH treated groups.

Male Rat Model for LH Activity

The testosterone production by Leydig cells in testes is regulated by LH. LH stimulated increase in testosterone production can be used to evaluate LH like activity of investigational drugs.

Procedure

Male Wistar rats weighing 200-250 g and 3-4 month old are used. The interstitial tissue (containing Leydig cells) obtained from wet dissection of testes is incubated at 32°C for 1 h in 2 ml of Kreb's - Ringer bicarbonate buffer containing 0.2% glucose at pH 7.4. The tissue is further incubated with different concentrations of drug/vehicle/LH (100 ng/ml) in an atmosphere of O_2 + CO_2 (95:5). The incubation tubes are then placed in ice and total volume made up to 1 ml with Kreb's-Ringer Bicarbonate glucose buffer. The tissue is now homogenized using a sonicator. The homogenate is used for testosterone estimation by radioimmunoassay. Addition of LH or drugs with LH like activity significantly increases the testosterone synthesis as compared to control.[26]

Granulosa Cell Culture for Effects of FSH and LH

The granulosa cells from the ovarian follicles of rats when challenged with gonadotropins in culture show increased secretions of steroidal hormones, the estradiol and progesterone. These hormones can be estimated in culture medium to evaluate the gonadotropin like activity of test drug.

Procedure

The rats undergo hypophysectomy at the age of 23 days. The granulosa cells are obtained from the ovaries on day 26 using a needle and syringe. The collected cells are washed with serum free medium thrice. After each wash cells are separated by centrifugation (200 g, 10 min). Finally, the cells are suspended in 1:1 mixture of DMEM and Ham's F12 containing gentamicin, glutamine and sodium bicarbonate. After checking for cell viability with trypan blue, culture is established in multiwell plates at a concentration of 2×10^5 cells/ml. The culture is maintained at 37°C under 5% CO_2 atmosphere. To evaluate for the activity of drug the medium is supplemented with vehicle/drug/FSH/LH. The medium is collected at 48 h with addition of fresh medium. The medium is collected again after 48 h and the levels of estradiol and progesterone are measured by radioimmunoassay. The supplementation of medium with FSH (1-100 ng/ml) or LH (30 ng/ml) leads to significantly higher levels of estradiol, progesterone by 96 h of culture as compared to control.[27]

OXYTOCINS

Oxytocins are agents that increase the force and frequency of uterine contractions. Apart from this, they also cause milk ejection reflex and with higher doses, they produce reduction in blood pressure.

Isolated Uterus

Isolated uterus of virgin guinea pigs is very sensitive to oxytocin and is used to determine the oxytocic activity of the unknown compounds. In contrast to guinea pig uterus, isolated rat uterus is less sensitive, but it does not show spontaneous contraction in solution containing low calcium and glucose concentrations.[28]

Procedure

Female Wistar rats weighing 120 to 200 g are used. Eighteen to 20 h prior to the experiment, animals are injected (i.m.) with 100 mg of estradiol benzoate. One horn of the uterus is dissected out and suspended in De Jalon's solution, maintained at 32°C in tissue bath 10 ml in volume, bubbled with 95% oxygen and 5% carbon dioxide. Suspended tissue is allowed to rest for 30-60 min. Dose response curve of standard oxytocin and the test compounds are obtained. The potency of the test compound is evaluated by 2+2 assay.

Modifications

Apart from rat uterus, Berde et al.[29] used the rat uterus *in situ*, the cat uterus *in vitro* and the cat uterus in situ for the evaluation of synthetic analogues of oxytocin.

Stimulation of Myometrium

An improved bioassay for the testing of oxytocic compounds by the use of myometrium layer preparations has been developed to test the oxytocic activity of synthetic analogues in comparison to oxytocin.

Procedure

The vitality of the tissue is found for more than 8 h. The sensitivity of the bioassay is found in the region of 10^{-11}mol/l oxytocin. The maximum of the stimulation of muscle strips varies from 5×10^{-5} IU/ml to 10^{-4} IU/ml oxytocin in the organ bath. Various doses of synthetic hormone analogues are added to the organ bath and the contractions of the myometrium strips are recorded. The calculation of the results is afforded planimetrically and by measuring of the concentration-maximum during the testing period.[30]

Potency ratios of the test preparations are compared to standard by 2+2 assay.

Chicken Blood Pressure

Administration of oxytocin causes transient fall in blood pressure in chicken and also in other birds in a dose dependent manner, and this response is used to evaluate oxytocic property of unknown preparation.

Procedure

White Leghorn chickens (1.2 to 2.0 kg) are anesthetized by sodium pentobarbitone (200 mg/kg, i.v.). Ischiadic artery is cannulated and connected to polygraph. Baseline blood pressure is usually between 100 and 120 mm Hg. The crural vein is cannulated for injections of the test preparations. Different doses of oxytocin used as standard are chosen which cause fall of 20 to 40 mm Hg. Two doses of standard and test are selected and result is evaluated by 4-point assay.[31]

Milk Ejection Method

This is a sensitive method and shows the milk ejecting properties of oxytocic compounds.

Procedure

Female rabbits weighing 1.5 to 2 kg are anesthetized with urethene (700 mg/kg) or by pentobarbitone (40 mg/kg). One of 6 ducts of rabbit nipples are cannulated and connected to polygraph. Jugular vein is isolated for injecting test compound and standard. Time interval of the doses is kept at 3 to 10 min. Two doses of standard and test drugs are taken. Oxytocic potency ratios of the test preparations are evaluated by 2+2 assay.[32]

Modifications

Apart from rabbits, rats can also be used for this experiment. Female rat (300 g) in 3-21st day post-parturition is used. They are anesthetized with pentobarbital and tip of one teat is connected to the polygraph. Both standard and test compounds are injected through jugular/femoral vein.[33] Tindal and Yokoyama[34] recommended the use of guinea pigs applying the similar procedure but the injection of standard and test is given into the internal saphenous artery.

VASOPRESSIN

Vasopressin is structurally related to oxytocin. It is extracted from animal posterior pituitary. Vasopressin has both antidiuretic and vasopressor effects and is the main hormone regulating the body fluid osmolality.

Vasopressor Activity

Vasopressor activity can be demonstrated in animal by blocking response of other pressor substances in the body.[35]

Procedure

Male Wistar rats (300 g) are anesthetized with 1.75 mg/kg of urethane anesthesia (s.c.). After half an hour, the trachea of the animal is cannulated. Simultaneously, one femoral vein and one carotid artery are cannulated for drug injections and for the measurement of blood pressure respectively. Heparin (2,000 U/kg) is injected through the venous cannula. Dibenamine, which is going to block other pressor substances, is injected twice (i.v.) at 10 min interval at the concentration of 1 mg/kg. The basal blood pressure obtained is about 50 mm Hg. Different doses of vasopressin are injected and there is a dose dependent increase in blood pressure. Two selected doses from standard as well as test are repeatedly administered to obtain the Latin square design and potency ratio is calculated using 2+2 point assay.

Modifications

Apart from rats, rabbits can also be used.[36] Knape and van Zwieten[37] used pithed rat to study vasoconstrictor activity of vasopressin after pretreatment with various drugs.

Vasopresser Activity in Guinea Pig Ileum

Procedure

Guinea pigs of either sex (0.5 to 1 kg) are sacrificed under ether anesthesia. Ileum is dissected out and cut into 2 to 3 cm pieces. Pieces of guinea pig ileum are suspended in an organ bath. The contractions of ileum in response to the standard and test drugs are measured by a strain gauge transducer. Potency ratios are calculated using 2+2 point assay.[38]

Antidiuretic Activity

Various tests in water loaded rat model were developed by Burn[39] to demonstrate antidiuretic activity of vasopressin.

Procedure

Wistar or Sprague Dawley rats of either sex (140 to 250 g) are used for the experiment. One preliminary test is carried out with the saline solution instead of the test preparation. 0.1 ml of saline per 100 g body weight is injected (i.v.). Any rat showing undue excitement or frequent micturition or stress is not taken for the main test. Food and water are not given during the tests. Animals are divided into various groups of standard or test drug, each comprising of 6 animals. Animals are weighed and placed in separate chambers. They are given warmed water through Ryle's tube and urine of each animal is collected. Rats are provided total water load equivalent to 8% of the animal's body weight.

Urine during the first 5 min after injection is discarded and the same is collected at an interval of 15 min until the excreted urine volume becomes greater than 30% of the total water load. The potency ratio is calculated from 2+2 point assay.

Modifications

Hydrated conscious dogs were used to test the antidiuretic activity of vasopressin by van Dyke et al.[40]

Hereditary Model (Brattleboro Strain)

These animals have genetic deficiency of vasopressin synthesis. Schmale et al.[41] observed a single base deletion in the vasopressin gene, which ultimately causes diabetes insipidus in Brattleboro rats.

Procedure

Animals are placed in metabolic cages provided with a wire mesh bottom and a funnel to collect the urine. Stainless-steel sieves are placed in the funnel to retain the feces. Animals are given standard diet and water ad libitum. Fifteen hours prior to the experiment, food and water are withdrawn. For screening procedures, two groups of three animals are used for one dose of the test compound. The test agent is given orally dissolved in 5 ml of water/kg body weight. Two groups of 3 animals receive 1 g/kg urea orally. Additionally, 5 ml of 0.9% NaCl solution per 100 g body weight are given by gavage. Urine excretion is recorded after 5 and 24 h. Sodium content is determined by flame photometry.

THYROID HORMONES

Thyroid gland secretes two hormones thyroxine and tri-iodothyronine, commonly called as T4 and T3, respectively. Various bioassays are following to screen thyroid hormone analogues for their activity.

IN VITRO METHODS

Lipogenic Enzyme Assay

Fish of body weight 20 ± 2.0 g are collected from fresh water bodies. Liver samples are collected and are pooled as well as minced with ice-cold Hank's balanced salt solution (HBSS). Samples are centrifuged and a known quantity of the liver samples are transferred to separate culture flasks containing ^{14}C-acetate in 2 ml culture medium (HBSS) and various concentrations (10^{-7}, 10^{-8} or 10^{-9} M) of test agents and standard (thyroxine). Medium without hormone serves as control group. Samples are incubated at 30°C in a shaking water bath for 8 h. Post-incubation, samples are washed in HBSS to remove unbound ^{14}C-acetate. Samples are stored at –20°C for analysis of ^{14}C-acetate incorporation into lipids. Similar experiments without ^{14}C-acetate are done to assay lipogenic enzymes. Major lipogenic enzymes are measured in the liver samples and the values are expressed as IU/mg protein. Absorbance is recorded by using spectrophotometer. Lipids are extracted from the liver tissue. Extracted lipids are separated by thin layer chromatography (TLC). Lipids of interest are collected from the TLC plate and placed in a separate scintillation vials containing 5 ml of scintillate fluid and 0.2 g of 1, 4 bis (2-15-phenyloxazolyl) benzene/liter. Activity is counted in scintillation counter and expressed as cpm/mg tissue.[42]

Tadpole Tail Culture Method

The tadpole (*Xenopus laevis*) is a valuable model for thyroid hormone actions as the chemical structure of thyroxine and T3 in *Xenopus* are similar to mammalian thyroid hormones. The process of metamorphosis in tadpole is dependent on the availability of thyroid hormones from developing thyroid gland. Moreover, each tissue responds directly and independently to thyroid hormones in organ culture.

Procedure

Tadpole tails are cultured according to the procedure described by Tata et al. (1991).[43] Staged tadpoles are first treated with Steinberg's solution (10 mm Hepes, 60 mM NaCl, 0.67mM KCl, 0.34 mM $Ca(NO_3)_2$, 0.83 mM $MgSO_4$, pH 7.4) containing gentamicin (70 µg/ml) and streptomycin (200 µg/ml). Twenty-four hours later tadpoles are anesthetized in water containing 0.01% amino ester benzoic acid and 6 mm of the tail is cut and transferred to 1 ml of Steinberg's solution containing antibiotics and 5 µg/ml insulin in falcon tissue culture dishes. The drug treatment is instituted 24 h later with change of culture medium every 48 h. The length of each tail is measured every 24 h and a comparison between the control and test groups is made.

IN VIVO METHODS

Thyroidectomy

Pharmacological evaluation of thyroid hormones and analogues are mainly performed in thyroidectomized rats. Bomskov et al.[44] described the methods of thyroidectomy in various animal species such as guinea pigs, rats and mice.

Procedure

Neck fur of the animal is removed with electric clippers and the area is disinfected. A median incision of 2 cm is made upwards from the sternum. On both sides, large salivary glands and maxillary lymph nodes are pushed to the side to make muscles covering the trachea visible. This muscle is split. The isthmus of the thyroid glands is separated from trachea and blood vessels are ligated. Alternatively, thyroid can be removed by electrocauterization.[45]

Iodine Release Inhibition

^{131}I release from thyroid gland is inhibited by thyroxine and the degree of inhibition is dose dependent.[46] This activity is used to compare the potency of thyroid hormone derivatives with standard thyroxine.

Procedure

Male Sprague Dawley rats (200 to 240 g) are fed with normal diet with or without supplementation of 0.03% propylthiouracil. ^{131}I is administered (i.p.) and food is withheld for 8 h before and 24 h after the ^{131}I injection. Thereafter, the radioactivity over the thyroid region is determined 40 h later under light ether anesthesia. This value is taken as a zero time and after this reading, diet is changed to the diet containing 0.03% propylthiouracil and various doses of standard and test preparations are injected (s.c.) at 24 h intervals for a total of four doses.

After last 4 doses, percent zero counts of the remaining ^{131}I is plotted against logarithm of the dose and potency ratios of unknown are calculated from this curve.

Antigoitrogenic Activity

Administration of the exogenous goitrogenic compounds block thyroid hormone secretion resulting in reduced thyroid hormone level in circulation. This stimulates the secretion of thyroid stimulating hormone (TSH), which induces the enlargement of the thyroid gland. By the administration of thyroxine or other thyroid derivatives, thyroid gland hyperplasia can be prevented.

Procedure

Male Sprague-Dawley rats (150 to 180 g) are divided into various groups, each comprising of 8 to 10 animals. During treatment period, 0.1% thiouracil is added to food. After 2 weeks, rats are administered test or the standard drug (thyroxine) subcutaneously at the dose of 10 to 40 mg/kg. Animals in the control group receive thiouracil diet and saline injection only and are fed normal diet. Rats are sacrificed after 2 weeks. Thyroid gland is dissected out and weighed.

Weight of the thyroid gland is increased by 2 to 3 times by thiouracil diet and the size is reversed to normal in dose dependent manner by thyroidal substances.[46] Dose response curve of standard and test compounds are plotted and potency ratio is calculated.

Reduction in Tensile Strength

Short-term treatment with thyroid hormone decreases tensile strength of connective tissue in a dose dependent manner. This activity can be used to evaluate the thyroid hormone derivatives.

Procedure

Male Sprague Dawley rats (100 to 120 g) are administered various doses of thyroid hormone subcutaneously. After 24 h, animals are sacrificed and the tensile strength of the distal femoral epiphyseal plates, tail tendons or skin strips is measured by the following methods.

a. *Measurement of tensile strength of femoral epiphyseal plates*: After sacrificing the animal, the hind legs are stretched at the hip joints and fastened at the column femoris. Longitudinal tension results in rupture of the femoral epiphyseal cartilage. The ultimate load of the femoral epiphyseal plate is registered by an instrument at an extension rate of 5 cm/min.[47] Single injection of thyroid hormone results in decrease in tensile strength in a dose dependent manner.
b. *Measurement of tensile strength of tail tendons*: After sacrificing the animal, the tail is amputated at the base and tail skin is removed. Single tendons are pulled out from the dorsal and ventral bundles and kept in normal saline. Tendons of the same diameter (0.25 mm) are selected and tendons of the same vertebral insertion are tested alternatively. The tendons are fixed in special clamps at a distance of 2 cm and immersed in a bath with physiological saline. Stress-strain curves and ultimate loads are determined with an Instron[46] instrument with an extension rate of 5 cm/min.[48]
c. *Measurement of tensile strength of skin strips*: The animal is sacrificed and the back is shaved and a skin flap of about 5 × 5 cm is removed. The skin flap is placed between 2 pieces of plastic material with known thickness and the actual thickness of the excised skin is measured by calipers. Two dumb-bell shaped specimens are cut with a special punch in perpendicular direction to the body axis. They are fixed between the clamps of an Instron[46] instrument. Stress-strain curves and ultimate loads are registered at a strain rate of 5 cm/min. From stress-strain curves, the values of ultimate load and extension are registered.[49]

   Dose response curve of different doses of test compounds and standard are established and potency ratio is calculated.

PARATHYROID HORMONE

Parathyroid hormone (PTH) acts chiefly on bone and kidney by regulating calcium and phosphate passage. Processes that are regulated by parathyroid hormone includes the absorption of calcium from the gastrointestinal tract, the deposition and mobilization of bone calcium and the control of excretion of calcium in urine, feces, sweat and milk.

IN VITRO METHODS

Tissue Culture Assay

The tissue culture technique is based on the method described by Fell and Weiss et al.[50] for the study of PTH induced bone resorption *in vitro*. For 2+2 assay design, 40 mice, 6 to 9 day old are required. The mice near the same age and size from two or three complete liters are chosen. The calvaria are dissected out under sterile conditions. The bone samples are pooled immediately into culture fluid at room temperature. The calvaria are cleaned and trimmed in order to get a symmetrical bone sample consisting of two parietal bones. This is halved along the sagittal suture and the halves are placed on wire table in each of the pair of culture vessels inside a petridish unit. Two halved calveria per pair of culture dishes are needed when the volume of culture fluid is 2 ml. Thereafter, petridishes are kept in incubator at 37°C with 5% CO_2 in air for 10 min. After 3 days, culture fluid is removed with a sterile Pasteur pipette and is retained for analysis. Fresh medium containing PTH derivatives are then added to one of the pair of culture vessels, the other receiving medium without PTH, to serve as the control. Experiment is terminated after 3 days and the medium from each culture vessels is numbered at the beginning of the experiment and various doses of test compounds are alternated throughout all the dishes.

Samples of rat serum and medium are directly placed into Auto Analyzer cups and stored at 4°C until analyzed. A technicon Auto Analyser is used for estimation of calcium and phosphate. When tissue culture media are being analyzed, a sample of medium without serum from the batch of media, which is used for the experiment, is run at the beginning and end of each set of samples.

IN VIVO METHODS

Increase in Serum Calcium

Administration of parathyroid extract results in increase in serum calcium level in animals. Dogs, rabbits and rats can be used as animal models. However, healthy rats are insensitive to parathyroid hormone but sensitivity can be increased by parathyroidectomy.

Procedure

Parathyroidectomy is performed in anesthetized male Wistar rats (200 to 250 g) by cauterization. After a recovery period of 1 week, blood is withdrawn by retro-orbital puncture. Various doses of test and standard preparations are given (s.c.) to different groups comprising of 6 to 8 animals. Retro-orbital puncture is performed again after 21 hours. Blood samples from all the groups are collected and centrifuged and finally calcium is determined in the serum by flame photometry.[51]

Mean values of the increase in serum calcium are plotted against log dose of the test preparations and standard. Thereafter, potency ratio is calculated.

Modifications

Treatment with parathyroid hormone in normal rats and in rats with osteoporosis induced by pregnancy and lactation under a low calcium diet show increase in whole body calcium and skeletal mass was found by Hefti et al.[52]

Decrease in Serum Phosphate Level

This method involves the decrease in serum phosphate following the injection of parathyroid hormone.

Procedure

Male Wistar rats (150 to 200 g) are fed normal diet for 2 weeks before the experiment. During the experiment, animals are only allowed to have water. Blood sample (0.6 ml) is taken out from each animal of different groups given test and standard preparations. It is centrifuged for 10 min and 0.2 ml of sample serum of each animal is added to 6 ml of 10% trichloroacetic acid. Again, this preparation is centrifuged and 5 ml of aliquot is used for the estimation of inorganic phosphorus. Serum phosphorus is measured initially and 3 h after subcutaneous administration of various doses of test and standard.[53]

Dose response curve of test drug and standard preparations is established to calculate the potency ratio.

cAMP Release

Parathyroid hormone and its derivatives cause release of cAMP from adult bone and this can be measured in a perfusion system of isolated rat femora.

Procedure

Femur is removed from five-week-old Wistar rats under anesthesia. Adhering muscles are cleaned from the bone. A hole is made at the nutrient foramen below the femoral neck. Thereafter, a 21-gauge needle is inserted through the hole to avoid the leakage of the perfusate. The bone is then placed in an apparatus for liver perfusion and perfused at a flow rate of 1 ml/5 min by a pump with Krebs-Ringer bicarbonate continuously gassed with 95% O_2 and CO_2 and containing 1 mg/ml glucose. Once the perfused bone is assembled, the bone is allowed to equilibrate for 45 min. Samples are collected into a chilled tube for determination of basal cAMP levels. Then various doses of the test preparations or the standard are injected for 5 min. In the perfusate, cAMP in the perfusate is measured by radioimmunoassay.[54] Dose response curve of test and standard preparations are obtained to calculate the potency.

Modifications

Activation of plasma membrane adenylatecyclase in canine renal cortex by parathyroid hormone was measured by Nissenson et al.[55] Saito et al.[56] established a new biological assay where eleven day old chick embryonic femur is labeled with ^{45}Ca *in vitro*. t1/2 is calculated from the sequential release of labeled calcium into the medium. Parathyroid hormone reduces the t1/2 indicating enhanced bone resorption. Docherty and Heath[57] used osteosarcoma cells for an *in vitro* bioassay determining cAMP formation.

Cytochemical Bioassay

This method has been developed to determine agonist and antagonist activities of parathyroid hormone analogue.[58]

Procedure

Renal Cytochemical Assay

Kidney segments from guinea pigs are maintained in non-proliferative organ culture for 5 h using Trowell's T8 medium. The medium is changed before exposure to various doses of standard and test drug for an additional 8 min. To test the antagonistic activities, each segment is exposed to a single concentration of hPTH- (1-84) (106 fmol/l) or to hPTH-(1-34) (255 fmol/l) in the presence or absence of the analog being tested. The segments are then stored at –70°C in N-hexane before being sectioned at 16 μm on a cryostat. The sections are then examined for their glucose-6-phosphate dehydrogenase activity. The precipitated formazane activity is then quantified in the cells of the distal convoluted tubules by means of a microdensitometer (585 nm).

For Metatarsal Cytochemical Assay

Metatarsals of young female Wistar rats (50 to 100 g) are removed and are maintained individually in non-proliferative organ culture in 5 to 15 ml of Trowell's T8 medium (pH 7.8) in presence of 95% O_2 and 5% CO_2 at 37°C for 5 h. After the culture period, the medium is discarded and each metatarsal is exposed to fresh medium containing a low priming dose of PTH (0.5 fg/ml) for 8 min followed by exposure to known concentrations of standard PTH or various concentration of PTH analogues for 8 min. The metatarsals are then briefly dipped in a 5% solution of polyvinyl alcohol and chilled immediately in N-hexane at –70°C.

Each bone is sectioned by cryostat. The sections are then examined for their glucose-6-phosphate dehydrogenase activity in a similar way described in renal cytochemical assay. The enzyme activity of each section is measured in 10 individual hypertrophic chondrocytes or osteoblasts lining the metaphyseal trabeculae by scanning and integrating micro-densitometry at a wavelength of 585 nm. Dose response curves are tested for linearity and parallelism and potency ratios against standard is calculated.

ADRENAL STEROIDS

Adrenal glands lie at the superior poles of two kidneys and are composed of two distinct parts- adrenal medulla and adrenal cortex. The adrenal cortex releases a large number of steroids into the circulation. The hormonal steroids may be classified as:

a. Glucocorticoids, having important effect on intermediary metabolism.
b. Mineralocorticoids, having principally salt-retaining activity.

Both natural and synthetic corticosteroids are used for diagnosis and treatment of disorders of adrenal function. They are also used in the treatment of a variety of inflammatory and immunologic disorders.

GLUCOCORTICOIDS

IN VITRO METHODS

Receptor Binding Assay

The relative-binding affinities for the glucocorticoid receptor present in rat liver or thymus cytosol can be measured by competitive displacement of [^{3}H]-dexamethasone.

Procedure

Male Wistar rat (130 to 150 g) is adrenalectomized under ether anesthesia. After two days of adrenalectomy, liver is surgically removed and homogenized in phosphate buffer containing 50 mM Tris HCl, 1 mM EDTA, 2 mM dithiothretol, 10 mM Na_2MnO_4 and 10% glycerol (pH 7.4). The homogenate is centrifuged for 1 h at 10.500 g at 4°C and supernatant is collected. The cytosol is mixed with 5 nM [^{3}H]-dexamethasone in presence or absence of competitors and incubated for 2 h at 4°C. The reaction is terminated by the addition of hydroxyapatite to separate the receptor steroid complex from the free [^{3}H]-dexamethasone. The radioactivity bound to the receptors is determined by liquid scintillation spectrometry.[59] IC_{50} values are estimated by probit analysis.

Modifications

Apart from the rat liver, cytosol can be prepared from other organs such as cultured hepatoma cells, from normal human lymphocytes, thymocytes from rat thymus gland, from human leukemic lymphoid cell line, from rat and human lung.[60-65] Transient co-transfection of receptor cDNA and suitable receptor genes were used to study human glucocorticoid receptor function using CV-1 mammalian cell line. Various natural and synthetic steroids have been analyzed to see whether they can activate gene expression through glucocorticoid receptors.

Transactivation Assay

Transactivation assay is useful in determining steroid agonistic and antagonistic properties.[66] The transactivation assay is based on the principle that steroid receptor proteins act as ligand regulated tanscriptional activators. After-binding of hormone, the steroid receptor interacts with hormone responsive elements (HREs) of hormone regulated genes, thereby inducing a cascade of transcriptional events.[67]

The transactivation assay determines the agonist and also the antagonistic potency of a given compound by induction or inhibition of reporter gene activity.[68]

Procedure

CV-1 cells and COS-1 for transient transfection are grown in DMEM supplemented with 10% fetal calf serum, 4 mmol/l L-glutamine, penicillin and streptomycin. Stable and transient transfections are performed by using Lipofectin Reagent according to the procedure of Flegner et al.[69]

Stable transfections are carried out as described by Fuhrmann et al.[70] For transient transfections, 1 × 10^6 COS-1 or CV-1 cells are harvested onto 100 mm dishes one day prior to transfection. After 24 h, when cells become about 80% confluent, cells are washed twice with 1 ml Opti-MEM per dish to prepare for transfection. For each dish, 5 μg pHGO (hGR expression plasmid) and 5 μg pM MTV-CAT are diluted with 1 ml of Opti-MEM. Next, the DNA and the Lipofectin Reagent dilutions are combined in a polystyrene snap-cap tube to obtain 2 ml of transfection solution per dish, gently mixed and incubated at room temperature for 5 min and added to the washed cells. After 5 h, the transfection solution is replaced by 6 ml DMEM containing 10% fetal calf serum.

After 24 h of transfection, transiently transfected cells are trypsinized, pooled and replated onto 60 mm dishes at a density of 4.5 × 10^5 per dish to study the effect of glucocorticoids analogues. Stably transfected cells are seeded onto 6-well dishes (1 × 10^5 cells/dish). Cells are cultured in medium supplemented with 3% charcoal stripped FCS and appropriate hormones for 48 h. Cells are cultured in 1% ethanol and act as negative controls for reporter gene incubation.

CAT Assay

By freezing and thawing (37°C water bath) for at least three times, transiently transfected cells and stably transfected cells are disrupted. Protein concentrations of the cell extracts are determined according to the method of Bradford.[71] The CAT assay is performed by the method of Gorman et al.[72] After the cells are centrifuged for 15 min at 4°C, the supernatants are separated for enzyme assay. The assay mixture contains (final vol 180 ml) 100 ml of 0.25 M Tris-HCl, 20 ml of cell extract, 1 mCi of [^{14}C] chloramphenicol and 20 ml of 4 mM acetyl co-enzyme A. Controls contain CAT instead of cell extract. All the reagents except coenzyme A are preincubated together for 5 min at 37°C. After equilibration is reached at this temperature, the reaction is started by adding coenzyme A and is terminated by 2 ml cold ethyl acetate. The organic mixture is dried and is taken up in 30 ml of ethyl acetate and spotted on silica gel thin layer plate. The plate is developed in a mixture of chloroform: methanol (95:5). The spots are cut and transferred to the counting vials. Data are expressed as the amount of chloramphenicol acetylated by 20 ml of the extract. Concentration-response for CAT induction is established to determine the potency of test hormone. Dexamethasone (10^{-10} to 10^{-6}mol/l) is used as a standard.

Inhibition of Cell Growth

Human fibroblasts are grown in Eagle's Minimum Essential Medium supplemented with 10% fetal calf serum. The cultures are buffered by the addition of $NaHCO_3$ to the medium and are maintained on 5% CO_2 and 95% air in an incubator. Cells are subcultured in 25 cm^2 culture flask. Treated cultures receive test compounds dissolved in 95% ethanol while control cultures receive ethanol alone. With the addition of 10 μl aliquots of these solutions, the final concentration of ethanol (0.063%) does not affect cell growth in control cultures. Designating the day of drug addition as day 0, cells are harvested and are counted on day 5 when the cells are still in logarithmic phase growth. Cells are trypsinized (1:250 trypsin) and are scraped from the culture flask. The results are expressed in terms of percentage of control cell growth.

This expression is obtained by dividing the difference in cell counts between day 5 and day 0 cultures, which have been treated with drug.

Tyrosine Aminotransferase Activity

Glucocorticoid induces tyrosine aminotransferase synthesis in hepatoma tissue culture cells.[73]

Procedure

Hepatoma tissue culture cells are grown at a density of about 8×10^5 cells/ml. Before centrifugation, cells are washed 3 times at 0°C with buffer. After centrifugation, cell pellets are resuspended in serum free medium containing 0.1% BSA and 0.1% $NaHCO_3$. Standard (dexamethasone) and test steroids of different concentrations are added to the supernatant of cell suspension. After 16 h of incubation at 37°C, the cells are harvested and tyrosine aminotransferase is determined. The cells are washed twice and then disrupted with an ultrasonicator. The enzyme is assayed at 37°C by conversion of p-hydroxyphenylpyruvate to p-hydroxybenzylaldehyde.

Enzyme specific activity is expressed in milliunit of tyrosine aminotransferase/mg of cell protein. Standard dose response curve is drawn and potency of test preparation is calculated.

IN VIVO METHODS

Adrenalectomy in Rats

Majority of the studies regarding the evaluation of the physiological role and pathological effect is done in adrenalectomized animal.

Procedure

Sprague Dawley or Wistar rat (120 to 150 g) of either sex is first anesthetized in a closed vessel containing ether. The dorsal fur is shaved and the rat is placed on a wooden block on its abdomen with fore and hind limb well extended. In this position, the spine tends to arch which is a useful landmark for skin incision. A transverse incision of about 5 mm long is made in the midline at the costovertebral angle. To remove the left adrenal gland, the skin is retracted to the ventral side and the lumber muscles are incised just superior and anterior to the splenic shadow. Now the gland is visible just below the incision. The adrenal gland along with the periadrenal fat is removed. Any remnants of the capsule to which cortical tissue may adhere are removed.

After surgical removal of the left gland, the animal is turned around and the right gland is removed through skin incision. A small incision is made through the lumber muscles above and anterior to the lumbocostal artery near the costal margin. With the help of curved forceps, liver is elevated which covers the adrenal gland on this side; and thereafter, the gland along with periadrenal fat and the mesentric attachments is removed. The skin is closed by skin clip. The entire procedure is done within a short period of time so that additional ether anesthesia is not to be given. The animals become normal within a few minutes following the surgery.[74]

Adrenal and Thymus Gland Atrophy

When corticosteroid is administered repeatedly, it is going to produce both central and peripheral effects. In immature rat, thymus gland involution is seen. Adrenal gland atrophy is observed when ACTH secretion from pituitary is inhibited.

Procedure

Immature male Sprague Dawley rats are used for this experiment. Animals are injected different doses of test drug subcutaneously daily for 6 days. Standard hydrocortisone is given daily at the dose of 0.05 mg per animal. Vehicle is injected to the control group in similar frequency. On 7th day, all animals are sacrificed and the adrenal and thymus gland weight is determined.

The degree of reduction of the weight of thymus gland represents the degree of catabolic activity of the test compounds. Involution of the adrenal glands is a measure of the ability of the compound to inhibit the secretion of ACTH from pituitary. From the dose response curves of these two parameters of the standard, the potency of the test compound is compared.

Decrease in Eosinophillic Cell Count

Reduction in eosinophillic cell count occurs in animals as well as in man by glucocorticoids. By this phenomenon, glucocorticoid effect can be quantitated in adrenalectomized mice *in vivo*.

Procedure

Male albino mice (20 to 25 g) are adrenalectomized and they are maintained at 28°C with 1% NaCl in place of drinking water. Fifteen milligram pellets of deoxycorticosterone acetate (DOCA) are implanted at the time of operation. Steroids are dissolved in benzyl alcohol or mixed with sesame oil. Three days after the operation, the mice receive 5 μg of epinephrine subcutaneously and after 4 h, various concentrations of test substance are given. Blood samples are obtained from tail before and 3 h after the steroid injection.[75]

Potency ratio of the test compound is calculated from the dose response curve of the standard.

Liver Glycogen Test

It is a simple and specific test for evaluation of glucocorticoid activity.

Procedure

Male Sprague Dawley rats (140 to 160 g) are adrenalectomized and given standard laboratory diet and 1% NaCl instead of drinking water. On the 4th postoperative day, food is withdrawn; and on the 5th day of operation, drinking fluid is withdrawn. Animals are given test compound by a single subcutaneous injection dissolved in sesame oil. After 7 h, rats are sacrificed under anesthesia and liver is dissected out. Liver is perfused with double distilled water to remove blood. Following this, liver is weighed and put into the flasks containing hot 30% potassium hydroxide and digested on a hot plate. The digest is diluted and aliquot is assayed for liver glycogen by an anthrone procedure.[76]

Calibration curves are established using glucose as a standard. Three doses of test compound and of standard are given to the animals in order to find dose response activities. From mean values, dose response curves are established for each compound and potency ratio is calculated from standard curve.

MINERALOCORTICOIDS

IN VITRO METHODS

Receptor-binding Assay

For mineralocorticoid receptor-binding assay, rat kidney preparations and radioactive-labeled aldosterone are used.

Procedure

Kidney is dissected out from adrenalectomized rats and homogenized in phosphate buffer solution containing 10 mM Tris, 0.25 M saccharose and HCl, pH 7.4. Supernatant is obtained after centrifugation at 0°C for 10 min at 8000 g. RU 28362 is added at the concentration of 0.001 M to the aliquot in order to inhibit binding of aldosterone to the glucocorticoid receptor. The aliquot is again centrifuged at 10.500 g for 60 min. The cytosol (supernatant) is removed and kept for incubation at 0°C with different concentrations of test compounds and [^{3}H]-aldosterone (5 nM). Nonspecific binding is determined in presence of 1 mM aldosterone.

By the help of charcoal-dextran technique, free [^{3}H]-aldosterone is separated after 1 h or 24 h of incubation. Supernatant is centrifuged and concentration of bound ligand is determined by liquid scintillation counter. The following parameters are calculated:

a. Total binding of [^{3}H]-aldosterone
b. Nonspecific binding
c. Specific binding: Total binding—nonspecific binding
d. % inhibition: 100—specific binding as percentage of the control value.

Binding potency of the test compounds is evaluated as the relative-binding affinity with respect to the standard.[77]

Modifications

Mineralocorticoid receptor-binding assay can also be done in the supernatant of rabbit kidney or rat kidney slices. Arizza et al.[78] cloned the transfected monkey kidney cells with plasmids containing the human mineralocorticoid receptor.

IN VIVO METHODS

Electrolyte Excretion

Sodium retention and potassium excretion is increased by mineralocorticoids. This property can be used to estimate mineralocorticoid activity of the unknown compound.

Procedure

Male Sprague Dawley rats (140 to 160 g) are adrenalectomized and are given normal laboratory diet and 1% NaCl instead of plain water. Food and NaCl are withdrawn on the 4th postoperative day. Next day, each animal is given water by Ryle's tube followed by 0.9% NaCl orally and injected with test compounds suspended in vehicle. To collect the urine, each animal is anesthetized by ether and the bladder is evacuated. The animals are kept in cages for 4 h and then further they are anesthetized with the same anesthetic agent and are removed from the cages. Urine volume is measured and diluted. Appropriate dilutions are analyzed for sodium with a flame photometer. Deoxycorticosterone acetate is used as a standard.[79]

Potency ratio of the test compound is calculated by comparing the dose response curve of the test drug with that of the standard.

Modifications

Both sodium and potassium concentration were estimated by Simpson and Tait[80] in urine and the sodium to potassium ratio is used as a index of mineralocorticoid activity of the test compound. Nikisch et al.[81] infused glucocorticoid substituted adrenalectomized rats with saline glucose containing aldosterone. The sodium and potassium concentration of urine in 1 h fractions are calculated.

ANDROGENS

The principal circulating androgen in men is testosterone. Androgens are responsible for male sexual differentiation *in utero* and male pubertal changes. The clearest indication for the administration of testosterone is male hypogonadism.

IN VITRO METHODS

Receptor-binding Assay

Prostate, from Wistar male rats (150 to 200 g) castrated 24 h before sacrifice, are removed. They are minced and homogenized in three volumes of Tris-HCl buffer, pH 7.4 (20 mmol/l) containing EDTA and dithiothreitol (1.5 mmol/l) each. The homogenate is centrifuged at 1,05,000 g for 1 h to obtain the cytosol fraction.[82] Cytosol (2 ml) is preincubated with [^{3}H]-5 alpha dihydrotestosterone (2×10^{-9} mol/l) at 0°C for 30 min to ensure equal concentration of the label in all parallely processed samples. Aliquot portions (150 μl) of cytosol labeled with [^{3}H] dihydrotestosterone are labeled to the dry residue of tested steroid, mixed and incubated at 0°C under shaking for 2 h. For standard (dihydrotestosterone) and test 2.5, 5, 10, 20×10^{-9} mol/l concentrations are taken. Separation of free and bound ligands and the determination of the-binding characteristics are carried out by a polyacrylamide gel electrophoresis method of Krieg et al.[83]

Modifications

Tezon et al.[84] studied the influence of androgen and antiandrogens on androgen receptors, which are distributed intracellularly in the rat epididymis.

The use of tritiated 7 alpha, 17 alpha-dimethyl-19-nor-testosterone for the assay of androgen receptors was recommended by Schilling and Liao.[85]

Sebum Secretion Test in Rat

Androgens are known to have an effect on sebaceous gland in rat as described by Archibald and Shuster et al.[86] A bioassay for androgenic and non-androgenic steroids is developed on the basis of this effect. The sebum secretion rate stimulated by androgenic hormones is found parallel to increasing dose of androgenic steroids. This bioassay system can be used to evaluate various androgenic and anti-androgenic substances for their activity.

Procedure

Measurement of sebum secretion in rat

The procedure of surface lipid extraction and measurement of sebum secretion rate were depicted by Archibald and Shuster et al. Pre-pubertally castrated male rats are used, when they reached a weight of 150-200 g and age of 6 to 24 weeks. They are anesthetized with ether in glass jar. The anesthetized rats are suspended by the forepaws and immersed in 300 ml of solvent (an ethanol-ether mixture which gave a 90-94 % extraction of surface lipid) with the head extended so that the ears remain above the surface of the solvent. After 60 sec the rats are gently lifted up and down 6 times and transferred to a second volume of solvent for a further 30 sec. The rats are dried with a hot air blower and returned to the cage. The solutions are filtered into weighed aluminium cups and evaporated to dryness in a fume cupboard. The cups were then re-weighed. The minimum 2 extractions are required for the same rat for lipid extraction. The quantity of lipid recovered from each extraction is calculated as a percentage of total lipids removed from each rat.

By subsequent dipping at different time intervals it is shown that up to 4 days after the first lipid extraction the rate of accumulation of lipid is found linear; after this it tends to flatten off. It is therefore possible to measure the sebum secretion rate from surface lipid accumulation during the first 4 days after an initial defatting and four-day sebum collections are made in all assays.[87]

Bioassay Method of Androgens

The response to increasing concentration of androgenic steroid daily is measured at intervals for a month. The slope of the dose-response curves increases rapidly until the 17th day after which it increased very little. In all subsequent assays a 13 to 17 day collection of sebum is therefore made.

The sebum secretion rate is shown to increase in dose of androgenic steroids and vice versa. This bioassay can be used to assess the androgenic potential of unknown compounds.[88]

IN VIVO METHODS

Castration Procedure

Castration is best performed in young male rats weighing not more than 60 g. Under ether anesthesia, a small transverse incision is given in the skin on the ventral site over the symphysis.

Testis present in the scrotum is gently pushed into the abdominal cavity. The abdomen is then opened and with the help of forceps, the testis with the epididymis is pulled out from the wound. The ductus deferens with the testicular vessels is separated and the testis together with the epididymal fat pad is removed with the help of a fine scissors. The same procedure is performed on the other side. The skin wound is closed with wound clips. The animal recovers immediately with no bleeding.[89]

Chicken Comb Method

Growth of capon comb by androgen has been a popular method to evaluate androgenic activity. This method is useful for the isolation and structural elucidation of natural androgens.

Procedure

Single comb White Leghorn chicks (2 to 3 day old) are used for the experiment. At the beginning of the assay, the sum of the length and height of each comb is calculated. Chickens are distributed in different groups, each comprising of 8 animals. Chickens are injected with various doses of standard (olive oil as vehicle) and the test preparations intramuscularly daily for 5 consecutive days. Twenty-four hours after the last injection, chickens are sacrificed and comb size is determined by excision. Growth of the comb is expressed as the sum of length and height in millimeters.[90]

The mean values of each group are calculated and plotted as dose response curve for the test compound and the standard in order to calculate the potency ratio of the unknown.

Modifications

Newly hatched chicks of either sex can be used to study growth of the combs after systemic and local administration.

Growth of Secondary Sex Organs

Androgens have a dose dependent effect on male secondary sex organs. The growth of ventral prostate, seminal vesicles and musculus levatorani is dependent on androgen.

Procedure

Castrated immature male Sprague Dawley rats are used for the experiment. The rats are administered various doses of test preparations and standard (testosterone) in 0.5 ml of 0.5% carboxymethylcellulose orally or subcutaneously in 0.2 ml of sesame oil suspension daily over a period of 10 days. Controls receive the vehicle only. Each group is comprised of 8 to 10 animals. On the 11th day all rats are euthanized and seminal vesicles, ventral prostate and levato rani muscle are carefully dissected and weighed. Body weight of each animal is noted at the beginning and the end of the experiment.[91]

The ratio of the organ weight/body weight is calculated for each organ and for each animal. Mean values are calculated for each group and dose response curves are established for each organ. Potency ratios are calculated by comparing the test with standard.

Nitrogen Retention Test

Positive nitrogen balance can be induced by anabolic agents in living organisms.

Procedure

Castrated rats (25 day old) are kept untreated till the body weight becomes 300 g with normal laboratory chow. Thereafter, animals are given liquid-diet force feeding regime. Besides carbohydrates and fat, it contains casein and brewer's yeast as nitrogen source. At the beginning of the experiment, rats are given 10 ml per day and this is increased to 26 ml per day. This feeding is continued for 30 days with simultaneous administration of various doses of test and standard preparations. Twenty-four hour urine specimens are collected 3 times weekly and analyzed for total nitrogen.

Greatest daily retention of sodium and total nitrogen retention is calculated for each test and standard group.[92]

Modifications

Apart from rats, monkey (*Macaca mulatta*) can also be used as an experimental animal for sodium retention study.[93]

Change in β-glucuronidase Activity

There is an alteration in the testosterone levels in experimental animals with the change in kidney β-glucuronidase activity. It is, therefore, suggested that β-glucuronidase activity can be used as an assay of androgens.[94]

Procedure

Male Wistar rats (100 day old) are used for this study. The rats are maintained under a regulated 12:12 h light and dark schedule and are provided food and water ad libitum. Animals are randomly divided into different groups of control, standard and treated, each comprising of 6 to 8 animals. Control is injected with normal saline (0.9% NaCl) and experimental groups are given various doses of standard and test preparations (s.c.) for three alternate days. On the 7th day, animals are euthanized by decapitation. Blood is collected and kidneys are dissected out.

Determination of β-glucuronidase Activity

Approximately 100 mg of kidney tissue is homogenized in 100 mM acetate buffer (pH 4.5) and stored at –20°C until assayed. The homogenate is made up to 10 ml with the same buffer. An aliquot of 0.3 ml homogenate is incubated at 37°C for 90 min with 0.1 ml of 0.005 M phenolphthalein β-glucuronidase and 0.6 ml of 0.1 M acetate buffer (pH 4.5). The incubation is terminated by placing the tubes in boiling water bath for 1 min and 1.5 ml distilled water. Absorbance is measured at 540 nm on a synthetic spectrophotometer.

PROGESTERONE

Progesterone is produced by corpus luteum and converts the uterine epithelium from proliferative to secretory phase. It is necessary for successful implantation of the ovum.

The clinical uses of the progestational agents are ill-defined apart from contraception and postmenopausal hormone replacement therapy. Following are the well-established models to screen progestational agents.

IN VITRO METHODS

Receptor-Binding Assay

Preparation of Cytosol

Female New Zealand white rabbits weighing approximately 3 kg are injected (s.c.) with 50 mg estradiol benzoate in sesame oil daily for 4 days. On day 5, the animals are anesthetized with sodium pentobarbitone, the uteri are excised and placed immediately in ice-cold TESHMo (10 mM Tris-HCl, pH 7.4, 1.5 mM EDTA, 15 mM thioglycerol, 10 mM sodium molybdate) buffer. All subsequent procedures are performed at 0 to 4°C. The uteri are weighed, mixed and homogenized with a Polytron homogenizer in 4 vol of TESHMo. Following centrifugation at 10.500 g for 1 h, supernatant (cytosol) is passed over phosphocellulose prior to chromatography on any other resin. The nonadsorbed fraction is collected and used for subsequent experiments.

Determination of Progesterone Binding to the Receptor

In some experiments, cytosol is labeled overnight with 10 mM [^{3}H] progesterone at 4°C. Free steroid is removed by mixing the sample with 1.33 vol. of a charcoal suspension (0.5% dextran: 0.5% charcoal, v/v) and incubating for 10 min on ice followed by centrifugation at 5,000 g for 10 min.

During chromatography of progesterone receptor without bound steroid, receptor concentration is determined at selected point by Seat chard analysis of the binding of [^{3}H]-progesterone (0 to 20 mM) ± 100 M excess progesterone. At all steps in the procedure, binding is estimated by incubation with 10 mM [^{3}H]-progesterone ± 100 M excess progesterone, in triplicate. Receptor concentration is expressed as [^{3}H]-progesterone bound (p mol/mg protein).[95]

Modifications

The binding of progesterone agonist and antagonist to the progesterone receptor from calf uterus was characterized by Hurd and Moudgil et al.[96] Different DNA-binding properties of the calf uterine estrogen and progesterone receptors were explained by different dimerization constants.[97] Mutation of the progesterone receptor was found to be responsible for species specificity and has been used for the evaluation of agonistic and antagonistic activity.[98]

IN VIVO METHODS

Clauberg Test in Rabbits (McPhail Test)

Clauberg et al.[99] first described the histological changes of the endometrium in rabbits that are pretreated with estrogen and after treated with progestational compounds and McPhail systemically examined the test and introduced scores for the changes of endometrium.[100]

Procedure

Immature female rabbits (550 to 650 g) are administered daily injections (s.c.) of 5.0 mg of estradiol benzoate in sesame oil solution per animal for a period of 6 days. Thereafter, rabbits are given various doses of test compounds and the standard for the next 5 days. Control group receives either the vehicle or estradiol benzoate only. Animals are sacrificed on the 15th day of the experiment and both the horns of the uterus are removed and fixed in 10% formalin. For histological examinations, sections are made from the middle part of the each horn.

Increase in uterine weight is compared in control and treated groups by the following scoring system:

0—ramification of uterine mucosa, no proliferation

1—slight proliferation of mucosa

2—medium proliferation with slight additional ramification of uterine mucosa

3—pronounced proliferation of mucosa

4—pronounced proliferation as well as pronounced ramification.

The scores are arranged from each group, mean values are obtained and are plotted for dose response curve in order to calculate the potency ratio.

Modifications

Direct injection of progesterone can also be given in the uterine segment. This is performed in immature rabbits primed for 6 days with estrogen. On the 7th day, the upper middle segment of each horn of the uterus is ligated without disturbing the circulation. Test agent of various doses is injected into the lumen of one segment and in the opposite horn, only vehicle is injected. After three days, animals are sacrificed and sections of horn are evaluated histologically according to McPhail scores.[101]

Endometrial Carbonic Anhydrase

Progesterone enhances endometrium carbonic anhydrase activity. Measurement of carbonic anhydrase activity in the rabbit endometrium can be used to evaluate compounds having progesterone like activity.

Procedure

Immature female rabbits are used and are given estrogen and progestin treatment as described in Clauberg test. After sacrificing the animals, the uteri are opened longitudinally and endometrium is dissected, weighed and homogenized. After centrifugation, carbonic anhydrase activity is measured by colorimetric method.

Mean values of carbonic anhydrase activity/g wet tissue are calculated and dose response curve of test and standard are plotted to calculate the potency ratio.[102]

Rat Decidualization Model

This model measures the progestational activity of the compounds in the uterus. The target cells are the endometrial stromal cells, which undergo a progestin dependent proliferation and differentiation that is required for normal embryo implantation and maintenance.

This response is very specific for progestin and is used to evaluate the compounds having progesterone like activity.

Procedure

Adult female Sprague Dawley rats (200 to 250 g) are ovariectomized. Ovariectomies are performed 10 days prior to treatment. Upon arrival, the rats are randomized to groups of 5 to 6 animals each. The standard and test preparations are administered once daily for 7 days orally by gavage (0.5 ml). Approximately 24 h following the final treatment, rats are euthanized by CO_2 asphyxiation. The uteri are removed, trimmed of fat and the decidualized (D) and control (C) horns are weighed separately. The decidual response is expressed as D/C.[103]

Rat Uterine C3 Model

Female Sprague Dawley rats (50 day old) are ovariectomized. The ovariectomies are performed 8 days prior to the treatment. The rats are randomly divided into various groups, each consisting of 6 animals. The rats are treated once daily for 2 days per orally in a volume of 0.5 ml or s.c. injection in the nape of the neck (0.2 ml) with either the standard or test preparations or vehicle. On the second day of the treatment, the animals are also treated with 17 alpha-ethinyl estradiol (EE) (0.08 mg/kg body weight) orally by gavage. Approximately 24 h after the final treatment, the animals are euthanized by CO_2 asphyxiation. The uteri are then removed, stripped of remaining fat and mesentery, weighed and snap frozen on dry ice.

The total RNA is isolated from the uteri using the Trizol Reagent. To find the potencies of the test preparations, northern blot analysis is performed with RNA that are separated in a 1% agarose gel containing 1% formaldehyde. The 28S rRNA is quantified with ethidium bromide stained gels. cDNA probes are labeled with a ^{32}P-dCTP using the Radiprime random primer DNA labeling kit. C3 mRNA is quantified using a phosphorimager and normalized to 28S rRNAlization in rodents.[104]

Rat Ovulation Inhibition Model

Progestins function at the level of hypothalamus to block the LH surge associated with ovulation. This activity of progestins has been utilized to develop a method to evaluate unknown compounds having progestational activity.

Procedure

Random cycling mature female rats weighing 180 to 200 g are used for the experiment. Animals are synchronized for estrous with 2 mg/rat of luteinizing hormone-releasing hormone (LH-RH) (in PBS containing 0.1% BSA) s.c. at 09:00 h and again at 16:00 h. Animals are allowed to rest for 8 days prior to the administration of the test compounds. Animals are then divided into various treatment group, each comprising of 7 to 9 animals. From the morning of the ninth day following LH-RH treatment, the rats are treated with standard and test preparations orally once a day for 4 consecutive days. The animals are euthanized in the morning following the last treatment. Oviducts are removed, placed between two glass slides and are viewed through a dissecting microscope to count ova. The animals presenting ova in the oviduct are also recorded.[105]

ESTROGENS

The dramatic actions of estrogen in the maintenance of female reproductive tissues are well known. Pharmacological intervention using a variety of steroidal and nonsteroidal estrogens is widely practiced for contraception, for hormonal control of prostatic carcinoma and for alleviation of many of the serious sequelae of menopause. This wide array of important therapeutic actions has sustained a high level of interest in the continued development of new estrogens.

IN VITRO ASSAY

Receptor Binding Assay

Cytosol Preparation

Adult female Wistar rats (200 to 250 g) are ovariectomized and five days later uteri are removed and washed with cold saline. All the procedures are carried out at 4°C. One gram of the tissue is homogenized in 1 ml phosphate buffer. The homogenate is centrifuged at 10.500 g for 90 min and the supernatant is used as estrogen receptor-binding cytosol.

Competition Experiment

Ten microlitre of [^{3}H]-estradiol (final conc. 5×10^{-8}mol/l) and 10 µl of unlabeled estradiol for the standard curve or 10 µl of the test substances in appropriate concentrations are added to 40 µl of the cytosol. Each sample is incubated for 120 min at 4°C. Postincubation unbound estrogens are adsorbed by incubating with 0.5 ml of a suspension of dextran coated charcoal in Tris buffer (0.01 M, pH 7.5) containing 1.5 mM EDTA and 10% glycerol for 10 min at 4°C. After centrifugation for 5 min at 15,000 rpm, an aliquot of the supernatant is withdrawn and counted for radioactivity. The relative-binding affinity is evaluated according to the method of Bouton and Raynaud.[106]

Recombinant Yeast and Beta-galactose Assay

The recombinant (BJ-ECZ) yeast strain contains a reported gene with two estrogen responsive elements upstream from the yeast proximal cytochrome C1 promoter fused to the Lac Z gene. These yeast cells are transfected with rtER or hER expression vectors. The activation of the reporter gene is strictly dependent on the presence of estrogen receptor and estrogens and results in the production of galactosidase (beta-Gal).

Four independent colonies are incubated at 30°C in a shaking incubator at 300 rpm for 36 h. About 100 ml of yeast suspension (0.6 OD_{600}) is distributed in each well of conical bottomed 96 well plates. After 4 h of incubation at 30°C in presence of test compounds, plates are centrifuged and the media is discarded. Fifty microliter of lyticase solution is added to each well, and the plates are incubated at room temperature for 30 min. About 100 ml of 0.1% triton × 100 is added to each well. Plates are then centrifuged at 10.500 g for 10 min and 100 ml of supernatants are transferred to flat bottomed 96 well microtitration plates and 20 ml of O-nitrophenyl β-D-galactopyranoside substrate is added to each well. The enzymatic reaction is performed at 30°C for 1 h. The reaction is stopped by adding 50 ml of 1 mol/l Na_2CO_3 and the OD_{405} is read after 5 min equilibration. The beta-galactosidase units are defined as OD_{405}/mg protein/min of enzymatic reaction.[107]

Alkaline Phosphatase Assay

Cell Culture

The Ishikawa cell line is maintained in Eagle's Minimum Essential Medium (MEM) containing 10% (v/v) fetal bovine serum (FBS) supplemented with antibiotics, glutamine and sodium pyruvate. On the day of the experiment, cells are harvested and plated in 96 well plate (2×10^4 cells/200 µl) in phenol red free DMEM/F-12 medium supplemented with 5% FBS stripped of endogenous estrogen with dextran-coated charcoal. On the day of the experiment, 2 µl of the test compound is added. Dose response is performed in 1/5 serial dilution. After 48 h of the treatment, the plates are rinsed with 200 µl Tris/HCl 0.1 ml/l, pH 7.4 and cells are lysed by adding 20 µl Tris/HCl 0.1 mmol/l, pH 9. Now the plates are placed at -80°C for at least 15 min followed by thawing at room temperature for 5 to 10 min. This freeze and thaw cycle can be omitted with loss of about 15% of detectable ALP activity. The plates are placed in ice and 50 µl of ice-cold solution containing 5 mM p-nitro phenyl phosphate, 0.24 mM $MgCl_2$ and 1 M diethanolamine (pH 9.8) is added. Plates are warmed to room temperature and the yellow colour from the production of p-nitrophenol is allowed to develop. Plates are monitored at 405 nm in an enzyme-linked immunosorbent assay plate reader.[108]

Dose response experiments are analyzed mathematically by nonlinear regression method. The sigmoidal dose response curve is used as a model. The EC_{50} is calculated from log EC_{50}.

IN VIVO METHODS

Castration of Female Rats

Ovariectomy is usually done in immature female rats weighing less than 60 g. The whole procedure is performed under ether anesthesia. A single incision is made in the skin of the back. A small puncture is then made over the site of the ovary, which can be seen through the abdominal wall embedded in a pad of fat. With the help of fine forceps, fat around the ovary is removed without rupturing the ovarian capsule. The ovary together with the fallopian tubes is removed with a single cut by a pair of fine scissors. Usually, no bleeding is observed. The ovary of the other side is removed in a similar way. The skin wound is closed by one or two clips. The animals recover immediately.

Vaginal Cornification

Immature female rats (approx. 55 g) are ovariectomized and kept for about 1 week on standard laboratory diet and water ad libitum. The test compounds are administered in 0.5% solution of carboxymethylcellulose or in cotton-seed oil either orally or subcutaneously in various doses. Estradiol is used as standard and each group comprises of 10-20 animals. The compounds are given twice daily for two consecutive days at the gap of 8 h interval. Vaginal smears are taken on third day afternoon and on fourth day morning with the help of spatula or cotton swabs moistened with saline. Smears are transferred to a glass slide and evaluated microscopically according to the following scores:

0—diestrous stage, mainly leukocytes and a few epithelial cells are present
1—metestrous stage, mixture of leukocytes and epithelial cells
2—proestrous stage, nucleated or nucleated plus cornified cells
3—estrous stage, cornified cells only

Animals showing score 2 or 3 are considered to be positive. The number of positive animals in each group is recorded. ED_{50} value is calculated by using various doses of the test drug.[109]

Modifications

The sensitivity of the assay can be enhanced by local application of estrogen into the vagina of castrated animals.

Increased Uterus Weight

Estrogen enhances the weight of the uterus when it is given repeatedly in a dose dependent manner in castrated female rats.

Procedure

Immature female Wistar rats (55 g) are ovariectomized and divided into various groups, each comprises of 6 to 8 animals. Animals are administered with various doses of test and standard compounds simultaneously for seven days. The test compound is administered in 0.5% solution of carboxymethylcellulose or in cotton-seed oil. Control animals are given vehicle only. On the 8th day, the animals are sacrificed and uterine weight is determined.[110]

Dose response curve of test and standard compounds are obtained to find out the potency ratios.

Modifications

Rubin et al.[111] used albino mice who are administered the oil solution of hormone (s.c.). Twenty-four hours after the injection, animals are sacrificed and uterine as well as body weight are taken. The uterine ratio is calculated by dividing the uterine weight (mg) by body weight (g), multiplied by 100.

In addition to uterus weight, Branhan et al.[112] studied luminal and glandular epithelium height in cross sections of the uterus horns of rats by histological means.

Chick Oviduct Method

Administration of natural or synthetic estrogen enhances the oviduct weight of young chicken in a dose dependent manner.

Procedure

Seven-day-old chicks are given subcutaneous injections of various doses of test compounds and standard twice daily for 6 days. Six to ten chicks are used for each group. On the day after the last injection, the animals are sacrificed and body as well as oviduct weight is determined.

The ratio of oviduct weight/body weight is calculated for each animal. Mean values of test and standard groups are plotted to get dose response curve in order to calculate the potency.[113]

REFERENCES

1. Foster CM, Borondy M, Padmanabhan V, et al. Bioactivity of human growth hormone in serum: validation of an in vitro bioassay. Endocrinology 1993;132:2073-82.
2. Nederman T, Sjodin L. The quantitation of human growth hormone by a radioreceptor assay using an established human cell line. J Biol Stand 1987;15:199-211.
3. Mayumi Ishikawa, Atsuko Nimura, Reiko Horikawa, Noriyuki Katsumata, Osamu Arisaka, Mitsufumi Wada, Masaru Honjo, And Toshiaki Tanaka. A Novel Specific Bioassay for Serum Human Growth Hormone. J Clin Endocrinol Metabol 2000;85(11):4274-9.
4. Wada M, Uchida H, Ikeda M, Tsunekawa B, Naito N, Banba S, et al. The 20-kilodalton (kDa) human growth hormone (hGH) differs from the 22-kDa hGH in the complex formation with cell surface hGH receptor and hGH-binding protein circulating in human plasma. Mol Endocrinol 1998:12(1):146-56.
5. Strasburger CJ , Wu Z, Pflaum CD, Dressendorfer RA. Immunofunctional assay of human growth hormone (hGH) in serum: a possible consensus for quantitative hGH measurement. J Clin Endocrinol Metab 1996;81:2613-20.
6. Marx W, Simpson ME, Evans HM. Bioassay of the growth hormone of the anterior pituitary. Endocrinology 1942;30:1-10.
7. Carrillo A, Rising R, Tverskaya R, Lifshitz F. Effects of exogenous recombinant human growth hormone on an animal model of suboptimal nutrition. J Am Coll Nutr 1998; 17: 276-81.
8. Greenspan FS, Li CH, Simpson ME, et al. Bioassay of hypophyseal growth hormone: The tibia test. Endocrinology 1949;45:445-63.
9. Collins EJ, Baker VF. Growth hormone and radiosulphate incorporation: a new assay method for growth hormone. Metabolism 1960;9:556-60.
10. Jeffcoate SL, Bacon RA, Beastall GH, et al. Assays for prolactin: guidelines for the provision of a clinical biochemistry service. Ann Clin Bio Chem 1986;23:638-51.
11. Segaloff A. Prolactin. In: Dorfman RI (Ed). Methods in Hormone Research. Vol II, Chapter 18, New York and London: Academic Press, 1962;609-15.
12. Bergman AJ, Meites J, Turner CM. A comparison of methods of assay of the lactogenic hormone. Endocrinology 1940;26:716-22.
13. Haynes RC. The activation of adrenal phospholipase by the adrenocorticotropic hormone. J Bio Chem 1958;233:1220-2.
14. Mountjoy KG, Robbins LS, Mortrud MT, et al. The cloning of a family of genes that encode melanocortin receptors. Science 1992;257:1248-51.
15. Kapas S, Orford CD, Barker S, et al. Studies on the intracellular mechanism of action of alphamelanocyte-stimulating hormone on rat adrenal zona glomerulosa. J Mol Endocrinol 1992;9:47-54.
16. Penhoat A, Jaillard C, Saez JM. Corticotropin positively regulates its own receptors and cAMP response in cultured bovine adrenal cells. Proc Natl Acad Sci USA 1989;86:4978-81.
17. Munson PJ, Rodbard D. Ligand: a versatile computerized approach for characterization of ligandbinding systems. Anal Biochem 1980;107:220-9.

18. Thompson RE, Fisher JD. Correlation of preparative history and method of assay of corticotropin with clinical potency. Endocrinology 1953;52:496-509.
19. Roe JH, Kuether CA. The determination of ascorbic acid in whole blood and urine through the 2, 4-dinitrophenylhydrazine derivative of dehydroascorbinic acid. J Bio Chem 1943;147:399-407.
20. Vogel HG. Evaluation of synthetic peptides with ACTH activity. Acta Endocrinol (Kbh) Suppl 1965; 100: 34-8.
21. Pekkarinen A. Bioassay of corticotropin preparations with the international working standard on living guinea pigs. Acta Endocrinol Suppl 1965;100:35-40.
22. Wang XN, Greenwald GS. Hypophysectomy of the cyclic mouse. II. Effects of follicle-stimulating hormone (FSH) and luteinizing hormone on folliculogenesis, FSH and human chorionic gonadotropin receptors, and steroidogenesis. Biol Reprod 1993;48:595-605.
23. Hardy MP, Kelce WR, Klinefelter GR, Ewing LL. Differentiation of Leydig cell precursors in vitro: a role for androgen. Endocrinology 1990;127:488-90.
24. Sriraman V, Rao VS, Sairam MR, Rao AJ. Effect of deprival of LH on Leydig cell proliferation: involvement of PCNA, Cyclin D3 and IGF-1. Mol Cell Endocrinol 2000;162:113-20.
25. Sriraman V, Jagannadha Rao A. Evaluation of the role of FSH in regulation of Leydig cell function during different stages of its differentiation. Mol Cell Endocrinol 2004;224:73-82.
26. Cooke BA, Janszen FH, Clotscher WF, Van der Molen HJ. Effect of protein-synthesis inhibitors on testosterone production in rat testis interstitial tissue and Leydig-cell preparations. Biochem J 1975;150:413-8.
27. Taylor CC, Terranova PF. Lipopolysaccharide inhibits in vitro luteinizing hormone-stimulated rat ovarian granulose cell estradiol but not progesterone secretion. Biol Reprod 1996;54:1390-6.
28. Holton P. A modification of the method of Dale and Laidlaw for the standardization of posterior pituitary extract. Br J Pharmacol 1948;3:328-34.
29. Berde B, Doepfner W, Konzett H. Some pharmacological actions of four synthetic analogues of oxytocin. Br J Pharmacol 1957;12:209-14.
30. Cornely M, Rimpler M. A bioassay for the testing of the oxytocic effect of hormone analogues of the neurohypophysis and the pineal body. Z Geburtshilfe Perinatol 1985;189:103-11.
31. Coon JM. A new method for the assay of posterior pituitary extracts. Arch Intern Pharmacodyn Ther 1939;62:79-99.
32. van Dyke HB. Some features of pharmacology of oxytocin. In Caldeyro-Barcia, Heller H (Eds): Oxytocin: Intern Sympos Montevideo. London, Pergamon Press. 1961:48-67.
33. British Pharmacopoeia, Vol II. Biological assay of Oxytocin. Appendix XIV C: A 171 1988.
34. Tindal JS, Yokoyama A. Assay of oxytocin by milk ejection response in the anaesthetized lactating guinea pig. Endocrinology 1962;71:196-202.
35. Dekanski J. The quantitative assay of vasopressin. Br J Pharmacol 1952;7:567-72.
36. Vogel G, Hergott J. PharmakologischeUntersuchungeniiber O-Methyl-tyrosin 2-lysin-8-vasopressin. Arzneim Forsch/Drug Res 1963;13:415-21.
37. Knape JT, van Zwieten PA. Vasoconstrictor activity of vasopressin in the pithed rat. Arch Int Pharmacodyn Ther 1988;291:142-52.
38. Simson A. The secretion of the posterior lobe of the hypophysis after the administration of drugs. J Pharmacol 1933;49:375-86.
39. Burn JH. Estimation of antidiuretic potency of pituitary (posterior lobe) extract. Quart J Pharmacy 1931;4:517-29.

40. van Dyke HB, Adamsons K, Engel SL. Pituitary hormones. Aspects of the biochemistry and physiology of the neurohypophyseal hormones. Rec Progr Hormone Res 1955;11:1-41.
41. Schmale H, Richter D. Single base deletion in the vasopressin gene in the cause of diabetes insipidus in Brattleboro rats. Nature 1984;308:705-9.
42. Varghese S, Oommen OV. Thyroid hormones regulate lipid metabolism in a teleost Anabas testudineus (Bloch). Comp Biochem Physiol B Biochem Mol Biol 1999;124:445-50.
43. Tata JR, Kawahara A, Baker BS. Prolactin inhibits both thyroid hormone-induced morphogenesis and cell death in cultured amphibian larval tissues. Dev Biol 1991;146:72-80.
44. Bomskov C. Die chirurgischenMethodoen der Schildrusemforschung. In Methodik der Hormonforschung. Band 1, George Thieme Verlag, Leizig 1937:143-55.
45. Grossie J, Hendrich CE, Turner CW. Comparative methods for determining biological half life (t1/2) of L-thyroxine in normal, thyroidectomized and methimazole treated female rats. Proc Soc Exp Biol Med 1965; 120:413-5.
46. Perry WF. A method for measuring thyroid hormone secretion in the rat with its application to the bioassay of thyroid extracts. Endocrinology 1951;48:643-50.
47. Wiberg GS, Carter JR, Stephenson NR. The effects of various goitrogens on the determination of the relative potency of thyroid by the goiter prevention assay. Acta Endocrinol 1964;45:370-80.
48. her L, Schramm H, Vogel G. Uber die antagonistische Wirkung von Trijodthyronin und Progesteron auf den Prednisoloneffekt am Epiphysenknorpel. Acta Endocrinol 1963;42:29-38.
49. Vogel HG. Influence of desmotropic drugs on viscoelastic properties of tail tendons in rats. Acta Thera Peutica 1989;15:239-52.
50. Vogel HG. Stress relaxation in rat skin after treatment with hormones. J Med 1973; 4: 19-27. Fell HB, Weiss L. The effect of antiserum alone and with hydrocortisone on foetal mouse bones in culture. J Exp Med 1965;121:551-60.
51. Collip JB, Clark EP. Further studies on the physiological action of a parathyroid hormone. J Biol Chem 1925;64:485-507.
52. Hefti E, Trechsel U, Fleisch H, et al. Increase of whole body calcium and skeletal mass in normal and osteoporotic adult rats treated with parathyroid hormone. Clin Sci 1982;62:389-96.
53. Tepperman HM, Heureux MV, Wilhelmi AE. The estimation of parathyroid hormone activity by its effect on serum inorganic phosphorus in the rat. J Biol Chem 1947;168:151-65.
54. Sugimoto T, Fukase M, Tsutsumi M, et al. Additive effects of parathyroid hormone and calcitonin on adenosine 3', 5'-monophosphate release in newly established perfusion system of rat femur. Endocrinology 1985;117:1901-5.
55. Nissenson RA, Abott SR, Teitelbaum AP, et al. Endogenous biologically active human parathyroid hormone: Measurement by a guanyl nucleotide amplified renal adenylatecyclase assay. J Clin Endocrinol Metab 1981:52:840-6.
56. Saito M, Kawashima K, Endo H. The establishment of a new biological assay system for simultaneous measurement of bone resorption and bone mineralization in organ culture of chick embryonic femur. J Pharmacobiodyn 1987;10:487-93.
57. Docherty HM, Heath DA. Multiple forms of parathyroid hormone like proteins in a human tumor. J Mol Endocrinol 1989;2:11-20.
58. Goltzman D, Henderson B, Loveridge N. Cytochemical bioassay of parathyroid hormone: characteristics of the assay and analysis of circulating hormonal forms. J Clin Invest 1980;65:1309-17.

59. Raynaud JP, Ojasoo T, Bouton MM. Receptor-binding as a tool in the development of new bioactive steroids. In Ariens EJ (Ed): Drug Design, Vol VIII, New York: Academic Press, 1979:169-214.
60. Rousseau GG, Schmitt JP. Structure activity relationships for glucocorticoids-I: Determination of receptor-binding and biological activity. J Steroid Biochem 1977;8:911-9.
61. Steiner AE, Wittliff JL. A whole cell assay for glucocorticoid-binding sites in normal human lymphocytes. Clin Chem 1985;31:1855-60.
62. Lefebvre P, Danze PM, Sablonniere B, et al. Association of glucocorticoid receptor-binding with 90K non-steroid-binding component is stabilized by both steroidal and non-steroidal antiglucocorticoids in intact cells. Biochemistry 1988;27:9186-94.
63. Srivastava D, Thompson EB. Two glucocorticoids-binding sites on human glucocorticoid receptor. Endocrinology 1990;127:1770-8.
64. Druzgala P, Hochhaus G, Bodor N. Soft drugs-10. Blanching activity and receptor-binding affinity of a new type of glucocorticoid: loteprednoletabonate. J Steroid Biochem Mol Biol 1991;38:149-54.
65. Rohdewald P, Mollmann HW, Hochhaus G. Affinities for glucocorticoids receptors in the human lung. Agents Actions 1985;17:290-2.
66. Spencer RL, Young EA, Choo PH, et al. Adrenal steroid type I and type II receptor-binding: Estimates in vivo receptor number, occupancy and activation with varying level of steroid. Brain Res 1990;514:37-48.
67. Thompson EB, Tomkins GM, Curran JF. Induction of tyrosine transaminase activity by conversion of p-hydroxyphenyl-pyruvate to p-hydroxybenzaldehye. Anal Biochem 1966;16:385-401.
68. Dorfman RI. Corticoids. In Dorfman RI (Ed): Methods in Hormone Research, Vol II, Bioassay. New York and London: Academic Press, 1962:325-65.
69. Flegner PL, Gadek TR, Holm M, et al. Lipofection: a highly efficient, lipid mediated DNA-transfection procedure. Proc Natl Acad Sci 1987;84:7413-7.
70. Fuhrmann U, Bengtson C, Repenthin G, et al. Stable transfection of androgen receptor and MMTVCAT into mammalian cells: inhibition of CAT expression by antiandrogens. J Steroid Biochem Mol Biol 1992;42:787-93.
71. Bradford MM. A rapid and sensitive method for the quantitation of microgram quantities of protein utilizing the principle of protein dye-binding. Anal Biochem 1976;72:248-54.
72. Gorman CM, Moffat LF, Howard BH. Recombinant genomes which express chloramphenicol acetyltransferase in mammalian cells.Mol Cell Biol 1982;2:1044-51.
73. Thompson EB, Tomkins GM, Curran JF. Induction of tyrosine α-ketoglutarate transaminase by steroid hormones in a newly established tissue culture cell line. Proc Natl Acad Sci 1966;56:269-303.
74. Grollman A. Biological assay of adrenal cortical activity. Endocrinology 1941;29:855-86.
75. Speirs RS, Meyer RK. A method of assaying adrenal cortical hormones based on a decrease in circulating eosinophil cells of adrenalectomized mice. Endocrinology 1951;48:316-26.
76. Stafford RO, Barnes LE, Bowman BJ, et al. Glucocorticoid and mineralocorticoid activities of D3 fluorohydrocortisone. Proc Soc Exp Biol Med 1955;89:371-4.
77. Pasqualini JR, Sumida CH. Mineralocorticoid receptors in target tissue. In Pasqualini JR (Ed): Receptors and Mechanism of Action of Steroid Hormones. Part II. New York and Basal: Marcel Dekker, Inc, 1977:399-511.
78. Arriza JL, Weinberger C, Cerelli G, et al. Cloning of human mineralocorticoid receptor complementary DNA: structural and functional kinship with the glucocorticoid receptor. Science 1987;237:268-75.

79. Kagawa CM, Shipley EG, Meyer RK. A biological method for determining small quantities of sodium retaining substances. Proc Soc Exp Biol Med 1952;80:281-5.
80. Simpson SA, Tait JF. A quantitative method for the bioassay of the effect of adrenal cortical steroids on mineral metabolism. Endocrinology 1952;50:150-61.
81. Nickisch K, Beier S, Bittler D, et al. Aldosterone antagonists. 4. Synthesis and activities of steroidal 6, 6-ethylene -15, 16-methylene 17-spirolactones. J Med Chem 1991;34:2464-68.
82. Starka L, Hampl R, Kasal A, et al. Androgen receptor-binding and antiandrogenic activity of some 4, 5-secoandrostanes and ring B cyclopropanoandrostanes. J Steroid Biochem 1998;17:331-4.
83. Krieg M, Steins P, Szalay R, et al. Characterization of specific androgen receptor in rat prostate cytosol by agar gel electrophoresis: in vivo and in vitro studies. J Steroid Biochem 1974;5:87-92.
84. Tezon JG, Vazquez MH, Blaquier JA. Androgen controlled subcellular distribution of its receptor in the rat epididymis: 5 alpha-dihydrotestosterone-induced translocation is blocked by anti-androgens. Endocrinology 1982;111:2039-45.
85. Schilling K, Liao S. The use of radioactive 7 alpha, 17 alpha-dimethyl-19-nortestosterone (Mibolirone) in the assay of androgen receptors. Prostate 1984;5:581-8.
86. Archibald A and Shuster S. The bioassay of androgens and anti-androgens using sebum secretion in the rat. Proc R Soc Med. 1969;62(9):887–888.
87. Archibald A and Shuster S. The measurement of sebum secretion in the rat. Br.J. Derm. 1970;82,146.
88. Archibald A, Shuster S. Bioassay of androgen using the rat sebaceous gland. J Endocr 1967; 37, xxii.
89. Dorfman RI. Androgens and anabolic agents. In Dorfman RI (Ed): Methods in Hormone Research. Vol IIA. Chapter 4. New York and London: Academic Press, 1969:151-220.
90. Frank RT, Klempner F, Hollander R, et al. Detailed description of technique for androgen assay by the chick comb method. Endocrinology 1942;31:63-70.
91. Eisler M. Animal techniques for evaluating sex steroids. In Nodine JH, Siegler PE (Ed): Animal and clinical pharmacologic techniques in drug evaluation. Chicago: Year Book Medical Publisher, Inc, 1964:566-73.
92. Staford RO, Bowman BJ, Olson KJ. Influence of 19-nortestosterone cyclopentyl–propionate on urinary nitrogen of castrate male rat. Proc Soc Exp Biol Med 1954;86:322-6.
93. Stucki JC, Forbes AD, Northam JI, et al. An assay for anabolic steroids employing metabolic balance in the monkey: The anabolic activity of fluoxymesterone and its 11-keto analogue. Endocrinology 1960;66:585-98.
94. Malarvizhi D, Mathur PP. Renal β-glucuronidase activity is a bioassay of serum testosterone levels in rats. Indian J Exp Biol 1996;34:582-3.
95. Lamb DJ, Bullock DW. Hydrophobic interaction chromatography of the rabbit uterine progesterone receptor. J Steroid Biochem 1983;19:1039-45.
96. Hurd C, Moudgil VK. Characterization of R5020 and RU486-binding to progesterone receptor from calf uterus. Biochemistry 1988;27:3618-23.
97. Skafer DF. Different DNA-binding by calf uterine estrogen and progesterone receptors results from differences in oligomeric states. Biochemistry 1991;30:6148-54.
98. Garcia T, Benhamou B, Gofflo D, et al. Switching agonistic, antagonistic and mixed transcriptional responses to 11 beta substituted progestins by mutations of the progesterone receptor. Mol Endocrinol 1992;6:2071-8.
99. Clauberg C. Das Hormon des Corpus luteum. Zentralbl Gynakol 1930b;54:7-19.
100. McPhail MK. The assay of progestin. J Physiol 1934;83:145-56.

101. Tamaya T, Motoyama T, Ohono Y, et al. Local progestational and antiprogestational effects of steroids and their metabolites on the rabbit uterus. Jpn J Fertil Steril 1979;24:48-51.
102. Lutwak-Mann C. Carbonic anhydrase in the female reproductive tract. Occurrence distribution and hormonal dependence. J Endocrinol 1955;13:26-38.
103. Abrahamsohn PA, Zorn TMD. Implantation and decidualization in rodents.J Exp Zool 1993;266: 603-28.
104. Brown EO, Sundstrom SA, Komm BS, et al. Progesterone regulation of estradiol induced rat uterine secretory protein, complement C3. Biol Reprod 1990;42:713-9.
105. Schubert C, Donath J, Michna H, et al. The antiovulatory activity of progesterone antagonists is not correlated to their antiprogestational potency in the rat. J Steroid Biochem Mol Biol 1996;59:75-82.
106. Bouton MM, Raynaud JP. The relevance of kinetic parameters in the determination of specific-binding to the estrogen receptor. J Steriod Biochem 1978;9:9-15.
107. Petit F, LeGoff P, Cravedi JP, et al. Two complementary bioassays for screening the estrogenic potency of xenobiotics: Recombinant yeast for trout estrogen receptor and trout hepatocyte cultures. J Mol Endocrinol 1997;19:321-35.
108. Littlefield BA, Gurpide E, Markiewicz L, et al. A simple and sensitive microtiter plate estrogen bioassay based on stimulation of alkaline phosphatase in Ishikawa cells: estrogenic action of delta 5 adrenal steroids. Endocrinology 1990;127:2757-62.
109. Allen E, Doisy EA. An ovarian hormone: preliminary report on its localization, extraction and partial purification and action in test animals. J Am Med Ass 1923; 81:819-21.
110. Emmens CW. Estrogens. In Dorfman RI (Ed): Methods in Hormone Research, Vol IIA, Chapter 2, New York and London: Academic Press, 1969:61-120.
111. Rubin BL, Dorfman AS, Black L, Dorfman RI. Bioassay of estrogens using mouse uterine response. Endocrinology 1951;49:429-39.
112. Branhan W, Zehr DR, Sheehan DM. Differential sensitivity of rat uterine growth and epithelium hypertrophy to estrogens and antiestrogens. Proc Soc Exp Biol Med 1993;203:297-303.
113. Tullner WW, Hertz R. The effect of 17-alpha-hydroxy-11-desoxycorticosterone on estrogen stimulated chick oviduct growth. Endocrinology 1956;58:282-3.

CHAPTER

40

Antidiabetic Agents

INTRODUCTION

The pancreas is an organ composed of (98%) exocrine and (2%) endocrine cells. Islets of Langerhans, which form the endocrine part of pancreas, consist of four types of cells α-cells, β-cells, δ-cells and PP-cells, which secrete glucagons, insulin, somatostatin and pancreatic polypeptide.

Glucose stimulates the β-cells to release insulin, which then promotes glucose uptake and storage in various tissues. Diabetes mellitus is a disease characterized by derangement in carbohydrate, protein and fat metabolism caused by the complete or relative insufficiency of insulin secretions and/or insulin action.

Two major types of diabetes, one associated with insulin deficiency called type-I or insulin-dependent diabetes mellitus (IDDM) and the other associated with insulin resistance called

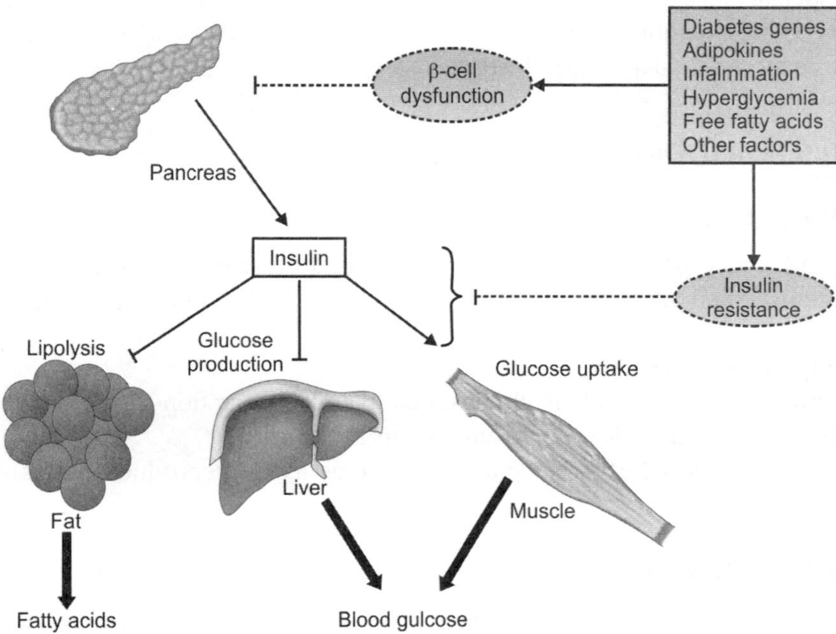

Figure 40.1: Pathophysiology of hyperglycemia

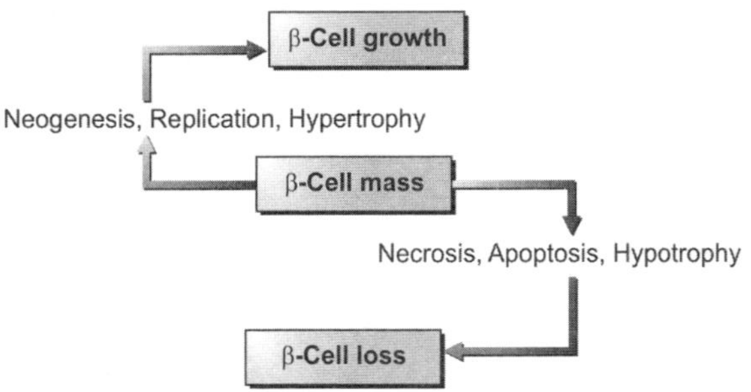

Figure 40.2: Factors regulating β-cell mass

type-2 or noninsulin-dependent diabetes mellitus (NIDDM). Type-1 is associated with a specific and complete loss of pancreatic β-cells. Type-II diabetes is the most common type and is associated with obesity, hyperinsulinemia and insulin resistance. Insulin resistance may be due to the defect at receptor level or at the postreceptor level. This defect may be in the effector cell or in the β-islet cell causing insulin resistance.

The β-cell mass is the overall balance of β-cell growth and β-cell loss, depending on the four mechanisms[1] as follows (Fig. 40.1):

1. Replication of existing differential β-cells.
2. Neogenesis of β-cells from precursors located in the pancreatic ductal epithelium.
3. β-cell size.
4. β-cell death.

In the 1980s, von Mering was working on the absorption of fat from the intestine after removing the pancreas of a dog. The animal developed polyuria and polydipsia and was found to have diabetes mellitus. Many experiments on rabbits and dogs followed, although history has given a special place to Marjorie, one of the dogs used by Banting and Best in their seminal experiments on the isolation and purification of insulin in the 1920s.[2] Marjorie is probably the most famous experimental animal in history.

MODELS FOR IDDM

Chemically-induced Diabetes

Chemically induced Type-I diabetes is the most commonly used animal model of diabetes. Chemical agents which produce diabetes can be classified into three categories, and include agents that:

- Specifically damage β-cell
- Cause temporary inhibition of insulin production and/or secretion
- Diminish the metabolic efficacy of insulin in target tissues.

In general, chemicals in the first category are of interest as they reproduce lesions resembling IDDM.

Alloxan-induced Diabetes

Alloxan, a cyclic urea analog, was the first agent in this category, which was reported to produce permanent diabetes in animals.

Mechanism of Action

The mechanism by which it induces diabetes is not very clear. Alloxan is a highly reactive molecule that is readily reduced to diuleric acid, which is then auto-oxidized back to alloxan resulting in the production of free radicals. These free radicals damage the DNA of β-cells and cause cell death. Second mechanism proposed for alloxan is its ability to react with protein SH groups, especially the membrane proteins like glucokinase on the β-cells, finally resulting in cell necrosis. However, there are major species differences in response to alloxan.

Procedure

Rabbits weighing 2–3 kg are used. Alloxan is infused via the ear marginal vein at a dose of 150 mg/kg for 10 min. About 70% animals become hyperglycemic and uricosuric. The remaining animals either die or are temporarily hyperglycemic.

When rats of Wistar or Sprague-Dawley strain each weighing 150–200 g are used, alloxan is injected s.c. in the dose of 100–175 mg/kg. In male Beagle dogs weighing 15–20 kg, alloxan is injected i.v. at a dose of 60 mg/kg. Alloxan has been given to nonhuman primates, like monkeys and baboons in the dose of 65–200 mg/kg i.v. to induce diabetes. All the animals, which are given alloxan, receive glucose and regular insulin for one week and food ad libitum. Thereafter, single daily dose of 28 IU insulin is administered s.c. The blood glucose level shows triphasic change, first a rise at 2 h, followed by hypoglycemic phase at 8 h, and finally an increase at 24 h probably due to depletion of β-cells of insulin.

Modifications

Diabetes can be induced in neonatal Sprague-Dawley rats by intraperitoneal injection of 200 mg/kg alloxan on days 2, 4, or 6.

Drawbacks:

- High mortality in rats
- Causes ketosis in animals due to free fatty acid generation
- Diabetes induced is reversible
- Some species like guinea pigs are resistant to its diabetogenic action.

Alloxan has been almost completely replaced by Streptozotocin (STZ) for inducing diabetes because of these drawbacks.[1-4]

Streptozotocin-induced Diabetes

STZ [2-deoxy-2-(3-methyl-3-nitrosourea) 1-D-glucopyranose] is a broad-spectrum antibiotic, which is produced from *Streptomyces achromogens*. Rakieten et al. first described the diabetogenic property of STZ.[5]

Mechanism of Causing β-cell Damage

- By process of methylation
- Free radical generation and
- Nitric oxide production.

Procedure

STZ induces diabetes in almost all species of animals. Diabetogenic dose varies with species and the optimal doses required in various species are: rats (50–60 mg/kg, i.p. or i.v.), mice (175–200 mg/kg i.p. or i.v.) and dogs (15 mg/kg, for 3 days). The blood glucose level shows the same triphasic response as seen in the alloxan treated animals, with hyperglycemia at 1 h, followed by hypoglycemia, which lasts for 6 h, and stable hyperglycemia by 24–48 h after STZ administration.

Modifications
Multiple low dose of STZ also induces diabetes by causing immune mediated pancreatic insulitis in rats. It has also been shown to have diabetogenic effect on the golden hamsters when given i.p at a dose of 50 mg/kg. Cyclosporin-A when given with STZ enhances its diabetogenic efficacy. STZ combined with complete Freund's adjuvant: each of CFA, incomplete Freund's adjuvant, *Mycobacterium butyricum* (component of CFA), *Listeria monocytogenes*, or endotoxin administered 24 h prior to STZ (25 mg/kg) and then repeated in the three subsequent weeks, all produce hyperglycemia. Fasting for 48 h (24 h prior to and 24 h subsequent to the STZ injection) also produces hyperglycemia. Neither four administration of CFA nor of STZ alone result in persistent hyperglycemia.

Advantages and Disadvantages
STZ has almost completely replaced alloxan for inducing diabetes because of:
- Greater selectivity towards β-cells
- Lower mortality rate
- Longer or irreversible diabetes induction
- However, guinea pigs and rabbits are resistant to its diabetogenic action.[5-9]

Hormone-induced Diabetes Mellitus

Dexamethasone, a long-acting glucocorticoid, is used to produce NIDDM. NIDDM form of diabetes is produced when dexamethasone is administered at a dose of 2–5 mg/kg i.p. twice daily over a number of days in rats.

Besides rat models, other experimental models using guinea pigs and rabbits are also reported for the study of diabetes using corticoids.[11,12] In these models, corticotrophin is used to stimulate adrenal cortex that results in hormonal imbalance causing steroid diabetes.[13,14]

Insulin Antibodies-induced Diabetes

Giving bovine insulin along with CFA to guinea pigs produces anti-insulin antibodies. Intravenous injection of 0.25–1.0 ml guinea pig anti-insulin serum to rats induces a dose dependent increase in blood glucose levels up to 300 mg%. This unique effect to guinea pig anti-insulin serum is due to neutralization of endogenous insulin by the insulin antibodies. It persists as long as the antibodies are capable of reacting with insulin remaining in the circulation. Slow i.v. infusion or i.p. injection prolongs the effect for more than a few hours. However, large doses and prolonged administration are accompanied by ketonemia, ketonuria, glycosuria and acidosis and are fatal to the animals. After lower doses, the diabetic syndrome is reversible after a few hours.[15]

Diabetes-induced by Viral Agents

Viruses are thought to be one of the etiologic agents for IDDM. Viruses may produce diabetes mellitus by:
- Infecting and destroying of β-cells in pancreas
- A less infecting or cytologic variant producing a comparable damage by eliciting immune autoreactivity to the β-cells
- Viruses producing systemic effect, not directly affecting the β-cells.

Various human viruses used for inducing diabetes include RNA picornoviruses, Coxsackie-B4 (CB4), encephalomylocarditis (EMC-D and M variants), Mengo-2T, as well as two other double stranded RNA viruses, reovirus and lymphocytic choriomeningitis virus (LMCV, Armstrong variant) (Table 40.1). Primary isolates of these human pathogenic agents are, generally, not pancreatotrophic or ilytic to mouse β-cells and must be adapted for growth either by inoculation into suckling mice, or by passage in cultured mouse β-cells.[16,17]

Table 40.1: Susceptible mouse strain

Virus	*Susceptible mouse strain*
EMC–D or M variant	SJL/J
	SWR/J
	DBA/1J
	DBA2J
	BALB/cCUM
Mengo–2T	SJL
	C57BL/6J
	CBA/J
	C3H/HCJ
	AKR/J
	CE/J
CB4	SJL/J
	SWR/J
Reo	SJLj
Kilham rat virus	BB –DR

Surgically-induced Diabetes

Induction of diabetes mellitus can be achieved through the surgical removal of all or part of the pancreas. In partial pancreactectomy more than 90% of the organ must be removed to produce diabetes. Depending on the amount of intact pancreatic cells, diabetes may range in duration from a few days to several months. Total removal of the pancreas results in an insulin-dependent form of diabetes, and insulin therapy is required to maintain experimental animals. The portion of the pancreas usually left intact following a subtotal pancreatic resection is typically the anterior lobe or a portion thereof.

Disadvantages

1. Surgical removal of pancreas results in loss of α- and δ-cells in addition to β-cells. This causes loss of counter-regulatory hormones, glucagon and somatostatin.
2. There is a loss of the pancreatic enzymes necessary for proper digestion, therefore, the diet for pancreatectomized animals must be supplemented with these pancreatic enzymes.
3. The total resection of the pancreas in rat is very difficult to achieve and the development and severity of the diabetic state appear to be strain specific.

The use of pancreatectomy in combination with chemical agents, such as alloxan and STZ, produces a stable form of diabetes mellitus in animals, such as cats and dogs, that does not occur when each procedure is applied independently. The combination therapy reduces the organ damage associated with chemical induction and minimizes the interventions, such as enzyme supplementation, necessary to maintain a pancreatectomized animal.[18,19]

Genetic Models

The NOD Mouse

Non-obese Diabetic (NOD) mice are an inbred strain of albino mice developed by Makino and coworkers, in Japan. It is derived from breeding Jcl:ICR (Swiss mice) progenitors, and NOD mice represent the product of over 80 generations of sib matings. Over the first 20 generations of sib matings, the strain was being maintained as a normoglycemic control line to match with another line being selected for impaired glucose tolerance (NON strain). Once spontaneous development of IDDM was observed in a female of the control NOD strain at F20, development of frank hyperglycemia and glycosuria rather than normoglycemia, it became the selected phenotype.[20]

The BB Rat

Spontaneous diabetes in the BB Wistar rat was initially diagnosed in 1974 by the Chapel brothers at the Biobreeding Laboratories commercial breeding facility in Ottawa, Ontario, Canada, in a noninbred but closed outbred colony of Wistar rats. It was decided to name this syndrome BB after the initials of the breeding lab. The clinical presentation of diabetes in the BB rat is similar to that of its human counterpart. Marked hyperglycemia, glycosuria, and weight loss occur within a day of onset and are associated with decreased plasma insulin that if untreated will result in ketoacidosis within several days. Like the NOD mouse, the BB rat is one of the few rodent models in which significant ketosis occurs in the absence of obesity. Unlike most NOD mouse colonies, both sexes of BB rats are equally affected.[21]

WBN/KOB Rat

Wistar Bonn/Kobori (WBN/KOB) rats show hyperglycemia and glucosuria by the age of 5 month. Degeneration of islet in size and number is evidenced by the age of 3 months.[22] Other changes observed are fibrinous exudation, deterioration of exocrine pancreatic tissues and demyelination by the age of 4 months.[14]

Cohen Diabetic Rat

Cohen diabetic rat is an excellent hyperglycemic rat model characterized by insulin resistance.[23] In this model, high blood glucose level, high insulin level, glucosuria and other diabetic complications are evidenced in rats on high sucrose diet.[14,24]

Other Diabetogenic Compounds

Other diabetogenic compounds used for the study of diabetes are dithizone[25] or goldthioglucose[26] or monosodium glutamate.[27] Chelators like dithizone, 8-(p-toluenesulfonylamino)-quinoline (8-TSQ), and 8- (benzenesulfanylamino)-quinoline are reported to used in the study of diabetes in experimental animals.[28] Dithizone, used in a single dose of 40-100 mg/kg by intravenous route, produce hyperglycemia in rats, cats, rabbits, golden hamsters and mice. In rabbits dithizone injected, produce hyperglycemia characterized by triphasic glycemic reaction; hyperglycemia after 2 h of injection followed by a normal blood glucose level for 8 h and permanent hyperglycemia after 24–72 h.

MODELS FOR NIDDM

Neonatal STZ Model of NIDDM (Chemically-induced Diabetes)

Neonatal rats of Wistar or Sprague-Dawley strain are treated with STZ (80–100 mg/kg i.p.) at birth or within the first 5 days following birth. There is severe pancreatic β-cell destruction, accompanied by a decrease in pancreatic insulin stores and a rise in plasma glucose levels. However, in contrast to adult rats treated with STZ, the β-cells of the treated neonates partially regenerate. Following an initial spike in plasma glucose the STZ treated neonatal rat becomes normoglycemic by 3 weeks of age. In the next few weeks, the β-cell number increases mainly from the proliferation of cells derived from ducts, the extent, depending upon both the age at which the animal is treated with STZ and the species of the treated rat.[29,30]

Other Chemically-induced NIDDM Models

Agents used for induction of NIDDM in rabbits include adrenaline (0.1 mg/kg s.c.). The peak hyperglycemic effect is noticed at 1 h and lasts up to 4 h. The increase in blood sugar levels is found to be 120–150 mg/100 ml. Oral hypoglycemic agents can be screened by this method. Diabetes can also be induced in animals with chelating agents 8-hydroxy quinoline and biphenyl thio carbazine. EDTA has been reported to be diabetogenic in partially depancreatized rats. Injection of an antiserum produced against ox insulin in guinea pigs or sheep causes diabetes in mice. Diabetes is associated with acute insulin deficiency and the animals exhibit marked hyperglycemia and ketonuria. It is, however, temporary in nature. This model does not have serious toxic side effects like other models, but induces mild pancreatitis in rats. Administration of thiazides, chlorthiazide, hydrochlorthiazide, diazoxide and furosemide, produced hyperglycemia and glycosuria in experimental animals, including rabbits, rats and mice. Diazoxide is found to be effective either alone or in combination with other drugs.[15]

Genetic Models of NIDDM

Monogenic Models of Obesity and NIDDM

The defining phenotypes of the monogenic rodent models include obesity, hyperinsulinemia, transient or sustained hyperglycemia and hyperlipidemia.

Animal models used are as follows:

Yellow Mouse (The Agouti Mouse)

The agouti mouse is believed to have first appeared in China, where it was treated as a curiosity because of its brilliant hair color. The agouti locus was identified as a result of studies on coat color pigments, and was named after the South American rodent *Dasyprocta agouti,* which has a banded pattern of hair color. Hyperinsulinemia, hyperglycemia, insulin resistance and NIDDM in males are found around 4–5 weeks of age.[31-37]

Obese and Diabetic Mouse
The obese (ob) mutation was detected in noninbred mouse stock and was subsequently maintained in the C57Bl/6J strain. The diabetes (db) mutation occurred in the C57BL/KSJ inbred strain. Both ob and db are autosomal recessive with full penetrance. Obese phenotype is characterized by extreme insulin resistance, glucose intolerance, and mild hyperglycemia, and, therefore, exhibits many of the characteristics of NIDDM. At 20–28 days fasting and fed states, both the number and size of pancreatic β-cells are increased. Hyperinsulinemia is accompanied by decreased glucose tolerance. Serum insulin eventually reaches a peak and then falls. Improvement and normalization of blood glucose tolerance, stabilization of serum insulin level and decrease in body weight follow this. In the db phenotype mouse, plasma insulin increases by 10 days and peaks at 6–10 times the normal by 2–3 months, when animals are severely hyperglycemic. Insulin levels drop rapidly to near normal values at the time when islets are hyperplastic and hypertrophic. Progressive degranulation and necrosis follow this, and the islet insulin content becomes greatly reduced. Glucose-induced insulin secretion is severely decreased and there is a rapid rise in blood glucose to over 22 mM up to 5–8 months of age.[32,38]

Tubby Mouse
The tub mutation arose spontaneously in a mouse colony at the Jackson Laboratory, and the tubby colony was bred from a single C57BL/6J male. Tubby mice are characterized by slowly developing obesity. Although hyperinsulinemia, hyperactivity of the islet β-cells and β-cell degranulation are conspicuous features of these animals, hyperglycemia is not observed, and the obesity syndrome does not normally progress to severe diabetes. Both, females and males develop mild hypoglycemia and hyperinsulinemia at 12 weeks, but then become euglycemic. The hyperinsulinemia persists, increasing in severity with age, and ultimately, is associated with insulin resistance.[31-39]

Fat Mouse
The fat (CPE ^{fat}) mutation was discovered in a HRS/J inbred mouse colony at the Jackson Laboratories. Inheritance is autosomal recessive. Animals develop obesity at 6–8 weeks of age. Males develop hyperglycemia by 7–8 weeks and then they return to normal. Chronic hyperinsulinemia is present in both sexes from weaning, and is associated with hypertrophic and hyperplastic pancreatic islet cells.[31-39]

Zucker Diabetic Fatty Rat (ZDF)
These arose from the inbreeding of a substrain of fa/fa rats that exhibited hyperglycemia. In this strain all males develop obesity, insulin resistance and overt NIDDM between 7 and 10 weeks of age, by which time their average plasma glucose exceeds 22 mM. Females are also obese and insulin resistant, but do not become diabetic.[31-40]

Wdf/Ta-Fa Rat
The WDF/Ta-fa rat, commonly referred to as the Wistar fatty rat, is a genetically obese, hyperglycemic rat established by the transfer of the fatty *(fa)* gene from the Zucker rat to the Wistar Kyoto rat. [41-43] The Wistar fatty rat exhibits obesity, hyperinsulinemia, glucose

intolerance, hyperlipidemia, and hyperphagia similar to Zucker rats being, however, more glucose intolerant and insulin resistant than Zucker rats. Hyperglycemia is usually not observed in females, but can be induced by addition of sucrose to the diet. Kobayashi and coworkers[44] found an increase of insulin sensitivity by activation of insulin receptor kinase by pioglitazone in Wistar fatty rats (*fa/fa*). Sugiyma and coworkers[45] found a reduction of glucose intolerance and hypersecretion of insulin in Wistar fatty rats after treatment with pioglitazone for 10 days.[46]

The WDF/Ta-fa rat is genetically modified rat model also known as the Wistar fatty rat. It is generated by injecting fatty (fa) gene from the Zucker rat to the Wistar Kyoto rat.[41-43] It is characterized by obesity, insulin resistance, glucose intolerance, hyperphagia and hyperlipidemia.[44-46]

Other spontaneous diabetic rat models reported in the literature are ESS-rat,[47,48] OBESE SHR rat[49-51] and BHE rat.[52]

Koletsky and JCR: LA-Corpulent Rats

The obese, spontaneously hypertensive, Koletsky rat strain develops obesity, hyperlipidemia and proteinuria with kidney disease. Several substrains have been developed from Koletsky rats, including the SHR/N-cp, LA/N-cp, and JCR: LA-cp strains. JCR: LA–cp rat develop marked hyperinsulinemia by 5–6 weeks of age and decreased glucose uptake. The hyperinsulinemia effectively maintains virtual normoglycemia, but this results in marked islet hyperplasia, and islets occupy 15–20% of the total pancreatic volume in 9-month-old cp/cp male rats.[53,54]

Polygenic Models of Obesity and NIDDM

No single gene has been demonstrated to be involved in the majority of patients with obesity and/or NIDDM. The overall contribution of single gene defects to the total NIDDM population is small and only 10% of the genetic risk factors for NIDDM are known. The more common forms of NIDDM probably result from interaction between the environment and several gene defects, each of which when expressed individually has little effect on glucose tolerance. Therefore, polygenic animal models represent human condition more closely.

Animal strains used are as follows:

New Zealand Obese (NZO) Mouse

Bielschowsky and Bielschowsky first described the NZO mouse. NZO mouse is hyperphagic, obese, hyperglycemic, hyperinsulinemic, insulin resistant, and mildly glucose intolerant. NZO mice become overtly obese by 8–10 weeks of age and reach their maximal weight (males) of 70 g at 12 months. Hyperinsulinemia and hyperglycemia develop early (by 4 weeks), and pancreatic insulin stores are increased at this time. Glucose intolerance decreases continuously with age and body weight.[55]

Diabetic db/db Mice

The Diabetic db/db Mice is a unique mice model derived from mice of the strain the C57BL/KsJ strain having spontaneous recessive mutation in leptin receptor gene, i.e. C57BL/6J db/db.[56] It is characterized by high blood glucose level up to 20–25 mmol/l[57]obesity and nephropathy.[58] Mutations on the leptin receptor result in an obese phenotype identical to that of *ob* mice.[59,60] In the *db/db* mouse strain observe abnormal splicing because the Ob-Rb transcript contains a premature stop codon.[61,62] Insulin level is high and insulin receptors are significantly low.[63]

Japanese KK Mouse

The KK mouse belongs to the Kasukabe (K) group of mouse strains. These mice show hyperinsulinemia, nonfasting hyperglycemia and glucose intolerance. They have insulin resistance due to defect in both the insulin receptor and postreceptor signal transduction systems, including glucose uptake, pentose pathways and impaired insulin sensitive phosphodiesterase in fat cells.[32]

Nagoya-Shibata-Yasuda (NSY) Mouse

NSY mouse was established as an inbred strain from a JcL: ICR mouse colony by selective breeding for glucose intolerance. Spontaneous diabetes develops in 98% of males and 30% females by 48 weeks of age. NSY mice do not become obese, but exhibit fasting hyperinsulinemia, and pancreatic insulin content at 36 weeks of age.[64]

PBB/Ld Mouse

The PBB/Ld mouse originated from pet store stock, selected on the basis of black coat color. They develop apparent obesity by 3–4 months and obese animals exhibit hyperlipidemia, hyperinsulinemia, mild hyperglycemia and reduced tolerance to glucose load.[65]

Otsuka-Long-Evans-Tokushima Fatty Rat (OLEFT)

Kawano and co-workers established the OLEFT rat strain by selectively inbreeding members of a normal colony of Long Evans rats, which developed polyuria, polydypsia, hyperinsulinemia, persistent hyperglycemia, hypertriglyceridemia and mild to moderate obesity. Obesity is evident approximately 2 weeks after weaning. There is a late onset hyperglycemia (after 18 weeks of age) associated with marked glucose intolerance. Diabetes develops in 80–100% of males by 25 weeks of age, females do not show any disability till 40 weeks of age.[66]

Goto-Kakisaki Rat

The GK rat was developed by Goto and Kakisaki through the selection of 18 rats from the local Wistar stock that were slightly glucose intolerant. These hyperglycemic animals were mated and inbred until, after 30 generations, the diabetic state became stable in subsequent generations. The GK rat is one of the best-characterized animal models of spontaneous nonobese NIDDM, since it exhibits similar metabolic, hormonal and vascular disorders to the human disease. This includes fasting hyperglycemia, pronounced glucose intolerance, peripheral and hepatic insulin resistance, impaired glucose-induced insulin secretion and late complications, such as neuropathy and nephropathy.[67]

Chinese Hamster

Mier and Yerganian first reported a diabetic syndrome in the Chinese hamster (*Cricetulus griseus*). Prediabetic hamsters are hyperphagic from birth and develop hyperglycemia, polydypsia and glycosuria early, but they do not become obese.[68]

Djungarian (Siberian) Hamster

An extremely high incidence of spontaneous diabetes has been reported in Djungarian hamsters (*Phodopus sungorus*).[69]

South African Hamster

The South African Hamster (*Mystromys albicandatus*) also develops diabetes without obesity. The degree of hyperglycemia and glucose intolerance varies with age of onset, incidence, and degree of severity in different colonies. Diabetic animals are characterized by polydypsia, glucosuria and ketonuria.[31]

Animal Models of NIDDM with Unknown Hereditary and Environmental Component

A number of models of NIDDM have been developed, as a result of the observation that animals taken from their natural environment developed diabetes mellitus when fed normal laboratory diet.

Sand Rat

Psommomys obesus is a small rodent (gerbil), indigenous to the desert regions of the Middle East where access to food and water is limited. They exhibit a genetic predisposition to the development of NIDDM cataracts, when fed standard high calorie laboratory diet ad libitum.[66]

Spiny Mice

The development of diabetes has been studied in two species of spiny mouse, *Acomys russates* and *A. cahirinus*. Both, males and females have congenital hyperplasia of pancreatic islets, with high insulin content. When laboratory bred *A. cahirinus* exhibits a moderate weight gain on a fat diet, accompanied by hyperglycemia but neither hyperlipidemia nor ketonuria. *A. russates* become obese on either a regular or fatty diet, but do not exhibit hyperglycemia or hyperlipidemia.[70]

Tuco-tuco

The tuco-tuco (*Ctenomys talarum*) were observed at 3 months of age, many of these animals developed cataracts. The ones with cataracts were hyperglycemic and were also mildly obese.[71]

Polygenic animal models produced by hybrid crosses

- BSB (C57BL/6J × Mus spretus)
- AKR/J × SWR/J Model
- GK crosses: GK × Fisher 344 strain, GK × nondiabetic Brown Norway rat.[72]

TRANSGENIC AND KNOCK-OUT ANIMALS

The genes controlling various aspects of metabolism and insulin secretion are manipulated to produce animal models of diabetes mellitus.

The genes that are manipulated to cause insulin resistance correspond to:

1. Insulin receptor
2. Insulin receptor substrate 1 and 2
3. Glucose transporters
4. Hexokinase II
5. Tumor Necrosis Factor-α (TNF-α)
6. Fatty acid-binding Protein 2
7. RAS associated with diabetes (Rad).

The genes that are manipulated to cause defective insulin secretion correspond to:

1. GLUT-2
2. Glucokinase
3. Hepatic Nuclear Factors

4. Islet Amyloid polypeptide.

Genes that increase body fat:

1. Knock out of uncoupling proteins
2. Knock out of β_3-adrenergic receptors.[73,74]

Gene Targeting and Transgenic Techniques

Gene targeting is the process by which single gene is disrupted in an embryonic stem cell and then transmitted along the germ line. This process leads to 'knockout animals'. The transgene is randomly incorporated into the host genome and some offspring will, therefore, express the modified gene.

The female mouse or rat (superovulate) is allowed to mate. The subsequent day, single cell zygotes are collected and maintained in culture for few hours. A genetic construct (insulin gene) is then injected into pronucleus of zygote and the construct integrates itself into the genome of the zygote, which results into the over-express insulin in adult life. The insertion of metallothionein promoter will enhance transgene expression when heavy metals are administered *in vivo* (Fig. 40.3).

Knockout Animals

Knockout animals are produced by using a genetic construct that will disrupt normal gene. Construct is developed, which contains DNA sequence homologues to the target gene but that are disrupted or contain a deletion. These are injected into embryonic stem cells (ES) and will undergo recombination with the normal gene, causing it to be 'knocked out'. ES cells are injected into pre-implantation mouse embryos and transferred to the oviducts of

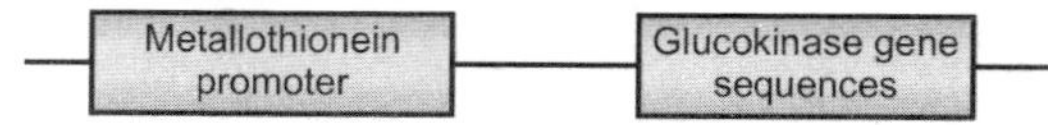

a. Single cell zygotes obtained from superovulated female mouse or rat after mating.

b. A gene construct is produced in which the gene of interest (e.g. glucokinase) is injected into pronucleus of zygote.

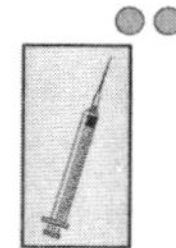

c. Some constructs will integrate with genome of the zygote of host DNA to allow the expression of the gene.

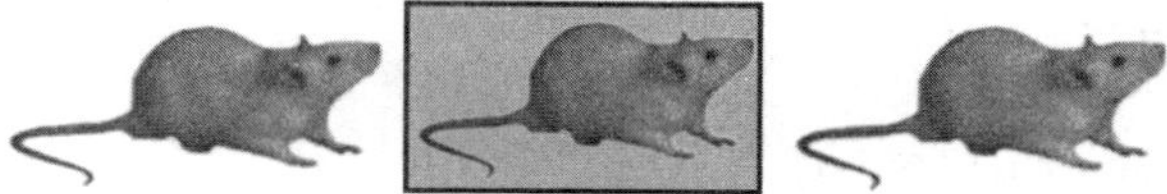

d. Pregnancies are allowed to go to term and off spring tested for transgene expression. In this example, the shaded mouse over-expresses the glucokinase gene. The presence of a metallothionein promoter will enhance transgene expression when heavy metals are administered *in vivo*

Figure 40.3: Producing transgenic animals that over express a gene

pseudopregnant mice and allowed to develop to term. ES cells contribute to the germ line of the offspring, selective breeding will allow the production of mice that are either heterozygous or homozygous for the knockout.

This approach has been used to produce a large number of animals to understand the pathogenesis of Type 1 and Type 2 diabetes.[75,76]

Miscellaneous Models

Invertebrate Animal Model

The silk worm *Bombyx mori* provides an excellent diabetes model alternative to conventional mammalian diabetes models owing to its various advantages like low maintenance cost, ease of experimentation and no ethical issues. In this model, high glucose diet, i.e. 10% glucose is fed to the silk worm for 3 days in the presence and absence of test drug and intervention by test drug is observed by comparing the blood sugar level, body size, weight and other parameters between normal, control and treatment silk worm groups.[14,77]

Diet-induced Metabolic Dysregulation

This model mimics the diabetes induced by metabolic dysregulation due to diet. In this model, hyperglycemia is induced in Baboon (*Papio hamadryas* sp.) by feeding them with high sugar, high fat diet (73% Purina Monkey Chow 5038 (a grain-based meal), 7% lard, 4% Crisco, 4% coconut oil, 10.5% flavored high fructose corn syrup, and 1.5% water) after 12 h fasting. High blood glucose level is demonstrated after 2 months of high glucose and lipid diet along with other diabetic changes like increased blood level of glycosylated hemoglobin (HbA1c), lipids and adipokines.[14,78]

NORMOGLYCEMIC ANIMAL MODELS

Rabbit Model

Rabbits are the animals of choice for this model as they have been used for standardization of insulin for many years and also for the ease in handling.

Procedure

Mixed breed rabbits of either sex weighing 3–4.5 kg are chosen and divided into groups of 4–5. For the evaluation of the insulin and insulin like compounds, food is stopped a day earlier to the experiment; while for the evaluation of hypoglycemic agents, the animals have free access to normal diet till the experiment. The test drug is given orally through gavage in the dose of 1 ml/kg in 0.4% starch suspension. Control group receives only the vehicle. Different doses are tried on other groups. Blood is withdrawn from the ear vein immediately before, and 1, 2, 3, 4, 5, 24, 48, and 72 h after treatment. Blood glucose is determined in 10 µl blood samples using the hexokinase enzyme method. Blood sugar values are plotted against time.[79]

Rat Model

Procedure

Male Wistar rats of 180–240 g body weight are chosen and fed on standard diet. They are divided into groups of 4–7. The test drug is given orally or i.p. in various doses suspended in 0.4% starch suspension. Control group receives only the vehicle. Blood is withdrawn from the tip of the tail immediately before, and 1, 2, 3, 5, and 24 h after administration of the test compound. Blood glucose is determined in 10 µl blood samples with hexokinase enzyme method. Average blood sugar values are plotted versus time or each dosage.

Modifications

Male guinea pigs (pirbright white) can be used instead of rats, each weighing 250–380 g. Blood is withdrawn by puncturing ear veins before and 1, 3, and 5 h after administration of the test compound or the vehicle.[79]

Dog Model

Procedure

Male beagle dogs weighing 15–20 kg, fed normal diet, are chosen. Food is stopped 18 h prior to the administration of the test compound that is given orally or i.v. in various doses. Control animals receive only vehicle. Blood is collected at various intervals up to 48 h. Blood glucose is determined with hexokinase enzyme method and plasma insulin with a radioimmunological method.[79]

Modifications

Pancreatectomized dogs up to 2–3 years prior to the study are given dry feed with 2–3 g pancreatic enzymes. Insulin is substituted with a single daily s.c. dose of 32 IU insulin (long acting); Vitamin D is given i.m. at a dose of 1 ml every 3 months. On the day before the study, animals receive 32 IU of short-acting insulin. This is given along with the food and test compound. Test compound is given as oral suspension in tap water. Blood glucose is determined before and up to 6 h after treatment at hourly intervals. Control animals receive only tap water.[79]

Diabetes is also induced in dogs by a single i.v. dose of 60 mg/kg of alloxan. Then 1000 ml of 5% glucose with 10 IU insulin is infused via jugular vein daily for one week and standard diet ad libitum. Then, a single dose of 28 IU of the shorter-acting insulin is given daily and the animals are fed commercial diet. On the day before the study, the dogs receive 28 IU of the short acting insulin. This insulin is given at the same time as food and test compound. The test drug is given as oral suspension in tap water. Blood glucose is determined before and up to 6 h after treatment at hourly intervals. Control animals receive tap water only.[79]

IN VITRO METHODS ON ISOLATED ORGANS, CELLS AND MEMBRANES

Isolated Pancreas of Rat

The *in vitro* perfusion of isolated pancreas helps us in studying the effect of the drug on insulin, glucagon and somatostatin secretion without interference from other organ changes.

Procedure

Animals used are male Wistar rats weighing 200–250 g. The animals are fed ad libitum. The pancreas is removed under pentobarbital (50 mg/kg i.p.) anesthesia. Once the pancreas is removed, through a portal vein cannula, Krebs-Ringer bicarbonate buffer with 2% bovine albumin and 5.5 mmol/l glucose is perfused at a rate of 1.75 ml/min. The temperature of the perfusion fluid is kept at 37.5°C and the pressure at which it is perfused is about 100 mmHg. The perfusate is collected every minute for 30 min. After the first 5 min of perfusion, test compound is added till the 15th min (conc. of test compound being 0.05–0.5 mM). From 16th min till 30th min, glucose of 5.5 mM and 16.6 mM is perfused. The samples collected are stored at –20°C. Hormones insulin, glucagon and somatostatin are estimated radioimmunologically. At least 3 experiments per concentration are performed. The effect of the test compound, whether it increases or decreases the secreted hormones of pancreas in response to elevated glucose level, is compared with the control.[80]

Isolated Rat Pancreatic Islets

Procedure

Two male Wistar rats weighing 200–250 g act as donors of pancreas, which is removed under pentobarbital anesthesia. The islets are obtained by the collagenase method and collected under a stereomicroscope. In every test, up to 10 chambers each with 15 islets are perifused. Cut-off microfuge tubes, sealed with Tuohy-Borst adapters, serve as perfusion chambers. Two thick-walled, small diameter Teflon catheters are passed through the adapter into the chamber. One of the catheters extends to the bottom of the chamber and acts as the perifusate inlet; the other extends to the lower edge of the adapter cone and acts as outlet. The latter is connected to a multichannel peristaltic pump, which delivers the perifusate to a fraction collector. The chamber volume is 0.15 ml. The perifusate flow rate is 0.1 ml/min. The perifusate consists of Krebs-Ringer bicarbonate buffer with 1.0 mmol/l glucose, 0.25% bovine albumin and 5 mmol/l theophylline. The storage vessels for the perifusate, the chambers and the inlet catheters are immersed in a water bath of 37°C. After a pre-perifusion phase of one hour, the perifusate is collected every minute for 46 min. From the 2nd until the 18th min, the test compound is added at concentrations between 0.1 and 2.5 μmol/l, and from the 34th to the 46th min, the glucose concentration is raised to 20.0 mol/l. Insulin is determined by radioimmunological methods. The determination is done immediately after the end of an experiment.[81]

Modifications

Free cell suspensions from mouse pancreatic islets have been tried, where the response to glucose is lower than that of intact isolated islets. Long term monolayer culture of adult rat islet of Langerhans as an experimental model for studying chronic modulation of α-cell function has been performed.[82]

Isolated Rat Liver

Procedure

Male Wistar rats weighing 200–250 g are anesthetized with 150 mg/kg hexobarbital i.p. after which the liver is removed from the animal, it is washed with 100 ml heparinized (5 IU/ml) physiological saline solution at 37°C for 3 min through the portal vein. The preparation is then transferred to perfusion apparatus, where portal vein cannula is attached to tubing containing the oxygenated medium. Perfusion is done with Krebs-Ringer bicarbonate buffer with 25% bovine erythrocytes, 1.6% bovine serum albumin, and 22.5 mmol/L Na-L-lactate at a rate of 30 ml/min. Seventy ml are used for recirculation over 2 h. The test compound is added to the perfusate medium in a concentration of 40–100 µmol/l. A variable CO_2/O_2 mixture, the ratio of which is dependent on the pH value of the perfusate is used for gassing. The perfusate is bubbled with 70 ml gas mixture/min. To avoid foam formation, a detergent has to be added to the perfusate. The samples for analyses are withdrawn by catheter.[83]

Isolated Hepatocytes

Procedure

Male Wistar rats weighing 200–300 g act as donors. The hepatocytes are then isolated by collagenase method from the liver. The isolated hepatocytes are suspended in 3.0 ml of Krebs-Ringer bicarbonate buffer containing 4% bovine albumin (pH 7.4). The cell suspension is preincubated for 15 min at 37°C in a Dubnof metabolic shaking incubator gassed with CO_2.

The following substrates are added in various combinations and each sample is incubated for 60 min:

1. Alanine, fructose, glycerol, lactate, pyruvate (10 mM), or
2. Palmitate (0.5 mM as sodium palmitate bound to albumin). Test drugs are added in concentrations between 0.05 and 5.0 mM. At the end of the 60 min incubation period, 0.2 ml of 70% $HClO_4$ is added into the medium to stop the reaction. The reaction mixture is then centrifuged, and the supernatant obtained is used to determine the intermediate metabolites. Glucose is assayed by the glucose-oxide method, lactate, pyruvate, acetoacetate and α-hydroxybutarate by enzymatic methods.[84]

Modifications

Instead of isolated hepatocytes, cultures of Hep G2 cells can be used. The Hep G2 cell line is a minimal deviation of human hepatoma that maintains the liver cell morphology and function. Hep G2 cells express insulin receptors, display a number of metabolic responses to insulin and insulin-like growth factor-I and have been used in various studies. Troglitazone (cs-045) was found to increase glycogen synthase-I activity I Hep G2 and BC3H-1 muscle cell.[85,86]

Fructose-2,6-bisphosphate Production in Rat Hepatocytes

Glycogenesis in hepatocytes is regulated by the cytosolic level of fructose-2,6-bisphosphate. Insulin increases fructose-2,6-bisphosphate by inhibiting fructose-2,6-biphosphatase through phosphorylation. If the drug increases the insulin secretion or acts like insulin, it should increase fructose-2,6-bisphosphate level.

Procedure

10^6 cells/ml suspension of hepatic cells is perfused with Hanks 10 mM HEPES buffer solution (pH 7.5, containing 0.5% BSA, and 1 mM palmityl oleate) at 37°C for 10 min. The cells are centrifuged at 40 g for 15 sec, and the supernatant is discarded. To the remainder, the same buffer and various concentrations of test compound are added and the mixtures are then incubated at 37°C for 10 min. The reaction is stopped by cooling on ice. The mixture is centrifuged at 170 g at 4°C for 60 sec. The pellet is homogenized with buffer solution containing 1 mM EGTA and 10 mM $MgCl_2$. After heating at 80°C for 20 min, the homogenate is mixed with an equal volume of 400 mM Tris-HCl buffer (pH 7.5) and the mixture is centrifuged at 17,500 g at room temperature for 5 min. In the supernatant, fructose-2,6-bisphosphate is measured by adding a solution of 54 mM Tris-HCl, 1 mM Fructose-6-phosphate, 0.2 mM NADH, 7.5 mM dithiothreitol, 0.5 mM EDTA, 0.01 U phosphofructokinase, 0.4 U aldolase, 1 U glycerine-3-phosphate dehydrogenase, and 3 U trisphosphate isomerase. The concentration of fructose-2,6-bisphosphate in the sample solution is measured by colorimetry and compared with the reaction rate of a known concentration of fructose-2,6-bisphosphate.[86-89]

Isolated Target Tissue: Muscle

Perfused Hind Limb in Rats

Procedure

Female Wistar rats weighing 170–230 g are used. They are fasted for 48 h before experiment. They are anesthetized by intraperitoneal injection of 50 mg/kg pentobarbital. After identification of aorta, a ligature is placed around it above the origin of the renal vessels and then tied. The aorta is incised between the left renal and iliolumbar vessels and a No. 18 polyethylene catheter, filled with 0.85% NaCl containing 200 U of heparin/ml, is introduced and passed up to a point midway between the iliolumbar vessels and the aortic bifurcation and after flushing with heparin-NaCl solution, it is tied in place. The vena cava is cannulated with a No. 16 needle that is secured in position, such that its tip is at the same level as the aortic catheter. The needle is connected to vinyl tubing. The preparation is then transferred to a perfusion apparatus. Aortic cannula is attached to tubing containing oxygenated medium. Perfusion medium consists of Krebs-Ringer bicarbonate buffer with 25% bovine erythrocytes, 4% bovine serum albumin, and 10 mmol/l D-glucose. It is perfused at a rate of 8 ml/min and 70 ml is used for recirculation over 2 h. The test compounds are added in a concentration of 40–100 mmol/l to the perfusate medium. The ratio of CO_2/O_2 bubbled, depends on the pH value of the perfusate and is bubbled at a rate of 70 ml gas mixture/min. To avoid foam formation, a detergent (14 ml/ml 0.1% Genapol PF-10) is added to the perfusate.[90,91]

MODELS TO STUDY INSULIN SECRETION FROM β CELLS

Insulin Secreting Cell Lines

Insulin secreting cell line culture provides an excellent *ex vivo* diabetic model alternative to conventional animal models. In this model, the HIT cell line is used to assess the insulin secretary and inhibitory activity of test drug. INS-1cells and INS-2 cells from parental RINm5f cells is another model used to study diabetes. In this model, glucose transport activity of test drug is observed and compared with standard anti diabetic formulations available in the market.

Another *ex vivo* model reported in the literature is genetically engineered insulin-secreting human liver cell line, i.e. betacyte (HEP G2ins/g cell), which is responsive to glucose.[92-97]

Muscle Cell Lines

BC_3H1 Myocytes

The BC_3H1 cell line is a nonfusing spontaneously and reversibly differentiating mouse muscle cell line derived from a mouse neoplasm. BC_3H1 myocytes have electron microscopic features of both smooth and skeletal muscle cell, but they have nicotinic acetylcholine receptors and an action potential more like that of a skeletal muscle cell.

BC_3H1 myocytes are cultured to confluence in 100 mm dishes over 10–14 days in Dulbecco's Modified Eagle's Medium (DMEM) added with 15% Process serum Replacement-I, 25 mM glucose (added 18 h before the experiment). Cells are rinsed and pre incubated at 37°C for 20 min in Dulbecco's phosphate buffered saline with 0.1 mM $CaCl_2$ and 1 mg/ml BSA, then treated with buffer (control) or agonists in the buffer for 30 min.

Test compound can be studied on this cell line for:

- Its direct effect on glucose transport
- Insulin-induced decrease of 5'-nucleotidase activity in skeletal muscle membranes
- Glucose transport associated with diacylglycerol-like activation of protein kinase C.[98,99]

L_6 Muscle Cells

They are cultured myogenic cell lines, cultured from thigh of a 1-day-old rat. It has features of skeletal muscle cell. They are grown in 75 cm^2 flasks in Ham's F-10 medium containing 15% horse serum, 2.5% fetal calf serum, 0.87% glutamine, 0.87% penicillin-streptomycin, and 7.5% $NaHCO_3$ at 37°C in a 5% CO_2 atmosphere. After 2–4 days, the cells are in a monolayer, confluent, aligned, and fused, but no myotubes are present. The medium is changed and test substances are added and are used to study glucose uptake.[100]

C_2C_{12} Cells

It is a mouse skeletal muscle cell line isolated from dystrophic mouse muscle. The cells are seeded in a 100 mm diameter, collagen coated, tissue culture dishes at 5×10^4 cells/ml and plated in growth medium consisting of DMEM containing 20% fetal bovine serum, 0.5% chick embryo extract, and 1% penicillin/streptomycin. Cells are grown in this medium to confluence between 75–85% and then induced to differentiate by transferring them to DMEM supplemented with 2% adult horse serum and 1% penicillin/streptomycin.[101]

In Vitro Assays for Insulin or Insulin-like Substances on Adipocytes

Isolated Adipocytes Preparation

The uptake of (^{3}H) glucose into fat cells and incorporation of this radiolabelled glucose in the lipids can measure insulin or insulin-like activity.

Procedure

Epididymal fat pads are removed from male Wistar rats weighing 160–180 g. The fat pads are cut into pieces and incubated for 20 min at 37°C with 1 mg/ml collagenase in KRHB (Krebs-Ringer bicarbonate buffer), 25 mM HEPES/KOH, (pH 7.4), 0.1 mM glucose, 1% w/v BSA (bovine serum albumin). Through 100 mm Nylon screen the cell suspension is filtered and washed 3 times by flotation (accumulation of a thin cell layer on top of the medium after centrifugation at 1000 g for 1 min in a swing-out rotor) with KRHB without glucose, and finally, suspended in the same solution. The suspension is adjusted to a final titer of 4×10^5 cells/ml.[102,103]

Rat Adipocytes Primary Culture

Insulin resistant adipocytes are generated *in vitro* by incubating freshly isolated cell in the primary culture with 25 mM glucose and 10 mM insulin, for 20 h at 37°C under slow shaking. When assayed for insulin stimulated glucose transport, these adipocytes show decreased insulin sensitivity and decreased insulin responsiveness.

3T3 Adipocytes

These cells were isolated from an established mouse fibroblast line, 3T3. These subclonal sublines accumulate large amounts of triglycerides when the cells are in the resting state. These cells have been used for the study of insulin-sensitizing agent. 3T3-L1 cells are grown in DMEM containing 25 mm glucose, 10% FCS and antibiotics. Almost 80–90% of these cells become confluent and differentiated (express the adipocyte phenotype). They are washed two times with KRHB and then incubated in the same buffer with test compound.[104,105]

Assays for Lipid Synthesis in Isolated Adipocytes

The assays measure the insulin stimulated glucose transport and conversion into lipid products like fatty acids, triglycerides and phospholipids. At low glucose concentration (0.1 mM), when the glucose transport is rate limiting, majority of the radiolabelled appears in the glycerol backbone. At higher concentrations (2 mM), when transport is not rate-limiting, 2/3rd of the label is incorporated into the fatty acids of the lipids. These lipids are then measured.

Procedure

Adipocytes are incubated with D-(3-^{3}H) glucose (0.55 mM concentration) and the cells are lysed. Toluene based scintillation cocktail is added to separate the lipids formed from the water-soluble products. After phase separation, radioactivity incorporated into the lipids is determined by liquid scintillation counting directly without removal of the lipid phase.

Incorporation of D-(3-^{3}H) glucose into toluene-extractable acylglycerides is measured after incubation of adipocytes with 1 ml KRPB in the absence or presence of test compound. Before measuring the radioactivity of (3-^{3}H), the reaction is started by adding 0.1 ml (3-^{3}H) glucose (2 μci/ml), 0.1 mM, 0.4 ml Krebs-Ringer bicarbonate buffer 2-fold, and 0.3 ml of substance with test compound to 0.2 ml of adipocyte suspension to scintillation vials. The scintillation vials are placed under a stream of CO_2 for 10 sec, then closed and placed in a very slowly shaking water bath (37°C). After incubation for 90 min, the reaction is terminated by the addition of 10 ml of toluene-based scintillation cocktail. The vials are mixed vigorously using vortex and subsequently left standing for 2–4 h to allow phase separation. The (3-^{3}H) radioactivity is determined with a liquid scintillation counter. Blank values obtained from a typical reaction mixture containing buffer and (3-^{3}H) glucose, but not containing adipocytes and the test compounds, have to be included in each experiment. Since, the lipid synthesis increases in basal state (quality of cell decreases with time), it is recommended to set up to basal incubation for every 20–25 test mixtures. The blank values are subtracted from the values measured for the corresponding set of test mixtures to correct for 3-^{3}H radiation originating from the aqueous phase.[105]

In Vitro Assays of Glucose Transport in Adipocytes

Adipocytes are incubated with 0.2 mM D-(V-^{14}C) glucose for 20 min. Cells are then centrifuged on silicon oil, removed and counted for radioactivity. This assay measures the total insulin-stimulated glucose uptake, transport and metabolism irrespective of whether the glucose is utilized via the oxidative or nonoxidative pathway.

Glucose Uptake by the Isolated Diaphragm from Mice and Rats

This model is useful for the study of the effects of insulin and insulin-like substances on muscle tissue.

To Study Glycogen Synthesis

Diaphragms are obtained from male Sprague-Dawley rats weighing 70–100 g. The diaphragms obtained are divided into two equal pieces. The hemidiaphragms are incubated in Krebs-Henseleit buffer, gassed with 95% O_2/5% CO_2 and with 5 mM (U-^{14}C) glucose (0.5 mci/ml), insulin or the compound to be tested. After 30 min, the hemidiaphragms are blotted on tissue and frozen in liquid nitrogen. The powdered tissue is dissolved by heating for 45 min at 100°C in 30% KOH (1 ml/100 mg tissue) before ethanol is added to a concentration of 70%. After freezing at -20°C, the samples are centrifuged at 2000 g for 10 min. The glycerin pellets washed 3 times with 70% ethanol before the amount of ^{14}C labeled glycogen is determined by liquid scintillation counting. Total glycogen is determined after hydrolysis to glucose (1 N HCL at 100°C for 3 h).[106]

To Study Glucose Transport

Freshly dissected rat diaphragms are incubated for 30 min at 37°C in HEPES-buffered saline (25 mM HEPES, 120 mM NaCl, 5 mM KCl, 1.5 mM $CaCl_2$, 1 mM $MgCl_2$, 5 mM glucose, 0.5 mM sodium pyruvate, 1.5 mM KH_2PO_4, pH 7.4) under constant bubbling with 95% O_2/5% CO_2. The diaphragms are then washed two times with the same buffer without glucose, and incubated further for 30 min in 5 ml of the above buffer with test compound or insulin. Glucose transport is initiated by addition of 50 ml of 10 mM 2-(1-^{3}H) deoxyglucose (10 mci/ml) in the absence or presence of 25 mM cytochalasin B (control). After 15 min, the diaphragms are rinsed four times with ice-cold buffer containing 10 mM glucose, 25 mM cytochalasin B, then blotted with filter paper and homogenized. Portions of the homogenate are used for protein determination. Samples of the supernatant in a volume of 1 ml are centrifuged at 10,000 g for 15 min and mixed with scintillation cocktail and counted for radioactivity. Glucose transport (dpm/mg of protein) is calculated as difference between diaphragm associated radioactivity measured in the absence (total uptake) and presence of cytochalasin (nonspecific uptake).[105]

To Study Glycogen Synthase Activity

Intact hemidiaphragms obtained from male Wistar rats are incubated in DMEM (10 ml/hemidiaphragm) with test compounds or insulin and 5 mM glucose at 37°C and constantly bubbled with O_2: CO_2 (95:5). The homogenate is prepared by blotting and freezing the diaphragms in liquid nitrogen. Frozen diaphragms are grounded in a porcelain mortar and then homogenized at 0°C in 10 vol of 25 mM tris/HCl (pH 7.4), 100 mM NaF, 5 mM EDTA, 0.1 mM PMSF. The homogenate is centrifuged (10,000 g, 20 min). The supernatant is used for glycogen synthase assay. Ten microliters of diaphragm homogenate is added to 200 ml of 25 mM Tris/HCl (pH7.4), 50 mM NaF, 10 mM EDTA (preincubated at 30°C) containing either 0.1 or 10 mM glucose-6-phosphate. The reaction is initiated by supplementing 0.2 mM (U-^{14}C) UDP-glucose (10 mci) and terminated after 15 min by addition of 2.5 ml of ice-cold 66% ethanol and filtration over pre-wetted Whatman GF/C glass fiber disks. The filters are washed, dried and counted for radioactivity. Blanks are assayed by adding the homogenate to tubes containing the complete reaction mixture plus ice-cold ethanol. The fractional velocity, as parameter for the portion of glycogen synthase active *in vivo* (l-form) toward the total enzyme contents (l- + d-forms) at the point of homogenization, is calculated as ratio between the activities measured at 0.1 (l-form) and 10 mM glucose-6-phosphate (l-+ d-forms).[106]

Insulin Receptor-binding Assays

Subcutaneous adipose tissue is obtained from the abdomen of patients undergoing gasteroenterological surgery. The adipose tissue is finely chopped and incubated for 90 min at 37°C in a HEPES buffer (pH 7.4), containing human serum albumin (25 g/l) and collagenase (0.5 g/l). The isolated adipocytes are subsequently washed five times in a HEPES buffer containing 50 g/l human albumin. The diameters, surface and volume are calculated for every cell. Insulin receptor-binding studies with isolated human adipocytes are performed in a 300 μl cell suspension containing about 1×10^5 cells/ml in a HEPES buffer (10 mmol/l HEPES, 50 g/l human albumin (pH 7.4) at 37°C. The iodine-labeled ligand (I^{125} Tyr^{A14}-monoiodinated insulin, specific activity about 350 mCi/mg) in a final concentration of 20 pmol/l is incubated with increasing amounts of unlabeled human insulin and insulin derivative to be tested. The reaction is stopped by adding 10 ml of chilled 0.154 mol/l NaCl and subsequent centrifugation with silicon oil. Nonspecific-binding is measured by incubating tracer in the presence of a large excess of unlabeled insulin. For association studies, the ^{125}I-labeled ligand is incubated for different period (1–240 min) and the reaction is terminated as described above. At each time point, the nonspecific-binding is measured and substracted subsequently from the data for total-binding. Dissociation rates are determined by first incubating isolated adipocytes at 37°C with either (^{125}I) TyrA14- insulin, or the test compound labeled in the same position for 90 min to achieve steady-state-binding conditions. Each incubation mixture is then centrifuged for 60 sec. The adipocytes are rapidly washed twice, by diluting with buffer to the original volume at 4°C and centrifugation and aspirations are repeated. After the third aspiration, the cells are diluted to the original volume with buffer alone or native insulin or the insulin derivative to be tested at a final concentration of 0.2 mmol/l at 22°C. The reaction is stopped at various times between 10 and 180 min and cell-associated radioactivity is determined.[107,108]

Modifications

Insulin receptor-binding assays have been done on receptors prepared from the membranes prepared from the rat liver.[109] The studies have also been done on solubilized purified insulin receptors from livers of Zucker fatty rats and Sprague-Dawley rats with dietary obesity.[110] Receptor-binding and tyrosine kinase activation by insulin analogues, in the human hepatoma HepG2 cells[72] have been studied. Binding of insulin derivative to human insulin receptor overexpressed on a transfected Chinese Hamster ovary cell line has also been studied.[112]

An ideal antidiabetic agent is one which normalizes all of the metabolic disturbances which occur in the diabetic patient. Diabetes, which is due to some degree of insulin deficiency, can be-induced experimentally by removal of source or action of insulin.

Screening of antidiabetic agents must take into consideration methods for discovering activity as well as definitive studies. Selection of physiologic end point for screening a large number of chemicals for preliminary activity is of prime importance. Historically and because diabetes is diagnosed by tests of glucose tolerance, attention has been generally directed to glucose metabolism. Although diabetes is a complicated disease involving all aspects of the intermediary metabolism, changes in blood glucose level are a convenient and useful tool in screening for antidiabetic agents.

The most useful screening method is based on depression of blood sugar values in intact animals, since the intact animal theoretically possesses all the mechanisms involved in blood regulation.

EXPERIMENTAL MODELS FOR DIABETIC COMPLICATIONS

The uncontrolled blood glucose level affects different body organ which causes some of the undesirable effects which include microvascular complications such as retinopathy (which can lead to blindness), nephropathy (ultimately kidney failure) and painful neuropathy (which can lead to amputations). In addition, macrovascular complications of diabetes include coronary artery disease, atherosclerosis, hypertension, and stroke. The micro and macrovascular complications observed in the diabetic population result from the actions of various pathological factors and pathways functioning independently or in combination.[113-115]

Some specific experimental models commonly used for screening of diabetic complications like cardiomyopathy, nephropathy and retinopathy are also reported. Models for cardiomyopathy and nephropathy are given below. Models for retinopathy are explained in detail in Chapter 41.

Diabetic Cardiomyopathy

Cardiovascular complications are leading cause of morbidity and mortality related to uncontrolled diabetes. Initially, increased coronary artery disease was considered as major risk for failing heart, but risk of developing heart failure remained one of the major health problem which was independent of coronary artery disease. One of the study reveals that diabetic patients with normal coronary artery suffered from heart failure suggesting that other etiologies are involved. Similarly, other studies have shown that diabetic patients with normal blood pressure, body weight, serum lipid profile and coronary artery developed heart failure. This research led to coin the term 'diabetic cardiomyopathy', which has been defined as ventricular dysfunction occurring in diabetes patients in the absence of coronary artery disease and hypertension.[116,117]

High glucose regulates structural and functional changes of cardiomyocytes via the activation of several signal transduction pathways, including impaired calcium homeostasis, activation of the renin-angiotensin system and increased oxidative stress.[118-123]

The heterozygous Ins2+/- Akita Diabetic Mouse

The Ins2Akita/+ (Akita) mouse is a model of type 1 diabetes, characterized by a point-mutation causing proinsulin misfolding with subsequent endoplasmic reticulum stress leading to beta-cell apoptosis. This affects folding of proinsulin in the endoplasmic reticulum, leading to endoplasmic reticulum stress, proteotoxicity in pancreatic β-cells, and cell loss. The Ins2WT/C96Y mouse provides an ideal nonobese model of type 1 diabetes that is based on a mutation described in human diabetes, while being free of potential confounding effects of STZ-induced type 1 diabetes. Moreover, Ins2WT/C96Y mice have several advantages over inbred mouse strains that require STZ treatment, including a better defined etiology, along with a more pronounced and durable hyperglycemia.

In Ins2Akita/+ (Akita) mouse, cardiomyopathy is characterized by early diastolic dysfunction in the absence of systolic dysfunction. It has been studied that the diastolic dysfunction in Ins2Akita/+ mice could be brought about by a number of factors, including elevated levels of β-MHC isoform and reduced SERCA2a levels, which may have contributed to the impaired relaxation of the LV.

Lipotoxicity may arise from myocardial triacylglycerol accumulation, increased oxidation of long-chain fatty acids, and increased production of ceramide and DAG, important markers of lipotoxicity in the heart. In addition, mitochondrial functions are impaired and the expressions of mitochondrial encoded genes are reduced. The elevated levels of fatty acids, triglycerol, ceramides, DAG, as well as lipid depositions in the Ins2Akita/+ hearts strongly suggest myocardial lipotoxicity as the dominant mechanism of the diastolic dysfunction in Ins2Akita/+ mice.[124-126]

OVE26 Mouse Model

OVE26 mouse is a model of type 1 diabetes. OVE26 mouse model shows severe and consistent diabetes, and has an early onset. It can survive for more than a year without insulin treatment, direct damage is specific to the pancreatic β-cell and breeding is simple. Overexpression of the Ca^{2+} binding protein calmodulin in pancreatic β-cells led to insulin deficient diabetes in first week after birth producing cell damage remains to be completely understood.[127]

OVE26 mice show cardiac abnormalities, which include reduced cardiomyocyte contractility, degenerating mitochondrial morphology and reduced mitochondrial glutathione content. Freshly isolated OVE26 diabetic cardiomyocytes had reduced contractility compared to control FVB myocytes. Several studies have shown impaired peak shortening, prolonged time to peak shortening, prolonged time to 90% re-lengthening and reduced velocities of shortening and re-lengthening.[128]

OVE26 diabetic hearts showed several distinguishable ultrastructural abnormalities like swollen mitochondria, mottled matrices and broken mitochondrial membranes with impaired pyruvated-supported mitochondrial state 3 respiration. Mitochondrial content is increased in OVE26 hearts and proteomic analysis showed induction of several proteins involved n the biogenesis of mitochondria. It is very well evident important role of oxidative stress in OVE26 hearts. In OVE26 diabetic hearts, reduced levels GSH, increased catalase expression and increased malondialdehyde levels are found. OVE26 diabetic hearts showed impaired intracellular Ca^{2+} handling, reduced activity of sarcoendoplasmic reticulum Ca^{2+}-ATPase 2a, impaired Ca^{2+} release and uptake from sarcoplasmic reticulum, and reduced Na^{2+}-Ca^{2+} exchanger expression.[129]

Diabetic Nephropathy

Diabetic nephropathy is one of the microvascular complications after chronic diabetes and is the major cause of morbidity and mortality in patients with type 2 diabetes. End-stage renal disease has been increased drastically worldwide in patients suffering from type 2 diabetes during the past two decades, and diabetes is associated with worse survival rate in patients undergoing dialysis. Despite the high prevalence of diabetic nephropathy, around 40% of all diabetic patients are at risk of developing end-stage kidney failure, and genetic studies indicate grave risk for diabetic nephropathy.[130] A large number of pool of genes have been identified in the onset and progression, but still are weak predictors of nephropathy in patients with type 2 diabetes. Experimental models of type 2 diabetes with nephropathy may offer a key to a better understanding of this complication in a multifactorial disease such as type 2 diabetes.[131]

Increased blood glucose level causes the nephropathy via different pathogenic mechanism like changes in hemodynamic mechanisms, activation of protein kinase C, aldose reductase pathway, increases level of cytokines and oxidative stress.[132-137]

Insulin-2 Akita Mouse

Akita mice develop type 1 diabetes because of the spontaneous mutation in Ins-2 gene. The mutation leads to the misfolding of insulin protein, which is toxic to pancreatic β-cell. Therefore, the ability of β-cell to secrete insulin is mainly decreased. The Ins-2 Akita mutation, which is autosomal dominant, was originally found in C57BL/6 mice in Akita, Japan.

Heterozygous mice develop significant hyperglycemia as a result of severe insulin deficiency at 3–4 weeks of age. A male suffers considerably worse insulin deficiency compared to female. Mice with Ins-2 Akita mutation exhibit modest levels of albuminuria and mild-to-moderate glomerular mesangial expansion. However, Akita mice develop higher levels of hyperglycemia, albuminuria, blood pressure, and more consistent structural changes of kidney compared with STZ-induced diabetic nephropathy. In one of the study, Gurley et al. 2006, have found that renal phenotype of Akita mice depend largely on their genetic background strains, which suggest that genetic factors might influence susceptibility to diabetic nephropathy in Akita mice which is the same in human disease. Thus, mice having Ins-2 Akita mutations have significant advantages as a model of type 1 diabetes.[138,139]

BTBR ob/ob Mice

When the ob/ob mutation is crossed with BTBR background, the mice are initially insulin resistant with elevated insulin levels, pancreatic islet hypertrophy and marked hyperglycemia by 6 weeks of age. They are largely resistant to significant lowering of blood glucose by insulin administration. The kidney phenotype of these mice shows early loss of podocytes and onset of proteinuria, both of which are detectable by 8 weeks of age.

Glomerular hypertrophy marked expansion of mesangial matrix, mesangiolysis, and capillary basement membrane thickening have been identified in this model. These features model morphologically mimics early human DN, and by 18 weeks of age, these mice model have progressive, advanced DN with features of marked proteinuria, more extensive mesangial expansion, mesangiolysis, persistent podocyte loss, and basement membrane thickening. Like other mice with leptin deficiency, these mice are infertile and breeding mice in sufficient numbers for interventional studies is labor intensive and expensive.[140,141]

eNOS Deficient Mice

Endothelial dysfunction is present in diabetes and is associated with impaired vascular nitric oxide (NO) synthesis. A number of polymorphisms in the endothelial NO synthase gene (eNOS), located on human chromosome 7, have been linked to renal vasculopathies. There are currently two models of diabetic nephropathy dependent on genetic deletion of endothelial nitric oxide synthase (eNOS–/–). eNOS provides the principal means by which nitric oxide is generated in the vasculature; NO is in turn a major regulator of vascular tone. Reduction of NO availability has been considered a major mechanism for the development of diabetic complications involving the vasculature, including diabetic nephropathy.[142]

The eNOS–/–/*db/db* mouse is a model of type 2 diabetes generated by backcrossing of eNOS knockout mouse on the C57/B6 background with *db/db* mouse on the C57BLKS/J background. The eNOS–/–/lepr *db/db* double-knockout mice exhibit obesity, hyperglycemia, hyperinsulinemia, hypertension, dramatic albuminuria, and decreased GFR. These mice develop histopathological features of DN-like human disease such as mesangial expansion, glomerular basement thickening, mesangiolysis, focal segmental and nodular glomerulosclerosis, nodules, fibronectin accumulation in glomeruli, arteriolar hyalinosis, minimal tubulointerstitial fibrosis, and microaneurysms.[143,144]

In second model, eNOS deficiency has been introduced in streptozotocin induced type I diabetes in eNOS–/– mice of C57BL/6 background. Although C57BL/6 mice are resistant to development of diabetic nephropathy; however, eNOS deficiency was found to be sufficient to induce development of features of advanced diabetic nephropathy, including hypertension, albuminuria, mesangial matrix expansion, mesangiolysis and mesangial nodule formation, and renal insufficiency. Like eNOS–/–/db/db mice, this model also offers a means to study mechanisms underlying advanced diabetic nephropathy, but several important pitfalls needs to be considered.[145]

Podocyte Specific Insulin Receptor Knockout Mouse

A recent study shows that a mixed mouse strain (with C57BL/6, 129/Sv, and FVB backgrounds) with podocyte specific deletion of insulin receptors using both podocin and nephrin promoters to drive cre-recombinase directed excision of the receptor. Furthermore, loss of podocyte insulin responsiveness in the intact perfused glomerulus results in glomerular pathology with a number of features characteristic of diabetic nephropathy (DN), including increased matrix production, glomerulosclerosis, thickening of the glomerular basement membrane, and, with time, podocyte apoptosis. These mice develop proteinuria and were reported to develop histologic features of DN despite maintaining normal insulin levels and normoglycemia. Features of DN exhibited by these mice included increased podocyte apoptosis at 8 weeks of age, detected at a time when significant proteinuria was becoming established, podocyte foot process effacement, and increased mesangial matrix.[146,147]

REFERENCES

1. Baily CC, Baily OT. Production of diabetes mellitus in rabbits with alloxan: a preliminary report. J Am Med Ass 1943;122:1165-6.
2. Dunn JS, McLetchie NGB. Experimental alloxan diabetes in the rat. Lancet 1943;11:384-7.
3. Lenzen S, Panten U. Alloxan: History and mechanism of action. Diabetologia 1988;31:337-42.
4. Kodoma T, Iwase M, Nunoi K, et al. A diabetes model induced by neonatal alloxan treatment in rats. Diab Res Clin Pract 1993;20:183-9.
5. Rakieten N, Rakieten ML, Nadkarni MV. Studies on the diabetogenic action of Streptozotocin (NSC 37917). Cancer Chemotherapy Rep 1963;29:91-8.
6. Povoski SP, McCullough PJ, Zhou W, et al. Induction of diabetes mellitus in Syrian golden hamsters using stored equilibrium solutions of Streptozotocin. Lab Anim Sci 1993;43:310-4.
7. Ar'Rajab A, Ahren B. Long term diabetogenic effect of streptozotocin in rats. Pancreas 1993;8:50-7.
8. Wright JR Jr, Lacy PE. Synergistic effects of adjuvants, endotoxin and fasting on induction of diabetes with multiple low doses of streptozotocin in rats. Diabetes 1988;37:112-8.
9. Chattopadhyay S, Ramanathan M, Das J, et al. Animal models in experimental diabetes mellitus. Indian J Exp Biol 1997;35:1141-5.
10. Ogawa A, Johnson JH, Ohneda M, et al. Roles of insulin resistance and Beta-cell dysfunction in dexamethasone-induced diabetes. J Clin Invest 1992;90:497-503.
11. Ingle DJ. The production of glycosuria in the normal rat by means of 17-hydroxy-11-dehydrocorticosterone. Endocrinology 1941;29:649-52.
12. Abelove WA, Paschkis KE. Comparison of the diabetogenic action of cortisone and growth hormone in different species. Endocrinology 1994;55:637-54.
13. Ingle DJ, Li CH, Evans HM. The effect of adrenocorticotropic hormone on the urinary excretion of sodium, chloride, potassium, nitrogen and glucose in normal rats. Endocrinology 1946;39:32-39.
14. Kumar S, Singh R, Vasudeva N. Acute and chronic animal models for the evaluation of anti-diabetic agents. Cardiovasc Diabetol 2012;11:1-13.
15. Moloney PJ, Coval M. Antigenicity of insulin: diabetes-induced by specific antibodies. Biochem J 1955;59:179-85.
16. Yoon JW. The role of viruses and environmental factors in the induction of diabetes. Current Top Microbiol Immunol 1990;164:95-123.
17. Szopa TM, Titchener PA, Portwood ND, et al. Diabetes mellitus due to viruses—some recent developments. Diabetologia 1993;36:687-95.
18. Duff GL, Murray EGD. The pathology of the pancreas in experimental diabetes mellitus. Am J Med Sci 1945;210:81-95.

19. Kaufmann F, Rodriguez RR. Subtotal pancreatectomy in five different rats strains incidence and course of development of diabetes. Diabetologia 1984;27:38-43.
20. Leiter EH. NOD mice and related strains: origins, husbandry, and biology. In: Heiter EH, Atkinson MA (Eds). NOD mice and related strains: Research Applications in Diabetes, AIDS, Cancer, and other Diseases, Austin: RG Landes, 1998:1-15.
21. Chappel CI, Chappel WR. The discovery and the development of the BB rat colony; and animal model of spontaneous diabetes mellitus. Metab: Clin and Exp 1983;32:8-10.
22. Yagihashi S, Wada RI, Kamijo M, et al. Peripheral neuropathy in the WBN/Kob rat with chronic pancreatitis and spontaneous diabetes. Lab Invest 1993;68:296-307.
23. Cohen AM, Teitelbaum A, Saliternik R. Genetics and diet as factors in the development of diabetes mellitus. Metabolism 1972;21:235-40.
24. Velasquez MT, Kimmel PL, Michaelis OE. Animal models of spontaneous diabetic kidney disease. FASEB J 1972;4:2850-59.
25. Hansen WA, Christie MR, Kahn R, et al. Supravital dithizone staining in the isolation of human and rat pancreatic islets. Diabetes Res 1989;10:53-57.
26. Heydrick SJ, Gautier N, Olichon-Berte C, et al. Early alteration of insulin stimulation of PI 3-kinase in muscle and adipocyte from gold thioglucose obese mice. Am J Physiol Endocrinol Metab 1995;268:604-12.
27. Sartin JL, Lamperti AA, Kemppainen RJ. Alterations in insulin and glucagon secretion by monosodium glutamate lesions of the hypothalamic arcuate nucleus. Endocr Res 1985;11:145-55.
28. Goldberg ED, Eshchenko VA, Bovt VD. The diabetogenic and acidotropic effects of chelators. Exp Pathol 1991;42:59-64.
29. Blondel O, Bailbe D, Portha B. Relation of insulin deficiency to impaired insulin action in NIDDM adult rats given streptozotocin as neonates. Diabetes 1989;38:610-7.
30. Weir GC, Clore ET, Zmachinski CJ, et al. Islet secretion in a new experimental model for noninsulin-dependent diabetes. Diabetes 1981;30:590-5.
31. Mordes JP, Rossini AA. Animal models of diabetes. Am J Med 1981;70:353-60.
32. Fiedorek FT. Rodent genetic models for obesity and noninsulin-dependent diabetes mellitus. In: Leroith D, Taylor SL, Olefsky JM (Eds). Diabetes Mellitus. Philadelphia: Lippincott-Raven Press, 1996;604-35.
33. York DA. Lessons from animal models of obesity. Endocrinol Metab Clin North Am 1996;25:781-800.
34. Elbein SC. The genetics of human noninsulin-dependent (Type 2) diabetes mellitus. J Nutr 1997;127: 1891S-6S.
35. Groop LC. The molecular genetics of noninsulin-dependent diabetes mellitus. J Intern Med 1997;241:95-107.
36. Bonner-Weir S, Leahy JL, Weir GC, et al. Induced rat models of noninsulin-dependent diabetes mellitus. In: Shafrir E, Renold AE (Eds). Frontiers in Diabetes Research. Lessons from animal models, Vol-II, London: John Libbey and Co, 1988:295-320.
37. Siracusa LD. The agouti gene: turned on to yellow. Trends Genet 1994;10:423-8.
38. Coleman DL. Obese and diabetes, two mutant genes causing diabetes-obesity syndromes in mice. Diabetologia 1978;14:141-8.
39. Coleman DL, Eicher EM. Fat (fat) and tubby (tub): two autosomal recessive mutations causing obesity syndromes in the mouse. J Hered 1990;81:424-7.
40. Peterson RG, Shaw WN, Neel MA, et al. Zucker diabetic fatty rat as a model for noninsulin-dependent diabetes mellitus. ILAR News 1990;32:16-9.
41. Ikeda H, Shino A, Matsuo T, et al. A new genetically obese-hyperglycemic rat (Wistar fatty). Diabetes 1981;30:1045–50.

42. Kava RA,West DB, Lukasik VA, Greenwood MRC. Sexual dimorphism of hyperglycemia and glucose tolerance in Wistar fatty rats. Diabetes 1989;38:159–63.
43. Velasquez MT, Kimmel PL, Michaelis OE. Animal models of spontaneous diabetic kidney disease. FASEB J 1990;4:2850–59.
44. Kobayashi M, Iwanshi M, Egawa K, et al. Pioglitazone increases insulin sensitivity by activating insulin receptor kinase. Diabetes 1992;41:476–83.
45. Sugiyama Y, Taketomi S, Shimura Y, et al. Effects of pioglitazone on glucose and lipid metabolism in Wistar fatty rats. Arzneim Forsch/Drug Res 1990;40:263-7.
46. Vogel HG. Drug discovery and evaluation; Pharmacological assays. Third edition, Heidelberg, Berlin: Springer-Verlag; 2007.
47. Tarrés MC, Martínez SM, Liborio MM, et al. Diabetes mellitus en unalínea endocrinada de rata. Mendeliana 1981;5:39-48.
48. Dumm CLAG, Semino MC, Gagliardino JJ: Sequential changes in pancreatic islets of spontaneously diabetic rats. Pancreas 1990;5:533-9.
49. Koletsky S: Pathologic findings and laboratory data in a new strain of obese hypertensive rats. Am J Pathol 1975;80:129-42.
50. Russell JC, Graham S, Hameed M: Abnormal insulin and glucose metabolism in the JCR:LA-corpulent rat. Metabolism 1994;43:538-43.
51. Friedman JE, Ishizuka T, Liu S, Farrell CJ, Bedol D, Koletsky RJ, Kaung HL, Ernsberger P. Reduced insulin receptor signaling in the obese spontaneously hypertensive Koletsky rat. Am J Physiol Endocrinol Metab 1997;273:1014-23.
52. Berdanier CD. Metabolic abnormalities in BHE rats. Diabetologia 1974;10:691–95.
53. Koletsky S. Obese spontaneously hypertensive rats, a model for study of atherosclerosis. Exp Mol Pathol 1973;19:53-60.
54. Takaya K, Ogawa Y, Hiraoka J, et al. Nonsense mutation of leptin receptor in the obese spontaneously hypertensive Koletsky rat. Nature Genet 1996;14:130-1.
55. Bielschowsky M, Bielschowsky F. A new strain of mice with hereditary obesity. Proc Univ Otago Med Sch 1953;31:29-36.
56. Tartaglia LA, Dembski M, Wenig X, et al. Identification and expression cloning of a leptin receptor, OB-R. Cell 1995;83:1263-71.
57. Like AA, Lavine RL, Poffenbarger PL, ChickWI. Studies on the diabetic mutant mouse. VI Evolution of glomerular lesions and associated proteinuria. Am J Pathol 1972;66:193–224.
58. Gardner K. Glomerular hyperfiltration during the onset of diabetes mellitus in two strains of diabetic mice (C57BL/6J db/db and C57BL/KsJ db/db) Diabetologia 1978, 15:59–63.
59. Li C, Ioffe E, Fidahusein N, Connolly E, Friedman JM. Absence of soluble leptin receptor in plasma from dbPas /dbPas and other db/db mice. J Biol Chem 1998;10078–82.
60. Lee GH, Proenca R, Montez JM, Carroll KM, Darvishzadeh JG, Li JI, Friedman JM. Abnormal splicing in the leptin receptor in diabetic mice. Nature 1996;379:632–35.
61. Friedman JF, Halaas JL. Leptin and the regulation of body weight in mammals. Nature 1998;395:763–70.
62. Coleman DL, Hummel KP. Effects of parabiosis of normal with genetically diabetic mice. Am J Physiol 1969;217:1298-304.
63. Raizada MK, Tan G, Fellows RE. Fibroblastic cultures from the diabetic db/db mouse. Demonstration of decreased insulin receptors and impaired responses to insulin. J Biol Chem 1980;255:9149-55.
64. Ueda H, Ikegami H, Yamato E, et al. The NSY mouse, a new animal model of spontaneous NIDDM with moderate obesity. Diabetologia 1995;38:503-8.

65. Hunt CE, Lindsey JR, Walkley SU. Animal models of diabetes and obesity, including the PBB/Ld mouse. Fed Proc 1976;35:1206-17.
66. Kawano K, Hirashima T. Spontaneously diabetic rat, OLEFT as a model for NIDDM in humans, In: Shafrir E (Ed). Lessons from Animal Diabetes VI, Boston: Birkhauser, 1996;225-50.
67. Goto Y, Suzuki KI, Sasaki M, et al. GK rat as a model of nonobese noninsulin-dependent diabetes mellitus, selective breeding of over 35 generations. In: Shafrir E, (Ed). Frontiers in diabetes research. Lessons from animal Diabetes II, Boston: Birkhauser 1988;301-3.
68. Frankel BJ. Diabetes in Chinese hamster. In: Shafrir E (Ee). Lessons from animal Diabetes VI, Boston: Birkhauser 1996;2:267-98.
69. Voss KM, Herberg L, Kem HF. Fine structural studies of the islets of Langerhans in the Djungarian Hamster (Phodopussungorus). Cell Tissue Res 1978;191:333-42.
70. Shafrir E, Adler JH. Enzymatic and metabolic responses to affluent diet of two diabetes prone species of spiny mouse, Acomyscahirinus and Acomysrussatu. Int J Biochem 1983;15:1439-46.
71. Wise PH, Weir B, Hime JM, et al. The diabetic syndrome in the tuco-tuco (Ctenomystalarum). Diabetologia 1972;8:165-72.
72. Bray G, Bouchard C. Genetics of obesity, research directions. FASEB J 1997;11:937-45.
73. Accilli D. Insulin receptor knock-out mice. Trends Endocrinol Metab 1997;8:101-11.
74. Patti ME, Kahn CR. Lessons from transgenic and knock-out animals about NIDDM. Trends Endocrinol Metab 1996;7:311-4.
75. Rees DA, Alcolado JC. Animal models of diabetes mellitus. Diabetic Med 2005;22:359-70.
76. Pellegrino Masiello. Animal models of type 2 diabetes with reduced pancreatic beta-cell mass. Int J Biochem Cell Biol 2006;38:873-93.
77. Matsumoto Y, Sumiya E, Sugita T, et al. An Invertebrate Hyperglycemic Model for the Identification of Anti Diabetic Drugs. PLoS ONE 2011;6(3):e18292.
78. Higgins PB, Bastarrachea RA, Lopez-Alvarenga JC, et al. Eight week exposure to a high sugar high fat diet results in adiposity gain and alterations in metabolic biomarkers in baboons (Papio hamadryas sp.). Cardiovascular Diabetology 2010;9:71.
79. Geisen K. Special pharmacology of the new sulfonylurea glimpiride. Drug Res 1988;38:1120-30.
80. Grodsky GM, Heldt A. Method for the in vitro perfusion of the pancreas. In: Larner J, Pohl SL (Eds) Methods in Diabetes Research Vol I, Laboratory Methods, Part B, New York: John Wiley and Sons, 1984;137-46.
81. MalaisseLagai F, Malaisse WJ. Insulin release by pancreatic islets. In Larner J, Pohl SL, (Eds). Methods in Diabetes Research Vol I, Laboratory Methods, Part B, New York: John Wiley and Sons, 1984;147-52.
82. Lernmark A. The preparation of and studies on, freecell suspensions from mouse pancreatic islets. Diabetologia 1974;10:431-8.
83. Ross BD. Perfusion techniques in biochemistry. A laboratory manual in the use of isolated perfused organs in biochemical experimentation. Oxford: Clarendon Press, 1972;135-220.
84. Berry MN, Friend DS. High yield preparation of isolated rat liver parenchymal cells; A biochemical and fine structural study. J Cell Biol 1969;43:506-20.
85. Seglen PO. Preparation of rat liver cells. In: Prescott DM, (EDs). Methods in Cell Biology, Vol-XIII. New York: Academic Press, 1976;71-98.
86. Ciaraldi TP, Gilmore A, Olefsky JM, et al. In vitro studies on the action of CS-045, a new antidiabetic agent. Metabolism 1990;39:1056-62.

87. Podskalny JM, Takeda S, Silverman RE, et al. Insulin receptors and bio-responses in a human liver cell line (Hep G2). Eur J Biochem 1985;150:401-7.
88. Mori K, Kaku K, Inoue H, et al. Effects of tolbutamide on fructose-2,6-bisphosphate formation and ketogenesis in hepatocytes from diabetic rats. Metabolism 1992;41:S706-10.
89. Mourn K, Inoue Y, Emoto M, et al. CS-045 a new oral antidiabetic agent, stimulates fructose-2, 6-bisphosphate production in rat hepatocytes. Eur J Pharmacol 1994;254:257-62.
90. Richards CS, Uyeda K. The effect of insulin and glucose on fructose-2, 6-bisphosphate in hepatocytes. Biochem Biophys Res Commun 1982;109:394-401.
91. Daniels EL, Lewis SB. Acute tolbutamide administration alone and combined with insulin enhances glucose uptake in the perfused rat hindlimb. Endocrinology 1982;1840-42.
92. Santerre RF, Cook RA, Crisek RMD, et al. Insulin synthesis in a clonal cell line of simian virus 40-transformed hamster pancreatic beta cells. Proc Natl Acad Sci USA 1981;78:4339-43.
93. Masuda K, Okamoto Y, Tuura Y, et al. Effects of troglitazone (CS-045) on insulin secretion in isolated rat pancreatic islets and HIT cells: an insulinotropic mechanism distinct from glibenclamide. Diabetologia 1995;38:24-30.
94. Asfari M, Janjic D, Meda P, et al. Establishment of 2-mercaptoethanol dependent differentiated insulin-secreting cell lines. Endocrinology 1992;130:167-78.
95. Simpson AM, Tuch BE, Swan MA, Tu J Marshall GM. Functional expression of the human insulin gene in a human hepatoma cell line (HEP G2). Gene Therapy 1995;2:223-31.
96. Tuch BE, Beynon S, Tabiin MT, et al. Effect of cell toxins on genetically engineered insulin-secreting cells. J Autoimmun 1997;10:239-44.
97. Chaudry IH, Sayeed MM, Baue AE. The effect of insulin on glucose uptake in soleus muscle during hemorrhagic shock. Can J Physiol Pharmacol 1975;53:67-73.
98. Ruderman NB, Houghton CR, Hems R. Evaluation of the isolated perfused rat hindquarter for the study of muscle metabolism. Biochem J 1971;124:639-51.
99. Cooper DR, Vila MC, Watson JE, et al. Sulfonylurea stimulated glucose transport association with diacylglycerol like activation of protein kinase C in BC3H1 myocytes. Diabetes 1990;39:1399-407.
100. Rogers BJ, Standaert ML, Pollet RJ. Direct effects of sulfonylurea on glucose transport in the BC3H1 myocytes. Diabetes 1987;36:1292-6.
101. Davidson MB, Molnar IG, Furman A, et al. Glyburide stimulated glucose transport in cultured muscle cells via protein kinase C mediated pathway requiring new protein synthesis. Diabetes 1991;40:1531-8.
102. Mcmahon DK, Anderson PA, Nassar R, et al. C2C12 cells: biophysical, biochemical and immuno-cytochemical properties. Am J Physiol 1994;266:C1795-802.
103. Renold AE, Martin DB, Dagenais YM, et al. Measurement of small quantities of insulin like activity using rat adipose tissue: A proposed procedure. J Clin Invest 1960;39:1487-98.
104. Moody AJ, Stan MA, Stan M, et al. A simple free fat cell bioassay for insulin. Horm Metab Res 1974;6:2-16.
105. Ishizuka T, Cooper DR, Hernandez H, et al. Effects of insulin on diacylglycerol-protein kinase C signaling in rat diaphragm and soleus muscle and relationship to glucose transport. Diabetes 1990;39:181-90.
106. Standing VF, Foy JM. The effect of glibenclamide on glucose uptake in the isolated rat diaphragm. Postgrad Med J 1970;Dec suppl:16-20.
107. Muller G, Weid S, Wetekam EM, et al. Stimulation of glucose utilization in 3T3 adipocytes and rat diaphragm in vitro by the sulfonylureas glimepiride and glibenclamide, is correlated with modulations of the cAMP regulatory cascade. Biochem Pharmacol 1994;48:985-96.
108. Volund A, Brange J, Drejer K, et al. In vitro and in vivo potency of insulin analogues designed for clinical use. Diabet Med 1991;8:839-47.

109. Robertson DA, Singh BM, Hale PJ, et al. Metabolic effects of monomeric insulin analogues of different receptor affinity. Diabet Med 1992;9:240-6.
110. Koch R, Weber U. Partial purification of the solubilized insulin receptor from rat liver membranes by precipitation with concanavalin A. Hoppeseylers Z Physiol Chem 1981;362:347-51.
111. Hurrell DG, Pedersen O, Kahn CR. Alteration in the hepatic insulin receptor kinase in genetic and acquired obesity in rats. Endocrinology 1989;125:2454-62.
112. Drejer K, Kruse V, Larsen UD, et al. Receptor-binding and tyrosin kinase activation by insulin analogues with extreme affinities studied in human hepatoma HepG2 cells. Diabetes 1991;40:1488-95.
113. He Z, King GL. Microvascular complications of diabetes. Endocrinol Metab Clin North Am 2004; xi-xii;33:215-38.
114. Beckman JA, Creager MA, Libby P. Diabetes and atherosclerosis: epidemiology, pathophysiology, and management. JAMA 2002;287:2570-81.
115. Kato M, Castro NE, Natarajan R. MicroRNAs. Potential mediators and biomarkers of diabetic complications. Free Radic Biol Med 2013;64:85-94.
116. Regan TJ, Moschos CB, Weisse AB. MI with normal coronaries in toxic cardiomyopathy. Circulation 1977;55(4):679.
117. Fein FS. Diabetic cardiomyopathy. Diabetes Care 1990;13(11):1169-79.
118. Clark RJ, et al. Diabetes and the accompanying hyperglycemia impairs cardiomyocyte calcium cycling through increased nuclear O-GlcNAcylation. J Biol Chem 2003;278(45):44230-7.
119. Lebeche D, Davidoff AJ, Hajjar RJ. Interplay between impaired calcium regulation and insulin signaling abnormalities in diabetic cardiomyopathy. Nat Clin Pract Cardiovasc Med 2008;5(11):715-24.
120. Flack JM, Hamaty M, Staffileno BA. Renin-angiotensin-aldosterone-kinin system influences on diabetic vascular disease and cardiomyopathy. Miner Electrolyte Metab 1998;24(6):412-22.
121. Cai L, Kang YJ. Oxidative stress and diabetic cardiomyopathy: a brief review. Cardiovasc Toxicol 2001;1(3):181-93.
122. Maritim AC, Sanders RA, Watkins JB. 3rd, Diabetes, oxidative stress, and antioxidants: a review. J Biochem Mol Toxicol 2003;17(1):24-38.
123. Wold LE, et al. Metallothionein alleviates cardiac dysfunction in streptozotocin-induced diabetes: role of Ca^{2+} cycling proteins, NADPH oxidase, poly(ADP-Ribose) polymerase and myosin heavy chain isozyme. Free Radic Biol Med 2006;40(8):1419-29.
124. Bugger H, et al. Tissue-specific remodeling of the mitochondrial proteome in type 1 diabetic akita mice. Diabetes 2009;58(9):1986-97.
125. Boudina S, et al. Mitochondrial energetics in the heart in obesity-related diabetes: direct evidence for increased uncoupled respiration and activation of uncoupling proteins. Diabetes 2007;56(10): 2457-66.
126. Chavali V, Tyagi SC, Mishra PK. Differential expression of dicer, miRNAs, and inflammatory markers in diabetic Ins2+/- Akita hearts. Cell Biochem Biophys 2014;68(1):25-35.
127. Epstein PN, Overbeek PA, Means AR. Calmodulin-induced early-onset diabetes in transgenic mice. Cell 1989;58(6):1067-73.
128. Duan J, et al. Impaired cardiac function and IGF-I response in myocytes from calmodulin-diabetic mice: role of Akt and RhoA. Am J Physiol Endocrinol Metab 2003;284(2):E366-76.
129. Ye G, et al. Metallothionein prevents diabetes-induced deficits in cardiomyocytes by inhibiting reactive oxygen species production. Diabetes 2003;52(3):777-83.

130. Breyer MD, et al. Mouse models of diabetic nephropathy. Journal of the American Society of Nephrology 2005;16(1):27-45.
131. Raptis A, Viberti G. Pathogenesis of diabetic nephropathy. Exp Clin Endocrinol Diabetes 2001;109(Suppl 2):S424-37.
132. Ziyadeh FN, Wolf G. Pathogenesis of the podocytopathy and proteinuria in diabetic glomerulopathy. Curr Diabetes Rev 2008;4(1):39-45.
133. Nagai Y, et al. Temporary angiotensin II blockade at the prediabetic stage attenuates the development of renal injury in type 2 diabetic rats. J Am Soc Nephrol 2005;16(3):703-11.
134. Kunisaki M, et al. Normalization of diacylglycerol-protein kinase C activation by vitamin E in aorta of diabetic rats and cultured rat smooth muscle cells exposed to elevated glucose levels. Diabetes 1994;43(11):1372-77.
135. Tilton RG, et al. Prevention of hemodynamic and vascular albumin filtration changes in diabetic rats by aldose reductase inhibitors. Diabetes 1989;38(10):1258-70.
136. Sharma K, Ziyadeh FN. Hyperglycemia and diabetic kidney disease: the case for transforming growth factor-β as a key mediator. Diabetes 1995;44(10):1139-46.
137. Vasavada, Agarwal N and R. Role of oxidative stress in diabetic nephropathy. Adv Chronic Kidney D 2005;12(2):146-54.
138. Gurley SB, et al. Impact of genetic background on nephropathy in diabetic mice. Am J Physiol-Renal Physiol 2006;290(1):F214-22.
139. Qi Z, et al. Characterization of susceptibility of inbred mouse strains to diabetic nephropathy. Diabetes 2005;54(9):2628-37.
140. Hudkins KL, et al. BTBR Ob/Ob mutant mice model progressive diabetic nephropathy. J Am Soc Nephrol 2010;21(9):1533-42.
141. Lindström P. The physiology of obese-hyperglycemic mice [ob/ob mice]. Scientific World J 2007;7:666-85.
142. Nakagawa T. Uncoupling of the VEGF-endothelial nitric oxide axis in diabetic nephropathy: an explanation for the paradoxical effects of VEGF in renal disease. Am J Physiol Renal Physiol 2007;292(6):F1665-72.
143. Brosius FC, et al. Mouse models of diabetic nephropathy. J Am Soc Nephrol 2009;20(12):2503-12.
144. Mohan S, et al. Diabetic eNOS knockout mice develop distinct macro-and microvascular complications. Lab Invest 2008;88(5):515-28.
145. Surwit RS, et al. Diet-induced type II diabetes in C57BL/6J mice. Diabetes 1988;37(9):1163-67.
146. Welsh GI, et al. Insulin signaling to the glomerular podocyte is critical for normal kidney function. Cell Metab 2010;12(4):329-40.
147. Hale LJ, et al. Insulin directly stimulates VEGF-A production in the glomerular podocyte. Am J of Physiol Renal Physiology 2013;305(2):F182-8.

CHAPTER

41

Diabetic Retinopathy

INTRODUCTION

Diabetes mellitus is a heterogeneous disorder defined by the presence of hyperglycemia. Diagnosis criteria for diabetes mellitus include (1) a fasting plasma glucose >126 mg/dl, (2) symptoms of diabetes plus a random plasma glucose > 200 mg/dl, or (3) a plasma glucose level > 200 mg/dl after an oral dose of 75 g of glucose. Hyperglycemia in all cases is due to a functional deficiency of insulin action, which may be either due to a decrease in insulin secretion by the β-cells of the pancreas or insulin resistance. Majority of cases of diabetes are regarded as primary processes for which individuals have a genetic predisposition and are classified as either type I or type II. Type I diabetes mellitus is characterized by autoimmune β-cell destruction leading to severe insulin deficiency.

In contrast to Type I diabetes mellitus, Type II diabetes mellitus is 10 times more common, has stronger genetic component, occurs commonly in adults, increases in prevalence with age and is associated with increased resistance to the effects of insulin.

The diabetic patient is susceptible to a series of complications that cause morbidity and premature mortality. Diabetic retinopathy is one such complication that is associated with long-standing diabetes. It remains as one of the leading cause of blindness. Diabetic retinopathy has been understood as a microvascular complication, the pathogenesis of which is not completely understood. Microscopically, the basement membrane appears to be thickened with increased amounts of collagen and decreased amounts of proteoglycan. In conditions of high circulating levels of sugar, glucose nonenzymatically reacts with amino groups in proteins to form Advanced Glycation End Products (AGEs). AGEs bind to matrix components of basement membrane, specific receptors on macrophages, and endothelial cells to initiate a cascade of release of cytokines, which in turn affect the proliferation, and function of vascular cells (Fig. 41.1).

Diabetic retinopathy can be classified in different ways, but there are three main types:

a. Background retinopathy: There are tiny swellings in the blood vessel walls. These blebs (micro aneurysms) appear as small red dots on the retina. There are tiny yellow patches of hard exudates (proteins from the blood) on the retina. Dots and blots of hemorrhage appear on the retina (Figs 41.2A and B).
b. Maculopathy: In maculopathy, the hemorrhages, exudates and swellings of the first stage occur in the macula. This may interfere with vision, particularly for reading and seeing fine details (Fig. 41.3).

c. Proliferative retinopathy: The fundamental characteristics of proliferative retinopathy are new vessel formation and scarring. The stimulus for neovascularization may be retinal hypoxia secondary to capillary or arterial occlusion (Fig. 41.4).

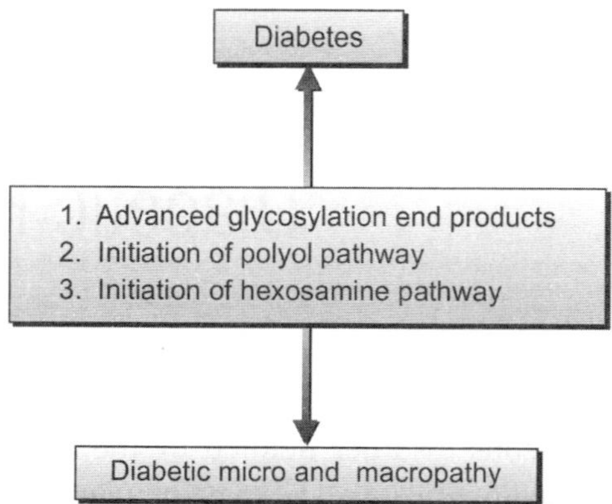

Figure 41.1: Etiopathology of diabetic retinopathy

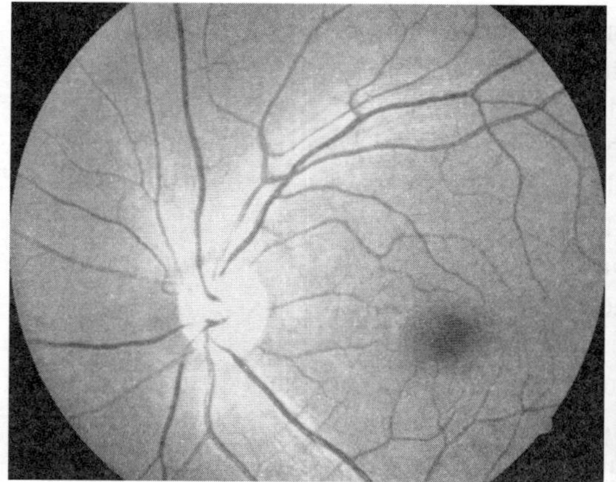

Figure 41.2A: Normal human retina

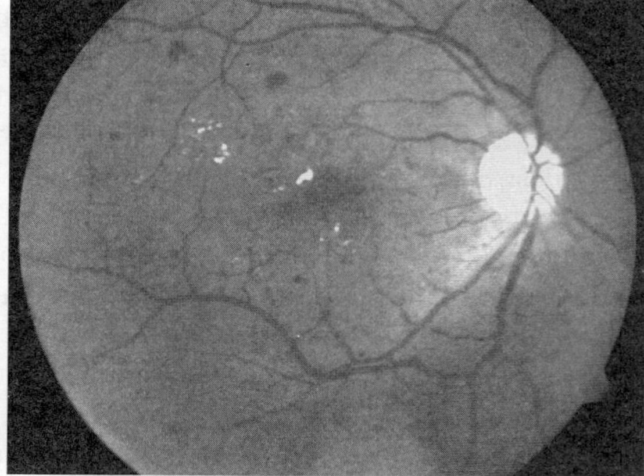

Figure 41.2B: Background diabetic retinopathy with characteristic microaneurysms and hard exudates

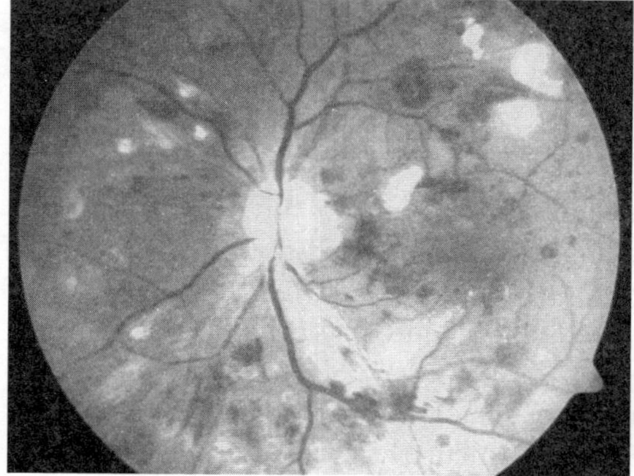

Figure 41.3: Diabetic maculopathy

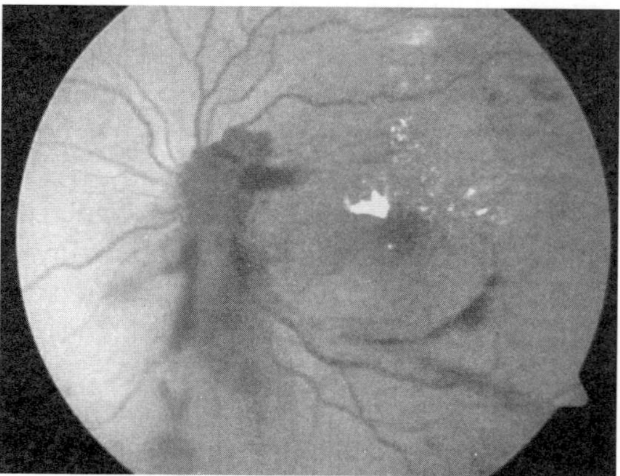

Figure 41.4: Proliferative retinopathy

Diabetic retinopathy occurs in two distinct stages: non-proliferative and proliferative. Nonproliferative retinopathy is characterized by microaneurysms of the retinal capillaries, appearing as tiny red dots. This background retinopathy has often been documented as the earliest clinically detectable sign of diabetic retinopathy. Further there is a loss of pericytes that surround and support the capillary walls leading to increased vascular permeability and leaking of fat. This progresses to formation of hard exudates in areas of macula. Macular edema describes the condition where retinal blood vessels can develop tiny leaks. When this occurs, blood and fluid seep from the retinal blood vessels, and fatty exudates deposit in the retina. This causes swelling of the retina and is called diabetic macular edema leading to reduced or blurred vision.

The above-mentioned preproliferative stage often worsens to a more severe proliferative stage. Proliferative retinopathy describes the changes that occur when new, abnormal blood vessels begin growing on the surface of the retina. This abnormal growth is called neovascularization. If these abnormal blood vessels grow around the pupil, glaucoma can result from the increasing pressure within the eye. These new blood vessels have weaker walls that may break and bleed, or cause scar tissue to grow. These complications may cause retinal detachment and finally severe vision loss, blurred and distorted images including blindness.

MAGNITUDE OF DISEASE

Diabetic retinopathy is emerging as one of the important causes of blindness in both developing and developed countries. In 2013, there are more than 382 million (or 8.3% of Adults) people suffering from diabetes, and it is being projected that the number of diabetic patients will reach 592 million, or one adult in 10, will have diabetes in 2035. This equates to approximately three new cases every 10 sec or almost 10 million per year.[1] India is also plagued by the condition and it is expected that the country will have over 50 million cases by 2025. Diabetic retinopathy, a complication of diabetes occurs in patients of both type 1 and type 2. Recently, it has been shown that nearly all type 1 and 75 percent of type 2 diabetes will develop diabetic retinopathy after 15 year duration of diabetes.[2] In a clinic population of a cohort of 6792 type 2 diabetic patients attending a diabetes center in south India, the prevalence of diabetic retinopathy was found to be 34.1 percent.[2]

PRESENT THERAPY FOR DIABETIC RETINOPATHY

Currently, there is no specific drug therapy for diabetic retinopathy. The sole management lies in surgery. Surgical treatment is decided, after taking into account the stage of the disease and the specific problem that requires attention. The retinal surgeon relies on several tests to monitor the progression of the disease and to make decisions for the appropriate treatment. These include fluorescein angiography, retinal photography and ultrasound imaging of the eye. Focal photocoagulation (focal laser treatment for sealing specific leaking blood vessels) or Scatter (pan-retinal) photocoagulation (laser treatment over a wide area of retina) are the two oft-used approaches for the management. Other management approaches include intraocular steroid injection, cryotherapy and vitrectomy. However, these management options suffer from drawbacks as laser photocoagulation burns and destroys part of the retina that itself can result in some permanent vision loss. Treatment may cause mild loss of central vision, reduced night vision, and decreased ability to focus. Some people may lose their peripheral vision. It may also lead to ocular neovascularization. Rare complications of laser photocoagulation that may cause severe vision loss include vitreous hemorrhage, traction retinal detachment, and accidental laser burn of the fovea.

Management of diabetic retinopathy remains a challenge with very few modalities available. There is a paucity of pharmacological approaches towards its management. Some of the molecules that have come into fore are tabulated (Table 41.1) and have substantial role to play in both prevention and therapeutics. Therefore, screening of new molecules in preclinical and clinical studies against models of diabetic retinopathy, takes prime importance.

Table 41.1: Novel molecules for prevention of diabetic retinopathy

S.No.	*Novel molecule*	*Putative mechanism of action*
1	Vitamin C	Antioxidant, Prevents protein glycosylation
2	Vitamin E	Antioxidant, Prevents protein glycosylation
3	Acetyl-L-carnitine	Antioxidant
4	Magnesium	Role unclear
5	Ginkgo biloba	Antioxidant

IN VITRO MODELS

Retinal Endothelial Cell Culture

The capillaries of the retina constitute a barrier (Blood Retinal Barrier, BRB) between the systemic circulation and retina that physiologically functions to regulate the passage of blood borne solutes, compounds, amino acids, and glucose from blood to retina. Histologically, BRB comprises of microvascular endothelial cells (also known as Inner BRB) and retinal pigment epithelial cells (also known as Outer BRB). Chronic exposure to hyperglycemia, as in diabetes and its associated complications such as diabetic retinopathy, has been recently reported to alter the physiology of BRB, especially inner BRB.[3]

Primary cell cultures of retinal endothelial cells are being extensively used to study the physiology, pathogenesis and putative therapeutic interventions for diabetic retinopathy. The retinal endothelial cells isolated from human, murine or bovine vessels are seeded on a reconstituted basement membrane extracellular matrix in the absence or in the presence of the substance under test, and the efficacy of the test substance to inhibit formation of a capillary-like network is observed and quantified by digital image analysis.[4]

Primary Cell Cultures of Bovine Retinal Endothelial Cells

Bovine retinas are the source of capillaries used to isolate cells for primary culture. Cow eyes can be obtained from a local abattoir. Primary bovine retinal endothelial cell (BREC) cultures are established from fresh calf eyes. Under sterile conditions, the retinas are isolated and washed in Dulbecco's modified Eagle's medium (DMEM) and pieces of adherent retinal pigment epithelial cells are removed. The retinas are transferred to an enzyme solution containing pronase (100 μg/ml), collagenase (500 μg/ml) and DNase (70 μg/ml) and incubated with shaking at 37°C for 20 min. After incubation, the retinal digest is passed through 210 and 50 μm nylon mesh and the microvessels trapped on top of the 50 μm mesh are collected in DMEM by centrifugation. The fragments are resuspended in DMEM with 15% fetal calf serum (FCS), 20 μg/ml endothelial growth supplement, heparin (100 μg/ml) and antibiotic-antimycotic solution, plated and grown on fibronectin coated dishes in low glucose DMEM, at 37°C with 5% CO_2. To determine the effect of high glucose, BREC can be grown in low (5.5 mM) or high (25 mM) D-glucose medium up to 48 h.[5,6]

Cell Line of Retinal Capillary Endothelial Cells

A conditionally immortalized retinal capillary endothelial cell line can be grown and maintained in DMEM with low glucose, containing 10% fetal bovine serum (FBS), 100 U/ml penicillin G, 100 U/ml streptomycin in humidified atmosphere composed of 95% air and 5% CO_2 at 33°C. Cells are grown to approximately 40-50% confluence and incubated in regular DMEM containing 5.5 or 25 mM glucose at 37°C. Control experiments can be performed using mannitol to test the effect of high osmolarity on various intracellular paradigms like GLUT1 expression.[5]

Retinal Neural Cells

During the event of pathogenesis of diabetic retinopathy, methylglyoxal and glyoxal are intermediates of AGEs. These substances in conjunction with other factors such as oxidative stress, induce apoptosis of retinal neurons. Studies conducted on retinal neural cells provide crucial information with regard to diabetic retinopathy.[7]

E1A-NR3 is a rapidly proliferating rat retinal precursor cell line that has been used in several studies to study the expression of various retinal and neuronal markers. The rat retinal cell line E1A-NR is maintained in DMEM containing 10% FCS, 2 mM glutamine, 1% nonessential amino acids, and 1%vitamins.

Immunocytochemistry studies can be conducted by growing the cells on glass coverslips coated with collagen IV (5 μg collagen IV/ml 0.05 M HCl for 60 min). Monoclonal mouse antihuman antibodies can be added directly to the cell cultures and appropriately incubated. After washing the cells are fixed with 4% paraformaldehyde. FITC-conjugated antibodies can be used and the cells can be viewed with a fluorescence microscope.

Apoptosis assays are conducted on retinal neural cells to demonstrate the influence of various stresses on cell viability and functionality. The cells are seeded and when they are subconfluent, glyoxal, methyl glyoxal, or hydrogen peroxide is added to the culture medium. After incubation, the supernatant is removed and the detached cells are collected. Adherent cells are collected after trypsin treatment. Adherent and detached cells are pooled, washed with PBS containing 1% horse serum, and subjected for apoptosis assays like fluorescence activated cell sorting (FACS), terminal deoxynucleotidyl transferase biotin-dUTP nick end labeling (TUNEL).[7]

Retinal Pigmented Epithelium (RPE) Cell Line

Human Retinal pigmented epithelium (HRPE) cell line is widely used to screen drugs having protective effect on diabetic retinopathy. High blood glucose in diabetes is associated with increased intracellular soluble adenylyl cyclase (sAC), and intracellular cAMP levels in HRPE cells which results in impairment of integrity of HRPE cell line barrier.

In this model, HRPE cell line is treated with high glucose concentration (25 mM) to mimic the hyperglycemic condition in the absence or presence of the test drug. The efficacy of test drug is assessed by measuring its ability to reverse drop in the transepithelial electrical resistance (TEER) due to high glucose concentration.[8]

EX VIVO MODELS

The effect of chronic hyperglycemia on retinal vasculature can also be studied *in vivo*, using *ex vivo* models. The colony of Goto Kakizaki (GK) rats shows persistent hyperglycemia after six weeks of age. Six month to one year old diabetic rats are used for the study. They are fed normal rat chow ad libitum and maintained in temperature controlled facilities with 12 h light-dark cycles. Glucose concentrations are routinely measured on tail blood samples using a glucose monitor.

To study changes associated with diabetic retinopathy, the rats are sacrificed by decapitation and their eyes are quickly removed. Retinas are isolated and wrapped in aluminum foil, frozen on liquid nitrogen and stored at -80°C until used. The study is conducted on membrane fraction of the retina from diabetic GK rats. Total retina homogenates from diabetic rats is obtained by tissue lysis in 10 mM Tris-HCl, 1 mM EDTA, 250 mM sucrose, protease inhibitors, pH 7.4, at 4°C and mechanical disruption using a homogenizer (50-60 strokes). The samples are centrifuged at 9,000x g to remove nuclei, mitochondria and unlysed cells, and recentrifuged at 1,00,000x g for 75 min to obtain the total cell membranes. The membrane pellet is resuspended in 10 mM Tris-HCl, 1 mM EDTA, pH 7.4 containing protease inhibitors, 0.5% sodium deoxycholate (DOC) and 1% Triton X-100. The samples are then centrifuged at 14,000x g to remove the unsoluble fraction.

Using standard techniques of Western, Northern blot, RT-PCR, protein changes in the basement membrane can be qualitatively and quantitatively assessed.[5]

IN VIVO MODELS

Diabetic Retinopathy in Streptozotocin Induced Diabetic Rats

Healthy adult Wistar rats of either sex weighing between 250-300 g are maintained on standard laboratory chow and tap water under 12 h light: dark cycles. Diabetes is induced by single injection of streptozotocin (50-70 mg/kg, ip).[9]

The control group is simultaneously administered equal volume of vehicle (3 mM citrate buffer, pH 4.5). After 10 days, the plasma glucose of the animals is monitored and rats with plasma glucose > 300 mg/dl are included in the study. After two weeks, diabetic retinopathy can be studied in the rats. The following paradigms can be evaluated to assess the etiology, pathogenesis, preventive and therapeutic interventions in this model:

a. **Proliferative diabetic retinopathy** is assumed to develop because vasogenic factors are released from retinal areas that are ischemic and hypoxic secondary to occlusion of the retinal vascular bed. Vascular occlusion in diabetic retinopathy may be due to the deposition of periodic acid Schiff positive glycoprotein compounds in the retinal vascular walls.

Periodic acid Schiff staining and immunohistochemistry helps to investigate the expression of laminin, fibronectin, type VI collagen and VEGF in areas of retinal capillary closure.

b. **Blood sugar monitoring:** Blood glucose level of normal, control and experimental groups of rats can be estimated periodically. Around 0.05 ml of blood is withdrawn from the tail vein by tail puncture and applied to the strip. The blood glucose levels are recorded using digital glucometer.
c. **Blood HbA1c, Hb-AGE measurements:** According to the method of Al-Abed et al. (1999),[10] under light ether anesthesia, whole blood of rats is collected from tail vein into heparinized tubes. Hemolysates are prepared and purified hemoglobin is prepared in the standard method. Hemoglobin content is measured by Drabkin's reagent and the quantity of HbA1c is measured by using a standardized chromatography method. AGE-modified hemoglobin (Hb-AGE) can be measured by an AGE-specific ELISA.
d. **Antioxidant activity:** The retina is homogenized in 50 mM PBS, under cold conditions using hand homogenizer for the estimation of Thiobarbituric acid reacting substances (TBARS), antioxidant enzymes (reduced glutathione, catalase and superoxide dismutase).
e. **Fluorescein angiography:** Clinical presentation of the pathology can be monitored by fluorescein angiography. Fluorescent dye is injected into the leg vein of the rat. The dye travels through the body including the eyes. With special camera, meant for the purpose of photography of the retina, the retinal vessels are observed and photo documented as the dye flows through the retinal vessels.[11]
f. **Visualization of vessel leakage:** Increased vascular permeability is a useful marker and can be assessed after 2 weeks of induction of hyperglycemia. The dye Evans blue, which has the property of plasma albumin binding, is used to study the blood trajectory and vessel leakage, if any. Briefly, the following protocol is followed. Under deep anesthesia, rats weighing approximately 200 g are kept on a warming plate (37°C, 20 min) before injection of 200 μl of 2% (wt/vol) Evans blue dissolved in sterile physiological solution through the femoral vein. The animals are returned to the warming plate for 20 min before sacrificing. Retinas are rapidly isolated and stored in 10% formaldehyde, flat mounted,and immediately viewed and photographed under fluorescent light (excitation filter 546 nm, barrier filter 590 nm). Modifications of the standard protocol are also widely applied. Retinal vascular leakage can also be measured by intravenously injecting FITC-BSA. After induction of anesthesia, the rats receive tail vein injections of 100 mg/kg FITC-bovine serum albumin and the animals are sacrificed 20 min later, and their eyes are removed, embedded in OCT medium, and snap-frozen in liquid nitrogen. The plasma is simultaneously collected and assayed for fluorescence with a fluorescence spectrophotometer based on standard curves of FITC-BSA in normal rat plasma. Frozen retinal sections (6 μm thick) are collected and viewed with fluorescence microscope. Quantification of FITC-BSA fluorescence intensity indicates the vascular leakage.[12]

Diabetic Retinopathy in Streptozotocin-induced Diabetes in C57Bl/6 Mice

Male C57Bl/6 mice weighing 20-25 g (5-6 weeks old) are randomly assigned to nondiabetic control or diabetic groups. Diabetes is induced by a single intraperitoneal injection of streptozotocin at (180 mg/kg). Control animals receive an equivalent dose of the drug vehicle (citrate buffer at pH 4.6). The mice are caged individually and allowed food and water ad libitum. Blood glucose level has to be measured fortnightly. Diabetic animals with blood glucose levels between 20 and 30 mM are included in the study.[13]

Feit-Leichman et al. (2005), induced diabetes in C57Bl/6J mice of 7 to 10 weeks with 5 consecutive injections of streptozotocin @ 55 mg/kg.[14] The blood levels were maximum at 4 weeks after the STZ treatment.

Diabetic Retinopathy in Galactose Fed Rat model

Feeding with galactose is another method to induce hyperglycemia. In this model, blood aldohexose concentration is elevated in the animal and other biochemical parameters such as concentrations of insulin, glucose, fatty acids, and amino acids remain unaltered. The monitoring of animals can be done up to 28 months as galactose-fed rats have a longer life span as compared to other diabetic models.

Method: In this model, weanling Sprague-Dawley rats are used; normal control group is fed with laboratory chow plus 50% starch, diabetic control group is fed with 50% D-galactose, and treatment group is fed with 50% D-galactose with test drug for 4 to 8 months and then changes by addition of test drug are measured and compared with control groups.[15]

Nondiabetic Models of Proliferative Retinopathy

Proliferative retinopathy can also be induced in animals by inducing neovascularization in the ocular region. Proliferative retinopathy is induced mainly by two methods: (i) by introduction of ischemia to the eyes, such as oxygen-induced retinopathy (OIR) or retinal occlusion; and (ii) by direct injection or genetically induction of the angiogenic factor, VEGF, into the ocular region.

In OIR model one week old neonatal mice are kept in a 75% oxygen chamber for five days and then returned to room air. Vessel loss in the central area of retina, which is associated with hypoxic challenges, is observed immediately at this time. Neovascularization extending from the inner retina into the vitreous begins at two days after the return to room air, peak is observed on third week, and is gradually regressed and spontaneously resolved by fourth week.[16]

DR can also be induced by producing ischemia in the retina using retinal occlusion models; by unilateral ligation of pterygopalatine artery (PPA) and external carotid artery (ECA),[17] branch retinal vein occlusion,[18] and elevating the intraocular pressure (IOP).[19] In these occlusion models, reduced thickness of retinal cell layers, increased apoptotic cells, reduced a-wave, b-wave, and OPs amplitudes of the ERG are evidenced.

Transgenic Models of Spontaneous Retinopathy

HLA-A29 Mice

Humans inheriting the class I major histocompatibility allele HLA-A29 are at a markedly increased relative risk of developing eye diseases. The human MHC class I specificity HLA-A29 has been recorded in over 95.8% patients of chorioretinopathy. Transgenic mice expressing HLA-A29 molecules have been developed as an animal model for retinopathy.[20]

For constructing the transgene, HLA-A*2902 cDNA (A29c) is obtained from patient suffering from bird shot chorioretinopathy (BSCR). The *SalI–Hind* III cDNA insert is cloned into pBluescript II SK expression vector (Stratagene). After digestion, the purified insert is inserted into pBSK-SP19 containing the H-2K^b promoter and the simian virus 40 poly(A) addition site. The resultant recombinant gene is excised by *XhoI* and *NotI* and used to generate HLA-A29 transgenic mice. Briefly, the protocol for producing transgenic mice is described here.

Procedure: The DNA fragments are purified free of vector DNA by preparative agarose gel electrophoresis and microinjected into fertilized (C57BL/6×SJL) × BALB/c oocytes. Embryos surviving microinjection are reimplanted into oviducts of pseudopregnant females, and offsprings are tested for the integration of the transgene by Southern blot analysis of tail-derived DNA digested by *ClaI* and *BamHI* with the use of a 0.9-kb fragment containing the simian virus 40 poly(A) addition site as a probe.[20] The descended mice can be utilized to conduct studies on retinopathy.

Spontaneous Hypertensive Rats (SHR)

Inflammation has an important role in the pathogenesis of diabetic retinopathy. The main secondary risk factor associated with DR is hypertension. Genetic hypertension in early retinal inflammation in experimental diabetes has been studied by Silva et al. 2007.[21]

They induced diabetes in both fully hypertensive rats and rats developing hypertension along with the age matched control normotensive Wistar Kyoto (WKY) rats. They concluded that the developing hypertension and fully developed hypertension lead to earlier development of inflammation in diabetic retina.

Procedure: Spontaneous hypertensive rats of 12 weeks age (fully hypertensive) and 4 weeks age (developing hypertension) are administered 50 mg/kg streptozotocin intravenously. After 20 days the rats are sacrificed to collect the retina and the changes in the retinal expression of inflammatory parameters can be evaluated.

Spontaneous diabetic rodent models: There are some strains of rodents which are reported to show spontaneous hyperglycemia used in the study of DR including db/db mice,[22] Non-obese diabetic (NOD) mice,[23] Akita (Ins2^{Akita}) mice,[24] Zucker diabetic fatty rats,[25] Otsuka long-Evans Tokushima fatty rats,[26] Goto-Kakizaki rats,[27] Diabetic Torii rats.[28]

Transgenic Vascular Endothelial Growth Factor; Kimba Mouse Model

Role of vascular endothelial growth factor (VEGF) in the pathogenesis of DR instigated Shen et al. 2006, to investigate whether transgenic mice with moderate VEGF expression in photoreceptors (trVEGF029) developed changes similar to diabetic retinopathy and whether retinopathy progressed with time.[29]

Evaluation of human $VEGF_{165}$ ($hVEGF_{165}$), serum glucose levels; changes in the density of retinal vasculature and changes similar to diabetic retinopathy such as retinal leukostasis, capillary endothelial cell and pericyte loss and number of acellular capillaries, suggested that an early short-term elevation in $hVEGF_{165}$ expression leads to progressive retinopathy. Mice can be generated by the following method.

Procedure: Mice are generated through microinjection of a DNA construct containing $hVEGF_{165}$ gene (pcDNA.opsin.VEGF) driven by a truncated mouse rhodopsin promoter confining transgene expression to the eye. Backcrossing with C57BL/6J mice produces fifth and sixth generation heterozygous mice and age matched wild type littermates. These mice demonstrate moderate elevation of $hVEGF_{165}$, limited neovascular changes and minimal retinal damage; and help in the examination of early pathological changes.[29,30]

Akimba mice model: Akimba mice is an ideal model created by crossing of Akita mice with Kimba mice, (Ins2AkitaVEGF+/−) and has the advantage that it inherits the diabetic phenotypes from their parental strains and show hyperglycemia and retinal neovascularization at the same time.[31]

Monkey Model of DR: Monkey provides a good model in eye research, as the ocular structures of monkeys are similar to that of humans. Some of the reported monkey models are Hyperglycemic DR model,[32] VEGF-induced proliferative retinopathy[33] and Spontaneous diabetes[34,35] in obese rhesus monkeys.

In Hyperglycemic DR model, pancreatectomy or STZ injections are used to induce hyperglycemia in monkeys[32] and retinal changes due to hyperglycemia are measured. In VEGF-induced proliferative retinopathy model, human recombinant VEGF in pellet is implanted into the vitreous cavity of the animal to mimic the inflammatory changes associated with natural DR.[33] In Spontaneous diabetes model hyperglycemia occurs spontaneously in obese rhesus monkeys.[34,35]

In monkey models morphological changes in retina like BRB break down, vascular tortuosity are observed after 2 weeks of implantation. However these models are not used widely and not validated due to many demerits like ethical issues, lack of proliferative retinopathy, high cost, longer duration of study, etc. Other animal models reported for the study of DR are dog,[36-38] rabbit,[39] cat,[40-42] and swine.[43,44]

Rat model of streptozotocin-induced diabetes is one of the most widely accepted models for long-term studies. Retinal lesions seen in rats have similarity to the initial process of DR in man.[20] However, mice can be genetically manipulated and provide the opportunity to study the molecular pathways in the development of diabetic retinopathy. Transgenic mice help in the examination of individual factors, which contribute, to early stages of diabetic retinopathy and to test early therapeutic interventions. The models described above vary from each other in some aspect or the other having their own advantages and disadvantages. The selection of the appropriate experimental model therefore has a prime importance in execution of one's study.

Zebrafish Model of DR

Zebrafish is an important tool to study visual development and impairments. They are proving to play important role in the study of etiology, pathogenesis, preventive and therapeutic interventions in DR owing to their very small size, large breeding size, easy to handle and similarity to those seen in human. The distinctive pattern of the mammalian retinal cell layers, ranging from ganglion cell layer to retinal pigment epithelium, is observed in zebrafish.[45] They have a short life span and a large breeding size, which in turn allow a shorter experimental turnover time. Moreover, a number of studies showed that genes of interest can be specifically induced, deleted, or overexpressed in zebrafish, allowing mechanistic studies of diseases.[46]

DR can be studied in zebrafish via direct elevation of glucose in the surrounding as well as angiogenesis without the involvement of glucose and by genetic manipulation.

Glucose-induced Diabetic Model of DR

In this model, hyperglycemia is induced in zebrafish by immersing the fish in 2% glucose solution and water every other day for one month. After one month animal is sacrificed, eyes are dissected and pathological changes are observed and compared between control (untreated zebrafish) and treated zebrafish group.

Method: In this model, adult zebrafish are acclimated to standard laboratory conditions; 14 h light and 10 h dark cycle, 28°C temperature are selected for screening. The acclimated fish are placed in 2% glucose solution and water alternate days for one month under standard conditions of laboratory. After a period of one month fish are anesthetized by 0.04% tricaine methanesulfonate solution environment. Anesthetized fish are decapitated by a sharp blade and blood glucose readings are collected immediately. Whole eyes are dissected, and incubated for fixation in 4% formaldehyde solution for 1 week. The fixed eyes are equilibrated in phosphate-buffered saline solution containing 30% sucrose at 4°C for overnight and sectioned. The sectioned retinal tissues are labeled with 4,6-Diaminidino-2-phenyloindole (DAPI) and images are viewed under fluorescence microscopy. Various morphological changes like thickness of the inner plexiform layer (IPL) and inner nuclear layer (INL) are measured and comparison is done between normal, treated (administered test drug) and control group (untreated zebrafish) to detect any change by the test drug in the pathogenesis of disease.[47]

Angiogenesis model for study of DR in Zebrafish: Two models are reported to study angiogenesis in zebrafish environmentally and transgenic-induced models.

Hypoxia-induced retinal angiogenesis in zebrafish: In this model, retinal neovascularization is induced by keeping the fli-EGFP-Tg zebrafish in hypoxic aquaria where the air saturation is gradually reduced to 10% (820 bbp) over a course of 2 to 3 days. Zebrafish is exposed in this hypoxic environment for different time points with a maximal period of 15 days. After 12 days of hypoxic challenge, neovascularization is observed in the retina evident by increased number of branch points, sprouts, and vascular area as well as reduced intercapillary distance.[48]

Transgenic Zebrafish model: Retinal angiogenesis can also be induced in zebrafish via transgenic approach. Zebrafish carrying $vhl^{-/-}$ mutation displays an upregulation of hypoxia-inducible factor, which in turns triggers VEGF production and expression of the VEGF receptors. However, this model is not commercially available, which limits its use in the field even though severe neovascularization and proliferative retinopathy are observed.[47-50]

REFERENCES

1. http://www.eatlas.idf.org/; data published in the latest edition of the IDF Diabetes Atlas, launched on World Diabetes Day 2013.
2. Rema M, Pradeepa R. Diabetic retinopathy: an Indian perpective. Indian J Med Res 2007;125: 297-310.
3. Grant MB, Afzal A, Spoerri P, Pan H, Shaw LC, Mames RN. The role of growth factors in the pathogenesis of diabetic retinopathy. Expert Opin Investig Drugs 2004;13:1275-93.
4. Rezzola S, Belleri M, Gariano G, Ribatti D, Costagliola C, Semeraro F, et al. In vitro and ex vivo retina angiogenesis assays. Angiogenesis 2014;17:429-42.

5. Fernandes R, Carvalho AL, Kumagai A, Seica R, Hosoya K, Terasaki T, et al. Down regulation of retinal GLUT1 in diabetes by ubiquitinylation. Mol Vis 2004;10:618-28.
6. Kowluru RA, Atasi L, Ho YS. Role of mitochondrial superoxide dismutase in the development of diabetic retinopathy. Invest Ophthalmol Vis Sci 2006;47:1594-9.
7. Kniep EM, Roehlecke C, Ozkucur N, Steinberg A, Reber F, Knels L, et al. Inhibition of apoptosis and reduction of intracellular pH decrease in retinal neural cell cultures by a blocker of carbonic anhydrase. Invest Ophthalmol Vis Sci 2006;47:1185-92.
8. Pavan B, Capuzzo A, Forlani G. High glucose-induced barrier impairment of human retinal pigment epithelium is ameliorated by treatment with Goji berry extracts through modulation of cAMP levels. Exp Eye Res 2014;120:50-4.
9. Bosco AA, Lerario AC, Santos RF, Wajchenberg BL. Effect of thalidomide and rosaglitazone on the prevention of diabetic retinopathy in streptozotocin-induced diabetic rats. Diabetologia 2003;46:1669-75.
10. Al-Abed Y, Mitsuhashi T, Li H, Lawson JA, Fitzgerald GA, Founds H, et al. Inhibition of advanced glycation endproduct formation by acetaldehyde: role in the cardioprotective effect of ethanol. Proc Natl Acad Sci USA 1999;96:2385-90.
11. Yotsumoto T, Naitoh T, Sakuya T, Tanaka T. Effects of specific antagonists of angiotensin II receptors and captopril on diabetic nephropathy in mice. J Pharmacol 1997;75:59-64.
12. Shyong MP, Lee FL, Kuo PC, Wu AC, Cheng HC, Cheng HC, et al. Reduction of experimental diabetic vascular leakage by delivery of angiostatin with a recombinant adeno-associated virus vector. Mol Vis 2007;13:133-41.
13. Cox OT, Simpson DAC, Stitt AW, Gardiner TA. Sources of PDGF expression in murine retina and the effect of short term diabetes. Mol Vis 2003;9:665-72.
14. Feit-Leichman RA, Kinouchi R, Takeda M, Fan Z, Mohr S, Kern TS, Chen DF. Vascular damage in a mouse model of diabetic retinopathy: relation to neuronal and glial changes. Invest Opthalmol Vis Sci 2005;46:4281-7.
15 Robison WG Jr, Jacot JL, Glover JP, Basso MD, Hohman TC. Diabetic-like retinopathy: early and late intervention therapies in galactose-fed rats. Invest Ophthalmol Vis Sci 1998;39(10):1933-41.
16. Smith LE, Wesolowski E, McLellan A, et al. Oxygen-induced retinopathy in the mouse. Invest Ophthalmol Vis Sci 1994;35:101-11.
17. Ogishima H, Nakamura S, Nakanishi T, et al. Ligation of the pterygopalatine and external carotid arteries induces ischemic damage in the murine retina. Invest Ophthalmol Vis Sci 2011;52:9710-20.
18. Zhang H, Sonoda KH, Qiao H, Oshima T, Hisatomi T, Ishibashi T. Development of a new mouse model of branch retinal vein occlusion and retinal neovascularization. Jpn J Ophthalmol 2007;51:251-7.
19. Inokuchi Y, Shimazawa M, Nakajima Y, et al. A Na+/Ca2+ exchanger isoform, NCX1, is involved in retinal cell death after N-methyl-D-aspartate injection and ischemia-reperfusion. J Neurosci Res 2009;87:906-17.
20. Szpak Y, Veiville JC, Tabary T, Naud MC, Chopin M, Edelson C, et al. Spontaneuos retinopathy in HLA-A29 transgenic mice. Proc Natl Acad Sci USA 2001;98:2572-6.
21. Silva KC, Pinto CC, Biswas SK, Lopes de Faria JB, Lopes de Faria JM. Hypertension increases retinal inflammation in experimental diabetes: A possible mechanism for aggravation of diabetic retinopathy by hypertension. Curr Eye Res 2007;32:533-41.
22. Midena E, Segato T, Radin S, di Giorgio G, Meneghini F, Piermarocchi S, et al. Studies on the retina of the diabetic db/db mouse. I. Endothelial cell-pericyte ratio. Ophthalmic Res 1989;21:106-11.

23. Makino S, Kunimoto K, Muraoka Y, Mizushima Y, Katagiri K, Tochino Y. Breeding of a non-obese, diabetic strain of mice. Jikken Dobutsu 1980;29(1):1-13.
24. Barber AJ, Antonetti DA, Kern TS, Reiter CE, Soans RS, Krady JK, et al. The Ins2Akita mouse as a model of early retinal complications in diabetes. Invest Ophthalmol Vis Sci 2005;46(6):2210-8.
25. Danis RP, Yang Y. Microvascular retinopathy in the Zucker diabetic fatty rat. Invest Ophthalmol Vis Sci 1993;34(7):2367-71.
26. Lu ZY, Bhutto IA, Amemiya T. Retinal changes in Otsuka long-evans Tokushima Fatty rats (spontaneously diabetic rat)-possibility of a new experimental model for diabetic retinopathy. Jpn J Ophthalmol 2003;47(1):28-35.
27. Miyamoto K, Ogura Y, Nishiwaki H, Matsuda N, Honda Y, Kato S, et al. Evaluation of retinal microcirculatory alterations in the Goto-Kakizaki rat. A spontaneous model of non-insulin-dependent diabetes. Invest Ophthalmol Vis Sci 1996;37(5):898-905.
28. Shinohara M, Masuyama T, Shoda T, Takahashi T, Katsuda Y, Komeda K, et al. A new spontaneously diabetic non-obese Torii rat strain with severe ocular complications. Int J Exp Diabetes Res 2000;1(2):89-100.
29. Shen WY, Lai C-M, Graham CE, Binz N, Lai YKY, Eade J, et al. Long-term global retinal microvascular changes in a transgenic vascular endothelial growth factor mouse model. Diabetologia 2006;49:1690-701.
30. Lai C-M, Dunlop SA, May LA, Gorbatov M, Brankov M, Shen W-Y, et al. Generation of transgenic mice with mild and severe retinal vascularisation. Br J Opthalmol 2005;89:911-6.
31. Rakoczy EP, Ali Rahman IS, Binz N, Li CR, Vagaja NN, de Pinho M, et al. Characterization of a mouse model of hyperglycemia and retinal neovascularization. Am J Pathol 2010;177(5):2659-70.
32. Tso MO, Kurosawa A, Benhamou E, et al. Microangiopathic retinopathy in experimental diabetic monkeys. Trans Am Ophthalmol Soc 1988;86:389-421.
33. Ozaki H, Hayashi H, Vinores SA, Moromizato Y, Campochiaro PA, Oshima K. Intravitreal sustained release of VEGF causes retinal neovascularization in rabbits and breakdown of the blood-retinal barrier in rabbits and primates. Exp Eye Res 1997;64 (4):505-17.
34. Johnson MA, Lutty GA, McLeod DS, Otsuji T, Flower RW, Sandagar G, et al. Ocular structure and function in an aged monkey with spontaneous diabetes mellitus. Exp Eye Res 2005;80(1):37-42.
35. Kim SY, Johnson MA, McLeod DS, Alexander T, Otsuji T, Steidl SM, et al. Retinopathy in monkeys with spontaneous type 2 diabetes. Invest Ophthalmol Vis Sci 2004;45(12):4543-53.
36. McLeod DS, Crone SN, Lutty GA. Vasoproliferation in the neonatal dog model of oxygen-induced retinopathy. Invest Ophthalmol Vis Sci 1996;37(7):1322-33.
37. Kobayashi T, Kubo E, Takahashi Y, Kasahara T, Yonezawa H, Akagi Y. Retinal vessel changes in galactose-fed dogs. Arch Ophthalmol 1998;116(6):785-89.
38. Takahashi Y, Wyman M, Ferris F 3rd, Kador PF. Diabetes like preproliferative retinal changes in galactose-fed dogs. Arch Ophthalmol 1992;110(9):1295-302.
39. Drago F, La Manna C, Emmi I, Marino A. Effects of sulfinpyrazone on retinae damage induced by experimental diabetes mellitus in rabbits. Pharmacol Res 1998;38 (2)97-100.
40. Hatchell DL, Toth CA, Barden CA, Saloupis P. Diabetic retinopathy in a cat. Exp Eye Res 1995;60(5):591-93.
41. Linsenmeier RA, Braun RD, McRipley MA, et al. Retinal hypoxia in long-term diabetic cats. Invest Ophthalmol Vis Sci 1998;39(9):1647-57.

42. Mansour SZ. Reduction of basement membrane thickening in diabetic cat retina by sulindac. Invest Ophthalmol Vis Sci 1990;31(3):457-63.
43. Umazume K, Barak Y, McDonald K, Liu L, Kaplan HJ, Tamiya S. Proliferative vitreoretinopathy in the Swine-a new model. Invest Ophthalmol Vis Sci 2012;53 (8):4910-6.
44. Lee SE, Ma W, Rattigan EM, et al. Ultrastructural features of retinal capillary basement membrane thickening in diabetic swine. Ultrastruct Pathol 2010;34 (1):35-41.
45. Goldsmith P, Harris WA. The zebrafish as a tool for understanding the biology of visual disorders. Semin Cell Deve Biol 2003;14 (1):11-8.
46. Collery RF, Cederlund ML, Smyth VA, Kennedy BN. Applying transgenic zebrafish technology to study the retina. Adva Exp Med Biol 2006;572:201-7.
47. Gleeson M, Connaughton V, Arneson LS. Induction of hyperglycaemia in zebrafish (Danio rerio) leads to morphological changes in the retina. Acta Diabetol 2007;44 (3):157-63.
48. Cao R, Jensen LDE Söll I, Hauptmann G, Cao Y. Hypoxia-induced retinal angiogenesis in zebrafish as a model to study retinopathy. PLoS One 2008;3 (7);e2748.
49. Rooijen E van, Voest EE, Logister I, et al. Von Hippel-Lindau tumor suppressor mutants faithfully model pathological hypoxia-driven angiogenesis and vascular retinopathies in zebrafish. Dis Models Mech 2010;3(5-6):343-53.
50. Lai AKW , Lo ACY. Animal Models of Diabetic Retinopathy: Summary and Comparison. J Diab Res 2013;2013: 29 pages. Article ID 106594, doi:10.1155/2013/106594.

CHAPTER

42

Ocular Toxicity

INTRODUCTION

Many substances are regularly used that are capable of damaging the eyesight. The eyes represent a valuable asset to people and the sense of vision is critical for normal functioning of an individual. They are in danger of accidental or intentional exposure to chemical preparations. This can occur at any step during the production, transportation, use and disposal of these preparations. In the mid-twentieth century, the aftermath of chemical warfare research and the hazards of unsafe cosmetics justified the need of public protection. Thus, the Draize eye test[1] became the standard method endorsed by the government of various countries to evaluate the safety of materials meant for use in or around the eyes. The test involves a standardized protocol for instilling agents on to the cornea and conjunctiva of rabbits. In the past few years, the ethical concerns over and the cost involved in the use of animals in research, has led to active development in the field of alternative testing for ocular toxicity assessment.

IN VIVO IRRITATION TESTING

An *in vivo* test to study the eye irritation potential of chemicals was developed in 1944 by Draize et al,[1] and became the famous Draize test. This was based on the original work of Friedenwald et al.[2] For years, the Draize test has been used as the animal test to identify human eye irritants. For the pharmaceutical industry, eye irritation testing is performed when the material is intended to be put into the eye as a means or route of application or for ocular therapy. The test has been modified by regulatory agencies around the world in terms of numbers of animals to be used, dose to be applied, scoring of the parameters and evaluation of the results, but the basis of the test procedure remains constant.

Procedure

For the test, usually six albino rabbits are used. 0.1 ml of the liquid or 0.1 g of solid test substance is instilled into the lower conjunctival sac of one of the eyes of each rabbit; the eyelids are held together for a few seconds and then released. The other eye of the animal serves as control. The test eye is not washed. Both the eyes are examined at 1, 24, 48, 72 h after treatment for the degree or extent of opacity of the cornea, the redness on the iris, and the chemosis and discharge on the conjunctiva. A numerical score as is shown in Table 42.1 is assigned subjectively for

Table 42.1: Eye irritation test: grading values for ocular lesions

Description of lesion	*Value*
1. Cornea	
A. Opacity, degree of density	
• No opacity	0
• Scattered or diffuse areas of opacity, but details of iris clearly visible	1
• Easily discernible translucent areas, details of the iris slightly obscured	2
• Opalescent areas, no details of iris visible, size of pupil barely discernible	3
• Opaque cornea, iris invisible through opacity	4
B. Area of cornea involved	
• One quarter (or less), but not zero	1
• Greater than one quarter	2
• Greater than one half	3
• Greater than three quarters, up to complete area	4
Score = Part A × Part B × 5 – Maximum score = 80	
2. Iris	
A. Normal	0
• Folds above normal, congestion, swelling circumcorneal injection, iris still reacting to light (sluggish reaction, but positive)	1
• No reaction to light, hemorrhage, gross destruction	2
Score = Part A × 5 – Maximum score = 10	
3. Conjunctiva	
A. Redness (refers to palpebral conjunctiva)	
• Blood vessels normal	0
• Blood vessels hyperemic (injected)	1
• Diffuse, crimson color, individual, vessels not easily discernible	2
• Diffuse vessels, beefy red	3
B. Chemosis (lids and nictitating membranes)	
• No swelling	0
• Any swelling above normal (includes the nictitating membranes)	1
• Obvious swelling with partial eversion of lids	2
• Swelling with lids half-closed	3
• Swelling with lids more than half-closed	4
C. Discharge	
• No discharge	0
• Any amount different from normal (does not include small amounts observed in inner canthus of normal animals)	1
• Discharge with moistening of lids and hairs adjacent to lids	2
• Discharge with moistening of the lids and hairs of considerable area around eye	3
Score = (Parts A + B + C) × 2 – maximum score = 20	

Source: Draize JH, Woodard G, Calvery HO. J Pharmacol Exp Ther 1944; 82: 377-90. With permission.

each of these parameters at the different time periods of examination. Each animal is graded separately, and the scores for the different parameters are added. The total score for each animal does not exceed 20. The treated eye may be washed at the 24 h period if considered appropriate to show whether washing with water results in decrease or increase in irritation. If there is no evidence of irritation at 72 h, the study may be terminated. If residual injury is present, examination of the eyes may be prolonged. Extended observation, e.g. at 7 and 21 days may be necessary if there is persistent corneal involvement or other ocular irritation in order to determine the progress of the lesions and their reversibility or irreversibility. However, the observation period normally need not exceed 21 days after instillation.

On comparing the scores for each of the rabbit, if only two or three rabbits show a positive effect, the test is considered as inconclusive and is repeated with a new set of animals. If four or more rabbits are positive in response, the test is considered positive.

The Draize test has been a subject of controversy both in the animal rights group and the scientific community. The test has been criticized on the dose volume, use of rabbit as model, number of animals, the infliction of pain to animals, and the subjective nature of assessment giving rise to variable interpretation.

There are a few modifications, which have been proposed and adapted for the Draize test. These modifications have been targeted at making the tests more accurate in predicting human responses and at reducing both the use of animals and the degree of discomfort or suffering experienced by them.

A modification of the standard Draize procedure is the **Low-Volume Eye Test (LVET)** in which only 0.01 ml or 0.01 g of the test substance is applied directly to the cornea instead of the conjunctival sac, and the eyelids are not held shut following treatment.[3] Several studies have shown that the LVET more accurately predicts human ocular exposure, good correlations being obtained between LVET results and the human response.[4,5] The LVET can be successfully conducted with three rabbits rather than six usually used.[6]

Over the years, it has been proposed that topical anesthetics be administered to the eyes of rabbits prior to their use in the test to decrease the pain inflicted to the rabbit. However, use of anesthetics can interfere with test results and thus compromise scientific validity and/or advantages of using anesthetic remain inconclusive. Irrigation of the eye at various times after dosing is another measure proposed to decrease animal suffering. Alternatively, use of sodium fluorescein dye and/or slit lamp has also been proposed for evaluation of the changes in the eye to decrease the subjectivity of evaluations.

Humane and scientific concerns regarding the use of the animals in toxicology and the subjective nature of the Draize test that leads to inter- and intra-laboratory variations has prompted active research for the replacement of animal testing for toxicity evaluation. One of the approaches to the above is the prediction of ocular toxicity from pre-existing data. The data on ocular irritation published in the literature and/or contained in computer databases may be evaluated for investigating the probable toxicity of a new chemical. However, these strategies suffer from the drawbacks of limited information available, discrepancies in scoring, variability and lack of strict reproducibility making interlaboratory comparisons very difficult. From these databases, only a broad classification of the chemical as irritant or non-irritant can be concluded. Computer modeling developed on the basis of computer databases is another approach proposed. But this also suffers from the drawback similar to that of databases.

Prediction of toxicity from physical/chemical data is an alternative widely employed. It is assumed that compounds having extreme pH (< 3 or > 12) are severe irritants and does not require animal testing. Comparisons have been made between dermal and ocular irritation data under the hypothesis that if a material is irritating to the skin, it will also be irritating to the eye. It was found that the degree of correlation between the two was dependent upon the *in vivo* classification scale used.[7] The correlation between the two tests was better if the compound was classified as irritant or non-irritant than when compound was classified as non-, mild, moderate or severe irritant.

IN VITRO METHODS

The next approach is the use of *in vitro* methods for evaluation of toxicity. The major parameters scored in the *in vivo* test are corneal opacity, inflammation and cytotoxicity. While no single test can cover all the three parameters, individual tests can address some of these end points. It seems probable to use a battery of these validated tests as screens for toxicity evaluation thereby reducing animal experimentation, which may be used only for the final and crucial premarket testing of products for regulatory requirements.

Opacity Tests

Corneal opacity is the most heavily weighted component of the Draize score. Several *in vitro* tests have been developed that assess opacity.

Isolated Rabbit Eye

The method was first introduced by Burton et al.[8] and modified by Price and Andrews[9] with the end points of the assay being opacity, corneal thickness and fluorescein dye retention.

Rabbits with a normal eye and corneal thickness are selected for the study and killed by overdose of sodium pentobarbitone. The eyes are enucleated and lightly supported by clamps within temperature-regulated (32°C) chambers and warm isotonic physiological saline is dripped continuously over the cornea at a rate of 0.1-0.15 ml/min for 45-75 min. Slit lamp examination is repeated for observation of any corneal changes; and if no change is found, the eye is used for further experimentation. 0.1 ml of the test solution is dripped over the cornea for 10 sec or 0.1 g powder is sprinkled on the corneal surface and left for 10 seconds. The test substance is washed off with physiological saline and effects of treatment are assessed at intervals of 1 h over a period of 4 h by slit lamp examination. The eyes are observed for: (i) generalized or patched opacities that represent severe tissue damage, (ii) changes in the thickness of the surface epithelium and objective measurement of any swelling of the corneal stroma using a slit lamp with a corneal pachymeter attachment. Mild to moderate irritants result in some loss of surface epithelium and swelling of the stroma. For scoring system, please refer Price and Andrews,[9] and (iii) changes in the epithelial layers and in penetrability that can be detected by applying 2% fluorescein sodium to the surface of the eye for a few seconds and then rinsing off with the isotonic salt solution. This procedure is followed when required.

The advantages of the method are that no living animal is subjected to pain. Also, two eyes are available for test from a single animal. The eyes may be taken from rabbits used for other tests not relevant to the eye. Changes are observed in cornea, which is a specialized nonvascular structure essential for the proper functioning of the eye and is undisturbed in the whole eye organ preparation. This test has been validated with a wide range of compounds, with good correlations being established between *in vitro* effects and *in vivo* irritancy.[9] The effects of liquid test substances were more successfully predicted *in vitro* as compared to solid test agents. However, one serious drawback of this technique over assessment in a live animal is that it cannot indicate the degree of discomfort caused by the test material entering the eye.

Isolated Chicken Eye (ICE) Test

Based on the above method, Prinsen and Köeter (1993) described a protocol for isolated chicken eye test.[10] The components of the test method were more or less same except for the dose-volume of the test substance, which was modified for the chicken eye. The parameters considered are corneal swelling, corneal opacity, and flourescein retention. The method is being used since 1993 without any significant change. The method has been evaluated by National Toxicological Program Interagency Centre for the Evaluation of Alternative Toxicological Methods (NICEATM) and the Interagency Coordinating Committee on the Validation of Alternative Methods (ICCVAM).[11]

Intact chicken heads are transported from the slaughterhouse to the laboratory within 2 h in the humidified boxes so as to prevent the damage due to transportation and dessication. The eyes are excised without damaging the cornea. The eyes are mounted on a stainless steel clamp individually with corneas in a vertical position. The eyes are then transferred to a superfusion apparatus. The corneas are moistened with isotonic saline, which is supplied at a rate of 0.10-0.15 ml/min through a bent stainless steel tube attached to a peristaltic pump. The corneal integrity is again examined under slit lamp microscope to exclude damaged corneas from the test. Once the eyes are examined and approved they are equilibrated for 45 to 60 min before dosing. A single dose of the test substance (30 μl for liquids and 30 mg for solids) is applied to cover the whole cornea for 10 sec. Corneas are rinsed with 20 ml isotonic saline. Mean values for corneal swelling, corneal opacity and flourescein retention are evaluated at regular intervals up to 4 h post treatment.[11]

Advantage of the test includes the availability of the test system. Chicken eyes can be obtained easily as they are widely consumed by the people worldwide. The removal of eyes compared to bovine and porcine eyes is much easier. Moreover, chicken cornea are comparable to rabbit cornea structurally. The changes in the opacity are more easily observed due to black iris of the chicken eye.

Other investigators have experimented with the technique using enucleated eyes of cattle and pigs held by clamps in suitable chambers containing a suitable medium.[10,12]

Bovine Corneal Opacity-Permeability (BCO-P) Test

The method was developed by Sina and Gautheron.[13] The corneas are obtained from an abattoir as target tissue. They are dissected free of the bovine eye and mounted in plastic holders, which allow access to both sides of the corneas. The isolated corneas are allowed to equilibrate in culture medium containing 1% serum for 1 h. Then, the posterior chamber is filled with fresh culture medium containing 1% serum and the anterior chamber is filled with test substance in either medium or polyethylene glycol 400. After an appropriate exposure period, the exposure medium is replaced with fresh medium, and the opacity of the treated cornea is measured relative to control without removal of the corneas from the holders. This measurement is done in an opacitometer (which is similar to a dual beam spectrophotometer), with a control cornea in one compartment and the treated one in another. The difference in light transmission is a measure of the chemically induced increase in opacity of the treated cornea.

It was found that the correlation between the opacity measurement and *in vivo* Draize score was very good. This model also allows the assessment of recovery from injury, by simply continuing incubation of the cornea in fresh medium after taking the initial opacity reading. Readings taken at various times thereafter would give an indication of reversibility of the lesion.

One modification of this technique includes filling up of the posterior chamber with fresh medium after taking opacity readings. The anterior compartment is filled with sodium fluorescein in buffer. After 90 min of incubation period, the amount of dye in the posterior chamber is determined spectrophotometrically at 490 nm. Since, the epithelial layers of the cornea form a barrier resistant to chemical penetration, the amount of dye penetrating through the cornea to the posterior chamber is directly proportional to the degree of damage to the epithelium.

The limitation of the method, however, is the difficulty in assessment of the compound that is hydrophobic or insoluble, a weak irritant, as well as the agents that cause minimal *in vivo* irritation initially (24 or 36 h) but induce increasing irritation at a later stage over a period of time.

Eyetex™ Assay

This is another assay for alternative measurement of the corneal opacification. It is a complete nonbiological test. This method stems from the observation that transparency of the cornea depends on the hydration and organization of proteins and that the presence of high molecular weight aggregates of protein cause opacity. The test uses a "proprietary reagent" of a soluble protein matrix from the jack bean, which turns opaque when an appropriate test substance causes alterations in the hydration/organization of the soluble protein, thereby reducing light transmission through a cuvette placed in a simple spectrophotometer. The change in light transmission is equated with a standard curve provided in the kit relative to *in vivo* eye irritancy scores. The correlations of Eyetex data with *in vivo* data are conflicting as some investigators showed good correlations while others showed the correlations to be poor. The correlation was not good when alcohol-containing formulations were tested. Another potential drawback of this assay is that if a chemical exerts its irritant effects by a mechanism other than protein precipitation or coagulation, the test would give false results.[13]

EpiOcular™ Assay

EpiOcular™ corneal model is a three dimensional tissue construct of normal human derived epidermal keratinocytes, cultured to form a stratified squamous epithelium, and models the human corneal epithelium. The EpiOcular™ tissue construct models the top epithelial layer only and not the stromal and endothelial layers of the cornea. The test is based on the hypothesis of Maurer and Jester (2002) that the level of ocular irritation is related to the extent of initial injury.[14]

It estimates the potential ocular irriation of a test article when exposed topically. To measure the ocular irritation potential of any test material the time taken to reduce tissue viability by 50% [ET_{50}] is considered. Relationship between the ET_{50} of a test material and nature and extent of histological changes that occur is established by this method. As the depth and severity of the tissue damage increases the tissue viability decreases progression and types of changes associated with tissue damage helps in distinguishing the degrees of ocular irritation. *In vivo* ocular irritation potential of a test article is directly related with its *in vitro* potential for cytotoxicity and tissue penetration.[15,16]

Long-term Corneal Culture Assay

Raabe et al. 2005 has proposed the long-term corneal culture as an *in vitro* model to evaluate eye irritation and post-treatment recovery after chemical exposures. The method is modification of the previously published method.[17,18]

Porcine eyes are obtained from the abattoir. The eyes are disinfected. Corneas are dissected out leaving a 3-5 mm circular rim of sclera intact, and cultured within 24 h of sacrifice. Corneas are suspended in 24 well plates wells with epithelial side facing the bottom of the well filled with Hank's Balance Salt Solution (HBSS). An agar/gelatin/M-199 mixture is added to the endothelial cavity to support the corneal architecture drop by drop and allowed to gel till the cavity is completely filled and the gel solidifies. Corneas are inverted and transferred to large deep well dishes. The M-199 culture medium is added to each dish so that the limbal conjunctivae are covered with medium and corneal epithelium exposed to air. The dishes are then incubated at 37°C, 5% CO_2 and 90% RH for 24 h prior to dosing. The corneas are moistened by brief immersion in the medium every 2.7 h using a modified plate rocker. The corneas are treated either with SLS, ethanol and water (control) after 24 h of initiating the cultures. The exposure time ranged between 2-10 min. The surface of the corneas is rinsed with PBS till they are free from the test substance. They are again transferred to fresh wells and cultured for varying time points. The observations both visual and microscopic are made daily. After the incubation, the corneas are fixed, embedded, sectioned and stained for histological examination. Corneas can be cultured upto 96-120 h with normal morphology. SLS and ethanol-induced damage in porcine corneas exhibited histological similarities with observations made in other *ex vivo* models. The cornea exhibited re-epithelialization after exposure to ethanol. Thus, the model demonstrates the potential for further optimization of evaluating recovery of damaged corneas.[17]

Cytotoxicity Tests

Majority of the alternatives to Draize test assess cellular toxicity *in vitro*. This assay involves the use of immortalized cell lines of different origin and examines dye inclusion/exclusion/leakage as indices of membrane integrity. Usually, these methods are simple, straightforward, and relatively rapid, with defined end points, which can be reproducibly and accurately measured.

The disadvantages are that these assays do not provide information on the mechanism by which a chemical causes irritation and, therefore, any correlation with *in vivo* data for one group of compounds may be due to chance and may not hold for another type of chemical.[13]

The dyes that are used include: neutral red or fluorescein diacetate which enters only viable cells, and either gets localized in the cells or leaks out back from the damaged plasma membrane; propidium iodide and ethidium bromide that can enter only the damaged cell and stain the DNA but are large enough to be excluded from the viable cells; and trypan blue that stains the proteins in nonviable cells by entering through the damaged cell membranes.

HCE-T TEP Assay

For assessing the eye irritation potential of chemicals and formulations HCE-T TEP assay is being evaluated by ICCVAM to be used as a Draize Alternative Test Method.[19]

The method is used for evaluating the human eye irritation potential of water-soluble chemicals and formulations within the irritation range referenced by Draize. It measures the dose-dependent efficacy of any test material on fluorescein transepithelial permeability (TEP) in human corneal epithelial cells (HCE-T). An HCE-T cell line has been used to develop a three dimensional *in vitro* model of human corneal epithelium.[20] These cells are grown at the air-liquid interface on a collagen membrane in serum free medium which stratify and differentiate forming an epithelial barrier like in the human eye. These cells are treated with the test material. Addition of sodium fluorescein to the culture and consequent measurement of the concentration of fluorescein present in the medium determines damage to the epithelial cell barrier.

Another example of a dye penetration assay is the method developed by Tchao et al.[21] Madin-Darby Canine Kidney cells (MDCK) are grown on a filter and form tight junctions upon confluency, forming two separate compartments. Fluorescein is placed in the inner chamber and the passage of dye through the cell sheet to the other chamber is monitored. When an intact monolayer covers the filter, the passage of fluorescein is restricted. If a chemical damages the cells, extensive leakage of fluorescein occurs. Sina and Goutheron[13] found that the assay correctly identified only the severe irritants. Mild and moderate compounds, as well as some severe irritants (which presumably act by a mechanism other than junction disruption), showed no increased penetration. Besides, MTT dye reduction assay is also used as a cytotoxic test to study cellular metabolism.[22] Uridine uptake study has also been proposed as one of the methods.[23]

The cytotoxicity assays can be used as a complementary assay in a battery of tests to screen a compound *in vitro* for its irritation potential.

Inflammatory Tests

Inflammation is another important aspect of Draize test. Few *in vitro* tests have been developed that can produce an inflammatory response. Inflammation is a complex event and is difficult to mimic a similar response in an *in vitro* system. However, the right type of cells can release chemotactic factors and/or inflammatory mediators such as histamine, serotonin, prostaglandin, thromboxane, and leukotrienes which can be quantitated indirectly via their chemotactic effects on neutrophils or by direct assay using high performance liquid chromatography (HPLC).

Bovine Corneal Cup Model

The model is developed by Elgebaly and colleagues[24] on the basis that chemotactic factors are released from a variety of tissues in response to injury. In this assay, corneas (bovine, rabbit or human) are put into temperature-controlled plastic holders such that the epithelial surface forms the inside of a cup. Physiological medium with or without a test substance is pipetted onto the cup. Following an appropriate incubation period, the released chemotactic factors associated with inflammation are removed with the medium for subsequent interaction with isolated neutrophils. In the assay, the isolation or identification of chemotactic response of the neutrophils is the end point of assay. In a modification of this assay by Benassi et al.[25] the inflammatory mediators released from mast cells (histamine, serotonin, leukotrienes) are derivatised by fluorescamine prior to their quantitation by HPLC.

In isolated rat vaginal tissue, Dubin et al.[26] have attempted to quantify and associate the release of eicosanoids with inflammation, measuring the cellular release of prostaglandin (PGE_2, PGF_2, 6-keto PGF_1) and thromboxane B_2 in the medium by using HPLC with fluorescence or radioimmunoassay (RIA).

These techniques, however, require extensive interlaboratory validation with a broad range of known or potential ocular irritants.

Chorioallantoic Membrane (CAM) Assay or The Hen's Egg Test-Chorioallantoic Membrane Test (HET-CAM)

In this assay, the vascularized respiratory membrane surrounding the embryonic chicken within an egg is used as the site of irritant activity.

Fertile eggs, on day 0 are incubated at 37°C. On day 3, the shell is penetrated in two places. First, near the pointed end of the egg a small opening is ground and the shell membrane is exposed. Through the opening, a needle is inserted and 1.5 to 2 ml of albumen is removed and discarded. A rectangular window is made on the wall of the egg. A distinct false air space is seen below the window. The fluid content of the egg is present at the floor of the air space and the shell dust that results from cutting of window sinks into the fluid. The window is covered with a transparent tape. On the 14th day, the tape over the window is removed and a Teflon ring (10 mm internal diameter) is placed on the CAM. The ring serves as a marker of the test and as a container for holding the test substance. Forty ml of the test sample is placed in the ring and the window is resealed with tape. The eggs are further incubated for 3 days and on the 17th day of incubation the tape is removed, the window is enlarged and the CAM is observed for the extent of necrosis.[27]

HET-CAM is a similar technique.[28] The eggs to be treated are first candled in order to discard the defective eggs and only fresh, fertile eggs are used for the test. Eggs weighing less than 50 g and more than 60 g, are also rejected. For the assay, the eggs are put in incubator trays with large ends up and put in an incubator at 37.5°C and 62.5% relative humidity where the trays rotate automatically. The eggs are candled on the 5th day and each day thereafter to discard the nonfertile eggs. On day 10 of incubation, the shell is scratched around the air cell by a dentist's rotary saw and then pared off. The vascular CAM is exposed after removal of the inner egg membrane. The liquid test substance is dropped onto the membrane in a volume of 0.2 ml; and the solid test substance (0.1 g) is applied on the vascular chorioallantois and irrigated after 20 sec with 5 ml of warm water. In every case, a series of four eggs are used; two eggs treated with vehicle only, serves as controls. After application of the test substance, the CAM, the blood vessels, including the capillary system, and the albumen are examined and scored for irritant effects (hyperemia, hemorrhage, coagulation) at 0.5, 2 and 5 min after treatment.

A modification of this assay, the CAM Vascular Assay (CAMVA), is carried out in the same manner, but vascular changes constitute the lesion, a positive test being indicated by hemorrhage, obstruction, or narrowing of blood vessels 30 min after applying the test substance to the CAM of a 14-day-old fertilized hen's egg.

The CAM assay has been validated, but the results are mixed. High number of false positive results have been obtained; the scoring is again subjective in nature like the *in vivo* test; the tissue under investigation has little anatomical similarity to the cornea; the test substance may be toxic to the embryo; there is no evidence for inflammatory response; circulating neutrophils are absent in chicken embryo; and at the embryonic stage, the immune response is not completely developed.[29] Therefore, this assay also will not be a very useful alternative for the replacement of Draize test.

The *in vitro* assays described above measure different end points. Therefore, a single test measuring a single end point cannot be used as an alternative to Draize test. Each test can only be used together in a battery of tests to evaluate the ocular irritation potential of a new chemical. Also, many of these tests are not validated; results in interlaboratory variations; and good correlations do not exist with the *in vivo* test. It does not appear in the near future that either single or a group of these tests can completely replace the Draize test.

The regulatory authorities worldwide consider the Draize eye irritancy test among the most reliable methods currently available for evaluating the safety of a substance in and around the eye; and that to-date there are no alternatives of equivalent efficacy. Continued use of Draize test for the evaluation of ocular irritancy potential is not due to a shortage of potentially useful alternative methods, since more efforts have probably been put into the development of alternatives to the Draize test than in seeking replacements to all other *in vivo* test put together. However, no test, combination of tests, or testing strategy has yet been developed which meets all of the requirements of the regulatory authorities.

Active research is going on globally in the field of development of *in vitro* alternatives to Draize test and also sincere efforts are underway for their validation. These tests can definitely be used as prescreens to the final determination of irritation potential by Draize test.

REFERENCES

1. Draize JH, Woodard G, Calvery HO. Methods for the study of irritation and toxicity of substances applied topically to the skin and mucous membranes. J Pharmacol Exp Ther 1944;82:377-90.
2. Friedenwald JS, Hughes WF, Hermann H. Acid-base tolerance of the cornea. Arch Ophthalmol 1944;31:279-83.
3. Griffith JF, Nixon GA, Bruce RD, et al. Dose-response studies with chemical irritants in the albino rabbit eye as a basis for selecting optimum test conditions for predicting hazard to the human eye. Toxicol Appl Pharmacol 1980;55:501-13.
4. Freeberg FE, Nixon GA, Reer PJ, et al. Human and rabbit eye responses to chemical insult. Fundam Appl Toxicol 1986;7:626-34.

5. Williams SJ. Changing concepts of ocular irritation evaluation: pitfalls and progress. Food Chem Toxicol 1985;23:189-93.
6. Bruner LH, Parker RD, Bruce RD. Reducing the number of rabbits in the low-volume eye test. Fundam Appl Toxicol 1992;19:330-5.
7. Gad SC, Walsh RD, Dunn BJ. Correlation of ocular and dermal irritancy of industrial chemicals. J Toxicol-Cutan Ocular Toxicol 1986;5:195-213.
8. Burton ABG, York M, Lawrence RS. The in vitro assessment of severe eye irritants. Food Cosmet Toxicol 1981;19:471-80.
9. Price JB, Andrews IJ. The in vitro assessment of eye irritancy using isolated eyes. Food Chem Toxicol 1985;23:313-5.
10. Prinsen MK, Koeter HBWM. Justification of the enucleated eye test with eyes of slaughterhouse animals as an alternative to the Draize eye irritation test with rabbits. Food Chem Toxicol 1993;31:69-76.
11. http://iccvam.niehs.nih.gov/methods/ocutox/ocutox.htm.
12. Whittle E, Basketter D, York M, et al. Findings of an interlaboratory trial of the enucleated eye method as an alternative eye irritation test. Toxicol Methods 1992;2:30-41.
13. Sina JF, Gautheron PD. Ocular toxicity assessment in vitro. In: Gad SC (Ed). In vitro Toxicology. New York: Raven Press Ltd, 1994:21-46.
14. Maurer JK, Jester JV. Extent of initial corneal injury as the mechanistic basis for ocular irritation: key findings and recommendations for the development of alternative assays. Regul Toxicol Pharmacol 2002;36:106-17.
15. Blazka ME, Diaco M, Harbell JW, Raabe H, Sizemore A, Wilt N, et al. EpiOcular™ human cell construct: tissue viability and histological changes following exposure to surfactants. Presented at the 5th World Congress on Alternatives and Animal Use in the Life Sciences. Berlin, Germany, 2005;21-26.
16. Curren R, Harbell J, Trouba K. The EpiOcular™ Model Protocol, Performance and Experience. Regul Toxicol Pharmacol 2002;36:106-17.
17. Raabe H, Bruner L, Snyder T, Wilt N, Harbell J. Optimization of an in vitro long term corneal culture assay. Presented at the 5th World Congress on Alternatives and Animal Use in the Life Sciences, Berlin, Germany 2005;21-6.
18. Foreman DM, Pancholi S, Jarvis-Evans J, McLeod D, Boulton ME. A single organ culture model for assessing the effects of growth factors on corneal re-epithelialization. Exp Eys Res 1996;62:555-64.
19. http://iccvam.niehs.nih.gov/methods/ocutox/hce.htm.
20. Kruszewski FH, Walker TL, Dipasquale LC. Evaluation of a human corneal epithelial cell line as an in vitro model for assessing ocular irritation. Toxicological Sci 1997;36:130-40.
21. Tchao P, Cotovio J, Dossou KG, et al. Assessment of surfactant cytotoxicity: comparison with the Draize eye test. Int J Cosmet Sci 1989;11:233-48.
22. Gay R, Jadlos S, Marenus K. The living dermal equivalent (LDE) as an assay for ocular irritation potential. Presented at the 7th Annual CAAT Symposium, 1989.
23. Shopsis C, Sathe S. Uridine uptake inhibition as a cytotoxicity test: Correlations with the Draize test. Toxicology 1984;29:195-206.
24. Elgebaly SA, Forouhar F, Kreutzer DZ. In vitro detection of cornea-derived leukocytic chemotactic factors as indicators of cornea inflammation. In: Goldberg AM (Ed). Alternative methods in toxicology. New York: Mary Ann Liebert 1987;6:257-68.

25. Bennasi CA, Angi MR, Salvalaio L, et al. Ocular irritancy evaluated in vivo by conjunctival lavage technique and in vitro by bovine eyecup model. In: Goldberg AM (Ed). Alternative methods in toxicology. New York: Mary Ann Liebert 1987;5:235-42.
26. Dubin NH, Ghodgaonkar RB, Parmley TH. Differential response of in vitro vaginal tissue to various test agents. In Goldberg AM (Ed). Alternative methods in toxicology. New York: Mary Ann Liebert, 1988;5:153-8.
27. Leighton J, Nassauer J, Tchao R. The chick embryo in toxicology: an alternative to the rabbit eye. Food Chem Toxicol 1985;23:293-8.
28. Leupke NP. Hen's egg chorioallantoic membrane test for irritation potential. Food Chem Toxicol 1985;23: 287-91.
29. Bagley DM, Waters D, Kong BM. Development of a 10-day chorioallantoic membrane vascular assay as an alternative to the Draize rabbit eye irritation test. Food Chem Toxicol 1994;32:1155-66.

CHAPTER

43

Phototoxicity

INTRODUCTION

Many systemic, therapeutic agents photosensitize human skin to solar or artificial sources of UV radiation (UVR). The phototoxic potential of an agent is often only noted during clinical trials late in product development. Withdrawal of an agent at this stage is extremely costly to the manufacturer and although various animal skin phototoxicity models exist, there is increasing ethical pressure to develop alternative methods.[1]

The solar energy has been considered essential for the development and evolution of life on earth. It can produce photobiological effects on microorganisms, plants, animals and humans. The portion of the solar spectrum containing the biologically most active region is from 290 to 700 nm. The UV part of the spectrum includes wavelengths from 200 to 400 nm. The most relevant spectral regions are UVB (290-320 nm) and UVA (320-400 nm). Shorter wavelength radiation (λ = 290 nm) is efficiently filtered by the atmosphere, mainly by the stratosphere ozone layer and does not reach the earth's surface. Sunlight containing radiation of longer than 400 nm has much lower biological effectiveness. The most thoroughly studied photobiological reactions that occur in skin are induced by UVB. UVB represents approximately 1.5% of the solar energy received at the earth's surface; it elicits most of the known chemical phototoxic and photoallergic reactions. The visible portion of the spectrum, representing about 50% of the sun's energy received at the sea level, includes wavelengths from 400 to 700 nm. Visible light is necessary for such biological events as photosynthesis, vision, the regulation of circadian cycles and melanogenic effects. The various models used for screening of phototoxicity are given in Table 43.1.

Table 43.1: Various models used for screening of phototoxicity

In vivo models	*Photosensitization models*	*In vitro assays*
• Rabbit Dorsal Surface Method • Guinea Pig Dorsal Surface Model • Mouse Ear Swelling Model • Rabbit Ear Model • Hairless Mouse Model	• Guinea Pig Dorsal Surface • Armstrong Assay • Photo Hen's Egg Test (PHET)	• Photohemolysis • Photosensitized Candida Albicans Growth Inhibition • Photodegranulation of Mast Cells • Photo-Basophil-Histamine Release Test • Histidine Photodegradation

The intensity of irradiation used in phototoxicity testing is determined with a light meter, which provides output as watts/m^2. The shelves on which the animals are tested during the exposure periods are normally adjustable in order to control the dose of light to the exposure area. The irradiation from fluorescent lights will somewhat vary from day to day, depending on temperature, variations in the current, etc. The dose the animals receive is generally represented as joules/cm^2. One joule is equal to 1 watt/sec. Therefore, the dose of light is dependent on the period of exposure.[2]

$$\text{Period of exposure} = \text{W sec/J}$$

Three protocols for assessing topical phototoxicity potential in rabbit, guinea pig and mouse are discussed here.

Rabbit Dorsal Surface Method

The traditional method uses rabbit for phototoxicity testing.[3] A brief procedure has been described here. Eight adult female New Zealand white rabbits, 6 for each test and 2 for positive control are used. Animals are acclimatized at least for 7 days prior to the study. Animals are given free access to commercial laboratory feed and water. A dose of 0.5 ml of test drug in liquid form or 500 mg in solid form or semisolid dosage is applied to each test site. A liquid substance is used undiluted. For solids the test article is moistened with water (500 mg test article/0.5 ml water or another suitable vehicle) to ensure good contact with the skin. The positive control material is a lotion containing 1% 8-methoxypsoralen. The animals are weighed on the first day of dosing. The fur of the test animal is clipped from the dorsal area of the trunk using a small animal clipper, then shaved to clean the dorsal trunk with a fine blade clipper one day prior to the dosing. On the day of dosing, the animals are placed in a restrainer to prevent licking. One pair of patch (approximately 2.5 × 2.5 cm) per test article is applied to the skin of the back, with one patch on each side of the backbone. A maximum of two pairs of patches, at least 2 inches apart, are applied to each animal. The patches are secured to the skin by means of an occlusive tape for the 2 h exposure period. Following exposure the occlusive tape as well as the patches on the right side of the animal, are removed. The left side of the animal is covered with an opaque material. The animal is then exposed to approximately 5 J/cm^2 of UVA (320-400 nm). After exposure to the UVA light, the patches on the right side of the animal as well as the occlusive tape are replaced. The tape is again removed approximately 23 h after the initial application of the test article. Residual test article is carefully removed, using water or another suitable vehicle. Animals are examined for signs of erythema and edema, and the responses scored at 24, 48 and 72 h, after the initial test article application, according to the Draize reaction grading system. Any unusual observation and mortality is recorded. The data from the irradiated and nonirradiated sites are evaluated separately. The scores from erythema, scar formation and edema at 24, 48 and 72 h, are added for each animal. The values are then divided by 3, yielding six individual score. The mean of the six individual animal irritation score represents the mean primary irritation score (maximum score = 8, as in the primary dermal irritation study).

Guinea Pig Dorsal Surface Model

This protocol uses guinea pig for phototoxicity testing.[4] Ten young adult male Hartley guinea pigs (300 to 500 g) are divided into two groups. Four animals are used as irradiation controls and 6 animals for material treatment. All the animals are acclimatized at least for 5 days prior to the study. Animals are given free access to food and water. The test assumes that material is in solution form. The most volatile, nonirritating organic solvent such as ethanol, acetone, dimethylacetamide, or some combination is used. There can be upto four sites per animal, each measuring 1.5 × 1.5 cm (2.25 cm^2). In general, one side is selected for a vehicle control, and another for positive control [8-methoxypsoralen (8-MOP), 0.005% in ethanol]. A dose of 0.025-0.05 ml is applied using a micropipette or HPLC Hamilton syringe to each site. Animals are weighed on the first day of dosing. Approximately 48 h prior to the treatment, the hair is removed from a 6 × 8 cm area on the back with a fine clipper. The animals are dosed as described above. Test areas are separated to prevent mixing of test solutions after application. No patches or wraps are used. Immediately after dose application, the animals are placed in a restrainer while keeping the sites uncovered. Prior to irradiation, the heads of the animals are covered to prevent eye damage from the light exposure. Thirty minutes after dosing, animals are exposed to a nonerythmogenic dose of light in the UVA band (peak intensity between 335 and 365 nm). The dose of light should be 9 or 10 J/cm^2 for UVA and 0.1-0.3 J/cm^2 for UVB. Immediately after the light exposure, the animals are wiped clean if necessary and returned to the respective cages. Animals are inspected and scored at 24 h and 48 h post-exposure according to the following scoring scale: 0, no reaction; 1, slight erythema; 2, moderate erythema; 3, severe erythema, with or without edema.

This scoring scheme is similar to that used for dermal sensitization scoring, whereas the scoring method for the rabbit model discussed previously is that for dermal irritation studies. Any unusual clinical sign during exposure should be noted. The following descriptive parameters are calculated from the data.

$$\text{Phototoxicity irritation index} = \frac{\text{Number of positive sites}}{\text{Number of exposure sites}} \times 100$$

$$\text{Phototoxicity severity index} = \frac{\text{Total of scores}}{\text{Total of observations}}$$

Mouse Ear Swelling Model

The method is used for topical phototoxicity testing.[5] In this female BALB/c mice are used and divided into two or three groups if positive control is included. Five mice each for solvent/irradiation controls and for test material treatment are used. Five animals are used for positive control (8-MOP). Animals should be juvenile, weighing 20 to 25 g. Animals are acclimatized at least 5 days prior to the experiment. Animals are given free access to food and water. This test assumes that material is in solution form. Generally, the most volatile and non-irritating organic solvent like ethanol, acetone, dimethylacetamide or some combination is used. For treatment each ear in each mouse in a group is treated with the same solution. A dosage of 8-10 μl is applied on each side of the ear using a micropipette. Animals are weighed on the first day of dosing. Approximately 48 h prior to treatment, the ears are inspected and animals assigned to treatment groups. Animals with swollen or damaged ears are excluded from the test. Preliminary ear thickness measurements are taken by vernier caliper. On the day of dosing, animals are placed in specially designed restrainers and the animals are dosed as described previously. No patches or wraps are used. Thirty to 60 min after dose application, the animals are exposed to a nonerythmogenic dose of light in the UVA band (150 W short-arc UV solar simulator with internal 1 mm UG-11 and WG 320 filters with peak intensity between 290 and 410 nm). Irradiation in W/cm^2 is determined using a radiometer with an appropriate UVA or UVB detector. Light is between 5 and 7 J/cm^2 for UVA and 0.2-0.4 J/cm^2 for UVB. Only the right ear is exposed. The left ear is protected from light by the researcher's hand. Immediately after light exposure, the animals are wiped clean if necessary and returned to respective cages. Ear thickness measurements are taken at 24, 48 and 72 h post-dosing using a handheld dial micrometer. The ear is positioned so that the contact plates of the micrometer can be placed towards the outer edge of the ear. The spring-loaded lever of the micrometer is slowly released until the plates come in contact with the surface of the ear as judged visually. Care is taken so that the plates do not close too quickly or tightly on the ear, causing compression of any edema that might be present. Two measurements are taken at adjacent sites on each ear and the average ear thickness is determined. Changes in ear thickness from the pretreatment baseline are calculated and expressed as mm × 10^{-2}. A statistically significant (paired t-test) increase in ear thickness in the irradiated ears vs. the nonirradiated ears within the test article treated groups is considered sufficient evidence for phototoxicity, provided that there is not a statistically significant change in the control group.

This method has obvious advantages over the guinea pig and rabbit dorsal surface models already described. The animals are less expensive to obtain and maintain, and the test is very objective and reliable.

ALTERNATIVE DESIGNS IN THE *IN VIVO* METHODS

Rabbit Ear Model

There are at least two *in vivo* alternatives to this traditional test. The first uses just the ear of the rabbit. The rabbit ear provides a site, which is of sufficient size with uniform thin skin without a thick, hairy coat, thus, offering advantages over the whole body rabbit and mouse models. The external surface of the pinna is shaved with clippers and radiation is delivered using a xenon arc solar simulator with multiple liquid light guides (Solar Light Co, Philadelphia, PA) adjusted to provide intensity steps varying by 40%. Depending on the test situation, exposures range from 0.5 to 12 min. In the absence of phototoxic agents or sunscreens, a 1 minute exposure generally produces detectable erythema from the midrange light guides. The intensity of the erythema is graded and corresponds with the radiation flux.[6]

Hairless Mouse Model

In this method, the dorsal skin thickness is measured using vernier skinfold calipers. In this way, the degree of dermal edema induced by phototoxic agents is measured readily and is not subjected to the problems of visual assessment of erythema as in rodent skin.[7]

Advantages and Disadvantages

The classic and alternative methods share common advantages and disadvantages. They have no appreciable false negative results. These are easy to perform and relatively inexpensive. On the other hand, the disadvantages of the method are that the photometers must be carefully calibrated to control UV exposure, results are subjective rather than objective, and significant amount of test material is required.

PHOTOSENSITIZATION MODELS

Guinea Pig Dorsal Surface

This method uses dermal exposure without any adjuvant to increase the response.[8] Young adult female Hartley guinea pigs, weighing between 300 to 400 g are used. The females are preferred because the aggressive social behavior of males may result in considerable skin damage that might interfere with the interpretation of the challenge reactions. Animals that show poor growth or illness in any way are not used because illness markedly decreases the response. Animals with skin marked or scarred from fighting are avoided. The guinea pigs are quarantined and observed for at least 2 weeks to detect any illness prior to the study. The guinea pigs are randomly assigned to a test group of 10 animals and negative control group of 6 animals. If a pretest group is necessary then animals, as needed for that group, are also randomized. The test and control group guinea pigs are weighed 1 week prior to dosing (day-7), on the day of dosing (day-0) and weekly thereafter.

If pre-test is necessary, then several animals are exposed to different concentrations of test substance dissolved in acetone. This is used to determine the topical dermal irritation threshold concentration on the skin that is exposed to UVB and UVA irradiation sequentially and on the skin that is exposed to UVA irradiation alone. The hair of these animals is clipped over the whole dorsal region. A volume of 0.2 ml of each test concentration is applied twice to each guinea pig: (i) at the nuchal region and (ii) the dorsal lumbar region. Thirty minutes after application, the treated nuchal sites are irradiated with sunlamp [fluorescent "sunlamp" of tubes (UVB irradiation): type of tubes Westinghouse FS40; skin distance, 15 cm; dose, measured and calculated at time of exposure; (exposure time, 30 min; emission, 285-350 nm) emissions (UVB for 30 min)], while the lumbar sites are shielded with elastoplast tape. After the UVB exposure the tape is removed from the lumbar region, and both the treated nuchal sites and lumbar sites are irradiated with black light [fluorescent 'black light' tubes (UVA irradiation): type of tubes, GE F40 BL; skin distance, 10 cm; dose measured and calculated at time of exposure; exposure time, 30 min; emission, 320-450 nm; a pane of window glass (3 mm thick) is used to eliminate passage of radiation of lower than 320 nm] emissions (UVA) for 30 minute. Thereafter the animals are returned to their respective cages after the UVA exposure. Twenty-four hours after the initial exposure to the test substance, the nuchal and lumbar skin sites are scored for erythema formation. A concentration is chosen for induction application that causes a mild or weak erythema response at the nuchal sites. If the substance does not cause erythema response then the highest concentration level that is practical should be used for the erythema induction. The highest concentration of the test substance that is nonirritating to the lumbar sites is used for challenge application. Two lower concentrations of the test substance, prepared by serial dilution from the highest concentration are also used for the challenge application.

Days 0, 2, 4, 7, 9, and 11 are used for induction stage. The hair in an area of approximately 3 × 3 cm is clipped from the nuchal region of each test and control group guinea pig. A volume of 0.2 ml of a relatively high concentration of the test substance in either acetone or ethanol is applied to the shaved nuchal region of each test group guinea pig. The concentration will be the highest level that can be well tolerated locally by the guinea pig, as determined by a pretest for dermal irritation. Then a volume of 0.2 ml of solvent (acetone or ethanol) is applied to the shaved nuchal region of each control group guinea pig. Thirty minutes after application, the treated nuchal sites of test and control guinea pigs are irradiated with sunlamp emissions for 30 min and black light emissions for 30 min, successively. The lumbar region of the back is shielded from the light sources during the irradiation procedures with elastic bandage, which is wrapped around the torso of each animal. The clipping, topical exposures to test substance and irradiation procedures are repeated six times during a 12-day period (induction days are 0, 2, 4, 7, 9, and 11). The day 32 is a challenge day. The elicitation of contact photosensitivity is performed on 21 day from the last sensitizing (induction) exposure. The hair of the dorsal lumbar region of each of 10 test group and 3 of 6 control group guinea pigs is clipped for the first time. Three different concentrations of the test substance using the solvent used for induction, as determined from the pre-test, are applied topically to this region; test and control animals are treated alike. Each concentration is applied to the right and left side of the dorsal midline. The torso of each test and control guinea pig is wrapped in Saran Wrap (1 layer thick) after the test chemical is applied. The Saran Wrap is held in place at the ends with athletic adhesive tape. The same tape is used to shield the left side of each animal from the UVA light source. Thirty minutes after application, the right side of each animal is exposed to nonerythmogenic (> 320 nm) UVA emissions for 30 min. The radiation is passed through a pane of window glass 3 mm thick in order to eliminate passage of radiation lower than 320 nm. After black light exposure, all animals are unwrapped, returned to their respective cages, and placed in a darkened room for 24 h. If the test substance leaves a colored residue the excess test material is removed by washing with a suitable solvent at 24 h so that the area of challenge skin can be evaluated accurately. All the test sites, both irradiated and nonirradiated, are scored and interpreted 24 and 48 h after the initial test substance application and subsequent exposure to black light irradiation. The erythema is scored as follows: 0, no erythema; 1, minimal, but definite erythema; 2, moderate erythema; 3, considerable erythema; 4, maximal erythema.

If the test substance is judged a nonphotosensitizing agent after the challenge application, a second and final challenge application is performed on each test animal 7 days after the initiation of the first challenge dose. Controls from the first challenge application are rechallenged because they have been exposed to the test substance and are no longer true negative (naive) controls. The three remaining naive control group animals (not used for the first challenge) are challenged for comparison to the re-challenge of test group animals. The procedure used for the first challenge application is used for the second challenge application. Either the same procedure will be used or new concentrations of test substance, including reshaving, the same patching method and the same duration of exposure is used. Observations are again made 24 h and 48 h after the second challenge application and skin reactions are recorded. The negative control group of animals, having received no previous photosensitive (induction) exposure, serves to identify any phototoxic or primary irritant (nonphototoxic) substances. An erythema score of one or more is considered a positive response.

Armstrong Assay

This method originally published by Ichikawa et al[9] introduced the use of adjuvant in a photosensitization test system in guinea pig. The assay has been recommended by the Cosmetic, Toiletries, and Fragrances Association (CTFA). This assay uses UVA light (320-400 nm) in the induction and challenge phase. The UVA lights are commonly known as "black lights" ("BLB" fluorescence-type bulbs). However, the selection of the light source is critical because the range of wavelengths emitted by the bulb is controlled by the phosphor coating and different manufacturers use different phosphors to produce BLB lights. There may even be different phosphors used by the same manufacturer with no code on the bulbs to indicate the type of phosphor being used. The General Electric BLB emits effective energy only at wavelength longer than 350 nm, whereas the entire spectrum between 250 and 350 nm is covered by Sylvania BLB bulb. Less than 2% of the energy emitted by General electric BLB light is between 250 and 350 nm, whereas 42% of the energy from the Sylvania BLB light falls in this range. There are known photoallergens that require the energy contained in the spectrum below 345 nm for activation, and thus give false negative results if the incorrect light source is used. The best precaution is to determine the emission spectrum of the lights, which are to be used in the assay.[10]

It is necessary to determine the total energy being emitted by the lights in order to calculate the proper J/cm2 exposure. An International Light Model 700 provides a relatively inexpensive means of measuring the light energy when fitted with a cosine-corrected UVA detector (W150s quartz diffuser, UVA-pass filter SEL015 detector). The device has a peak sensitivity of 360 nm and width of 50 nm. A bank of eight bulbs is readily prepared by bolting together two industrial four-bulb (48" long) reflectors. Two sets of these will allow 40 animals to be treated at one time. The lights are allowed to warm 30 min before use. They are turned off just before the animals are placed under them and then turned back on. The light intensity is measured at several locations at the level of the top of the backs of the animal and the correct exposure time is then calculated. The lights are adjusted between 4 and 6 inches above the back and 10 J/cm^2 is the proper exposure. The Hill Top Chamber provides a good patching system in this assay. A volume of 0.3 ml is used. Suitable animal restrainers for holding the animals during the patching and the exposure to the light as well as in providing excellent occlusion should be used. The majority of hair is removed from the intended patching site with a small animal clipper fitted with a No. 40 blade. The assay frequently requires the complete removal of hair using a depilatory cream, which is applied and left in contact with the skin for not more than 15 min. It must be washed away completely with a stream of warm running water. The animals are dried with a towel and the inside of the cages wiped clean of any depilatory cream before putting the guinea pigs. When required, the epidermis is partially removed by tape stripping. The skin must be completely dry otherwise the stripping will be ineffective. An approximately 8 inches long tape strip is used. Starting at one end of the rope, it is placed against the skin and rubbed with the finger to adhere firmly. It is then pealed away, taking with it some dry epidermis cells. A new section of the tape is then applied to the skin and the procedure repeated four or five times. The skin will have a shiny appearance due to the leakage of moisture from the dermis. The tape should not be jerked away from the skin because this can cause the rupture of dermal capillaries.

The potential of the animal to respond to a sensitizer is enhanced by the injection of Freund's complete adjuvant (Calbio-chem-Behring, San Diego, CA, or Difco, Detroit, MI). The adjuvant is diluted 1:1 with sterile water before use. The injections must be given by intradermal route. In the Armstrong assay, a pattern of four 0.1 ml injections is given just prior to the first induction patching in the nuchal area. All four injections should fit under the edge of the area to be covered by the Hill Top chamber. It is advisable to perform the skin stripping operation before the injections as the adjuvant can leak onto the skin and prevent effective removal of the epidermis. The test site(s) is exposed to the UVA light after 2 h of occlusion. The animal is left in the restrainer and the dental dam above the test site to be exposed is cut and the patch removed. Excess material is wiped from the site to be exposed and the remaining parts of the animals are covered with aluminum foil. All patches are removed after the light exposure step, the patched areas wiped free of excess material, and the animals are returned to the cage. The grading is similar to as described earlier.

With the exception of water it is desirable to use a vehicle for the induction, which is different from the one used at the challenge. Because the controlled animals in the Armstrong assay are sham treated (including any vehicle), one can patch the test and controlled animals with vehicle at the challenge if the same vehicle is to be used for both the induction and the challenge. It is advantageous to use a vehicle, which dissolves the test compound and is inert.

Assay Procedure

For Irritation/Toxicity Pretest (8 animals)

Day 0: The hair from the lumbar region is removed by clipping and depilation. Two concentrations are applied on each animal on adjacent left side/right side locations for a total of four dose concentrations. The patches are occluded for 2 h (+ 15 min). The right side is exposed to 10 J/cm^2 of UVA light after removing the patches on the right side. The remaining patches and excess material are removed after the exposure to light. Day 1: All test sites are graded 24 h (± 1 h) after removal of all patches (24 h grade). Day 2: The grading is repeated 48 h (± 2 h) after removing the patches (48 h grade).

For Induction (20 tests + 10 sham controls + any rechallenge controls)

Day 0: All test and control animals are weighed. The hair from the nuchal area is removed with clippers and depilatory cream. The epidermis is removed by stripping four or five times with tape. Four 0.1 ml id. injections of a 1 : 1 dilution of Freund's complete adjuvant are made in an area to be covered by the patch. This area is covered on the test animals with a Hill Top Chamber, which has 0.3 ml of test material preparation. The sham controls are patched with water or solvent on the patch. Occlusion with dental dam is done, and animals are restrained in a holder for 2 h (± 15 min). The patches are removed and the non-patched areas are covered with foil, and are exposed to 10 J/cm^2 of UVA light for 30 min. On day 2, 4, 7, 9, and 11 the activities of Day 0 are repeated with the following exceptions. Animals are not weighed and not injected with adjuvant. The patch is removed when the original induction site becomes too damaged but it is kept in the nuchal area. Depilation may not be needed at each induction. For challenge, 20 tests + 10 sham control animals (9-13 days after last induction exposure) are required. On day 0: All the animals are weighed, the lumbar region is clipped free of hair, and depilated. The skin is not stripped. Each animal is patched with a pair of adjacent patches (one on the left side and one on the right side) containing 0.3 ml of a nonirritating concentration of test material on a Hill Top Chamber. The patches are removed from the right side and the remaining animal is covered with foil. The right side is exposed to 10 J/cm² of a UVA light. The remaining patches are removed and any excess material is cleaned. On day 1, all challenge sites either exposed or unexposed to light (24 h ± 1 h) are graded after removal of the patches (24 h grade) and recorded separately. On day 2, the grading is repeated at 48 h (± 2 h) after removal of the patches (48 h grade). All or selected animals are rechallenged with the same or a different test material 7-12 days after the challenge. Ten new sham treated controls and naive test sites on all animals are used following the same procedure as used in the challenge. The number of positive responders is determined (number of animals with a score >1 at either the 24 or 48 h grading or with a score 1 unit higher than the highest score in the control). The average score is determined at 24 and 48 h for the test and control groups using face values. The data for the sites exposed to light are kept separate from the data unexposed to light.

The Armstrong assay has been found to give responses similar to human in the guinea pig: positive responses for 6-methyl coumarin and musk ambrette. A major disadvantage is that the procedure is time consuming with six induction exposures. The procedure is very stressful on the animals because of the injection of adjuvant and the multiple skin strippings and depilation.

The recommended positive control is musk ambrette. Tetrachlorosalicylanilide (TCSA) also gives positive results, but it should be noted that this material is reported to be an allergen without UV light activation. Animals are induced with a 10% w/v solution of musk ambrette in acetone and sham controls are patched with acetone alone. The Hill Top Chamber is used for all patch studies.

The Photo Hen's Egg Test (PHET)

As an alternative to the rabbit eye test (Draize test) hen's egg test (HET), was introduced by toxicologists as a screening model for mucocutaneous toxicity.[11-13] Neumann et al employed the yolk sac blood vessel system (YS) of the incubated hen's egg in combination with UV irradiation as a new valid and inexpensive screening model for phototoxicity.[14-18]

Fertile white Leghorn eggs are incubated in horizontal position at 37.5°C and relative humidity 65%. At 3 days of incubation all eggs are candled in order and defective eggs are discarded. A hole is made into the eggshell and 5 ml of egg white is removed to lower the embryo and its surrounding yolk substance. Afterwards a 1.5 × 2.5 cm window is sawed out of the shell. Eggs are covered by a wax sheet and replaced back in the incubator. At day 4 of incubation, only eggs with normally developed embryos and YS are used for testing. The PHET has a 2 × 2 factorial test designs with the factors "irradiation" and "substance application" and the levels "yes" and "no". PHET is established to investigate phototoxic reactions; the yolk sac blood vessel system of the incubated hen's eggs is exposed only to nontoxic concentrations of the test substances and to a nontoxic UVA dose (5 J/cm²) concurrently. At day 4 of the incubation period, test group is exposed to a test substance, immediately followed by an irradiation with 5 J/cm² UVA.

Physiological salt solution (PSS) may be used as vehicle. Serving as controls, three additional test groups exposed only to PSS and 5 J/cm^2 UVA or to PSS or to a test substance alone. Readings performed 24 h after irradiation. During this observation period, the morphological parameters such as membrane discoloration (MD), hemorrhage (HR) were monitored via a macroscope and graded following a four point scale:

Level 0: No visible MD or HR

Level 1: Just visible MD or HR

Level 2: Visible MD or HR, structures are covered partially

Level 3: Visible MD or HR, structures are covered totally

The test parameters MD and HR as well as embryo lethality are summarized in morphology and a lethality index (Table 43.2). Using these indices, the relative phototoxic potential of an assumed photosensitizer compared to other well-known photosensitizers can be calculated.

Table 43.2: Photo hen's egg test

Relative lethality: Lethality rate of the interaction group (Li) minus the average lethality rate of controls LC = (lc1 + lc2 + lc3)/3 Relative lethality L = Li _ Lc Relative lethality L (%) = L × 100
Relative hemorrhage I and II: Sums of the hemorrhage (HR) levels of the interaction group HRG1i and HRG2i: Frequencies of level 0 HR + level 1 HR = HRG1i Frequencies of level 2 HR + level 3 HR = HRG2i Sums of the hemorrhage (HR) levels of the controls: Frequencies of (level 0 HR + level 1 HR = HRG1c Frequencies of level 2 HR + level 3 HR = HRG2c Relative hemorrhage I (HR I) = HRG1i–[(HRG1c)/3] Relative hemorrhage II (HRII) = HRG2i–[(HRG2c)/3]
Sums of the membrane discoloration (MD) levels of the interaction group MDG1i and MDG2i: Frequencies of level 0 MD + level 1 MD = MDG1i Frequencies of level 2 MD + level 3 MD = MDG2i
Sums of the membrane discoloration (MD) levels of the controls: Frequencies of level 0 MD + level 1 MD = MDG1c Frequencies of level 2 MD + level 3 MD = MDG2c
Membrane discoloration: Relative membrane discoloration I (MD I) = MDG1i–[(MDG1c)/3] Relative membrane discoloration II (MD II) = MDG2i–[(MDG2c)/3]

IN VITRO ASSAYS

Photohemolysis

Photohemolysis is quantified in two ways: (a) by the release of hemoglobin, through the absorbance of the supernatants (after centrifugation) at 540 nm; (b) by the decreasing number of intact red blood cells, which is proportional to the optical density at 650 nm. An intrinsic limitation of this test system is that it detects photosensitization only at the cell membrane level. Hence, false negative predictions must be expected for compounds acting via photodamage to

DNA or other biological targets different from the membrane components. This assay is rapid and easy to perform.[19]

Photosensitized *Candida albicans* Growth Inhibition

Candida albicans growth inhibition is evaluated as the diameter of the yeast free zone.[20,21] Such inhibition is assumed to indicate injury to DNA.

The test compound is dissolved in ethanol, DMSO or acetone. A known volume of a 0.05-10% solution is applied to 7.5 mm filter discs. The latter is transferred to Sabouraud agar plates where a suspension of a fresh culture of *C. albicans* has been evenly spread. The plates (duplicate samples) are exposed to UVA radiation (1 mW/cm^2). The controls are kept in the dark and the vehicle alone. After exposure is complete, the diameter of the yeast free zone is measured. The pathogenicity of this species is a drawback of this assay.

Photodegranulation of Mast Cells

Phototoxicity is frequently associated with urticaria and histamine release from the skin mast cells. The release of histamine is measured by means of spectrophotometric methods[22] or by radioactive mediator (^{3}H-serotonin) resulting from mast cell degranulation, in the supernatant.[23]

Photo-Basophil-Histamine Release Test

Suspensions of human leucocytes are used in this case as the model system, and photosensitized release of histamine from the cells to the supernatant (measured spectrofluorimetrically after derivatization) serves as an end-point for identifying phototoxic drugs.[24]

Histidine Photodegradation

Solutions of tiaprofenic acid in 10% propylene glycol in PBS (0.01 M, pH 7.4) are mixed with the same amount of L-histidine monochloride solution (0.61 mM) in PBS. These mixtures are bubbled with oxygen and irradiated with the light of psoralens and ultraviolet A radiation (PUVA) unit (365 nm, 16 mW/cm^2). When irradiation is complete, the samples are incubated in the dark at room temperature for 30 min. Histidine is determined by a modified Pauly reaction. For this, 200 µl of test solution is made up to 2 ml with PBS; 200 µl of 1% sulfanilic acid in 0.87 N HCl and 200 µl of 5% sodium nitrite are added and the mixture is left for 10 min; 0.6 ml of 20% sodium carbonate is then added, followed by the addition of 2 ml of ethyl alcohol after 2 min. The OD of the final solution is read at 530 nm in a spectrophotometer against a control; the remaining histidine is measured from a standard curve.[25]

REFERENCES

1. Ferguson J. Fluoroquinolone photosensitization: A review of clinical and laboratory studies. Photochem Photobiol 1995;62:954-8.
2. Lambert J, Warmer W, Kornhauser A. Animal models for phototoxicity testing. Toxicol Methods 1996;2:99-114.
3. Marzulli FM, Maibach HI. Perfume phototoxicity. J Soc Cosmet Chem 1970;21:685-715.

4. Nilsson R, Maurer T, Redmond N. A standard protocol for phototoxicity testing: Results from an interlaboratory study. Contact Dermatitis 1993;28:285-90.
5. Gerberick GF, Ryan CA. A predictive mouse ear swelling model for investigating topical phototoxicity. Food Chem Toxicol 1989;12:813-9.
6. Marks R, Gabriel KL, Hershman RJ, et al. The rabbit ear as an animal model for phototoxicity and photobiology studies. J Am College Toxicol 1986;5:606.
7. Lowe NJ. Cutaneous phototoxicity reactions. Br J Dermatol 1986;115:86-92.
8. Harber LC, Shalita AR. The guinea pig as an effective model for the demonstration of immunologically mediated contact photosensitivity. In: Maibach H (Ed). Animal Models in Dermatology. Edinburgh, UK:Churchill-Livingstone, 1975:90-102.
9. Ichikawa H, Armstrong RB, Harber LC. Photoallergic contact dermatitis in guinea pigs: Improve induction technique using Freund's complete adjuvant. J Invest Dematol 1981;76:498-501.
10. Cole CA, Forbes PD, Davies RE. Different biological effectiveness of blacklight fluorescent lamps available for therapy with psoralens plus ultraviolet. J Am Acad Dermatol 1984;11:599-606.
11. Draize HJ. Intracutaneous sensitization test on guinea pigs. In Apraisal of the Safety of Chemicals in Food, Drugs and Cosmetics, Association of Food and Drug Officials of the United States, Austin, Texas, 1959.
12. Duffy PA. Irritancy testing-a cultured approach. Toxicol In Vitro 1989;3:157-8.
13. Rosenbruch M. Toxizita¨tsuntersuchungen am bebru¨teten Hu¨hnerei, Derm Beruf Umwelt 1990;38:5-11.
14. Freeman RG, Murtishaw W, Knox JM. Tissue culture techniques in the study of cell photobiology and phototoxicity. Invest Dermatol 1970;54:164-9.
15. Maier K, Schmitt-Landgraf R, Siegmund B. Development of an in vitro test system with human skin cells for evaluation of phototoxicity. Toxicol In Vitro 1991;5/6:457–61.
16. Neumann NJ, Hö lzle E, Lehmann P, Rosenbruch M, Klaucic P, Plewig G. Photo hen's egg test: a model for phototoxicity. Br J Dermatol 1997;136:326-30.
17. Neumann NJ, Klaucic A, Hö lzle E, Lehmann P. Evaluation of the phototoxic potential of ciprofloxacin in the photo hen's egg test. Arch Dermatol Res 1995;287:384.
18. Neumann NJ, Hö lzle E, Wallerand M, Vierbaum S, Ruzicka S, Lehmann P. The photoprotective effect of ascorbic acid, acetylsalicylic acid, and indomethacin evaluated by the photo hen's egg test. Photodermatol Photoimmunol Photomed 1999;15:166-70.
19. Kahn G. Fleischaker B. Red blood cell hemolysis by photosensitizing compounds. J Invest Dermatol 1971;56:85-90.
20. Daniels F. A simple microbiological method for demonstrating phototoxic compounds. J Invest Dermatol 1965;44:259-63.
21. Kavli G, Volden G. The Candida test for phototoxicity. Photodermatology 1984;1:204-7.
22. Sik RH, Paschall CS, Chignell CF. The phototoxic effect of benoxaprofen and its analogs on human erythrocytes and rat peritoneal mast cells. Photochem Photobiol 1983;38:411-5.
23. Gendimenico GJ, Kochevar IE. Degranulation of mast cells and inhibition of the response to secretory agents by phototoxic compounds and ultraviolet radiation. Toxicol Appl Pharmacol 1984;76:374-82.
24. Przybilla B, Schwab-Przybilla U, Ruzicka T, et al. Phototoxicity of nonsteroidal anti-inflammatory drugs demonstrated in vitro by a photo-basophil-histamine-release test. Photodermatol 1987;4:73-8.
25. Figueiredo A, Fontes Ribeiro CA, Goncalo M, et al. Experimental studies on the mechanisms of tiaprofenic acid photosensitization. J Photochem Photobiol B1993;18:161-8.

CHAPTER

44

Anti-asthmatic Agents

INTRODUCTION

Asthma is a complex inflammatory airway disease characterized by airflow obstruction that remains leading cause of hospitalization and death worldwide. In Asthma the airway occasionally constricts, becomes inflamed, and is lined with excessive amounts of mucus, often in response to one or more triggers. These episodes may be triggered by such things as exposure to an environmental stimulant (or allergen), cold air, warm air, moist air, exercise or exertion, or emotional stress. In children, the most common triggers are viral illnesses such as those that cause the common cold. This airway narrowing causes symptoms such as wheezing, shortness of breath, chest tightness and coughing. Between episodes, most patients feel well but can have mild symptoms and they may remain short of breath after exercise for longer periods of time than the unaffected individual. The symptoms of asthma, which can range from mild to life threatening, can usually be controlled with a combination of drugs and environmental changes. Patients usually have reduced forced expiratory volume in one second (FEV_1) as well as reduced airflow. Other features, characteristic of asthma but not unique to the disease are airway inflammation and bronchial hyperresponsiveness.[1]

Short-term relief is most effectively achieved with bronchodilators, agents that increase airway caliber by relaxing airway smooth muscle and of these the α-adrenoreceptor stimulants (α_2-agonists) are the most widely used. Theophylline, a methyl xanthine drug, and antimuscarinic agents (e.g. ipratropium bromide) are also used for reversal of airway constriction. Long term control is most often achieved with an anti-inflammatory agent such as an inhaled corticosteroid (e.g. budesonide) or an inhibitor of mast cell degranulation, e.g. cromolyn or nedocromil sodium. Of the several drugs currently available neither clinicians nor patients are completely satisfied with their effects. There is no doubt that there is an urgent need of new and effective drugs, which are able to treat or even possibly cure the allergic inflammation.

To mimic bronchial asthma in animals, a wide variety of animal models have been developed. The use of an appropriate model could help us to develop new chemical entities for the treatment of human allergic disorders in a more predictable way. There have been many attempts to develop and characterize animal models that approximate human allergy or asthma. Each model has its own inherent advantages and shortcomings and unfortunately, no model is identical to the conditions found in human disease. Nonetheless, the development of relevant animal models continues in anticipation that they will aid in the examination of underlying processes that contribute to asthma or allergy, or will assist in the identification of novel therapies that can be used to treat these diseases.

Animal systems that accurately reflect disease pathophysiology continue to be essential to the development of new therapies for asthma. In this review, the pre-clinical *in vitro* and *in vivo* models that recapitulate many of the features of asthma are described. Specifically, the pro's and con's of the standard models are discussed and recently developed systems designed to more accurately reflect the complexity of both diseases are reflected. The new models of asthma described herein demonstrate that improved clinical understanding of the diseases and better preclinical models is an iterative process that will hopefully lead to therapies that can effectively manage asthma.

IN VITRO MODELS

Binding Assays

Histamine Receptor Assay

This method evaluates the affinity of test compound to histamine H_1 receptor. This is done by measuring their inhibitory activities on the binding of ^3H pyrilamine (H1 antagonist) to guinea pig brain plasma membrane preparation.

Male guinea pig weighing 300-600 g is sacrificed by CO_2 necrosis. The brain is homogenized in ice-cold Tris buffer (pH 7.5, 1 g in 30 ml buffer) and homogenate is centrifuged for 10 min at 4°C at 50,000 g. Supernatant is discarded and pellet is resuspended in buffer, centrifuged again. The pellet obtained after centrifugation is re-suspended in Tris buffer (1 g/5 ml) and aliquots of 1 ml are frozen at -70°C. In a shaking bath maintained at 25°C 50 ul^3H pyrilamine (2×10^{-9} M), 50 ul test compound (10^{-5}-10^{-10} M) and 100 ul membrane suspension from guinea pig whole brain (10 mg/ml) per sample are incubated for 30 min. Incubation buffer used is TrisHCl buffer (50 mM, pH 7.5). With 11 conc. of ^3H pyrilamine ($0.1\text{-}50 \times 10^{-9}$ M) saturation experiments are performed. Total binding is determined in the presence of incubation buffer, non-specific binding in presence of mepyramine (10^{-5} M). By rapid vacuum filtration through glass fiber filters reaction is stopped. Subsequently the membrane bound is separated from the radioactivity. The retained membrane bound radioactivity on the filter is measured after addition of 3 ml scintillation cocktail/sample in liquid scintillation counter.[3]

The parameters calculated are total binding of ^3H pyrilamine, non-specific binding and specific binding (total binding–non-specific binding) and % inhibition of ^3H pyrilamine binding (100- specific binding as % of control value).

The dissociation constant (Ki) and IC_{50} value of test compound are determined from experiment of ^3H pyrilamine Vs non-labeled drug by computer-supported analysis of the binding data.

Cell Culture Method

CULTEX Technique

The CULTEX technology is a new experimental system for cultivation and exposure of cells intermittently at the air/liquid interface with ultrafine particles, gases, or mixtures of both which fixedly flows. Studies on cytotoxicity of air contaminants such as gaseous or particulate compounds and complex mixtures have traditionally used animal experiments because of the difficulties in exposing cell cultures directly to these substances. This technique has enhanced the efficiency of *in vitro* studies, and allows direct exposure of the bronchial epithelial cells.

CULTEX technique uses a transwell membrane technique for direct exposure of complex mixtures like sidestream cigarette smoke at the air/liquid interface. Before exposure, the bronchial epithelial cells are washed with PBS and then transferred from the companion plate to the cell exposure unit. The factors influencing the susceptibility of human bronchial epithelial cells (e.g. gas flow rate or duration of exposure) are studied and the cells are finally exposed for one hour to clean air or different concentrations of sidestream smoke. To achieve homogeneous aerosol distribution above the cell cultures, a specially designed exposure top can be adapted to the CULEX unit to allow direct exposure. Incubation intervals and cell preparation for analysis are the same for cells exposed to the test atmosphere and the air/liquid controls. The test group bronchial epithelial cells are incubated with the test drug for 24 hr and then exposed for 1 h to different concentrations of sidestream smoke.[4] The biological parameters that can be estimated in the control and treated groups are number of cells, metabolic activity and glutathione concentration. Also cell viability measurements in the control and test groups can be carried out by using the WST assay and electronic cell counting.[5]

WST Assay

Briefly, in the WST assay the cells are transferred from the cell exposure vessels to conventional companion plates containing 2 ml of fresh RPMI medium per well. Five hundred microliters of medium with 100 ml of WST-1 dye is layered on the attached cells and removed after 1 hr of incubation. Aliquots of 100 µl are transferred into a 96 well microplate for measuring their absorbance at 450 nm/630 nm using a microplate reader. Additional cells from the same membrane are trypsinized by adding 500 µl trypsin/EDTA solution on top of the monolayer. After 4 min of incubation at 37°C, the enzymatic activity is stopped after adding 25 µl of trypsin inhibitor (10,000 BAEE units/mg protein). The cells are gently suspended and 100 µl of the suspension diluted in 9.9 ml CASYton. Aliquots are analyzed with an electronic cell counter.

Thus, CULTEX technique enables treatment of bronchial epithelial cells with sample atmospheres for subsequent *in vitro* assays. The introduction of these cultivation and exposure techniques offers new testing strategies for the toxicological evaluation of a broad range of airborne and inhaled compounds.

Tests in Isolated Organs

Spasmolytic Activity in Guinea Pig Lungs

Several autacoids such as histamine and leukotrienes induce bronchoconstriction. Histamine causes bronchoconstriction by activating H^1 receptors. It is an important mediator of immediate allergic and inflammatory reactions. Calcium ionophores induce the release of leukotrienes via the 5-lipoxygenase pathway that cause potent bronchoconstriction. Using this method, drugs are tested for their capability of inhibiting bronchospasm induced by histamine or calcium ionophore.

Albino guinea pigs of either sex, weighing 300 to 450 g, are sacrificed with an overdose of ether. The chest is opened and the lungs are removed and cut into strips of 5 cm each and placed into a physiological saline solution. Thereafter, the lungs are mounted in an organ bath containing a nutritive solution. The nutritive solution has following components in percent of anhydrous salts: NaCl 0.0659, $NaHCO_3$ 0.0252, KCl 0.046, $CaCl_2$ 0.005, $MgCl_2$ 0.0135, NaH_2PO_4 0.01, Na_2HPO_4 0.008, glucose 5%, pH 8. The bath is bubbled with carbogen and maintained at 37°C. Under a preload of 0.5 to 3 g, the tissue is left to equilibrate for 30 to 60 min. Prior to the testing, carbachol is added to the bath to test the lung strip's ability to contract. Twenty minutes later two pre-values are obtained by adding the spasmogen to the bath and recording contractile force at its maximal level. Following a 20 min equilibration period the spasmogen is administered again. The spasmogens commonly used are histamine dihydrochloride (10^{-6} g/ml for 5 min), Ca-inophore (10^{-6} g/ml for 5 min), leukotine C_4 and D_4 (10^{-8} g/ml for 10 min). Five minutes thereafter the test compound is administered. The contractile dose is determined isometrically. The percentage inhibition of spasmogen-induced contraction by the test drug is calculated.[6]

Vascular and Airway Responses to the Isolated Lung

The model provides the opportunity of simultaneous registration of pulmonary vascular and airway responses to drugs.

Sprague Dawley rats (300 to 350 g) are anesthetized intraperitoneally with pentobarbitone sodium (50 mg/kg). The trachea is cannulated and the animal is maintained on artificial respiration. Rat is heparinized with 1,000 units of heparin and rapidly exsanguinated by withdrawing blood from the carotid artery. Lung is exposed by median sternotomy and a ligature is placed around the aorta to prevent systemic loss of blood. Lung is removed and suspended in a warmed (39°C), humidified (100%) water-jacketed chamber. The pulmonary artery is also catheterized. An external heat exchanger is used to maintain temperature of the perfusate solution (Krebs-Henseleit), which is placed in a reservoir and mixed constantly by a magnetic stirrer. Lungs are perfused using a peristaltic roller pump at a flow rate of 8 to 14 ml/min to maintain pulmonary arterial pressure of 15 mmHg. Pulmonary arterial pefusion pressure, airway pressure and reservoir blood level are continuously monitored, electronically averaged and recorded with the help of a polygraph. Changes in pulmonary arterial pressure and airway pressure after injection of test compounds are measured in mmHg and compared with baseline values.[7]

Reactivity of the Isolated Perfused Guinea Pig Trachea

This model is best suited to study the mechanism by which the epithelium affects the reactivity of tracheal musculature. The effect of histamine, calcium ionophores, bradykinin, leukotrienes and potassium channel openers can be studied using this method. Contractile agonists can be added either to the extraluminal (serosal) or the intraluminal (mucosal) surface.

Albino guinea pigs of either sex (300 to 550 g) are sacrificed by CO_2 narcosis. The entire trachea is dissected out and cut into individual rings, 12 to 15 rings are tied together with silk threads and mounted in an organ bath containing Krebs-Henseleit buffer solution. The solution is pumped at a rate of 30 ml/min through the lumen. The tissue is maintained at 37°C under a tension of 0.5 g and gassed with carbogen. Responses of the tracheal musculature are obtained by changes in inlet-outlet pressure between the side holes of indwelling catheters. Both the catheters (inlet and outlet) are connected to the positive and negative sides respectively of a differential transducer. Isometric contractions are recorded via a transducer connected to a polygraph. After 45 min equilibration, spasmogens are added. The spasmogens commonly used are carbachol (2×10^{-7} g/ml) histamine dihydrochloride (10^{-7} g/ml), Ca-inophore (10^{-6} g/ml), leukotine C_4 and D_4 (10^{-8} g/ml). When the contraction has reached maximum (initial spasm) the standard drug [(isoprenaline (1 ng/ml), aminophylline (10 ng/ml)] is administered. The bronchial responses are allowed to plateau and are recorded. The tissue is washed thoroughly and control contractions are induced again after adding spasmogen. After obtaining the initial contraction again, the test drug is added and the contractile force is recorded to its maximal level. A 15 min washing time is observed during the experiment.

Responses are quantified as change in pressure in cm of water. EC_{50} values are determined from least square analysis of a logrit model and presented using 95% confidence intervals.[7] From dose-response curves ED_{50} values can be calculated and the percent inhibition of spasmogen-induced contractions is calculated.[8]

IN VIVO MODELS

Bronchospasmolytic Activity in Anesthetized Guinea Pigs

Changes in air volume of a living animal in a closed system consisting of the respiratory pump, the trachea and the bronchi are registered using this method. Also reservoir permitting measurement of volume or pressure of excess air can be measured. A decrease in the volume of inspired air and increase in the volume of excess air is induced by bronchoconstriction. Contraction of bronchial smooth muscles results on administration of spasmogen. The method permits the evaluation of bronchospasmolytic effect by measuring the volume of air, which is not taken up by the lungs after bronchospasm.

Guinea pigs of either sex (250 to 500 g) are anesthetized with 1.25 g/kg urethane intraperitoneally and it is ensured that there is no spontaneous respiration. The trachea is cannulated, one arm is connected to a respiratory pump and the other to a Statham P23 Db transducer. The animal is artificially ventilated at a frequency of 60 strokes/min. Excess air, not taken up by the lungs, is measured and recorded in a polygraph. The jugular vein is cannulated for test drug administration and carotid artery for blood pressure measurement. Each animal is placed in a plastic container of 15 l volume. An aerosol of 0.25% histamine solution at 180 mmHg pressure is sprayed. The exposure time is 5 min. The test drug is administered orally 1 h before the exposure. The spasmogen challenge is repeated. Unprotected animals fall on their sides, asphyxiated. ED_{50} is calculated and the results are expressed as percent inhibition of induced bronchospasm over the control agonistic responses.[9]

Arachidonic Acid or PAF-induced Respiratory and Vascular Dysfunction in Guinea Pigs

Thromboxane and prostacyclin are the products of arachidonic acid metabolism. Thromboxane leads to brochoconstriction and thrombocytopenia whereas prostacyclin leads to reduction in systolic and diastolic pressure.

Male guinea pigs (300 to 600 g) are anesthetized with 60 mg/kg pentobarbitone sodium (intraperitoneally). Jugular vein is cannulated for administration of a spasmogen/test compound. Both carotid arteries are cannulated and one is connected to a pressure transducer for measuring blood pressure and the other is used for blood withdrawal. The trachea is connected to a respirator (70 to 75 strokes/min). Excess air, not taken up by the lungs, is conducted to a transducer with bronchotimer, which translates changes in airflow to an electric signal. Changes in airflow and arterial blood pressure are recorded continuously. Animals receive multiple intravenous injections of the same dose of arachidonic acid (60 μg/kg) until two bronchospasms of equal intensity are obtained. The test compounds are administered intravenously and the spasmogen is given again. Percent inhibition or increase of bronchospasm, reduction of blood pressure, thrombocytopenia and hematocrit following test drug administration are calculated in comparison to control values before drug treatment. For the reduction of blood pressure both the magnitude and the duration are determined.[10]

Anaphylactic Microshock in Guinea Pigs

In the anaphylactic response, histamine is released from various sites. Antihistamines are useful in various anaphylactic manifestations such as bronchial asthma and serum sickness. Introduction of a foreign protein in the body can produce microshock. A microshock is apparently one that is interrupted before death, and is repeatable.

Guinea pigs (200 to 300 g) are sensitized with subcutaneous injection of egg albumin. After three weeks the animals are exposed to an aerosol of 5% albumin in an exposure chamber. They are removed from the chamber as soon as they become dyspneic. If not removed at that moment, they die. The time from the commencement of exposure to severe dyspnea, the preconvulsion time, is noted which serves as a measure of the severity of the shock. If no signs of shock are seen after 6 min, the animal is regarded as protected and the preconvulsion time is taken as infinite. The degree of protection (p) is calculated from the formula:

$$p = [1 - (C/T)] \times 100$$

C and T are preconvulsion time of the control and treated animals respectively.

After a control exposure the guinea pig is treated with a drug. After another 4 to 7 days, it is again given a control exposure.[11,12] Animals with C below 40 sec and above 165 sec are excluded.

Serotonin Aerosol-induced Asphyxia in Guinea Pig

Guinea pigs when exposed to an aerosol containing serotonin, develop constriction of the bronchi, which, if sufficiently large causes asphyxia.

Guinea pigs (200 to 300 g) are placed in an anesthetic box and 2% serotonin aerosol is introduced by means of a compressor. Animals exposed to the aerosol behave in a characteristic manner and show progressive signs of difficulty in breathing, convulsion and death. By observation, experience is gained so that the pre-convulsion time can be judged accurately, and is quiet constant if the guinea pigs are not used frequently. As soon as the preconvulsive breathing commences, the animals are placed in fresh air. An infusion pump injects the test drug within 1 min. Alternatively, the animal is treated orally or subcutaneously with the test drug. The percent protection afforded by the drug is calculated from the formula

$(1\text{-}T_1/T_2) \times 100$ where T_1 is the mean of the control preconvulsion time 2 days before, and 2 days after the administration of the drug and T_2 is the preconvulsion time determined with the administration of the drug.[13,14]

Histamine-induced Bronchoconstriction in Anesthetized Guinea Pigs

Respiratory parameters such as respiratory frequency and respiratory amplitude can be measured in guinea pigs by plethysmograph. Bronchodilatory drugs attenuate the decrease in respiratory amplitude and the reflectory increase of respiratory frequency after histamine inhalation. Additional respiratory parameters can be recorded using Fleisch tube and a catheter inserted into the pleural cavity. In addition, using this method antagonism against bradykinin-induced bronchoconstriction or the bronchodilator effects of potassium channel openers can also be evaluated.

Guinea pigs of either sex weighing 400 to 600 g are anesthetized with 70 mg/kg pentobarbital intraperitoneally and the trachea, jugular vein and carotid artery are cannulated. Animal is maintained on artificial respiration (60 strokes/min). The guinea pigs are placed inside a whole body plethysmograph box and tracheal, venous and arterial catheters are connected to onset ports in the wall of the plethysmograph box. The tracheal port is connected to the respirator. Airflow rate into and out of the plethysmograph is measured using a differential pressure transducer. Tidal volume and transpulmonary pressure are measured. Signals from the airflow, tidal volume and transpulmonary pressure are fed into an online computer system for calculation of pulmonary resistance (PR) and dynamic lung compliance (LC). Systemic arterial pressure is measured using a Statham pressure transducer. Heart rate is computed from pressure pulses. Intravenous injection of histamine (0.5 to 2.0 µg/kg) leads to decrease in LC and increase in PR by 200% compared to baseline values. After 5 min interval, challenges are repeated yielding the same increase in pulmonary resistance during the whole experimental duration. After three reproducible responses the test compound is administered intravenously 1 min before histamine injection. Inhibition of histamine-induced bronchoconstriction by test compound is recorded and ED_{50} is calculated. Further, the time required for histamine antagonism is evaluated.[12]

Pneumotachography in Guinea Pigs

Pneumotachograph allows simultaneous measurements of several respiratory and circulatory parameters in anesthetized guinea pigs. Its use is based on the principle of the Fleisch tube.

Guinea pigs (300 to 400 g) are anesthetized intraperitoneally with 1.5 g/kg urethane. The animals are fixed at the upper extremities on a heated operating table. The trachea is cannulated. A thin plastic catheter is inserted into the esophagus and the tip is located inside the thorax to register intrathoracic pressure. Further, the cephalic vein of one side and carotid artery of the other side are cannulated. The tracheal cannula is connected to the pneumotachograph. The pneumotachograph is connected to a differential pressure transducer. One side of another pressure differential transducer is connected with the esophageal catheter and the other side remains open to room air. For recording of arterial pressure a Gould pressure transducer is used. The signals of airflow and esophageal pressure are monitored using an oscilloscope. Using an analog computer various respiratory and circulatory parameters are measured.

Pulmonary mechanics like airway resistance, dynamic compliance and end respiratory work can be measured.

Each animal serves as its own control. For each individual experiment the data of the last 5 min before the first substance application are averaged and used as controls. The response values after substance application are then expressed as percentages of the control.[6]

Microshock in Rabbits

Although the guinea pig has been favored for screening antihistaminic agents because of its sensitivity to histamine, the rabbit may serve as a suitable model when a second species is desired.

Rabbits (200 to 300 g) are placed in a glass aquarium 61 × 30.5 × 30.5 cm with its open side down on a smooth rubber surface, having a hole connected to a nebulizer. Each rabbit is placed in a separate chamber and subjected to an aerosol of 0.2% histamine aerosol. In small doses rabbit exhibits shock symptoms in gradual succession. The first sign is the drawing in of the abdominal walls to assist in breathing. The movements become stronger, the respiration becomes slower and deeper or more rapid and shallow. In the latter case the animal's head moves rapidly to and fro. At this stage, the animal has to be removed from the chamber. Otherwise the sequelae in quick succession are seen, e.g. gasping for air, convulsions, urination, cyanosis and possibly death. In order to prevent desensitization, an interval of 8 days or more is interposed between tests. The test drug is administered intraperitoneally 30 min before the experiment. The time at which the animal has to be removed from the chamber is recorded.[15-17] The percent protection offered by the drug is calculated using the formula

$$(1-T_1/T_2) \times 100$$

where

T_1 = control preconvulsion time

T_2 = preconvulsion time after administration of the drug.

Bronchial Hyperactivity in Guinea Pigs

Inhalation of histamine or other spasmogens can induce symptoms like asphyctic convulsions resembling bronchial asthma in guinea pigs. The challenging agents are applied as aerosols produced by an ultrasound nebulizer. Early symptoms are increased breathing frequency, forced inspiration and finally anaphylactic convulsions. Antagonistic drugs can delay the occurrence of these symptoms. Preconvulsion time can be measured.

Male albino guinea pigs (300 to 400 g) are used. The inhalation cages consist of three boxes each ventilated with airflow of 1.5 l/min. The animal is placed into box A to which the test drug or the standard is applied using an ultrasound nebulizer which provides an aerosol of 0.2 ml solution of the test drug injected in an infusion pump within 1 min. Alternately, the animal is treated orally or subcutaneously with the test drug or the standard. Box B serves as sluice through which the animal is passed into Box C. There, the guinea pig is exposed to an aerosol of 0.1% solution of histamine hydrochloride provided by an ultrasound nebulizer. Time until appearance of asphyctic convulsions is measured. Then, the animal is immediately removed from the inhalation box. Percent increase of preconvulsion time is calculated versus controls. ED_{50} (50% increase in preconvulsive time) is also calculated.[18]

Airway Microvascular Leakage in Guinea Pigs

Evans Blue dye can be used to study plasma exudation in guinea pig airways *in vivo*. The antagonism against bradykinin and platelet-activating factor (PAF)-induced microvascular leakage and vagal stimulation-induced airway responses can be studied using this method.

Guinea pigs (380 to 600 g) are anesthetized with urethane (1.5 g/kg, intraperitoneally). The trachea, jugular vein and carotid arteries are cannulated. Jugular vein is cannulated for the administration of test compounds and carotid artery for the measurement of blood pressure. The animal is maintained on artificial respiration (60 strokes/min). Lung resistance is measured as an index of airway function and monitored throughout the experiment. Transpulmonary pressure is measured using a pressure transducer with one side attached to the catheter inserted into the right pleural cavity and the other side attached to the intratracheal cannula. Airflow is measured using a pneumotachograph. The test compound is given intravenously. Ten minutes later, Evans Blue dye is injected intravenously for 1 min. After 1 min, bronchoconstriction and microvascular leakage is induced by injection of bradykinin or PAF or vagal stimulation. Six minutes after induction of leakage the thoracic cavity is opened and a cannula is inserted into the aorta through a ventriculotomy. Perfusion is performed with 100 ml (0.9%) saline at a pressure of 100-120 mmHg in order to remove the intravascular dye from the systemic circulation. The right ventricle is opened and perfused with 30 ml saline.

The lungs are also removed. The tissues are blotted dry and weighed. Evans Blue dye is extracted in 2 ml of formamide and measured in a spectrophotometer at 620 nm. Evans Blue dye concentration, expressed as ng/mg tissue as well as lung resistance are compared by statistical means between treated groups and controls receiving the challenge only.[19-21]

Airway Inflammation in Mice

Balb/c mice sensitized with ovalbumin and challenged by repeated exposure to ovalbumin yields marked eosinophilia in bronchoalveolar lavage (BAL) fluid. It has also been seen that eosinophil influx varies dramatically in mice of the different stains. Strains such as 129/SV, CBA belong to non- or low-responder. Strains such as SWR, FVB, C57BL/6 respond to antigen challenge with a marked increase of eosinophils both in the BAL and in the lung tissue.[22,23]

Balb/c mice, used for this study are subcutaneously implanted with heat-coagulated egg white. Fourteen days later the mice are challenged intratracheally with heat-aggregated ovalbumin. Test drug is administered subcutaneously, intraperitoneally or orally. Forty-eight hours after antigen challenge, bronchoalveolar lavage fluid is collected from animals of both groups and total number of eosinophils, neutrophils and eosinophil peroxidase activity are assessed. The animals are then sacrificed and histopathological evaluation is carried out. Based on the results of histopathological study and BAL fluid examination, protection that is offered by the test drug is evaluated.[24,25]

Innovation in Model Development

The lack of translation from preclinical to clinical studies of new asthma compounds and biologics is of particular importance to the severe and/or therapy-resistant asthma group, where new effective therapies for improved asthma control are crucial. The challenge is to develop models that more accurately recapitulate the asthmatic airway for mechanistic studies, target identification and validation, and efficacy and safety testing. Addressing this will require a multidisciplinary, collaborative and innovative approach.

Biomimetic Models

The opportunities afforded by tissue engineering, coupled with advances in bioreactor and scaffold design, have resulted in several tissue-engineered human airway equivalents becoming available. Although these have added valuable insight into the pathophysiology of the disease, they are still too simplistic to mimic important *in vivo* features, such as fully functioning immune and/or circulatory system.[26]

Microfluidics

Tissue engineering is a rapidly evolving science and tissue engineers have embraced the challenge of building complexity into their models. Although there might still be some way to go in recapitulating *in vitro* entire immune or circulatory systems, steps are being made. Advances in the emerging field of microfluidic lab-on-a-chip technologies, combined with tissue engineering, offers great opportunity in this regard. Microfluidics provide many advantages over current macroscopic techniques and have been used to microfabricate successfully blood vessels, muscles, brain, kidney and liver for basic research and drug discovery.[27.]

In silico modelling

In silico modelling has the potential to change the way drugs develop, and accelerate the drug discovery process. These approaches are forming the newest wave of modelling tools in asthma research and drug development. Numerous models have been developed to study basic events, such as molecular interactions (ligand–receptor), whole-organ functions (e.g. bronchoconstriction and aerosolized drug deposition in the lung), and even virtual patients.[28]

Precision cut lung slices

Ex vivo precision cut lung slices (PCLS) from human lung also offer exciting opportunities for increasing understanding of asthma development and progression, and bridge the gap between cell culture and isolated tissue preparations and animal studies. Despite this, however, PCLS approaches are rarely adopted. Originally developed for toxicological purposes, PCLS have been successfully adapted to study airways disease and have several advantages over current *in vivo* approaches. The main focus of their use has been to assess airway smooth muscle responses, including hyperresponsiveness, remodeling and bronchoconstriction in response to several stimuli, such as allergens, pharmacological challenge and infection. Recently, PCLS has been used to investigate the response of airways to drugs used in the treatment of asthma, where these models are already identifying alternative treatment strategies as potential future asthma therapies; however, these are yet to be tested clinically.[29]

Transgenic Approaches

Genetically modified animals, especially mice, are considered important models in basic research to define specific pathways for drug discovery, mechanistic studies and target identification and/or validation. They have been extensively used in asthma, with numerous 'off-the-shelf' transgenic mice and species-specific probes and reagents commercially available, which enable researchers to suppress, switch off or upregulate a single molecular signalling pathway specifically. However, it is questionable how useful these models are for studying a disease that is associated with several molecular and cellular pathways that function synergistically or independently of each other.[30]

DISCUSSION

Animal models of asthma are necessary and irreplaceable for the further understanding of the pathophysiological mechanisms and preclinical evaluation of new treatments. Since all allergic diseases are characterized by early and late phase symptom's models of both phases are available. Furthermore, it is also necessary to investigate mediators and cells involved in early and late phase of an allergic reaction. Additionally, the increased airway responsiveness should also be modeled. In animals, inflammatory changes should be induced that result in pathological changes including remodeling.

A murine model for asthma presents numerous advantages when compared with the use of other animal species. This model offers the opportunity to explore mechanisms of allergic reactions because of the existence of numerous immunological reagents specific for murine cytokines, adhesion molecules, etc. Murine models have provided fundamental information regarding certain features of asthma such as involvement of lymphocytes. Because mice are extremely useful for immunological studies, a suitable murine model of allergic pulmonary inflammation can be invaluable to study drug effect on it. There are certain transgenic or knock out strains available. On the other hand, because of considerable physiological dissimilarities with primates, the ability to extrapolate murine findings to humans will be difficult.

The rat has received considerable attention during recent decades. Experimental data suggest that the most characteristic features of human asthma including pathological changes can be duplicated in rats. Certain strains such as Brown Norway rats produce IgE as the major anaphylactic antibody. Since a large number of corresponding immunological reagents are available the role of cytokines and chemokines in allergic inflammation can also be studied in a rat model. In contrast to guinea pigs, allergic sensitization requires use of adjuvant such as alum or *Bordetella pertussis*. Another disadvantage of this species is that early phase bronchoconstriction cannot be induced via inhalation of the antigen. It should be given intravenously. The rat also offers economic advantage.

The guinea pig was or perhaps is still the most popular animal model of allergic reactions. The benefits are the pragmatic benefits of economy and ease of animal handling to the features, which allergen-induced bronchoconstriction and human bronchial asthma have in common. Such features include the bronchoconstrictor response to antigen contact, the hyper-responsiveness of the airway to mediators and the eosinophilic nature of allergic bronchial inflammation. However, the scarcity of inbred strains is a disadvantage with regard to studying genetic influence.

The hamster is seldom used in asthma research. Its oral mucosa is well suited for intravital microscopy and therefore for studying microcirculation. It is sometimes employed for testing *in vitro* effect of kinins. The rabbit provides an interesting animal model. This species can demonstrate early and late phase responses with accumulation of eosinophils, BHR is also observed. A further advantage of this species is the production of IgE. Rabbits are small, docile animals and relatively without danger of desensitization. The sheep represents a species, in which sensitization to Ascaris occurs naturally. The antigen response consists of an early and a late phase bronchoconstriction. The latter is accompanied with cell infiltration. Dogs can be sensitized by natural exposure to Ascaris, but other antigens can also immunize them.

In asthma research, little attention has been paid to domestic pigs or mini- or micropigs. From an anatomical point of view, pigs have several similarities to humans. The real handicap with pigs is their size. Monkeys demonstrate an IgE mediated early and late phase respiratory response to antigen. They have shown BHR. Monkeys are considered to have an immune system very similar to that of humans in comparison to mice, rats and guinea pigs.

CONCLUSION

In summary, it should be emphasized that any animal model will have both strengths and weaknesses and its value in answering particular research questions must be evaluated with respect to its relevance to human diseases. Unfortunately, this relevance becomes more difficult to determine when the cause of the underlying disease is unclear, or potentially complex as in asthma. Thus many species have been utilized in the development of animal model of asthma including mice, rats, guinea pigs, ferrets, hamsters, rabbits, dogs, sheep, pig, horses and nonhuman primates. Each possesses certain advantages and disadvantages as a model of asthma. Therefore, certain caveats must be recognized in using animal systems. It must however, be appreciated that animals are only surrogates. Results from such studies may be compared with information obtained from experiments performed with human materials in order to minimize or even to avoid faulty extrapolations. It is also important to recognize that no single model is sufficient to draw conclusions on the therapeutic value of new chemical entities. Prudent employment of well-designed animal models can provide valuable information on drug effects. Advances in new technologies, including tissue engineering, imaging and in silico modelling, can provide researchers with new opportunities for innovative model development. Integrating these technologies in existing preclinical testing programs is crucial to accelerating the development of more predictive but fewer animal models and a fundamental shift in the way that asthma research and drug development is carried out.

REFERENCES

1. Tai A, Ranganathan S. Optimizing medications for poorly controlled asthma. Am J Respir Crit Care Med 2007;176:520-1.
2. Martin BL, Caruana-Montaldo B, Craig T. Comprehensive management of asthma. Drugs of Today 1997;33:149-60.
3. Hill SJ, Emson PC, Young JM. The binding of 3H mepyramine to histamine H1 receptor in guinea pig brain. J Neurochem 1978;31:997-1004.
4. Knebel JW, Ritter D, Aufderheide M. Exposure of human lung cells to native diesel motor exhaust: Development of an optimized in vitro test strategy. Toxicol In Vitro 2001;16:185-92.
5. Piperi C, Pouli AE, Katerelos NA, et al. Study of the mechanisms of cigarette smoke gas phase cytotoxicity. Anticancer Res 2003;23:2185-90.
6. Kleinstiver PW, Eyre P. Evaluation of lung parenchyma strip preparation to measure bronchoactivity. J Pharmacol Methods 1979;2:175-85.

7. Allen DA, Schertel ER, Bailey JE. Reflex cardiovascular effects of continuous prostacyclin administration into an isolated in situ lung in the dog. J Appl Physiol 1993;74:2928-34.
8. Baersch G, Frolich JC. A new bioassay to study contractile and relaxant effects of PGE2 on perfused guinea pig trachea. J Pharmacol Toxicol Methods 1996;36:63-8.
9. Miura M, Belvisi MG, Barnes PJ. Modulation of nonadrenergic noncholinergic neural bronchoconstriction by bradykinin in anesthetized guinea pigs in vivo. J Pharmacol Exp Ther 1994;268:482-6.
10. Lefort J, Vargaftig BB. Role of platelets in aspirin-sensitive bronchoconstriction in the guinea pig: Interactions with salicylic acid. Br J Pharmacol 1978;63:35-42.
11. Chand N, Diamantis W, Nolan K, et al. Azelastine inhibits acute allergic dyspnoea in a conscious guinea pig asthma model. Res Commun Mol Pathol Pharmacol 1994;85:209-16.
12. Vitkun SA, Foster WM, Bergofsky EH, et a!. Large and small airway responses to bronchoconstrictors in the guinea pig and the ferret. Lung 1990;168:249-57.
13. De Bie JJ, Henricks PA, Cruikshank WW, et al. Modulation of airway hyperresponsiveness and eosinophilia by selective histamine and 5-HT receptor antagonists in a mouse model of allergic asthma. Br J Pharmacol 1998;124:857-64.
14. Konno S, Adachi M, Matsuura T. Bronchial reactivity to methacholine and serotonin in six inbred mouse strains. Arerugi 1993;42:42-7.
15. Ali S, Mustafa SJ, Metzger WJ. Adenosine receptor mediated bronchoconstriction and bronchial hyperresponsiveness in allergic rabbit model. Am J Physiol 1994;266:L271-7.
16. Ali S, Mustafa SJ, Metzger WJ. Modification of allergen-induced airway obstruction and bronchial hyperresponsiveness in the allergic rabbit by theophylline aerosol. Agents Actions 1992;37:168-70.
17. Harris JO, Bice D, Salvaggio JE. Cellular and humoral bronchopulmonary immune response of rabbits immunized with thermophilic actinomyces antigen. Am Rev Respir Dis 1976;114:29-43.
18. Rogers DF, Boschetto P, Barnes PJ. Plasma exudation: Correlation between Evans Blue dye and radiolabelled albumin in guinea pig airways in vivo. J Pharmacol Methods 1989;21:309-15.
19. Aoki S, Bouberkeur K, Kristersson A, et al. Is allergic airway hypersensitivity of the guinea pig dependent upon eosinophil accumulation in the lung. Br J Pharmacol 1988;94:365-71.
20. Chand N, Nolan K, Diamantis W, et al. Repeated aeroallergen challenge induces lung dysfunction but not bronchial hyperresponsiveness in conscious guinea pigs. Agents Actions 1992;37:184-7.
21. Perretti F, Manzini S. Activation of capsaicin sensitive sensory fibers modulates PAF-induced bronchial hyperresponsiveness in anesthetized guinea pigs. Am Rev Respir Dis 1993;148:927-31.
22. Mitchell HW, Turner DJ, Gray PR, et al. Compliance and stability of the bronchial wall in a model of allergen-induced lung inflammation. J Appl Physiol 1999;86:932-7.
23. Waserman S, Xu LJ, Olivenstein R, et al. Association between late allergic bronchoconstriction in the rat and allergen stimulated lymphocyte proliferation in vitro. Am J Respir Crit Care Med 1995;151:470-4.
24. Hessel EM, Van Oosterhout AJ, Hofstra CL, et al. Bronchoconstriction and airway hyper responsiveness after ovalbumin inhalation in sensitized mice. Eur J Pharmacol 1995;293:401-12.
25. Temann UA, Geba GP, Rankin JA, et al. Expression of IL-9 in the lungs of transgenic mice causes airway inflammation, mast cell hyperplasia and bronchial hyper responsiveness. J Exp Med 1998;188:1307-20.
26. Nichols JE, Cortiella, J. Engineering of a complex organ: progress toward development of a tissue-engineered lung. Proc Am Thorac Soc 2008;5:723-30.

27. Song JW, et al. Microfluidic endothelium for studying the intravascular adhesion of metastatic breast cancer cells. PLoS ONE. 2009;4,e5756.
28. Van de Waterbeemd H, Gifford E. ADMET in silico modelling: towards prediction paradise? Nat Rev Drug Discov 2003;2:192-204.
29. Ressmeyer AR, et al. Characterisation of guinea pig precision-cut lung slices: comparison with human tissues. Eur Respir J 2006;28:603-11.
30. Kaiko GE, Foster PS. New insights into the generation of Th2 immunity and potential therapeutic targets for the treatment of asthma. Curr Opin Allergy Clin Immunol 2011;11:39-45.

CHAPTER

45

Cell-Based Assays in High-Throughput Screening of Drugs

ABSTRACT

Drug discovery is a complex process which is aimed to develop drug candidates with all desired pharmacological and pharmacokinetic properties with minimal side effects. With the advancement of combinatorial chemistry, genomics, proteomics and bioinformatics which necessitate a very rapid screening strategy for lead identification and optimization. Conventional animal models become obsolete due to its high cost, low throughput and moral issues. Over the past two decades, high-throughput screening (HTS) assays has emerged and matured as a platform in the early stage of drug discovery in the pharmaceutical industry. More than half of the HTS assays are being replaced with cell-based assays for target validation and ADMET (absorption, distribution, metabolism, elimination and toxicity) in the early drug discovery processes. In this review, different types of cells, culture systems (2D, 3D and microfluidic cell culture), detection methods and its recent advancements in cell based HTS are discussed with successful examples in commercial development of new drugs.

BACKGROUND

Cell-based high-throughput screening (HTS) assays have been developed to provide more relevant *in vivo* biological information for drug discovery processes. Historically, drug screening greatly relies on animal models as proxies for human beings in drug target validation and ADMET (absorption, distribution, metabolism, elimination and toxicity) but because of its low throughput and moral issues, the animal models are being replaced with cell-based HTS assays to accelerate early-phase drug discovery.[1]

TYPES OF CELL-BASED ASSAYS

Cell-based assays for HTS mainly include three types:

- *Second messenger assays*: This is based on the principle that it monitors signal transduction following activation of cell surface receptors. In this assay, fluorescent molecules that respond to intracellular Ca2+ concentrations, membrane potential, pH, etc. are being used to assay receptor/ion channel activation.[2,3]

- *Reporter gene assays*: This assay monitor cellular responses at the transcription or translational level, e.g. Quantification of G-protein coupled receptor (GPCR) internalization using GPCR-green fluorescent protein hybrids.[4]
- *Cell proliferation/cytotoxicity assays*: The overall cell growth or death in response to external stimuli or stress is evaluated using this assay, e.g. Virus-induced cytopathic effects on cell proliferation monitored by following the reduction of tetrazolium salt to formazan quantified by measuring absorbance at 410 nm.[5]

COMPONENTS OF CELL-BASED HTS ASSAYS

The components of cell-based HTS assays include:

- Cells - Sources and types
- Devices for culturing cells
- Detection system to quantify cell/cellular activities.

Cells—Sources and Types

Primary cells: Primary cells are the cells that have been freshly isolated from a living organism and maintained for growth *in vitro*. These cells closely mimic the physiological state of cells *in vivo* and generate more relevant data representing living systems. The cell types most frequently found in primary cell culture are epithelial cells, fibroblasts, keratinocytes, melanocytes, endothelial cells, muscle cells, hematopoietic and mesenchymal stem cells.

Disadvantages: They have a limited life span in culture, difficult to grow and transfect.[6]

Immortalized cell lines: Immortalized cells are the cells whose growth characteristics have been altered to grow continuously and divide indefinitely *in vitro*, e.g. HEK293 cells derived from human kidney, HeLa cells are human epithelial cells from a fatal cervical carcinoma transformed by human papilloma virus 18 (HPV18).[7] They are cheap, easy to grow, reliable and reproducible, and hence widely used for drug screening assays.

Disadvantages: Significant mutations and altered biological characteristics in the immortalization process will make them different from those of the native/normal cells.[6]

Human cancer cell lines: These cells are derived from human cancers and they are widely used for anticancer drug screening in pharmaceutical research, e. g. NC160, a panel of 60 human tumor cell lines (NC160) representing 9 tissue types for screening potential new anti-cancer agents.[8] The presence of mutations in these cell lines may affect the experimental outcome.

Cancer stem cells: Cancer stem cells may be genetically raised from oncogenic transformation of either stem cells or progenitor cells. They can be isolated from tumors and have the capability to self renew, differentiate and regenerate a phenotype of the original tumor,[9] e.g. Phase II screening of new drugs in ovarian cancers and malignant melanoma.[10]

Mesenchymal stem cells (MSCs): MSCs (MSCs, also known as bone marrow stromal cells or skeletal stem cells) are multipotent stem cells that can differentiate into chondrocytes (cartilage cells), osteoblasts (bone cells) or adipocytes (fat cells)—making them ideal candidates for tissue engineering. MSCs can contribute to the regeneration of bone, cartilage, muscle and tendons. It has also been shown that—when transplanted systemically into animals—they are able to migrate to the sites of the injury, e.g. Human MSCs derived osteoblasts for testing purmorphamine.[11]

Embryonic stem cells (ESCs): These cells exhibit an almost unlimited proliferative capacity in culture and maintain their pluripotent potential to differentiate into all cell lineages in the body.These cells can serve as better cell models for both drug efficacy and toxicity screening, e.g. Human embryonic stem cell derived cardiomyocytes for electrophysiological drug screening.[12]

Induced pluripotent stem cells (iPSCs): iPSCs are pluripotent cells artificially derived from somatic cells (Fibroblasts and other adult cell types) by inducing a small set of powerful pluripotency genes. Their previous somatic cell properties are lost and are similar to human ESCs in terms of morphology, growth properties, gene-expression profiles and differentiation potential. iPSCs derived from patients with specific diseases have been considered as a new tool in drug discovery.

Devices for Culturing Cells

The majority of cells cultured *in vitro* grow as monolayers on an artificial substrate. Hence, the substrate must be correctly charged to allow cell adhesion, or to allow the adhesion of cell-derived attachment factors that will allow cell adhesion and spreading. Therefore, the normal cells need to be spread out on a substrate to proliferate and inadequate spreading due to poor adhesion or overcrowding will inhibit proliferation.[13,14] However, the hemopoietic cell lines, rodent ascites, tumors and a few other selected cell lines such as small-cell lung cancer,[15] many transformed cell lines grow in suspension and can be independent of surface charge on the substrate.

The factors which govern the choice of culture vessel include:

1. The cell mass required,
2. Whether the cells grow in suspension or as a monolayer,
3. Whether the culture should be vented to the atmosphere or sealed,
4. The frequency of sampling,
5. The type of analysis required, and
6. The cost.

The vessels used for adherent cultures and suspension cultures are given in Figure 45.1.

TYPES OF CELL CULTURE SYSTEMS

Conventional 2D Culture Systems

It is well documented that the cells grown on 2D surfaces do not mimic true *in vivo* physiology. Though 2D cell-based assays in multiwall plates together with automated operation are widely used in drug screening, 2D assays may result in errors in predicting tissue-specific responses due to the loss of native morphology and limited cell-cell and cell-matrix interaction. This is overcome by the development of 3-dimensional (3D) cell cultures.

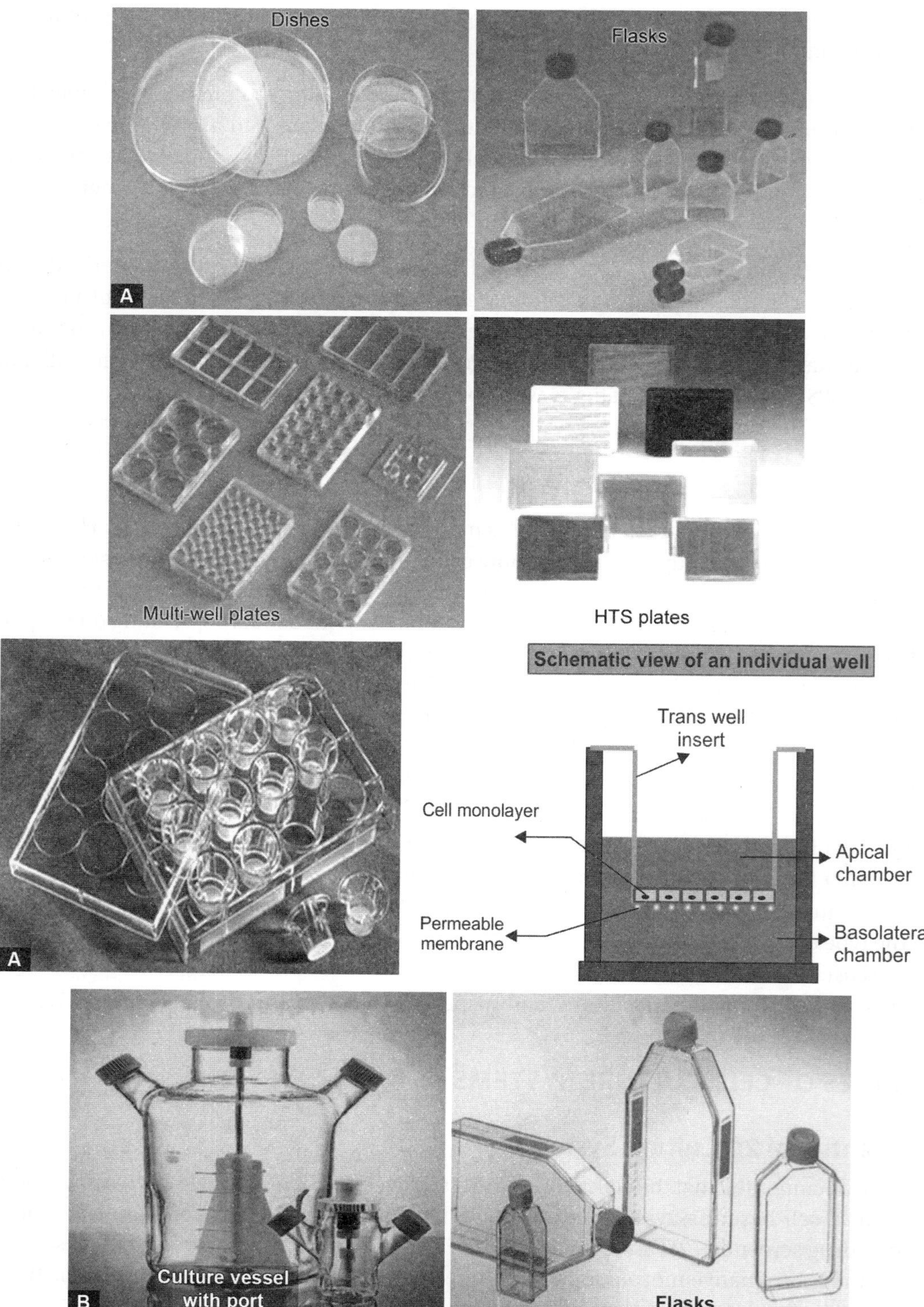

Figure 45.1: Types of vessels for human cell cultures: (A) Adherent culture system; (B) Suspension culture system (Ref. www.sigmaaldrich.com)[16] (*For color version see Plates 22 and 23*)

3D Culture Systems

The cells grown on 3D scaffolds are demonstrated to show similar in vivo morphology with intimate cell-cell and cell-ECM (extracellular matrix) interaction.[1] The 3D scaffold provides another direction for cell-cell interactions, cell migration and cell morphogenesis which are critical in regulating cell cycle and tissue functions.[1] In addition, 3D cell cultures provide not only the templates for cells to adhere and grow but also allow the distribution of nutrients and metabolites thus enabling long-term cell culture *in vitro*.[17] It holds promise for being more predictive of in vivo responses to drug treatments.

Numerous studies have documented that cell response to drugs in 3D cultures are distinct from those in 2D cultures, which highlights the advantages of using 3D-based models.[18-20] Therefore, it is having a greater potential to become a superior platform for drug development to bridge the 2D monolayer cell culture systems and the animal models.

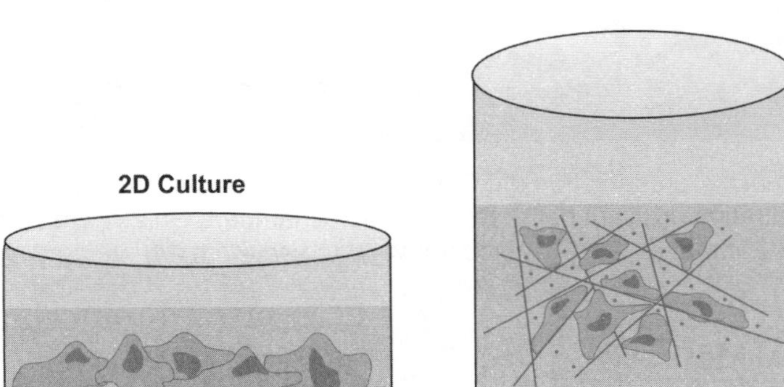

Figure 45.2: Schematic representation of 2D vs 3D cultures (*For color version see plate 23*)

3D Microfluidic Cell Cultures

3D microfluidic cell culture systems offer a biologically relevant model to conduct micro-scale cell based research and applications in drug screening. Various natural and synthetic hydrogels have been incorporated into microfluidic cell culture systems to support cells in 3D.[1] A variety of 3D microfluidic cell culture models have been developed.[21,22] Vickerman et al. (2008) developed a microfluidic platform capable of mimicking the in vivo microenvironments by integrating fluidic microenvironments and 3D microenvironments using microinjection of gel solution containing cells. An open lumen-like structure was created when human adult dermal microvascular endothelial cells were cultured on this microfluidic platform for up to 7 days.

DETECTION METHODS

Detection methods used in cell-based HTS assay fall into two groups:
1. Electrochemical methods
2. Optical methods

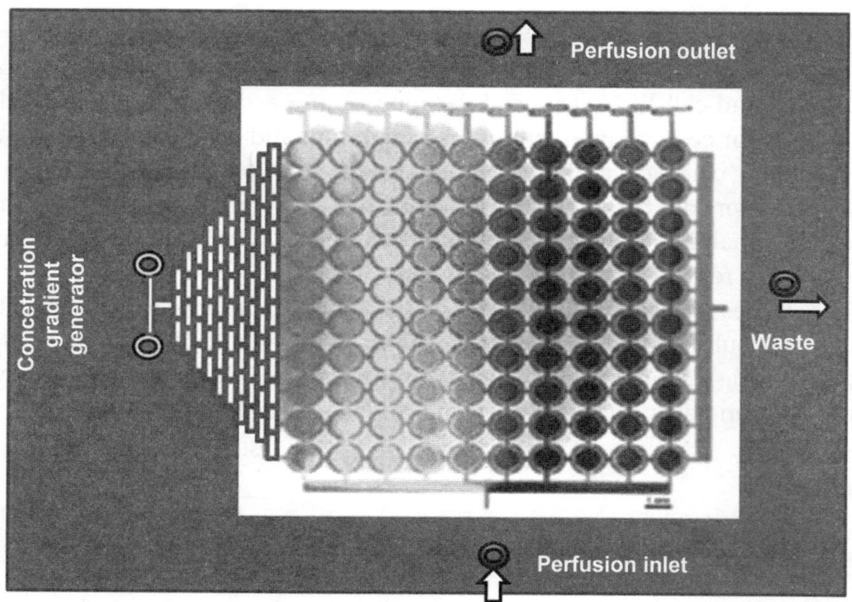

Figure 45.3: Schematic representation of 3D microfluidic culture system. Microfluidic cell culture array showing concentration gradient generator and microchambers On 2×2 cm device (*Adapted from Hung et al 2005*[23] *& Zang et al, 2012*[1]) *(For color version see Plate 24)*

Electrochemical Methods

The detection method by electrochemical technique is based on:

A. Cellular activity and function,

B. Cellular barrier behaviour, and

C. Recording/stimulation of electric potential of electrogenic cells.

Methods based on Cellular Activity and Function

The cell viability of a living cell can be measured as a function of electron generation and charge transfer caused by redox reaction and changes of ionic composition, e.g. the tumor cells when attached to a specialized electrode exhibit an irreversible voltammetric response, which is related to the oxidation of guanine and thus the oxidation peak can be used to investigate the exogenous effect to study anti-tumor drug sensitivity.

In addition, the cellular activities can be measured using conventional potentiometry and amperometry methods. The potentiometric method utilizes either ion-selective electrode (ISE) or gas-sensing electrode (GSE) coated with a layer of cells to monitor metabolic products during cell growth,[24] e.g. screening of toxins by ISE. This is achieved by integrating cells with a K+ selective film wherein a change in potential caused by the ion accumulation or depletion on the electrode can be measured. This method requires a very stable reference electrode which limits the application of potentiometry sensors.

Amperometric methods are widely used for the determination of pH, dissolved oxygen or glucose as a measure of cellular biochemical changes. The application of this approach in HTS cell based assays is limited due to many uncontrollable environmental factors.

Method based on Cellular Barrier

In general, cells with insulating properties would significantly increase the electrode impedance.[25,26] This has been exploited to study the biological status of cells including cellular viability, morphology, cell number, cell apoptosis and cell adhesion using electrochemical impedance spectroscopic techniques, e.g. A novel electrical impedance sensor array integrated into the bottom of a microtiter plate has been specially designed for the quantitative detection of living cells. Real-time assessment of cytotoxicity and acute toxicity can be achieved using this device.[26]

Method based on the Recording/Stimulating of cellular electrical potential

Electrogenic cells and tissues such as heart, muscle, pancreas beta and nerve cells are capable of generating bioelectrical signals when they are grown in culture on microelectrode arrays or on field effect transistors in response to any neuroactive compounds added to the culture medium. Such signals can be used to test drugs against critical diseases such as cardiac arrhythmia, hypertension, Parkinson's disease, diabetes, depression and neuropathic pain.[27] A nanoelectronic biosensor was developed based on single-wall carbon nanotubes (SWCNTs) to measure non-invasive detection of cellular activities of electrogenic cells with high throughput, high sensitivity, easy handling and the capacity of long-term cell culture.

Disadvantages of Electrochemical Methods of Detection

- No specific information can be obtained on cellular activities directly related to certain cell functions, biomarkers or signalling pathways which are essential for better understanding of mechanisms of cytotoxicity and action of drugs.
- Not suitable for 3D cell cultures which requires cell direct contact with the electrode.

Optical Methods

The optical methods of detection include, colorimetric, luminescent or fluorescent methods.

Colorimetric Method

The colorimetric method of detection relies on the color change of the growth medium after cell metabolites react with chemical agents, e.g. Assays using ruthenium dye[28] and alamar blue have been developed.[29] These types of assays are basically employed to study the effect of test drugs on cell proliferation or cellular viability. However, ruthenium dye and alamar blue (Resazurin) (Fig. 45.4A) are not being used in HTS measurements because of its low sensitivity and reproducibility.

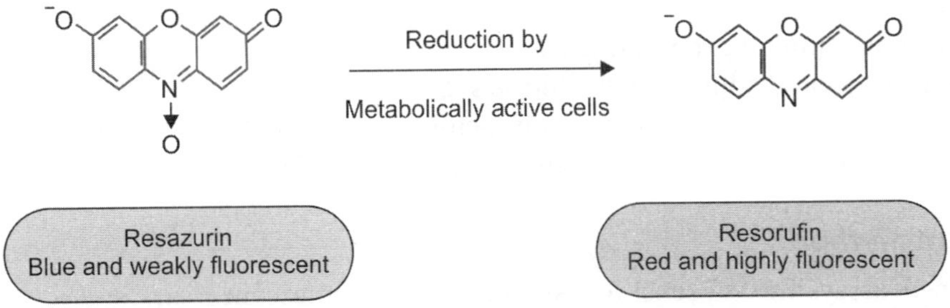

Reduction by
Metabolically active cells
Resazurin
Blue and weakly fluorescent
Resorufin
Red and highly fluorescent

Figure 45.4A: Principle of cell viability/toxicity assay using alamar blue

A spectrum of assays using tetrazolium salts such as MTT [3-(4,5-Dimethylthiazole-2-yl)-2,5-diphenyltetrazolium bromide] and the variants of this assay using MTS [3-(4,5-dimethylthiazol-2-yl)-5-(3-carboxymethoxyphenyl)-2-(4-sulfophenyl)-2H-tetrazolium) and XTT [2,3-bis-(2-methoxy-4-nitro-5-sulfophenyl]-2H-tetrazolium-5-carboxanilide) are also available commercially (Fig. 45.4B).

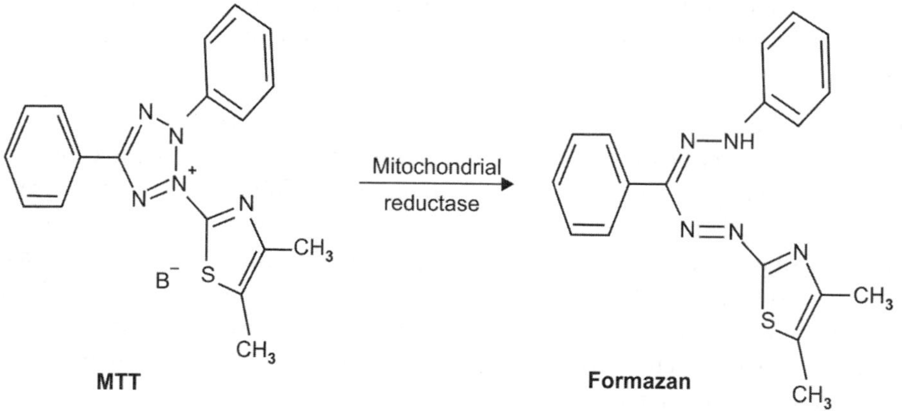

Figure 45.4B: Principle of cell viability/toxicity assay using tetrazolium salt (MTT)

Limitations

- Multiple additions of chemicals at pre-scheduled time points which interfere or disrupt the targeted cells
- Time consuming and laborious
- Insufficient to obtain dynamic data which can provide more information about the effects of drugs on cells
- Requires expensive robotic arms for HTS application
- Low sensitivity.

Luminescent Method

This assay is based on the principle that the oxidation of luciferin catalyzed by luciferase produces light that is detected by an illuminometer or optical microscope, allowing observation of biological processes.[30] This reaction may be mediated by ATP or calcium ions, e.g. Luciferase assays for kinase activity in which luciferase is widely used as a reporter in cells expressing a luciferase gene under the control of a promoter if interest to assess its transcriptional activity.[31]

Limitations

- Its application is limited to end-point assay
- Requires cell lysis and addition of luciferase substrate
- Luminescent intensity is affected by many factors, such as luciferin absorption, availability of co-factors, pH and transparency of culture media or buffer.

Fluorescent Method

The fluorescent assays are very sensitive as compared to luminescent assays, and very easy to be miniaturized for HTS applications and thus enable the measurement of cell activities, pathway activation, toxicity and phenotypic cellular responses of exogenous stimuli. The fluorescent methods for cell based assays were initially developed using small, highly-fluorescent, organic molecules to monitor ion concentrations, membrane potential and as intracellular substrates for reporter genes. These conventional fluorescent molecules have been replaced with photo-unstable quantum dots (QDs). QDs are semiconductor nanocrystals and are photo-chemically stable, provide narrow and adjustable emission. These QDs can be excited by light of any wavelength shorter than that of the emission peak.[32]

For example, two fluorescent proteins fused with a peptide linker comprising a caspase-3-cleavage site is being used to study the activation of caspase-3 or apoptosis in live cells.[33]

RECENT DEVELOPMENTS IN 3D CELL-BASED HTS ASSAYS FOR DRUG DISCOVERY

3D Cell-Based Fluorescence Assays

This assay enables the real-time analysis of cell proliferation based on fluorescence read-outs from a fluorometer and the fluorescence signals are generated from cells cultured on conventional 96-well plates. The lack of sensitivity and accuracy, high fluctuating background signals mediated by change in pH, culture environment and other autofluorescent components in the medium render it unreliable for assessing cytotoxicity or cell proliferation. These limitations can be overcome by culturing GFP-expressing cells in a PET scaffold in a modified well which significantly reduces background noises and increases the total cell number per unit area. Such a 3D culture significantly improves a background noise and provides a 20-fold higher cellular fluorescence. This kind of assays has been successfully employed to study cytotoxicity effects of chemicals, cancer drugs and Chinese herbal medicines in early-stage drug discovery process.[1]

Microfluidic Cell-Based Assays

Microfluidics refers to the science and technology that allows one to manipulate tiny amounts (10-9 to 10-6 liter) of fluids using microstructures with characteristic dimensions on the order of tens to hundreds of micrometers. This technology has been emerged as a promising tool. Its unique design paves the way to create a more in vivo–like cellular microenvironment in vitro. It can be fully automated for HTS assays with improved data quality, reduced assay time and cost.

A digital microfluidics (DMF) has emerged as an alternative to conventional format of enclosed micro-channels in which nano-liter sized droplets are manipulated on an open surface of an array of electrodes, e.g. the first time lab-on-a-chip platform has been developed by Barbulovic-Nad et al. (2010)[34] which is capable of implementing all steps required for complete mammalian cell culture. This is a very promising technique for improvising HTS via well-controlled fluid handling without the need for complex robotics.

CELL-BASED HTS IN COMMERCIAL DRUG DEVELOPMENT

The global market for cell-based assays in drug discovery was estimated as $6.2 billion in 2010 and it is expected to increase at an annual growth rate of 11.6% to nearly $10.2 billion in 2015.[1] There has been a growing interest in drug discovery to use cell-based assays for lead identification and optimization since they provide more relevant physiological information than biochemical assays. Hence, now it becomes an integral part of successful drug discovery processes. The successful examples of cell based HTS in commercial drug discovery is given in Table 45.1.

Table 45.1: Examples of cell-based HTS in commercial drug discovery

Name of the drug (US trade name; Company)	Indication	Target class	Type of assay employed	Year FDA approval	Reference
Eltrombopag (Promacta; GlaxoSmithKline)	Thrombocytopenia	Cytokine receptor	Cell-Based Luciferase reporter assay	2008	Duffy et al., 2001[35]
BMS-790052 (Daclastavir;Bristol-Myers Squibb)	Hepatitis C	HCV-NS5A	Cell-based replicon screening method	Phase III	Lee C, 2011[36]
Bortezomib (Velcade; Millinium Pharmaceuticals)	Myeloma	Protease	Cell-Based assays using NC160	2003	Paull KD,1989[37]

CONCLUSION AND PERSPECTIVES

The advancement of combinatorial chemistry, genomics, proteomics and bioinformatics necessitate the development of a very rapid screening strategy for lead identification and optimization. Conventional animal models become obscure due to its high cost, low throughput and moral issues. Hence, in order to meet the high screening attrition rate in lead identification and optimization, HTS assays have been emerged as a potential platform in early drug development program. Today, more than half of the HTS assays are replaced with cell-based assays. However, the conventional 2D static cell culture systems have many limitations which restrict its use in cell proliferation and cytotoxicity studies. This can be overcome by the development of cell-based 3D culture with fluorescent detection. Such system is fast, sensitive and physiologically more relevant which can be used to bridge the gap between biochemical assays and animal tests. The recent advances in 3D cell culture with microfluidic technology coupled with stable fluorescent probes offer a great advantage of long-term study of drugs in an *in vivo* like 3D environment and flow fields. This would enable more effective screening and exploration of new drugs for their health benefits.

REFERENCES

1. Zang R, Li D, Tang IC, et al. Cell-based assays in high-throughput screening for drug discovery. Int J Biotechnol Wellness Ind 2012;1:31-51.
2. Denyer J, Worley J, Cox B, Allenby G, Banks M. HTS approaches to voltage-gated ion channel drug discovery. Drug Discov Today 1998;3:323-32.
3. Gonzales J, Oades K, Leychkis Y, Harootunian A, Negulescu P. Cell based assays and instrumentation for screening ion channel targets. Drug Discov Today 1999;4:431-9.

4. DeBasio R, Guiliano K, Zhou L, Demarest K. Quantification of G-protein coupled receptor internalization using G-protein coupled receptor-green fluorescent protein conjugates with the Array Scan TM high -content screening system. J Biomol Screening 1999;4:75-86.
5. Bedard J, May S, Barbeau D, Yuen L, Rando R, Bowlin T. A high throughput colorimetric cell proliferation assay for the identification of human cytomegalovirus inhibitors. Antiviral Res 1999;41:35-43.
6. Ebert AD, Svendsen CN. Human stem cells and drug screening: opportunities and challenges. Nat Rev Drug Discov 2010;9:1-6.
7. Henrietta Lacks, 1951. http://www.microbiologybytes.com/LabWork/lacks/lacks1. htm
8. Shoemaker RH. The NCI60 human tumor cell line anticancer drug screen. Nat Rev 2006;6:813-23.
9. Sabisz M, Skladanowski A. Cancer stem cells in drug resistance and drug screening: can we exploit the cancer stem cell paradigm in search for new antitumor agents? In: Cancer stem cells theories and practice. Ed Stanley Shostak, ISBN 978-953-307-225-8, 472 pages, Publisher: In Tech 2011. 424-44.
10. Salmon SE, Meyskens FL Jr, Alberts DS, Soehnlen B, Young L. New drugs in ovarian cancer and malignant melanoma: in vitro phase II screening with the human tumor stem cell assay. Cancer Treat Rep 1981;65:1-12.
11. Wu X, Ding S, Ding Q, Gray NS, Schultz PG. A small molecule with osteogenesis-inducing activity in multipotent mesenchymal progenitor cells. J Am Chem Soc 2002;124:14520-1.
12. Caspi O, Itzhaki I, Kehat I, et al. In vitro electrophysiological drug testing using human embryonic stem cell derived cardiomyocytes. Stem Cells Dev 2009;18:161-72.
13. Folkman J, Moscona A. Role of cell shape in growth control. Nature 1978;273:345-9.
14. Danen EH, Yamada KM. Fibronectin, integrins, and growth control. J Cell Physiol 2001;189(1):1-13.
15. Carney DN, Bepler G, Gazdar AF. The serum-free establishment and in vitro growth properties of classic and variant small cell lung cancer cell lines. Recent Results Cancer Res 1985;99:157-66.
16. http://www.sigmaldrich.com
17. Luo J, Yang ST. Effects of three-dimensional culturing in afibrous matrix on cell cycle, apoptosis, and MAb production by hybridoma cells. Biotechnol Prog 2004;26:306-15.
18. Smitskamp-Wilms E, Pinedo HM, Veerman G, Ruiz vanHaperen VW, Peters GJ. Postconfluent multilayered cell line cultures for selective screening of gemcitabine. Eur J Cancer 1998;34:921-6.
19. Fischbach C, Chen R, Matsumoto T, et al. Engineering tumors with 3D scaffolds. Nature Methods 2007;4:855-60.
20. Suna T, Jackson S, Haycock JW, MacNeil S. Culture of skin cells in 3D rather than 2D improves their ability to survive exposure to cytotoxic agents. J Biotechnol 2006;122:372-81.
21. Vickerman V, Blundo J, Kamm R. Design, fabrication and implementation of a novel multi-parameter control microfluidic platform for 3-D cell culture and real time imaging. Lab Chip 2008;8:1468-77.
22. Toh YC, Zhang C, Yu H. A novel 3D mammalian cell perfusion culture system in microfluidic channels. Lab Chip 2007;7:302-9.
23. Hung PJ, Lee PJ, Sabounchi P, Lin R, Lee LP. Continuous perfusion microfluidic cell culture array for high-through put cell-based assays. Biotechnol Bioeng 2005;89:1–8.
24. Ding L, Du D, Zhang X, Ju H. Trends in cell-based electrochemical biosensors. Curr Medicinal Chem 2008;15:3160-70.
25. Chen SYC, Hung PJ, Lee P. J Microfluidic array for three dimensional perfusion culture of human mammary epithelial cells. Biomed Microdevices 2011;13:753-8.

26. Yeon JH, Park JK. Cytotoxicity test based on electrochemical impedance measurement of HepG2 cultured in microfabricated cell chip. Anal Biochem 2005;341:308–15.
27. Hogg D, Boden P, Lawton G, Kozlowski R. Drug Discov World 2006;7:83.
28. Wodnicka M, Guarino RD, Hemperly JJ, Timmins MR, Stitt D, Pitner JB. Novel fluorescent technology platform for highthroughput cytotoxicity and proliferation assays. J Biomol Screen 2000;5:141-52.
29. O'Brien J, Wilson I, Orton T, Pognan F. Investigation of the Alamar Blue (resazurin) fluorescent dye for the assessment of mammalian cell cytotoxicity. Eur J Biochem 2000;267:5421–6.
30. Durick K, Negulescu P. Cellular biosensors for drug discovery. Biosens Bioelectron 2001;16:587-92.
31. Wischhusen J, Melino G, Weller M. p53 and its family members – reporter genes may not see the difference. Nat Cell Death Different 2004;11:1150–2.
32. Beske OE, Goldbard S. High-throughput cell analysis using multiplexed array technologies. Drug Disc Today 2002;7(18Suppl):S131-S135.
33. Xu X, Gerard AL, Huang BC, Anderson DC, Payan DG, Luo Y. Detection of programmed cell death using fluorescence energy transfer. Nucleic Acids Res 1998; 26(8):2034-35.
34. Barbulovic-Nad I, Au SA, Wheeler AR. A microfluidic platform for complete mammalian culture. Lab Chip 2010;10:1536-42.
35. Duffy KJ. Hydrazinonaphthalene and azonaphthalene thrombopoietin mimics are nonpeptidyl promoters of megakaryocytopoiesis. J Med Chem 2001;44:3730-45.
36. Huang CP, Lu J, Seon H, et al. Engineering microscale cellular niches for three-dimensional multicellular co-cultures. Lab Chip 2009;9:1740-8.
37. Lee C. Discovery of Hepatitis C virus HS5A inhibitors as a new class of anti-HCV therapy. Arch Pharm Res 2011;34:1403-7.

INDEX

Page numbers followed by *f* refer to figure and *t* refer to table

B

C

H

I

J

K

L

M

P

Q

R

S

T

U